AF853987

Health Science Fundamentals

Fourth Edition

TEACHER'S WRAPAROUND EDITION

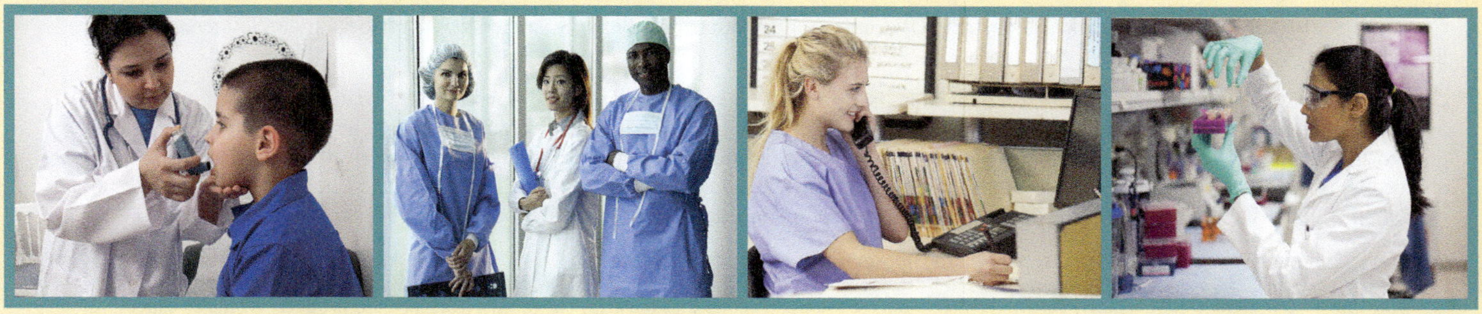

Pearson

Cover art: Shutterstock, Joshua Resnick/Shutterstock, Dragana Gordic/Shutterstock, SofikoS/Shutterstock, Prostock-studio/Shutterstock, leaf/123rf.com

Copyright © 2024, 2020, and 2016 by Pearson Education, Inc. or its affiliates, 221 River Street, Hoboken, NJ 07030. All Rights Reserved. Manufactured in the United States of America. This publication is protected by copyright, and permission should be obtained from the publisher prior to any prohibited reproduction, storage in a retrieval system, or transmission in any form or by any means, electronic, mechanical, photocopying, recording, or otherwise. For information regarding permissions, request forms, and the appropriate contacts within the Pearson Education Global Rights and Permissions department, please visit www.pearsoned.com/permissions/.

Acknowledgments of third-party content appear on the appropriate page within the text.

Unless otherwise indicated herein, any third-party trademarks, logos, or icons that may appear in this work are the property of their respective owners, and any references to third-party trademarks, logos, icons, or other trade dress are for demonstrative or descriptive purposes only. Such references are not intended to imply any sponsorship, endorsement, authorization, or promotion of Pearson's products by the owners of such marks, or any relationship between the owner and Pearson Education, Inc., or its affiliates, authors, licensees, or distributors.

Library of Congress Cataloging-in-Publication Data

Cataloging-in-Publication Data is available on file at the Library of Congress.

1 2022

Pearson

ISBN-10: 0-13-808280-4
ISBN-13: 978-0-13-808280-2

Contents

Chapter 3
Finding the Right Occupation for You 45

Chapter 4
Employability and Leadership 71

Chapter 8
Teamwork 171

Chapter 9
Effective Communication 183

Chapter 15 Mental Illness 425

Chapter 16 Nutrition 445

List of Procedures

Chapter 20 • Medical Assisting and Laboratory Skills

Chapter 21 • Therapeutic Techniques and Sports Medicine

Chapter 22 • Responsibilities of a Dental Assistant

Introduction

The Teacher's Wraparound Edition for *Health Science Fundamentals* is a comprehensive guide to the student edition text. In addition to providing instructors with essential information about how to use the student edition in the classroom, it includes exclusive material such as additional activities, vocabulary, discussion topics, and suggestions for ways to customize lessons for tiered learning.

The Teacher's Wraparound Edition presents instructors with teaching tips and other relevant content directly alongside the full-page view of the student text. Instructors can see exactly what the student sees while referencing the information they need to manage the classroom and promote learning.

The Teacher's Wraparound Edition includes the following features and elements:

- **Advance Preparation:** A table is included on the opening page of each chapter with suggestions for steps instructors may take to prepare for the class.
- **Customized Instruction Overview:** These list the pages where teachers can look for instructional materials customized for different levels of learning.
- **Focus and Engage:** Each chapter begins with a "bell-ringer" activity to start the class off and to help focus the students' attention on the content to come. Corresponding text helps teachers expand on that activity.
- **Discuss:** These discussion topics relate directly and indirectly to the content on the current page.
- **Reinforce and Review:** Topics covered in the previous section, or in previous chapters, that instructors may want to review before continuing are provided.
- **Teaching Tips:** These items help explain the content and provide additional information for instructors to use in the classroom.
- **Customized Instruction Boxes:** These include accommodations and additional activities for More Advanced, Less Advanced, English Language Learners, Special Needs, and At-Risk Students.
- **Activity Boxes:** These original activities are not in the student edition textbook.
- **Teamwork Activity Boxes:** These original activities are designed to promote teamwork, cooperation, and leadership skills.
- **Figure Focus:** Every figure in the student edition has a corresponding Figure Focus feature in the Teacher's Wraparound Edition, to provide answers to the figure prompts and questions, and provide additional information for discussion and instruction.
- **Feature Focuses:** Every feature and box in the student edition has a corresponding feature in the Teacher's Wraparound Edition, to provide answers, discussion prompts, and additional teaching tips.
- **End-of-Section/End-of-Chapter Activities:** Answers, additional teaching tips, discussion points, and supplemental activities relating to the end-of-chapter activities are provided.

Preview of the Teacher's Wraparound Edition

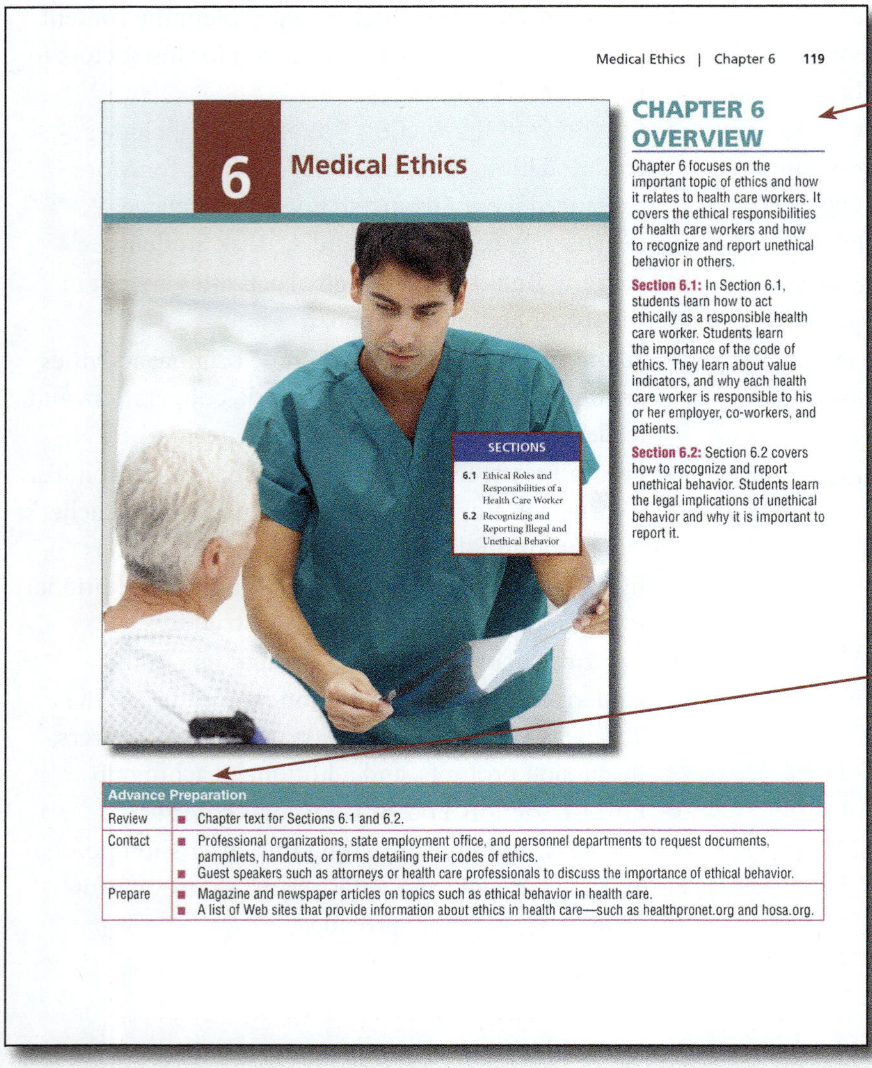
Medical Ethics | Chapter 6 119

6 Medical Ethics

SECTIONS

6.1 Ethical Roles and Responsibilities of a Health Care Worker

6.2 Recognizing and Reporting Illegal and Unethical Behavior

CHAPTER 6 OVERVIEW

Chapter 6 focuses on the important topic of ethics and how it relates to health care workers. It covers the ethical responsibilities of health care workers and how to recognize and report unethical behavior in others.

Section 6.1: In Section 6.1, students learn how to act ethically as a responsible health care worker. Students learn the importance of the code of ethics. They learn about value indicators, and why each health care worker is responsible to his or her employer, co-workers, and patients.

Section 6.2: Section 6.2 covers how to recognize and report unethical behavior. Students learn the legal implications of unethical behavior and why it is important to report it.

Advance Preparation	
Review	▪ Chapter text for Sections 6.1 and 6.2.
Contact	▪ Professional organizations, state employment office, and personnel departments to request documents, pamphlets, handouts, or forms detailing their codes of ethics. ▪ Guest speakers such as attorneys or health care professionals to discuss the importance of ethical behavior.
Prepare	▪ Magazine and newspaper articles on topics such as ethical behavior in health care. ▪ A list of Web sites that provide information about ethics in health care—such as healthpronet.org and hosa.org.

Each chapter includes a **Chapter Overview**, which presents the main topics of the chapter.

The **Advance Preparation** table provides suggestions for steps teachers may take to prepare for the class.

Each chapter begins with an activity to start the class off and to help focus the students' attention on the content to come. **Getting Started** text helps teachers expand on that activity.

Introduce the Section includes information on the chapter that can be used to introduce content to come.

The **Customized Instruction Overview** table lists the pages where teachers can look for instructional materials customized for different levels of learning.

Customized Instruction boxes contain accommodations and additional activities for More Advanced Students, Less Advanced Students, English Language Learners, Special Needs Students, and At-Risk Students.

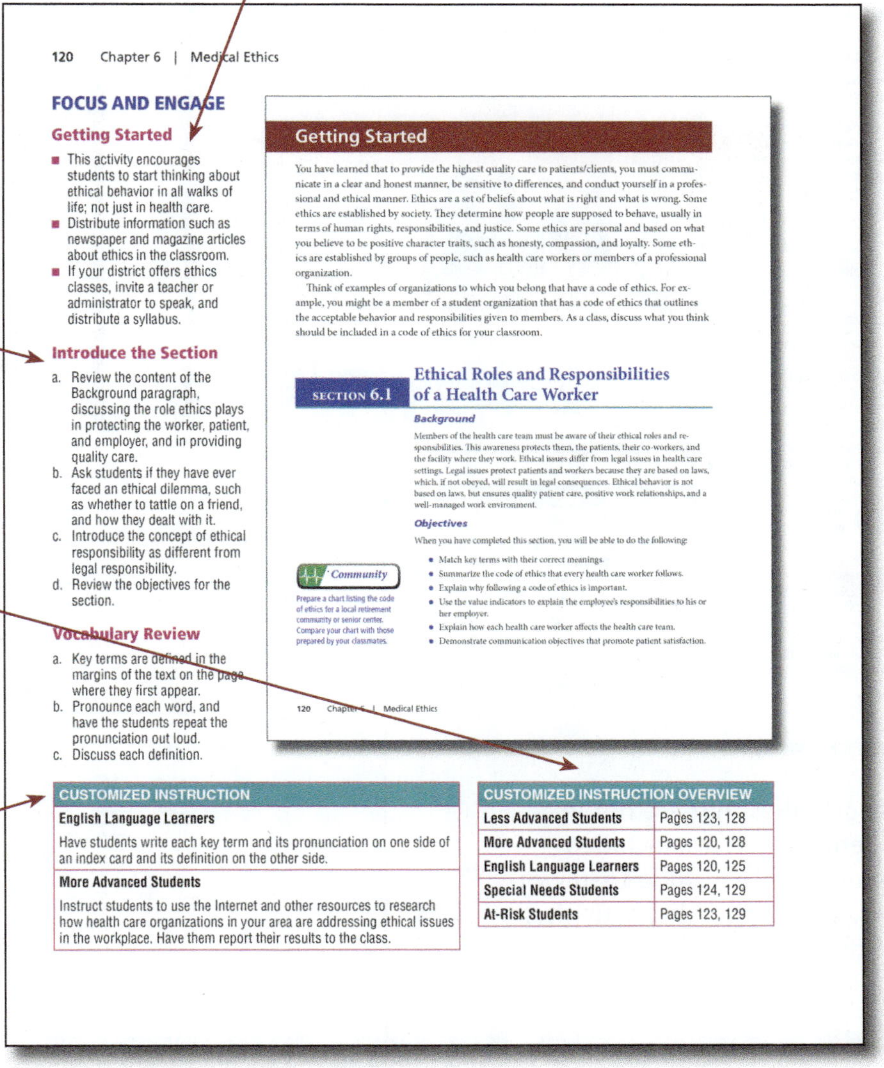

120 Chapter 6 | Medical Ethics

FOCUS AND ENGAGE

Getting Started

- This activity encourages students to start thinking about ethical behavior in all walks of life; not just in health care.
- Distribute information such as newspaper and magazine articles about ethics in the classroom.
- If your district offers ethics classes, invite a teacher or administrator to speak, and distribute a syllabus.

Introduce the Section

a. Review the content of the Background paragraph, discussing the role ethics plays in protecting the worker, patient, and employer, and in providing quality care.
b. Ask students if they have ever faced an ethical dilemma, such as whether to tattle on a friend, and how they dealt with it.
c. Introduce the concept of ethical responsibility as different from legal responsibility.
d. Review the objectives for the section.

Vocabulary Review

a. Key terms are defined in the margins of the text on the page where they first appear.
b. Pronounce each word, and have the students repeat the pronunciation out loud.
c. Discuss each definition.

Getting Started

You have learned that to provide the highest quality care to patients/clients, you must communicate in a clear and honest manner, be sensitive to differences, and conduct yourself in a professional and ethical manner. Ethics are a set of beliefs about what is right and what is wrong. Some ethics are established by society. They determine how people are supposed to behave, usually in terms of human rights, responsibilities, and justice. Some ethics are personal and based on what you believe to be positive character traits, such as honesty, compassion, and loyalty. Some ethics are established by groups of people, such as health care workers or members of a professional organization.

Think of examples of organizations to which you belong that have a code of ethics. For example, you might be a member of a student organization that has a code of ethics that outlines the acceptable behavior and responsibilities given to members. As a class, discuss what you think should be included in a code of ethics for your classroom.

SECTION 6.1 Ethical Roles and Responsibilities of a Health Care Worker

Background

Members of the health care team must be aware of their ethical roles and responsibilities. This awareness protects them, the patients, their co-workers, and the facility where they work. Ethical issues differ from legal issues in health care settings. Legal issues protect patients and workers because they are based on laws, which, if not obeyed, will result in legal consequences. Ethical behavior is not based on laws, but ensures quality patient care, positive work relationships, and a well-managed work environment.

Objectives

When you have completed this section, you will be able to do the following:

- Match key terms with their correct meanings.
- Summarize the code of ethics that every health care worker follows.
- Explain why following a code of ethics is important.
- Use the value indicators to explain the employee's responsibilities to his or her employer.
- Explain how each health care worker affects the health care team.
- Demonstrate communication objectives that promote patient satisfaction.

Community

Prepare a chart listing the code of ethics for a local retirement community or senior center. Compare your chart with those prepared by your classmates.

120 Chapter 6 | Medical Ethics

CUSTOMIZED INSTRUCTION
English Language Learners
Have students write each key term and its pronunciation on one side of an index card and its definition on the other side.
More Advanced Students
Instruct students to use the Internet and other resources to research how health care organizations in your area are addressing ethical issues in the workplace. Have them report their results to the class.

CUSTOMIZED INSTRUCTION OVERVIEW	
Less Advanced Students	Pages 123, 128
More Advanced Students	Pages 120, 128
English Language Learners	Pages 120, 125
Special Needs Students	Pages 124, 129
At-Risk Students	Pages 123, 129

Teaching Tips help explain the content and provide additional information for teachers to use in the classroom.

Every feature and box in the student edition has a corresponding feature in the Teacher's Wraparound Edition to provide answers, discussion prompts, and additional teaching tips.

Each captioned figure in the student edition has a corresponding **Figure Focus** feature. It gives answers to the figure prompt and question and provides additional information for discussion and instruction.

End-of-chapter materials include answer keys, additional teaching tips, discussion points, and supplemental activities.

178 Chapter 8 | Teamwork

Teaching Tips

- Emphasize the importance of team communication.
- Review the components of effective communication:
  - Active listening
  - Giving and receiving feedback
  - Checking for comprehension
- Emphasize the importance of a communication network.

Apply It

- If necessary, have students review the sample careers discussed in Chapter 3. They should focus on the Therapeutic Services, Diagnostic Services, Health Informatics, and Support Services pathways.
- This will have them better understand the various roles of health care team members.
- They might also want to review the Patient Care Partnership (Patient's Bill of Rights) discussed in Chapter 5.

Figure Focus

8.2 How do strong communication skills help a health care team provide better service to the patient?

Answer: Strong communication skills among team members ensures that ideas, concepts, knowledge, and information regarding a patient's care are shared with the appropriate resources.

TEAMWORK

Divide the class into small groups. Have each person write one positive comment about each of the other members of the group. Share the comments.

- Learning good communication skills so you can share ideas, concepts, and knowledge
- Performing your duties to the best of your abilities

Team Communication

Effective interpersonal communication is vital to the smooth functioning of any team. (**Figure 8.2**) Team members should be skilled in active listening, giving and receiving feedback, and checking for comprehension.

It is also important for a team to develop an effective communication network. For example, team members should establish who relays information to whom within the team. The team must work to share relevant information in the most efficient way possible.

Some other important communication practices for a health care team include the following:

- A clear and effective system of recording patient information
- A regularly scheduled meeting for members to discuss patient's progress
- A regularly scheduled meeting to evaluate the team's function and development
- A procedure for communicating with other groups inside or outside the health facility

As with communication skills for interacting with patients, quality of care is also dependent upon the skills used for team discussions. When preparing for a specific practice or procedure, one member of the team may be called upon to complete research and present the findings, particularly if a new diagnosis has been identified or new practice is being implemented. As the team member doing the research, it is important to plan and prepare an effective presentation for the rest of the team as though it were for a large audience.

Teams can also learn to communicate better and practice dealing with emotional and stressful situations such as trauma and chronic and terminal illness using role play, providing valuable experience in a lower stakes situation.

Apply It

Form teams of five. A new patient has been admitted to your hospital and her care has been assigned to your team. What channels of communication will you follow to provide the best quality care possible? Create a poster that illustrates the tools and resources you will use to communicate information to all those involved in her care.

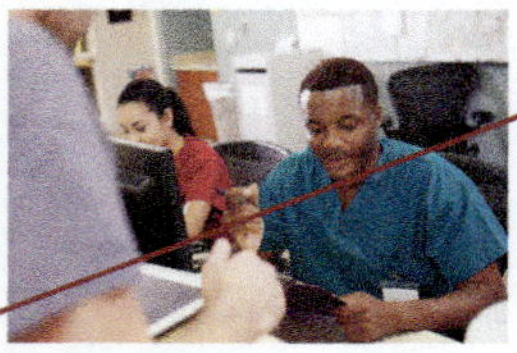

Figure 8.2
How do strong communication skills help a health care team provide better service to the patient?

Conflict Resolution

Health care team members represent a variety of skills, professional backgrounds, and opinions. In addition, interdisciplinary collaboration can be complex. With these types of dynamics, conflict between team members is inevitable.

178 Chapter 8 | Teamwork

CUSTOMIZED INSTRUCTION

More Advanced Students

More advanced students might assume they should alwa
situations where they must be subordinate to others in gr
so that they can understand the dynamics from a team m

English Language Learners

As a group, have students discuss what techniques a tea
barriers between members. Have students create a list of
language barriers that any type of team could follow. The
all members understand the goal and their individual resp
speaking clearly (and more slowly), using a translation di
exercising patience and understanding if something need

Original activities that are not in the student edition are included throughout. These include teamwork activities, critical-thinking activities, and hands-on activities.

Understanding Health Care Systems | Chapter 2 43

CHAPTER 2 REVIEW

Chapter Review Questions

1. Under what three circumstances might ambulatory care be preferable and why? (2.1)
2. Name one health care provider and explain how they provide medical care. (2.1)
3. What are we trying to do to contain the high costs of health care? (2.2)
4. Explain several ways in which we are addressing personal wellness issues. (2.1)
5. Name three government agencies that provide health services. What does each agency do? (2.1)
6. How do the policies of managed care help to provide quality care for patients? (2.1)
7. What are the benefits of an organizational chart in a health care facility? (2.1)
8. Explain the four major services in health care. (2.1)
9. How does the Healthcare Effectiveness Data and Information Set help patients/clients? (2.2)
10. What are some of the costs that third-party payers might require a patient/client to pay? (2.2)

Activities

1. Choose a facility such as a general hospital, specialty hospital, rehabilitation center, or clinic. Visit the facility, research its Web site, or call the facility to identify the different departments in the facility and its line of authority. Then, create a diagram that shows the relationship of health care professionals within that facility.
2. Create a pie chart that shows the National percentage of the health care expenditures for:
   - Nursing care
   - Other residential care
   - Prescription drugs
   - Home health
   - Dental care
   - Physician/clinical
   - Other professional
   - Hospital

   Describe how these health services expenditures impact the economy.
3. Working in teams of three or four, select a section from the Affordable Care Act. Analyze the impact of the section at the national, state, and local levels. Report your findings to the rest of the class or submit the report to the teacher.
4. Identify the governing agency at the national, state, and local level responsible for regulating the section selected in Activity 3 from the Affordable Care Act. Add this information in the report for Activity 3.
5. Research hazardous waste removal and recycling services available for hospitals in your area. Create a proposal for how your local hospital could save money and better protect the environment.
6. Research the various governmental regulations and guidelines that hospitals must adhere to from entities such as the World Health Organization, Centers for Disease Control and Prevention, Occupational Safety and Health Administration, U.S. Food and Drug Administration, Joint Commission, and National Institute of Health. Prepare a brief presentation on one of these for your class.

Case Studies

1. A patient's colonoscopy procedure will cost \$3,350. There is a co-pay of \$30 and the co-insurance is 20%. The annual deductible is \$1,000, of which the patient has met \$325. What amount will the patient have to pay?
2. An elderly man is leaving the hospital after receiving care for his broken leg. He lives with his family, but he is alone all day while his family works. What kind of care will the man need after he leaves the hospital? What type of facilities might you recommend to this patient?

Underst... 43

CHAPTER 2 REVIEW

Chapter Review Questions

1. Answer: Ambulatory care is preferable for rehabilitation, outpatient surgery, and day care because it allows a patient to return home.
2. Answer: Answers will vary but should include one of the following:
   - General hospitals: provide a range of diagnostic, medical, surgical, and emergency care services.
   - Convalescent care facilities: care for elderly people needing nursing services.
   - Ambulatory care: physicians with different specialties provide patient with immediate care for many different illnesses.
   - Physician and dental offices: care that promotes wellness and diagnose illness.
   - Rehabilitation centers: provide physical therapy, and hydrotherapy.
   - Home health agencies: provide care in the home for patients who need health services but not hospitalization.
   - Senior day care: care to the elderly who are able to live at home with their families but need care when the family is away.
3. Answer: To control the high costs of health care, managed care is promoting preventive care, primary care doctors, specialty doctors, urgent care facilities, and preadmission authorization requirement for hospitalization.
4. Answer: Preventive care, such as routine physicals, well-baby care, immunizations, and wellness education helps keep patients healthy. Wellness education stresses the importance of good nutrition, weight control, exercise, and healthy living practices. Health education programs, wellness centers, weight-control programs, fitness centers, health food distributors, and health care organizations all promote wellness and preventive care.
5. Answer: Answers will vary but should include three of the following: U.S. Public Health Service performs research, prevents drug and alcohol abuse, prevents and controls diseases, checks the safety of food and drugs, plans ways to deliver health services, and makes quality care affordable and available; State psychiatric hospitals serve the mentally ill; State university medical centers provide training, health care, and conduct medical research; State public health services provide health education materials; U.S. Department of Health and Human Services protects the health of all American by providing vital human services; The National Institute of Health conducts and supports medical research; Centers for Disease Control and Prevention monitors and prevents disease outbreak include bioterrorism; The Food and Drug Administration assures the safety of foods, cosmetics, pharmaceuticals, and biological devices; The Occupational Safety and Health Administration imposes safety and health legislation to prevent injury, illness, and death in the workplace; The Agency for Healthcare Research and Quality works to improve health care; County hospitals provide care to the ill and injured who require financial assistance.
6. Answer: Preventive care promotes wellness that will include ways to prevent illness, urgent care is for non-emergencies that require prompt treatment and is less expensive than emergency care, and outpatient care instead of in-hospitalization stays.
7. Answer: The benefits of an organization chart in a health care facility is that it shows the chain of command, lists supervisors, and lists the areas of responsibility for all employees.

PART I
Becoming a Health Care Worker

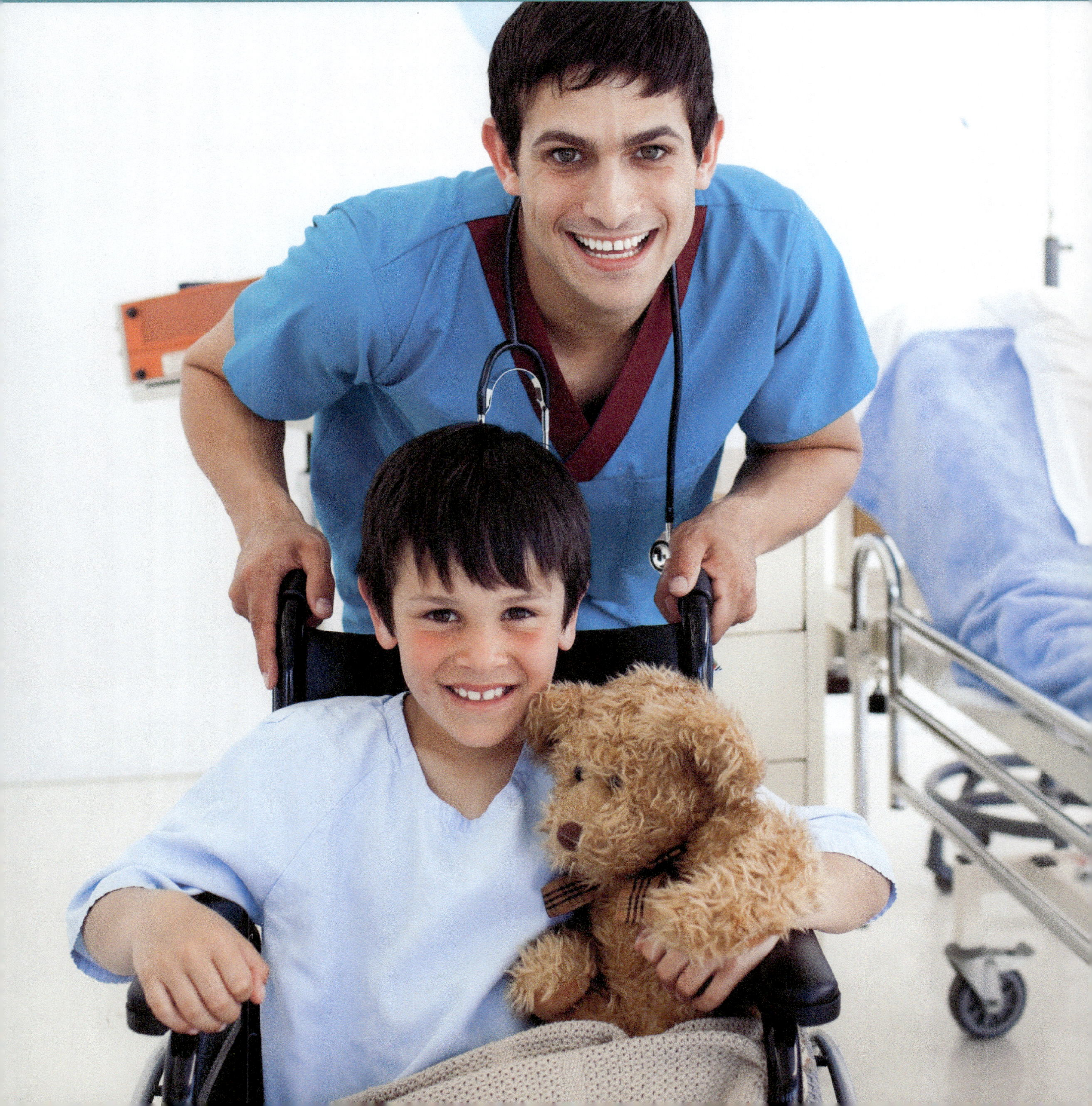

1 Introduction to Being a Health Care Worker

SECTIONS

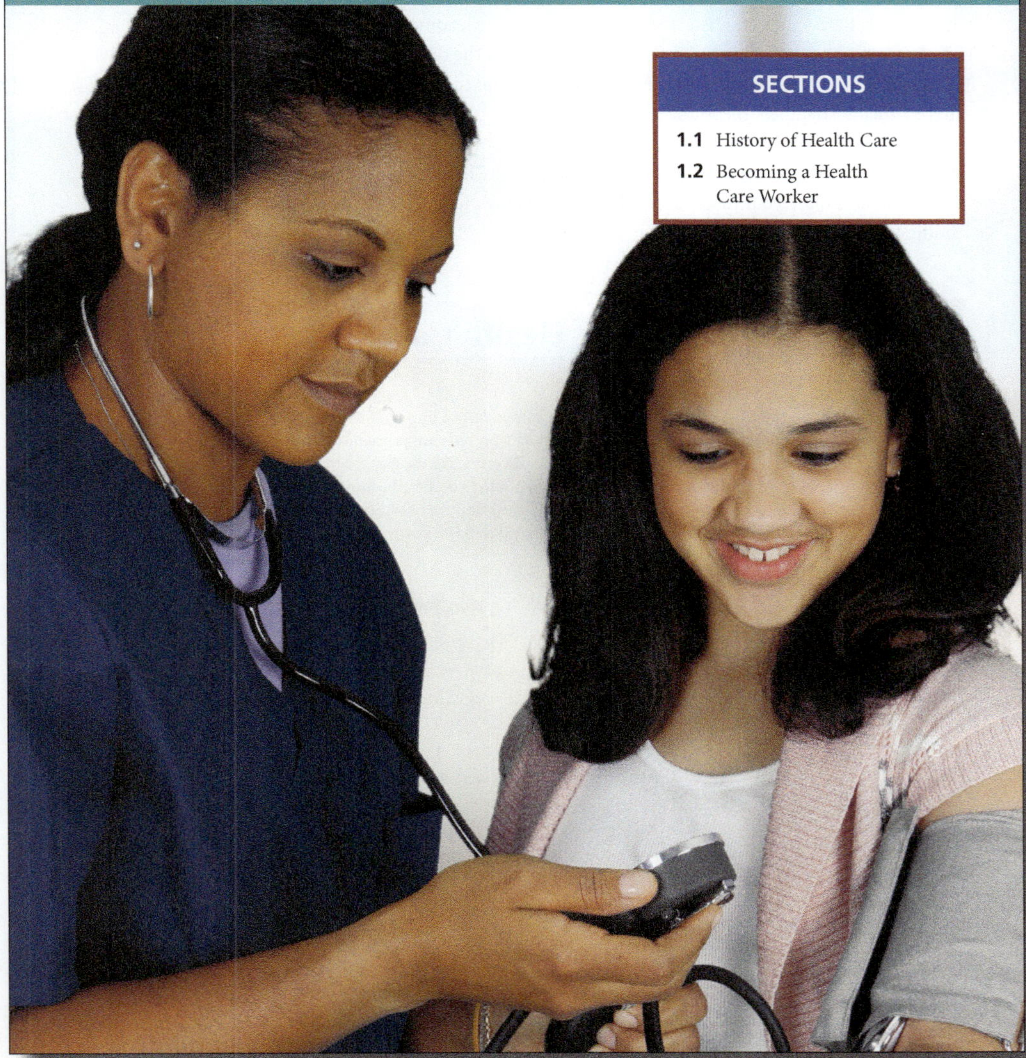

CHAPTER 1 OVERVIEW

Chapter 1 provides an introduction to what it means to be a health care worker.

Section 1.1: The first section, "History of Health Care," is a history of health care from primitive times through today. It covers people, practices, and discoveries that have had an impact on health care through the ages, and also looks at what we can expect in the 21st century.

Section 1.2: Section 1.2, "Becoming a Health Care Worker," introduces the educational and personal requirements for being a successful health care worker. Key topics include the importance of health care education, personal hygiene, standards of behavior, and confidentiality.

Advance Preparation	
Review	■ *Health Science Fundamentals* textbook, chapter text for Sections 1.1 and 1.2.
Contact	■ Guest speakers to discuss their personal experiences in health care education, or health care training programs available in your area. ■ Guest speakers to discuss trends in health care. ■ Human Resources departments at local hospitals or clinics to request information about job skill requirements.
Prepare	■ Magazine and newspaper articles on topics such as medical advances. ■ Videos from local libraries or public television stations on the history and trends in health care. ■ Books or articles about famous scientists or others who have had an impact on health care. ■ Pamphlets or brochures about health care training programs in your area. ■ A list of Web sites that provide information about the history of health care, scientists responsible for health care discoveries, and health care trends, such as nlm.nih.gov and mla-hhss.org.

FOCUS AND ENGAGE

Getting Started

- The opening activity introduces health care as the opportunity to cure or prevent illness and disease.
- Allow at least 10 minutes to complete the activity.
- To save time, you might have students work in groups.
- Encourage students to use their existing knowledge.
- You may want to have students select the disease at the beginning of the chapter, and then complete the exercise at the end.

Introduce the Section

a. Review the content of the Background paragraph, explaining that the concept of health care has been around since primitive times.

b. Explain that understanding the history of health care will help students understand and appreciate health care today.

c. Ask students to imagine whether current health care workers could have practiced in earlier times. Point out resources, such as technology and transportation, that might not have been available in the past.

d. Discuss the objectives for the section.

Vocabulary Review

a. Key terms are defined in the margins of the text on the page where they first appear.

b. Pronounce each word, and have the students repeat the pronunciation out loud.

c. Discuss the definition of each word.

Getting Started

As you will learn in this chapter, many people have contributed to finding the causes and cures of illness, injuries, and other disabling conditions. Others have identified different body parts and their functions. Some notable discoveries include Louis Pasteur's identification of the process that makes milk safe for human consumption. This process is called pasteurization, in honor of the founder. Bartolommeo Eustachio discovered the tube leading from the ear to the throat, an important finding that was named Eustachian tube after the discoverer. Others include the Salk vaccine to prevent polio (named after Dr. Jonas Salk) and the Roentgen Ray (now called x-ray) after Wilhelm Roentgen, the founder.

Assume you could find a cure for, or identify a cause of, a disease or illness such as cancer, childhood arthritis, hepatitis C, autism, or asthma. Write the condition and cure (or cause) on a 3 × 5 card, and share your discovery with the class. Why did you choose this particular disease or condition?

SECTION 1.1 History of Health Care

Background

Health care has developed and changed throughout history. Knowing the history of health care helps you understand current procedures, practices, and philosophies. The experiences and discoveries of the past led to the advances of today. Today's achievements could not have occurred without the trials and errors of the past. When you understand the primitive beginnings of medicine, you appreciate the advances made during the past 5,000 years.

Objectives

When you have completed this section, you will be able to do the following:

- Match key terms with their correct meanings.
- Identify scientists and explain what they contributed to medicine.
- Choose one era in the history of health care and explain how health care technology changed.
- Discuss advances in medicine in the twentieth century.
- Research and report on advances in medicine for the twenty-first century.
- Explain the origin of medical ethics and the impact of medical advances on ethics.
- Compare health care in the past with health care in the twentieth and twenty-first centuries.
- Explain current trends in health care.

4 Chapter 1 | Introduction to Being a Health Care Worker

CUSTOMIZED INSTRUCTION OVERVIEW	
Less Advanced Students	Pages 13, 14
More Advanced Students	Pages 8, 26
English Language Learners	Pages 5, 21
Special Needs Students	Pages 15, 18
At-Risk Students	Pages 16, 21

Early Beginnings

Primitive human beings had no electricity, few tools, and poor shelter. Their time was spent protecting themselves against **predators** and finding food. They were **superstitious** and believed that illness and disease were caused by supernatural spirits. In an attempt to heal, tribal doctors performed ceremonies to **exorcise** evil spirits. One such ceremony involved an early form of **trephining**, whereby the tribal doctor would remove part of the cranium, with a primitive tool, to exorcise demons. They also used herbs and plants as medicines. Some of the same medicines are still used today. Here are some examples:

- Digitalis comes from the foxglove plant. Today it is given in pill form, **intravenously**, or by injection to treat heart conditions. In early times, people chewed the leaves of the foxglove plant to strengthen and slow the heartbeat.
- Quinine comes from the bark of the cinchona tree. It controls fever, relieves muscle spasms, and helps prevent malaria.
- Belladonna and atropine are made from the poisonous nightshade plant. They relieve muscle spasm, especially in gastrointestinal (GI) pain.
- Morphine is made from the opium poppy. It is an effective medication for treating severe pain. It is addicting and used only when nothing else will help.

Medicine in Ancient Times

The Egyptians were the earliest people to keep **accurate** health records. They were superstitious and called upon the gods to heal them. They also learned to identify certain diseases. In the Egyptian culture, the priests acted as physicians. They used medicines to heal disease, learned the art of splinting fractures, and treated disorders by bloodletting with the use of leeches. Their primary function is to drain blood, since pooled blood around a wound can threaten the healing of tissue. Interestingly, today, leeches are being used as a treatment to help heal skin grafts and restore blood circulation.

The ancient Chinese, from as early as the Stone Age, were the first to use primitive acupuncture therapies. These early medical pioneers learned to treat a variety of illness and disease with stone tools. Their methods eventually developed into the advanced practice of Chinese acupuncture, still in common use today.

To the ancient Greeks, medicine was considered an art and not just a profession. Physicians had a noble and sacred mission, often housed in sacred temples of healing. They were the first to study the causes of disease and to determine that illnesses may have natural, rather than spiritual, causes. They kept records on what they observed and what they thought caused illness. The Greeks understood the importance of searching for new information about disease. This research helped eliminate superstition. In addition, Greeks further developed the use of massage and herbal therapies.

primitive
(PRIM i tiv)
Ancient or prehistoric.

predators
(PRED uh ters)
Organisms or beings that destroy.

superstitious
(soo per STISH uhs)
Trusting in magic or chance.

exorcise
(EK sawr sahyz)
To force out evil spirits.

trephining
(TRAY fin ing)
Surgically removing circular sections (of bone, for example).

intravenously
(in truh VEE nuhs lee)
Directly into a vein.

accurate
(AK yer it)
Exact, correct, or precise.

Introduction to Being a Health Care Worker | Chapter 1 5

TEACH

Discuss

- Discuss how advances in health care have improved quality of life, such as increased life expectancies and pain relief.
- Point out some health care methods that were once considered state-of-the-art that are now known to be useless or even harmful, such as bloodletting or not taking baths.

Reinforce and Review

- If necessary, review historical time periods and civilizations to help students visualize the context.
- For example, describe prehistoric or primitive eras, ancient civilizations, as well as the dark and middle ages.

Teaching Tips

- Introduce the basic concept of health care in the context of primitive society.
- Remind students that primitive people had no knowledge or understanding of how the body works.
- Review the medicines that were used in primitive times that are still in use today, and point out that they are all derived from plants.
- Discuss how superstition played an important role in early health care.
- Point out that there are still health care superstitions around today, such as "An apple a day keeps the doctor away."

ACTIVITY

Have students write a short story about a superstition that involves health or health care.

CUSTOMIZED INSTRUCTION

English Language Learners

Have students write each key term and its pronunciation on one side of an index card and its definition on the other side.

Teaching Tips

- Review illness and disease and how they were viewed from the early beginnings to the twentieth century.
- Compare the ways different ancient civilizations practiced health care.
- Emphasize the work of Hippocrates. Remind students how early in history he lived and worked, and that the Hippocratic Oath is still used today.

Figure Focus

1.1 Hippocrates is considered the father of medicine. How did Hippocrates and other Greek and Roman physicians help to develop health care as we know it today?

Answer: The Romans were the first to organize medical care. They organized hospitals for the care of the sick. Physicians were paid by the government. The Greeks observed and measured the effects of disease. They determined that some disease was caused by lack of sanitation, which the Romans addressed by developing a sanitation system.

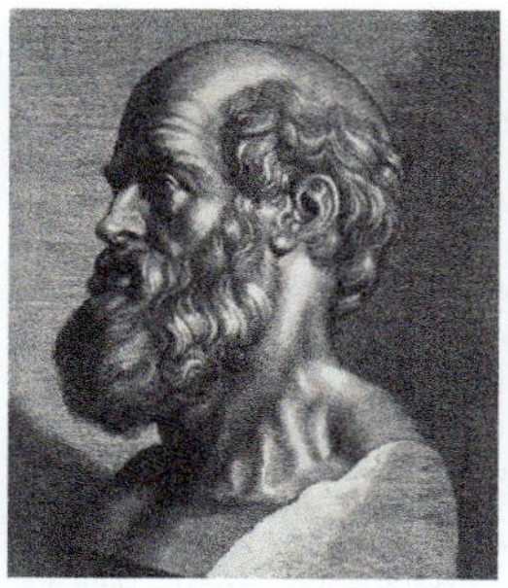

Figure 1.1
Hippocrates is considered the father of medicine. How did Hippocrates and other Greek and Roman physicians help to develop health care as we know it today?

anatomy
(uh NAT uh mee)
The science dealing with the structure of humans, animals, and other living organisms.

observation
(ob zur VEY shuhn)
Act of watching.

symptom
(SIMP tuhm)
A sign or indication of something.

ethics
(ETH iks)
A system of moral principles.

convents
(KON vents)
Establishments of nuns.

monasteries
(MON uh ster ees)
Homes for men following religious standards.

custodial
(kuh STOH dee uhl)
Marked by watching and protecting rather than seeking to cure.

epidemics
(ep i DEM iks)
Diseases affecting many people at the same time.

vaccines
(VAK seenz)
A weakened bacteria or virus given to a person to build immunity against a disease.

During ancient times, religious custom did not allow bodies to be dissected. The father of medicine, Hippocrates (ca. 469–377 b.c.), based his knowledge of **anatomy** and physiology on **observation** of the external body. (**Figure 1.1**) He kept careful notes of the signs and **symptoms** of many diseases. With these records he found that disease was not caused by supernatural forces. Hippocrates wrote the standard of **ethics** called the Oath of Hippocrates. This standard is the basis for today's medical ethics. Physicians still take this oath.

The Greeks observed and measured the effects of disease. They found that some disease was caused by lack of sanitation. The Romans learned from the Greeks and developed a sanitation system. They brought clean water into their cities by way of aqueducts (waterways). They built sewers to carry off waste. They also built public baths with filtering systems. This was the beginning of public health and sanitation.

The Romans were the first to organize medical care. They sent medical equipment and physicians with their armies to care for wounded soldiers. Roman physicians kept a room in their houses for the ill. This was the beginning of hospitals. Public buildings for the care of the sick were established. Physicians were paid by the Roman government. It is interesting to note that the Roman physician wore a death mask. This mask had a spice-filled beak, which the Romans believed protected them from infection and bad odors.

The Dark Ages (a.d. 400–800) and the Middle Ages (a.d. 800–1400)

When the Roman Empire was conquered by the Huns (nomads from the north), the study of medical science stopped. For a period of 1,000 years, medicine was practiced only in **convents** and **monasteries**. Because the Church believed that life and death were in God's hands, the monks and priests had no interest in how the body functioned. The primary treatment was prayer. Medication consisted of herbal mixtures, and care was **custodial**. Monks collected and translated the writings of the Greek and Roman physicians.

Terrible **epidemics** caused millions of deaths during this period. Bubonic plague (the black death) alone killed 60 million people. Other uncontrolled diseases included smallpox, diphtheria, syphilis, and tuberculosis. Today, these illnesses are not always life threatening. Scientists have discovered **vaccines** and medications to control these diseases. It is important to remember that some diseases can become epidemic if people are not vaccinated.

Science Link

Lyme Disease

If not for modern day medicine and scientific research, the United States may have experienced an epidemic situation with Lyme disease.

The first case of Lyme disease was reported in Old Lyme, Connecticut, in 1975. Since then, cases of Lyme disease have been reported in most parts of the United States. The disease can be detected by a blood test and treated with antibiotics. If caught early enough, Lyme disease may cause little or no complications.

Lyme disease is caused by a bacteria carried by ticks. The ticks contract the bacteria by biting a mouse or deer infected with Lyme disease. Humans contract the disease if bitten by an infected tick. Initial symptoms may include a rash around the area of the bite and flu-like symptoms, including, chills, fever, fatigue, and body aches. If the infection is not treated, it can cause severe joint pain and neurological deficiencies and even heart-related problems.

Meningitis (inflammation of the tissues around the brain and spinal chord), Bell's palsy (loss of muscle tone in the face), and numbness in limbs are some of the more severe effects of Lyme disease. In the most severe cases, paralysis can occur.

Create a historical timeline showing the spread of Lyme disease from 1975 to the present in 10-year increments. Calculate the number of cases by state for each period (some will not have reported any cases) and the percentage of the total cases reported for each state on the timeline.

Create a second timeline that shows the various treatments and their outcomes used as they are developed and adopted.

Why is it beneficial to study the history of health care and how it has progressed into modern day medicine and health care practices?

The Renaissance (a.d. 1350–1650)

The Renaissance period saw the rebirth of learning. During this period, new scientific progress began. There were many developments during this period:

- The building of universities and medical schools for research
- The search for new ideas about disease rather than the unquestioning acceptance of disease as the will of God
- The acceptance of **dissection** of the body for study
- The development of the printing press and the publishing of books, allowing greater access to knowledge from research

These changes influenced the future of medical science.

Apply It

Divide into groups, each responsible for creating a timeline and researching medical discoveries, inventions, and people of a specific era.

After researching, each group should prepare and present a paper on their findings to the class.

dissection
(di SEK shuhn)
Act or process of dividing, taking apart.

The Sixteenth and Seventeenth Centuries

The desire for learning that began during the Renaissance continued through the next two centuries. During this time, several outstanding scientists added new knowledge. Here are some examples:

- Leonardo da Vinci studied and recorded the anatomy of the body. See da Vinci's depiction of the human body in **Figure 1.2**.

Introduction to Being a Health Care Worker | Chapter 1 7

Science Link—Lyme Disease

- Discuss the factors that might contribute to any epidemic.
- Point out how Lyme disease is transmitted, and why it is difficult to prevent and diagnose.

Why is it beneficial to study the history of health care and how it has progressed into modern day medicine and health care practices?

Answer: Research based on what we have learned in the past has ensured that epidemics are much less common today. The syndrome known as Lyme disease was recognized after a series of cases occurred in towns in southeastern Connecticut in 1975 (including the town of Lyme). But physicians had been treating related ailments for over 75 years. Doctors in Connecticut were able to use the information accumulated through the years to develop a treatment and help stem the epidemic. Medical history provides us with building blocks for research.

Teaching Tips

- Point out the lack of education, as well as creative and scientific advancement during the Dark Ages, and how it adversely impacted health care.
- Compare the Renaissance, with its renewed emphasis on education, to the Dark and Middle Ages.

Apply It

- Depending on class size, more than one group can work on the same era.
- For example, you could assign separate groups an era or century instead of the entire period of history.
- Likewise, you could have groups select one or two people to research. Allow class time for all of the groups to present their prepared papers.

Teaching Tips

- Focus on the scientists who made advances during the sixteenth and seventeenth centuries.
- Point out that some of these scientists may have been considered mad, or heretics, for their ideas.
- Discuss quackery. Ask students if there are any practices today that might seem like quackery?
- Point out that infection is still a leading cause of death.

Figure Focus

1.2 Human body as depicted by Leonardo da Vinci. How does the figure illustrate Leonardo da Vinci's contribution to the medical field?

Answer: Leonardo da Vinci studied and recorded the anatomy of the body.

Teaching Tips

- Note that during the eighteenth century, students were taught about medicine and health care using techniques similar to those in use today.
- Review the men and women who made contributions to the field during the eighteenth century.

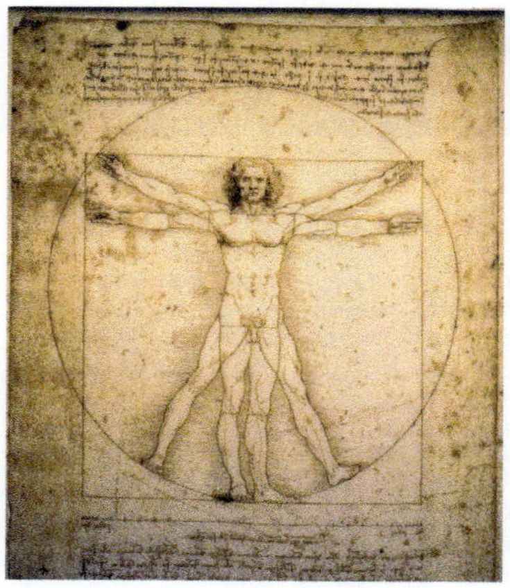

Figure 1.2
Human body as depicted by Leonardo da Vinci. How does the figure illustrate Leonardo da Vinci's contribution to the medical field?

physiology
(fiz ee OL uh jee)
The branch of biology dealing with the functions and activities of living organisms and their parts.

quackery
(kwak uh ree)
Practice of pretending to cure diseases.

stethoscope
(STETH uh skohp)
Instrument used to hear sound in the body (e.g., heartbeat, lung sounds, bowel sounds).

respiration
(res pu REY shuhn)
The inhalation and exhalation of air, or breathing.

- William Harvey used this knowledge to understand **physiology**, and he was able to describe the circulation of blood and the pumping of the heart.
- Gabriele Fallopius discovered the fallopian tubes of the female anatomy.
- Bartolommeo Eustachio discovered the tube leading from the ear to the throat (Eustachian tube).
- Antonie van Leeuwenhoek invented the microscope, establishing that there is life smaller than the eye can see. Van Leeuwenhoek scraped his teeth and found the bacteria that causes tooth decay. Although it was not yet realized, the germs that cause disease were now visible.

In addition, apothecaries, early pharmacies, started in this time. In medieval England, these apothecaries engaged in a flourishing trade in drugs and spices from the East.

Despite these advances, mass death from childbed fever, **quackery**, and disease continued. The causes of infection and disease were still not understood. Interestingly, infections are, even today, one of the leading causes of death.

The Eighteenth Century

Many discoveries were made in the eighteenth century that required a new way of teaching medicine. Students not only attended lectures in the classroom and laboratory, but also observed patients at the bedside. When a patient died, they dissected the body and were able to observe the disease process. This led to a better understanding of the causes of illness and death. Also, in the eighteenth century a wider range of students was studying medicine. In 1849, Elizabeth Blackwell (1821–1910) became the first female physician in the United States. The study of physiology continued, and more new discoveries were made:

- René Laënnec (1781–1826) invented the **stethoscope**. The first stethoscope was made of wood. It increased the ability to hear the heart and lungs, allowing doctors to determine if disease was present.
- Joseph Priestley (1733–1804) discovered the element oxygen. He also observed that plants refresh air that has lost its oxygen, making it usable for **respiration**.
- Benjamin Franklin's (1706–1790) discoveries affect us in many ways. His discoveries include bifocals, and he found that colds could be passed from person to person.
- Edward Jenner (1749–1823) discovered a method of vaccination for smallpox. Smallpox killed many people in epidemics. His discovery saved millions of lives. His discovery also led to immunization and to preventive medicine in public health.

8 Chapter 1 | Introduction to Being a Health Care Worker

CUSTOMIZED INSTRUCTION

More Advanced Students

Leonardo da Vinci is not the only artist who studied medicine and science, or scientist who studied art. Encourage more advanced students to learn more about the relationship between medicine and the arts, and the people who crossed from one to the other. They can report their findings to the class.

The Nineteenth and Twentieth Centuries

Medicine continued to progress rapidly, and the nineteenth century was the beginning of the organized advancement of medical science. Important events during the nineteenth and twentieth centuries include the following:

- Ignaz Semmelweis (1818–1865) identified the cause of childbed fever (puerperal fever). Large numbers of women died from this fever after giving birth. Semmelweis noted that the patients of midwives (women who delivered babies but were not physicians) had fewer deaths. One of the differences in the care given by the physicians and the midwives was that the physicians went to the "dead room," where they dissected dead bodies. These physicians did not wash their hands or change their aprons before they delivered babies. Their hands were dirty, and they infected the women. Semmelweis realized what was happening, but other physicians laughed at him. Eventually, his studies were proved correct by others, and handwashing and cleanliness became an accepted practice. Today, handwashing is still one of the most important ways that we control the spread of infection.
- Louis Pasteur (1822–1895), known as the "Father of **Microbiology**," discovered that tiny **microorganisms** were everywhere. Through his experiments and studies, he proved that microorganisms cause disease. Before this discovery, doctors thought that microorganisms were *created by* disease. He also discovered that heating milk prevented the growth of bacteria. **Pasteurization** kills bacteria in milk. We still use this method to treat milk today. He created a vaccine for rabies in 1885.
- Joseph Lister (1827–1912) learned about Pasteur's discovery that microorganisms cause infection. He used carbolic acid on wounds to kill germs that cause infection. He became the first doctor to use an **antiseptic** during surgery. Using an antiseptic during surgery helped prevent infection in the incision.
- Ernst von Bergmann (1836–1907) developed **asepsis**. He knew from Lister's and Pasteur's research that germs caused infections in wounds. He developed a method to keep an area germ-free before and during surgery. This was the beginning of asepsis.
- Robert Koch (1843–1910) discovered many disease-causing organisms. He developed the culture plate method to identify pathogens and also isolated the bacterium that causes tuberculosis. He also introduced the importance of cleanliness and sanitation in preventing the spread of disease.
- Wilhelm Roentgen (1845–1923) discovered x-rays in 1895. He took the very first picture using x-rays of his wife's hand. His discovery allowed doctors to see inside the body and helped them discover what was wrong with the patient.

microbiology
(mahy kroh bahy OL uh jee)
The branch of biology dealing with the structure, function, uses, and modes of existence of microscopic organisms.

microorganisms
(mahy kroh AWR guh niz uhms)
Organisms so small that they can only be seen through a microscope.

pasteurization
(PAS chuh rahyz ay shuhn)
To heat food for a period of time to destroy certain microorganisms.

antiseptic
(an tuh SEP tik)
Substance that slows or stops the growth of microorganisms.

asepsis
(uh SEP sis)
Sterile condition, free from all germs.

Teaching Tips

- Review the important developments that occurred during the nineteenth and twentieth centuries, and the people responsible for them.
- Emphasize the development of techniques that kill germs, such as antiseptic and asepsis.

Discuss

- Discuss the development of treatments for pain.
- Emphasize the importance of the development of asepsis and pain relief for the advancement of surgery.
- Discuss the discovery of viruses.
- Review the list of diseases caused by viruses.
- Ask students if they think treating the mind is the same as treating other parts of the body, such as the heart or the lungs.

- Paul Ehrlich (1854–1915) discovered the effect of medicine on disease-causing microorganisms. His treatment was effective against some microorganisms but was not effective in killing other bacteria. His discoveries brought about the use of chemicals to fight disease. In his search to find a chemical to treat syphilis, he completed 606 experiments. On the 606th experiment, he found a treatment that worked.

anesthesia
(an uhs THEE zhuh)
Loss of feeling or sensation.

Before the nineteenth century, pain was a serious problem. Surgery was performed on patients without **anesthesia**. Early physicians used herbs, hashish, and alcohol to help relieve the pain of surgery. They even choked patients to cause unconsciousness to stop pain. Many patients died from shock and pain. During the nineteenth and twentieth centuries, nitrous oxide (for dental care), ether, and chloroform were discovered. These drugs have the ability to put people into a deep sleep so that they do not experience pain during surgery. The knowledge of asepsis and the ability to prevent pain during surgery are the basis of safe, painless surgery today.

Scientists and physicians kept learning from the discoveries of the past. They continued to study and research new ways to treat diseases, illness, and injury. Some of the most important discoveries in the late 19th and 20th centuries included:

- Gerhard Domagk (1895–1964) discovered sulfonamide compounds. These compounds were the first medications effective in killing bacteria. They changed the practice of medicine by killing deadly diseases.
- In 1892 in Russia, Dmitri Ivanovski discovered that some diseases are caused by microorganisms that cannot be seen with a microscope. They are called viruses. These viruses were not studied until the electron microscope was invented in Germany. These are some of the diseases caused by viruses:
    - Poliomyelitis
    - Rabies
    - Measles
    - Influenza
    - Chicken pox
    - German measles
    - Herpes zoster
    - Mumps

psychology
(sahy KOL uh jee)
The science of the mind or of mental states and processes.

psychiatry
(si KAHY ut tree)
The practice or science of diagnosing and treating mental disorders.

- Sigmund Freud (1836–1939) discovered the conscious and unconscious parts of the mind. He studied the effects of the unconscious mind on the body. He determined that the mind and body work together. This led to an understanding of psychosomatic illness (physical illness caused by emotional conflict). His studies were the basis of **psychology** and **psychiatry**.
- Sir Alexander Fleming (1881–1955) found that penicillin killed life-threatening bacteria. The discovery of penicillin is considered one of the most important discoveries of the twentieth century. Before penicillin was discovered, people died of illnesses that we consider curable today, including pneumonia, gonorrhea, and blood poisoning.
- Jonas Salk (1914–1995) discovered that a dead polio virus would cause immunity to poliomyelitis. This virus paralyzed thousands of adults and children every year. It seemed to attack the most active and athletic people.

10 Chapter 1 | Introduction to Being a Health Care Worker

It was a feared disease, and the discovery of the vaccine saved many people from death or crippling.

- In contrast to Salk's virus, Albert Sabin (1906–1993) used a live polio virus vaccine, which is more effective. This vaccine is used today to immunize babies against this dreaded disease.
- Francis Crick (1916–2004) and James Watson (born 1928) discovered the molecular structure of DNA, based on its known double helix. Their model served to explain how DNA **replicates** and how hereditary information is coded on it. This set the stage for the rapid advances in molecular biology that continue to this day. In 1962, they won the Nobel Prize in Medicine for this discovery.
- Christian Barnard (1922–2001) performed the first successful heart transplant in 1968.
- Ben Carson (born 1951) continues to be a pioneer in separating Siamese twins and performing hemispherectomies, surgeries on the brain to stop seizures.

replicate
(REP li kate)
To reproduce or make an exact copy.

The discovery of methods to control whooping cough, diphtheria, measles, tetanus, and smallpox saved many lives. These diseases kill unprotected children and adults. It is important for everyone to be immunized. Immunizations are available from doctors, clinics, hospitals, and public health services.

The Twenty-First Century

Our society is discovering new approaches to medical care every year. Patients/clients are being taught more about wellness, and they are learning more about self-care. The word healthy no longer just refers to a person's physical health. It also refers to a person's emotional, social, mental, and spiritual wellness. To help patients achieve this kind of holistic health, the medical community has become more open to alternative and complementary methods of care. People now go to ayurvedic practitioners, Chinese medicine practitioners, chiropractors, homeopaths, hypnotists, and naturopaths to help meet their medical needs.

Nurses and technicians are visiting patients/clients at home or caring for them in an ambulatory care setting. Just a few years ago, patients were admitted to the hospital for surgery and recovered in the hospital over a period of several days. Today, many patients enter the hospital, have surgery, and are sent home the same day.

Doctors are now often practicing telemedicine. **Telemedicine** includes consultative, diagnostic, and treatment services. Health care providers now use electronic communications to send important medical information to a patient or another health care provider. This has improved patient care by supplying health providers and patients with quicker access to information and greater opportunities for communication.

telemedicine
(TEL uh med uh sin)
Using electronic communications to exchange medical information from one site to another for the health and education of the patient or health care provider.

Introduction to Being a Health Care Worker | Chapter 1 11

Teaching Tips

- Continue reviewing the people who contributed to advancements in medicine.
- Remind students that many of these developments are fairly recent.
- Ask if they know of any relatives, such as grandparents or great-grandparents, who contracted a disease such as polio.
- Note that there are still outbreaks of whooping cough, measles, and other diseases every year.
- Point out that in many parts of the world, immunizations for these diseases are scarce.
- Introduce the concept of wellness and discuss ways wellness care is implemented, such as exercise and diet.

ACTIVITY

As a class, discuss medical treatments used today that might be considered alternative care.

Teaching Tips

- Review ongoing developments.
- You may want to emphasize some advancements that you have witnessed in your own lifetime:
  - Organ transplants
  - Technology such as MRI, pacemakers, and CAT
  - Identification of genetic markers

Language Arts Link—Medical Treatments: From Ancient Times Through Present Day

- Review the alternative and complementary methods of care discussed on p. 11.
- Remind students about your school's Internet policy before having them go online to find information.
- Emphasize that they should use reputable Web resources, such as sites sponsored by the government or educational institutions.
- Remind them to keep a list of sources to use for a bibliography.
- If students do not have access to the Internet, be sure to direct them to other resources, such as books, periodicals, or videos.
- You may want to have students draft an outline or story web to organize their ideas for the report.
- For evaluation, you should verify that the information is correct and in the correct order, and you should mark spelling and grammatical errors.

recipient
(ri SIP ee uhnt)
One who receives.

noninvasive
(non in VEY siv)
Not involving penetration of the skin.

geriatric
(jer ee A trik)
Pertaining to old age.

People are living longer and are usually healthier. New inventions and procedures have changed medicine as we once knew it. Here are some examples:

- The possibility of eliminating disabling disease through genetic research
- The ability to transplant organs from a donor to a **recipient**
- The ability to reattach severed body parts
- The use of portable and handheld computers to aid in diagnosis, accurate record keeping, and research
- The ability to use **noninvasive** techniques for diagnosis
- The advancement in caring for the unborn fetus
- The rediscovery and the medical profession's greater acceptance of alternative medicine and complementary medical practice including acupuncture, acupressure, herbal therapy, and healing touch
- The ability to monitor patient health using automated monitoring equipment, even remotely using wearable devices
- The ability to communicate more easily with patients and have them collect information on their own health using mobile apps

Every day, science makes new progress. We are living in a time of great advancement and new understanding in medicine. People are living longer, creating a need to better understand **geriatric** medicine. In addition, new types of facilities such as assisted living centers are being developed to better meet the physical, emotional, and mental needs of senior citizens.

Language Arts Link

Medical Treatments: From Ancient Times Through Present Day

As you read in this chapter, medical practices, beliefs, and equipment have changed significantly over time. Some practices that have been used for thousands of years are still in use today. They are often integrated with Western medicine and are known as Complementary and Alternative Medicine (CAM).

Select two CAM practices and create a timeline showing when each was first introduced, how the practice has continued to be used, and how it has or has not been altered. To complete your assignment, gather relevant information from multiple print and digital sources using advanced searches effectively. Integrate the information gathered into the timeline description. Include information on ancient civilizations, the Dark Ages, the Middle Ages, the Renaissance, and the 16th–21st centuries in your timeline. Include citations for the sources used. When you are done creating your timeline, organize, compile, and write ideas into a summary report. Include a title for your report and a thesis statement (a sentence stating your main ideas) in the opening paragraph.

Proofread your work to see if you can improve it by making it clearer, more concise, or more interesting to read. Check the spelling and grammar and correct any errors. Be sure to cite any sources that you use in the format required by your instructor. Exchange reports and timelines with a classmate. Provide feedback and corrections as necessary. Read your classmate's comments and revise your report and timeline as necessary.

12 Chapter 1 | Introduction to Being a Health Care Worker

ACTIVITY

One of the results of improvements in health care is that people are living longer. This also means there are more older people to care for. Make a two-column chart or table. In column one, list positive benefits of a longer lifespan. In column two, list negative drawbacks. Discuss this issue as a class.

The Advancement of Nursing

In the nineteenth century, nursing became an important part of medical care. In 1860, Florence Nightingale (1820–1910) attracted well-educated, dedicated women to the Nightingale School of Nursing. (**Figure 1.3**) The graduates from this school raised the standards of nursing, and nursing became a respectable profession.

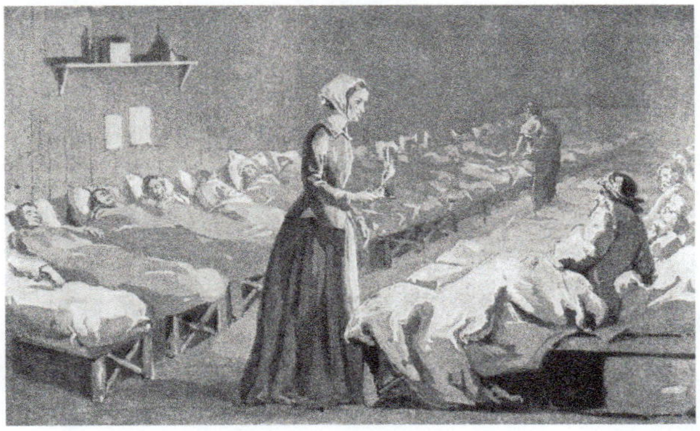

Figure 1.3
Florence Nightingale, founder of modern nursing. What effect did Florence Nightingale's work have on the medical field?

Before this time, nursing was considered unsuitable for a respectable lady. The people giving care to patients were among the lowest in society. As Florence Nightingale was to say, nursing was left to people "too old, too weak, too drunken, too dirty, or too bad to do anything else."

Florence Nightingale came from a cultured, middle-class family who opposed her interest in caring for the ill. However, she convinced her father to give her money to live, and she gained experience by volunteering in hospitals. During the Crimean War, she took a group of 38 women to care for soldiers dying from cholera. More soldiers were dying from cholera than from war injuries. She became a legend while she was there because of her dedication to nursing.

After the war she devoted much of her life to preparing reports on the need for better sanitation and construction and management of hospitals. Her primary goal was to gain effective training for nurses. The public established a Nightingale fund to pay for the training, protection, and living costs of nurses. This was established in recognition of her services to the military during the Crimean War.

She also designed a hospital ward that improved the environment and care of the patients. Prior to this time, patients were crowded into small areas that were often dirty. The ward that she designed allowed for a limited number of beds, permitted circulation of air, had windows on three sides, and was clean.

Introduction to Being a Health Care Worker | Chapter 1 13

Teaching Tips

- Discuss the historical development of the practice of nursing.
- Review the people who contributed to the development of nursing.

Figure Focus

1.3 Florence Nightingale, founder of modern nursing. What effect did Florence Nightingale's work have on the medical field?

Answer: Florence Nightingale established nursing as a respectable profession, encouraged better training for nurses, and improved the hospital environment.

CUSTOMIZED INSTRUCTION

Less Advanced Students

Less advanced students may have trouble differentiating between the many people who have contributed to advancements in medicine and health care. Encourage them to keep a chronological list of names, dates, and contributions as a study guide. Alternatively, have them focus on one or two people, or one or two time periods.

Figure Focus

1.4 What are the benefits of working as part of a caregiver team?

Answer: Student answers will vary, but this is a good opportunity to discuss the benefits of teamwork.

Discuss

- Review the ways patient care today is different from patient care in the past, such as:
  - Caregiver teams
  - Licensed vs. unlicensed caregivers
  - Use of technology

Teaching Tips

- Review the advances of the twentieth and twenty-first centuries.

During this same time, Clara Barton (1821–1912) served as a volunteer nurse in the American Civil War. After the war, she established a bureau of records to help search for missing men. She also assisted in the organization of military hospitals in Europe during the Franco-Prussian War. Barton campaigned for the United Sates to sign the Treaty of Geneva, which produced relief for sick and wounded soldiers. These experiences led her to establish the American Red Cross in 1881 and to serve as its first president.

Another step forward in the field of nursing was contributed by Lillian Wald (1867–1940). She was an American public health nurse and social reformer. She established the Henry Street Settlement in New York to bring nursing care into the homes of the poor. This led to the Visiting Nurse Service of New York. Today, visiting nurse services are found in most communities.

Patient Care Today

Nursing care has changed significantly throughout the years. Patients have been cared for by teams that included a registered nurse as team leader, a licensed vocational nurse or practical nurse (LVN/LPN) as a medication nurse, and a nursing assistant who provided personal care. In primary care nursing, which followed team nursing, all patient care was provided by a registered nurse.

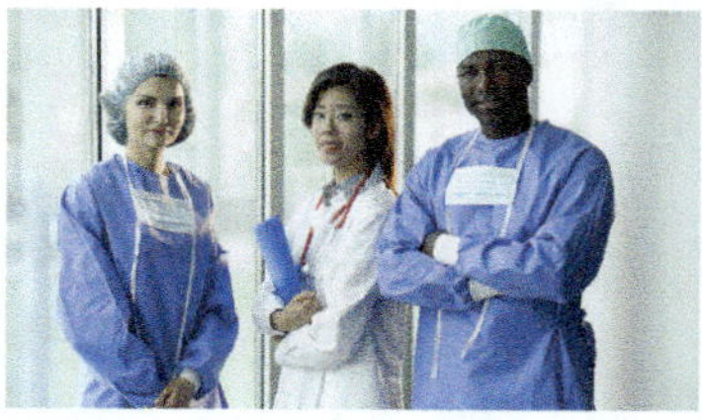

Figure 1.4
What are the benefits of working as part of a caregiver team?

phlebotomy
(fluh BOT uh mee)
Practice of opening a vein by incision or puncture to remove blood.

Today, unlicensed assistive caregivers are part of the patient caregiver team. (**Figure 1.4**) There are many titles and new job descriptions for these positions, including clinical partner, service partner, nurse extender, health care assistant, and patient care assistant. These new positions extend the role of entry-level employees. The nurse assistant performs additional tasks, such as **phlebotomy** and recording an electrocardiogram (EKG). Employees from departments other than nursing learn patient care skills. Environmental service workers and food service workers may help with serving food and providing some routine patient care. The registered nurse delegates patient care tasks according to the training and expertise of the assistive personnel.

Because of the scientific and technological advances in health care, the role of the nurse has evolved into one that requires more technology skills. This has created a need for a complex mix of the technologically savvy nurse and the holistic caregiver. Never before has it been more important to maintain the art of nursing, which includes compassion, comfort, and the ability to see the patient as an individual and a member of a family and a community.

14 Chapter 1 | Introduction to Being a Health Care Worker

CUSTOMIZED INSTRUCTION

Less Advanced Students

Less advanced students may benefit from the opportunity to draw a poster depicting their experience as a patient or caregiver, or to record it on a tape, disc, or as an audio file.

Language Arts Link

Historical Contributions

Today, we would never expect a health care professional to examine us with a wooden stethoscope or for surgery to be performed without anesthesia, but, as you learned in this chapter, that wasn't always the case.

Select a medical device, procedure, or person that made an important contribution to health care. Integrate and evaluate multiple sources of information presented in diverse formats and media to learn more about your topic. Record related details and facts that you find. Use citations for the sources you are using in the format required by your instructor.

When you have all of your information, organize, compile, and write ideas into a summary report. Include the details and facts that were found. Include the years in which the device or procedure was used and for what purpose. If you select a person, include the contribution made, the purpose, and whether it is in use today. If it's still being used today, have there been any significant changes? Be sure to proofread your work to see if you can improve it by making it clearer, more concise, or more interesting to read. Check the spelling and grammar and correct any errors. Exchange reports with a classmate. Provide feedback and corrections as necessary. Read your classmate's comments and revise your report as needed.

A Look Back and an Overview of the Future

In the twentieth and twenty-first centuries, medicine has made great strides in improving health care. During these centuries, we have experienced many changes, including these:

- Antibiotics for bacterial diseases
- Improved life expectancy
- Organ transplants
- Healthier hearts (reduced smoking, better diets)
- Dentistry without pain
- Noninvasive diagnosis with computers (CAT, MRI)
- End of smallpox
- Childhood immunizations
- New understanding of DNA and genetics
- Control of diabetes with the discovery of insulin
- Decline in polio.
- Medical machines, such as those for kidney dialysis and the heart-lung machine
- Test tube babies
- HMOs as an alternative to private insurance
- Development and growth of hospice care

Apply It

Investigate recent health care issues, developments, or technologies and their implications. Then create a newscast as medical reporters covering current trends in health care. After appropriate research, each reporter can use charts or live interviews to help present the topic. Video tape the newscast and play it to the class.

Introduction to Being a Health Care Worker | Chapter 1 15

Language Arts Link—Historical Contributions

- Have students select an approved topic. It may be something covered in this chapter, or something the student discovers on his or her own.
- You may want to have a list of topics available.
- You may want to assign a minimum and maximum length.
- You may want to have students draft an outline or story web to organize their ideas for the report.
- Remind students about your school's Internet policy. Emphasize that they should use reputable Web resources, such as sites sponsored by the government or educational institutions.
- Remind them to keep a list of sources to use for a bibliography.
- If students do not have access to the Internet, be sure to direct them to other resources, such as books, periodicals, or videos.
- For evaluation, you should verify that the information is correct and in the correct order, and you should mark spelling and grammatical errors.

CUSTOMIZED INSTRUCTION

Special Needs Students

Prepare a list of devices, procedures, and people that contributed to helping those with visual, hearing, speech, or other physical impairments.

Apply It

- Before students begin their investigative reporting, as a class, discuss current and recent health care issues, technologies, and developments.
- Encourage teams to assign roles to each member and work together to achieve the goal.
- For example, each team might have a project manager responsible for collecting the work from others. There might be a researcher, writer, and illustrator.
- Reports may be made in writing or delivered to the class orally.
- Encourage students to use multimedia in their presentations, such as posters and artwork, or presentation graphics software.

Career Connect

- Explain what a biotechnology company is, and what it does.
- Discuss what it means to develop a pharmaceutical product.
- Discuss people who participate in the process, including researchers, managers, and marketers.
- If a tour is not possible, request a guest speaker, or a presentation you can display on the process of inventing and bringing a new pharmaceutical to market.
- An alternative activity might be to ask the students to research these positions on a company's Web site, or by contacting the company directly.

Teaching Tips

- Review the possibilities of the future.
- Introduce the concept of medical ethics.
- Discuss new developments that might raise ethical dilemmas:
  - Stem cell research
  - Human egg donation
  - Euthanasia
- Point out that medical ethics is not a new problem.
- Refer back to the information about Hippocrates to show how health care workers have grappled with ethical questions throughout history.

What's New?—New Vaccines

- Define vaccine.
- Review the types of vaccines and the diseases they prevent.
- Ask students if they know what vaccines they have received during their lives.

Career Connect

If there is a biotechnology company in your community, ask for a group tour that focuses on the different processes necessary for inventing a new pharmaceutical product and getting it to market.

If there is no biotechnology company in your community, complete an Internet search of a leading company to identify the process that is used to develop a new pharmaceutical product.

The future of medicine holds many promises for better health. Current and future research will hopefully provide advances in the following:

- Cure for HIV, AIDS, and the Ebola virus
- Decrease in the cases of malaria, influenza, leprosy, and African sleeping sickness
- Gene editing therapy may bring a cure for genetically transferred diseases (e.g., Tay-Sachs, muscular dystrophy, multiple sclerosis, cerebral palsy, Alzheimer's, lupus)
- Improved treatment for arthritis and the common cold
- Isolation of the gene that causes depression
- Use of electronics to allow disabled persons to walk
- Nutritional therapy to decrease the number of cases of schizophrenia
- Stem cell technology and cloning may allow hospitals to grow tissue and organs from samples taken from transplant recipients themselves, avoiding rejection issues

Medical Ethics

Advancement in medicine creates new problems. How will the recipient of an organ be chosen? Who will be allowed to receive experimental drugs? How will the creation of in vitro embryos be ethically managed? Is it ethical to provide continuing confidentiality about AIDS patients, or should they be required to report their condition? Does a terminally ill patient have the right to assisted death (euthanasia)? Is editing the genetic code of a patient safe or ethical? Are vaccines used for immunization tested rigorously enough to prove their safety? There are many questions now, and there will be more questions in the future as health care changes and technology continues to advance.

What's New?

New Vaccines

In the eighteenth century, Edward Jenner discovered a method of vaccination for smallpox that helped to end the epidemic. In the twenty-first century, doctors and scientists continue to do research to develop vaccines for diseases and illnesses.

While today's adults received only a few vaccines for illnesses such as measles, mumps, and rubella, when they were children, today's children are offered a variety of vaccines. One such vaccine is Varivax. This vaccine helps to prevent, or at least lessen, the effects of chicken pox. In previous generations, children had to suffer the uncomfortable symptoms of this virus. The vaccine gives today's children some degree of protection.

Other new vaccines now offered to children are Gardasil and Cervarix, which were developed to protect girls from getting cervical cancer when they get older, and Menactra and Menveo, vaccines developed to prevent children from getting meningitis.

How might these new vaccines affect people's lives and the cost of health care?

16 Chapter 1 | Introduction to Being a Health Care Worker

How might these new vaccines affect people's lives and the cost of health care?

Answer: Patients will spend less time being sick with common and sometimes serious diseases, such as chicken pox, meningitis, and cervical cancer. This may reduce the cost that people have to spend on health care. In addition, life expectancy for both children and adults will continue to increase as deadly diseases such as meningitis and cervical cancer are prevented with vaccines.

CUSTOMIZED INSTRUCTION

At-Risk Students

Have students write a definition of the word *ethics* on one side of an index card. On the other side, ask them to write two examples of ethical behavior in the classroom. Ask them to share with the class.

Summary

You have learned that the science of health care has grown and developed over the last 5,000 years. These changes increased the average life expectancy. Our standards of living improved with the progress of medical science. The dedication of the many scientists discussed in this section is responsible for the improvements in health care that we enjoy today. Their research is the foundation of the high technology that is developing in medicine.

Section 1.1 Review Questions

1. What did early human beings believe caused illness and disease?
2. Who were the first people to organize medical care?
3. Name two ways that medical progress was made during the Renaissance period.
4. Which discoveries in the nineteenth and twentieth centuries led to safer surgeries?
5. How does technology continue to improve medical care today?
6. Explain how society's view of women in medicine has changed over the years.

Becoming a Health Care Worker

SECTION 1.2

Background

A health care worker is a well-trained professional whose top concern is patient welfare. Health care workers must have a thorough knowledge of current health procedures. They must maintain a professional appearance and practice professional behavior. They must also safeguard the confidentiality of patient information. You must keep in mind all of these standards of behavior as you become a health care worker.

In addition, health care workers must realize that careers in this field are emotionally and physically demanding. Long hours, strenuous activity, and difficult situations, such as dealing with death and critically ill patients, can cause exhaustion and stress for caregivers. Knowing how to prepare for such circumstances can assist the health care worker to be the most productive caregiver.

Objectives

When you have completed this section, you will be able to do the following:

- Match key terms with their correct meanings.
- Discuss the importance of proper health care training.
- Describe the proper appearance for a health care worker.
- Discuss standards of behavior.
- Discuss the importance of confidentiality when working with patient records.

Introduction to Being a Health Care Worker | Chapter 1 17

Section 1.1 Review Questions

1. Answer: Early human beings believed that illness and disease were caused by supernatural spirits.
2. Answer: The Romans were the first to organize medical care. They sent medical equipment and physicians with their armies to care for wounded soldiers. Roman physicians kept a room in their houses for the ill. This was the beginning of hospitals.
3. Answer: During the Renaissance period, medical progress was made by:
   - The building of universities and medical schools for research
   - The search for new ideas about disease rather than the unquestioning acceptance of disease as the will of God
   - The acceptance of dissection of the body for study
   - The development of the printing press and the publishing of books, allowing greater access to knowledge from research
4. Answer: During the nineteenth and twentieth centuries, nitrous oxide (for dental care), ether, and chloroform were discovered, which led to safer surgeries.
5. Answer: Doctors are now often practicing telemedicine. Health care providers may now e-mail, fax, or telephone important medical information to a patient or another health care provider. Telemedicine has improved patient care by supplying health providers and patients with quicker access to information and greater opportunities for communication.
6. Answer: Florence Nightingale created the Nightingale School of Nursing, raised the standards of nursing, and made nursing a respectable profession. Clara Barton established the American Red Cross, and Lillian Wald created the Visiting Nurse Service of New York.

FOCUS AND ENGAGE

Introduce the Section

a. Review the content of the Background paragraph, focusing on the three key points of becoming a health care worker.
b. Explain why it is important to have a thorough knowledge of current health procedures, behave and appear professionally, and respect confidentiality.
c. Ask students to reflect on their own experiences with health care workers, and whether they were professional in both behavior and appearance.
d. Discuss the objectives for the section.

Vocabulary Review

a. Key terms are defined in the margins of the text on the page where they first appear.

b. Pronounce each word, and have the students repeat the pronunciation out loud.

c. Discuss the definition of each word.

TEACH

Discuss

- Present brochures, books, or pamphlets about health care training programs available in your area, such as technical schools and colleges or universities.
- Discuss the similarities and differences among associate's, bachelor's, master's, and doctoral degrees, including the amount of time and money involved with obtaining them.
- Point out to students that becoming a health care entrepreneur requires studying business, in addition to health care education.

Teaching Tips

- Review the different types of training available, including professional development.
- Point out the differences between secondary and postsecondary studies.
- Ask students to discuss their educational goals.
- Emphasize the importance of cleanliness in stopping the spread of viruses, as well as in projecting a professional appearance.

Health Care Education

professional
(pro FESH uh nuhl)
One who is paid for their work.

accredited
(a KRED dit ted)
Attested and approved as meeting prescribed standards.

When you start considering a career as a health science **professional**, there are many things to think about; these include the educational requirements, along with other factors, such as how much money you will make. When you have decided to become a health professional, it is important to research and choose a quality health care education program that fits your interests. Technical, community, or four-year colleges in your area may have **accredited** health care programs. These programs offer a variety of degrees, including:

- Certification, where a person is certified as being able to competently complete a job, usually by passing an examination
- Associates degree, usually awarded after completion of a 2-year program
- Bachelor's degree, usually awarded after completion of a 4-year program
- Master's degree, a post-graduate degree awarded after completion of a 5- to 6-year program
- Doctoral degree, or doctorate, a post-graduate degree that is the highest certificate of membership in the academic community

Depending on the type of health professional you wish to be, there will be different licensing requirements. A license is issued by a governmental entity and allows the individual to provide health care or related services.

Visit Web sites of schools that offer health care education to see which program appeals to you most. Visit each college and talk to students before you enroll. You may also talk to health professionals in local clinics or hospitals to find out where they received their education.

After enrolling in a health care program, be sure to work hard at your studies. Health care information can be complicated and detailed. It is important for you to learn all procedures correctly, so you can provide the best treatment to patients.

Health care procedures and knowledge change all the time. Even after you are employed as a health care professional, it is important for you to continue your education. Take any training sessions that are provided by your health care facility. Read professional journals to learn about new health breakthroughs. Discuss procedures with other health care professionals in your facility, to make sure you are all providing the most up-to-date treatment.

Continuing education credits (CEUs) are required for maintenance of certification or advancement in many positions. This is to ensure that health care professionals stay current on developments in their fields to provide the best patient care.

entrepreneur
(ahn truh pruh NUR)
A person who organizes and manages a business.

In the health care field, there is a rise among multicompetent workers. Multicompetent workers are trained in one field or occupation and then receive additional education to work in a second field or occupation. In addition, another opportunity in health care professions is that of the **entrepreneur**. The entrepreneur organizes, manages, and assumes the risks of a business. In the health care field, entrepreneurs often work under the direction of a physician or dentist.

18 Chapter 1 | Introduction to Being a Health Care Worker

CUSTOMIZED INSTRUCTION

Special Needs Students

You may want to have information about the availability of opportunities for special education in health care for special needs students. For example, you may want to provide brochures or contact information for schools in your area that offer such instruction.

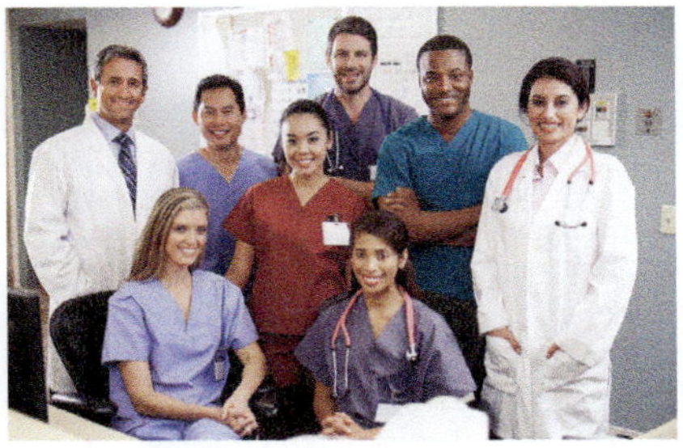

Figure 1.5
Health care workers should be well-groomed and professional. Why do the health care workers in the photograph appear professional?

Appearance and Hygiene

A professional **appearance** makes a statement about your **commitment** to patient care. A well-groomed and well-dressed staff signals that everyone in the facility is interested in the welfare of the patient. (**Figure 1.5**) A clean appearance reassures patients who may be anxious and sick that the staff is efficient, professional, and capable of providing necessary medical service. The following are **recommendations** for maintaining a well-groomed, professional appearance that meet industry expectations:

1. Dress according to your facility's dress code, including uniform. This usually means that clothes will be clean, neat, and in good repair. They should not be of extreme fashion.
2. Keep jewelry to a minimum (e.g., watch, stud earrings, and a ring). Jewelry can cause injury to the patient and the professional (if the patient grabs on to it), as well as transmit germs. Body piercings do not indicate a professional appearance, and can cause infections.
3. Wear your name badge every day, and make sure patients/clients can clearly see it. People need to be able to relate to you, and to call you if they need you. It also helps them identify who is assisting them.
4. Wear clean and appropriate shoes every day.
5. Keep your hair clean.
6. Follow rules of good **hygiene**:
   a. Brush your teeth at least twice a day.
   b. Floss daily.
   c. Use mouthwash or breath mints.
   d. Bathe daily.
   e. Use unscented deodorant. Remember that odors can be offensive to patients who are ill and nauseated and some patients may be allergic to perfumes and deodorant.
   f. Wear your hair up and off your collar. You do not want your hair to fall on a patient when working with them.

appearance
(uh PEER ents)
The way someone or something looks.

commitment
(kuh MIT ment)
A pledge or promise.

recommendations
(rek uh men DAY shuns)
Suggestions.

hygiene
(HI jean)
The practice of keeping clean.

Community

Present a fashion show of what to wear (or not wear) in a professional setting. The narrator can provide information as to why the look is appropriate or inappropriate. The student models will represent each look. This can be videotaped, or you may be able to present your fashion show at a local long-term care facility or hospital.

Introduction to Being a Health Care Worker | Chapter 1 19

Teaching Tips

- Review the importance of personal hygiene for the health care worker. Relate it to wellness, as well as to professionalism.
- Display or handout codes of behavior and/or dress policies obtained from health care facilities.
- Ask students to list reasons why these policies and codes are important.
- Ask students to suggest possible ramifications of an unprofessional appearance.
- Point out that some people may be allergic to scented products, such as deodorant, perfume, and even hairspray.
- Discuss the difference between recommendations and requirements in terms of personal appearance and hygiene, but emphasize that workers must use their best judgment at all times.
- Ask students what they think might happen to workers who do not follow a facility's dress code.

Figure Focus

1.5 Health care workers should be well-groomed and professional. Why do the health care workers in the photograph appear professional?

Answer: The staff is well-groomed. They are wearing uniforms and clothing appropriate to their jobs. Their hair and clothes are neat and clean while they are working. A professional appearance makes a statement about your commitment to patient care. A well-groomed and well-dressed staff signals that everyone in the facility is interested in the welfare of the patient. A clean appearance reassures patients who may be anxious and sick that the staff is efficient, professional, and capable of providing necessary medical service.

Community

- Allow time to plan how each "model" will dress and to write a script for the narrator.
- Video-taping the fashion show provides the opportunity to deliver copies to senior centers, long-term care facilities, or hospitals.
- If you cannot tape the event, have students contact a facility to inquire about performing live.

ACTIVITY

Call students' attention to the Community project on this page. Then ask them to page through their books to see other community service projects that are suggested. Discuss with them that community service is a donated service or an activity that is intended to benefit the public. Encourage them to use the community service examples in their books, along with their own experiences and ideas, to develop additional community service projects that they can carry out to benefit others.

Teaching Tips

- Point out to students that maintaining their appearance on the job shows respect for their chosen professions.
- Review the gender-specific guidelines.
- Review the standards of behavior.
- Ask students to provide examples of each standard.
- Discuss the problems that can arise from poor behavior in the workplace.
- Emphasize that the consequences of poor behavior may result in losing the job.

Reinforce and Review

- Reinforce the concepts of standards, policies, and codes.
- Remind students that different types of health care facilities may have different standards, policies, and codes.
- Point out that standards, policies, and codes for appearance and dress must be followed when participating in all clinical-type experiences.

Apply It

- You might want to prepare index cards with a personal characteristic and an occupation ahead of time, if possible.
- Have teams select a card at random.
- You may want to put a time limit on the role-play.

Female

7. Keep makeup conservative (e.g., no dark, heavy makeup).
8. Do not use perfume or cologne, for the same reason as you would use unscented deodorant.
9. Keep nails short, clean, and bare or only use light-colored nail polish. Long nails can scratch a patient. Polish can cover up dirt and can chip and contaminate a patient's wound or dressing.

Male

10. Do not use cologne or strong aftershave, for the same reason as you would use unscented deodorant.
11. Keep beard or mustache neatly trimmed.
12. Shave daily. No stubble!

Standards of Behavior

As a health care worker, you should always behave professionally. By practicing the following set of behaviors and adhering to the established policies and procedures of the employer, you show respect for patients and your fellow health care workers:

1. Maintain a calm, **courteous** manner.
2. Listen carefully when patients or other health care workers are speaking with you.
3. Monitor patients appropriately, in order to ensure their safety.
4. Manage your time effectively and perform tasks efficiently and carefully.
5. Do not gossip about patients or other health care workers.
6. Do not use coarse or offensive language.
7. Do not practice horseplay or other dangerous behaviors.
8. Watch for hazardous situations and correct any hazards that you see.
9. Follow all safety procedures that are required by your health care facility.
10. Always be punctual as you perform your duties.

courteous
(KUR tee us)
Polite.

Apply It

Refer to the "Personal Characteristics" section. In pairs or teams of three, select a health care profession (such as doctor, EMT, or dental hygienist) and role-play a situation in which you demonstrate one of the personal characteristics listed. Have the class identify which characteristic you are portraying.

Personal Characteristics

In addition to professional behavior, health care workers who exhibit the following personal characteristics will be more involved and interested in the welfare of their patients and in being able to solve problems as a critical part of the medical team. Health care workers must be:

1. Caring—demonstrating kindness and concern for others
2. Empathetic—the ability to understand and share what another person is thinking or feeling
3. Compassionate—sympathy for what another person is experiencing with a desire to help
4. Honest—the quality, condition, or characteristic of being fair, truthful, and morally upright

20 Chapter 1 | Introduction to Being a Health Care Worker

5. Dependable—to be reliable or trustworthy
6. Willing to learn—the openness to admit that you don't know the answer or that you are willing to accept help in understanding a situation more fully
7. Patient—the ability to put up with waiting, delay, or provocation without becoming annoyed or upset, or to act calmly when faced with difficulties
8. Accepting criticism—the ability to deal with disapproval or a suggestion that something can be improved
9. Enthusiastic—excited interest in or eagerness to do something
10. Self-motivated—energetic, ambitious, and able to get things done without being directed by others
11. Tactful—ability to avoid giving offense; an intuitive sense of what is right or appropriate
12. Competent—the ability to do something well, measured against a standard, especially ability acquired through experience or training, following the facility's established policies and procedures
13. Responsible—accountability; the state of being accountable to somebody or for something
14. Discrete—the good judgment and sensitivity needed to avoid embarrassing or upsetting others
15. Team players—somebody who works cooperatively; a member of a group who cooperates with other people and who subordinates personal interests in order to come to a consensus and achieve a common goal
16. Ethical—demonstrating a strong sense of moral principles and itegrity
17. Positive—ability to see the situation in the best light; ability to demonstrate optimism
18. Critical thinkers—the ability to think about a problem from multiple viewpoints or angles and solve problems
19. Adaptable—the ability to adjust to changing or challenging situations and maintain quality care
20. Proactive—the ability to show initiative and recognize when something needs to be done and respond without being asked to
21. Respectful of the chain of command—the understanding that the personnel structure is in place to mitigate problems and should be followed unless absolutely necessary
22. Customer service—can treat patients in a way that makes them feel respected and that they are getting a good value for their money

Personal Goals

Wanting or needing something can be a strong motivator, which encourages you to set goals and make decisions that will lead to your happiness and well-being. A goal is a plan to obtain something. You might set a goal to obtain a specific thing—such as a new jacket or a special phone. You might set a goal to achieve a position—such as soloist in the chorus or soccer team captain. Goals help you focus on what is really important to you and what you are willing to work for.

Long-term goals are plans that help you focus on what you want a year from now, or even 5 or 10 years from now. Short-term goals can be achieved in a shorter amount of time. For example, improving your tennis serve is a short-term goal you may be able to achieve within a few weeks or a few months. Becoming certified to work as a pharmacist is a long-term goal that will take years to achieve.

List two or three short-term goals for yourself. What steps will you need to take to achieve your goals?

Body Language

Every move that we make sends a message. Positive messages come from good eye contact, smiling, and paying close attention to who we are interacting with. Negative messages can portray you as hostile, combative, and unwilling. Below are guidelines on how to avoid negative body language and send positive messages:

1. Make eye contact with patients as they enter the health care facility. This will make them feel welcome.
2. **Maintain** eye contact as you **converse** with patients. This will let them know you are interested in hearing what they have to say.

maintain
(meyn teyn)
Keep up.

converse
(KUHn vurs)
Talk, have a conversation.

Introduction to Being a Health Care Worker | Chapter 1 21

CUSTOMIZED INSTRUCTION

At-Risk Students

Have students select three of the personal characteristics listed in the text and write it on one side of an index card. On the other side, they should provide an example of how they demonstrate the characteristic at home, in school, or in their community.

English Language Learners

Ask students to comment on differences—if any—in body language in their country of origin vs. here in the United States. For example, does making eye contact send a positive or negative message in their country of origin?

Teaching Tips

- Read the personal characteristics out loud, and provide examples or definitions.
- Emphasize that exhibiting these characteristics will result in respect and admiration from co-workers, supervisors, and patients. This may lead to job promotions and raises.
- Remind students that the standards of behavior, personal characteristics, and personal goals are not limited to health care occupations; they will serve the students well in any situation.
- Read the list of body language characteristics out loud.
- Ask students to volunteer to demonstrate each one of the body language characteristics.
- They may also demonstrate "negative" body language characteristics. For example, not making eye contact, or fiddling with their hair or face.

Personal Goals

- Emphasize the difference between short-term and long-term goals. Have students compare and contrast differences in pursuing short-term and long-term goals.
- Ask students to share one of their personal short-term goals with the class, and explain why the goal is short-term rather than long-term.
- Discuss steps to take to achieve short-term goals.

TEAMWORK

Have students perform a skit exhibiting the consequences of good and bad behavior in the workplace. Advise them to incorporate as many of the standards of behavior and personal characteristics as possible.

Teaching Tips

- Display a privacy form from a health care facility.
- Point out that confidentiality is a very important topic that is covered in more detail in Chapter 5, "Understanding Your Legal Obligations."
- Emphasize that confidentiality is not just a recommendation, but is mandated by law.
- Discuss ways in which confidentiality can help a patient, such as allowing a patient to discuss personal and private matters with a health care provider.
- Also discuss how breaching confidentiality can hurt patients, caregivers, and health care facilities. For example, an employer might fire an employee if they find out confidential information about a health care problem.

stance
(stans)
The way you stand.

3. Smile. Let people know that you're friendly.
4. Keep an open **stance**. Crossed arms or hands indicate an unwillingness to listen or a barrier in communication.
5. Give your full attention to one patient at a time, even when you have multiple tasks (e.g., telephone, other patients).
6. Keep your hands away from your mouth when speaking. This makes it a more "open" exchange.
7. Sit or stand at eye level with patients as you converse. Avoid standing over patients when conversing.

Maintaining Confidentiality

confidentiality
(kon fuh den chee AL uh tee)
A promise to keep certain information secret.

Maintaining the **confidentiality** of medical records is critical. Medical records contain private information that must not be shared with people who are not involved in the patient's health care. If some private information gets into the wrong hands, it may be used to damage the patient's personal reputation or financial well-being.

reprimanded
(REP ree man did)
Punished.

Each patient signs a confidentiality form before receiving treatment. This form is a legally binding document that promises that the medical facility will protect patient information. Any health care worker who does not follow procedures to ensure patient confidentiality may be **reprimanded**.

Language Arts Link

Managing Your Time

Industry expectations of professional conduct include the ability to manage your time. Managing your time successfully is a matter of organizing and prioritizing what you need to get accomplished. Two handy tools for managing your time are to-do lists and planners. Writing or inputting for short time frames such as is used in the to-do lists, typically for a day or two, and routinely over extended time frames, as in the weekly/monthly planners, should include a range of specific tasks and purposes. Follow a multistep procedure as described below and analyze the results of the work you proposed to complete.

To-do lists: Sometimes it is helpful to write down all the things you have to do. That way you can prioritize what you have to take care of immediately and what can wait. Sometimes the process of writing your tasks down makes them seem more manageable. And, you get the satisfaction of crossing each task off as you complete it!

Weekly/monthly planners: Having a big picture of all your classes, appointments, and social obligations in one place is a great way to organize your time. Write down what you have to do—and where you have to be—for each day of the week. You can create a calendar page on the computer. Or, sketch it out using a ruler and paper.

Create a to-do list for tasks you need to complete for the next month. Sometimes it's most productive to just brainstorm all of the things you need to do and then prioritize them later. Once you've completed your draft to-do list, reorganize the list ranking things according to importance.

Either create a calendar page on the computer, or draw one on a paper using a ruler and pencil. (You can also find blank calendar pages on the Internet. Search on key words such as "Calendar.") Fill in all of your classes, appointments, and social commitments. If you have a paper due or a big test coming up, mark that on your calendar, too.

22 Chapter 1 | Introduction to Being a Health Care Worker

Language Arts Link—Managing Your Time

- Point out that working in health care is usually fast-paced and often unpredictable.
- Discuss the importance of staying organized and focused in order to accomplish all of the tasks you are responsible for.
- For the To Do list, students may want to handwrite the list, or use a word-processing program. They might prioritize the list based on the date when a task must be done, or based on the importance of the task.
- For the Planner, students should use an actual calendar or date book.
- Point out that there should be some overlap between the two. For example, if there is an exam scheduled, it should be on the calendar, and studying for the exam should be on the To Do list.
- Evaluate the projects based on completeness, proper spelling and grammar, and organization.

As a health care worker, you should learn your health care facility's policies and procedures related to confidentiality. Carefully follow these procedures to protect patient privacy.

Summary

In this section, you learned the professional appearance of a health care worker shows his or her commitment to patient care and the practice of professional behavior shows respect to patients. Confidentiality is an important part of staying within legal boundaries, and, as a health care worker, it is your responsibility to ensure patient confidentiality by learning your facility's policies and procedures.

Section 1.2 Review Questions

1. How do you determine which health care education best matches your interests?
2. Why is proper health care training important?
3. List the recommendations for maintaining a well-groomed, professional appearance.
4. List five standards of behavior and list five personal characteristics for health care workers.
5. Why is it important to use positive body language?
6. As a health care worker, why is it important to learn your facility's policy and procedures related to confidentiality?

Career-Ready Practices

You are the office manager for a dental office. Patients are seen by appointment only and through your efficient scheduling system, patients rarely have to wait more than a few minutes to see their dentist or dental hygienist. Today, though, one of your hygienists is caught in a huge traffic jam and will be late getting to work. Her first patient, who had arrived on time and has already been waiting almost 30 minutes, became agitated and demanded that he get in to be seen immediately. The receptionist comes to you to help solve the problem. With a partner, role-play the scenario with one person being the patient and the other person being the office manager. How do you think the office manager should handle the problem?

Keep in mind that career-ready individuals recognize that such problems can arise in the workplace and they are prepared to take the appropriate action to address them. As the health care workers analyze the problem, they soon discover the root cause of the problem and may quickly realize there could be multiple options for solutions. Examining possible ... ahead of time can ... service

Section 1.2 Review Questions

1. Answer: Determine which level degree you want, visit the Web sites of each school you are interested in, visit each school and talk to enrolled students, and talk to health care professional about their education.
2. Answer: Proper health care training is important so that you can provide the best care and treatment for patients.
3. Answer: Recommendations for maintaining a well-groomed, professional appearance include the following:
   - Dress according to your facility's dress code (neat, clean, and in good repair).
   - Keep jewelry to a minimum (e.g., watch, stud earrings, and a ring).
   - Wear your name badge every day, in view of patients/clients.
   - Wear clean and appropriate shoes every day.
   - Keep your hair clean.
   - Follow the rules of good hygiene (brush your teeth and floss daily, use mouthwash or breath mints, bathe daily, use unscented deodorant, wear your hair off your collar).
   - Females should keep makeup conservative, refrain from using perfume, and keep nails short, clean, and bare.
   - Males should refrain from using cologne or strong aftershave, keep beards or mustaches neatly trimmed, and shave daily (no stubble).
   - See also the Career-Ready Practice annotation on p. 26.
4. Answer: There are more than five standards of behavior and they include:
   - Maintain a calm, courteous manner.
   - Listen carefully when patients or other health care workers are speaking with you.
   - Monitor patients appropriately, in order to ensure their safety.
   - Perform tasks efficiently and carefully.
   - Do not gossip about patients or other health care workers.
   - Do not use coarse or offensive language.
   - Do not practice horseplay or other dangerous behaviors.
   - Watch for hazardous situations and correct any hazards that you see.
   - Follow all safety procedures that are required by your health care facility.

   The personal characteristics for health care workers include: empathy, honesty, dependability, willingness to learn, patience, acceptance of criticism, enthusiasm, self-motivation, tact, competence, responsibility, discretion, team player
5. Answer: Body language sends a message and it is important to use positive body language so that patients have faith in your ability to care for them. Smiling, eye contact, and paying attention to the person you are interacting with are example of positive body language.
6. Answer: If a person's private, confidential information gets into the wrong hands, it could be used to damage the person's reputation or financial well-being so it is important to learn your facility's policy and procedures related to confidentiality.

CHAPTER 1 REVIEW

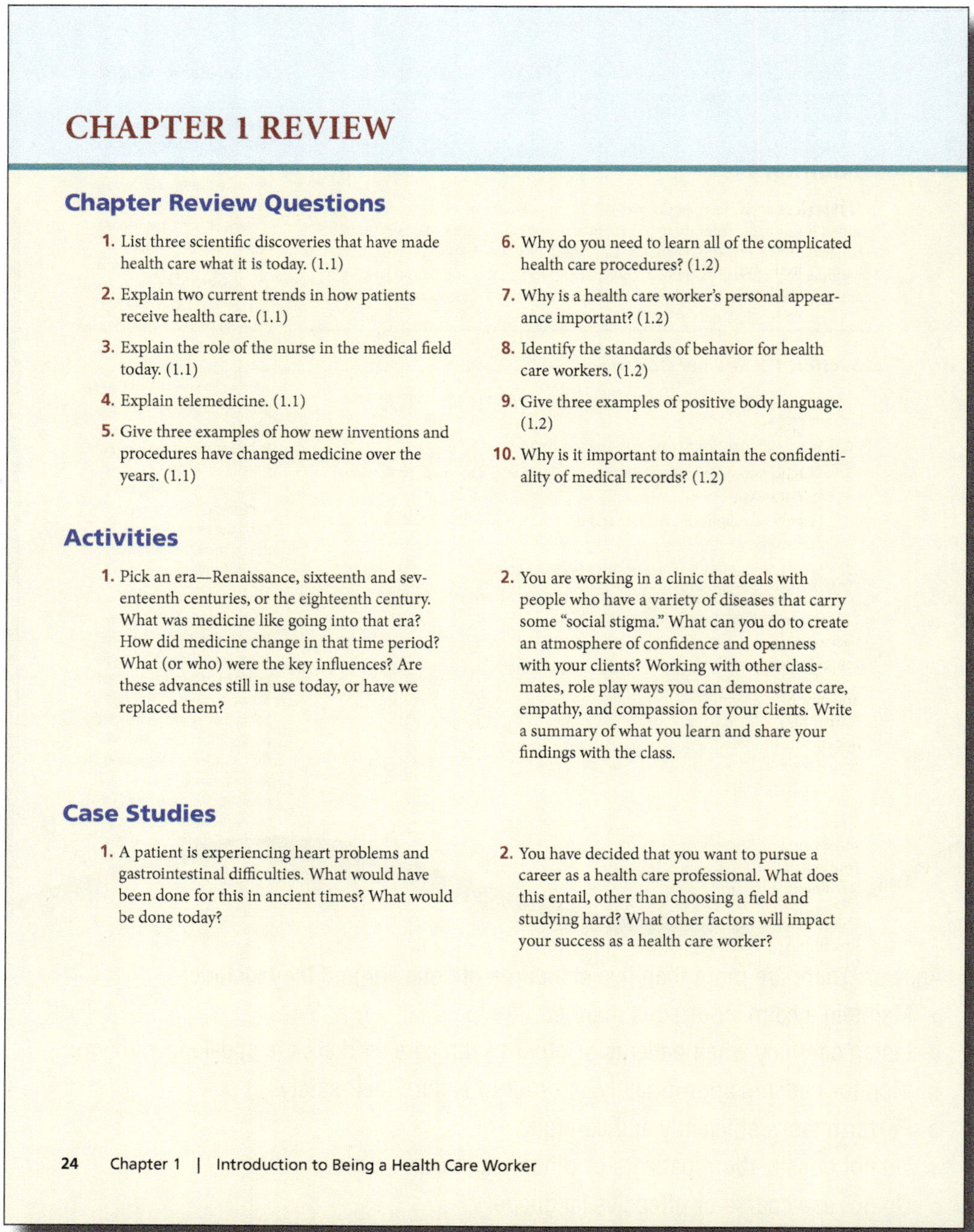

CHAPTER 1 REVIEW

Chapter Review Questions

1. List three scientific discoveries that have made health care what it is today. (1.1)
2. Explain two current trends in how patients receive health care. (1.1)
3. Explain the role of the nurse in the medical field today. (1.1)
4. Explain telemedicine. (1.1)
5. Give three examples of how new inventions and procedures have changed medicine over the years. (1.1)
6. Why do you need to learn all of the complicated health care procedures? (1.2)
7. Why is a health care worker's personal appearance important? (1.2)
8. Identify the standards of behavior for health care workers. (1.2)
9. Give three examples of positive body language. (1.2)
10. Why is it important to maintain the confidentiality of medical records? (1.2)

Activities

1. Pick an era—Renaissance, sixteenth and seventeenth centuries, or the eighteenth century. What was medicine like going into that era? How did medicine change in that time period? What (or who) were the key influences? Are these advances still in use today, or have we replaced them?
2. You are working in a clinic that deals with people who have a variety of diseases that carry some "social stigma." What can you do to create an atmosphere of confidence and openness with your clients? Working with other classmates, role play ways you can demonstrate care, empathy, and compassion for your clients. Write a summary of what you learn and share your findings with the class.

Case Studies

1. A patient is experiencing heart problems and gastrointestinal difficulties. What would have been done for this in ancient times? What would be done today?
2. You have decided that you want to pursue a career as a health care professional. What does this entail, other than choosing a field and studying hard? What other factors will impact your success as a health care worker?

24 Chapter 1 | Introduction to Being a Health Care Worker

Chapter Review Questions

1. Answer: There have been many scientific discoveries that have made health care what it is today, including vaccines, dissection of the body, microorganisms, pasteurization, antiseptic, asepsis, x-rays, anesthesia, morphine, DNA, organ transplantation, and limb reattachment.
2. Answer: Telemedicine has improved patient care by supplying health providers and patients with quicker access to information and greater opportunities for communication. Health care providers may now e-mail, fax, or telephone important medical information to a patient or another health care provider.
3. Answer: Today, the role of the nurse has changed into a more technological role and holistic caregiver because of scientific advances in health care. Also, unlicensed assistive caregivers are part of the patient caregiver team, not just nurses.
4. Answer: Telemedicine is using electronic communications, such as e-mail, fax, telephone, or video to exchange medical information from one site to another for health care and education of the patient or health care provider. In addition, telemedicine can provide consultative, diagnostic, and treatment services. This method has improved patient care by supplying health providers and patients with quicker access to information and greater opportunities for communication and care.
5. Answer: Examples of how inventions and procedures have changed medicine over the years include:
   - The possibility of eliminating disabling disease through genetic research
   - The ability to transplant organs from a donor to a recipient
   - The ability to reattach severed body parts
   - The use of computers to aid in diagnosis, accurate record keeping, and research
   - The ability to use noninvasive techniques for diagnosis
   - The advancement in caring for the unborn fetus

TEAMWORK

Form study groups to prepare for the Chapter 1 Review. Assign the groups to include all levels of achievers. Encourage the groups to meet outside of class to prepare, and provide time in class for them to work together.

CHAPTER 1 REVIEW

Thinking Critically

1. **History of Medicine**—If you created a timeline in the Language Arts link refer back to that. Or, create a timeline that shows the major advancements in medicine from ancient times through the twentieth century. What do you consider to be the single most important development and why?
2. **Professionalism**—If you exhibit a professional look and demeanor that models industry expectations, your clients and colleagues will have more confidence in you. Why is this? Give specific examples of positive and negative behaviors and appearance factors.
3. **Confidentiality**—You are expected to always keep confidentiality in mind, particularly when working in areas to which clients have access. What are three specific steps that you can take that would help maintain confidentiality?
4. **Solving Problems**—Your success as a health science professional will require you to apply critical-thinking and leadership skills, work in a team effectively to build a consensus, and adapt to changing conditions. How will you achieve these goals? What areas do you think you will need to work on the most?

Portfolio Connection

Planning and preparing for a career is a process that allows you to look back on your experiences and learn from them. You can evaluate the things in your past that worked for you and those that did not.

You now have an opportunity to create a file that reflects what you learn. This file is called a *career portfolio*. Your portfolio will contain documents that show what you have learned during your vocational preparation. Your work will show the abilities and skills you gain throughout your training.

You will also create a job search packet that helps you identify ways to share your portfolio with schools or potential employers. Developing your portfolio provides a chance to express the positive results of your learning experiences in a professional manner.

> **PORTFOLIO TIP**
>
> As you build your portfolio, remember that you will want to show how your strengths have helped you, and how you have learned and changed from previous experiences. This will be invaluable when presenting yourself to a potential employer.
>
> It will showcase your ability to deal with new situations and to learn from your mistakes.

Think about a time when you surprised yourself by accomplishing something that you were not sure you could do. What caused you to try it when you were unsure about it? What went well in that experience? What would you do differently? Explain your answers in a short paper. Your explanation must clearly identify your self-evaluation and show how you would approach uncertain experiences in the future.

This assignment helps you review and evaluate your past experience. Some of the future assignments for your portfolio will require a similar process, with a focus on your college and career preparation. Turn in this assignment to your instructor. When you create your portfolio in Chapter 2 your instructor will return it to you.

Introduction to Being a Health Care Worker | Chapter 1 25

- The rediscovery and the medical profession's greater acceptance of alternative medicine and complementary medical practice

6. Answer: You must learn all complicated health care procedures in order to efficiently and effectively treat and care for your patients.
7. Answer: A health care worker's appearance is important because it makes a statement about commitment to patient care and reassures the patient that the staff is professional and capable of providing medical service.
8. Answer:
   - Maintain a calm, courteous manner.
   - Listen carefully when patients or other health care workers are speaking with you.
   - Monitor patients appropriately, in order to ensure their safety.
   - Perform tasks efficiently and carefully.
   - Do not gossip about patients or other health care workers.
   - Do not use coarse or offensive language.
   - Do not practice horseplay or other dangerous behaviors.
   - Watch for hazardous situations and correct any hazards that you see.
   - Follow all safety procedures that are required by your health care facility.

ACTIVITY

Have students write a letter to a health care training facility requesting information about admissions requirements.

9. Answer: Three examples of positive body language include smiling, eye contact, and paying close attention to the person you are interacting with.
10. Answer: If a person's private, confidential information gets into the wrong hands, it could be used to damage the person's reputation or financial well-being so it is important to learn your facility's policy and procedures related to confidentiality.

Activities

1. You may want to make sure the eras are distributed evenly, so that not all students are working on the same era. You may want to specify a length for the written response, such as at least 1½ pages.
2. Make sure students understand the word *stigma*. Encourage students to be creative with this activity.

Case Studies

1. Students should refer to Section 1.1 to find the answer to this question. If necessary, advise them to use a medical dictionary to learn the meaning of gastrointestinal.
2. Advise students to use this opportunity to think about themselves and their own goals.

Thinking Critically

1. Remind students to use research to support their thoughts and ideas. Answers should include a thesis statement and specific examples to support the thesis.
2. Student answers will vary, but should refer to specific factors discussed in the text.
3. Student answers will vary.
4. Encourage students to be honest about the areas that they need to work on.

Portfolio Connection

- Be sure students understand the concept and purpose of a career portfolio.
- Career portfolios are covered in Chapter 3.
- The purpose of this written activity is to help students start a self-evaluation, which in turn will help them develop their career goals.
- Explain that the experience they write about in this exercise does not have to relate specifically to health care.
- Check to make sure that students have completed the assignment.

CUSTOMIZED INSTRUCTION

More Advanced Students

More advanced students may want to research the legal implications of breaching confidentiality in your state, or contact a local hospital to ask them about their own policies on confidentiality. They can present their findings to the class.

2 Understanding Health Care Systems

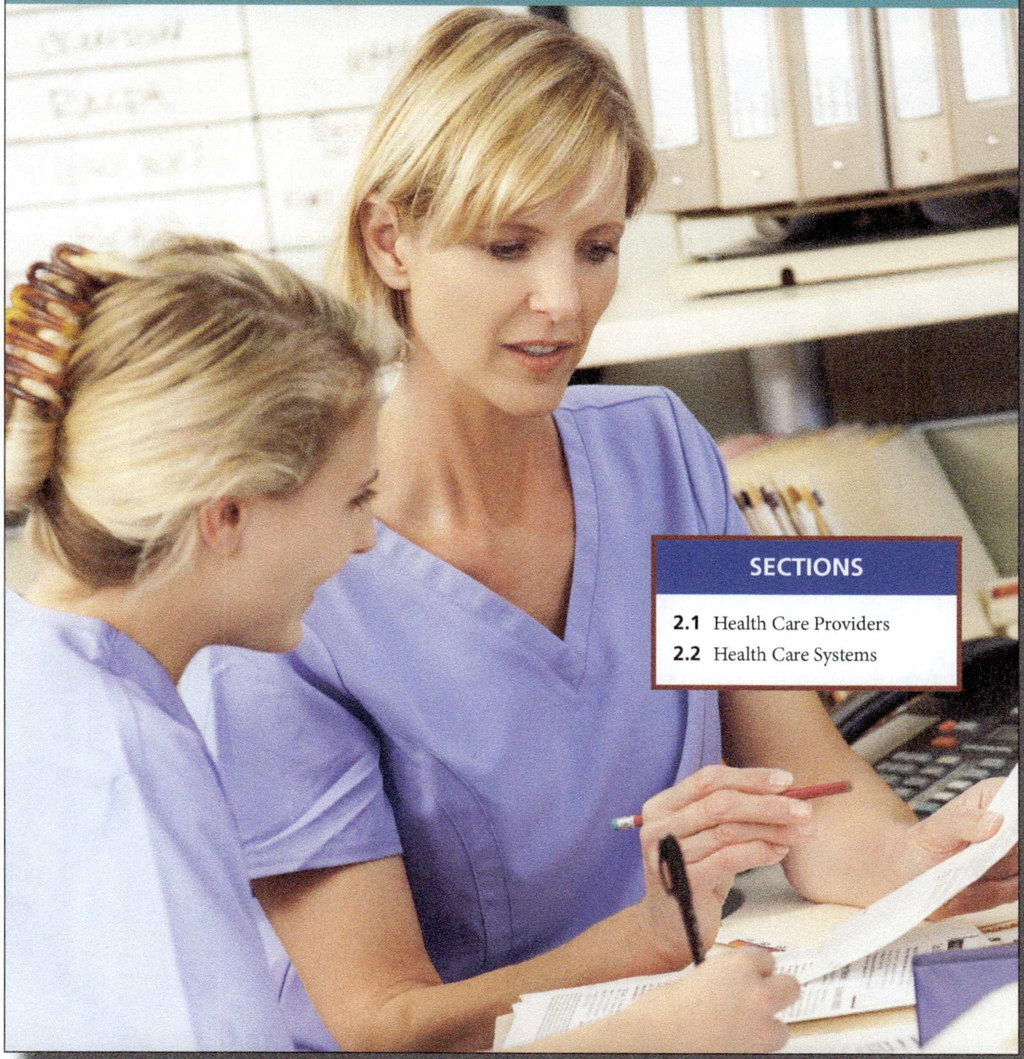

SECTIONS

CHAPTER 2 OVERVIEW

Chapter 2 introduces students to the types of health care delivery systems and providers that are used in the United States.

Section 2.1: The first section covers health care providers such as private hospitals and government agencies. It also introduces concepts such as managed care, wellness, and preventive care.

Section 2.2: This section covers health care systems with an emphasis on cost control and containment. Key topics include health care reform, types of health care insurance, health care payments, and the Healthcare Effectiveness Data and Information Set.

Advance Preparation	
Review	■ Cognitive Mapping form, Student Activity Guide, chapter text for Sections 2.1 and 2.2.
Contact	■ Volunteer agencies to request pamphlets or other information. ■ Guest speakers to explain how their organizations function. ■ Local hospital or clinic to arrange a tour.
Prepare	■ Magazine, newspaper, and online articles on topics such as health costs, health insurance, wellness, and preventive care. ■ A list of volunteer, government, and other health agency Web sites—such as redcross.org, who.int, and hhs.gov.

FOCUS AND ENGAGE

Getting Started

- Use the Cognitive Mapping activity to illustrate the interaction between departments in a hospital.
- Allow at least 15 minutes to complete the activity.
- To work as a class, draw the form on the board.
- You may want to have the students complete the form at the beginning of the chapter, and then again at the end to gauge their knowledge.

Introduce the Section

a. Review the content of the Background paragraph, explaining the role of health care providers in the United States.

b. Explain that understanding the different types of health care provider systems will help students make career decisions.

c. Discuss the objectives for the section.

Vocabulary Review

a. Key terms are defined in the margins of the text on the page where they first appear.

b. Pronounce each word, and have the students repeat the pronunciation out loud.

c. Discuss the definition of each word.

Getting Started

Use the Cognitive Mapping form from Chapter 2 in the Student Activity Guide, or create your own. Put "hospital" in the center circle, and then fill in the four extending circles. Each circle will have one hospital department and the main activity that occurs in that department and what the department's responsibilities are. Share your information with the rest of the class.

SECTION 2.1 Health Care Providers

Background

The health of individuals in a community can have an impact on the economic and social well-being of the entire community. It is the responsibility of every health care worker to help patients/clients solve their health problems. Since the health care industry has many delivery systems, it is important for future health care workers to be aware of health care agencies and facilities, their delivery systems, their organizational structure, and the major services they provide. When you understand how health care facilities and agencies serve the public, you will become a resource person for members of your community.

Nearly everyone sometime during their life accesses the health care system. In 2015, health care expenditures were $3,243 billion, more than $10,000 per person. Nearly 13% of the population works in health care with more than 20% of the workforce employed in health care in some communities. These statistics describe the impact of health services on the economy; the impact of those that receive compensation as a health care worker, the businesses generated by the use of heath care services, and the amount of resources spent on health care services.

Businesses

Health care providers are business organizations. Businesses provide goods and services to consumers. A business may function for profit, or not-for-profit. A health care provider may be a corporation, such as a hospital, or a sole proprietor, such as a doctor who practices alone. Some health care providers are privately-owned. Many times, however, they are public corporations, owned by shareholders and managed by a board of directors. Some health care providers are part of larger public corporations that manage many health care providers. Businesses are responsible to the communities in which they operate.

What responsibilities does a health care provider have to the community?

Objectives

When you have completed this section, you will be able to do the following:

- Match key terms with their correct meanings.
- Research a volunteer agency.
- Define managed care.
- Define ambulatory care.
- Understand the role of government agencies in providing health care.
- List six types of outpatient care and the type of treatment given.
- Define wellness and preventive care.
- Be able to use or read an organizational chart.
- Give two reasons why the organization of health care facilities is important.
- Explain a chain of command.
- List and define the major services in health care.
- Identify two departments in each major service.

28 Chapter 2 | Understanding Health Care Systems

Businesses

Discuss various businesses in your community and the ways they support the community. For example, a local bank might offer higher interest rates on savings accounts for area students. Or, a local hardware store might sponsor little league baseball teams. Health care providers have responsibilities such as health care and wellness education, serving as a link between residents and the appropriate health/social services, and providing access to quality health care services.

CUSTOMIZED INSTRUCTION OVERVIEW	
Less Advanced Students	Pages 29, 40
More Advanced Students	Pages 30, 35
English Language Learners	Pages 29, 32
Special Needs Students	Pages 33, 38
At-Risk Students	Pages 32, 33

Types of Health Care Providers

There are several **facilities** and agencies that provide medical care. Some are familiar, and others may be new to you. The following descriptions will help you understand the differences among the many providers of medical care.

General hospitals do not specialize in any one type of medical treatment; rather, they provide a wide range of **diagnostic**, medical, **surgical**, and emergency care services. (**Figure 2.1**) General hospitals are staffed by professional physicians, surgeons, nurses, and support staff to provide inpatient care to those who need close monitoring and outpatient care to those who need treatment but not constant monitoring.

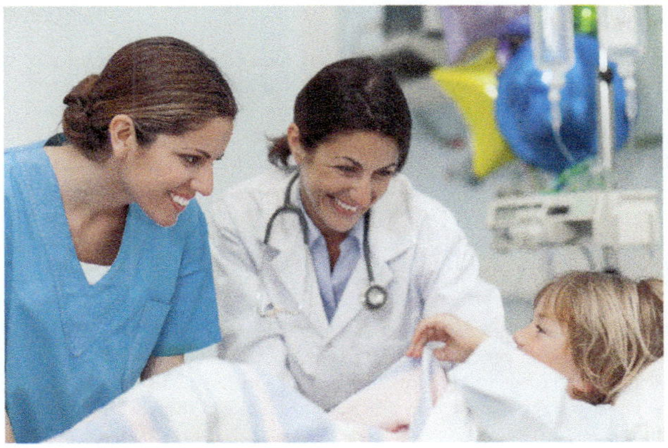

Figure 2.1
General hospitals are facilities where patients are hospitalized for a short time, ranging from a few days to a few weeks. What are the benefits of having many types of health professionals in one place?

Specialty hospitals provide inpatient continuity of care for clients with persistent, recurring diseases or complex medical conditions that require long-term stays (often over a month) in an acute care environment. These may include **chronic** diseases, pulmonary or physical rehabilitation, wound care, and **psychiatric** problems. Specialty hospitals are not nursing home facilities or transitional units. One example of a specialty hospital is St. Jude's Children's Research Hospital, which specializes in treating children with catastrophic diseases.

Convalescent care (e.g., nursing home, long-term care) facilities generally engage in **geriatric** care—care for elderly people needing nursing services and assistance with personal care and daily living activities. These facilities also care for physically ill or injured people of all ages who require an extended **convalescence** for recovery. Many of these facilities focus on rehabilitation, or optimizing the functional status of the client so that they may return to the community. The staff includes nurses; nursing aides and assistants; physical, occupational, and speech therapists; recreational assistants; and social workers.

facilities
(fuh SIL i teez)
Places designed or built to serve a special function (e.g., hospital, clinic, doctor's office).

diagnostic
(dahy uhg NOS tik)
Pertaining to the determination of the nature of a disease or injury by examining (e.g., using x-ray and laboratory tests).

surgical
(SUR ji kuhl)
Repairing or removing a body part by cutting.

chronic
(KRA nik)
Continuing over many years and for a long time (e.g., chronic illness).

psychiatric
(sahy kee A trik)
Pertaining to the mind.

geriatric
(jer ee A trik)
A branch of medicine that deals with the problems and diseases of old age and aging people.

convalescence
(kon vu LES nts)
The gradual recovery of health and strength after illness.

Understanding Health Care Systems | Chapter 2 29

TEACH

Discuss

- Show pamphlets and brochures from different providers.
- Ask students to reflect on their own experiences with different types of health care providers.
- Remind students that health care providers are business organizations: some are for-profit businesses, while others are non-profit.
- Ask students to name a business organization and describe the nature and type of business organization that it is, including whether it is non-profit or for-profit, sole-proprietor or owned by shareholders, public or privately owned.
- Discuss how the state of the economy, both locally and globally, affects business organizations, including health care providers.
- Point out that health care facilities and agencies exist to serve the public.
- Discuss the responsibilities of a health care provider to the community in which it conducts business.
- If students are willing, ask them to list types of providers they have visited or consulted in the past.
- Alternatively, ask students to name providers in the community, such as local hospitals, clinics, or agencies such as the Red Cross.

Reinforce and Review

- Review the history of health care covered in Chapter 1.
- Remind students that the current health care systems evolved over time, and will continue to evolve to meet the needs of the community.

CUSTOMIZED INSTRUCTION

Less Advanced Students

Provide additional time for less advanced students to learn the vocabulary.

English Language Learners

Have students write each key term and its pronunciation on one side of an index card and its definition on the other side.

Figure Focus

2.1 General hospitals are facilities where patients are hospitalized for a short time, ranging from a few days to a few weeks. What are the benefits of having many types of health professionals in one place?

Answer: Benefits include having access to different types of care all under one roof, and professionals can easily consult with each other on patient care and treatment.

TEAMWORK

Prepare a bulletin board or other display using brochures, posters, and other information obtained from agencies, providers, or the Internet.

Teaching Tips

- Review the types of health care providers listed on this page and the next.
- Emphasize the role each organization plays in the health care delivery system.
- Provide examples of how each type of provider or agency delivers care.
- For example, point out how a doctor's office differs from a hospital or rehabilitation center.

ACTIVITY

Write the types of health care agencies or providers on slips of paper. Have students randomly select one type. The student should then explain to the class the type of service and delivery system his or her selection offers.

ambulatory
(AM buhlu tor ee)
Serving patients who are able to walk.

specialties
(SPESH uhl teez)
Fields of study or professional work (e.g., pediatrics, orthopedics, obstetrics).

outpatients
(aout PAY shunts)
Patients/clients who do not require hospitalization but are under a physician's care.

occupational therapy
(ock you PAY shun l)
Helps to give people skills for the job of living satisfying lives, such as dealing with job-related injuries.

recreational therapy
(rek ree A shun l)
Uses play, recreation, and leisure activities to improve physical, cognitive, social, and emotional functioning; the primary goal is to develop lifetime leisure skills.

hydrotherapy
(hi dro THER a pee)
Treatment that uses water therapy for disease or injury.

prosthetics
(pros THE tiks)
Artificial parts made for the body (e.g., teeth, feet, legs, arms, hands, eyes, breasts).

Nursing homes can differ from extended care facilities. Nursing home facilities are places of residence for people who require constant nursing care and have significant problems with activities of daily living.

Extended care facilities are designed to care for those who need assistance with activities of daily living or with medical needs. An extended care facility is needed when someone has a condition that is likely to last for a long period of time or for the rest of his or her life, like moderate Alzheimer's.

There are also *independent living* and *assisted living facilities.* For older individuals with an active lifestyle, independent living offers the opportunity to remain independent in a home of their own that's typically located on a campus with health care professionals on staff and facilities/activities designed specifically for older individuals. Assisted living bridges the gap between independent living and extended care or nursing homes.

Ambulatory *care/clinics* offer medical care—including diagnosis, observation, treatment, and rehabilitation—that does not require an overnight admission to a hospital or other health care facility. In other words, the patient is still "ambulatory." In most ambulatory care facilities, several physicians with different **specialties** combine their practices. This allows the patient/client to receive immediate care for any of a variety of illnesses. Ambulatory care can be delivered at a physician's office, in a designated area of a hospital, and in urgent care centers. Through this type of care, patients/clients are more likely to remain at home throughout treatment and recovery, thus avoiding costly stays in a hospital or other medical facility.

Physician and dental facilities provide care that promotes wellness and diagnosis of illness. Simple surgery, bone setting, counseling, and administration of drugs take place here. Diagnostic services, such as laboratory tests and x-rays, might also take place. Physicians and dentists may provide care in an ambulatory care setting.

Rehabilitation centers provide **outpatient** care for clients who require physical or **occupational therapy**, **recreational therapy**, **hydrotherapy**, and other therapies (such as speech or hearing therapy) for loss of function in mobility or the activities of daily living. Patients/clients may receive **prosthetics** and learn how to use adaptive devices.

Industrial health care centers are located in large companies and industrial facilities. They provide health care services, including basic examinations and emergency or urgent care, for the staff and employees of the business. In addition, many industrial health care centers teach accident prevention and safety.

School health services are found in educational institutions. They provide emergency care in case of accidents or sudden illnesses. School nurses also provide medication dosing, and monitor children with chronic childhood diseases and problems such as diabetes, asthma, and cognitive impairment.

30 Chapter 2 | Understanding Health Care Systems

CUSTOMIZED INSTRUCTION

More Advanced Students

Have students explore the health services provided by your school district. Have them prepare a poster that illustrates the services and share with the class. If possible, display the posters elsewhere in the school.

Health maintenance organizations (HMOs) are a type of managed care organization. HMOs stress wellness (preventive health care). This helps avoid unnecessary major medical expenses. They provide health services that include basic medical services, **immunizations**, basic checkups, and education.

Essential community providers (ECPs) provide services to predominately low-income, medically under-served individuals. As part of the Affordable Care Act (ACA), health insurance companies that offer plans on the health insurance marketplace are now required to include in their network a number of ECPs, such as federally qualified health centers, Ryan White HIV/AIDS providers, critical access hospitals, etc.

Home health care agencies provide care in the home for patients/clients who need health services but not hospitalization. Services include nursing, physical therapy, personal care (bathing, dressing, etc.), and homemaking (e.g., housecleaning, food shopping, and cooking). Home health care workers provide care for all ages, from infants to the elderly.

Tele-health care offers medical services through the use of electronic information and telecommunications technologies. It is a way to provide health care, including consultations, procedures, and examinations, to remote areas or communities that do not have full-time health care providers.

Senior day care provides for elderly people who are able to live at home with their families but need care when the family is away. Services typically include activities, **rehabilitation**, and contact with others as well as administration of medications and assistance with mobility.

Hospices are important in our health care system. Hospices provide end-of-life care to those patients expected to live six months or less. The number one diagnosis for hospice patients is cancer. Health professionals and volunteers provide medical services and psychological and spiritual support to both the patient and their family. The goal of hospice is to make the patient as comfortable as possible by controlling pain and providing comfort.

Government Agencies

In the United States, the federal, state, and local governments provide health services. These services are funded by taxes. They are responsible for giving direct health care, safeguarding our food and water supplies, and promoting health education.

The World Health Organization (WHO), an agency funded by the United Nations, was founded in 1948. It is concerned with world health problems and publishes health information, compiles statistics, and investigates serious health problems.

U.S. Department of Veterans Affairs (VA) hospitals are federally supported and provide care for veterans who served in the armed forces.

immunizations
(im yuh nuh ZEY shuhns) Substances given to make disease organisms harmless to the patient; may be given orally or by injection (e.g., tetanus, polio).

rehabilitation
(ree huh BIL i tey shuhn) Process that helps people who have been disabled by sickness or injury to recover as many of their original abilities for activities of daily living as possible.

Apply It

Form two groups. One will explore the services offered by a genetic counseling center; the other will focus on an optical center. Create a list of these services and present the information to the class.

Apply It

In teams of three to five, research one of the health-related government agencies discussed on this page and the next. Create a slide show presentation with at least 10 slides that summarizes the regulations and guidelines set forth by the agency and how it contributes to the overall health and wellness of our nation.

Teaching Tips

- Direct students to the Web sites of federal government agencies for more information, starting with health.gov, and also:
  - hhs.gov
  - nih.gov
  - cdc.gov
  - fda.gov
- Also, direct students to the sites of the state and local government agencies in your area. Alternatively, display pamphlets and brochures from these agencies.

Apply It

- You may need to adjust the size of the groups, depending on the number of students in the class.
- You may want to have a list of health providers ready for the students to use.

Apply It

- You may need to assign each health care service to a team instead of having the teams research all five areas.

ACTIVITY

Have students select one of the government agencies discussed in the text and research at least one career within it. They will create a "help wanted" ad for the selected career that includes a description, education requirements, special training or certification requirements, and salary range. Post the ads on a class bulletin board.

Career-Ready Practices

- Students create a table that lists and describes at least five volunteer opportunities with local health care providers. You might consider compiling the lists into a single master list for all students to review.
- This activity gives students real-world experience in applying the following Career-Ready Practice: Act as a Responsible and Contributing Citizen and Employee.
- For more information on the Career-Ready Practices, visit careertech.org/career-ready-practices.

Career-Ready Practices

Health care providers of all types and sizes often rely on volunteers to provide some of the services needed by members of the community. Volunteers are unpaid workers who are looking for ways to help others and contribute to the greater good.

Explore the volunteer opportunities in your area with local health care providers. For example, you might volunteer to read to residents at a nursing home, develop a Web site for a local health care clinic, or teach CPR and first aid at your community center. Create a table that lists and describes at least five volunteer opportunities in your community and share it with the class.

Then, volunteer! Remember, career-ready individuals act as responsible and contributing citizens and understand the obligations of being a member of a community. They think about the consequences of their actions and act in ways that contribute to the betterment of their families, teams, workplace, and community.

communicable
(kuh MYOO ni kuh buhl)
Capable of passing directly or indirectly from one person or thing to another.

maternal
(MA ter nel)
Relating to the mother or from the mother.

licensing
(LAHY suhn sing)
Giving an agency or person permission to carry on certain activities and defining the activities they are authorized to do.

The *U.S. Public Health Service* is a federal agency whose mission is to protect, promote, and advance the health and safety of the nation. Their major responsibilities include disease control and prevention; biomedical research; regulation of food, drugs, and medical devices; mental health and drug abuse; and health care delivery.

State psychiatric hospitals serve the mentally ill.

State university medical centers provide training for health workers, give medical care, and conduct medical research.

State public health services provide health education materials. They are responsible for water and food purity, **communicable** disease control, alcohol and drug abuse control, **maternal** health, and **licensing** of various health agencies.

The *U.S. Department of Health and Human Services* (USDHHS) protects the health of all Americans by providing vital human services, especially to those least able to help themselves.

The *National Institute of Health* (NIH) is the world's leading agency for conducting and supporting medical research.

The *Centers for Disease Control and Prevention* (CDC) monitors and works to prevent disease outbreaks, including influenza, ebola, and bioterrorism. The CDC implements disease prevention strategies and maintains national health statistics.

The *Food and Drug Administration* (FDA) assures the safety of foods, cosmetics, pharmaceuticals, biological products, and medical devices.

The *Occupational Safety and Health Administration* (OSHA) imposes safety and health legislation to prevent injury, illness, and death in the workplace.

The *Agency for Healthcare Research and Quality* (AHRQ) works to improve the quality, safety, efficiency, and effectiveness of health care for all Americans by using research and technology to promote the delivery of the best possible care.

County hospitals provide care for the ill and injured, especially those patients/clients who require financial help in order to receive care.

A *laboratory* is a facility (which may be a government or private facility) that provides controlled conditions in which scientific research, experiments, and measurements can be performed. Laboratories can be found in hospitals, dental offices, schools, universities, industry, government, and military facilities.

Local *public health departments* provide services to local communities—focusing on the reporting of communicable diseases, public health nursing, health education, **environmental sanitation**, maternal and child health services, and public health clinics.

Senior centers have clinics that provide special services for geriatric patients (e.g., **podiatry** clinic, **hypertension** clinic, general medical care).

Centers for Medicare and Medicaid Services (CMS) administer programs established under Medicare and Medicaid, part of the USDHHS.

32 Chapter 2 | Understanding Health Care Systems

CUSTOMIZED INSTRUCTION

English Language Learners

For the Activity above, have students read their ad aloud to a partner.

At-Risk Students

In the Career-Ready Practices feature, students explore volunteer opportunities with health care providers in their community. Ask students to name a volunteer who they have interacted with recently. For example, the coach of a community soccer team or an assistant at the local library may be working on a volunteer basis. Ask students why they think the individual volunteers his or her time.

Not-for-Profit Agencies

Not-for-profit, organizations receive support from donations, gifts, membership fees, fundraisers, and **endowments**. They are not supported by the government, and many of the people who work for them are not paid. They raise funds for medical research and for public education about various health problems. Many of them focus on a particular disease or medical condition, such the following:

- American Cancer Society
- March of Dimes
- American Red Cross
- American Heart Association
- American Diabetes Association
- National Alliance on Mental Health
- National Association of People with AIDS
- National Coalition Against Domestic Violence
- American Lung Association

There are other non-profit health organizations, such as HOSA-Future Health Professionals (which is covered in Chapter 4) and the Joint Commission. All of these agencies and facilities help bring good health to individuals and communities. With growing concerns over racial disparities in medicine and economic inequality, organizations like these play an essential role in breaking down socioeconomic barriers to access medical care.

Managed Care: Quality Care and Managed Costs

Managed care is a system of health care in which patients agree to visit only certain doctors and hospitals, and in which the cost of treatment is monitored by a managing company, such as an HMO, another type of doctor/hospital network, or an insurance company. The managed care provider's goals are to provide quality care at reasonable costs. Certain programs help ensure quality care at minimal cost. One such program is the independent practice association (IPA). This is a group of health professionals, usually licensed physicians, who partner together and make their services available to insurance companies or other groups. This partnership allows for shared resources, such as managing their own offices, computer systems, and personnel. By having this contract, physicians can remain independent but can work with managed care systems and decrease costs.

Preventive care, such as routine physicals, well-baby care, immunizations, screenings for patients with specific risk factors, and wellness education, helps keep patients healthy. Wellness education stresses the importance of good nutrition, weight control, exercise, and healthy living practices. Health education programs, wellness centers, weight-control programs, fitness centers, health food distributors, and health care organizations all promote wellness and preventive care. Being healthy helps prevent serious illness and lowers medical costs.

environmental sanitation
(in VI run men tel sa ne TA shun)
Methods used to keep the environment clean and to promote health.

podiatry
(po DI u tree)
The diagnosis and treatment of foot disorders.

hypertension
(hi per TEN shun)
Elevation of the blood pressure.

endowments
(in DAU munts)
Gifts of property or money given to a group or organization.

Apply It

With a partner, research one of the not-for-profit agencies listed on this page. Gather information on their mission and/or responsibilities, the services they provide, and the individuals who typically use their services. Explore how health professionals in these agencies and in other health care organization develop and foster relationships within the community that promote health and wellness. Create a presentation about the agency and share with the class.

managed care
(MAN ijd kair)
A health care plan or system that seeks to control medical costs by contracting with a network of providers and by requiring preauthorization for visits to specialists.

Understanding Health Care Systems | Chapter 2 33

Teaching Tips

- Ask students if they have used a not-for-profit or volunteer agency, or if they know someone who has.
- Compare and contrast agencies that are not-for-profit with those that are for-profit.
- Discuss how fundraising helps support not-for-profit or volunteer organizations.
- Discuss volunteer opportunities that may be available to students, and how volunteer experience can help when looking for a job.

Apply It

- You may want to assign the not-for-profit agencies listed to teams to avoid duplication.

Teaching Tips

- Explain how managed costs, preventive care, and primary care providers all fit into the philosophy of managed care.
- Explain how managed care and ambulatory care help reduce the costs of health care.
- Discuss changes students or their families may have experienced first-hand, including the following:
  - Patients today may be more limited in choosing a provider.
  - Patients today spend less time in hospitals. Compare the hospital stay for new mothers then and now.
  - Patients today are more likely to be treated at outpatient facilities. List several procedures that now take place out of hospital, such as cataract surgery or hernia repair.
- Discuss resources available to people who are dealing with difficult circumstances. For example, individuals who have blood-borne diseases like HIV, people affected by mental health disorders, or those who are victims of domestic violence.
- Have students identify local resources in the community for helping individuals with challenges, in addition to national resources that can be accessed on the Internet.

CUSTOMIZED INSTRUCTION

Special Needs Students

For the Apply It activity on this page, some students may benefit from delivering an oral report or presentation rather than a written presentation.

At-Risk Students

Have students list on an index card three forms of preventive care they could apply to their daily living practices. These might include exercising, a healthy diet, and adequate sleep.

ACTIVITY

Call students' attention to the various types of health care providers identified on pp. 30–35. Have each student select a type of health care provider to research. Ask them to describe the provider and explain the range of services provided. Have a class presentation about health care providers.

TEAMWORK

Prepare and present a presentation about one aspect of preventive medicine, such as diet, exercise, or socialization.

Teaching Tips

- Ask students to think of specific ways ambulatory care lowers cost. If possible compare the cost of nursing care in a hospital with the cost of home care.
- Review the types of specialty care facilities and the types of care given in these facilities.

refer
(ri FER)
To send to.

obstetrics
(ub STE triks)
The branch of medical science concerned with childbirth.

orthopedics
(or tho PE diks)
The medical specialty concerned with correcting problems with the skeletal system.

chiropractic
(KI ruh prak tik)
The method of adjusting the segments of the spinal column.

audiology
(o dee A luh gee)
The study of hearing disorders.

urology
(yew RO le gee)
The study of the urine and urinary organs in health and disease.

Primary care providers may include family and general practice physicians, internists, nurse practitioners, and physician's assistants. This is "the family doctor"—usually the first contact a patient has for an undiagnosed condition. Primary providers care for all routine medical problems. They also **refer** patients/clients to specialists.

Specialty care is care given by a provider who is trained in one special area. Specialists usually limit their practice to treating one type of problem. Specializing gives them a broad knowledge of that area. A few specialties are:

- Surgery
- Podiatry
- **Obstetrics**
- **Orthopedics**
- **Chiropractic**
- **Audiology**
- **Urology**

Emergency care and *urgent care* provide different services. Emergency care is for life-threatening conditions that require hospitalization. These might include ambulance services, rescue squads, and helicopter or airplane rescue vehicles. Urgent care is for non-emergencies that require prompt treatment. Emergencies requiring hospital care are expensive. Excellent care is available in the urgent care setting, and costs are lower.

Ambulatory care, as discussed earlier, provides a variety of medical services, including diagnosis, observation, treatment, and rehabilitation, on an outpatient basis.

Organization

An efficient health care facility must be well organized. Organization improves the performance of health care workers and ensures that the facility delivers high-quality health care to patients/clients.

The most common organizational structure for health care organizations is a pyramid-shaped hierarchy, which defines the functions it carries out. (Figure 2.2)

Language Arts Link

Investigate Health Care Facilities

As you learned in this chapter, there are many different types of health care facilities. Working with a partner, select two different types of health care facilities in the community where you live. Integrate and evaluate multiple sources of information using the Internet, calling the facility, or referring to any available print information. Determine the services each facility offers, the specialized procedures, if any, if it is in-patient (overnight stays) or out-patient only, and whether short -term or long-term care is provided.

Produce clear and coherent writing to create a brochure or booklet for each facility appropriate to the potential audience, such as health care referring agencies and offices. Be sure to seek approval from each facility to ensure the information included is accurate and that you have permission to make copies for distribution. Be sure to proofread your work and cite any sources that you used. Check spelling and grammar and correct any errors.

34 Chapter 2 | Understanding Health Care Systems

Language Arts Link—Investigate Health Care Facilities

- You may want to provide a list of the facilities in your area.
- You may want to have students draft an outline, story web, or list questions they need to answer to organize their ideas.
- Remind students about your school's Internet policy before having them go online to find information. Emphasize that they should use reputable Web resources, such as sites sponsored by the government or educational institutions.
- Remind them to keep a list of sources to use for a bibliography.
- If students do not have access to the Internet, be sure to direct them to other resources, such as books, periodicals, or videos.
- For evaluation, verify that the information is correct and in the correct order, and you should mark spelling and grammatical errors.

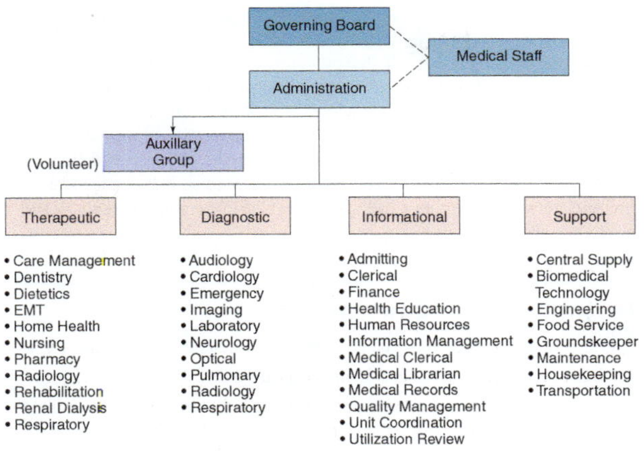

Figure 2.2
Sample organizational structure.

As you can see in Figure 2.2, each function within the organization is supported by a number of specialized departments. In general:

- **Therapeutic** services provide care over time.
- Diagnostic services are those used to identify a particular condition or disease, such as x-rays or blood tests.
- Informational services document and process information.
- Support services help to create a relaxing, healing, and supportive environment for patients.

Most health care organizations utilize an organizational chart that identifies the key management and supervisory positions assigned to its various functions. An organizational chart establishes a chain of command that helps to ensure communication among relevant parties and facilitates problem-solving. It is important for all workers in the health care organization to know to whom they should take questions, discuss problems, and pose suggestions. Bypassing a link in the chain causes misunderstanding and is unprofessional.

Health Care Regulatory Agencies

State and federal regulatory agencies for the health care industry set standards for health care, keep health care workers informed, and monitor facilities' and workers' compliance with laws that pertain to health care. As a health care worker, one of your first encounters with a health care regulatory agency will be for licensure. Based on your chosen profession, you will need to meet specific requirements set forth by the federal or state board that regulates that profession.

Quality Control

Increased public demand for high-quality health care and error reduction over the past 50 years has resulted in health care providers initiating ongoing efforts to deliver excellence in care. For example, medication errors have been reduced by requiring nurses to verify patients by name and birth date as well as arm band identification before administering the medications. Drug packaging bar codes read by scanners and documented into the electronic health record also help to minimize medication errors.

Quality control is achieved through a process of gathering and evaluating information about the health care services provided, as well as the measurable results achieved. The gathered information and results are then compared against accepted standards, often called benchmarks. Benchmarks used for quality control may be set on a local, state, or national level.

Quality control is achieved and maintained through formal, systematic evaluations. Overall patterns of care are evaluated and compared to benchmarks. When problems, or deficiencies, are identified, the benchmarks offer a standard for improvement.

What benchmarks do you use to evaluate your work in school?

therapeutic
(ther uh PYOO tik)
Pertaining to the treatment of disease or injury (e.g., physical therapy, radiology, diet, nursing).

Figure Focus

2.2 Sample organizational structure.

Explain each major service in health care and how they relate to each other in the organization. Discuss the importance of these services within an organization. Discuss the departments that are usually part of the major services.

Teaching Tips

- Discuss the effect of organizational systems on performance and quality in the workplace.
- Explain the hierarchy of a chain of command.
- Discuss the importance of knowing who is responsible for managing a department or staff.
- Ask students if they are part of a chain of command in any other aspects of their lives, such as at a part-time job or at home.
- Ask students to discuss the types of problems that might arise from breaking the chain of command.
- Explain to students that they will need to pay attention to all information provided by the state and federal agencies that regulate their chosen area of health care.
- Discuss how quality control affects health care.

ACTIVITY

A family tree is an organization chart that represents your family. Have students create a poster illustrating his or her family tree. Display the posters in the classroom, or on a bulletin board.

CUSTOMIZED INSTRUCTION

More Advanced Students

Have advanced students visit the Web site of a major health care provider such as a hospital. Students can learn about the number and type of departments, programs, and even about employment possibilities.

Summary

There are many facilities that help individuals with health problems. Health care facilities offer a variety of services, including therapeutic, diagnostic, information, and support. There are also agencies—some private, some funded by federal, state, or local governments—that help meet special needs. Most facilities and agencies have an organizational chart in place to help them identify and manage key functions and to establish a chain of command. Managed care, outpatient care, and ambulatory care are growing forms of care that emphasize wellness and preventive care.

Section 2.1 Review Questions

1. List two types of facilities that generally house patients for more than a day.
2. How do volunteer agencies help the medical field?
3. What can you determine by looking at an organizational chart for a facility?
4. How does ambulatory care help to meet the needs of patients?
5. What does preventive care mean?
6. Name and describe the activities of two government agencies that provide health care-related services.

Personal Wellness

Hospital Help

Hospitals are known for the diagnostic, medical, surgical, and emergency care services that they provide. However, many hospitals offer classes and support groups to educate patients and promote personal wellness. The instructional sessions cover a range of topics. For example, some classes help patients understand their diseases. Classes about cancer, diabetes, and arthritis can help patients anticipate symptoms and explore types of care.

Emotional support is offered in the form of support groups for bereavement, for patients with terminal illnesses, and for caregivers. These groups help patients and families deal with the mental and emotional stress that often comes with disease.

Not only do hospitals help with the difficulties associated with disease, they also offer classes on topics of daily health. Classes on exercise, men's and women's health, stress management, and nutrition are available. Expectant mothers can learn about pregnancy and parenthood through weekly classes. Hospitals reach out to communities to educate people and help keep them well. In a clear and effective manner, write a short essay that answers the questions below.

Why do you think hospitals offer these types of classes?

Why is it essential that all people have access to quality health care? What are the effects of either having or not having access to quality health care?

36 Chapter 2 | Understanding Health Care Systems

Section 2.1 Review Questions

1. Answer: The following facilities house patients for more than a day: general hospitals, specialty hospitals, convalescence care facilities, nursing homes, and extended care facilities.
2. Answer: Volunteer agencies help the medical field by raising funds for medical research and for public education about various health problems.
3. Answer: An organizational chart shows how each department fits into the system and identifies the line of authority. By looking at an organization chart, you can see who your immediate supervisor is, and it tells the areas of responsibilities for all of the employees and it establishes the chain of command.
4. Answer: With ambulatory care, the patient/client goes to a facility for care and returns home each day when their care has finished. This is comforting to patients that they can return home.
5. Answer: Preventive care keeps patients healthy. Preventive care includes routine physicals, well-baby care, immunizations, and wellness education.
6. Answer: Answers will vary but should include two of the following:
   - Veterans Administration hospitals provide care for veterans.
   - U.S. Public Health Service performs research, prevents drug and alcohol abuse, prevents and controls diseases, checks the safety of food and drugs, plans ways to deliver health services, and makes quality care affordable and available.
   - State psychiatric hospitals serve the mentally ill.
   - State university medical centers provide training, health care, and conduct medical research.
   - State public health services provide health education materials.
   - U.S. Department of Health and Human Services protects the health of all American by providing vital human services.
   - The National Institute of Health conducts and supports medical research.
   - Centers for Disease Control and Prevention monitors and prevents disease outbreak include bioterrorism.
   - The Food and Drug Administration assures the safety of foods, cosmetics, pharmaceuticals, and biological devices.
   - The Occupational Safety and Health Administration imposes safety and health legislation to prevent injury, illness, and death in the workplace.

Health Care Systems

SECTION 2.2

Background

The cost of health care has increased significantly over the years. It is important to understand the causes for the increase as well as methods providers use to help contain the costs. Every health care worker should also know the health care systems that help patients/clients afford the services they need. When patients/clients receive regular and complete care, they live healthier and happier lives.

Objectives

When you have completed this section, you will be able to do the following:

- Match key terms with their correct meanings.
- Explain recent health care reform legislation and how it has affected the way Americans access health care.
- Explain how health care providers have modified their practices to provide patients quality health care at a lower cost.
- Explain the purpose of the Healthcare Effectiveness Data and Information Set.
- Identify and differentiate the various health care systems.
- Compare and contrast health maintenance organizations and preferred provider organizations.
- Analyze and predict where and how certain factors—such as cost, managed care, technology, an aging population, etc.—may affect various health care delivery system models.

Health Care Reform

Health care reform has been—and continues to be—a hot topic on our nation's political, economic, and social agendas. The intent of health care reform is to identify ways to stem the rising costs of health care and make it more affordable and accessible to more people.

This is the premise on which recent comprehensive health reform, known as the Patient Protection and Affordable Care Act (PPACA), commonly called the Affordable Care Act (ACA), was built. The ACA was signed into law in March 2010. In a nutshell, the ACA (also referred to as ObamaCare for U.S. President Barack Obama, who signed it into law), required most U.S. citizens and legal residents to have health insurance coverage or else pay a fee. The fee or fine for not having insurance coverage was removed in 2018.

Many people already have health insurance through their employers, through government-sponsored programs such as Medicaid and Medicare, and through self-insured plans. For those who do not have insurance, the ACA created a "marketplace" for **subsidized** insurance plans that provide individuals, families, and small businesses with free or low-cost health insurance coverage.

subsidized
(SUB se dizd)
Having partial financial support from public funds.

Understanding Health Care Systems | Chapter 2 37

FOCUS AND ENGAGE

Introduce the Section

a. Review the content of the Background paragraph, explaining the concept of health care systems, and how they help people afford the services they need.

b. Explain why it is important to understand the different methods available for covering the costs of health care, both for individuals and organizations.

c. Ask students to reflect on their own experiences or that of their families paying for health care. Ask if they know whether or not they have health care insurance, and, if so, what type.

d. Discuss the objectives for the section.

- The Agency for Healthcare Research and Quality works to improve health care.
- County hospitals provide care to the ill and injured who require financial assistance.

Personal Wellness—Hospital Help

- Explain that as part of preventive care, many hospitals now have outreach programs for providing information and instruction to the community.
- Discuss programs that might be available in your community, such as CPR classes and health fairs.
- Ask students if they have ever taken advantage of such programs.

Why do you think hospitals have started to offer these types of classes? Why is it essential that all people have access to quality health care? What are the effects of either having or not having access to quality health care?

Answer: One trend of health care is to teach patients more about wellness. Doctors are more concerned than ever with wellness of the whole person (emotional, mental, social), not just the physical person. In addition, classes on exercise, stress management, and nutrition can help to prevent disease and lower health care costs. It is important that all members of society have access to proper health care.

TEAMWORK

Contact a local hospital and ask for a list of programs or classes, or look up the list on the Internet and print it.

Vocabulary Review

a. Key terms are defined in the margins of the text on the page where they first appear.

b. Pronounce each word, and have the students repeat the pronunciation out loud.

c. Discuss the definition of each word.

TEACH

Discuss

- Demonstrate how the costs of health care have grown over recent years by comparing the cost of a doctor's visit twenty years ago to the cost today.
- Discuss how this might impact patients making health care decisions, and ask students if they or anyone they know has ever had to make a health care decision based on cost.
- Ask students to consider reasons why health care workers should be aware of the high cost of care.
- Discuss why health care providers should or should not work to control or contain costs.
- Discuss the various types of input and output that health care systems have that provide feedback.

The premium you pay for a plan bought through the marketplace is based on your income, age, family size, geography, tobacco use, and the type of plan you buy. You cannot be denied coverage on the marketplace because of pre-existing conditions, health status, claims history, duration of coverage, gender, or occupation.

Supporters of the ACA say it increases the quality, accessibility, and affordability of health insurance, while it decreases health care costs and spending. But there are many others who believe the opposite. There is still much debate about the ACA its effectiveness.

lawsuits
(LA soots)
A legal action started by one person against another based on a complaint that the person failed to perform a legal duty.

systems
(SIS tems)
Coordinated bodies of methods or plans of procedure.

legislation
(le jus LA shun)
A law or body of laws.

bulk
(bulk)
A greater amount.

intervention
(in tur VEN shun)
The act of interfering to modify an outcome.

Quality Health Care Costs

Cost Containment

As you have learned, the high cost of health care has drawn much attention in recent years. Technological advances in the medical field, an aging population, and health-related **lawsuits** have all been factors in driving up the price of medical care and services offered by health care **systems**. Advanced equipment and technologies that health care providers use to make a more thorough diagnosis is often expensive to purchase and maintain. In addition, as the population continues to grow and age, the demand for this type of care increases.

A number of programs have been instituted to address health care costs. The federal government passed **legislation** in 1983—originally developed for Medicare payment systems and then modified for the general population—to regulate the price of medical care. The system ensures that the specific health care agency will have to pick up any extra costs after the government and patient have paid their part.

This legislation approved the grouping of medical conditions, the reasonable cost for each condition, and its standard treatment. These groupings are known as *diagnostic-related groupings* (DRGs). Some of the top groupings are normal newborn, heart failure, psychoses, cesarean section, angina pectoris, pneumonia, and hip/knee replacement.

Systems Theory

Any kind of system has input and output, along with a feedback loop. In a system such as a health care system, the input is information, materials, and human effort or energy. The output is the services provided to patients. Both positive and negative feedback affect the input that occurs next. For a system to work, there must be goals, and feedback must govern what continues to happen within the system. Adaptability to feedback is important in achieving goals.

DRGs help reduce unnecessary procedures and encourage self-care and home care. So, for example, a woman might wake up with a fever, sore throat, and ringing in her ears. She goes to an urgent care facility where she can be seen that morning and is diagnosed with strep throat. The standard diagnosis for strep is based on a throat culture (rapid strep test) and treatment is about 10 days of antibiotics. Based on the DRG, the facility will only be reimbursed by insurance or Medicare for a fee that falls within a specific range. The facility would not, on the other hand, be reimbursed for x-rays or a CAT scan for this condition.

Health care providers also promote lower health care costs by combining services, offering outpatient services, purchasing supplies in **bulk**, and emphasizing early **intervention** and preventive care.

38 Chapter 2 | Understanding Health Care Systems

CUSTOMIZED INSTRUCTION

Special Needs Students

Be sure to provide enough time for students with reading disabilities to read the section text thoroughly.

An often-overlooked part of managing health care costs is planning for effective handling and removal of medical waste. Effective recycling processes, where possible, can dramatically reduce costs while also lessening the impact on the environment.

Measuring the Performance of Care and Service

Under the direction of the National Committee for Quality Assurance (NCQA), the The Healthcare Effectiveness Data and Information Set (HEDIS) was developed to establish guidelines on the quality of health care given in this country. HEDIS is a tool used by more than 90 percent of the country's health plans to measure performance on important aspects of care and service. Because the HEDIS guidelines are so specifically defined, they make it possible to:

- Measure health plan performance
- Identify physicians and other providers who give high-quality medical care to their patients/clients
- Identify physicians and other providers who do not meet the quality care guidelines

Quality health care can be defined as the extent to which patients get the care they need in a manner that most effectively protects or restores their health. This means having timely access to care, getting treatment that medical evidence has found to be effective, and getting appropriate preventive care.

Health Care Payments

Health Insurance: Third-Party Payers

As you learned at the beginning of this section, most American citizens and legal residents have health insurance, which they can obtain through an employer-sponsored plan, self-insurance, a government-sponsored program, or the marketplace established by the Patient Protection and Affordable Care Act (PPACA). Insurance plans are called third-party payers. Insurance companies require the subscriber to pay a fee for insurance coverage and in return agree to pay for specific medical care.

Each insurance company determines what it will and will not pay for and how much it will pay. For example, many third-party payers require a **co-payment**. A co-payment is a set amount the subscriber pays for each medical service. This may be from $10 to $50 that a subscriber pays to the provider on the day that he or she visits a medical office or picks up a prescription.

Most insurance companies also have a **deductible**, an amount the subscriber must pay before the insurance begins to pay. For example, a subscriber may have to pay the first $250 of medical bills in a given year. Even after a subscriber pays the co-payment and the deductible, he or she may still have to pay a **co-insurance**. For example, a subscriber may be required to pay 20 percent of every medical bill. The subscriber must pay any fees that the insurance company does not pay.

Joint Commission

The Joint Commission is an independent non-profit organization that accredits and certifies more than 20,000 health care organizations and programs in the United States. Founded in 1951, it has established a set of performance standards designed to ensure that health care organizations provide "safe and effective care of the highest quality and value."

The Joint Commission offers accreditation to hospitals, home care providers, laboratories, nursing care centers, behavioral health centers, and ambulatory care centers.

With a partner, research health care organizations and programs in your community that have received the Joint Commission's Gold Seal of Approval.

Go online to the Web site jointcommission.org and research the patient safety standards established to enable health care facilities to earn accreditation. Determine if there are differences based on the types of facilities (i.e., hospitals, laboratories, home care, etc.).

co-payment
(koh PEY muhnt)
A set amount the subscriber pays for each medical service.

deductible
(di DUHK tuh buhl)
An amount the subscriber must pay before the insurance begins to pay.

co-insurance
(koh in SHOOR uhns)
A percentage the subscriber is required to pay of every medical bill.

Understanding Health Care Systems | Chapter 2 39

Teaching Tips

- Explain the Healthcare Effectiveness Data and Information Set, and how it helps to insure quality of care.
- If possible, display a set and examine the list of measures with the students.
- To explain how a third-party payment system works, have three students act as the three parties; one student is the patient who seeks and receives care, one the provider who delivers the care, and one is the insurer, who pays for the care.
- Be sure to explain the additional costs, such as the fee the patient pays the insurer, co-pays, and deductibles.Explain factors that have affected health care costs, such as advancements in technology and medical science, as well as costs of malpractice insurance.
- Discuss how the factors affecting health care provide feedback in a health care system.
- Discuss the relationship between lowering costs and maintaining the quality of care.
- Discuss why it is important to contain costs.
- Discuss why avoiding duplication of services is an effective way to reduce health care costs.
- Describe systems that health care providers and the government have put in place to control or lower costs.
- Provide an example of a diagnostic-related grouping and explain how such groupings help control costs.
- Explain the concept of the Patient Protection and Affordable Care Act.
- Point out that the ACA is a form of a national health plan system. Many countries have universal health care systems in place, including Canada, the United Kingdom, and Brazil.
- Discuss the pros and cons of such a system.

Joint Commission

- With a partner, students are to research health care organizations in their community that have received the Joint Commission's Gold Seal of Approval.
- Encourage students to visit the Joint Commission's Web site at jointcommission.org before they begin their research.
- They should review the programs that are eligible for accreditation and certification.
- You may want to assign student teams to specific programs or organizations.
- Make sure students can identify the official icon for the Gold Seal.

TEAMWORK

Research the cost of a medical procedure and compare how much a patient would pay with and without insurance, or with different types of insurance. Present your findings to the class.

Math Link—Metric Prefixes

- Explain the concept of out-of-pocket expenses.
- Explain how most insurers cover a portion—or percentage—of the total cost, leaving you to pay the remainder.
- Work through the first two examples with the class, then have them try the third example on their own. The answer is $82.25.

Why is it important to know how to figure out how much money any insurance company will pay for a medical procedure?

Answer: Patients may choose different ways to care for an illness or disease based on how much their third-party payer is willing to cover. Other patients may want to know how much they need to save for a particular procedure.

Teaching Tips

- Compare the delivery system of a health maintenance organization with a preferred provider organization.

claim
(kleym)
The formal request by an insurance policy holder to receive payment for services received or incurred.

fraud
(frawd)
Illegal process of filing a claim for insurance payment of services not actually received or incurred.

To use health insurance, a patient files a **claim**. Many times the health care provider will file the claim with the insurance company. Once the insurance company receives the claim, it is processed according to the particular plan purchased by the patient. Payment will be made to the provider or the patient, depending on how the claim is processed. The insurer will provide the patient with an Explanation of Benefits (EoB) form which details what was covered and what was denied, as well as why any denials occurred.

A problem in the insurance industry is that of **fraud**. Fraud is the process of filing a claim for services that were not actually received by the claimant or exaggerated by the claimant or provider. Fraud is illegal and can be considered a felony or misdemeanor. In order for payments to be processed correctly, the health care provider must submit claims to the insurer (or Medicare/Medicaid) using the appropriate medical coding, a system of codes meant to designate the diagnosis and reason for specific therapies/procedures. These codes allow health care providers and insurers to quickly and effectively understand the patient's needs but can create problems if entered incorrectly.

Math Link

Metric Prefixes

When trying to figure out how much you or a patient will have to pay when dealing with a third-party payer, knowing how to work with percentages can help. A third-party payer may require the subscriber to pay a certain percentage of every medical bill. In order to figure out how much a subscriber will have to pay, follow these steps:

Step 1: Convert the percentage to a decimal. You can do this by moving the decimal point to the left two spaces. For example, 10% would be .10 and 20% would be .20.

Step 2: Multiply the decimal by the amount of the medical bill.

Example 1

Mike is having surgery on his arm. The total cost of the procedure is $2,982. Mike's insurance requires a 15% coinsurance.

Step 1: 15% = .15

Step 2: 2,982 × .15 = 447.30

Mike would have to pay $447.30 for the surgery.

Example 2

Kelly needs to have a cavity filled. The total cost of the procedure is $350. Kelly's insurance pays 30% of the cost of any dental procedure.

Step 1: In this instance, first you need to find out how much Kelly is required to pay.

100%
– 30%
70%

70% = .70

Step 2: 350 × .70 = 245

Kelly would have to pay $245 to have the cavity filled.

Calculate percentages to solve this example. Andrew needs to have a mole removed from his back. The total cost of the procedure is $235. Andrew's insurance pays 65% of the cost of a medical procedure. How much would Andrew have to pay?

Why is it important to know how to figure out how much money an insurance company will pay for a medical procedure?

Complete a survey of four deferent third party payer types (private medical insurance, dental insurance, vision service plans) to determine the amount of co-pay required for three selected procedures for each insurance type. Average the co-pay by percentage to determine the typical percentage by plan for each procedure selected.

CUSTOMIZED INSTRUCTION

Less Advanced Students

For the Math Link feature, let less advanced students use a calculator to determine the out-of-pocket expenses.

Health Maintenance Organizations

Health maintenance organizations (HMOs) require members to pay a co-payment, or co-pay, for medical services. The member must get medical care from the physicians, labs, hospitals, etc. that agree to the fee the HMO is willing to pay. If the member gets medical care outside the HMO, he or she will have to pay for the care.

Preferred Provider Organizations

Physician groups and hospitals work together to give comprehensive health care at a reduced cost to various large companies and corporations. Employees of these companies contract with a preferred provider organization (PPO) and agree to see providers on the PPO list. If they see other providers, they pay a larger fee.

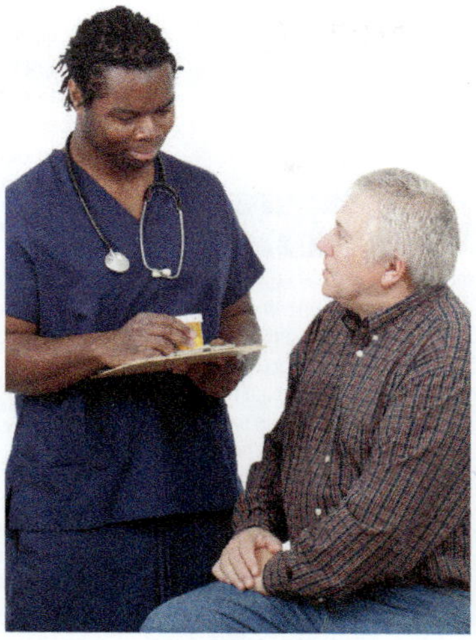

Figure 2.3
What kind of health care programs are available from the government for a person over 65?

Medicaid

Medicaid is a health insurance program provided by the state and federal government for low-income Americans. **Benefits** and **eligibility** are different in each state. People who are blind, disabled, or of low income are generally able to get Medicaid insurance.

Medicare

Medicare is a health insurance program provided by the federal government to people over the age of 65. Subscribers pay a monthly payment to the Social Security Administration. (Figure 2.3) Medicare consists of two parts. Part A covers in-patient care at hospitals, hospice care, and home health care. Part B helps cover medical services like doctors' services, outpatient care, and other medical services that Part A does not cover. In addition, Part B covers some **preventive** services. While most people get Part A without paying a monthly payment, Part B requires a **premium** each month. Some health care providers accept Medicare payments, or reimbursements, as payment in full for services; others charge more than Medicare pays. To cover the extra costs, many people buy a third-party payer insurance to cover all of their medical costs. There are many programs for Medicare recipients that provide care for a small co-payment.

TRICARE

TRICARE is a health care program for active duty service members, retirees, and their families. One part of TRICARE is called TFL (TRICARE for Life). This medical care is for Medicare-eligible uniformed services retirees age 65 or older. The plan also covers family members and survivors. This health program works with Medicare to provide service members additional health benefits.

benefits
(BEN a fits)
Payment and assistance based on an agreement.

eligibility
(e li ja BI la tee)
The quality or state of being qualified.

preventive
(pri VEN tiv)
Intended to keep from happening.

premium
(PREE mee uhm)
The periodic payment to Medicare, an insurance company, or a health care plan for health care or prescription drug coverage.

Teaching Tips

- Emphasize that Medicaid and Medicare are government programs, and then compare them by discussing who is eligible for coverage.
- Explain that when a health care provider charges more than Medicare pays for a service and does not accept the Medicare reimbursement as full payment, the patient owes the difference.
- Emphasize that it is often necessary to purchase supplement insurance, even when you are covered by Medicare. Mention the high cost of prescription medications.
- Discuss who is eligible for the TRICARE health care program.

Figure Focus

2.3 What kind of health care programs are available from the government for a person over 65?

Ask students to list the government programs that are available to people over 65. The responses should include Medicare, as well as TRICARE for those who served in the military.

ACTIVITY

Use the Internet or other resources to learn the eligibility requirements for Medicare and Medicaid.

Teaching Tips

- Explain Workers' Compensation. Discuss how Workers' Compensation is different from health care insurance programs offered by employers to employees.

Career Connect

- Encourage students to research the responsibilities of an insurance administrator and human resource/insurance manager.
- Have student prepare a list of questions to ask the guest speaker.

Section 2.2 Review Questions

1. Answer: Technological advances in the medical field, an aging population, and health-related lawsuits have all helped to drive up the price of medical care and affected health care systems.
2. Answer: Legislation was adopted that ensures that the specific health care agency will have to pick up any extra costs after the government and patient have paid their part.
3. Answer: Diagnostic-related groups help reduce unnecessary procedures and encourage self-care and home care.
4. Answer: HMOs require members to pay a co-payment for medical services. Members must get medical care from the physicians, labs, etc. that agree to the fee the HMO is willing to pay. Physician groups and hospitals work together to give comprehensive health care at a reduced cost to various large companies and corporations. Employees of these companies contract with a preferred provider organization (PPO) and agree to see providers on the PPO list. If they see other providers, they pay a larger fee.
5. Answer: Medicaid eligibility varies by state but people who are blind, disabled, or of low income are generally able to get Medicaid insurance.
6. Answer: Employees who are injured or die at work are covered by state workers' compensation laws. Workers' compensation also includes any illness that may result from the workplace.
7. Answer: The impact of those that receive compensation as a health care worker; the businesses generated by the use of heath care services; and the amount of resources spent on health care services.

Workers' Compensation

compensation
(kom puhn SEY shuhn)
Payment.

Workers' **compensation** is a state-mandated insurance program that provides compensation to employees who suffer job-related injuries and illnesses. Workers' compensation covers any job-related injury or illness. Employers are required to have workers' compensation insurance. Benefits include payment for lost wages and payment of medical bills.

Career Connect

Research health insurance companies with offices in your community. You can do this on the Internet or by contacting your local chamber of commerce. Select one and invite them to visit the class and discuss their responsibilities and the services provided.

Summary

Recent health care reform has affected the way many Americans access health care. Despite efforts to stem the tide of rising health care costs, prices have continued to rise due in part to technological advances, an aging population, and health-related lawsuits. However, health care providers and systems continue to help patients/clients receive affordable care. By encouraging less hospital time for the patient through outpatient services and early intervention, providers help keep costs low. In addition, health maintenance organizations and preferred provider organizations work with providers to offer patients/clients reduced costs. The federal and state governments also protect patients/clients by offering programs such as Medicaid, Medicare, TRICARE, and workers' compensation.

Section 2.2 Review Questions

1. List three causes of rising health care costs.
2. How are health care providers trying to reduce costs for their patients/clients?
3. What is the benefit of diagnostic-related groupings?
4. What is the difference between health maintenance organizations and preferred provider organizations?
5. Who is eligible for Medicaid?
6. When can a worker receive workers' compensation?
7. List three conditions and describe the impact of health services on the economy of a community.

42 Chapter 2 | Understanding Health Care Systems

CHAPTER 2 REVIEW

Chapter Review Questions

1. Under what three circumstances might ambulatory care be preferable and why? (2.1)
2. Name one health care provider and explain how they provide medical care. (2.1)
3. What are we trying to do to contain the high costs of health care? (2.2)
4. Explain several ways in which we are addressing personal wellness issues. (2.1)
5. Name three government agencies that provide health services. What does each agency do? (2.1)
6. How do the policies of managed care help to provide quality care for patients? (2.1)
7. What are the benefits of an organizational chart in a health care facility? (2.1)
8. Explain the four major services in health care. (2.1)
9. How does the Healthcare Effectiveness Data and Information Set help patients/clients? (2.2)
10. What are some of the costs that third-party payers might require a patient/client to pay? (2.2)

Activities

1. Choose a facility such as a general hospital, specialty hospital, rehabilitation center, or clinic. Visit the facility, research its Web site, or call the facility to identify the different departments in the facility and its line of authority. Then, create a diagram that shows the relationship of health care professionals within that facility.
2. Create a pie chart that shows the National percentage of the health care expenditures for:
   - Nursing care
   - Dental care
   - Other residential care
   - Physician/clinical
   - Prescription drugs
   - Other professional
   - Home health
   - Hospital

   Describe how these health services expenditures impact the economy.
3. Working in teams of three or four, select a section from the Affordable Care Act. Analyze the impact of the section at the national, state, and local levels. Report your findings to the rest of the class or submit the report to the teacher.
4. Identify the governing agency at the national, state, and local level responsible for regulating the section selected in Activity 3 from the Affordable Care Act. Add this information in the report for Activity 3.
5. Research hazardous waste removal and recycling services available for hospitals in your area. Create a proposal for how your local hospital could save money and better protect the environment.
6. Research the various governmental regulations and guidelines that hospitals must adhere to from entities such as the World Health Organization, Centers for Disease Control and Prevention, Occupational Safety and Health Administration, U.S. Food and Drug Administration, Joint Commission, and National Institute of Health. Prepare a brief presentation on one of these for your class.

Case Studies

1. A patient's colonoscopy procedure will cost $3,350. There is a co-pay of $30 and the co-insurance is 20%. The annual deductible is $1,000, of which the patient has met $325. What amount will the patient have to pay?
2. An elderly man is leaving the hospital after receiving care for his broken leg. He lives with his family, but he is alone all day while his family works. What kind of care will the man need after he leaves the hospital? What type of facilities might you recommend to this patient?

CHAPTER 2 REVIEW

Chapter Review Questions

1. Answer: Ambulatory care is preferable for rehabilitation, outpatient surgery, and day care because it allows a patient to return home.
2. Answer: Answers will vary but should include one of the following:
   - General hospitals: Provide a range of diagnostic, medical, surgical, and emergency care services.
   - Convalescent care facilities: Care for elderly people needing nursing services.
   - Ambulatory care: Physicians with different specialties provide patient with immediate care for many different illnesses.
   - Physician and dental offices: Care that promotes wellness and diagnoses illness.
   - Rehabilitation centers: Provide physical therapy and hydrotherapy.
   - Home health agencies: Provide care in the home for patients who need health services but not hospitalization.
   - Senior day care: Care for the elderly who are able to live at home with their families but need care when the family is away.
3. Answer: To control the high costs of health care, managed care is promoting preventive care, primary care doctors, specialty doctors, urgent care facilities, and preadmission authorization requirements for hospitalization.
4. Answer: Preventive care, such as routine physicals, well-baby care, immunizations, and wellness education helps keep patients healthy. Wellness education stresses the importance of good nutrition, weight control, exercise, and healthy living practices. Health education programs, wellness centers, weight-control programs, fitness centers, health food distributors, and health care organizations all promote wellness and preventive care.
5. Answer: Answers will vary but should include three of the following: The U.S. Public Health Service performs research, prevents drug and alcohol abuse, prevents and controls diseases, checks the safety of food and drugs, plans ways to deliver health services, and makes quality care affordable and available; state psychiatric hospitals serve the mentally ill; state university medical centers provide training, health care, and conduct medical research; state public health services provide health education materials; the U.S. Department of Health and Human Services protects the health of all Americans by providing vital human services; the National Institutes of Health conducts and supports medical research; the Centers for Disease Control and Prevention monitors and prevents disease outbreaks, including bioterrorism; the U.S. Food and Drug Administration assures the safety of foods, cosmetics, pharmaceuticals, and biological devices; The Occupational Safety and Health Administration imposes safety and health legislation to prevent injury, illness, and death in the workplace; the Agency for Healthcare Research and Quality works to improve health care; and county hospitals provide care to the ill and injured who require financial assistance.
6. Answer: Preventive care promotes wellness that will include ways to prevent illness, urgent care is for non-emergencies that require prompt treatment and is less expensive than emergency care, and outpatient care is available instead of in-hospitalization stays for those who do not need constant monitoring.
7. Answer: The benefits of an organizational chart in a health care facility are that it shows the chain of command, lists supervisors, and lists the areas of responsibility for all employees.

8. Answer: Therapeutic services provide care over time; diagnostic services are those used to identify a particular condition or disease, such as x-rays or blood tests; informational services document and process information; and environmental services help to create a relaxing, healing, and supportive environment for patients.
9. Answer: The Healthcare Effectiveness Data and Information Set helps patients/clients with its report card that measures health plan performance, helps identify physicians who give high-quality medical care to patients, and identifies those physicians who do not meet the quality care guidelines.
10. Answer: Third-party payers might require patients to pay co-pays, deductibles, or co-insurance.

Activities

1. You may want to have a list of facilities and contact information available. Students should create an organizational chart showing the departments and personnel in the facility.
2. Refer students to the www.cms.gov Web site. Search for National Health Expenditure Projections 2012-2022. Using the current year data, locate the percentage for each category listed for the activity. Create a pie chart using the percentages for each category.
3. Refer students to the www.hhs.gov/healthcare/about-the-law/index.html Web site. To simplify the assignment you can suggest they select from one of the categories on the left side of the page to complete their research, or they can investigate the entire law (although it is rather lengthy). The categories are: Pre-Existing Conditions, Young Adult Coverage, Cancellation & Appeals, Benefit Limits, and Preventive Care.
4. Students will research the various agencies at all levels to determine the responsible agency for the section selected.
5. Student answers will vary.
6. You may want groups of students to work together as a team doing research and presenting.

CHAPTER 2 REVIEW

Thinking Critically

1. **Managed Care**—We hear a lot today about the benefits and difficulties of managed care. What do you think exemplifies the best of managed care? How could we further improve the system? Give examples.
2. **Health Costs**—The costs of health care continue to increase. What do you think we can do to help contain these costs? Look at the problem from the perspective of the patient and the provider.
3. **Running the Organization**—Like any efficient corporation, each health care facility has a chain of command. Why is it important to follow this chain of command? Think of specific examples that show what might happen if you do not follow the chain of command.
4. **Working in Health Care**—Every community includes a variety of health care services. Many people living in the community work in this industry sector. In teams of two, complete research to determine the percentage of the population working in health care in your community and prepare a report that describes how the health services employment impacts the local economy.
5. **Access to Health Care**—While it is obvious that better health care improves patient outcomes, not everyone has the same level of access to quality health care. Why do you think this is? What steps can be taken to improve access? What are the effects of not having access to quality health care?

Portfolio Connection

Starting to determine which career best matches your interests and strengths can seem overwhelming. Taking a close look at your abilities can help you make better choices whenever you're faced with big decisions regarding the future. Before setting your goals, it's a good idea to think about what you enjoy doing most, what you're good at, and how challenges that lie ahead might impact your future.

Of course, understanding your basic personality is critical in helping you identify a career path. Are you methodical and detail-oriented? Do you prefer dealing with research to dealing with people? Are you more interested in building relationships? Are you a "doer" or a "thinker" . . . or both?

PORTFOLIO TIP

Remember the wide variety of health care settings in which you could work. Try to collect samples for your portfolio from as many settings as possible (hospital, clinic, doctor's office, home care, etc.) as you continue your studies.

Some companies use Myers-Briggs or other types of tests as one tool to help determine where a candidate might best fit in the organization. The Myers-Briggs Type Indicator, the most common, is a personality questionnaire designed to identify certain psychological differences according to the theories of Carl Gustav Jung, a Swiss psychiatrist credited for founding analytical psychology.

Study some of the basic questions used in personality testing. Then, create a list of your 10 strongest personality traits. Rate each on a scale of 1, 2, or 3, with 1 representing the strongest trait and 3 representing a milder trait. For example, you might thoroughly enjoy nurturing or taking care of people and would rate it a 1. You might also dislike competitive behavior, but you still compete in sports. You would rate that a 2.

Think about the careers we've touched on. This is early in the process, but which do you think would best suit you? Why? Articulate why it is important to do this type of analysis. Keep this in your portfolio. You will refer to it later on in the course. Put it in the personal section of your portfolio.

44 Chapter 2 | Understanding Health Care Systems

Case Studies

1. Students should use the skills they learned in the Math Link on p. 40 to calculate the patient's out-of-pocket expenses.
2. Advise students to act as a counselor or agency representative to consider and answer the two questions.

Thinking Critically (1–5)

- Remind students to use research to support their thoughts and ideas. Answers should include a thesis statement and specific examples to support the thesis.

Portfolio Connection

- Be sure students understand the concept and purpose of a portfolio.
- Refer students to a Web site or other resource for more information about Myers-Briggs or other personality tests (myersbriggs.org).
- Encourage students to create their list of personality traits in a word processing document and to format it attractively. Below the list, they should write about the careers they think best suit them and why. Remind them that this is an exploratory exercise and that they will most likely change their minds often about possible careers.

3 Finding the Right Occupation for You

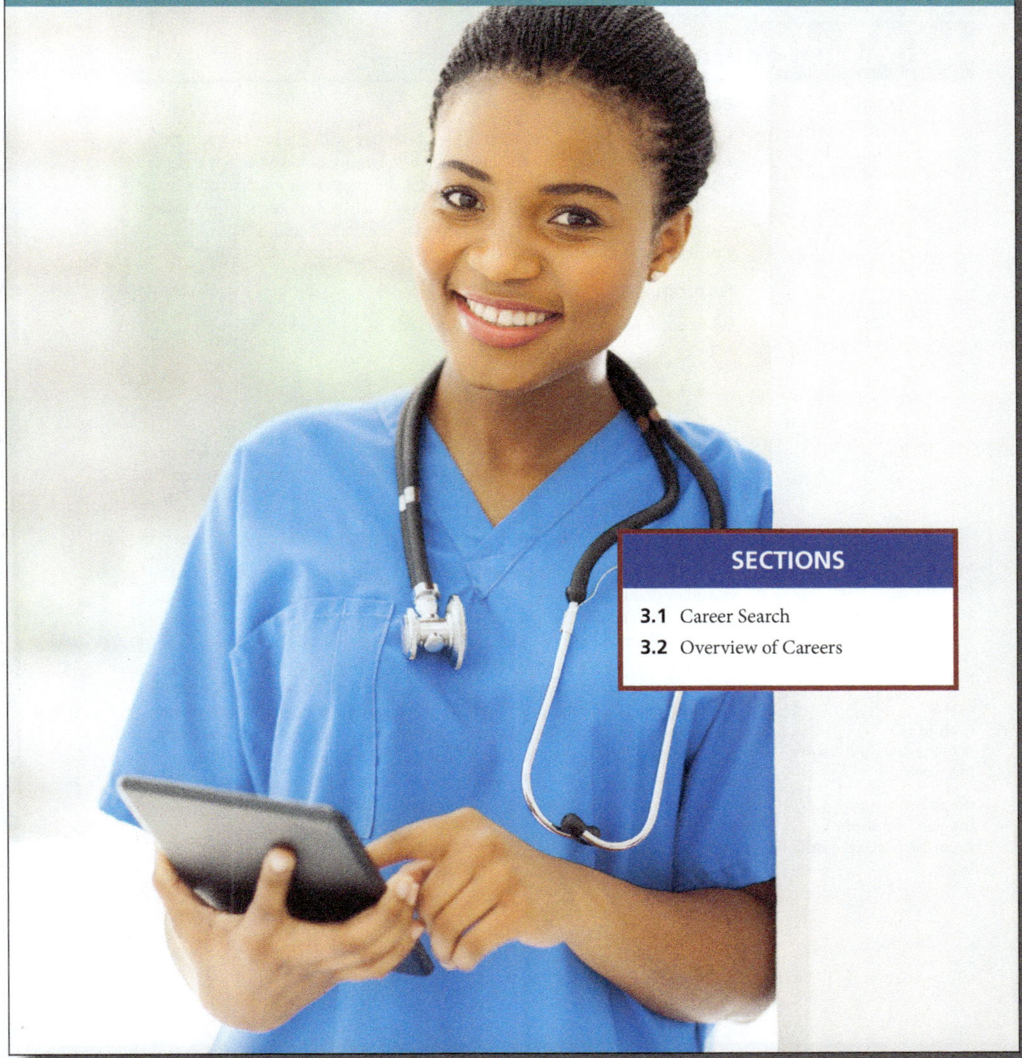

SECTIONS

CHAPTER 3 OVERVIEW

Chapter 3 provides students with a comprehensive look at how to find an occupation in the health science field. It covers methods for conducting a career search, and describes the multitude of occupations that are available.

Section 3.1: In Section 3.1, students learn how to begin a career search in the health industry. They learn techniques for identifying their interests, values, and abilities in order to develop a career plan, and they learn how to use career search resources such as books and Web sites.

Section 3.2: This section lists occupations in the Health Science career cluster and explores the five career pathways that fall under it. It includes examples of occupations in each pathway, along with typical responsibilities, and skills and education requirements.

Advance Preparation	
Review	■ Cognitive Mapping form, Student Activity Guide, chapter text for Sections 3.1 and 3.2.
Contact	■ Professional organizations, state employment office, and personnel departments at local health care facilities to request pamphlets, ■ Guest speakers to explain their occupations and the path they followed to reach their current position. ■ A career center to arrange a visit. ■ One or more health care departments to arrange a tour.
Prepare	■ Magazine and newspaper articles on topics such as health occupations, salary, and growth sectors—*Dictionary of Occupational Titles, Occupational Outlook Handbook, Encyclopedia of Careers.* ■ Web sites that provide information about health science careers—careertech.org, healthpronet.org, or hosa.org.

FOCUS AND ENGAGE

Getting Started

- Use the same Cognitive Mapping from as in Chapter 2.
- Allow at least 15 minutes to complete the activity.
- Students should add two professionals to each department that they had previously identified.
- If working in groups or as a class, have each student identify one process that the professional may perform.
- You may want to have the students complete the form at the beginning of the chapter, and then again at the end to gauge their knowledge.

Introduce the Section

a. Review the content of the Background paragraph, explaining the importance of understanding oneself in order to select an appropriate career.
b. Ask students if they have any personal experience looking for a job, and what resources they used.
c. Explain the concept of a career portfolio, and instruct students to bring a three-ring binder, three-ring pockets, and dividers to class.
d. Review the objectives for the section.

Vocabulary Review

a. Key terms are defined in the margins of the text on the page where they first appear.
b. Pronounce each word, and have the students repeat the pronunciation out loud.
c. Discuss the definition of each word.

Getting Started

Using the Cognitive Mapping form that you started in Chapter 2, fill in the two circles that extend from the department circles with health care professionals that work in each department. Briefly describe at least one task that each professional may perform.

SECTION 3.1 Career Search

Background

When you consider an occupation in the health care field, it is important to focus on your interests, values, and abilities. When you understand yourself, it is easier to select the right occupation. There are many different career opportunities in the health care field. Researching several careers will help you choose the right career for you. Learning how to use the resources for researching occupations will make it easier for you to choose a career.

Objectives

When you have completed this section, you will be able to do the following:

- Define interests, values, and abilities.
- List work-related values.
- Explain the importance of a career plan.
- Identify resources for occupational research.
- Complete an academic plan.

Interests

interests
(IN ter ists)
Something that concerns, draws the attention of, or arouses the curiosity of a person.

career
(kuh REER)
A profession; a person's life work.

occupation
(ok yuh PEY shuhn)
A person's job to earn a living.

Your **interests** are the subjects or activities that attract your attention and that you enjoy doing or learning about. If you are like most people, you will spend half your life or more working. So, choosing a **career** that will bring you satisfaction makes good sense. How can you know what will bring satisfaction? One way is to choose a career that gives you a chance to use and develop your interests. For example, if you like math and working with numbers, you might enjoy a career as a pharmacist. Or, if you enjoy being around children, you might want to pursue a career as a pediatrician or pediatric nurse.When you know your interests early in your career search, you can identify careers that use those interests. If you discover that many of the tasks associated with a particular **occupation** are not interesting to you, reconsider your choice, and research careers that use and build on your interests.

46 Chapter 3 | Finding the Right Occupation for You

TEACH

Discuss

- Ask students if they know the difference between a job and a career.
- Point out that career goals will require money management to pay for education and getting established in their chosen profession.
- Discuss the importance of job satisfaction as it relates to health occupations.

CUSTOMIZED INSTRUCTION OVERVIEW	
Less Advanced Students	Pages 47, 48
More Advanced Students	Pages 56, 58
English Language Learners	Pages 47, 50
Special Needs Students	Pages 52, 54, 65
At-Risk Students	Pages 48, 66

Values

A **value** is the importance that you place on various elements in your life. Money might be more important to you than leisure time. Working with people might be more important to you than what shift you work. Knowing what values you feel most strongly about helps you avoid **compromising** the things that are most important to you. Recognizing your values also helps you **prioritize** your work-related values, some of which are described below:

- **Job security.** Having a steady, long-term job.
- **Leisure time.** Having time outside of work.
- **Wages.** Being paid well for your work.
- **Recognition.** Having a job that commands the respect and admiration of others.
- **Creativity.** Having a job that allows you to express yourself or use your imagination.
- **Advancement.** Having opportunities for promotion and advancement to more challenging responsibilities.
- **Work environment.** Being able to work in a space where you are comfortable, such as outside, or in an office.
- **Flexibility.** Being able to choose your work schedule, such as 9 to 5 Monday through Friday or shift work.
- **Challenge.** Having the opportunity to perform difficult or important tasks.
- **Leadership opportunities.** Managing or supervising the work of other people.

Your work-related values can affect your career decisions. Make a list of these work values and any others you think of and put them in order of their importance to you. When you research an occupation, refer to your list often so you do not choose a job that conflicts with many of your values.

value
(VAL yoo)
The importance that you place on various elements in your life.

compromising
(KOM pruh mahyz)
Giving up something important.

prioritize
(prahy AWR i tahyz)
To put in order of importance.

leisure
(LEE zher)
Time free from the demands of work.

wages
(WEYJ s)
Money that is paid or received for work or services.

Apply It

Make a list of what you consider to be your five strongest abilities. Ask someone who knows you well—a family member, friend, or teacher—to create a list of what they consider your five strongest abilities. Then, compare the lists. How are they similar and how are they different? What does the other person's list tell you about yourself?

Abilities

An **ability** is something you do well or your talents. You have many abilities. Most people have both specific abilities—such as playing the guitar or repairing machines—and more general abilities that help them succeed in life, such as being a good listener or being able to to manage your resources well. It is much more pleasant to work in an occupation that uses your abilities. If you choose an occupation that is too far below your ability level, you will be bored. If it is too far above your ability level, you will be frustrated. It is important to evaluate your abilities as you embark on your career search.

ability
(uh BIL i tee)
Something a person does well.

Developing a Career Plan

Once you have identified your interests, values, and abilities, you have taken the first step in developing a career plan. A **career plan** is a tool that shows you how to achieve your career goals. You use it to identify your skills and interests, to find

career plan
(kuh REER plan)
A tool that shows you how to achieve your career goals.

Finding the Right Occupation for You | Chapter 3 47

CUSTOMIZED INSTRUCTION

Less Advanced Students

Be sure less advanced students understand the difference between interests, values, and abilities.

English Language Learners

Have students write each key term and its pronunciation on one side of an index card and its definition on the other side.

Reinforce and Review

- Review the types of health service providers covered in Chapter 2.
- Remind students that these are all potential employers.

Teaching Tips

- Discuss the importance of knowing your interests, abilities, and values in relation to career choice.
- Emphasize that ability is something you do well naturally while interests are things you like to do, but may have to work to learn.
- Explain that values are subjective, and are therefore neither right nor wrong.
- Point out that values can change, depending on the current circumstances or new developments, and that different people have different values.
- Discuss the way one value may have more importance than another value.
- For example, students probably value both money and job security. Ask them if they can identify which one is more important.
- Show students a sample career plan. If your school does not have a standard form available, you may download a free template from various education and career-oriented Web sites.

Apply It

- You may allow students time in class to complete the first part of this activity.
- Review the results of the entire activity in class.
- Discuss how the way we see ourselves might not always match up with the way others see us.

Teaching Tips

- Explain that a career self-assessment is a process that helps you identify your skills, interests, values, and abilities so that you can choose a career path that will bring you satisfaction.
- Make sure students understand that being truthful and honest in their assessment is essential. Otherwise, they will not get an accurate or realistic sense of the career paths that might be most suitable for them.
- Explain that a self-assessment is a tool designed to help you recognize your strengths and talents as well as your weaknesses. It is a tool that can provide you with a balanced and objective view of the jobs you might be suitable for and those that might not be as appropriate.
- Discuss the importance of conducting a thorough career search.
- Point out that being in the wrong job can be frustrating and stressful.
- Explain that there are a number of resources that can help in your career planning effort.
- Introduce the Career Clusters by displaying the careertech.org Web site on-screen and navigating through its various pages.

Figure Focus

3.1 Why is it important to work with someone objective when you develop a career self-assessment?

Answer: Someone who is objective can help you be honest and accurate about your skills and abilities.

a career that suits your skills and interests, and to determine the type of education and training you will need to succeed. Your career plan should be specific, realistic, and attainable. It should include a long-range career goal as well as a series of short-term milestones that will help you get there. Every once in a while, you should revisit your career plan and make adjustments or corrections. Your goals might change as you develop new interests and abilities, so your career plan will change, too.

Your instructor or counselor may have a form available for you to use in preparing your career plan. Most career plans include the following information: career self-assessment; a list of career planning resources; an academic plan aligned with a selected career; and a career outlook analysis.

Career Self-Assessment

A career self-assessment includes a prioritized list of skills, interests, and abilities. You have already learned the importance of knowing your interests and abilities. The career self-assessment is a series of questions that when answered honestly and objectively, helps you identify your specific skills, interests, and abilities. (Figure 3.1)

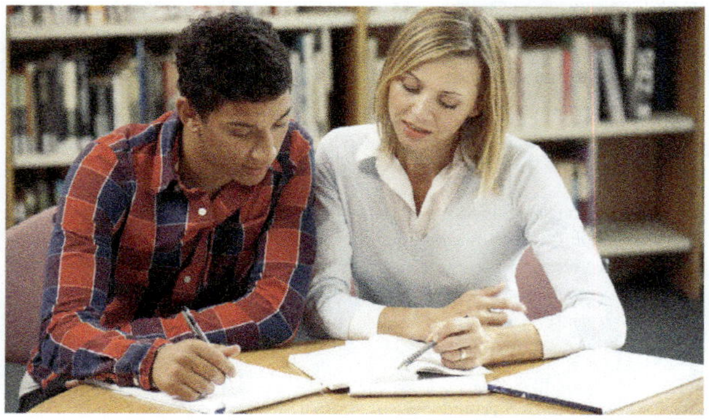

Figure 3.1
Why is it important to work with someone objective when you develop a career self-assessment?

Resources for Analyzing Careers

There are an overwhelming number of available career opportunities. How can you possibly identify the ones that match your skills, interests, and abilities? The 16 career clusters—developed by the National Association of State Directors of Career Technical Education Consortium (NASDCTEc)—are a good place to start. They can help you identify types of careers and specific jobs and help you pick out the ones that you might find interesting. They also show you the educational and skill requirements you might need and the path you might take to achieve the career of your dreams. The Health Science career cluster is covered in Section 3.2 of this chapter. You can find information about all the career clusters at careertech.org.

CUSTOMIZED INSTRUCTION

At-Risk/Less Advanced Students

In preparing their career self-assessments, help students identify their skills, achievements, and abilities if they are struggling with these. Their skills can be as simple as knowing the multiplication tables or being able to identify the seven continents. Their achievements can be passing a big test or getting their homework done on time. Their abilities can range from taking care of a younger sibling to running errands for an elderly relative. If you think it's appropriate, ask the teachers of their favorite subjects to assist in identifying skills and achievements.

Language Arts Link

Managing Stress

Studies have shown that job-related stress can affect your physical health and mental stability. While no job is completely stress-free, the importance of choosing a career that aligns well with your interests, values, and abilities will ensure the work you do has a positive impact on your quality of life. When in a stressful environment, regardless of job selection, it is helpful to know how to deal with stress to protect your mental, emotional, and physical health.

To prevent or manage stressful situations, plan for potential eventualities, stay organized, and manage your time well while on the job. Produce clear and coherent writing in paragraph form, using your prioritized values list, and explain how a career that does not match your most important values can cause stress. Analyze your explanation and consider why you believe this job would not work for you. Include your thoughts in the paragraphs that you produced for discussion. Participate effectively in a collaborative discussion with your class by presenting your information, findings, and supporting evidence clearly and persuasively.

In addition, your guidance and career counselors have books, computer programs, videos, and lists of useful Web sites that provide information about types of careers. School clubs and organizations may also have information about types of careers. A business club might invite a representative from the community to speak about his or her occupation. An organization such as Family, Career and Community Leaders of America (FCCLA) or Health Occupations Students of America (HOSA) has career-related projects and activities.

The U.S. Bureau of Labor Statistics (BLS) is a government agency responsible for tracking information about jobs and workers. Its Web site (bls.gov) includes information on the nation's job market, employment trends, demographics, productivity, etc. The BLS also publishes the *Occupational Outlook Handbook* (OOH). Available in printed and online editions, the OOH is a comprehensive and valuable resource that describes hundreds of occupations, including responsibilities, working conditions, education requirements, salary ranges, and job outlook.

Last, one of the best ways to learn about different careers is from someone who is employed. For example, you can job-shadow someone who has a job you find interesting. Job shadowing means to follow someone around at work for a day or part of a day. By job shadowing, you can see exactly what the responsibilities, tasks, and rewards are for a particular job. Informational interviews are also a good way to explore careers. An informational interview gives you the opportunity to sit down with someone who is employed in a career or industry that interests you. You can ask specific questions about the job responsibilities, see the work environment, and maybe even meet other people in the industry.

Finding the Right Occupation for You | Chapter 3 49

Language Arts Link—Managing Stress

- Define stress, describe the symptoms, and discuss how it can affect job performance as well as personal life.
- Point out that there are some careers that are known to induce higher levels of stress, such as air traffic controller.
- Discuss health occupations that might be particularly stressful.
- Remind students that a thesis statement is a sentence that explains the main idea, and that it will help them focus their thoughts for the essay.
- Encourage students to draft an outline, story web, or list questions they need to answer to organize their ideas for the essay.
- Emphasize that the essay is primarily an opinion piece, but that they should support their opinions using facts or real-life examples.
- For evaluation, you should verify that the essay relates to the thesis statement, that the student uses facts or real-life examples to support the thesis, and you should mark spelling and grammatical errors.

Teaching Tips

- Explain the importance of researching an occupation.
- Point out that researching and exploring various career resources helps students do the following:
  - Learn the specific duties associated with a job.
  - Match interests, values, and abilities with the actual job.
  - Learn what skills are needed for a job.
  - Learn which employers hire people for that job.
  - Identify whether a job offers growth potential.
- Demonstrate how to navigate the Bureau of Labor Statistics Web site (BLS.gov) and particularly the *Occupational Outlook Handbook*.
- Emphasize that talking to someone already holding the job can help students gain insight into the specific day-to-day responsibilities.

Teaching Tips

- If your school has an academic plan template, make sure each student has a copy.
- Some things that you might put in your personal academic plan include:
  - Goals beyond high school
  - Assessment of your skills, knowledge, and experience
  - Assessment of factors that will contribute to your success
  - Assessment of factors that might interfere with your success
  - Graduation requirements
  - Plan for achieving graduation
  - Plan for achieving goals beyond high school
  - A list of all the courses you have taken, when you took them, and your final grade

Career-Ready Practices

- Students develop an academic plan in this activity. Make sure they have a copy of a standard academic plan or direct them to a Web site from which they can download one for free.
- This activity gives students real-world experience in applying the following Career-Ready Practice: Plan Education and Career Path Aligned to Personal Goals.
- For more information on the Career-Ready Practices, visit careertech.org/career-ready-practices.

academic plan
(ak uh DEM ik plan)
A document that you use to set goals for the things you want to accomplish while you are in school.

Career-Ready Practices

Career-ready individuals take personal ownership of their own educational and career goals. They understand that meeting their goals will require time, effort, and commitment. They seek out counselors, mentors, and other resources to help them develop and act on a plan that will ensure they meet their career and personal goals.

Working with your instructor, a counselor, or a family member, develop an academic plan that starts now and takes you through high school graduation. If your school has a form for the plan, use it. Otherwise, use the Internet to locate a form that you might be able to use or adapt for your needs. Be sure to include your academic and career goals and an assessment of your skills, interests, and abilities. You can include your school report card or transcript, as well as a list of your co-curricular and community activities. Add the plan to your career portfolio. (Refer to the "Portfolio Connection" activity at the end of each chapter.)

Academic Plan

An **academic plan** is a document you use to set goals for the things you want to accomplish while you are in school. Your years in school teach you skills and information you need to get and keep a job, and provide an opportunity to prepare for a career. Think about this: Most companies will not hire an employee who has not graduated from high school. A growing number will not hire an employee who does not have a college degree or other post-secondary training. Developing strong academic skills can help you in any career you choose. An academic plan that is aligned with a selected career or career cluster will help you identify ways to meet the educational and training requirements and build the skills you need for the career of your choice.

Start your academic plan by writing a statement that describes your long-term ultimate goal. The goal should be specific and should include career, education, and lifestyle goals. For example, you might write: *I will be an occupational physical therapist living in California by the time I am 30 years old.*

Add short-term goals that define how you will gain the skills, knowledge, and experience that you need to achieve your ultimate goal. Include a timeline for achieving each one. For example, the occupational physical therapist might have the following short-term goals:

- Get an A in health class this semester
- Enroll in advanced science classes next semester
- Volunteer at a physical rehabilitation center this summer
- By the end of the school year, research colleges and universities in California that offer physical therapy degrees

Your instructors and school counselor can help you develop an academic plan. Some schools have forms you can use; if not, you can organize your plan in a way that maps your academic achievement and future plans. Most academic plans include goals in four basic areas:

- Career-related planning, skills, and experiences
- Academic preparation and planning
- School and community involvement
- Plans and goals for after high school

Career Outlook

job outlook
(job OUT look)
The expectation or prospect of a particular job in the future.

Your career plan should include an analysis of the outlook for the selected career or career cluster. A **job outlook** provides statistics and trends about whether the job is in an industry that is growing or shrinking. The *Occupational Outlook Handbook* published by the BLS is a comprehensive resource for trends in specific occupations. It provides statistics on projected employment, trends in the industry, and job prospects. The more you know about your selected occupation and the need and demand for workers in that occupation, the better prepared you are to set goals that will help you achieve career success.

50 Chapter 3 | Finding the Right Occupation for You

CUSTOMIZED INSTRUCTION

English Language Learners

With a partner, have students read aloud their list of questions before participating in the informational interview mentioned in the Apply It on the next page.

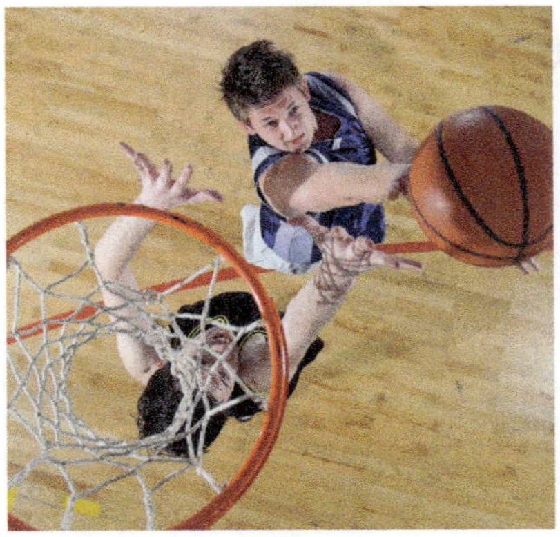

Figure 3.2
Why is it important to include co-curricular activities as part of your academic plan?

Developing a Career Portfolio

A **career portfolio** is a tool you will use to document, organize, and maintain the materials you collect and create as you plan your career. You have already begun to assemble your portfolio through the "Portfolio Connection" activities in Chapters 1 and 2 of this course. You will continue to add to your portfolio as you complete each activity in subsequent chapters. Completing this project demonstrates to college admissions officers and potential employers your ability to plan, organize, and create a final product that showcases your knowledge, skills, abilities, and interests. Compile, organize, and write out the various items and ideas into summaries for your portfolio, providing an easy to read and understand collection for potential reviewers.

Summary

In this section you learned that it is important to identify and evaluate your work interests, values, and abilities. You learned how to use this information when you choose a career, how to use many resources to research career possibilities, and the importance of developing a career plan.

Section 3.1 Review Questions

1. Explain the difference between interests and values.
2. List three work-related values.
3. Why is it important to choose an occupation that suits your abilities?
4. Identify two resources that could help you with occupational research.
5. What are some of the things you can learn from occupational research?
6. What are the benefits of a portfolio?

Apply It

Use the resources discussed in this section (career clusters at careertech.org and the *Occupational Outlook Handbook* from BLS.gov) to research health careers that interest you. Select one career that you'd like to learn more about and develop a list of at least 10 questions regarding it.

Then, set up an informational interview with someone who has the same job you selected. You can find potential candidates to interview at local hospitals and clinics, doctor and dental offices, urgent and ambulatory care centers, fitness centers, nursing homes, etc.

When you have completed the interview, write a paper explaining how the occupation you researched matches your interests, abilities, and values. Discuss aspects of the occupation that might not match your interests, abilities, and values. Determine if these would be a stressor for you and if so how you would manage this stress.

Career portfolio
A collection of materials that shows your knowledge, abilities, skills, and insights as they pertain to a particular occupation, business, or profession.

Figure Focus

3.2 Why is it important to include co-curricular activities as part of your academic plan?

Answer: Co-curricular activities help you build skills such as leadership and teamwork. They give you the opportunity to explore and develop your interests and abilities.

Apply It

- Encourage students to explore other resources to learn about a career that interests them.
- It might be helpful if you contact a hospital, clinic, or other care center beforehand to arrange for group informational interviews; for example, you might contact a hospital to see if a registered nurse could meet with students interested in that profession.
- In evaluating student papers, make sure they discuss how the occupation matches their interests, abilities, and values as well as where it doesn't match them, and how they could address those potential conflicts.

Teaching Tips

- Discuss the type of information that should be included in a career portfolio, and display a career portfolio.
- Explain that a career portfolio is a collection of information to help you fill out application forms or answer interview questions when looking for a job.
- A good career portfolio includes important dates as well as specific information about training and education.
- Point out that having such information immediately available in an interview demonstrates that the student is organized and prepared.

Section 3.1 Review Questions

1. Answer: Interests are what you like to do and what you do not like to do. Values are the importance that you place on various elements in your life.
2. Answer: Work-related values include job security, leisure time, wages, recognition, creativity, advancement, working environment, home life, responsibility, and management.
3. Answer: It is important to choose an occupation that suits your abilities because it will make your job more pleasant. If you choose an occupation that is below your abilities, you will be bored and if you choose an occupation that is beyond your abilities you will be frustrated.
4. Answer: Resources that could help with occupational research include the Career Clusters at careertech.org, the U.S. Bureau of Labor Statistics Web site (BLS.gov), the *Occupational Outlook Handbook*, school clubs and organizations, and informational interviews.

5. Answer: By conducting occupational research, you learn about the tasks to be performed, education required, working environment, job outlook, and salary.
6. Answer: The benefits of a portfolio is that it shows your mastery of career requirements to an employer, college, or higher-level training program. A portfolio also shows your own growth and accomplishments over time.

FOCUS AND ENGAGE

Introduce the Section

a. Review the content of the Background paragraph, explaining that it is no exaggeration to say that there are hundreds of careers in the health care field.

b. Explain that the careers discussed in this section are organized according to the five pathways within the Health Science Career Cluster.

c. Examples of careers within each pathway include brief information on job growth potential, as well as the educational requirements and typical responsibilities.

d. Discuss the objectives for the section.

Vocabulary Review

a. Key terms are defined in the margins of the text on the page where they first appear.

b. Pronounce each word, and have the students repeat the pronunciation out loud.

c. Discuss the definition of each word.

SECTION 3.2 Overview of Careers

Background

As you have learned, the health care field continues to evolve as health care reform, an aging population, and advances in medical technology bring about changes to the way patients access care as well as the manner in which it is provided. According to the Bureau of Labor Statistics, the health care and social assistance industry is one of the largest in the country, with nearly 22 million jobs, and it is projected to grow 13 percent by 2031. For those interested in a career in health care, this translates to a growing number and broader variety of job opportunities. Understanding how occupations within health care are categorized will help you in your career planning.

Objectives

When you have completed this section, you will be able to do the following:

- Define the key terms.
- Describe the Health Science career cluster and identify its pathways.
- Compare and contrast therapeutic, diagnostics, health informatics, support, and biotechnology research and development services.
- List and describe sample occupations within each Health Science pathway.

Career Clusters

In an effort to classify occupations within all major industries, the National Association of State Directors of Career Technical Education Consortium (NASDCTEc) developed 16 career clusters. The career clusters provide a structure for organizing specific jobs and industries into similar categories.

Within each of the 16 clusters are related job, industry, and occupation types known as **pathways**. Each pathway offers a variety of careers you might choose.

pathway
(PATH wa)
Related job, industry, and occupation types within a career cluster.

The 16 career clusters and their pathways help job seekers and individuals interested in specific careers to identify professions that best suit their interests and abilities. Through them, you can learn about the education and skills you will need to be effective in a specific job and career.

The Health Science career cluster is described as "planning, managing, and providing therapeutic services, diagnostic services, health informatics, support services, and biotechnology research and development." Employees in this cluster work in cities, suburbs, rural areas, and other communities to provide crucial services to a diverse client base. Individuals employed in these fields take on legal responsibilities, must have strong ethics, and often use their technical skills. Each of the five Health Science pathways includes a variety of different career areas.

52 Chapter 3 | Finding the Right Occupation for You

TEACH

Teaching Tips

- You might want to revisit the careertech.org Web site at this point and explore the Health Science career cluster.
- Review the Common Career Technical Core with performance elements, Knowledge & Skills Statements, and Plan of Study.
- Display the Career Cluster Frame and make a copy for each student. This shows different occupations that fall within each pathway.

CUSTOMIZED INSTRUCTION

Special Needs Students

Provide enlarged copies of the Career Cluster Frame to students with visual impairments.

They have been organized by similar functions, rather than job title specificity. As you consider your career, examine the functions within each cluster and compare the various health science careers for each. Following is a description of the five pathways in the Health Science career cluster:

- *Therapeutic Services:* Careers focus on changing the health status of the patient over time. Employees in this pathway work directly with the patient, providing care, treatment, counseling, and education information. Because they work one-on-one with patients, they must possess strong oral and written communication skills. Likewise, they use these skills to coordinate patient care among other team members. Examples of occupations in this pathway are physical therapist, respiratory therapist, athletic trainer, and dental hygienist.
- *Diagnostic Services:* Employees in this pathway use tests and evaluations to detect, diagnose, and treat disease, injuries, and other physical conditions. Diagnostic service workers must have strong oral and written communication skills with both patients and other professionals/departments in the health care facility. Because they are often responsible for positioning, transferring, and transporting patients, they must understand the principles of body mechanics. Furthermore, they must demonstrate knowledge of and be able to perform a given procedure—within their scope of practice—according to protocol. Examples of occupations in this pathway are medical lab technicians, pathologists, and radiology technicians.
- *Health Informatics:* This pathway covers many different levels of health care careers, including health care administrators who manage health care agencies; individuals who manage patient data and information; those who handle financial information; those who work on computer applications related to health care processes and procedures; and those who develop programs to guide excellence in health care delivery. Workers in this pathway must be able to evaluate and analyze health and medical information and employ methods for the confidential communication of it to the appropriate parties. This often involves a comprehensive understanding of information systems and managing the collection, processing, distribution, and storage of electronic data. Examples of occupations in this pathway are admitting clerk, health care administrator, medical librarian, and transcriptionist.
- *Support Services:* Employees in this pathway help to provide a safe, supportive environment for the delivery of health care. Careers range from entry level to management and include technical and professional occupations. Workers in this pathway must have strong organizational skills and be able to follow established procedures for tasks that ensure and promote safety and quality within the health care facility. They must know how to use and manage available resources. Problem-solving and decision-making skills are often called in to use to ensure legal, regulatory, and other guidelines are being followed. Examples of occupations in this pathway include dietary technicians, social workers, and hospital maintenance engineers.

Apply It

Split into teams of three to four students, with each team having a different color pad of sticky notes. Each team will have five minutes to write down as many health care occupations that they can think of. Write each occupation on a separate sticky note.

On a poster board or large sheet of paper, create headings for the five pathways within the Health Science career cluster. These are therapeutic services, diagnostics services, health informatics, support services, and biotechnology research and development. Each team will then post its occupations under the appropriate pathway.

Compare your posters. If necessary, refer to the Health Science Career Cluster Frame at http://www.careertech.org/sites/default/files/CCFrame-HealthScience.pdf. The frame lists sample occupations for each career cluster pathway.

Finding the Right Occupation for You | Chapter 3 53

Teaching Tips

- Review each of the pathways within the Health Science Career Cluster, and some of the professions in each pathway:
  - Therapeutic workers provide treatment using procedures.
  - Diagnostic workers prepare and perform tests to determine the cause of illness or the extent of injury.
  - Support Services or Environmental workers provide a therapeutic environment and repair and maintain equipment.
  - Health Informatics or Information workers keep permanent records for patient care and research.
  - Biotechnology Research and Development workers try to find new treatments, improve testing, or create new devices.
- It might be helpful to display the Career Cluster Frame on a screen or provide each student with a copy as they review the descriptions of the five pathways.
- Make sure students can differentiate between therapeutic services and diagnostic services.

Apply It

- Divide the class into an even number of groups.
- Come prepared with an equivalent number of pads of sticky notes.
- Provide a large sheet of paper or poster board for each team.
- Compare team posters to the Health Science Career Cluster Frame.

TEAMWORK

An alternative to the Apply It activity is to divide the class into five groups. Assign each group one of the pathways. Have the groups list as many occupations as they can in their assigned pathway. (You may want to impose a time limit.) Discuss the results as a class.

Teaching Tips

- Explain that the remainder of Section 3.2 examines the history and evolution of each of the pathways, and examples of different occupations within the pathway.
- Begin by reviewing the purpose of occupations in Therapeutic Services.

ACTIVITY

Have students select a career in the Therapeutic Services pathway other than those discussed in the text. They should use available resources such as the *Occupational Outlook Handbook*, BLS.gov, healthpronet.org, and hosa.org, as well as other books and Web sites to research and report on the career. They should include information such as the educational requirements, entry-level opportunities, salary range, potential employers, and opportunities for advancement. Encourage students to create a slide presentation on their selected career.

Apply It

- You may have students work in pairs on this project.
- Encourage students to use multimedia elements in their presentations.

Apply It

Research the history of the therapeutic services career pathway. How have careers in this pathway advanced over time? How do these health professionals develop and foster relationships within the community that promote health and wellness? Create a presentation or poster describing your findings.

Career Connect

Art/Music/Dance Therapist

A growing therapeutic field in health care is that of art/music/dance therapists. They are often referred to as recreational therapists. They provide recreation-based treatment for a variety of illnesses, diseases, and disorders using art, crafts, music, drama, and dance. They may work in a variety of settings with a variety of age groups. For more information about careers in art, music, and dance therapy, research the Web site for the National Council for Therapeutic Recreational Certification, nctrc.org.

- *Biotechnology Research and Development:* Careers in this pathway involve bioscience research and development as it applies to human health. Employes may work to find new treatments for diseases, improve diagnostic testing, or create new medical devices to assist the patient. Strong math and science skills are a must for workers in this pathway. Employees must be able to apply mathematical concepts and use statistical and scientific data in the research and development of biotechnological products. They must have a solid understanding of biotechnology areas, including recombinant DNA, genetic engineering, nanotechnology, and genomics. They must possess a basic understanding of laboratory procedures. They must also understand the ethical, moral, and legal issues related to biotechnology. Examples of occupations in this pathway are biomedical chemist, microbiologist, pharmacist, and toxicologist.

The rest of this chapter provides more in-depth discussion of each of the Health Science pathways and various occupations within each. As you will find, there is a broad range of career opportunities in health science in a variety of settings.

Therapeutic Services

Workers in therapeutic services are those caregivers whose primary responsibilities are providing care, treatment, counseling, and health education information directly to the patient. They are doctors, nurses, paramedics, and therapists. They are podiatrists, pharmacists, and veterinarians (physicians that care for animals). They are the assistants and technicians who work directly with patients to ensure their health care needs are being met.

In the early and mid-1900s, therapeutic services were focused primarily on occupational therapy, a form of therapy that promotes health and well-being through the performance of meaningful, everyday life activities, referred to as "occupations." It was used initially to treat patients with mental illness but quickly expanded to include those with physical illnesses as well. Notably, occupational therapy played an important role in treating patients affected by epidemics, such as polio, tuberculosis, and HIV/AIDS.

In the 1970s, legislation was passed that required public schools to provide therapeutic services to enable children with disabilities to participate in regular school settings. Since then, the types of therapeutic services available and the methods by which they are delivered have expanded significantly. Following is a sampling of occupations that fall under the therapeutic services pathway.

Respiratory Therapy/Respiratory Care Workers

Helping patients/clients with their breathing is a very important part of health care. Patients/clients may live without water or food for a few days. But without air, they will suffer brain damage within a few minutes and may die after nine minutes.

respiratory
(RES per uh tawr ee)
Pertaining to or serving for breathing.

Respiratory therapy workers and respiratory care practitioners evaluate, treat, and care for patients/clients of all ages who have breathing problems. Therapists test lung capacity and check blood for oxygen and carbon dioxide content. They give treatments and teach self-care to patients/clients with chronic respiratory

54 Chapter 3 | Finding the Right Occupation for You

CUSTOMIZED INSTRUCTION

Special Needs Students

For the Activity on this page, allow students to provide a written or oral report if desired.

problems. They also give emergency care for drowning, stroke, shock, heart failure, and other emergencies. Other duties may include keeping records and making minor repairs to equipment. (**Figure 3.3**)

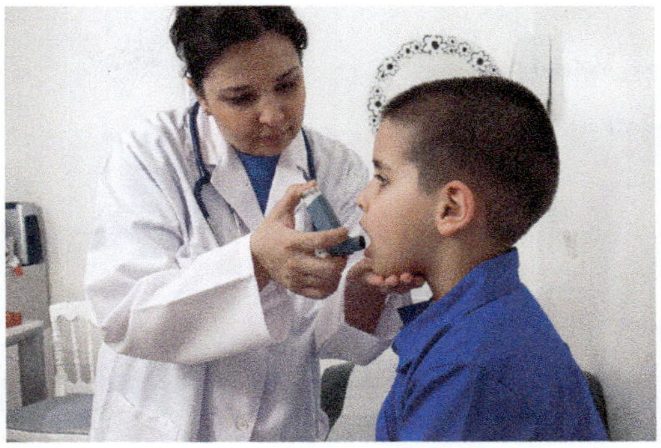

Figure 3.3
What tasks might a respiratory therapist have to complete?

Respiratory care workers work in acute care hospitals, **cardiopulmonary** laboratories, ambulatory care units, health maintenance organizations, home health agencies, and nursing homes. They work indoors and may be exposed to flammable gases and body fluids. Their jobs might require shift work and weekend work. They stand for long periods of time and carry or push equipment throughout the facility. (You can learn more about respiratory therapy and care at aarc.org, which is the Web site for the American Association for Respiratory Care.)

cardiopulmonary
(kahr dee oh PUHL muh ner ee)
Of, pertaining to, or affecting the heart and lungs.

Emergency Services Workers

Emergency service workers are the vital links between the community and the hospital. Paramedics and emergency medical technicians provide care for illnesses and injuries outside of hospitals and trauma centers. Because the lives of people depend on rapid, appropriate care in an emergency, paramedics and emergency medical technicians (EMTs) must be able to able to make decisions quickly and be very detail-oriented. They must be alert at all times for safety issues, as many emergency situations have environmental hazards present, such as downed power lines, burning vehicles, raging water, etc.

Paramedics and EMTs work in a variety of conditions and environments. They general work in shifts and must be able to lift heavy objects, move quickly, and work in life-and-death situations.

The National Registry of Emergency Medical Technicians is the professional organization (nremt.org/rwd/public) responsible for providing certification and licensing of emergency services workers. Certification and licensing also varies by state but usually includes a written as well as a skills examination.

Pharmacy Technicians

Pharmacy workers prepare and **dispense** medications prescribed by physicians, dentists, and other health care professionals. (**Figure 3.4**) They provide information to health care professionals and to the public about medications. Another important task is to review the medications that patients/clients are taking. This reduces the chance that the patient/client will have a drug interaction that can cause illness or an allergic reaction. Pharmacy workers also help in the strict control of distribution and use of government-controlled products, such as narcotics and barbiturates. Since vaccines and other drugs deteriorate, pharmacy workers are responsible for careful inventory control.

dispense
(di SPENS)
To distribute or pass out.

Finding the Right Occupation for You | Chapter 3 55

Figure Focus

3.3 What tasks might a respiratory therapist have to complete?

Answer: Test lung capacity, check blood for oxygen and carbon dioxide content, give treatments, teach self-care, keep records, and give emergency care.

Teaching Tips

- Discuss the general tasks and responsibilities of respiratory care workers and the typical settings in which they work.
- Review the description and tasks of a pharmacy assistant.
- Discuss what they think the workers in a pharmacy do.
- Ask students if they have ever used a pharmacy and to share their thoughts on interactions they've had with pharmacy workers.

ACTIVITY

Encourage students to visit a pharmacy and observe the pharmacy workers. Students should tell workers why they are there and what they are doing. They should take notes on how they interact with customers, the type of work they do, their appearance, and their behavior. Have them report their observations to the class.

Figure Focus

3.4 Pharmacy workers prepare and dispense medications. How do pharmacy workers help to ensure the safety of clients?

Answer: They provide information about medicines to health care professionals and the public. They also review the medicines that clients are taking.

Career-Ready Practices

- Students develop a wellness program for a business that should include at least five programs and initiatives. They should consider programs that benefit both the employee and the employer and be prepared to discuss these benefits when they present their posters.
- This activity gives students real-world experience in applying the following Career-Ready Practice: Attend to Personal Health and Financial Well-Being.
- For more information on the Career-Ready Practices, visit careertech.org/career-ready-practices.

Teaching Tips

- Review the description of nursing service workers.
- Remind students that nursing services offers a wide range of career opportunities.

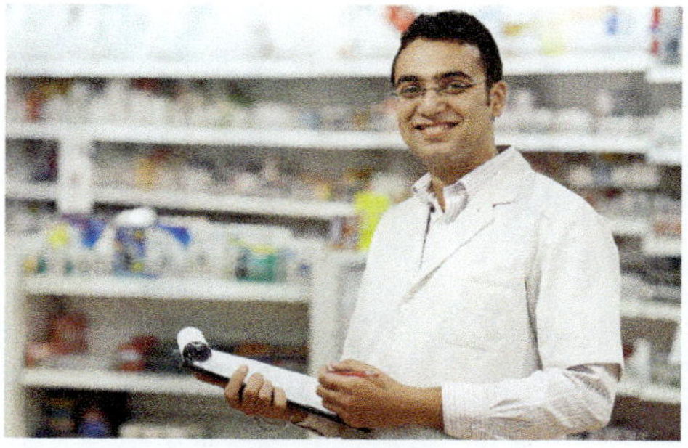

Figure 3.4
Pharmacy workers prepare and dispense medications. How do pharmacy workers help to ensure the safety of clients?

Pharmacy workers are employed in acute care hospitals, community pharmacies, grocery store pharmacies, health maintenance organizations, home health agencies, and clinics. A pharmacist may also work for state and local health departments, as well as for pharmaceutical manufacturers. They work indoors and may be required to work in a restricted environment, such as areas where sterile solutions are prepared. In large hospitals or community pharmacies, they may work in shifts. Their work requires lifting, carrying, pushing items, and climbing ladders in storage areas. They need good vision for close-up work. They stand for long periods of time and must take proper safety precautions when working with products that can be dangerous. (You can learn more about pharmacy care careers at aacp.org, the Web site for the American Association of Colleges of Pharmacy.)

Anesthesia Service Workers

Anesthesia is defined as the lack of pain or feeling. The process of anesthesia is completed by artificially causing the lack of pain or feeling by administering particular drugs. This process most often occurs during surgery or other similar procedures. A variety of health care providers can function in the field of anesthesia.

Career Connect

Mortuary science is the career pathway that focuses on the care of a person after death. Funeral directors, embalmers, and morticians are some of the career titles available in this field. Funeral directors assist families in planning memorial services and burials or cremations. Embalmers prepare the body for burial. The title *mortician* may also apply to a funeral director, depending on the job responsibilities at the particular mortuary or funeral home. These careers fall under the Health Science Therapeutic pathway.

Anesthesiologists are licensed physicians who administer drugs during surgery to eliminate pain or feeling during the operation. They also supervise nurse anesthetists who are registered nurses with advanced training to administer medications during procedures to provide anesthesia. There may also be anesthesia technologists/technicians whose responsibilities include the monitoring and maintenance of anesthesia equipment.

Anesthesia professionals typically work indoors within sterile environments in hospitals, physician offices, and outpatient clinics. They may work long hours, rotating shifts, and must be detailed-oriented. They must closely monitor the safety of the patient throughout the operative procedures. (You can learn more about anesthesia careers at aana.org, the Web site for the American Association of Nurse Anesthetists, and andasahq.org, the Web site for the American Society of Anesthesiologists.)

Nursing Service Workers

Nursing service workers provide many essential services. (**Figure 3.5**) They care for patients who are physically ill or disabled and provide preventive care (e.g., immunizations). They work in industry, community health agencies, general hospitals, long-term care facilities, government agencies, schools, educational institutions, visiting nurse associations, clinics, physicians' offices, ambulatory care units, homes, and health maintenance organizations. Nurses work indoors. They may have rotating shifts and work on weekends. Their work requires standing,

56 Chapter 3 | Finding the Right Occupation for You

CUSTOMIZED INSTRUCTION

More Advanced Students

Ask more advanced students to find out if your state has any special requirements or licensing processes for pharmacy workers, and to report on their findings to the class.

walking, lifting, and pushing patients, carts, and wheelchairs. They are exposed to unpleasant odors and body fluids.

Registered nurses are the primary point of contact for patients and their families. They conduct physical assessments, collaborate with physicians and other team members to develop a treatment plan, coordinate delivery of care, administer treatment and medications, operate equipment, and evaluate the outcome of care.

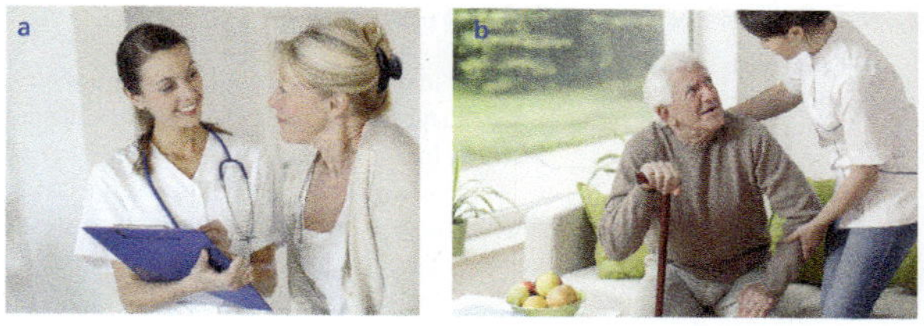

Figure 3.5
A nurse assistant (a) and home health aide (b) helping clients. What is the difference between a nurse assistant and a home health aid?

A licensed practical nurse (LPN) works under the direction of the registered nurse and physician to provide technical care, such as dressing wounds, collecting samples for testing, recording food and fluid intake/output, measuring and recording vital signs, and assisting patients with bathing, dressing, and personal hygiene.

Nurse assistants answer patient call lights, assist patients with personal hygiene, serve and collect food trays, provide snacks and fresh drinking water, transport patients in wheelchairs or stretchers or help them with walking, and tidy patients' rooms.

A home health aid does many of the same functions as a nurse assistant but works in the home of the patient. They assist patients of all ages who need more health care than their families can provide.

What's New?

Technology and Nursing Care

Advances in technology continue to shape the way nurses care for patients.

- Nurses now use tablet computers, wall-mounted PCs in patient rooms, and mobile carts to enter and retrieve data almost instantaneously without ever having to leave the patient's bedside. This data includes patient records, lab results, pharmaceutical data, care guidelines, and other clinical resources.
- Medical devices such as infusion delivery systems and ventilators assist nurses by signaling problems and helping to avoid errors.
- Monitoring systems allow nurses to obtain patient information. These include fetal monitors, which can show the heart rate of a baby still in the uterus; heart monitors that display the electrical rhythm and pattern of a patient's heart; and vital sign machines that automatically take the patient's blood pressure, pulse, and respiration. Even systems built into the hospital bed monitor a patient's weight or movement during sleep.
- Bar-coding and scanners are now being used to ensure safety in medication administration and protect against errors. Medications now come prepackaged with a bar code that the nurse scans before giving to a patient. A patient's armband, which is also bar-coded, is scanned before the medication is given to ensure the right medication and dosage.

What ways do you use technology in your own personal health care?

Figure Focus

3.5 A nurse assistant (a) and home health aide (b) helping clients. What is the difference between a nurse assistant and a home health aid?

Answer: A home health aide cares for patients/clients in their homes instead of in a health facility.

Teaching Tips

- Make sure students understand the differences in tasks among the nursing service workers discussed in the text.
- Point out that home health aides are in growing demand and the career is one of the fastest growing in the country. Reasons for the rapid growth include an emphasis on wellness; shorter hospital stays; and the desire to contain costs.

What's New—Technology and Nursing Care

- Ask students to consider how technology has changed health care.
- Discuss how nurses administered care and monitored patients before the technological advances discussed in the text.
- Discuss how communication was handled before cell phones or e-mail.

What ways do you use technology in your own personal health care?

Student answers will vary but might include GPS running apps that quantify your daily exercise routines; armbands and watches that can help you track your exercise, weight, nutrition and sleep habits; "smart" customizable walking/running shoes in which you can insert a chip that connects wirelessly to your iPod; and apps for tracking calories.

ACTIVITY

Imagine you work for an employment agency specializing in nursing service workers. Create a poster listing the skills and qualifications of your nurses in a way that would make health care facilities want to hire them.

ACTIVITY

The tasks performed by a nurse's assistant in a health care facility are similar to those performed by a home health aide. Write an essay explaining the differences between the two from a caregiver's point of view. Include your opinion on which you think is better for the patient. Be sure to support your opinion with facts or real-life examples.

TEAMWORK

In small groups, work together to think of a new technology that might help health care workers be more efficient or accurate. The technology might be based on something that already exists, such as handheld computer or cell phone, or it might be something completely new. Create an advertisement for your invention, including a picture, and a list of features.

Teaching Tips

- Introduce the Diagnostic Services pathway and review how it has evolved over the last century.
- Ask students if they know of anyone who has participated in a clinical trial.
- Review the careers listed in the Career Cluster Frame that fall under Diagnostic Services.
- Review the description of medical laboratory workers and the tasks they commonly perform.

ACTIVITY

Ask students to think up a slogan or saying to remind medical laboratory workers that they must work carefully and accurately or risk incorrect results. They should make a poster using the slogan and display in the classroom.

Apply It

- You may have students work in pairs on this project.
- Encourage students to use multimedia elements in their presentations.

Career-Ready Practices

In an effort to control health care and insurance costs and promote healthy lifestyles, many employers offer personal wellness programs to their employees. Wellness programs vary widely. Some employers subsidize memberships in fitness clubs or actually have a fitness center on-site for employee use. They might offer smoking cessation and diet counseling, health risk assessments, and sponsor screenings for mammograms, high blood pressure, diabetes, etc. Many serve healthier foods in their cafeterias, offer healthier vending machine choices, and have nutritionists present seminars on healthy eating.

In teams of four or five, develop a wellness program for a business. Include at least five activities and initiatives in the program and explain the benefits of each.

Keep in mind that career-ready individuals recognize the relationship between their personal health and their performance on the job. They take responsibility for their own personal health and engage in activities that contribute to their well-being.

Create a poster for the program and share with your class. Discuss the benefits of a wellness program for both the employer and the employee. With your instructor's permission, hang the posters around your school.

Diagnostic Services

Workers in diagnostic services are responsible for running tests and conducting evaluations that aid in the detection, diagnosis, and treatment of illnesses, diseases, injuries, and other conditions. They assess patients' health status, communicate with other health personnel and departments, and prepare and implement appropriate procedures. They are audiologists, lab technicians, pathologists, and radiologists. They administer mammograms, fit eyeglass lenses, and develop fitness programs that include exercise or activities designed to improve physical health.

Diagnostic services have changed drastically over the decades. It was only about 100 years ago that a heart attack was diagnosed in a living patient for the first time. The patient died two days later but the diagnosis was confirmed by an autopsy. Even so, doctors in the early 20th century had little incentive to diagnose heart disease and other illnesses because they simply did not have the means for treating them. Instead, their focus was on treating known infectious diseases, such as pneumonia, tuberculosis (TB), and diarrhea and enteritis, which (together with diphtheria) caused one third of all deaths.

Over the last century, though, doctors, scientists, and other researchers have revolutionized the way illnesses are detected, diagnosed, and treated. Findings from clinical research and scientific studies are quickly translated to practice, thanks in part to advances in technology and electronic communication. Medical education has improved and now emphasizes the importance of keeping up with literature and research findings. The growing use of inexpensive, portable, and easy-to-use diagnostic technology, such as MRIs, mammograms, and colonoscopies, has put greater emphasis on prevention. The types of diagnostic services available and how they are applied and delivered have grown rapidly. Following is a sampling of occupations that fall under the diagnostic services pathway.

Medical Laboratory Workers

Medical laboratory workers perform a variety of tests. (**Figure 3.6**) Typically, they look for changes that have occurred in the blood, urine, lymph, and body tissues. They identify increases or decreases in white or red blood cells, cross-match blood for transfusions, identify microscopic changes in cells, and determine the presence of parasites, viruses, or bacteria in the blood, tissue, or urine. These tests help the physician make an accurate diagnosis and correctly treat the patient.

Medical laboratory workers are employed by acute care hospitals, private laboratories, physicians' offices, clinics, ambulatory care units, health maintenance organizations, public health agencies, pharmaceutical firms, and research institutions. Their work requires walking, standing, reaching, stooping, lifting, and carrying of equipment. In addition, they need good eyesight for close work. They work indoors and may be exposed to unpleasant odors and body fluids and have frequent contact with water and cleaning solutions. Their jobs often require them to work shifts and weekends.

58 Chapter 3 | Finding the Right Occupation for You

CUSTOMIZED INSTRUCTION

More Advanced Students

Some home health aides help provide hospice care for terminal patients. Learn more about hospice care by researching the topic and writing a report. You might start at nhpco.org, the Web site for the National Hospice and Palliative Care Organization, or nahc.org, which is the site for the National Association for Home Care & Hospice.

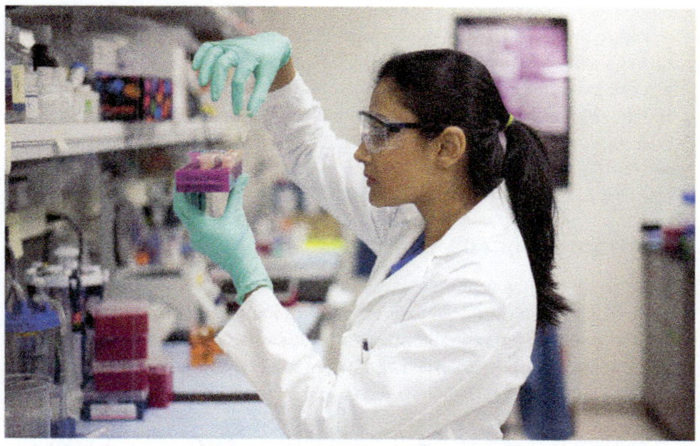

Figure 3.6
How do the tests that medical laboratory aides perform help the doctor?

Apply It

Research the history of the diagnostic services career pathway. How have careers in this pathway advanced over time? How do these health professionals develop and foster relationships within the community that promote health and wellness? Create a presentation or poster describing your findings.

Radiology Workers

Radiology workers operate x-ray equipment to take pictures of the internal parts of the body. (**Figure 3.7**) The x-rays provide information for the diagnosis and treatment of patients. For example, x-rays of the chest help detect lung diseases, such as lung cancer and tuberculosis. Some of the diseases or injuries that x-rays help diagnose or treat are ulcers, blood clots, cancer, and fractures. The use of imaging techniques like ultrasound and magnetic resonance imaging (MRI) is growing. Diagnostic medical sonographers use ultrasound equipment to obtain images of the body's tissues and organs. The term diagnostic imaging includes these procedures as well as x-ray techniques.

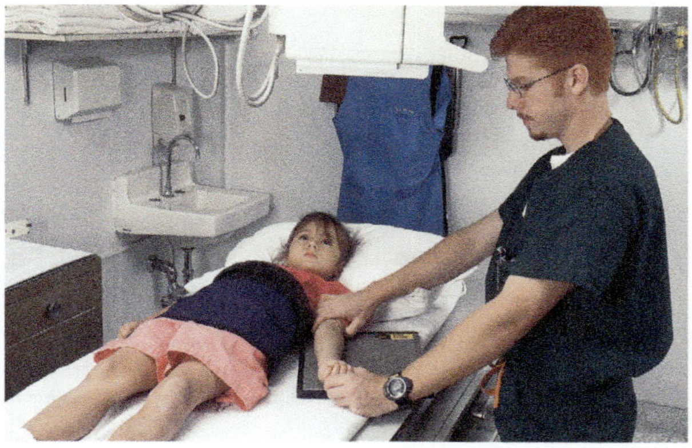

Figure 3.7
A radiologic technologist preparing to take an x-ray of a patient. What are some of the precautions that a radiologic technologists should take?

Finding the Right Occupation for You | Chapter 3 59

Figure Focus

3.6 How do the tests that medical laboratory aides perform help the doctor?

Answer: The tests help the doctor make an accurate diagnosis and correctly treat the patient.

Teaching Tips

- Ask students if they have ever had an x-ray, sonogram, or MRI.
- If so, ask them to describe their interaction with the radiology workers.
- If possible display an x-ray or MRI.

Figure Focus

3.7 A radiologic technologist preparing to take an x-ray of a patient. What are some of the precautions that a radiologic technologists should take?

Answer: Radiologic technologists may wear gloves, aprons, and film badges to protect themselves, and they may leave the room while the x-ray is being done.

ACTIVITY

Radiology workers may be exposed to radiation. Instruct students to write a brief report or create a presentation about the risks radiation poses to humans.

ACTIVITY

Students should look up the different radiologic disciplines—such as nuclear radiology, neuroradiology, gastrointestinal radiology, musculoskeletal radiology, or pediatric radiology—and select one they would like to know more about. They should research it using the Internet or books. In their research, they should find out what it involves and how it is different from other disciplines. Have them report their findings to the class.

Teaching Tips

- Review the tasks of an electrocardiographic technician.
- Review and explain the abbreviations/anagrams and terminology in this description:
  - EKG—eletrocardiogram
  - Holter monitor
- Point out the resource for more information.
- Review the responsibilities of an electroneurodiagnostic technologist.
- Review and explain the abbreviations/anagrams in this description:
  - END—electroneirodiagnostic technologist
  - EEG—electroencephalogram
  - EP—evoked potential
  - NCS—nerve condition study
  - PSG—polysomnograph (sleep study)

Radiology workers are employed in general hospitals, physicians' offices, trauma centers, chiropractic offices, private consulting offices, clinics, federal and state agencies, health maintenance organizations, and ambulatory care facilities. They work indoors and may be in confined areas. They wear protective gloves, aprons, and film badges because the hazards of radiation are present. Shift work and evening work may be part of their schedule. Their work requires the lifting and positioning of patients, standing during most of the shift, and pushing mobile equipment. They may be exposed to body fluids.

Electrocardiography Workers

Electrocardiography workers operate an EKG machine to record the electrical changes that occur during a heartbeat. (**Figure 3.8**) These recordings help physicians diagnose any irregularities or changes in the patient's heartbeat. These tests are done routinely after a certain age, before surgery, and as a diagnostic tool.

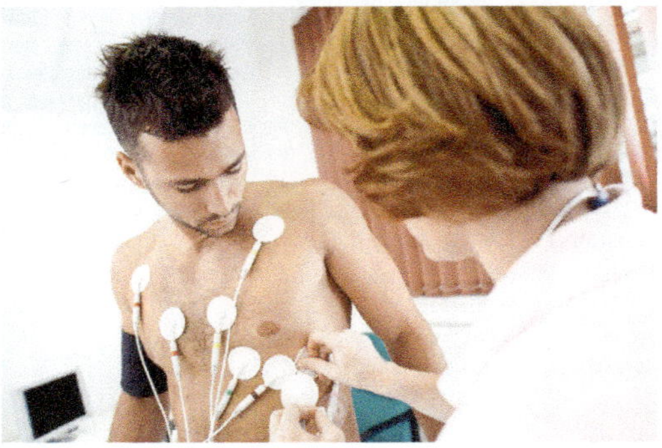

Figure 3.8
An EKG technician performing an electrocardiogram. Why does an EKG technician perform an electrocardiogram?

EKG technicians also apply Holter monitors. They work in acute care hospitals, clinics, private physicians' offices, health maintenance organizations, and ambulatory care facilities. They work indoors and may work shifts, evenings, and weekends. They spend a lot of their time standing and walking.

Electroneurodiagnostic (END) technologists use computers to record electrical impulses transmitted by the brain and the nervous system. They perform several different neurological tests including electroencephalograms (EEGs), evoked potentials (EPs), nerve conduction studies (NCSs), polysomnographs (PSG/sleep studies), and surgical monitoring. EEGs assist in the diagnosis of various brain disorders such as seizures, stroke, head trauma, and brain tumors. EPs are performed on patients with possible multiple sclerosis, brainstem tumors, and spinal cord problems. NCSs evaluate peripheral nervous system problems such as carpal tunnel syndrome.

Sleep studies are performed on patients to diagnose sleep disorders such as sleep apnea and narcolepsy. The brain, nerves and/or muscles can be monitored by END technologists during various brain and spinal cord surgeries. END technologists take medical histories, apply electrodes for the procedure being performed, record electrical impulses from the central and peripheral nervous systems, maintain equipment, and interact with patients to reduce anxiety during tests. They work in hospitals, neurologist's and neurosurgeon's offices, sleep centers, and psychiatric facilities. Some positions may require on-call duty, and sleep disorder technologists usually work evenings and nights.

60 Chapter 3 | Finding the Right Occupation for You

Figure Focus

3.8 An EKG technican perform an electrocardiogram. Why does an EKG technician perform an electrocardiogram?

Answer: An EKG technician performs an electrocardiogram in order to record the electrical changes that occur during a heartbeat. These recordings help physicians diagnose any irregularities or changes in the patient's heartbeat.

ACTIVITY

Have students make a chart comparing an EKG technician to an END technologist. They should compare job descriptions, responsibilities, requirements, and salary range. Have them discuss their chart with the class.

Health Informatics

Health informatics is one of the fastest-growing areas within health care. In a nutshell, it's a system for managing health information and getting the right information to the right person at the right time. Workers in the health informatics pathway collect, analyze, **extract**, and document information according to industry-based standards using information technology systems. They understand the sources, routes, and flow of information within the health care environment. They may have special skills and advanced training in computer programming and assist in the development of software that ensures delivery of high-quality and cost-effective care.

The field of health informatics got its start with sophisticated computer technology that allowed for the management of huge amounts of data. Emerging in the 1960s, health informatics began with development of the first standards for health care data reporting (established by the American Society for Testing and Materials). These included standards for "laboratory message exchange, properties for electronic health record systems, data content, and health information system security."

Soon thereafter, the idea of recording patient information electronically instead of on paper—known as the electronic medical record—was introduced and new standards for specific disciplines and services began taking shape. Bioinformatics, or the study of complex biological data, was introduced in the late 1970s. Health information technology continued to expand as professional associations and government agencies developed standardized formats for patient registration, orders, observation, discharge, insurance claims, and financial transaction messages.

Health informatics today is a complex and still developing field that offers a variety of career opportunities. Following is a sampling of occupations that fall under the health informatics pathway.

Apply It

Research the history of the health informatics career pathway. How have careers in this pathway advanced over time? How do these health professionals develop and foster relationships within the community that promote health and wellness? Create a presentation or poster describing your findings.

extract
(EK strakt)
Identify and take out or emphasize.

discharging
(dis CHAHRJ ing)
The act of releasing or allowing to leave.

Admitting Department Workers

Admitting department workers are responsible for the admitting and **discharging** of patients. They interview patients/clients for information necessary for accurate record keeping, assign rooms, prepare identification bands, and make sure admitting information is distributed to the appropriate parties. (Figure 3.9) The workers in the admitting department are usually the first hospital employees that the patient sees. Employees in this department help the patient feel confident about the hospital and the care that they will receive.

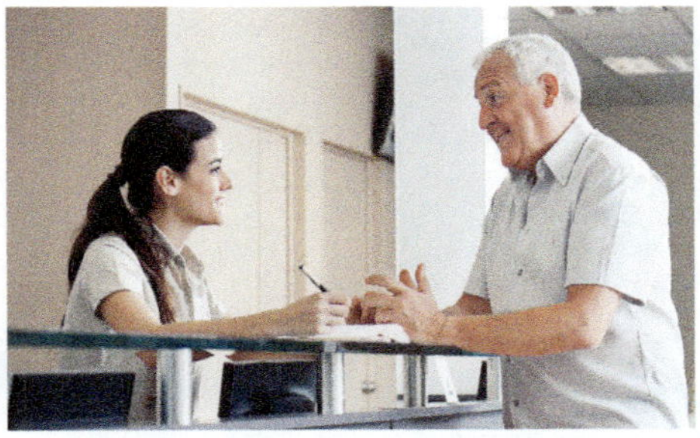

Figure 3.9
One of the many duties of an admitting clerk is interviewing patients/clients. What might be some questions an admitting clerk would ask when interviewing patients/clients?

Admitting workers are typically employed in hospitals and facilities that require overnight stays. They may assist with lifting patients and carrying their belongings. They may also push wheelchairs or stretchers. Their work is in an office environment. They may work shifts and evenings.

Finding the Right Occupation for You | Chapter 3 61

Teaching Tips

- Introduce the Health Informatics pathway and review how it has changed and evolved.
- Review the Knowledge & Skills Statements and Plan of Study for the Health Informatics pathway.
- Review the careers that fall under this pathway in the Career Cluster Frame.
- Point out that many of the positions in this pathway exist in industries other than health care.
- Discuss the role of admitting department workers and their typical tasks.
- Ask students why the position of an admitting department worker is so important to the overall quality of care given to patients/clients.

Career Connect

- Discuss how businesses of all types and sizes—not just those in health care—are following the trend to digitize their paper records and files.
- Point out that many of these businesses hire employees or contractors to convert paperwork into a digital format.
- Discuss the other types of technology-related jobs you might find in a health care facility or organization.
- Students are to review the sample careers in the Career Cluster Frame and identify those that involve information technology skills.

ACTIVITY

Contact a sleep clinic to request information about the type of sleep disorders they study, and the type of workers they employ. Many sleep clinics are affiliated with hospitals or universities. If you can find one locally, request a tour, or invite a representative to speak to the class.

Figure Focus

3.9 One of the many duties of an admitting clerk is interviewing patients/clients. What might be some questions an admitting clerk would ask when interviewing patients/clients?

Answer: An admitting clerk might ask about a person's symptoms, a person's health insurance carrier, or a person's health history.

TEAMWORK

In small groups, perform a skit demonstrating skills that might be required of an admitting clerk.

Teaching Tips

- Review the description of a health information technician and review the tasks they commonly perform.
- Point out that a health information technician may be responsible for highly confidential information. Discuss methods the technician might use to ensure confidentiality remains secure.

Figure Focus

3.10 Physicians, nurses, therapists, and insurance companies rely on health information technicians to maintain accurate medical records on their patients. Why is a health information technician an important position?

Answer: A health information technician is an important position because he or she organizes and pulls information about clients/patients so that staff members can access important health information about a client/patient quickly.

Career Connect

Health care regulations and the trend to convert medical paperwork into a digital format has driven the need for information technology jobs in the health care field. Individuals employed in information technology jobs build the bridges between people and technology. They design, develop, support, and manage hardware, software, multimedia, and systems integration services that allow you to have access to the Internet, operate your remote control device, and use your mobile devices. They are constantly working on cutting-edge technology aimed at making life easier for everyone. They are the computer technicians who build or repair computers used by doctors and nurses; the Web designers and administrators who develop and maintain the Web site for a health insurer; or the computer programmers who create applications for diagnosing illnesses.

Review the sample career specialties and occupations in the Health Science career cluster. Which ones involve information technology skills?

consultant
(kuhn SUHL tnt)
A person who gives professional or expert advice.

Health Information Technicians

Health information technicians organize and manage health information data. They ensure its quality, accuracy, accessibility, and security in both paper and electronic systems. (**Figure 3.10**) They use various classification systems to code and categorize patient information for insurance reimbursement purposes, for databases and registries, and to maintain patients' medical and treatment histories.

Another health career in this career cluster includes clinical account managers/technicians who manage the patient financial account with the health care provider. They coordinate and assist the patient with insurance and payment for care. Medical coders apply the proper diagnostic code for billing insurance and government payment programs for care. Health care administrators oversee the day-to-day operation of the hospital or practice providing care. Health educators teach patients about their diseases and disorders, treatment, and preventative care. A risk manager assesses situations within a facility to provide the safest environment for care and to minimize any potential risks to the facility.

Health information technicians are employed by acute care hospitals, long-term care hospitals, public health departments, manufacturers of medical record systems, and insurance companies.

Some may have a private practice as a **consultant**. Their work requires long periods of time working on a computer.

For up-to-date information about any of these and other health informatics careers, research the Bureau of Labor Statistics (bls.gov), or the American Health Information Management Association (ahima.org).

Medical Transcriptionists

Medical transcriptionists listen to voice recordings that physicians and other health care professionals make, and convert them into electronic reports. They may also review and edit medical documents created using speech recognition technology. Transcriptionists interpret medical terminology and abbreviations in preparing patients' medical histories, discharge summaries, and other documents.

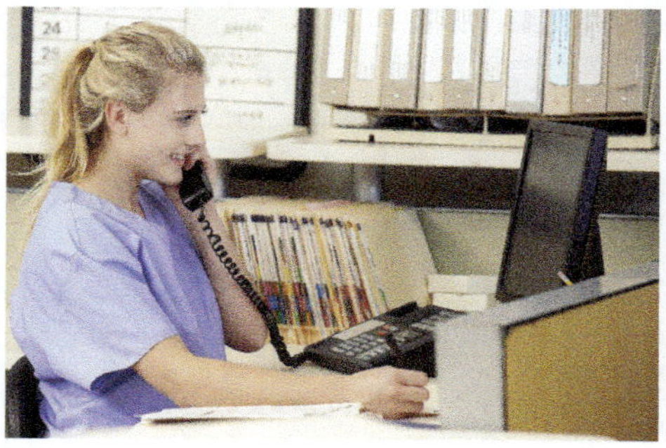

Figure 3.10
Physicians, nurses, therapists, and insurance companies rely on health information technicians to maintain accurate medical records on their patients. Why is a health information technician an important position?

62 Chapter 3 | Finding the Right Occupation for You

Apply It

- You may have students work in pairs on this project.
- Encourage students to use multimedia elements in their presentations.

Most medical transcriptionists work for hospitals, physicians' offices, and third-party **transcription** service companies that provide transcription services to health care establishments. Others are self-employed.

transcription
(tran SKYRAHYB)
A written copy.

Support Services

Those who work in support services perform functions that support the health care facility's core business activity, which is providing quality patient care. They work in non-clinical support departments, such as housekeeping, food services, facilities maintenance, and patient transportation.

Traditionally, employees in non-clinical support services do not have much, if any, direct interaction with patients. They might work in the billing department, which may or may not even be in the same building or complex of buildings; they work in the cafeterias or in the operations/utilities center where they have no interaction with patients.

Today, though, as health care organizations look for ways to implement and improve the concept of patient-centered care, they are taking steps to engage all employees in focusing on the best service possible to the patient/client.

Technology, too, is changing the way workers in support services do their jobs. For example, food service workers use smartphones or other handheld devices to process patient dietary requests, helping to cut down on food waste. Department managers use mobile technologies to perform routine tasks "on the go," enabling them to spend more time training and coaching employees and doing quality control checks.

Following is a sampling of career opportunities in the support services pathway.

Central Processing/Supply Workers

Central processing/supply workers supply various departments with equipment and materials. (Figure 3.11) The equipment must be in working condition. Malfunctioning equipment is life threatening. The workers keep an inventory of supplies and equipment and make sure they are properly packaged, cleaned, and sterilized. The workers in this department are key members of the health care team as other health care workers cannot give necessary care without proper tools and equipment. Central processing/supply workers are employed in acute care hospitals and large outpatient clinics. Lifting and moving articles and equipment are required. The workers stand on their feet for long periods of time and may be exposed to body fluids.

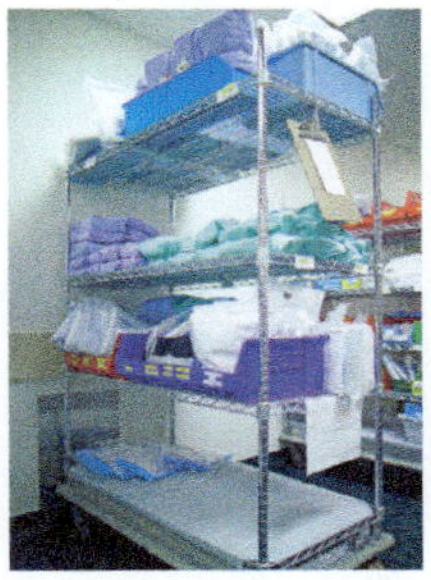

Figure 3.11
How do other health care workers depend on a central supply worker?

Housekeepers and Environmental Services Technicians

Housekeepers and environmental services technicians are responsible for the cleanliness of the environment. (Figure 3.12) Cleanliness helps prevent the spread of infection and creates a more pleasant environment for patients/clients, staff, and visitors. Some of their responsibilities include cleaning rooms, offices, labs, and other assigned areas; cleaning fixtures and equipment; disinfecting; moving furniture and fixtures; and reporting equipment that malfunctions.

Finding the Right Occupation for You | Chapter 3 63

Teaching Tips

- Review the description of a medical transcriptionist and review the tasks they commonly perform.
- Introduce the Support Services pathway and review how jobs in this area have changed from being more "behind the scenes" in terms of patient care to being totally engaged in providing the best service possible to the patient/client.
- Review the Knowledge & Skills Statements and Plan of Study for the Support Services pathway.
- Review the careers that fall under this pathway in the Career Cluster Frame.
- Review the description of central processing/supply workers and the tasks they perform.

Figure Focus

3.11 How do other health care workers depend on a central supply worker?

Answer: A central supply worker makes sure that important equipment is in working condition and delivers it to various departments. A central supply worker also properly packages, cleans, and sterilizes items for other health care workers.

Apply It

- You may have students work in pairs on this project.
- Encourage students to use multimedia elements in their presentations.

TEAMWORK

Divide the class into teams. Randomly select a career from the diagnostic services, therapeutic services, or health informatics pathway, and announce it out loud. Have each team write down how someone holding that position would depend on depend on a central supply worker.

Teaching Tips

- Discuss housekeepers and environmental services technicians and the tasks they perform.
- Emphasize that these positions are key for fighting infection and maintaining standards.

Figure Focus

3.12 A housekeeping attendant cleaning public areas, one of housekeeping's many duties. What are some of the other common duties of a housekeeping attendant?

Answer: A housekeeping attendant may load service carts; dust; vacuum; clean blinds, floors, furniture, and equipment; polish floors using a buffing machine; wash walls, ceilings, and windows; empty trash; scour sinks, tubs, and mirrors; disinfect bedsprings and unit equipment; replenish soap and towels; replace cubicle curtains and soiled draperies; report malfunctioning equipment; move furniture, equipment, and supplies; and turn mattresses.

Apply It

- Students are to explore the responsibilities and job duties of a selected occupation within the Support Services pathway.
- Their overview can be done in a word processing document or slide presentation.
- Make sure they address how the responsibilities and duties contribute to the overall quality of care provided to the patient/client.

Apply It

Research the history of the support services career pathway. How have careers in this pathway advanced over time? How do these health professionals develop and foster relationships within the community that promote health and wellness? Create a presentation or poster describing your findings.

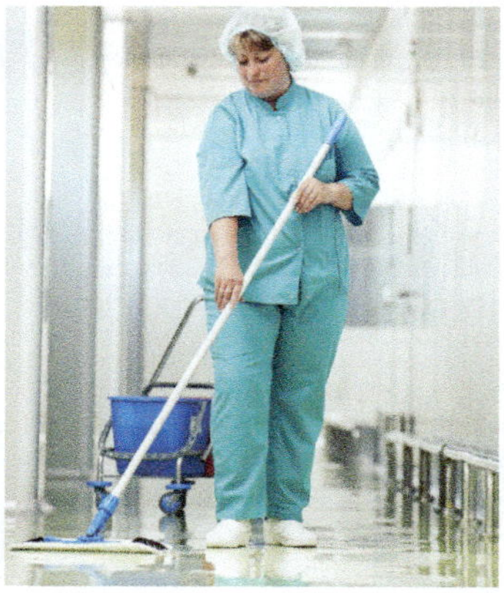

Figure 3.12
A housekeeping attendant cleaning public areas, one of housekeeping's many duties. What are some of the other common duties of a housekeeping attendant?

Apply It

Review the sample career specialties and occupations within the Support Services pathway by going to www.careertech.org/sites/default/files/CCFrame-HealthScience.pdf. Select one that interests you and research the responsibilities and typical job duties. Using your word processing or presentation software, create an overview of the occupation and explain how an employee working in that job contributes to the overall mission of providing the highest quality care possible to the patient. Make sure you summarize the responsibilities as they relate to following established guidelines, maximizing the use of resources, and implementing standards to maintain a high-quality health care facility.

They are employed in long-term care facilities, acute care hospitals, and clinics. They have frequent contact with water and cleaning solutions. They walk, stand, and stoop during their shift. They also push and pull equipment, climb on ladders when necessary, and may be exposed to body fluids. Their hours may include shift work and weekend work.

Food Service Workers

Food service workers are responsible for food preparation and providing nutritional care to clients. They plan special and balanced diets. They also distribute menus and prepare food trays for delivery to the patients. (**Figure 3.13**)

Food service workers are employed in acute care hospitals and in long-term care facilities. They generally work 40 hours a week and may work in shifts. The areas might be very warm, with much activity in a relatively small area. Some lifting, reaching, moving of equipment, and occasional bending are required. They walk and stand most of the shift.

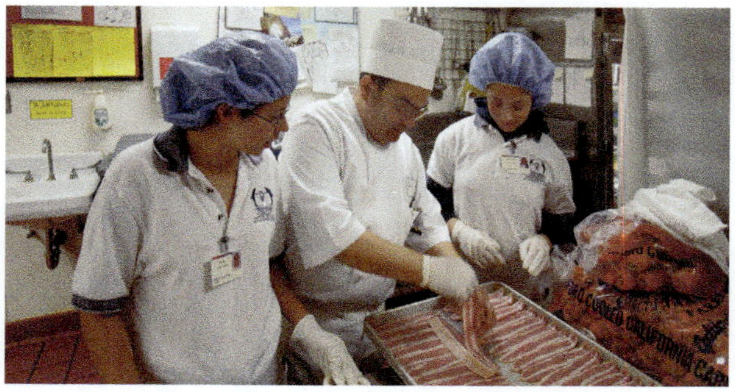

Figure 3.13
One of the many duties of a food service worker is preparing meals. What does a food service worker have to consider when preparing a meal for a patient/client?

Figure Focus

3.13 One of the many duties of a food service worker is preparing meals. What does a food service worker have to consider when preparing a meal for a patient/client?

Answer: A food service worker must prepare nutritional food that helps to create a balanced diet. In addition, a food service worker may have to make special accommodations such as preparing a soft or liquid diet for a patient/client. Some patients/clients may require less salt or fat in their diet than others.

ACTIVITY

Housekeepers and environmental services technicians can be hard and physically demanding jobs. Have students write an essay explaining why these positions provide an opportunity to get started in the health care industry. They should use facts or real-world examples to support their opinion.

Table 3.1 Other Support Services

Career	Responsibilities
Environment health advocate	Collect data regarding the environment (air, water, soil, food) to analyze for problems and suggest corrections to government officials and companies.
Food safety specialist	Ensure quality and safety of the food supply.
Industrial hygienist	Conduct health and safety evaluation in industrial or government facilities to minimize accidents.
Interpreter	Convert the translation of one language into another; may be oral or written, as in French into English or sign language for the deaf.
Mortician/funeral director	Arrange for preparation of the body and counsel families after death of a loved one; file legal documents for deceased.
Transport technician	Provide wheelchair or stretcher transportation of patient/client from one point to another (such as from hospital room to surgery).

Apply It

Research the history of the Biotechnology Research and Development career pathway. What are some of the careers you would find in this pathway? How have careers in this pathway advanced over time? How are these careers important to our society? Create a presentation or poster describing your findings.

Biotechnology Research and Development

Those who work in this pathway are involved in **bioscience** research and development as it applies to human health. They develop new treatments and medical devices designed to assist patients or improve the accuracy of diagnostic tests. They are medical scientists who conduct research to find causes of disease; toxicologists who study the adverse effects of chemicals on living organisms; or microbiologists who examine the organisms that cause infections.

bioscience
(BI o si ence)
Any science that deals with the biological aspects of living organisms.

When most people think about biotechnology, they think about DNA, genetics, and how living organisms can be manipulated to create new things. But humans have been using biotechnology for centuries. In the year 100, for example, the first insecticide was produced in China from powdered chrysanthemums.

Modern biotechnology began in the late 1800s with developments in the cross-breeding of plants to produce many varieties that had superior qualities. In the first half of the 20th century, biotechnology led to the discovery of the first cancer-causing virus and penicillin. By mid-century, the discovery that DNA carries the genetic code drove genetics to the forefront of biotechnology research. In 2003, we saw completion of the Human Genome Project (HGP), an international, collaborative research program that resulted in the complete mapping and understanding of all the genes of human beings (known as a "genome"). While HGP has helped scientists to identify, prevent, and treat many of the illnesses resulting from genetic malfunction, it has also made biology the science of the future and biotechnology one of the leading industries.

Apply It

The biotechnology research and development pathway is an exciting field that uses scientific information, technology, research, and hands-on skills to help solve medical problems, discover new treatments, and design new devices. What skills do you think are required to be successful in this pathway? Create a poster or presentation that demonstrates some of these skills. Include examples of technology that may be used in this field.

Epidemiologist

Epidemiologists study the occurrence and frequency of disease in large populations and determine the source and cause of infectious disease epidemics. For example, epidemiologists might study childhood obesity, avian influenza, or Ebola. They conduct research and seek solutions to reduce the risk and occur-

Finding the Right Occupation for You | Chapter 3 65

Teaching Tips

- Introduce the Biotechnology Research and Development pathway and discuss how it has evolved over the last half century.
- Review the Knowledge & Skills Statements and Plan of Study for the Biotechnology pathway.
- Review the careers that fall under this pathway in the Career Cluster Frame.
- Point out the many scientific innovations and developments in the biotechnology field.
- Review the descriptions of epidemiologists and biomedical engineers and their duties and responsibilities.

Apply It

- Before students begin their research, discuss that many health care professionals need to renew and maintain licensure and certification for health care professions.
- Remind students that requirements for licensure and certification may vary from state to state; if they are planning to look for work in another location, they can obtain other states' requirements to compare and contrast requirements.
- The Internet is a valuable tool for this type of research, but point out to students that it is a good idea to confirm licensure and certification requirements with printed information from the regulatory agencies.

CUSTOMIZED INSTRUCTION

Special Needs Students

Invite students who have special dietary needs or restrictions to share with the class the meals they eat in a typical day.

TEAMWORK

In small groups research environmental health issues facing your community. For example, there may be a hazardous waste site nearby, or a power plant that produces toxins. Create a presentation about the issue and deliver it to the class.

Teaching Tips

- Review the description of forensic pathologists and their duties and responsibilities.
- Point out the myriad TV shows about forensics and ask students if they think the shows accurately portray the job of forensic pathologist.

Apply It

- You may want to provide suggestions for health care occupations.
- Have students write down the questions and answers instead of just asking them.
- At the end of the exercise, discuss which questions helped the students identify the profession.

Language Arts Link—Self Assessment

- You may need to review the proper format for a personal business letter. If possible, have at least one on hand for display.
- Encourage students to write a rough draft of the letter, first.
- Remind students that a thesis statement is a sentence that explains the main idea, which in this case should describe the student's work-related values and needs.
- Emphasize that there is no right or wrong answer to this activity, but that the student should be honest and sincere.
- For evaluation, you should verify that the letter includes a thesis statement, and then supports it. You should mark spelling and grammatical errors. You may want to verify that the student used the proper formatting for a personal business letter.

Career Connect

Forensic Scientist/Technician

A detail-oriented career that utilizes critical-thinking skills, math and science, and problem-solving skills is that of a forensic scientist or technician. This professional may investigate a crime scene, looking for DNA as evidence using precise techniques. They collect specimens, such as blood or body fluids, clothing, fingernail scrapings, or other items that may contain DNA. They carefully process the sample and examine the cells so that they can determine the presence or absence of the DNA.

Forensic scientists and technicians may work for government agencies, private companies, or law enforcement. They may work in labs, outside in harsh environments, or in government facilities. An increasing number of companies who offer their DNA examination services to the public are available as well, using bodily fluids submitted by the customer.

rence of such diseases. Most epidemiologists are physicians and work in the community, universities, hospitals, laboratories, and government agencies such as the Centers for Disease Control and Prevention. Because many epidemiologists often work in the field, they may be exposed to infectious diseases, which is a risk associated with the job.

Biomedical Engineers and Chemists

Biomedical engineers apply engineering principles to the development of devices and procedures that help solve medical and health-related problems. For example, biomedical engineers might develop and evaluate prosthetics, cardiac pacemakers, or the laser system used for corrective eye surgery. Biomedical chemists work in laboratories to develop and test new therapeutic compounds and testing processes. Biomedical engineers and chemists are employed in a variety of work settings, including universities, hospitals, manufacturing, government regulatory agencies, and research facilities of companies and educational and medical institutions.

Forensic Pathologist

Forensic pathologists, also called medical examiners, are specially trained doctors who examine the bodies of people who died suddenly, unexpectedly, or violently. The forensic pathologist is responsible for determining the cause and manner of death. They determine this by studying the deceased individual's medical history, evaluating crime scene evidence, performing autopsies, and collecting medical and trace evidence from the body. Forensic pathologists are typically trained in toxicology, DNA technology, blood analysis, and firearms/ballistics.

Being employed in this occupation is demanding and not for the weak of heart (or stomach). Most forensic pathologists work in government and privately run laboratories, offices, and clinics. They also conduct work in the field at crime scenes or death sites. The job often requires long hours, traveling to and from crime scenes and death sites, and meeting the demands of many different agencies and parties.

Language Arts Link

Self Assessment

Being able to determine your likes, dislikes, and values is an important part of deciding your career path. Do you like working in a group or prefer working alone? Would you be willing to work the night shift at your local hospital or would the morning shift be better for you? No one but you can answer these questions.

Drawing on evidence from information you have analyzed, personal reflection, and research, create a letter for your teacher describing your work-related values, interests, and abilities. Include a thesis statement in the opening paragraph. List several (3–4) health care careers you believe may be right for you and, from multiple sources of information you have gathered, describe why these careers would be right for you.

Be sure to incorporate information on the major factors that would influence what career path you take. Be sure to proofread your work to see if you can improve it by making it clearer, more concise, or more interesting to read. Check the spelling and grammar and correct any errors.

66 Chapter 3 | Finding the Right Occupation for You

CUSTOMIZED INSTRUCTION

At-Risk Students

For the Language Art Links—Self Assessment, you may want to refer students to the Apply It activity on p. 47 of this chapter. Encourage them to use the list they created as an outline for their letter.

Table 3.2 Other Biotechnology Research Careers

Career	Responsibilities
Cell biologist	Study cell structure and function focusing on the treatment of disease.
Crime scene investigator	Collect evidence from crime scenes and analyze the data to provide to law enforcement for prosecution of crimes.
Pharmaceutical/clinical project manager	Oversee and manage the clinical trials of new drugs.
Quality control technician	Monitor product manufacturing to ensure that standards are met; makes recommendations to improve production process.

Apply It

Select a partner. Each of you should select a health care occupation that interests you, but do not share your choice with the other person. Using the Internet, library, or other resources, gather basic information on the occupation, such as typical responsibilities, education and certification requirements, work environment, salary, etc. Write the information on a piece of paper or record it in a word processing document.

Try to guess which occupation your partner selected by asking yes or no questions.

The Future of Health Care Occupations

As you have learned, the health care industry is one of the largest industries in the country, with nearly 22 million jobs projected for 2022. It is expected to generate almost 30 percent of new jobs from 2012–2022, which will make it the fastest growing industry overall during that time period. Furthermore, 13 of the 20 fastest growing occupations are in the health care field. The growing demand for health care workers is due in large part to a rapidly aging population. Other reasons include growth in the overall population, implementation of the Affordable Care Act, and advances in technology. While the outlook for health care careers is positive, many believe the supply of qualified workers will not meet the demand. For those who are interested in careers in the health science field, this presents a golden opportunity to pursue the job that fulfills their career goals.

Summary

In this section, you learned about the Health Science career cluster. There are five pathways within the cluster: therapeutic services, diagnostics services, health informatics, support services, and biotechnology research and development. Each pathway is an umbrella for related job, industry, and occupation types, several of which were introduced in this section.

Section 3.2 Review Questions

1. Which of the Health Science pathways do employees work directly with the patient, providing care, treatment, counseling, and education information?
2. Jobs in which the worker conducts tests and makes evaluations of a patient would fall under which Health Science pathway?
3. Understanding and managing the flow of information is the primary responsibility of workers in which Health Science pathway?
4. List three jobs/occupations that fall within the Support Services pathway.
5. What is the primary focus of workers in the Biotechnology Research and Development pathway?
6. Why would a business want to offer a personal wellness program to its employees?

Finding the Right Occupation for You | Chapter 3 67

Teaching Tips

- Discuss the statistics related to the growing need for health care workers in the United States.
- Emphasize that changes in health care occupations are ongoing, as new technology develops and more patients need health care.
- Ask students to predict other changes in health care and describe how they think those changes will impact the medical professional workforce.

Section 3.2 Review Questions

1. Answer: The Health Science pathway is Therapeutic Services.
2. Answer: These jobs would fall under the Diagnostic Services pathway.
3. Answer: It is the primary responsibility of workers in the Health Informatics pathway.
4. Answer: The three jobs/occupations discussed in this section are admitting department workers, health information technicians, and medical transcriptionists. Students may list others that appear on the Health Science Career Cluster Frame.
5. Answer: Workers in the Biotechnology Research and Development pathway are involved in bioscience research and development as it applies to human health. They develop new treatments and medical devices designed to assist patients or improve the accuracy of diagnostic tests. They conduct research to find causes of disease, study the effects of chemicals on living organisms, and examine the organisms that cause infections.
6. Answer: Businesses offer personal wellness programs to help control health care and insurance costs and promote healthy lifestyles. Employees who lead healthy lifestyles have better attendance records. They tend to have more energy and be more productive during a work day. Promoting wellness also demonstrates the company's commitment to the well-being of its employees.

CHAPTER 3 REVIEW

Chapter Review Questions

1. Answer: When choosing a career, consider your values, interests, and abilities.
2. Answer: A career plan is a tool that shows you how to achieve your career goals. It consists of a career self-assessment, which is a prioritized list of skills, interests, and abilities; a list of career planning resources; an academic plan aligned with a selected career; and a career outlook analysis.
3. Answer: Refer students to the www.ExploreHealthCareers.org Web page and then click on the *Is a Career in Health Right for You?* link. They can use the topics in the list to match with their own views. You can also direct them to interview different health care professionals to understand what it takes to work in the profession they have chosen.
4. Answer: Students can go on the Internet and enter *Health Science Pathway and Sample Career Specialties Chart* in the Search box. This one-page chart provides an extensive listing of the various careers within each pathway. Copies can be printed for student access or you can direct them to the site for review and career selection. Refer the students back to the www.ExploreHealthCareers.org Web page for details on each of the careers they have selected, to gather the information to complete this activity.
5. Answer: A job outlook can help you determine whether your selected career is in an industry that is growing or shrinking and what the demand will be for workers in that field.

CHAPTER 3 REVIEW

Chapter Review Questions

1. What three things should you consider when choosing a career? (3.1)
2. What is a career plan and what are its primary components? (3.1)
3. List at least two resources that can help you identify types of careers. (3.1)
4. What is the difference between an academic plan and a career plan? (3.1)
5. Why is it important to understand the outlook for your selected career? (3.1)
6. What factors are contributing to the rapid job growth in the health care sector? (3.2)
7. List and describe each of the five pathways within the Health Science career cluster. (3.2)
8. List two examples of how technology is used by workers in the health care field. (3.2)
9. What is the primary focus of those who have jobs in biotechnology research and development? (3.2)
10. Summarize the job outlook for those interested in pursuing a career in health care. (3.2)

Activities

1. As you learned in Section 3.1, a career plan is a tool that shows you how to achieve your career goals. Working with your teacher, a counselor, or a family member, develop a career plan that starts now. The plan may be part of an academic plan that you have already completed (see p. 50), or it may be a separate document. If your school has a form for the career plan, use it. Otherwise, develop the plan on a sheet of paper. Be sure to state a realistic and attainable long-term career goal that matches your skills, interests, and abilities. Also include short-term education and career goals that map out the steps you will take to achieve your ultimate career goal. Research the education, certification, licensing, and continuing education requirements for this career. Add the plan to your career portfolio.
2. In addition to careertech.org, there are many Web sites that provide information on the career clusters and their pathways. Open your Web browser and search for information on the Health Science career cluster. Identify three to four occupations that interest you most. In a word processing document, explain how your interests, values, and abilities fit well with the occupations you have chosen.
3. Divide into groups of two or three students. Each group should select a health care occupation and research and describe the regulatory agency or agencies that have authority over that occupation. In your research, identify the specific licensure or certification requirements for the occupation, including license or certificate renewal, and how one goes about fulfilling the requirements. Present your findings to the class in a clear, concise, and effective manner.
4. Select three careers for each of the five pathways and research health science careers within each system including: where work takes place (hospital, clinic, lab, private practice), education required (degree, license, certification), continuing education requirement, job outlook (decline, increase), average salary, and primary responsibilities. Create a presentation or poster that outlines what you learn about each of the careers:

Diagnostic systems
(Career)____________________
(Career)____________________
(Career)____________________

68 Chapter 3 | Finding the Right Occupation for You

6. Answer: Factors contributing to the rapid growth in the health care sector are the rapidly aging population, growth in the overall population, implementation of health care reform, and advances in technology.
7. Answer: The five pathways in the Health Science career cluster are: (1) Therapeutic Services, which focuses on changing the health status of the patient over time; (2) Diagnostic Services, which focuses on testing and evaluating to detect, diagnose, and treat disease, injuries, and other physical conditions; (3) Health Informatics, which focuses on evaluating and managing health and medical information and employing methods for the confidential communication of this information to the appropriate parties; (4) Support Services, which focuses on providing a safe, supportive environment for the delivery of health care; and (5) Biotechnology Research and Development, which focuses on bioscience research and development as it applies to human health.

CHAPTER 3 REVIEW

Therapeutic systems
(Career)________________________
(Career)________________________
(Career)________________________

Health Informatics systems
(Career)________________________
(Career)________________________
(Career)________________________

Support Services systems
(Career)________________________
(Career)________________________
(Career)________________________

Biotechnology Research and Development systems
(Career)________________________
(Career)________________________
(Career)________________________

Case Studies

1. Glenda needs to find a good job as soon as she graduates. She is sure she wants to work in the health care field but is uncertain as to how to find the right career. She must earn enough to pay for an apartment, a car, living expenses, and leisure activities. She wants a position that is well-respected, provides a clean environment, and offers potential for professional growth. She enjoys working with people and feels good when she is able to help others. List the steps Glenda should take to help her identify the best career options for her.
2. Sam is interested in helping people get better. He is good at encouraging people, and he is quite strong. He does not like to calculate numbers; however, he is detail-oriented when it comes to activities such as cleaning and organizing. Sam does not want to be behind a desk all day. He prefers a job that allows him to stand or walk. Based on this information, which careers in the Health Science career cluster would you suggest Sam research?

Thinking Critically

1. **Understanding Yourself**—You should use your abilities, interests, and values to help you choose a satisfying career. Why is it important to choose a career that aligns closely with these personal traits?
2. **Medical**—What are the overall responsibilities and goals of therapeutic versus diagnostic service positions? Explain these using a specific job in each pathway.
3. **Communication**—Most jobs that fall under the Health Science career cluster require strong oral and written communication skills. How do you think these skills would benefit you as a worker in the health care field?
4. **Technology**—The impact of technology on all areas of health care is tremendous. Select one of the five career pathways in the Health Science career cluster (diagnostic, therapeutic, health informatics, support services, or biotechnology research and development systems), and research and identify how a worker in that field would use technology on the job. What type of technological equipment would the worker use? Write a brief paper describing your findings.

Finding the Right Occupation for You | Chapter 3 69

8. Answer: Examples of how technology is used are:
   - Tablet and handheld computers and wall-mounted PCs that enable workers to enter and retrieve patient data almost instantaneously.
   - Monitoring systems that allow workers to obtain information on patients in real time and signal when problems occur.
   - Bar-coding and scanners that ensure safety in the administration of medication and protect against errors.
   - Computer applications and apps that enable workers to diagnose illnesses.
9. Answer: Those who work in biotechnology research and development focus on developing new treatments and medical devices designed to assist patients or improve the accuracy of diagnostic tests.
10. Answer: The outlook for those pursuing a career in health care is strong, as the health care industry is one of the largest in the country, with nearly 22 million jobs projected for 2022. It is expected to generate almost 30 percent of new jobs from 2012 to 2022, and 13 of the 20 fastest growing occupations are in the health care field.

Activities

1. Students are to develop a career plan to add to their career portfolio. Remind students that a career plan is a tool that shows them how to achieve their career goals. It consists of a career self-assessment, which is a prioritized list of skills, interests, and abilities; a list of career planning resources; an academic plan aligned with a selected career; and a career outlook analysis. If your school uses a career plan document, make copies available to students. Students will also need to create an academic plan if they have not already done so. Note that students could prepare an academic plan in the Career-Ready Practices activity on p. 50 of this chapter. You should also provide an academic plan template to help them prepare this document.

2. and 4. Encourage students to review lists they have already made of their interests, values, and abilities. Remind students to format their documents attractively and to proofread their work.

3. You may wish for students to summarize their findings in a brief document, and then compile all of the student reports into a master list.

Case Studies

1. Point out that students should focus on providing the steps Glenda should take to identify career options, not on recommending a career. Students should refer to Section 3.1 to find the information.
2. In this case, students should recommend a list of possible careers for Sam. Advise students to review the five pathways in the Health Science career cluster discussed in Section 3.2 as well as the descriptions of the responsibilities and tasks of various professions in each pathway.

Thinking Critically

1. Remind students to use honest self-evaluation to identify and list the personal traits that will guide their choices.
2. Answers should include a thesis statement and specific examples to support the thesis.
3. Students should answer that strong communication skills prevent misunderstandings, enable you to share your thoughts and ideas, and help establish a positive relationship with patients as well as those with whom you work.
4. Student answers will vary, but should include several examples with supporting evidence.

CHAPTER 3 REVIEW

Portfolio Connection

Now that you have learned about the Health Science career cluster and how to find information on different health care-related careers, you are ready to start assembling your official career portfolio. Remember that a career portfolio is a collection of materials that shows your knowledge, abilities, skills, and insights as they pertain to a particular occupation, business, or profession.

You can set up a portfolio using a three-ring binder or electronically on the computer, or both. A portfolio typically contains the following:

PORTFOLIO TIP

File portfolio items as soon as you complete them. Be sure to file the information in the appropriate section. Being able to file and store information is an important skill—at school, on the job, and at home—so that you can easily locate documents and information. You can modify them as needed. Keeping your portfolio current demonstrates your organizational skills and enables you to quickly access the materials that are important to your career search.

- Title page
- Table of contents
- Letter of introduction
- Academic plan
- Career plan
- Resume
- Sample projects
- Oral reports
- Technology skills
- Leadership activities
- Letter(s) of recommendation
- Advanced training or courses
- Certificates/licenses
- Skills check-off sheets
- Practical experience evaluation
- Evaluation of paid or unpaid time working in your career area
- Written reports and assignments in your career area
- Personal tips and reminders
- Final portfolio checklist

In the Personal tips and reminders section of the portfolio, add any advice or insights that will help you in your career. Be sure that this section can be removed before the portfolio is given to a prospective employer.

Ask your instructor to help you seek a job shadowing opportunity in one health career of your choice. As you will observe during your job shadowing experiences, no matter what career you choose, you will need to demonstrate decision-making and problem-solving skills. You can take some of the uncertainty and doubt out of decision-making and problem-solving by following the six-step process below.

1. Identify the decision to be made or the problem to be solved. Determine what goal you want to meet, or what goal is being blocked.
2. Consider all possible options. Try to think of as many as you can, and write them down. Don't just consider the obvious; some of the best options might seem odd at first. Consider your resources and what you are trying to achieve.
3. Identify the consequences of each option. Each option will have consequences—both positive and negative; and long-term and short-term.
4. Select the best option. Once you consider the options and identify the consequences, you have the information you need to make your decision or select the right solution.
5. Make and implement a plan of action. You must take steps to make your decision happen or resolve the problem.
6. Evaluate the decision or solution, and the process, and outcome. Did you achieve the goal you defined in step 1? Did you miss any possible options? Did you correctly identify the consequences? Did you make use of your resources? Was the outcome what you hoped for?

Assume you work in admissions and are having trouble getting information from an older patient being admitted. In your word processing program, write a plan on how you will address the issue using the six-step process.

70 Chapter 3 | Finding the Right Occupation for You

Portfolio Connection

- Allow time in class for students to assemble the portfolio and label the binder tabs.
- They should begin adding documents to their portfolio.
- Remind students that it is important to keep the documents in the portfolio neat and in good condition.
- Check to make sure that students have organized their portfolio correctly.
- Stress the importance of neatness and formatting portfolio documents in an attractive but professional manner.
- Suggest the use of electronic templates for creating documents.
- Explain that job shadowing allows you to follow an experienced worker through his or her work day to see the specific responsibilities and tasks required on the job.

4 Employability and Leadership

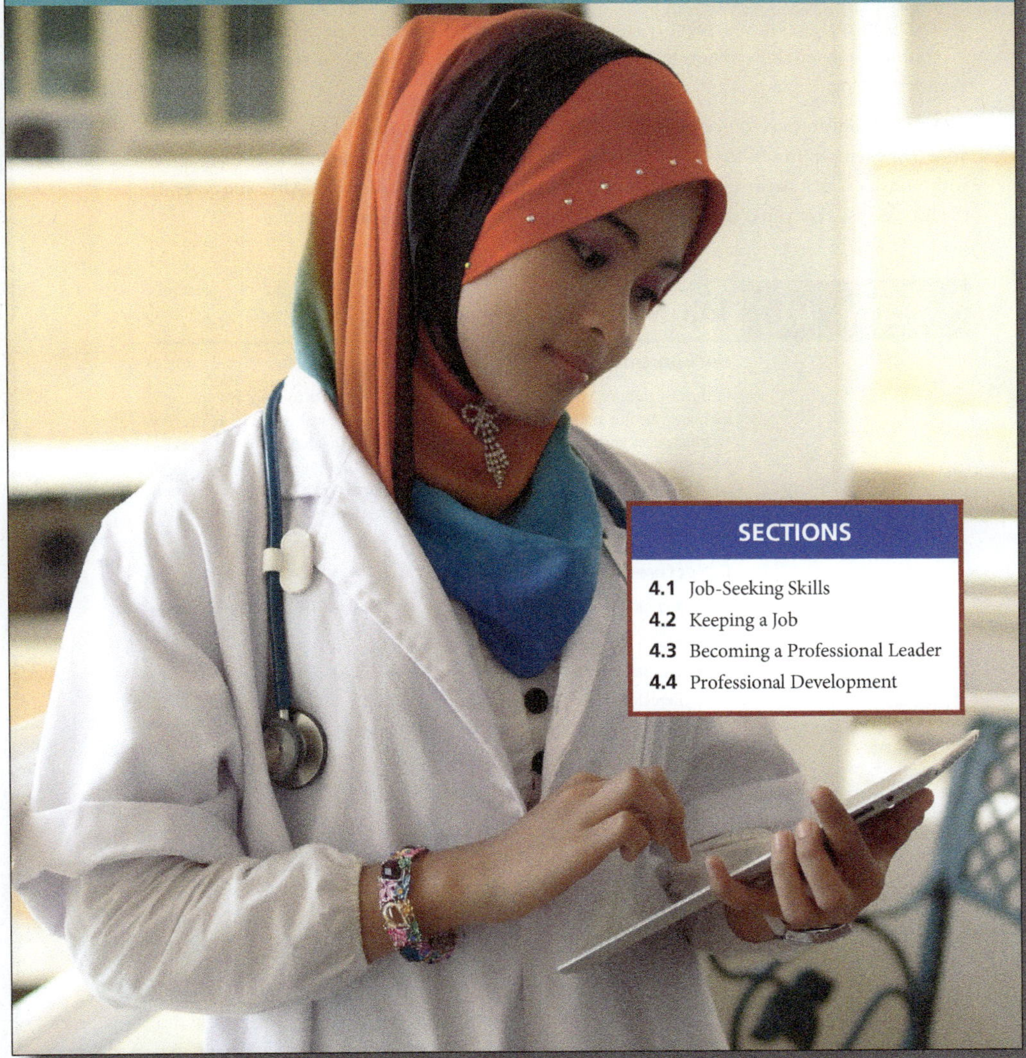

SECTIONS

CHAPTER 4 OVERVIEW

Chapter 4 builds on the employability skill introduced in Chapters 1 and 3 and covers the important topic of leadership.

Section 4.1: The first section focuses on specific methods for seeking employment, including where to look for job postings, how to prepare a cover letter and resume, and how to conduct oneself during an interview.

Section 4.2: This section covers the personal and professional characteristics required for keeping a job, including the responsibilities of an employer and an employee.

Section 4.3: In this section, students learn how to build leadership skills. Topics include joining a professional organization, taking part in professional competitions, and learning how to identify a leader.

Section 4.4: This section expands on the concept of professional development. It covers the importance of having a career plan, and continuing to keep pace with new developments in one's field.

Advance Preparation

- Review: Chapter text for Sections 4.1, 4.2, 4.3, and 4.4.

Contact:

- Health care employers in your area to request sample job listings and requirements.
- Guest speakers from human resources departments or career service agencies to discuss what they look for in a candidate.
- Guest speakers from professional organizations to discuss the importance of membership.
- Professional organizations to request pamphlets, brochures, or flyers.
- Programs or sponsors of professional development training to request pamphlets or brochures, or a calendar of class offerings.
- Organizations that might be willing to provide mentors for your students.

Prepare:

- Magazine and newspaper articles on topics such as interviewing skills and employment outlooks in the health care industry.
- Classified ads or other job or employer listings.
- Remind students to bring their career portfolios to class.
- A list of Web sites that provide information about careers in health care—for example, bls.gov, careertech.org, healthpronet.org, or hosa.org.

FOCUS AND ENGAGE

Getting Started

- This activity is designed to help students identify and prepare resources that would be helpful in managing a job search.
- Encourage students to think broadly about this. For example, if they do not have a computer with printer, they might be able to use library equipment or their school's computer lab. They will most likely need a supply of stationery and envelopes on which to print cover letters and resumes. If they land a job interview, they will not only need the proper attire, but also a means for getting to and from the interview.
- Assign the activity as homework, but allow time in class to review and discuss the finished projects.

Introduce the Section

a. Review the content of the Background paragraph, explaining the importance of making a strong and positive first impression.

b. Explain that the skills required for finding a job will come in handy throughout life.

c. Ask students to reflect on their own experiences looking for employment.

d. Discuss the objectives for the section.

Vocabulary Review

a. Key terms are defined in the margins of the text on the page where they first appear.

b. Pronounce each word, and have the students repeat the pronunciation out loud.

c. Discuss the definition of each word.

Getting Started

Searching for a job is hard work, requiring you to be organized, thorough, and resourceful. In addition, you will need all of the following skills:

- Communications skills to write job search materials, describe your strengths, and convey your interests nonverbally.
- Decision-making skills to identify job opportunities and to accept or turn down a job offer.
- Problem-solving skills to negotiate employment needs and improve your search materials or interviewing techniques.

As a class, brainstorm resources you think would be helpful for managing a job search. Be creative. For example, in addition to a computer with Internet access, you might think of a relative with a business that needs employees or a new outfit to wear on an interview. After you compile the list, discuss how you could effectively use each resource in a job search.

SECTION 4.1 Job-Seeking Skills

Background

In the last chapter, you learned about the tools you can use to identify careers that best match your skills, abilities, and interests. Now, you will explore the tools and resources you can use to land the job you desire. In addition to matching your skills, abilities, and interests to selected careers, keep in mind that potential employers also expect their staff to meet requirements such as punctuality, attendance, time management, communication, organizational skills, and productive work habits.

Objectives

When you have completed this section, you will be able to do the following:

- Match key terms with their correct meanings.
- List places to seek employment and explain the benefits of each.
- Explain different ways to contact an employer.
- Name the occasions when a cover letter is used.
- List the items required on a resume.
- Identify the items generally requested on a job application form.
- Write a cover letter and a resume.
- Complete a job application.
- List the dos and don'ts of job interviewing.
- Write a thank-you letter to a prospective employer.

72 Chapter 4 | Employability and Leadership

ACTIVITY

Write a personal essay describing either a positive or negative experience you had while looking for a job.

CUSTOMIZED INSTRUCTION

English Language Learners

Have students write each key term and its pronunciation on one side of an index card and its definition on the other side.

CUSTOMIZED INSTRUCTION OVERVIEW

Less Advanced Students	Pages 88, 94
More Advanced Students	Pages 75, 88
English Language Learners	Pages 72, 77
Special Needs Students	Pages 79, 91, 95
At-Risk Students	Pages 78, 89

Language Arts Link

Health Care Careers

For each career in the health care profession, the paths of study and job responsibilities will vary. For some careers, you will need additional certification or degrees.

Complete research for several health care careers that seem of interest from one of the following fields: radiology, dental care, or electronic medical records. Synthesize information from a range of sources to determine the skills needed for the field you selected. If possible, include interviews with someone currently practicing in the careers you selected. Ask how they became interested in this career; the education and certification, licensure, or degree requirements for entry into the career; continuing education requirements; and salary potential for a person working in this field.

After completing the research, create a chart or poster listing the careers you selected and compare and contrast the requirements for entry into the selected careers. Use technical terms, as appropriate, for your representation. Include citations for the sources used to obtain the information on the chart or poster.

Finding a Job

Managing a job search takes time and planning. In this chapter, you learn the steps to follow to conduct a successful job search.

Places to Seek Employment

There are many different ways to find career information and employment opportunities including:

- **Online resources.** The Internet is a great tool for finding career information. You can even use it to make contacts for networking. Some of the more effective online resources include:
  - *Company Web sites.* You can learn a lot about a company from its Web site, including what they do, the backgrounds of the people who work there, and who to contact in each department. Most sites also have a page listing job openings, with information on how to apply. Even if there are no openings that interest you, you can contact the human resources department to try to set up an informational interview.
  - *Government sites.* Like corporations, government agencies list information and job openings. There are also government Web sites that provide job listings.

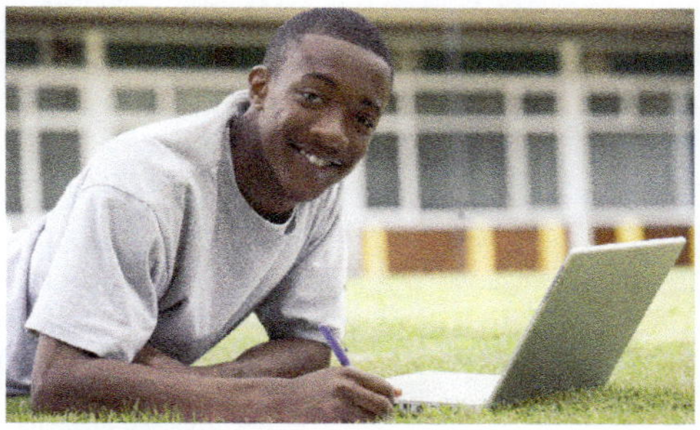

Figure 4.1
The Internet can save you time when you are searching for a job. How can online searches offer more job opportunities than are available in the newspaper or on a job bulletin board?

Language Arts Link—Health Care Careers

- You may want to provide a list of resources such as Web sites or local facilities that students can use to research this project.
- Remind students about your school's Internet policy before having them go online to find information.
- Emphasize that they should use reputable Web resources, such as sites sponsored by the government or educational institutions.
- Remind them to keep a list of sources to use for a bibliography.
- If students do not have access to the Internet, be sure to direct them to other resources, such as books, periodicals, or videos.
- For evaluation, you should verify that the information is correct, and you should mark spelling and grammatical errors.

TEACH

Reinforce and Review

- Review the Health Science Career Cluster and its pathways presented in Chapter 3.

Figure Focus

4.1 The Internet can save you time when you are searching for a job. How can online searches offer more job opportunities than are available in the newspaper or on a job bulletin board?

Answer: With the Internet, you can search by a specific profession, a specific type of facility, or a specific location. You can easily specify job criteria that enables you to narrow your search, thus allowing you to focus on only those jobs that meet your criteria.

Teaching Tips

- Emphasize that many employers use the Internet to post listings and accept resumes and applications online.
- Explain that there are benefits and drawbacks to using online resources to identify career opportunities and job leads. Some of the benefits are:
  - You can more easily and quickly find opportunities in other cities, other states, and other countries.
  - You can find background and financial information on potential employers through corporate Web sites as well as government media, and other independent Web sites.
  - You can submit an application or resume on a timely basis.
- Some drawbacks are:
  - The quality of information available on the Internet is not always current, reliable, accurate, or complete.
  - Because so many people use the Internet to search for and apply for jobs, employers are burdened with sorting through a flood of resumes.
  - The security of personal information you supply online may be jeopardized.

Teaching Tips

- Discuss the dynamics of networking. Students have probably engaged in networking without even realizing it. For example, has a friend ever referred you to a parent who needs a babysitter? What about an uncle whose grass you mowed and who then told his neighbors about you?
- Explain that the important thing about networking is building up the pool of specific individuals. You can get names through the following resources:
  - Teachers, friends, neighbors, relatives, and their friends
  - School- or community-based organizations, clubs, and associations
  - Community and public service agencies, such as resource center directors, librarians, and chambers of commerce
  - Human resource directors, public relations officials, or public information specialists at local businesses
  - Charities and other volunteer-run groups and the fundraising events they sponsor
  - Past employers
  - Your school's alumni group
- Ask students how many have attended a career or job fair. Ask those who have to talk about their experience. Did they find it helpful or productive? Then, you might want to suggest the following "dos" and "don'ts" about job fairs.
- Do:
  - Preregister and try to obtain a list of companies that will be present.
  - Research each company you hope to make contact with.
  - Be prepared to talk about your work experiences, skills, abilities, and education (including your current GPA).
  - Prepare specific questions for each recruiter and make sure you get his or her business card.
  - Practice successful interviewing skills, including a firm handshake, eye contact, a strong voice, and a positive attitude.
  - Bring copies of your resume including different versions of it if you are searching for different types of jobs.
  - Dress professionally, leaning toward the conservative, and wear comfortable shoes.
  - Ask about the company's hiring process, but don't ask too many questions about salaries, vacation time, and other benefits.
  - Take the initiative and ask about the next step in the process.
  - Follow up with each recruiter with a phone call or simple thank-you note.
- Don't:
  - Spend time with recruiters from companies that do not interest you.
  - Eliminate companies because they are recruiting for positions outside your field. Use the opportunity to network and expand your list of contacts.

- *Industry sites.* Many industries and industry associations have Web sites that list job opportunities. For example, if you are interested in a career as a social worker, you could look for positions on socialworkjobbank.com.
- *Online job agencies.* Online companies such as Monster.com or CareerBuilder.com list job openings and let you upload your resume for employers to look at. You can search these sites for jobs in a field or career that interests you. Some online agencies are specific to a certain industry, such as HEALTHeCAREERS.com, which posts job opportunities in the medical and health care fields. Be aware that some online agencies charge fees.
- *Social networking sites.* You can use social networking sites such as Facebook or LinkedIn to meet contacts and learn about jobs. There are groups for people in certain careers or who work for specific companies. Employers join these sites, as well. They look for potential employees based on the personal profile you create. That's an important reason for posting only information that would be appropriate for a potential employer to see!

networking
(NET wur king)
Sharing information about yourself and your career goals with personal contacts.

- **Personal contacts.** The people you already know can help you find job opportunities. Through **networking**, you can share information about yourself and your career goals with people you know already or new people you meet in your day-to-day activities. Hopefully, one of the contacts works for a company that is hiring or knows someone at a company that is hiring. The contact recommends you for the position. Employers like to hire people who come with a recommendation from someone they know and trust.
- **Career fairs.** An event such as a career or job fair is a great opportunity to meet representatives from many different companies. Companies set up booths where you can talk to representatives to learn more about the business, types of careers, and even available positions. Some companies use career fairs to collect resumes and set up interviews; some conduct interviews on the spot.

  Although many career fairs are general, which means there are companies from many different industries, there is a growing trend toward career fairs that focus on a specific industry. For example, at a health sciences career fair, you can meet representatives from companies in the health sciences industry.

  When you attend a career fair, assume you are being evaluated as a potential employee. You may be interested in collecting information for career planning, but the company representatives are looking for people to hire. Dress appropriately, be confident and outgoing, and be prepared to ask and answer questions.
- **Career center or employment agency.** A career center is an excellent place to start planning your career. Your school might have a career center that you can use free of charge. Career centers have job listings, research resources, and counselors who will help you identify jobs that match your skills and interests. They can also introduce you to former students who are now employed—giving you more opportunities for networking.

74 Chapter 4 | Employability and Leadership

An employment **agency** is similar to a career center. Some are sponsored by the state or local government. They provide job search resources and assistance free of charge.

Private employment agencies charge a fee to match employees with employers. Sometimes you pay the fee, and sometimes the employer pays the fee. Sometimes you pay even if you don't find a job.

They all have different policies, so be sure to ask before you sign a contract.

- **Internships.** Securing an internship with a company is often an effective place to pursue employment. Paid and nonpaid internships are many times available in companies. These internships provide the opportunity for the employer to get to know the intern or prospective employee without the demands and responsibilities of actual employment at first. The employer can see if the intern is suited to the company, as well as closely monitor the workplace behaviors exhibited by the intern.

  In addition, the intern can see how he or she interacts with the company employees and management. He or she can observe the operations of the business as they are being mentored during the internship. Internships can set someone apart from other prospective employees and provide real-world experience.

  If the internship is successful, future employment is possible. The internship mentor may be able to provide a positive recommendation with the internship company or recommend another company based on the intern's performance. Additionally, this work experience, whether paid or nonpaid, can be an advantage when other employment is sought.
- **Want ads.** Sometimes called classified ads, these are job listings for specific positions. They are printed in newspapers and magazines and posted online at newspaper and magazine Web sites. You can use the help wanted ads to find a specific job, but also to learn about career outlooks in your area. For example, you can identify companies that are hiring, industries that appear to have many openings —or very few—and salary ranges for listed jobs.

  Usually, there are many ads listed alphabetically. They may be organized into general categories, such as Medical, Professional, and Education. For example, if you are looking for a nursing position, you would look at the listings under Medical.

  Help wanted ad listings usually include a job title and a very brief description of the responsibilities and experience required. Sometimes they include information about wages and hours. There may be a phone number or e-mail address to contact for more information or to apply, or a mailing address where you can send a resume.

  Below is a list of some common abbreviations you might see in want ads.

appl.	**applicant**	immed.	immediately	incl.	included
asst.	assistant	exp.	experience	lic.	licensed
cert.	**certified**	FT	**full time**	N.A.	nurse aide
				PT	**part time**

agency
(EY juhn see)
An organization that helps people in a particular way.

applicant
(AP lih kent)
A person applying for a job.

certified
(SER ti fide)
A person who has received a certificate that shows he or she demonstrates understanding.

full time
(FUHL time)
Describes a job requiring between 32 and 40 hours per week.

part time
(PAHRT time)
Describes a job requiring fewer than 32 hours per week.

Employability and Leadership | Chapter 4 75

- Drop off your resume at the recruiter's table and walk away.
- Chew gum, play with your hair, or fidget.
- Use slang and filler words such as "um," "like," and "you know."
- Talk negatively about your school or previous jobs, companies, or supervisors.

Teaching Tips

- Explain that career centers or agencies have resources such as job listings, research resources, computers with Internet access, and counselors to help identify jobs that match your skills and interests.
- If your school has a career center, ask a representative to speak to the class about the resources available.
- Explain that many local and regional employers rely on help wanted ads in local media for two reasons:
  1. They want to avoid the flood of applications they typically receive when posting an opening on a major job site.
  2. They want locally based applicants so they don't have to pay relocation fees.
- Help wanted ads are suitable for finding local opportunities; often, applicants are familiar with the company. However, you might share that data from the U.S. Department of Labor indicates that a small percentage of job seekers obtain jobs through help wanted ads. That's why many career management consultants believe a career search that targets only advertised openings will likely miss more opportunities than it uncovers. Stress the importance of using various career search resources.

CUSTOMIZED INSTRUCTION

More Advanced Students

Have advanced students contact an employment agency and request a meeting with an employment counselor. Have them report back to the class the outcome of the meeting.

TEAMWORK

Ask students to bring in classified ads from newspapers and magazines for health care workers, and then use the ads to prepare a bulletin board or other display.

Teaching Tips

- Emphasize that a cover letter introduces the applicant to the potential employer.
- Explain that the cover letter is typically your first chance to make a good impression. In addition to telling the employer about the skills and abilities you can bring to the job and why the employer should consider you a qualified candidate, it represents your chance to highlight your individuality and personality. You do this not only through what you write, but also how you write it. Even the typeface (or font) and stationery you select can influence an employer's preconceptions about you.
- Point out that using the appropriate resume format is an indication to a potential employer of good judgment and/or following directions.
- Have students suggest keywords that could be used when applying for various positions, and discuss which ones would be best for particular jobs, and why.
- Explain that a resume provides a complete picture of the individual. It's a "snapshot image of your qualifications," meaning it captures in brief your qualifications, skills, and abilities.
- Explain that it's not uncommon for an employer to spend less than a minute reading a resume. In fact, if an employer has dozens of resumes to review, you can bet the ones that are long and overcrowded get tossed without much more than a glance.
- Explain the importance of being clear and concise and avoiding superfluous information. Remember, it's a resume, not an autobiography.

Preparing Job Search Materials

Now that you know where to look for health science career opportunities, you need to know how to make the contact and how to present yourself. Employers often consider hundreds of candidates for every job opening. Sometimes they shuffle through stacks of letters or field multiple phone calls and e-mail messages. How can you make a positive impression and show you are serious and qualified for the job? You can prepare professional, accurate job search materials, including a cover letter, resume, and list of references.

Cover Letter

cover letter
(KUH ver LEH tuhr)
A letter that introduces you to a potential employer.

A **cover letter** is sent along with your resume. It introduces you to a potential employer and highlights the qualities that make you suitable for the position you want. You need a cover letter when:

- You are applying for a job that is out of town
- You are answering a newspaper advertisement
- A potential employer requests a letter

Your cover letter is a sales letter. You want to sell yourself to the employer in order to get an interview. (A sample cover letter is shown **Figure 4.2**.) Consider these tips as you prepare your letter:

- Be neat
- Use proper spelling, punctuation, format, and grammar
- State where you heard about the job opening
- State what you are applying for and why you are qualified for this specific position
- Give a brief overview of your education, experience, and qualifications
- Refer to your portfolio and/or resume, along with work samples, skills lists, and evaluations
- Request an interview
- Give your address, e-mail address, and phone number

Resume

resume
(REZ oo mey)
A document that provides details about your work history and accomplishments.

A **resume** is a document that provides a snapshot image of your qualifications. It summarizes you, your skills, and your abilities. It is a statement of who you are, what you have done in your life, and what you hope to do next. Your resume may be the first communication between you and a potential employer. (See the example in **Figure 4.3**.) A resume includes the following:

- Your name, address, phone number, and e-mail address
- An objective that describes your career goal. It should be short and clear. You can have a general, long-term goal as your objective, or you can customize your resume for a specific position by using a short-term goal. For example, a general objective might be, "To work in veterinary care." A customized objective might be, "To work as a part-time assistant in a veterinary office."

76 Chapter 4 | Employability and Leadership

January 25, 2024

Mr. E. B. Burns
Director of Nurses
St. Joseph's Hospital
P.O. Box 123
Los Angeles, CA 90880

Dear Mr. Burns:

I am writing in response to your advertisement for a nursing assistant that appeared in the most recent issue of *Nurses World*. I am enclosing my resume for your review.

I graduated from Career Technologies High School this past December, where I took courses in physiology, nutrition, and communication. I have received my CPR certification and have also gained valuable experience working as a volunteer at Children's Hospital for the last three months.

I would welcome the opportunity to speak with you personally about the nursing assistant position. You can contact me by phone or e-mail using the information below.

Thank you for your time and consideration.

Mark Adams
888 Whitegate Avenue
Los Angeles, CA 90880
555-555-5555
markadams@mail.net

Figure 4.2
Sample cover letter to potential employer. When do you need to use a cover letter?

Mary Jane Rodgers

800 E. Oak Street, Conway, AR 72032 • 501-666-8340 (h) 501-620-9180 (c) • mjrodgers@mail.net

Career Plans	Complete 2-year Associate of Science Nursing Program Short-range: Nursing assistant Long-range: Complete a Bachelor of Science Program as a registered nurse
Experience	January 2022–present Henry's Hamburger Shop Conway, AR **Sales Clerk** • Food preparation • Counting inventory • Customer service • Operating a cash register and making change 2019–2020 June Allison Conway, AR **Babysitter** • Planning recreation for two children, 8 and 10 years of age • Meal preparation
Education	Currently enrolled at Hoover High School, Conway, AR; expect to graduate in June 2024.
Interests	Dancing, classical music, reading, skiing, member of Explorer Scouts Medical Post and Health Occupation Students of America
Skills and Strengths	Fluent in oral and written Spanish communication Proficient in Windows programs including Word, Excel, PowerPoint, and Outlook

Figure 4.3
Sample resume. How do the different sections of the resume organize a job applicant's information? Why is it helpful to list your interests?

Employability and Leadership | Chapter 4 77

Figure Focus

4.2 Sample cover letter to potential employer. When do you need to use a cover letter?

Answer: Use a cover letter when you apply for a job out of town, when you answer a newspaper advertisement, and when a potential employer requests a cover letter.

Discuss

- Review the components of a cover letter:
  - Return address
  - Date
  - Inside address
  - Salutation
  - Letter
  - Closing
- Remind students to include their contact information, such as phone number and e-mail.
- Emphasize the importance of proper grammar, format, and correct spelling.
- If possible, show students templates for a cover letter.

Figure Focus

4.3 Sample resume. How do the different sections of the resume organize a job applicant's information? Why is it helpful to list your interests?

Answer: Employers can easily differentiate between areas of information such as experience and education. You are more than just a worker, and listing your interests shows the other parts of your life that make you a whole person.

Teaching Tips

- Review the components of resume:
  - Name, address, and contact information such as phone number and e-mail address
  - Career goals
  - Work experience
  - Education
  - Volunteer experience
  - Awards and honors
  - Activities and interests
  - Skills
  - If possible, show students templates for a resume

CUSTOMIZED INSTRUCTION

English Language Learners

With a partner, have students read aloud either their own cover letter they write in the Activity on this page, or the cover letter in Figure 4.2.

ACTIVITY

Have students write a cover letter and exchange it with a classmate for evaluation.

Teaching Tips

- Discuss ways to format a resume. For example, emphasize the use of bullets or boldface to highlight important information.
- Point out that you should choose a format that highlights your experience and skills so they stand out to someone who might just glance at the resume quickly. You may also want to consider these tips:
    - Make it easy to read. Leave space between lines so it is not crowded or overloaded.
    - Use one, easy-to-read font, and apply different font styles and sizes for emphasis.
    - Bullets are effective for making lines of text stand out.
    - Use proper spelling, punctuation, and grammar.
    - Keep it to one page, if possible; two pages at the most.
- If possible display a blank job application form.
- Discuss the importance of filling out a job application neatly and thoroughly.
- Remind students that all of the information they need to fill out an application should be in their career portfolio.
- Explain that instead of leaving an item blank, it is appropriate to use the abbreviation N/A if a question is not applicable.

ACTIVITY

Have students obtain job applications from various businesses in the community. Place all of the applications in a location where students can review them. Select one application and make copies for the entire class to complete. Discuss how they filled in different parts of the application.

- Details about your education
- Your past work experience—paid or unpaid
- Honors you have earned
- Your personal interests
- Skills, strengths, and abilities
- References (always ask permission to use someone as a reference)
- List of all or your credentials and licensing, including dates
- Service learning, job shadowing, internships, and other work-based learning experiences

Resume Formats

There are many ways to organize and format a resume. Your word processing program comes with a selection of resume templates, or samples, that use a variety of styles and fonts.

Sometimes you will mail your resume in an envelope with a cover letter. Sometimes you will send it electronically by e-mail. Make sure it looks professional when it is printed, as well as when you view it on a computer. When submitting a resume electronically, it's best to save it in a format such as PDF or XPS, so that people can view the content in e-mail and on the Web, even if they don't have the same software you used to create it. These formats also maintain formatting, styles, and graphics.

Also, it's important to understand that many large employers use scanning software to review resumes that are submitted electronically. Resumes are scanned by a computer and sorted by how many **keyword** matches were found.

keywords
(KEE WUHRDZ)
Significant or descriptive words.

Adding appropriate keywords related to the advertised position, such as *detail-oriented* or *bilingual*, can make the difference in attracting the attention of a potential employer.

In addition to a resume, you may also want to have a portfolio of materials that showcase your work, including examples of projects, a writing sample, a recording of an oral report you might have given, and a summary of your leadership style and experience.

Job Application

Most employers require that you fill out an application form. A job application is a standard form you will fill out when you apply for a job. You might fill it out in person when you visit a potential employer, or you might fill it out online. It requires a lot of the same information that you put on your resume, such as your contact information, as well as details about your education and work experience.

Filling out an application form may seem simple, but a lot of people make mistakes or forget important information. On most applications, you will be required to provide the following:

78 Chapter 4 | Employability and Leadership

CUSTOMIZED INSTRUCTION

At-Risk Students

Tell students to think of a resume as a personal brochure. Using an 8½- by 11-inch piece of plain white paper folded in half, have them create a brochure about themselves. They can draw pictures or write about themselves or both. They should focus on their academic, community, and employment-related activities; for example, the subjects they take in school and their achievements in those subjects, extracurricular or volunteer activities, and any part-time jobs they've had. The front page or cover should include their name, address, and contact information. The inside should include their personal information, and the back can include names of important people in their lives.

- Your complete address with the ZIP code
- Your Social Security number (you can withhold this information until after you receive a job offer)
- Your phone number or a number where you can be reached
- A list of the schools you have attended, with dates
- A list of any special training that you have
- A prepared list of any past jobs, the address of the employer, the dates you worked there, and what your duties were
- A list of people who can give you a reference. Be certain that you have their addresses and phone numbers. Also be certain that you have asked permission to use them as a reference.

There are also other ways that you can prepare. Be sure that you:

- Carry a black pen—do not use a pencil.
- Read the application form all the way through before filling it out.
- Print unless you are told to write.
- Spell accurately.
- Answer every question. If there is a question that does not apply to you, enter "NA" (not applicable) in the space to show that you did not overlook the question.
- Recheck for errors.

Interview

The interviewer wants to be sure that you are the best fit for the job. She or he is assessing your skills from the time your resume was received. The interviewer's focus during the interview is to determine if your explanations and behaviors match the job requirements. The job interview helps you and the interviewer make important decisions regarding the position at stake. The interviewer decides if you are the best person for the position. You decide if the position is one you really want.

Interview Guidelines

Before you go on an interview, you should research the company. Human resource personnel suggest that you bring that research with you with specific items that you want to discuss highlighted. It shows interest in the company and your willingness to do some "upfront" work.

Follow these guidelines for a positive interview experience:

- Be well-groomed.
- Dress neatly and professionally (no jeans).
- Be on time.
- Turn off your cell phone.
- Greet the interviewer by name, and smile.

Employability and Leadership | Chapter 4 79

TEAMWORK

Have students create a resume and exchange it with a classmate for evaluation.

Teaching Tips

- Introduce the topic of the job interview.
- Emphasize that no matter how good a candidate looks on paper, he or she must make a positive impression at the interview.
- Explain that the interview is the applicant's opportunity to impress the employer, and sell him or herself as the best candidate for the job.
- Review the interview guidelines.
- Ask students to list reasons why an interview is important, such as giving the interviewer the opportunity to see how the applicant responds to questions.
- Ask students to think of additional guidelines, such as not smoking, not fidgeting, and being prepared with a question or two to ask the interviewer.

CUSTOMIZED INSTRUCTION

Special Needs Students

Some students may have trouble making eye contact during an interview. Have students practice looking at the interviewer's forehead or nose, instead.

Teaching Tips

- Discuss the importance of preparing for an interview.
- Review the potential interview questions, discussing the best ways to answer them.
- Discuss what happens after an interview.
- Review the sample interview rating scale, discussing behavior or responses that might result in excellent, average, or not acceptable scores.

Career-Ready Practices

- Emphasize to students that they can never practice interviewing too much.
- Remind them that the HOSA Handbook (www.hosa.org) provides information to help them develop their job-seeking skills and interviewing technique.
- If you have a career services center, ask a representative to act as the interviewer and conduct the interviews.
- Alternatively, you can act as the interviewer.
- If possible, videotape the interviews so students can see how they appear to others.
- This activity gives students real-world experience in applying the following Career-Ready Practice: Employ Valid and Reliable Research Strategies.
- For more information on the Career-Ready Practices, visit careertech.org/career-ready-practices.

Career-Ready Practices

With a partner, select a local business that interests you. You will stage a mock interview with one of you being the job candidate and the other being the interviewer representing the business. Each of you should prepare at least five questions to ask the other and then prepare answers to the questions you might be asked.

Remember, career-ready individuals use reliable research strategies to obtain information that can help them make decisions and evaluate the pros and cons of any given situation. They carefully consider the validity of the sources from which they obtain information.

Conduct your interview in front of the class and ask for feedback. Why is it important to be prepared for an interview?

- Shake hands firmly.
- Stand until asked to sit.
- Answer questions truthfully and sincerely.
- Be enthusiastic.
- Do not chew gum.
- Do not criticize former employers or teachers.
- Make eye contact with the interviewer when you talk.
- Do not talk about personal problems.
- When the interview is over, thank the interviewer and leave quickly.

Interview Preparation

Plan and prepare an effective presentation for the interview. The interviewer expects you to answer a variety of questions pertinent to the job for which you are applying. Be prepared to give at least three examples of your behavior in various situations. Each experience should describe the:

- **Situation.** What exactly happened?
- **Behavior.** What did you do?
- **Outcome.** What were the results?

Read the following questions and determine how to answer them:

- Tell me about the most difficult decision you made at school or work in the last few months.
- Tell me how you get along with people at school or work.
- Tell me about the most difficult job or school task you've done. Why was it difficult? How did you get past the difficulties?
- Explain a recent situation that demonstrates your ability to be a team player.

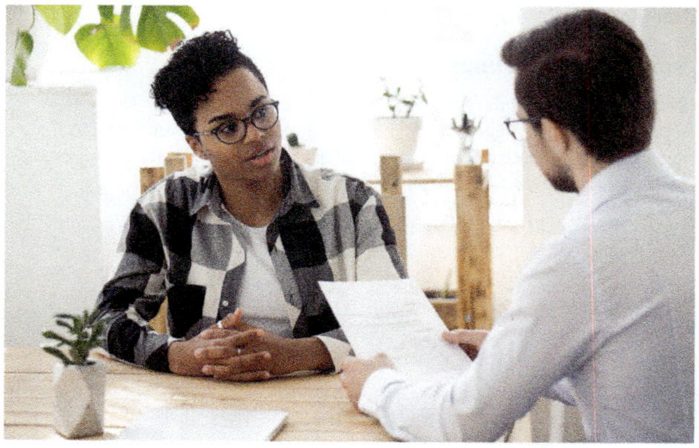

Figure 4.4
How does the expression, "You never get a second chance to make a first impression" relate to job interviews?

80 Chapter 4 | Employability and Leadership

Figure Focus

4.4 How does the expression, "You never get a second chance to make a first impression" relate to job interviews?

Answer: Student answers will vary, but this is a good opportunity to discuss how important it is to make a good first impression on a job interview.

- Describe a situation in which you had to work under pressure. What kind of pressure were you facing? How did you handle the situation? What was the outcome?
- Describe a situation where you had to be very flexible. How did your actions demonstrate your flexibility?

After the Interview

The interviewer may do a reference check to verify that your resume and application are honest and accurate. She or he may also rate your responses to help make a decision about which candidate is best for the job. The following is an example of an interview rating scale with topics.

	Excellent	Average	Not Acceptable
Appearance			
Manner			
Qualifications			
Experience			
Job fit			

After the interview, send a letter of thanks to the interviewer. This lets the interviewer know that you are interested in the position, and it may increase your chance of getting the job. You may also choose to send an immediate thank-you response via e-mail; follow up, however, by sending a thank-you letter in the mail, as well. Make sure you have a professional voice message on your cell phone when the perspective employer calls back.

Personal Wellness

Managing Stress

Job hunting can lead to concerns about where you will live, how much money you will earn, and what direction your career is taking. If these concerns cause you too much stress, they can affect your ability to present yourself well to prospective employers. Here are some tips to help manage the stress of job hunting:

- Stay organized. Keep a good supply of resumes and cover letters on hand. Make sure you have accurate directions and maps to employers you are visiting. Consider locating the place of the interview during a sample run before you go to the interview. Establish the time frame necessary for the drive.
- Use a schedule. Keep a clear and up-to-date schedule of all your appointments to avoid over-scheduling yourself. Have your schedule open in front of you when you make appointments for new and follow-up meetings and interviews.
- Join a job hunter's group. Groups offer good networking opportunities and emotional support.

Job hunting should be an exciting time. Managing the process so that you minimize stress can help you enjoy it and be successful.

Teaching Tips

- Emphasize the importance of following up an interview with a thank-you note.
- Discuss whether it is ever appropriate to use e-mail to write a thank-you note. For example, if the initial contact was made using the Internet, it may be appropriate. However, emphasize that it is always appropriate to write and mail a letter.

Personal Wellness—Managing Stress

- Discuss why job hunting may be stressful.
- Review the symptoms of stress, and how stress can be harmful.
- Review methods of combating stress during a job search.

Section 4.1 Review Questions

1. Answer: Through a help wanted ad, you can learn about career outlooks in your area by identifying the companies or industries that appear to have many listings. You can also learn about salary ranges.
2. Answer: Five resources include Web sites for companies, government agencies, specific industries, job agencies, and social networking sites; personal contacts; career fairs; career centers or employment agencies; and want ads.
3. Answer: A cover letter introduces you to a potential employers and highlights the qualities that make you suitable for a position whereas a resume is a comprehensive summary of your skills, experience, education, and achievements.
4. Answer: A job application form generally requests:
   - Your complete address with the ZIP code
   - Your Social Security number
   - Your phone number or a number where you can be reached
   - A list of the schools you have attended with dates
   - A list of any special training that you have
   - A prepared list of any past jobs including the address of the employer the dates you worked there, and what your duties were
   - A list of people who can give you a reference
5. Answer: After a job interview, you should send a thank-you note to the interviewer.

Summary

A successful job search requires identifying the appropriate resources for finding job opportunities, developing accurate and professional job search materials, and preparing for interviews. You can find job openings and opportunities through a variety of sources, including want ads in print publications and online, job fairs, career centers and employment agencies, corporate Web sites, and through your network of personal contacts. Applying for a job usually requires that you prepare a resume and complete an application. In many cases, you will also need to write a cover letter. If you are called for an interview with a potential employer, make sure you do your homework by researching the company and preparing answers to the questions you might be asked. After the interview, always follow up with a thank-you note.

Section 4.1 Review Questions

1. Other than the position being advertised, what can you learn about job opportunities by reviewing help wanted ads?
2. Name five resources where you can find job opportunities.
3. How is a cover letter different from a resume?
4. Identify the items generally requested on a job application form.
5. What kinds of follow up should you do after a job interview?

SECTION 4.2 Keeping a Job

Background

You spend a lot of time and effort learning the skills for a career in health care. You also put time and effort into finding and getting the job. Now that you have the job, you want to keep it. Employers look for specific things in an employee. The information in this section explains what these things are and how you can be a good employee.

Objectives

When you have completed this section, you will be able to do the following:

- Match key terms with their correct meanings.
- List four employer responsibilities.
- List four responsibilities of a good employee.
- Describe workplace goals.

82 Chapter 4 | Employability and Leadership

FOCUS AND ENGAGE

Introduce the Section

a. Review the content of the Background paragraph, explaining that being a good employee is more than doing a job.

b. Explain that in order to keep a job, you must meet all of the employer's expectations, but that it is also important that the employer meet your expectations.

c. Discuss the objectives for the section.

Vocabulary Review

a. Key terms are defined in the margins of the text on the page where they first appear.

b. Pronounce each word, and have the students repeat the pronunciation out loud.

c. Discuss the definition of each word.

Responsibilities

The Good Employer

An employer has responsibilities to you, and you have responsibilities to the employer. The good employer demonstrates:

- **Dignity**, by respecting each employee as an important member of the health care team. Providing a safe, clean working environment is an example of treating employees with dignity.
- **Excellence**, by encouraging personal and professional development, accountability, teamwork, and a commitment to quality health care. Supporting routine activities and providing the necessary materials that allow you to do the best possible job shows a dedication to excellence.
- **Service**, by establishing standards and guidelines directing appropriate, caring, compassionate health care to those dependent on the health care services. Providing clear guidelines for employees to follow gives the direction necessary to accomplish the job in a caring, compassionate manner.
- **Fairness** *and justice*, by establishing employee salaries and benefits that are fair and reliable. An employer who provides a reasonable salary for agreed-upon work and establishes a standard salary and benefit structure for all employees is striving to be a fair, equitable employer.

dignity
(DIG nih tee)
The quality of value and worth.

excellence
(EK sell ence)
The quality of having outstanding qualities.

service
(SUHR viss)
Caring for others.

fairness
(FAYR nes)
Applying good rules equally to all people.

organization
(or guh nuh ZAY shuhn)
Process of arranging items or tasks for the most efficient arrangement.

The Good Employee

As a good employee, you demonstrate:

- Dignity through communication and interpersonal effectiveness, by:
  - Being open, honest, and respectful
  - Listening actively and seeking understanding
  - Providing positive, helpful feedback
- Excellence through teamwork and accountability, by:
  - Creating an environment of continuous improvement
  - Trying new ways to improve performance, processes, and service
  - Seeking growth and development opportunities for you and others
  - Taking responsibility for individual and team actions, decisions, and results
  - Adapting to changing needs and learning new skills, knowledge, and behaviors
  - Asking for and being open to continuous feedback from your peers and supervisor regarding your performance
  - Seeking ways to manage time effectively and maintain **organization** of your workload
- Service through being flexible and customer focused, by:
  - Responding to the needs of those served and showing concern for meeting those needs
  - Responding quickly and effectively to problems that arise while providing service

Personal Goals in the Workplace

In addition to workplace goals that you and your supervisor set and review, think about your own goals. Consider your personal goals for having the job and what you want to, and can, accomplish and gain while you are working in the position for which you have been hired. For example, you may want to work as a nursing assistant to become familiar with health care procedures with a goal of going to school to become a registered nurse. Or you may choose to work in an assisted living facility with a goal of becoming confident in caring for older patients and clients so that you can pursue work as a home health care worker.

Employability and Leadership | Chapter 4 83

TEACH

Teaching Tips

- Ask students what they think makes a good employer.
- Ask students what they think makes a good employee.
- Discuss why it is important for both the employer and the employee to understand each other's responsibilities.
- Discuss the four responsibilities of a good employer.
- Point out that some of these responsibilities are mandated by law, such as treating all employees equally and fairly.
- Discuss the four responsibilities of a good employee.
- Ask students to think about and share qualities they possess that will help make them good employees.
- Discuss pride of work and accomplishment as it relates to a career in health care.
- Discuss why fostering a cooperative and team-oriented environment make both employers and employees happier and more productive.
- Ask students if they have ever lost a job, or if they know someone who has. Discuss the reasons why.

Personal Goals in the Workplace

Provide a general overview of the steps to setting and meeting a goal:

1. Identify the goal. Write down the goal using as much as detail as you can. Be positive.
2. Assess the goal. Determine if it is something you really want and if it is realistic and attainable.
3. Make an action plan for achieving the goal. What resources will you need?
4. Write down your action plan. Be as specific as possible.
5. Reevaluate your goals. Every once in a while, make sure they are still important to you and, if so, that you are on track to achieve them.

Teaching Tips

- Discuss how goals provide direction and motivation in the workplace.
- Ask students to discuss a list of short-term goals that can help them achieve their long-term career goals.

Apply It

- Allow time for students to prepare their presentations.
- Offer one or two points of immediate feedback after each team's presentation.
- Have a general discussion about the employability skills that were presented by the teams.

Figure Focus

4.5 Together Everyone Accomplishes More (TEAM). How does this saying help reinforce the benefits of teamwork?

Answer: When people cooperate as a team, they all benefit more than if they each worked individually.

- Fairness and justice:
  - Using equipment and supplies in an appropriate manner
  - Treating and responding to all people in the work environment with the same dignity, excellence, and service standards

Your roles and responsibilities as an employee are often similar to those you have in your life outside of work. For example, as a student, you most likely strive to learn new skills, knowledge, and behaviors. In your community, you may look for ways to provide positive, helpful feedback to address issues or solve problems. When you live up to your responsibilities in all areas of your life, you will be successful in any role in which you find yourself.

Apply It

In teams of four to five, prepare presentations for the class that demonstrate employability skills such as attendance, appearance, individual responsibility, professional conduct, and time management.

Workplace Goals

As an employee, you will have goals that you are expected to achieve. Some goals apply to all of the workers in your department, or there may be goals that are for everyone who works at the health care facility. One of your own workplace goals will be to perform the duties listed in your job description. Your job performance will be evaluated by your supervisor on a regular basis. In many work settings, you will meet with your supervisor before your performance review to set goals to help guide your work and motivate you to do your best on the job. Setting and achieving goals is a way to demonstrate that you are a good employee to your employer.

Be sure to understand all of the goals that are established for your position. In addition to your supervisor's review, you will want to monitor your own progress toward achieving these goals. Keeping notes is a helpful way to identify areas where you have been successful, as well as areas where you want to make improvements.

Figure 4.5
Together Everyone Accomplishes More (TEAM). How does this saying help reinforce the benefits of teamwork?

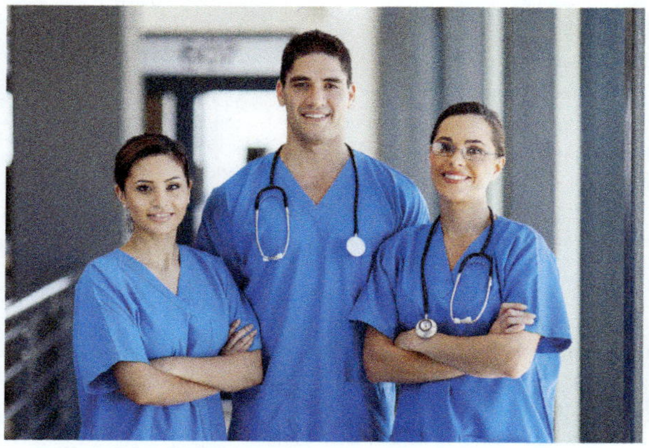

Teamwork and team building are essential if you and your fellow workers expect to accomplish your goals. (**Figure 4.5**) When you follow these guidelines, your job gives you a sense of accomplishment. Being able to keep a job until you are ready to leave builds your references for the future. Remember that each job you have becomes an important part of your professional experience, and you want it to be a positive experience.

Personal Wellness

Self-Evaluation

Evaluating your work helps you make sure you are doing the best job you can do. Self-evaluation can be as simple as keeping a journal in which you reflect on your work or more formal questionnaires that you fill out on a regular basis. Here are some tips to help you evaluate yourself effectively:

- Be honest. Tell yourself exactly how you think you are doing.
- Be specific. Don't simply say, "I'm doing well." Say, "I like the way I handled my boss's request to itemize the request list."
- Be constructive. Identify areas in need of improvement. Find a way to help yourself do a better job of the things you are struggling with. Don't say, "I am running meetings badly." Say, "I will ask my manager how I can run meetings more efficiently."
- Evaluate how your work decisions affect the population you are serving and your peers. Remember that patient needs should be the primary driver of all caregiver actions.

If you can evaluate yourself consistently and fairly, you are more likely to avoid the small problems that may lead to bigger problems later.

Evaluation by Others

Ask your peers to notify you if they observe any problems with your practice, or any other areas in need of improvement. Letting your peers know that you value their feedback will open a communication line and help you identify things you can improve upon before they become a problem.

Review the goals and comments from your annual review. Did any of the comments in the review indicate that you should change some of your work behaviors? Determine if you have taken steps to change these behaviors.

What should you do if, while you are evaluating your work, you discover you have done something unethical?

Summary

Once you acquire a job, you and your employer agree to work together to accomplish the goals of the job for which you have been hired. Your behavior reflects your attitude and values. Continually evaluate your actions using the Dignity, Excellence, Service, and Fairness/Justice criteria as a measure of your progress in the work environment. Be a team player by respecting your co-workers and encouraging them to do the best job they can do.

Section 4.2 Review Questions

1. How do employers demonstrate that they value dignity?
2. How do employees demonstrate excellence?
3. What are four employer responsibilities?
4. Define fairness.
5. What are four responsibilities of a good employee?
6. What can an employee do to demonstrate that they are service-focused?

Employability and Leadership | Chapter 4 85

Personal Wellness—Self-Evaluation and Evaluation by Others

- It can be difficult for people to evaluate themselves honestly and objectively.
- Point out that documenting their personal goals in the workplace and monitoring their progress toward those goals is a step of self-evaluation.
- You may want to have a list of questions students can use for self-evaluation.
- Emphasize that identifying areas in need of improvement is not intended to find things they are doing wrong, but a positive step toward a better performance.
- To practice, ask students to perform a self-evaluation of their work for this class. You may choose whether or not to collect the evaluations.
- Discuss the value of peer evaluations.
- Ask students to think about whether friends or classmates ever evaluate them, and whether or not it is helpful. Perhaps a friend has pointed out a clothing mismatch, or recommended a new hairstyle.

What should you do if, while you are evaluating your work, you discover you have done something unethical?

Answer: If you find you have done something unethical, talk to your manager at once.

Section 4.2 Review Questions

1. Answer: Employers demonstrate that they value dignity by respecting each employee as an important member of the health care team.
2. Answer: Employees demonstrate excellence by creating an environment of continuous improvement; trying new ways to improve performance, processes, and service; seeking growth and development opportunities for you and others; taking responsibility for individual and team actions, decisions, and results; adapting to changing needs and learning new skills, knowledge, and behaviors; and asking for and being open to continuous feedback from your peers and supervisor regarding your performance
3. Answer: The four responsibilities of a good employer are dignity, excellence, service, and fairness.
4. Answer: Fairness is applying good rules equally to all people.
5. Answer: The four responsibilities of a good employee are dignity, excellence, service, and fairness and justice.
6. Answer: An employee can demonstrate that they are service-focused by responding to the needs of those served and showing concern for meeting those needs and by responding quickly and effectively to problems that arise while providing service.

FOCUS AND ENGAGE

Introduce the Section

a. Review the content of the Background paragraph, explaining the concept of a professional organization.

b. Explain the difference between a job and a membership in a professional organization.

c. Discuss the objectives for the section.

Vocabulary Review

a. Key terms are defined in the margins of the text on the page where they first appear.

b. Pronounce each word, and have the students repeat the pronunciation out loud.

c. Discuss the definition of each word.

TEACH

Discuss

- Display pamphlets and brochures from professional and student organizations.
- Ask students if they are members of any club or organization, and what the benefits might be.
- Discuss the importance of making contacts and keeping up-to-date with new developments in the industry.

Reinforce and Review

- Review the information that should be included on a resume, including membership in professional organizations.
- Reinforce the importance of using contacts with other people to find employment.

SECTION 4.3 Becoming a Professional Leader

Background

Student and professional health care organizations enhance the delivery of compassionate, high-quality care by providing knowledge, skill, and leadership development. Committed students and professionals seek opportunities provided by these organizations to keep current and to provide patients with good-quality care.

Objectives

When you have completed this section, you will be able to do the following:

- Match key terms with their correct meanings.
- Name the three main benefits of being a member of a career and technical student organization.
- Name six benefits of being a member of a professional organization.
- Identify ways to find a professional organization.
- Identify steps to becoming a leader.
- Describe the goals and role of HOSA.
- Summarize why you plan to participate in a student and professional organization.

leadership
(LEED uhr ship)
Ability to influence or lead.

time management
(tahym MAN ij muhnt)
Planning scheduled tasks in order to use time in the most effective manner.

priority
(pry OR it ee)
A quality of importance; tasks of high priority are more urgent than items of low priority.

budget
(BUH jet)
An amount of money allocated for a particular purpose.

Membership in an Organization

Membership in your student or professional organization gives you an opportunity to gain occupational knowledge and skills. It also provides opportunities to develop leadership skills. Some of the skills that you learn include the following:

- Professional ethics
- Communication and interpersonal relations
- **Leadership** skills
- Ability to recognize and initiate change
- How to organize activities and people
- **Time management**
- Establishing **priorities**
- **Budgeting**
- Fundraising
- Current health issues

86 Chapter 4 | Employability and Leadership

Teaching Tips

- Review the skills learned from membership in a professional or student organization.

ACTIVITY

Contact a representative of a student organization and invite him or her to speak to your class.

HOSA

HOSA-Future Health Professionals is the only national career and technical student organization that exclusively serves middle, secondary and postsecondary/collegiate students in pursuit of careers in the health professions. From its early beginnings in 1976, the HOSA mission continues to be recruiting and retaining qualified students interested in health careers and providing members with personal, career and leadership development opportunities to be academic, college and career ready. HOSA serves as the health professions pipeline in response to the critical shortages facing the health industry. (Figure 4.6) Among HOSA's primary goals are to:

- Promote career opportunities in the health care industry
- Enhance and promote the delivery of quality health care to all people
- Encourage students and instructors to be actively involved in current health care issues, community service, and chapter activities

HOSA-Future Health Professionals
The student organization for health science students at the secondary, postsecondary, adult, and college levels.

Figure 4.6
The HOSA brand was adopted to serve as the marketing face of HOSA.

HOSA Competitive Events Program

HOSA provides many opportunities for students to learn and achieve. One such opportunity is the the National HOSA Competitive Events Programs. Competitions may occur at local, state, and national levels, with students advancing on to the next level by winning the previous one. HOSA offers many events divided into categories based on the curriculum. Competitive event categories include:

- Health Science:
  - Dental terminology
  - Medical spelling
  - Medical terminology
  - Knowledge Tests
    - Human Growth and Development
    - Pathophysiology
  - Medical Law and Ethics
  - Transcultural Health Care
  - Medical math
  - Medical reading
  - Pharmacology
  - Nutrition
- Health Professions Events:
  - Biomedical Laboratory Science
  - Clinical Nursing
  - Clinical Specialty
  - Dental Science
  - Home Health Aide
  - Medical Assisting
  - Nursing Assisting
  - Personal Care
  - Physical Therapy
  - Sports Medicine
  - Veterinary Science
- Emergency Preparedness:
  - CERT Skills
  - CPR/First Aid
  - EMT
  - Epidemiology
  - Life Support Skills
  - MRC Partnership

Apply It

In the HOSA Competitive Event Medical Assisting, students compete in completing patient registration and history forms. Working with a partner, interview each other or create patient scenarios for this activity. Then, complete the forms. Forms can be completed on the computer or written.

An electronic copy of the HOSA Medical Office Registration form in fillable PDF format is available from www.hosa.org. This fillable form simulates completing an electronic health record using an input screen on the computer.

Employability and Leadership | Chapter 4 87

Teaching Tips

- Review the meaning of HOSA and discuss its goals.
- Explain how skills competitions can help students gain knowledge as well as build confidence.
- Review the competitive event categories.
- Emphasize that participating in these competitions show qualities such as initiative, leadership, and an interest in doing well.
- Note that participation in this type of activity should always be added to a resume.
- Direct students to the Web site for HOSA (hosa.org), or a local chapter in your area, and allow them sufficient class time to explore it.

Figure Focus

4.6 The HOSA brand was adopted to serve as the marketing face of HOSA.

Discuss with the class benefits of being a HOSA member.

Apply It

- If possible, have students fill out forms both online and written.
- Emphasis that in written forms handwriting needs to be neat and clear.

Teaching Tips

- Review the requirements for participating in HOSA competitions.
- Review the code of conduct required for HOSA.

Apply It

- Provide students with professional journals or have them find them in the library.
- Guide students to use the Internet to identify professional organizations.

extemporaneous (ik stem puh REY nee uhs) Spoken or composed at the spur of the moment, without preparation or notes.

- Public Health
- Leadership Events:
  - **Extemporaneous** Health Poster
  - Extemporaneous Writing
  - Healthy Lifestyle
  - Interviewing Skills
  - Job Seeking Skills
  - Medical Photography
  - Prepared Speaking
  - Researched Persuasive Speaking
  - Speaking Skills
- Teamwork Events:
  - Biomedical Debate
  - Community Awareness
  - Creative Problem Solving
  - Forensic Medicine
  - Health Career Display
  - Health Education
  - HOSA Bowl
  - Medical Innovation
  - Parliamentary Procedure
  - Public Service Announcement
- Recognition:
  - Barbara James Service Award
  - Health Care Issues Exam
  - HOSA Happenings
  - MRC Volunteer Recognition
  - National Service Project
  - Outstanding HOSA Chapter
  - Outstanding State Leader

Apply It

Some professional organizations for health care workers are specific to a medical specialty, such as pediatrics or oncology. Other organizations are specific to types of occupations, such as nurse practitioners or medical assistants. With a partner, discuss career paths you are considering and research and identify professional organizations that will help you in your chosen professions.

Competition requirements include the following:

- Student must be an active HOSA member.
- Student must be identified as either a secondary student (currently enrolled in a high school) or a postsecondary student (graduate from high school or over 18 years of age).

Those who attend HOSA functions follow a strict code of conduct that includes competitive event dress codes. Experiencing the challenges, structure, and competition in HOSA teaches participants how to reach for and achieve their highest potential. In addition, HOSA offers many scholarship opportunities and leadership opportunities at the local, state, and national level. HOSA provides a unique program of leadership development, motivation, and recognition exclusively for students interested in pursuing careers in health professions.

88 Chapter 4 | Employability and Leadership

CUSTOMIZED INSTRUCTION

More Advanced Students

Have more advanced students contact a professional organization in your area to find out about upcoming events. He or she can then prepare a calendar of these events to share with the class.

Less Advanced Students

Have students think of an event they recently participated in—this can be an organized, competitive event, such as a soccer game, or something informal and more impromptu, such as contributing artwork to a school bulletin board or playing a video game with a few friends. Ask students to discuss the event and the skills used with the class.

Professional Organizations

Professional organizations help those who are employed keep current on the latest technology and trends in their industry or field of work. Being aware of the advantages offered through involvement in such organizations motivates health care workers to become active in the professional group for their chosen occupation.

There are numerous professional organizations for the health care worker. Most organizations have a local chapter, state chapter, and national chapter. Each supports the other, and all work toward common goals. Belonging to a professional organization provides the following benefits:

- Updates on new technological advances
- Communication with workers in other geographical areas
- Guidelines for meeting professional standards and, in some cases, accreditation, certification, and licensure in designated professions
- Shared resources
- Resources for employment opportunities
- Updates on current legislative issues
- Interaction with other health professionals
- Pooled money to accomplish changes for the good of the occupation/profession
- Power as a united group to encourage positive change
- Development of new ideas that support growth

You can find professional organizations by:

- Asking fellow employees
- Reading the bulletin boards at work
- Reading your professional journals
- Reading brochures
- Researching on the Internet
- Attending occupationally related inservice programs
- Checking the Occupational Outlook Handbook

Leadership

The leadership role is a very important part of the health care team. Health care is truly a "team effort" that requires cooperation and collaboration. Each team is guided by a team leader. This role may rotate through the team dependent upon the care to be provided. Leadership characteristics such as goal-setting and team building are critical for effective and efficient health services with optimum results.

Creating and maintaining an environment that fosters excellence is an important aspect of leadership. Employees working in this type of environment are more likely to strive to do their best and to be more satisfied with their job situation.

Career-Ready Practices

Career-ready individuals seek new methods, practices, and ideas from a variety of sources that they can apply to their own workplace. A professional organization is one such resource.

Joining a professional organization provides you with opportunities to learn more about your industry, strengthen your job skills, achieve accreditation or certification in your field, and expand your network of personal contacts. To an employer, it shows that you are motivated to look beyond the workplace to find new and innovative ideas that can help you and your organization be more productive.

One way that a professional organization helps its members is by distributing information about the industry through Web sites, newsletters, or magazines. Working in teams of three or four, select a health care career and create a two-page publication for a professional organization that would serve it.

Use the Internet to research current trends, policies, or events affecting the industry. Be sure to gather information on the organization's accreditation and certification procedures, if applicable, and how they prepare members to achieve the credentials necessary for certification and/or licensure in their field. Give the publication a suitable name, and write three or four articles that the members would find useful. Include pictures if appropriate. When your project is complete, print it to share with the class, or publish it on your class Web site.

Employability and Leadership | Chapter 4 89

CUSTOMIZED INSTRUCTION

At-Risk Students

At-risk students may feel intimidated by the prospect of joining a professional or student organization for any number of reasons. Or, there may be outside factors that prohibit them from joining. Make sure students are aware of the opportunities available at your school to become involved in an organization. Provide a list of student organizations and encourage them to learn about one or more that interests them. Contact a current member and ask him or her to share their experiences.

Teaching Tips

- Discuss the value of belonging to a professional organization.
- Explain that most professional organizations require members to pay annual dues.
- If desired, discuss the professional associations to which you or other teachers and staff belong and the benefits of your membership.
- Ask students to comment on any academic or youth associations to which they belong.
- Review the list of benefits provided by membership in a professional organization.
- Explain the concept of networking, or meeting other people with common interests who might be able to help you in your career.
- Review the ways of finding a professional organization to join.
- With the class, make a list of organizations available in your area.

Career-Ready Practices

- Discuss why an employer would encourage an employee to join a professional organization related to his or her area of work.
- Provide samples of information a member might receive from a professional organization (such as HOSA or an organization to which you belong).
- Encourage students to be creative in the format and design of their publication. Articles should be appropriate and of suitable content for the intended audience.
- This activity gives students real-world experience in applying the following Career-Ready Practice: Demonstrate Creativity and Innovation.
- For more information on the Career-Ready Practices, visit careertech.org/career-ready-practices.

Teaching Tips

- Discuss leadership, and why it is important for personal and professional growth and development.
- Emphasize that leadership is more than just a job title, such as Manager.
- Review the steps for becoming a leader.
- Discuss the quotes by Tom Peters. Ask students why they agree or disagree with his statements.
- Define the concept of a team as a group of people working together to achieve a common goal.
- Emphasize respect for others and an ability to listen and respond.
- Discuss the personal qualities that help an employee succeed as a member of a team. These include:
  - Integrity: Possessing and adhering to high moral principles or professional standards
  - Honesty: Being fair, truthful, and morally upright
  - Courtesy: Polite or considerate behavior toward others
  - Responsibility: Being accountable to somebody or for something
- Share with students the following suggestions on how to build strong team relationships.
  - If a problem or conflict arises among team members, be prepared to offer suggestions for solving it.
  - Avoid alienating others by placing the blame on everyone but yourself.
  - Use positive verbal and nonverbal skills. For example, do not use sarcasm or roll your eyes. Instead, listen carefully, ask questions, and make sure all team members understand the team's goal.
  - Follow through on the things you commit to doing.
  - Share credit for accomplishments and ideas.
  - Compliment others' talents, skills, and experience.

Leadership for Meetings

- Discuss leadership for meetings.
- Ask students to describe some examples of good leadership for meetings that they have experienced.

Becoming a leader in your occupational area takes time and patience. To become a leader you must take several important steps. These include the following:

- Developing a superior skill level
- Becoming a decision maker
- Being a good communicator
- Developing a balanced focus on tasks and people

Tom Peters, author of *A Passion for Excellence*, says:

"A leader is a . . .	**A leader is not a . . .**
cheerleader	cop
enthusiast	referee
nurturer	devil's advocate
coach	naysayer
facilitator	pronouncer"

A true leader unites people and works toward positive outcomes.

Leadership for Meetings

Meetings are a way for teams to communicate. Effective meetings require specific leadership:

- **Set goals.** These goals are based on topics that need to be covered.
- **Schedule.** Set a time and location for the meeting. Be firm about attendance. Prepare an agenda to share objective(s) before, or at the start of, the meeting.
- **Maintain control.** Begin on time. Assign a note-taker. Introduce each topic, guiding the team to focus and make decisions. If something cannot be resolved, set a time to address the issue. In concluding, all attendees should be aware of resulting duties.
- **Follow up.** After the meeting, send a memo with a brief summary. List action steps and a timeline for the team to achieve required follow-up. Thank attendees for their time and attention.

Teamwork

In the ideal workplace, all team members focus their efforts on outcomes that reflect the best possible plan of patient care. Team members respect each other and can expect the support of the team.

The team leader's responsibilities include knowing the strengths of his/her team members and facilitating the use of those strengths toward common goals. The leader is there to assist, encourage, monitor, and evaluate.

Good interpersonal relationships are fostered through positive attitudes toward each other. Interpersonal competency comes from being self-aware and using that self-awareness to relate to others. Respecting and valuing the input of your team members creates an environment in which each person gives individually to make a better whole. Practicing positive interactions encourages each team member to focus on team goals and quality outcomes.

To work effectively as part of a team, it's important to assist other team members when they need help and listen carefully when another team member is sharing ideas or beliefs. You must be able to respect the opinions of others even though you may not agree with them. This will enable you to stay open-minded and willing to compromise for the benefit of the patient when needed.

Also, avoid criticizing other team members and instead, support and encourage them whenever possible. Practicing good communication skills will help you share ideas, concepts, and knowledge so that you can perform your duties to the best of your abilities.

All team members work together to identify the needs of the patient, offer their opinions on the best type of care to serve the patient, and suggest additional health care professionals who might be able to assist with specific patient needs.

90 Chapter 4 | Employability and Leadership

To direct the input from various team members, the team leader must:

- Organize and coordinate the team's activities
- Encourage team members to share ideas and give opinions
- Motivate all team members to work toward established goals
- Assist with solving problems the team encounters and leads change
- Monitor the team's progress toward the goal and manages accountability
- Provide feedback to all team members on the effectiveness of the team

Leadership Skills

The professional leader has the basic knowledge and skills necessary to direct individuals and groups toward common goals.

The professional leader continually evaluates the individual members of the group and their goals. It is important for the leader to understand the different styles of leadership (democratic, where all team members have a voice in decision-making; laissez-faire, where the leader allows the team members to make decisions; and autocratic, where the leader makes the decisions and tells team members what to do) and modify her/his style to fit the needs of the group at any given time.

The professional leader convenes the group as needed and effectively conducts the meeting to gather input to ensure all members are recognized, valued, and participating to achieve the desired outcomes for the organization. The professional leader must also be able to effectively participate in meetings called to discuss issues, concerns, and other topics that contribute to a highly efficient and effective organization. The professional leader provides guidance to individual members of the group that facilitates functioning at the highest level of performance.

The professional leader promotes an environment that facilitates excellence in the individual and the group. This includes providing the tools necessary for success and acting as an advocate for the group as it interacts with other members of the health care team. In addition, a professional leader:

- Has strong interpersonal skills and respects the rights, dignity, opinions, and abilities of others
- Understands his or her own strengths and weaknesses
- Is driven, focused, and displays self-confidence and willingness to take a stand
- Is organized and communicates effectively and states ideas clearly
- Shows self-initiative and a willingness to work
- Completes tasks
- Shows optimism
- Is open-minded, balanced, and can compromise
- Motivates and inspires others while giving them their due credit
- Demonstrates leadership responsibilities that include goal-setting and team building

Apply It

In teams of six to ten, plan, prepare, and carry out a meeting following parliamentary procedure guidelines. Determine one or more topics to discuss. Assign a leader for the meeting and follow the steps listed in the "Leadership for Meetings" sidebar. After your meetings, as a class, discuss what made your meetings work well and what parts of the meetings and/or the teams' meeting behavior can be improved.

Apply It

Work in teams of two to three to create a list of three leaders in the medical field in the 19th, the 20th, and the 21st centuries. What made these people leaders?

Employability and Leadership | Chapter 4 91

Teaching Tips

- Ask students if they can think of a time when they exhibited leadership skills.
- Discuss the responses. Ask how they felt as a leader, and why they think they were effective.
- Discuss examples of ineffective leadership, such as someone who wants to be a bully, or someone who is not forceful enough.
- Emphasize the need for problem-solving skills to become an effective leader.

Apply It

- You may want to determine one or more topics to discuss and assign each to a team.
- Before students role-play their meeting skills, discuss basic rules that ensure an orderly and business-like meeting.
- Monitor students' meetings, offering guidance only if they are unable to move forward; note strengths and weaknesses for later discussion.
- Encourage students to evaluate their role-played meetings and share what they learned with the entire class.
- Have the class provide feedback on each team's meeting and what parts of the meetings and/or the teams' meeting behavior can be improved.

Apply It

- You may need to adjust the number of groups, depending on the number of students.
- Advise students to review Chapter 1, Section 1.1, for information about leaders who made historical contributions to medicine.
- Have students present their lists and explanations in a creative manner. For example, they may want to dress up as the leaders and perform a skit, or create a slide show.

ACTIVITY

Make a chart or graph comparing the qualities of someone who is a leader with someone who is not a leader. Make sure students understand that just because an individual does not exhibit leadership skills, he or she will still possess positive qualities.

CUSTOMIZED INSTRUCTION

Special Needs Students

Participating in meetings can be a challenge to students with vision or auditory impairments. In the Apply It activity on this page where teams role-play a meeting, make sure each team considers the needs of all its members and takes measures to ensure no one is excluded.

Summary

Participation in HOSA is an important part of your career development and professionalism. As a member, you are introduced to various health careers, develop a responsible attitude toward your community, develop knowledge and skills for the work world, and gain self-confidence.

Membership prepares you to be a leader in your chosen occupation; it also helps you prepare to become a valuable member of a professional organization when you join the workforce.

To become a leader you must develop superior skill levels, become a decision maker, be a good communicator, and develop a balanced focus on tasks and people.

Section 4.3 Review Questions

1. Name the three main benefits of being a member of a student health career and technical education organization.
2. Name six benefits of being a member of a professional organization.
3. Identify the four key steps to becoming a leader.
4. Define *HOSA*.
5. Provide three examples of "What a leader is . . ." and three examples of "What a leader is not . . .".
6. HOSA supports skills competitions. Name one event in each of the competitive skills categories.

Section 4.3 Review Questions

1. Answer: The benefits of being a member of a student health career and technical education organization include that it gives you an opportunity to gain occupational knowledge and skills, it provides opportunities to develop leadership skills, and it gives you the opportunity to interact with peers.
2. Answer: The benefits of a professional organization include:
   - Updates on new technological advances
   - Communication with people in other geographical areas
   - Shared resources
   - Resources for employment opportunities
   - Current legislative issues
   - Interaction with other health professionals
   - Pooled money to accomplish changes for the good of the occupation/profession
   - Power as a united group to encourage positive change
   - Development of new ideas that support growth
3. Answer: To become a leader, you must develop a superior skill level, become a decision maker, be a good communicator, and develop a balanced focus on tasks and people.
4. Answer: HOSA is the student organization for health occupation students at the secondary, postsecondary, adult, and college level.
5. Answer: A leader is a cheerleader, enthusiast, coach, facilitator, or nurturer. A leader is not a cop, referee, devil's advocate, naysayer, or pronouncer.
6. Answer:

   Health Science Events:
   - Behavioral health
   - Cultural diversities & disparities
   - Dental terminology
   - Human growth & development
   - Medical law & ethics
   - Medical spelling
   - Medical terminology
   - Medical math
   - Medical reading
   - Nutrition
   - Pathophysiology
   - Pharmacology

   Health Professions Events:
   - Biomedical laboratory science
   - Nursing assisting
   - Clinical nursing
   - Physical therapy
   - Dental science
   - Sports medicine
   - Home health aide
   - Veterinary science
   - Personal care
   - Pharmacy science
   - Medical assisting
   - Clinical specialty

   Emergency Preparedness Events:
   - CPR/First Aid
   - Emergency medical technician
   - MRC partnership
   - Public health
   - Life support skills
   - Epidemiology
   - CERT skills

   Leadership Events:
   - Researched persuasive writing and speaking
   - Extemporaneous writing
   - Health care photography
   - Extemporaneous health poster
   - Extemporaneous writing
   - Job-seeking skills
   - Prepared speaking
   - Interviewing skills
   - Speaking skills
   - Healthy lifestyle
   - Organizational leadership

   Teamwork Events:
   - Community awareness
   - Biomedical debate
   - Creative problem-solving
   - Forensic science
   - Health career display
   - Health education
   - HOSA bow
   - Public service announcement
   - Medical innovation
   - Parliamentary procedure

Professional Development

SECTION 4.4

Background

Being a member of a professional organization can help you keep up with changes in the workplace. There are many other resources you will want to tap to help you develop new skills and ensure that you stay up-to-date on changes and advancements in your field. Regardless of the profession you choose, you almost always have opportunities for improving your skills and learning more about your job. Seek out additional education and training to make sure you are prepared for changes and advancement opportunities that come your way.

Objectives

When you have completed this section, you will be able to do the following:

- Match key terms with their correct meanings.
- Explain the importance of maintaining professional competency.
- List five reasons why professionals need to learn and grow.
- Describe five resources for professional development.
- Explain how to revise a career plan.
- List three reasons people change careers.

Growing As a Professional

You don't stop learning just because you graduate from school. Health science professionals need to keep learning as long as they are in their profession. Education for people who have already begun their careers is called **professional development**.

professional development (pro FESS shun ul dee VEL up ment) Education for people who have already begun their careers to help them continue to grow.

Why should a health science professional always learn and grow? There are many reasons:

- **Ethical behavior demands it.** If you are to provide the best and most up-to-date service to your patients and clients, you need to learn the latest developments in your field. It would be unethical to offer outdated, substandard care. In fact, many licensed professionals, such as doctors, nurses, and EMTs, must participate in a specific number of hours of continuing education each year to maintain their license.
- **Technology changes.** Technology in the health science industry changes rapidly. Diagnostic equipment that was unavailable a generation ago is part of routine medical care now. Computers and software programs, as seen in Figure 4.7, continue to be more powerful and useful in all aspects of health care. Each of these changes in technology enables professionals to provide new services and better care to patients and clients, but only if professionals learn to use the technology effectively.

Employability and Leadership | Chapter 4 93

FOCUS AND ENGAGE

Introduce the Section

a. Review the content of the Background paragraph, explaining that learning does not stop once you graduate.
b. Explain that health care is a field that is constantly advancing and changing, and it is vital for health care employees to stay up-to-date.
c. Discuss the objectives for the section.

Vocabulary Review

a. Key terms are defined in the margins of the text on the page where they first appear.
b. Pronounce each word, and have the students repeat the pronunciation out loud.
c. Discuss the definition of each word.

TEACH

Discuss

- Ask students if they have any experience taking classes in any subject outside of school, such as lessons in a sport or music.
- Discuss what it would be like if a health care professional who graduated 30 years ago did not keep up with professional development.
- Explain that without continuing education, that person would not be aware of many major breakthroughs and advances in the field.
- Emphasize professional competency, and how important it is to stay current with new concepts and ideas.
- Review the reasons why professionals need to learn and grow.
- Point out that in addition to making a good employee, professional development also usually contributes to job satisfaction and self-worth.

Figure Focus

4.7 Computers have dramatically changed many health care jobs. Why do you think computers have changed how hospitals store and use medical records? What should a health care worker do if the technology isn't functioning properly?

Answer: Computers can store, organize, and retrieve lots of information very quickly, which affects the way employees work, the care they deliver, and the manner in which they communicate. If the technology malfunctions, the health care worker needs to report the problem and rely on manual back-ups, such as writing information on the chart.

Teaching Tips

- Review the resources students can use for professional development.
- Emphasize that Web sites can be valuable resources, but they must be evaluated to determine whether it is safe to visit the site and whether the information is reliable.
- Discuss blogs, establishing students' understanding of the fact that information on a blog is someone's opinion, even though the writing may be based on professional training and experience.
- Explain the concept of mentoring.
- Display brochures or pamphlets from some of the resources in your area, such as local colleges or universities or employer training courses.
- Make professional journals that list development opportunities available in your classroom.

Apply It

- Discuss the various types of mentor relationships in the workplace.

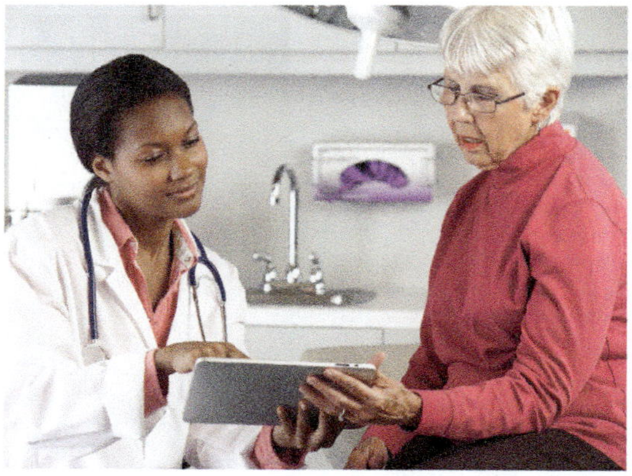

Figure 4.7
Computers have dramatically changed many health care jobs. Why do you think computers have changed how hospitals store and use medical records? What should a health care worker do if the technology isn't functioning properly?

- **Client needs change.** The population you serve as a health science professional is dynamic. An increase in the number of older people means you need to learn more about the health care needs of seniors. If you are a nurse, and a new disease or pathogen emerges and affects your patients, you need to learn how to treat patients with the new disease as best you can.
- **Responsibilities increase.** You probably want to advance in your career. As you advance, you will have new responsibilities at every stage. You need new skills to manage these responsibilities. For example, your position might grow and you might need you to know how to make a budget. If you have never have made a budget before, you need to learn how to make one.
- **Become more flexible.** By learning skills outside your own job, you are able to help your coworkers when they need it. You may learn that you like your new skills enough to move your career in a new direction.

Apply It

Not only will having a mentor help you, being a mentor can also benefit you. As you gain more experience, you may be asked to be someone else's mentor.

With a partner, role-play being the mentor and being mentored. What questions do you want to ask a mentor? What experiences can you share to help the person you are mentoring? Change roles at least once to experience both sides of the mentor equation.

mentor
(MEN tore)
A mentor is an experienced person who can offer advice and guidance.

Resources for Professional Development

There are many resources available for the professional development of people working in the health sciences:

- **Associations and Organizations.** Many professional associations and organizations provide meetings, courses, workshops, and other opportunities for professional development.
- **Employer Training Courses.** Many employers offer training courses that help develop employees. Employer programs often include workshops to improve management and communication skills and courses to help employees use new equipment and software.
- **Colleges and Universities.** Many colleges and universities offer classes that can help you learn more about your profession.
- **Journals and Blogs.** Professional journals help alert people to the latest developments in their fields. You will find many online journals and blogs on health care sites offering information and personal experiences that can provide insight into working in health care professions.
- **Mentors.** A formal or informal mentor relationship can help you in your professional development. (Figure 4.8) An experienced mentor can advise you when you are unsure about what to do in a specific situation. A mentor can also advise you more broadly about how to manage your career.

94 Chapter 4 | Employability and Leadership

- At some companies, the relationship may be casual and informal. You've simply formed the relationship because you trust the mentor and feel you can communicate freely with him or her.
- Some employers require that the arrangement be formalized through a contract that outlines both party's responsibilities.
- An increasing number of companies are establishing formal mentor programs in which personality tests are used to pair employees with other experienced workers who have volunteered to serve as a mentor for a certain period of time.

CUSTOMIZED INSTRUCTION

Less Advanced Students

Less advanced students might benefit from a mentor while still in school. Contact older students, teachers, or professionals who are willing to provide mentorship, and match them with willing students.

What's New?

Online Learning for Professional Development

Many schools, state agencies, and private companies offer distance learning courses in the health sciences. These courses are taught over the Internet. Offerings range from single classes that teach a particular skill, to entire programs, such as a Certificate of Leadership for Health Care Professionals. The programs are especially helpful to students who live in rural areas or in regions without access to a wide range of options in health science education.

Before you participate in any online learning program, make sure that the program you are interested in is offered by an accredited organization, so that your class work will be accepted by employers. The Web site of the United States Department of Education keeps a list of **accredited** institutions.

What might be one benefit and one difficulty of learning leadership skills through a distance-learning class?

accredited
(ah KRED it ted)
Approved and recognized by a governing body.

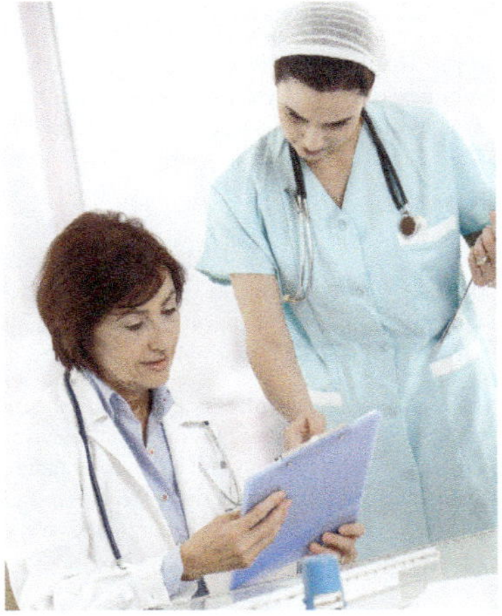

Figure 4.8
A mentor can help you develop professionally. Do mentors always have to be older than the person they are teaching?

Revising Your Career Plan

As you learned in Chapter 3, your career plan is a tool that shows you how to achieve your career goals. You use it to identify your skills and interests, to find a career that suits your skills and interests, and to determine the type of education and training you will need to succeed. Every once in a while, you should revisit your career plan and make adjustments or corrections. Your goals might change as you develop new interests and abilities, so your career plan will change, too.

ACTIVITY

Have students establish mentor-mentee relationships with younger students. Alternatively, have them practice mentoring skills with each other to inspire and teach.

ACTIVITY

Write a letter or e-mail to a college or university that offers courses in health care occupations and ask for a course catalogue. Highlight professional development courses in the catalogue. You may be able to access the course catalogue on the Internet.

What's New?—Online Learning for Professional Development

- Review the difference between an accredited and non-accredited program.
- Discuss how to determine whether a program offers certification.

What might be one benefit and one difficulty of learning leadership skills through a distance learning class?

Answer: A benefit might be that people could have access to more courses than they have at local institutions. A difficulty might be that a subject such as leadership might be difficult to study in the abstract, without anyone to lead.

Figure Focus

4.8 A mentor can help you develop professionally. Do mentors always have to be older than the person they are teaching?

Answer: No, a mentor can be younger, but he or she should have more experience than the person learning.

CUSTOMIZED INSTRUCTION

Special Needs Students

Most special needs students have education plans that have helped guide them through their school years. Relating the concept of a career plan to the concept of the education plan may help them understand how a career plan will help guide them professionally.

Teaching Tips

- Review reasons for revisiting a career plan annually.
- Discuss the importance of working with a supervisor or mentor when reviewing a career plan.
- Emphasize the importance of having concrete and achievable goals as part of your career plan.

Teaching Tips

- Review the reasons people change their career plans.
- Emphasize that a change may be small, or it may involve a complete switch from one pathway to another.
- Discuss reasons for changing careers completely:
  - Dissatisfaction
  - New skills
  - Relocation

Section 4.4 Review Questions

1. Answer: It is important to maintain professional competency to learn and grow. Professional development, education for people who have already begun their careers, helps them continue to grow.
2. Answer: Professionals need to learn and grow because ethical behavior demands it, technology changes, clients need change, responsibilities increase, and flexibility.
3. Answer: Resources for professional development include associations, employer training courses, colleges and universities, journals, and mentors.
4. Answer: To revise a career plan, meet with a supervisor or mentor, review any professional development experiences you have had over the past year, and evaluate those experiences. Then, make a new set of learning goals for the coming year, and find concrete ways to achieve those learning goals. Discuss specific work opportunities that can help you learn and apply what you need to know.
5. Answer: People change careers because they get tired and bored, careers become outdated or replaced, and for advancement in other careers.

With a supervisor or mentor, review any professional development experiences you have had over the past year, and evaluate those experiences. If necessary, make a new set of learning goals for the coming year, and list specific ways to achieve those goals. Discuss specific work opportunities that can help you learn and apply what you need to know.

Changing Careers

When you review your career plan, you might find that you are growing in a different direction than you expected. For example, you might discover that you enjoyed training people in a new skill, and would like to make training and teaching a focus of your career.

People change careers for other reasons, too. For example:

- Some people get tired, and simply need a change.
- Some careers become outdated, and are replaced.
- Some people decide that they have a better chance of advancing professionally in another career area.

If you decide you would like to change careers, use the same process to investigate your new career that you used to find your first one. You can research on your own, as well as seek the help of career counselors and career centers.

Summary

All health science professionals must maintain their proficiency through professional development. This also provides you with opportunities to learn new skills and keep up-to-date on ethical issues, technological changes, changing client needs, and changing responsibilities.

Associations, employer training courses, colleges and universities, journals, and mentors are all resources for professional development. Many workers find that as they develop new skills and learn more about their jobs and those of others in their workplace, they might decide to pursue a different job or new career altogether. As you grow, it is important to update your career plan and adjust your goals.

Section 4.4 Review Questions

1. Explain the importance of maintaining professional competency.
2. List five reasons why professionals need to learn and grow.
3. Describe five resources for professional development.
4. Explain how to revise a career plan.
5. Name two reasons that people might decide to change careers.

96 Chapter 4 | Employability and Leadership

CHAPTER 4 REVIEW

Chapter Review Questions

1. List the primary items required on a resume. (4.1)
2. Explain ways to contact an employer. (4.1)
3. How should you greet an interviewer? (4.1)
4. What is excellence? (4.2)
5. How do employers encourage good service? (4.2)
6. What is extemporaneous speaking? (4.3)
7. Identify ways to find a professional organization. (4.3)
8. What are six words Tom Peters uses to describe a leader? (4.3)
9. An experienced professional who can help you grow in your career is a(n)__________. (4.4)
10. A(n)__________ school is one that is approved and recognized by a governing body. (4.4)

Activities

1. Use the Internet, library, chamber of commerce directory, and other resources to identify companies or organizations in your community that you think might hire for the following occupations: medical diagnostic technician, physical therapist, medical information management specialist, and environmental scientist.
2. Pretend you are a doctor at a small medical practice. Describe your expectations of the office's staff for the following terms:
   Punctuality __________
   Attendance __________
   Time management __________
   Communication __________
   Organizational skills __________
   Productive work habits __________
3. You are ready for a job change and are looking for a career with opportunities for using your interest in advancing health care technology. List three health care fields where advancing technology use is extensive. For each field recognize and list three personal conditions that will be impacted by changing your employment.
4. In teams of four, take a turn at conducting a meeting to welcome a new member to the department. Each member when assigned to be the leader will draft an agenda for the meeting and conduct the meeting in an effective manner. The rest of the team will rate the leader on their effectiveness (clear concise directions, including all members in the introduction, making the new team member feel welcome and valued, etc.).
5. Working with a partner, create a list of job interview dos and don'ts for a specific health science career. Take turns role playing both "good" and "bad" interviews, with each taking turns as the interviewer and interviewee.
6. Using nursing careers as the example:
   - Identify the regulatory organization that grants credentialing for registering nurses and examine the specific preparation required for receiving a registered nurse designation, e.g., education, internship, examination, etc.
   - Identify the state or national organization that grants certification for nurse assistants and examine the specific preparation required for receiving the certification, e.g., education, internship, examination, etc.
   - Examine the role of the professional associations in the governance of registered nurse credentialing, including maintaining a current license and potential causes for having the license revoked.
   - Examine the role of the organization or agency in the governance of nurse assistant certification, including maintaining a current license and potential causes for having the license revoked.

Employability and Leadership | Chapter 4 97

CHAPTER 4 REVIEW

Chapter Review Questions

1. Answer: A resume includes: Your name, address, phone number, and e-mail address; career plans; details about your education; your past work experience—paid or unpaid; honors you have earned; activities you like; skills, strengths, and abilities; and references (always ask permission to use someone as a reference).
2. Answer: Ways to contact an employer include: E-mail—follow up on a job lead or contact an employment agency, or express interest in working for a particular employer by sending an e-mail with an attached resume; cover letter—a cover letter is a sales letter and gives you a chance to sell yourself; resume—a resume allows you to provide more information about yourself, skills, qualifications, etc.; and job application—a job application gives the employer needed information and also provides an opportunity to demonstrate that you are neat and well organized.
3. Answer: You should greet an interviewer by name, smile, shake hands firmly, and stand until asked to sit.
4. Answer: Excellence is the quality of having outstanding qualities.
5. Answer: Employers demonstrate good service by encouraging personal and professional development, accountability, teamwork, and quality health care.
6. Answer: Extemporaneous speaking is composed at the spur of the moment, without preparation or notes.
7. Answer: You can find professional organizations by asking fellow employees, reading the bulletin boards at work, reading your professional journals, reading brochures, attending occupationally related inservice programs, and checking the *Occupational Outlook Handbook*.
8. Answer: Tom Peters described a leader as a cheerleader, enthusiast, nurturer, coach, facilitator, and one who unites people and works toward positive outcomes.
9. Answer: Mentor
10. Answer: Accredited

Activities

1. Direct students to make a list of the names, addresses, and phone numbers of the companies.
2. Asking the students to put themselves in the role of the employer, maybe choosing a specific title such as doctor, hospital administrator, clinic manager, or ER head nurse might help them get a better sense of the importance of each item listed. The answers will vary and a discussion regarding the answers might prove valuable. You might also mention that practicing these traits at school will help them prepare for the workplace.
3. Use of technology in health care is advancing dramatically throughout the system. You might begin by giving several suggestions for further research such as diagnostic practices, electronic health records, distance treatments, pharmacology-immunotherapies and so forth. A Google search of advancing technological use in health care practices will provide a long list of sites for the students to explore.

Sample personal conditions might be an activity where students can collectively create a listing of traits to consider when making the career selection.

4. Refer the student teams to pages 90 (Teamwork) and 91 (Leadership Skills) and conduct a brief review before beginning the activity. Suggest using the lists from both sections for the team member evaluation of each leader.
5. Encourage students to dress the part on the day of the practice interviews.
6. Refer students to the site www.ExploreHealthCareers.org for general information about nursing credentialing and certification requirements. For specific state requirements refer the students to www.ncsbn.org (National Council of State Boards of Nursing) and insert the state in the Search box for state specific data.

Case Studies

1. Direct the students to page 91 (Leadership Skills) to help guide them with their response. It might also be beneficial if you could ask a representative from the local hospital Central Service department to review and discuss the students' answers with the class and offer some suggestions for resolving the conflict.
2. Direct the students to pages 90 (Teamwork) and 91 (Leadership Skills). Lead a brief review of the two sections and ask the students to use the information to guide their reports. Or you can form teams of eight students, each taking one of the roles listed in the activity. Assign one student as the lead sports rehabilitation technician and ask that she/he describe the process they would implement to complete the training. The team members can comment on the process described. Rotate the lead role among the team members.

CHAPTER 4 REVIEW

Case Studies

1. Staff working in Central Service is having conflicts related to equity of work assignments. Several of the team members believe they are working harder than one of the others and have submitted a written complaint asking for resolution regarding the discrepancy. You have just been promoted as head of the Central Service's department, and have been assigned to resolve the complaint. Describe how you would demonstrate the leadership skills, characteristics, and responsibilities of a leader, including goal-setting and team building, in guiding the team in the adoption and implementation of new equipment.
2. The Sports Medicine clinic where you are employed has just received several new pieces of equipment that are designed to more efficiently provide rehabilitative care for those patients with injuries received while participating in sporting events. The sports medicine team is comprised of sports medicine physicians, physician assistants, registered nurses, X-ray technologists, sports medicine physical therapists, athletic trainers, physical therapist assistants, and sports rehabilitation technicians. As the lead sports rehabilitation technician, you have been assigned to work with the equipment manufacturer for training on the use of the equipment. The clinic manager has observed that you have demonstrated leadership characteristics and skills such as goal-setting and team building and has asked that you lead the entire team as the clinic is reorganized around the use of the new equipment. Describe how you would demonstrate responsibilities of a good leader including goal setting and team building in guiding the team in the adoption and implementation of the new equipment.

Thinking Critically

1. **Relationships**—First impressions are important. Why do you think most employers refuse to read a resume past the first spelling error?
2. **Cause and Effect**—There are many ways to be a leader in the health science industry, but some are more effective than others. Brainstorm a list of leadership skills. Explain why a good leader is more likely to be a coach than a naysayer.

Portfolio Connection

The cover letter, resume, and thank-you letter are the primary tools for acquiring a career in health science. There are ways to make your application packet stand out from others. Here are some of them:

- Prepare each item perfectly so that it presents you as the best possible candidate.
- Include a job objective at the top of your resume—use key phrases that indicate your special talents and desires.
- Add a statement to your cover letter that tells about your values concerning client-centered care and about teamwork.
- Add a statement to your thank-you letter that indicates your confidence in being capable of doing the job and your interest in the position.

Rewrite your cover letter, resume, and thank-you letter samples with these additional elements. If possible, locate and fill out a job application. Place them in your portfolio.

Thinking Critically

1. Direct students to consider the type of impression a spelling error might make.
2. Explain the term *naysayer*. Answers should include a thesis statement and specific examples to support the thesis.

Portfolio Connection

- Review the importance of a cover letter, resume, and thank-you letter. Advise students to spend some time looking at sample cover letters and resumes to get ideas.
- You might have samples available in the classroom, or you can direct them to reference books or Web sites.
- Encourage them to use peer reviews when working on the documents. They can learn from each other while going through the process of writing and editing.
- Advise them to use a word processor for the cover letter and resume, but to handwrite the thank-you letter.
- Point out that if they have an electronic copy of a cover letter or resume, they can easily adapt it and print it for different applications, and update it as necessary.
- Check to make sure that students have completed the assignment and added it to their portfolio.

ACTIVITY

Sometimes it makes sense to keep more than one version of a resume on file. In case you are applying for different types of jobs, you could customize your resume by emphasizing different skills, experience, or education, or by using a different job objective. In this activity, prepare a second version of your resume, customized for a different position. Write a cover letter to go with the new resume.

5 Understanding Your Legal Obligations

SECTIONS

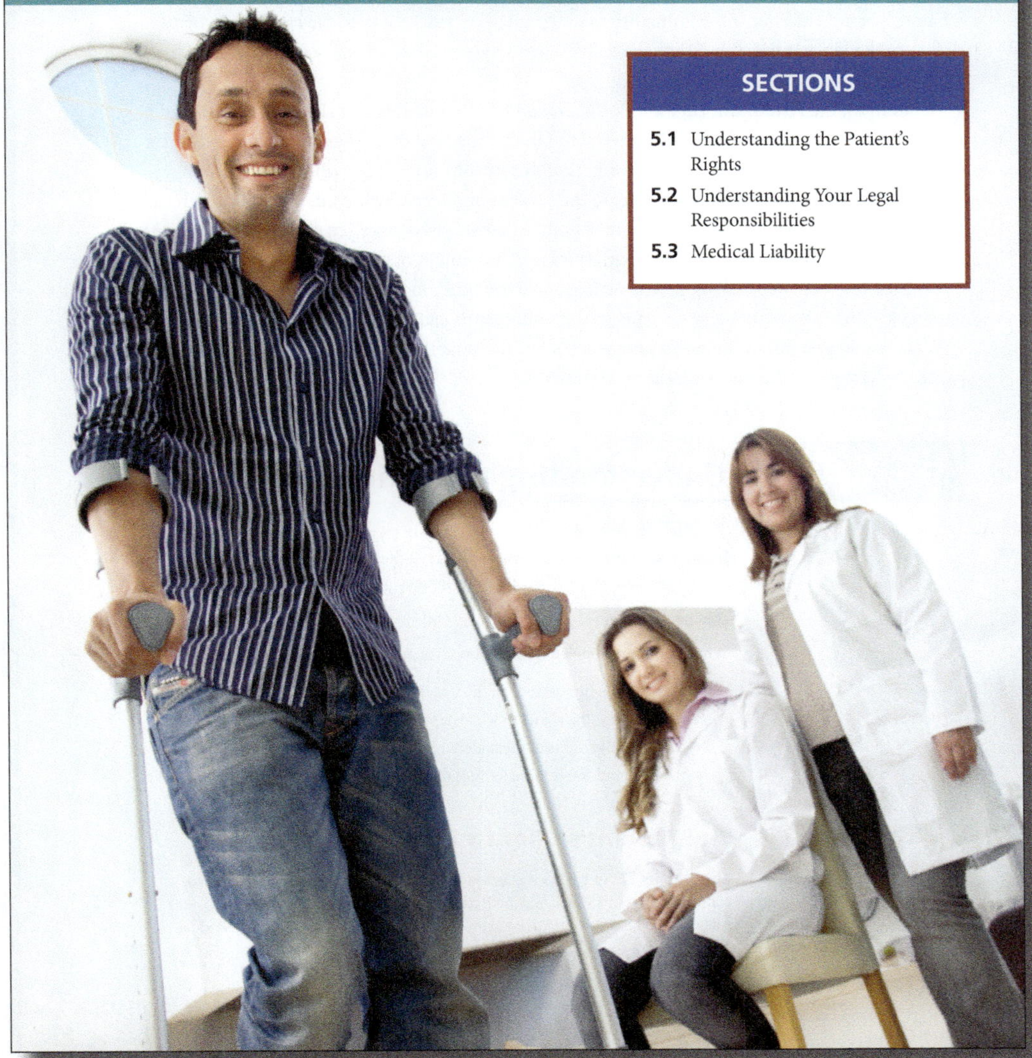

CHAPTER 5 OVERVIEW

Chapter 5 introduces the concept of an employee's legal obligations to an employer and to the patients.

Section 5.1: The first section focuses on the Patient's Bill of Rights, and covers the Nursing Home Reform Act of 1987.

Section 5.2: In Section 5.2, students learn about their legal responsibilities regarding the patient's rights and patient confidentiality. It covers resources for enduring legal compliance, the Health Insurance Portability and Accountability Act, as well as natural death guidelines and declarations.

Section 5.3: The final section covers medical liability. It explains malpractice and also discusses other legal issues, such as assault, negligence, and reasonable care.

Advance Preparation	
Review	■ Chapter text for Sections 5.1, 5.2, and 5.3, state regulations with scope of practice for health care workers, policy and procedure manual from a health care facility.
Contact	■ Health care facilities in your area to request copies of policies and procedures. ■ Guest speakers from human resources departments or legal departments to discuss legal obligations of a health care worker. ■ State regulators for information about licensing, certification, and registration of health care facilities and workers. ■ A medical facility to obtain an advance directive form.
Prepare	■ Magazine and newspaper articles on topics such as medical malpractice and patients' rights. ■ A list of Web sites that provide information about legal obligations for health care workers, such as hhs.gov, hosa.org, and your state's health and human services department.

FOCUS AND ENGAGE

Getting Started

- This activity encourages students to start thinking about confidentiality.
- Encourage students to make this activity personal—to put themselves in the position of the staff and then in the position of the patient.
- You might want to have students complete the activity at the beginning of the chapter and then again at the end to see how their responses change.
- This activity could be done in groups.

Introduce the Section

a. Review the content of the Background paragraph, explaining that legal obligations and responsibilities protect the employee as well as the patient and the employer.
b. Emphasize that the Patient's Bill of Rights is not a law, but rather a generally accepted policy.
c. Discuss the objectives for the section.

Vocabulary Review

a. Key terms are defined in the margins of the text on the page where they first appear.
b. Pronounce each word, and have the students repeat the pronunciation out loud.
c. Discuss the definition of each word.

Getting Started

As you will learn in this chapter, the right to privacy regarding health care practices and procedures as well as a patient's condition is a legal responsibility of the entire health care workforce. There are two documents that underscore this responsibility. The Patient's Bill of Rights outlines a patient's rights and responsibilities during a hospital stay. It assures that patients' needs are met in a fair, respectful, and non-discriminatory manner; gives patients a way to file complaints or address problems regarding the care they receive; encourages patients to take an active role in their health; and ensures confidentiality.

In addition, the Health Information Portability and Accountability Act (HIPAA) was signed into law in 1996. The law creates a national standard for medical privacy and gives patients greater control over their personal health information. If someone knowingly violates this law, they can be fined and imprisoned, depending on the severity and intent of the offense. You may recall from a recent visit to your doctor's or dentist's office that you were asked to sign a form declaring that you have been made aware of HIPAA. This is a requirement of the law.

Imagine that you are working part-time in a small medical office and can hear the staff discussing a patient. You know that patients in the waiting area can also overhear the conversation.

What would you do? Write down how you believe this situation should be handled. Be prepared to share your response with the rest of the class.

SECTION 5.1 Understanding the Patient's Rights

Background

Health care team members must be aware of their legal responsibilities. This awareness protects them, the patients, their co-workers, and their work facility.

Objectives

When you have completed this section, you will be able to do the following:

- Explain the importance of the Patient's/Client's Bill of Rights.
- Understand the rights to which a patient is entitled.
- Measure the rights of the patient against the needs of the health care facility.
- Understand the responsibilities of the patient in the health care process.

The Patient's/Client's Bill of Rights

The Patient's Bill of Rights was first adopted by the American Hospital Association (AHA) in 1973. It was revised in 1992 and then again in 1996 when it was renamed the Patient Care Partnership. While many states and individual

100 Chapter 5 | Understanding Your Legal Obligations

CUSTOMIZED INSTRUCTION

English Language Learners

Have students write each key term and its pronunciation on one side of an index card and its definition on the other side.

Special Needs Students

Special needs students may have first-hand experience being treated with respect, dignity, and sensitivity—or the opposite—by professionals. Ask them to share their experiences with the class.

CUSTOMIZED INSTRUCTION OVERVIEW

Less Advanced Students	Pages 101, 114
More Advanced Students	Pages 103, 109
English Language Learners	Pages 100, 102
Special Needs Students	Pages 100, 105
At-Risk Students	Pages 101, 114

health care institutions have tailored the AHA's original version to their patient community, the basic rights have remained unchanged.

The basic rights and responsibilities covered are summarized below.

High-quality hospital care. Patients have the right to care that is provided with skill, compassion, and respect. They have the right to know the identity of physicians, nurses, and others involved in their care, as well as when those involved are students, residents, or other trainees.

Involvement in your care. Patients have the right to be involved in decisions regarding their care. They are entitled to the opportunity to discuss and request information related to specific procedures and/or treatments, the risks involved, the possible length of recuperation, and the medically reasonable alternatives and their accompanying risks and benefits. It is of equal importance that the patient provides complete and accurate information about his or her health, health plan coverage, personal health care goals and values, who will make decisions if he or she is unable to (referred to as a **durable power of attorney**), and a **living will** or advance directive, if one exists.

A clean and safe environment. Patients have the right to receive care in a facility that adheres to strict guidelines regarding safety and cleanliness. If anything unexpected and significant happens during a stay in the facility, the patient has the right to be told what happened, and any changes in their care as a result.

Protection of privacy. State and federal laws protect the privacy of the patient's medical information, including any case discussion, consultation, examination, and treatment plan. The patient is entitled to receive a Notice of Privacy Practices that outlines how their information is used, disclosed, and safeguarded. They also have the right to review information pertaining to their medical care and must be informed of the procedures for obtaining a copy of this information.

Continuity of care. Patients have the right to expect reasonable **continuity of care** when appropriate, and to be informed of realistic patient care options that are available for when they leave the hospital. This includes information on self-care as well as referrals and caregivers outside the hospital.

Help with your bill and filing insurance claims. Patients have the right to be informed of the hospital's charges for services and available payment methods. The health care institution is responsible for filing claims for you with health care insurers and other programs such as Medicare and Medicaid. If a patient does not have health coverage, most providers will try to help the patient find financial help or make other arrangements.

Health Care Consumer Responsibilities

As a recipient of health care services, the consumer also has responsibilities of self-advocacy as a part of the health care team. Some of these responsibilities include:

- Be an informed consumer. Local health care facilities can provide health care navigators that can translate confusing terminology, procedures, and other care options.

Apply It

A bill of rights is a document that sets limitations in order to guarantee rights. As a class, hold a round-table discussion about the situations in which patients find themselves in hospitals and other health care settings.

Discuss the ways in which cultural, social and ethical issues affect consumers' needs and rights when they are patients or health care clients. Explain the benefits of a document such as a "bill of rights" for health care workers and patients.

durable power of attorney
(DYUR e bul pou r of e tur nee)
A type of advance medical directive in which legal documents provide the power of attorney (the authorization to act on someone else's behalf in a legal or business matter) to another person in the case of an incapacitating medical condition.

living will
(LIV ing will)
A will in which the signer requests not to be kept alive by medical life-support systems in the event of a terminal illness.

continuity of care
(KON te noo it tee of kaar)
Process by which the patient and the physician are cooperatively involved in ongoing health care management.

Understanding Your Legal Obligations | Chapter 5 101

TEACH

Reinforce and Review

- Review the codes of conduct for health care employees and employers.
- Reinforce the qualities and characteristics that make a good employee.

Teaching Tips

- Discuss the importance of protecting the rights of the patients in a health care facility.
- If possible, have your state's laws or regulations available for reference.
- Emphasize the need for cooperation and communication between the patient and the care givers.
- Point out that the Bill of Rights helps a facility understand and implement its responsibilities.
- Discuss the concept of continuity of care.
- Ask students to think of how a lack of respect for a patient's rights might negatively impact care, and how it might negatively impact the care facility. For example, it might lead to the revocation of a license to operate, or even legal action against the facility.

Apply It

- Before the round-table discussion, make sure students can identify cultural, social and ethical issues that could affect a person's needs as they relate to health care. These topics are discussed in detail in Chapter 6.
- Guide students to begin their round-table discussion, but encourage and allow them to carry out the discussion on their own.
- Be sure students address appropriate cultural, social and ethical issues that patients may encounter.

ACTIVITY

Create a chart with four columns. In the first column list the basic rights and responsibilities in a Patient's Bill of Rights. In the other columns, list how each item benefits the patient, the caregiver, and the health care facility.

CUSTOMIZED INSTRUCTION

Less Advanced/At-Risk Students

Make sure students understand what a bill of rights represents. Provide a copy of the U.S. Bill of Rights. Ask them to comment on the value of such documents in protecting the individual's rights.

Teaching Tips

- Remind students that the PPACA was signed into law in 2010. Through it, the health insurance "marketplace" was established to provide subsidized insurance plans that provide individuals, families, and small businesses with free or low-cost health insurance coverage. Discuss current changes in the law.
- Emphasize that the Omnibus Budget Reconciliation Act is specifically for nursing home facilities.
- Read the guidelines and the Resident's Bill of Rights out loud.
- Discuss reasons why the Patient's Bill of Rights might not have protected nursing home residents, making it necessary to pass OBRA.
- Point out that nursing home residents are typically more vulnerable than other patients.
- Ask students to share personal stories about members of their own families who have required nursing home care.

Career-Ready Practices

- Students may refer to the rights summarized on the previous page of the text or review other similar documents online.
- Make sure they keep in mind that a Patient's Bill of Rights should be designed to benefit not only the patient, but also the caregiver and the health care facility.
- This activity gives students real-world experience in applying the following Career-Ready Practice: Model Integrity, Ethical Leadership and Effective Management.
- For more information on the Career-Ready Practices, visit careertech.org/career-ready-practices.

Career-Ready Practices

A patient's bill of rights is an important tool that demonstrate's a health care provider's commitment to providing high-quality, ethical, and effective care to all patients/clients. Assume you have joined a team of physicians who are opening a private practice. You are charged with preparing the official Patient's Bill of Rights. Work in teams of three to four to create a document that explains these rights.

As a career-ready individual, it is important for you to understand how this document reflects on the integrity and commitment of the organization, and can positively impact the direction and actions of your team. You recognize the short-term and long-term effects it can have on productivity, morale, and organizational culture. When your document is complete, share it with the class.

- Communicate openly with health care providers.
- Actively participate in the health care provided or prescribed.
- Be respectful of health care providers. Concerns and problems with care should be reported to the appropriate team member in a timely manner.

Affordable Care Act Provides Additional Rights

With passage of the Patient Protection and Affordable Care Act (PPACA) in 2010, patients now have additional rights and protections related to health care coverage and insurance. These include the following:

- Insurers cannot discriminate against children with pre-existing conditions.
- Insurers cannot drop coverage due to an unintentional mistake on your application.
- Insurers cannot put a lifetime limit on the amount of coverage.
- When purchasing or joining a new health plan, consumers have the right to choose their own doctor from the plan's network of doctors.
- Insurers are banned from charging more for emergency services obtained at an out-of-network facility.
- Consumers who purchase or join a new plan are guaranteed the right to appeal insurance company decisions to an independent third party.
- Young adults are allowed to remain on their parent's health plan until their 26th birthday, unless they have coverage through an employer.
- If consumers join or purchase a new health plan, they will receive recommended preventive care with no out-of-pocket cost. This includes mammograms, colonoscopies, immunizations, and prenatal and new baby care.

Omnibus Budget Reconciliation Act

The Omnibus Budget Reconciliation Act (OBRA) was passed in 1987 to implement certain basic patient rights and guidelines for nursing home care facilities.

Nursing Home Reform Act

The OBRA guidelines suggest that:

1. Each resident be fully evaluated upon admission and each year after in regards to health, memory, hobbies, habits, etc.
2. A plan be created to maintain and possibly improve the resident's condition.
3. Patients have rights to a doctor and—if they can't find one on their own—the medical director of the nursing home will help them find one.
4. Patients have a right to be informed about treatment, and to refuse if desired.
5. Patients have a right to privacy and a right to complain without fear of reprisal.

OBRA also contains the Resident's Bill of Rights, which is similar to the Patient's Bill of Rights. This specifically addresses:

102 Chapter 5 | Understanding Your Legal Obligations

CUSTOMIZED INSTRUCTION

English Language Learners

With a partner, have students take turns reading aloud the Resident's Bill of Rights.

ACTIVITY

Have students obtain copies of the patient's bill of rights from at least two local health care agencies and compare them.

- Free choice of doctor, treatment, care, and participation in research
- Freedom from abuse and chemical or physical restraints
- Privacy and confidentiality of medical records
- Accommodation of needs and choice regarding activities, schedules, and health care
- The ability to voice grievances without fear
- Organization and participation in family/resident groups and in social, religious, and community activities
- Ability to manage their personal funds and use personal possessions
- Unlimited access to immediate family and can share room with spouse if both are residents
- Access to information about medical benefits, medical records, things wrong with the facility, and advocacy groups including ombudsman
- The ability to stay in the facility and not be transferred or discharged except for medical reasons, failure to pay, or if the facility cannot meet the patient's needs

Language Arts Link

Patient's Bill of Rights

Hospitals and all health care facilities that provide patient care must treat patients and their families with the highest degree of courtesy, respect, and professionalism. In this section, you were introduced to the basic rights and responsibilities covered in a Patient's Bill of Rights. The American Hospital Association's official Patient's Bill of Rights—now called the Patient Care Partnership—can be found at www.aha.org/advocacy-issues/communicatingpts/pt-care-partnership.shtml.

With a partner, create a Patient's Bill of Rights that is written in your own words for patients/clients in your age group. Think about the type of information you would find helpful and reassuring if you had to stay in a hospital. What should you expect from caregivers and hospital staff during your stay? What do they expect from you? The document should be easy to read and formatted attractively. Be sure to proofread your work to see if you can improve it by making it clearer, more concise, or more interesting to read. Check the spelling and grammar and correct any errors.

Exchange your Bill of Rights with another team. Provide feedback and suggestions to each other; then revise your document as necessary.

Summary

In this section, you learned that the Patient's/Client's Bill of Rights is a document originally written by the American Hospital Association outlining expected patient/client rights while in a hospital. Health care workers are legally bound to provide care as stated in the Patient's/Client's Bill of Rights. Remember that to receive the best health care, patients, or their families/surrogates, must be active participants in the process.

Understanding Your Legal Obligations | Chapter 5 103

Language Arts Link—Patient's Bill of Rights

- Note that this activity should be completed by pairs or teams of students.
- Remind students to review the summary of rights and responsibilities presented on p. 102.
- They should also visit the Web site for the Patient Care Partnership brochure. You may want to print a copy of the brochure for each team.
- Remind students to use their own words in writing their bill of rights. While they can use the Patient Care Partnership as a guide, they should not directly copy any of its content.
- Students may want to present their Bill of Rights in a word processing document, or in a presentation software program.
- Encourage students to show respect for each other during the peer review.
- Evaluate the projects based on creativity as well as on spelling and grammar.

CUSTOMIZED INSTRUCTION

More Advanced Students

Challenge more advanced students with the following activity: Contact a health care facility in your area and ask what type of resources the facility has for resolving disputes, grievances, and conflicts, and how they make this information available to patients. Prepare a report or presentation detailing the information, and present it to the class.

Section 5.1 Review Questions

1. Answer: The Patient's/Client's Bill of Rights is intended to improve the quality of health care by protecting the patient/client, as well as involving the patient/client in health care.
2. Answer: A designated surrogate or proxy decision maker can exercise the Bill of Rights on the patient's behalf.
3. Answer: The right to continuity of care is important to ensure the patient/client continues to receive the necessary treatment and care once he or she leaves the hospital.
4. Answer: Patients or surrogates should provide information about past illnesses, hospitalizations, medications, and other matters related to health status.
5. Answer: Under the Affordable Care Act, health insurers cannot:
   - Discriminate against children with pre-existing conditions.
   - Drop coverage due to an unintentional mistake on your application.
   - Put a lifetime limit on the amount of coverage.
   - Charge more for emergency services obtained at an out-of-network facility.

Section 5.1 Review Questions

1. Why is the Patient's/Client's Bill of Rights important?
2. If a patient lacks decision-making capacity, is legally incompetent, or is a minor, who can exercise the Bill or Rights on the patient's behalf?
3. Why is continuity of care an important patient right?
4. What should patients, or their surrogates, provide to the medical center in order to insure proper treatment?
5. Name two bans that the Affordable Care Act placed on health insurers.

SECTION 5.2 Understanding Your Legal Responsibilities

Background

Health care workers must be aware of their legal responsibilities for the protection of patients/clients, co-workers, employers, and themselves. Policies are in place to ensure that everyone working in a hospital practices and monitors legal behavior. Maintaining confidentiality is a key factor in staying within legal boundaries.

Apply It

Select a health care profession that interests you. Research and list the licenses, certifications, or registrations necessary for your chosen occupation.

Find out if there are additional educational or training requirements needed to move ahead in your chosen field.

Objectives

When you have completed this section, you will be able to do the following:

- Match key terms with their correct meanings.
- Explain why understanding legal responsibilities is important.
- Explain the importance of licensure, certification, and registration in helping improve quality health care.
- Summarize the importance of confidentiality in health care.
- Identify a law that helps ensure the confidentiality of medical information.
- Identify resources that can help you report illegal or unethical behavior.
- Understand elements of a contract.
- Explain the role of natural death guidelines and declarations.
- Describe the purpose and types of advance directives.

Patient/Client Rights

It is important for health care workers to remember that patients/clients have rights that represent not only moral and ethical issues, but also rights legislated by both federal and state governments. It is each health care worker's responsibility to recognize the importance of treating patients/clients with dignity.

104 Chapter 5 | Understanding Your Legal Obligations

FOCUS AND ENGAGE

Introduce the Section

a. Review the content of the Background paragraph, emphasizing that each facility has its own policies and procedures to protect everyone involved.
b. Point out that confidentiality is one of the most important legal responsibilities, but that there are others as well, such as certification and licensing.
c. Discuss the objectives for the section.

Vocabulary Review

a. Key terms are defined in the margins of the text on the page where they first appear.
b. Pronounce each word, and have the students repeat the pronunciation out loud.
c. Discuss the definition of each word.

TEACH

Teaching Tips

- Discuss the difference between job responsibilities and legal responsibilities.
- Discuss the difference between ethical and moral versus legal responsibilities.
- Ask students if they have ever had their confidence betrayed, and if so, how it made them feel, and whether there were any serious repercussions.

Apply It

- You may need to adjust the size of the groups, depending on the class size.
- Encourage students to find out whether there are different requirements in your state.

A list of patient/client rights is meaningless unless the person working with the patient understands and follows them. All health care workers must commit to giving the best possible care—which means complying with the professional standards of care for their particular profession.

Resources for Ensuring Legal Compliance

Policies, offices, and agencies exist to ensure that everyone working in a hospital practices and monitors legal behavior. An **ombudsman** is a social worker, nurse, or trained volunteer who makes certain that the patient/client is not abused and that the person's rights are secure. Most institutions have a designated office, officer, and phone number posted for the employee to use when reporting identified problems with patients rights or institutional practice.

Other systems help ensure that health care workers are properly trained, and regulated. **Licensure**, **certification**, and **registration** identify what a health care worker may or may not do. They determine the scope of practice for the health care worker. Controls help to improve the quality of care. Although not all health occupations require licensure, certification, or registration, it is important to be aware of these controls.

- *Licensure* is given by a governmental agency when a person meets the qualifications for a particular occupation.
- *Certification* is given to individuals who meet certain predetermined criteria and standards set for their occupation.
- *Registration* is a list of individuals on an official record who meet the qualifications for an occupation (e.g., registered nurse, registered dental assistant). Registered nurses are registered with the state in which they practice. (Figure 5.1)

ombudsman
(OM budz muhn)
A social worker, nurse, or trained volunteer who ensures that patients are properly cared for and respected.

licensure
(LIE sen sher)
A process by which a governmental agency or other authority gives permission to a person or health care organization to operate or to work in a profession.

certification
(ser tuh fi KAY shun)
A process by which an individual is evaluated and recognized as meeting certain predetermined criteria and standards.

registration
(rej uh STRAY shun)
A list of individuals on an official record who meet the qualifications for an occupation.

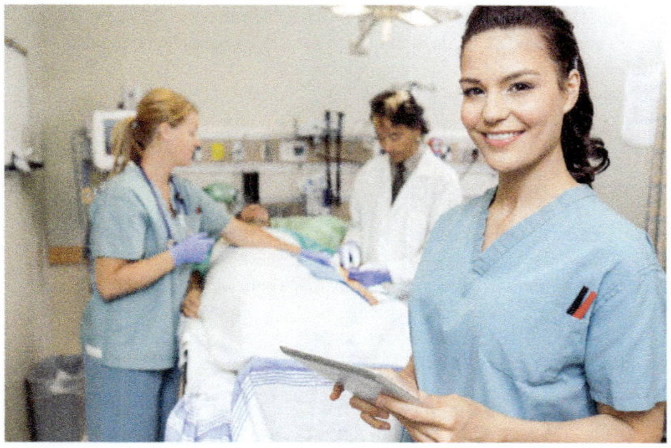

Figure 5.1
A registered nurse must be licensed to practice nursing. Why do you think states license nurses?

Understanding Your Legal Obligations | Chapter 5 105

Teaching Tips

- Review the resources for legal compliance.
- Discuss the role and importance of an ombudsman.
- Be sure to spend adequate time on licensing, certification, and registration requirements. Present handouts listing some of the licensing requirements for facilities and for care givers in your area.
- Emphasize the importance of understanding scope of practice—e.g., an RN (registered nurse) may do more procedures than an LPN/LVN (licensed vocational nurse); an LPN/LVN may do more than an NA (nurse assistant). Working out of the scope of practice can cause you to lose your job and/or your certification or licensure.
- You may also want to discuss some jobs or facilities that do not require licensing, certification, or registration.

Figure Focus

5.1 A registered nurse must be licensed to practice nursing. Why do you think states license nurses?

Answer: States license nurses to ensure that nurses are properly trained and educated before they practice.

CUSTOMIZED INSTRUCTION

Special Needs Students

Provide information about accommodations for special needs students in regards to licensing or certification.

Teaching Tips

- Discuss confidentiality. Give examples of when breaking a confidence is acceptable.
- Emphasize that breaching confidentiality leads to legal action, loss of job, etc.
- Note that there are exceptions for situations when there is a legal obligation to break the confidence.
- Point out that the age of consent for health care decisions is 18.
- Under 18, a parent or guardian makes health care decisions.
- Over 18, care givers cannot discuss the patient's care with anyone—even a parent or guardian—without signed consent from the patient.
- Ask students who might be 18 if they have ever signed a consent form so a care giver may discuss his or her health with a parent or guardian.
- Discuss the difference between and legal implications of written consent versus oral—spoken—consent.
- Review the Health Insurance Portability and Accountability Act, and why it is important.

Policies and Procedures

- Differentiate between policies and procedures.
- Ask students for examples of policies and examples of procedures.
- Discuss different policies and procedures in place in the classroom and in the school.
- Discuss why policies and procedures are important in the workplace.

Policies and Procedures

A policy is a principle, or rule, that guides decisions and actions in order to achieve as consistent an outcome as possible. A procedure is a series of steps also intended to achieve as consistent an outcome as possible, but for a specific task.

A health care facility develops and enacts policies and procedures to ensure patient safety and as a means of making sure that the facility is in compliance with legal requirements.

A policies and procedures manual includes descriptions of how to carry out all tasks, so workers have information to do their jobs properly. Policies and procedures are intended to provide guidance and information for workers.

Confidentiality

One of the most important aspects of patient/client care is confidentiality. Patient/client information is confidential. *Confidential* means "secret." Health care workers are obligated to protect and keep *all* patient/client information confidential. A good rule is to discuss a patient/client only when the discussion affects his or her care in some way; for example:

- When you find candy with the belongings of a diabetic
- When you find alcohol or medications with the belongings of a patient/client
- When patients discuss areas of stress in their personal life, such as financial problems or relationship problems

Even when a patient discusses information that does not pertain to his or her care, it is still subject to confidentiality. For example, a patient mentions that her sister is married to a local public official and has information about an upcoming ordinance that will affect property tax rates. This information is privileged communication and should be kept in confidence.

A medical facility, a physician, or a health care worker can be fined, sued, or lose his or her job for sharing *any* information about patients/clients with others, including family members. You must report any violation of patient confidentiality.

This *privileged communication* covers any personal or private information given by a patient/client to medical personnel that is **relevant** to his or her care. For example, a health care worker should consider all information in the patient chart as privileged communication.

Patients must provide **written consent** for many procedures affecting their care and for the release of medical information pertaining to their care. This includes *agreement*, usually written, given by a patient for surgery, experimental treatment, etc., after having been informed of the potential medical risks. It also includes any *legal document*, signed by the patient or his designee, stating that the patient understands any potential medical risks in surgery, experimental treatment, etc. Written consent is preferred because it is considered expressed consent, which is generally more legally defensible than implied consent.

relevant
(REL uh vuhnt)
Pertaining to, or having to do with, the patient/client.

written consent
(RIT en kon scent)
A person knowingly, without duress or coercion, clearly and explicitly consents to the proposed therapy in writing.

Health Insurance Portability and Accountability Act (HIPAA)
A law that includes regulations ensuring the privacy of patient information.

The Health Insurance Portability and Accountability Act (HIPAA)

A patient's medical information is protected by the **Health Insurance Portability and Accountability Act (HIPAA)**. This law regulates the sharing of medical information. Regulations in the act help ensure that a patient's medical information is kept secure and confidential. All employees of a health care system are required to comply with the HIPAA regulations that apply to their jobs. What kinds of information are protected by HIPAA? Here are a few examples:

- Information in medical records
- Conversations between health care providers about patient care or treatment (**Figure 5.2**)

- Health insurance information
- Patient billing information

As with a confidentiality violation of a patient's personal information, a violation of confidentiality regarding a patient's medical information must be reported.

Confidential communications are protected under law against any disclosure (forced or voluntary) over the objection of the patient. The rationale behind the rule is that a level of trust must exist between a physician and the patient so that the physician can properly treat the patient. If the patient were fearful of telling the truth to the physician because he or she believed the physician would report such behavior to others, then the treatment process could be far more difficult.

However, certain information may be considered **exempt**, such as suspected fraud, births and deaths, and illnesses and injuries caused by violence, including child abuse, drug abuse, communicable diseases, and sexually transmitted diseases (STDs). We know that, as the relationship between patients and health care professionals grows more complex, the definition of "privileged" or "confidential" information will be called into question.

exempt
(egg ZEM p t)
To be free or released from some liability or requirement to which others are subject.

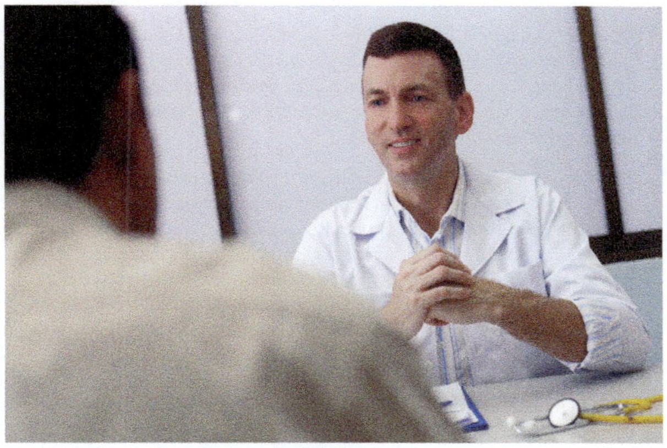

Figure 5.2
Information shared between physicians about a patient's care or treatment must be kept confidential. How does confidentiality show respect for the patient? What are the consequences of not respecting confidentiality protocols?

Understanding Elements of a Contract

As an informed health care worker, it is important to understand the elements of a contract. **Contracts** are legal documents that are often used to define the terms of patient care. It is key to remember that these contracts are geared to the needs of the patient—he or she is the **principal** concern. Examples include the document patients sign declaring that they have been made aware of the terms of HIPAA regulation, as well as advance directive documents declaring their preferences in accepting or refusing medical care under certain circumstances (discussed in the following section).

contracts
(KON trackt s)
A legally binding exchange of promises or an agreement between parties that the law will enforce.

principal
(prins si PULL)
First or among the first in importance or rank.

Teaching Tips

- Explain the concepts of privileged or confidential communications between a care giver and a patient, and discuss some exceptions, such as when illegal behavior is suspected.

Figure Focus

5.2 Information shared between physicians about a patient's care or treatment must be kept confidential. How does confidentiality show respect for the patient? What are the consequences of not respecting confidentiality protocols?

Answer: Confidentiality shows respect by treating the patient's condition as a personal matter and not just the job of the health care worker. An employee can be fired or put on notice if he or she does not follow protocols.

TEAMWORK

In small groups, perform skits depicting situations when it is wrong to break confidentiality, and when it might be right. Discuss the situations as a class.

Teaching Tips

- Review the elements of a contract, focusing on the three main elements:
  - Offer
  - Acceptance
  - Consideration
- Review the difference between an implied contract and an expressed contract.
- Allow adequate time to be sure students understand the concepts of legal documents, and why they are important.
- Emphasize that contracts are legally binding and that breaching a contract can result in legal action, such as a lawsuit.
- If possible, display examples of legal contracts or forms, pointing out the boilerplate content.
- Introduce the concept of death with dignity.
- Discuss natural death guidelines and declarations.
- If possible, have a handout of your state's laws governing natural death and declarations.
- Display an advance directive form.
- Discuss situations when an advance directive might be needed.
- Remind students that advance directives are contracts, with legal implications.

implied contracts
(im PLY d KON trackts)
Contracts in which some terms are not specifically stated, but are understood by the parties based on the nature of the transaction.

expressed contracts
(IK spres d KON trackts)
Contracts in which terms are written out in the document.

agent
(EY juh nt)
A person or business authorized to act on another's behalf.

directive
(de REK tiv)
Something that serves to guide or impel towards an action or goal.

legal disability
(LEE gull diss e BILL e tee)
A person has a disability for legal purposes if he or she has a physical or mental impairment which has a substantial and long-term adverse effect on his or her ability to carry out normal day-to-day activities.

minor
(MAHY ner)
Under the legal age of full responsibility.

Contracts are enforceable by law, and are composed of three main elements: offer, acceptance, and consideration. For a contract to be valid, one part must make an offer that the other party accepts. In many legal systems, consideration is also held to be a required component for a valid contract. Consideration means both parties bring something to the bargain specified in the agreement.

Contracts can be either implied or expressed. **Implied contracts** occur when some of the terms of the agreement are not expressed in words. An example in health care is when a patient goes to a hospital for treatment, he agrees that he will pay a fair price for the service. If he later refuses to pay for the treatment, he has breached the implied contract. **Expressed contracts** spell out the terms of the agreement in written form.

Contracts are typically made up of several parts, including boilerplate provisions and contract terms such as provisions or warranties describing what is agreed to in the contract. Parties to a contract may only take legal action for nonfulfillment of a term. Boilerplate provisions include any standardized language used in many similar contracts to govern how the contract will be administered.

Natural Death Guidelines and Declarations

For many years people were not allowed to make decisions about death with dignity. Today, new laws allow individuals to have a say in how they want to live their last days. Each state has adopted natural death guidelines and declarations that give direction to people about how to legally tell others their desire concerning end-of-life issues.

These documents ensure the individual the right to accept or refuse medical care. In the United States, every person is encouraged to prepare this document, which is called an "advance directive." Advance directives help ensure the right to accept or refuse medical care. Each state has slightly different laws that govern the interpretation of these documents. The advance directive is a written form designed to help patients communicate their wishes about medical treatment if they are unable to make decisions themselves. A formal contract will identify the **agent** or health care surrogate the patient has appointed to make decisions on his or her behalf. Then, the contract will specify the **directive**, which states the patient's wishes in the case of a terminal illness or irreversible condition. There may be additional specific requests, such as whether or not the patient wishes to be kept on life support, fed through a tube, or treated with antibiotics. The contract is then signed, witnessed by two competent adults who cannot benefit from the will, and notarized.

The advance directive takes effect when the patient is no longer able to make personal decisions about medical treatment, or if he or she is disabled. A person is considered to be under a **legal disability** if he or she is a **minor**, mentally incompetent, under the influence of drugs or alcohol, semi-conscious, or unconscious.

In the case of a minor, there is a legal mechanism that allows the minor to become emancipated. This means he or she is free from the authority of his or her parents or other legal guardians; in other words, they can make their own decisions.

108 Chapter 5 | Understanding Your Legal Obligations

Minors can be emancipated in a variety of ways—through marriage, pregnancy, economic self-sufficiency, educational degree/diploma, and military service, for example.

The agent appointed by the patient will have the authority to see that the patient's wishes are carried out. The agent is usually a spouse, adult child, relative, attorney/guardian, or other individual who the patient trusts completely.

Two common forms of advance directives are a living will and a (durable) power of attorney for health care.

Living Wills

A living will is a legal document prepared by a patient. This document gives instructions about the health care to be provided if the patient becomes terminally ill or falls into a permanent coma or persistent vegetative state. A living will is a way for the patient to make health care decisions before experiencing a health care emergency.

A living will specifies whether the patient wants to be kept on life-support machines. It specifies whether the patient wants tube feedings or artificial (IV) hydration if he or she is in a coma or persistent vegetative state.

It may also contain a Do Not Resuscitate (DNR) order. This order instructs any health care worker not to use cardiopulmonary resuscitation if the comatose or terminally ill patient experiences a life threatening event, such as a heart attack or stroke.

A living will should be on file with the patient's general health care provider. This information will be provided to any facility that is treating the patient. The physician providing treatment should add instructions from the living will to the patient's chart. Health care professionals must follow these instructions or risk legal action.

Health Care (Durable) Power of Attorney

Some patients may choose to legally appoint a health care power of attorney, or proxy. A health care proxy is a family member or close friend who is trusted to make health care decisions on behalf of the patient. A health care proxy may also be a doctor. However, a doctor who is a patient's proxy may not provide treatment and make health care decisions for the patient at the same time.

The health care proxy is asked to make decisions only when the patient can no longer think clearly or communicate. Therefore, it is important that the patient and health care proxy discuss potential medical situations and the patient's wishes for treatment before the patient becomes too ill.

The patient may also choose to write down instructions for treatment in a living will. In the event that the patient needs life support, the health care proxy works with physicians and other health care workers to carry out the patient's wishes or living will instructions.

Apply It

As a class, create a list of medical information that might be shared between a health care professional and a patient. Then, play an in-class version of *Law and Order*.

In teams of four, assign two students to be prosecutors who want evidence for a case, and two to be legal advocates who insist the information is covered under health care client privilege. Present your case to the class.

Apply It

Research the organizational policies and procedures at a health care facility in your community. Write a description of the issues and situations that the policies and procedures address. In your description, interpret at least three of the policies and explain why you think the facility provides those policies and procedures for its employees. Discuss your interpretations with a classmate.

Understanding Your Legal Obligations | Chapter 5 109

Teaching Tips

- Review the types of advance directives and the difference between them.
- Living will:
  - Lets a patient make his or her own health care decisions while he or she is able to do so.
  - Covers situations such as life support and do-not-resuscitate orders.
- Health care (durable) power of attorney:
  - Legally assigns the decision-making role to a specific person while the patient is not capable of making decisions.
  - The proxy makes decisions for the patient who cannot communicate.
  - May be combined with a living will.

Apply It

- Note that the first part of the activity involves the entire class, and the second part involves working in small groups.
- Point out that the role-playing should not be a trial, but rather arguing in front of a judge to get information made available.
- You may need to put a time limit on the activity.
- You may want to have some actual case law examples available for the class.

Apply It

- You may need to help students identify policies to interpret.
- Allow time for class discussion of the students' interpretations of policies.

ACTIVITY

Have students prepare a living will. You may wish to provide samples for them to review and use as reference.

CUSTOMIZED INSTRUCTION

More Advanced Students

Licensing and registration is not limited to individuals. Invite more advanced students to learn more about the licenses, certifications, or registrations necessary to operate different types of health care facilities. Have them focus on the requirements in your state, and report their findings to the class.

Teaching Tips

- Review the Patient Self-Determination Act.
- Discuss situations in which a living will or power of attorney might be overridden, such as when a patient is competent and alert and provides instructions directly to the physician.

TEAMWORK

As a class, discuss organ donation. Then, have students find out how they might make their intentions on organ donation known to others. They might discuss it with family members, fill out an organ donation form, or have a sticker attached to their driver's license.

A health care proxy becomes the patient's legal representative when the patient can no longer make decisions. In this situation, physicians and other health care workers must follow the instructions provided by the health care proxy. Other family members and friends do not have the legal right to override the decisions of the proxy.

If a patient recovers and is able to communicate, the patient then regains the right to make health care decisions. Health care workers must respect decisions made by the patient. The health care proxy cannot override these decisions.

Patient Self-Determination Act

The Patient Self-Determination Act (PSDA) was passed by Congress in November 1990 as an amendment to the Omnibus Budget Reconciliation Act of 1990. The law requires that most health care institutions (not individual doctors) inform a patient, at the time of admission or enrollment, of their rights, and the policies regarding advance directives in their state and in the institution itself. Patient rights include:

- The right to self-advocacy, including participating in and directing their own health care decisions
- The right to accept or refuse medical or surgical treatment
- The right to prepare an advance directive

The institution must also provide written notice about the following:

- Its policies with respect to recognizing advance directives
- Provisions for ongoing education to staff and the community on advance directives
- The prohibition of discrimination against a patient who does not have an advance directive

It is important to remember that even without a written change, a patient's wishes stated directly to the doctor generally carry more weight than a living will, health care power of attorney, or durable power of attorney, as long as the patient can decide and communicate his or her wishes.

Summary

In this section, you learned that confidentiality is an important part of staying within legal boundaries. When health care workers perform their duties within these boundaries, they help ensure the safety and welfare of everyone around them and help prevent both medical and legal problems. There are resources at your workplace to help you report unethical or illegal incidents

You also learned about the legal means by which patients can have a greater say in their final care, such as a living will or health care power of attorney.

Section 5.2 Review Questions

1. What systems help ensure that health care workers are properly trained and regulated?
2. What is an advance directive and what are the benefits of having an advance directive?
3. Summarize the importance of confidentiality in health care.
4. Identify a law that helps ensure the confidentiality of medical information.
5. In the hospital environment, what are the responsibilities of an ombudsman?
6. What are the differences between a living a will and the health care power of attorney?

Medical Liability

SECTION 5.3

Background

Understanding legal responsibilities ensures a safe work environment and prevents lawsuits. Health care workers must perform to the best of their abilities or risk legal repercussions. These repercussions can fall under criminal or civil law. **Criminal law** deals with crimes committed against the state. These include infractions such as stealing controlled substances from the hospital or stealing a patient's belongings.

Civil law covers **torts**, or wrongful acts that result in physical injury, property damages, or damages to a person's reputation for which the injured person is entitled to compensation. Torts are categorized as either intentional or unintentional (negligent). Health care workers need to understand the law as it applies to clinical (medical) negligence. Medical malpractice, one type of tort, can result from any mistake in medical treatment. For example, a health care worker mislabels a tissue sample, resulting in a misdiagnosis of breast cancer and a mastectomy.

criminal law
(KRI me nell loh)
Body of law that defines criminal offenses; deals with the apprehension, charging, and trial of suspected persons; and sets penalties applicable to convicted offenders.

civil law
(SI vel loh)
The body of law governing certain relationships between people, such as marriage, contracts, and torts (injuries).

tort
(TORT)
Under civil law, a wrong committed by one person against another.

Objectives

When you have completed this section, you will be able to do the following:

- Match key terms with their correct meanings.
- Explain the difference between civil law and criminal law.
- Explain scope of practice.
- Explain medical liability.
- Explain medical malpractice.
- List six common categories of medical malpractice.
- Provide examples of behaviors that are infractions of medical torts.

Understanding Your Legal Obligations | Chapter 5 111

Section 5.2 Review Questions

1. Answer: An ombudsman, licensure, certification, and registration are systems that help ensure health care workers are properly trained and regulated.
2. Answer: The advance directive contract is designed to help patients communicate their wishes about medical treatment at a time in which illness or injury makes them unable to make their wishes known. Advance directives help ensure the right to accept or refuse medical care.
3. Answer: One of the most important aspects of patient/client care is confidentiality. Patient/client information is confidential. Confidential means "secret." Health care workers are obligated to protect and keep all patient/client information confidential. A good rule is to discuss a patient/client only when the discussion affects his or her care in some way.
4. Answer: HIPAA is a law that helps ensure the confidentiality of medical information.
5. Answer: An ombudsman is a social worker, nurse, or trained volunteer who makes certain that the patient/client is not abused and that the person's rights are secure.
6. Answer: A living will is a legal document prepared by a patient. This document gives instructions about the health care to be provided if the patient becomes terminally ill or falls into a permanent coma or persistent vegetative state. A living will is a way for the patient to make health care decisions before experiencing a health-care emergency. The health care proxy (durable power of attorney) is asked to make decisions only when the patient can no longer think clearly or communicate. A health care proxy becomes the patient's legal representative when the patient can no longer make decisions.

FOCUS AND ENGAGE

Introduce the Section

a. Review the content of the Background paragraph, discussing the difference between criminal law and civil law, and defining malpractice and liability.
b. Emphasize that these laws ensure patient safety.
c. Discuss the objectives for the section.

Vocabulary Review

a. Key terms are defined in the margins of the text on the page where they first appear.
b. Pronounce each word, and have the students repeat the pronunciation out loud.
c. Discuss the definition of each word.

TEACH

Discuss

- Differentiate between criminal and civil law.
- Discuss ways in which laws apply to health care workers.
- Discuss professional standards of care and scope of practice.
- Emphasize that legal parameters have increased importance in emergency situations.

Reinforce and Review

- Point out that there are consequences for any illegal behavior on the part of a health care professional.
- Review the Patient's Bill of Rights and other legal, moral, and ethical obligations and responsibilities of a health care worker.
- Emphasize that each health care occupation has limits of authority and responsibility and that they must understand the particular limits for any health care profession in which they work.
- Discuss state statutes and administrative codes that apply to health care occupations.
- Point out that health care workers must be aware of care that would be considered reasonably prudent for that profession.

Teaching Tips

- Ask students to explain what it means to operate within the "scope of care."
- Ask students to describe emergency situations and discuss the legal implications of care that must be administered to patients in those situations.
- Discuss the concept of malpractice.
- Emphasize that malpractice leads to faulty care or neglect.
- Point out that malpractice does not necessarily refer to any specific action, but rather to any action that causes harm or neglect.

prudent
(PRU dent)
Careful or cautious.

scope of practice
(SKOHP uv PRAK tis)
A legal set of directives developed by a state board that governs practice for a health care professional.

Apply It

The scope of practice for a health care occupation is usually determined by a state board. Select an occupation that interests you and research your state's legal scope of practice for that occupation. Compile your findings with your classmates' and compare and contrast the scope of practice for different health care occupations.

malpractice
(mal PRAK tis)
Failure of a professional person, such as a physician, to render proper services through ignorance or negligence or through criminal intent, especially when injury or loss follows.

liable
(LAHY uh bul)
Legally responsible.

diagnosis
(die ug NO sis)
The identification of a medical condition.

informed consent
(in FORMD kun SENT)
The legal condition in which a person agrees to terms, after he or she understands all the facts and implications of an action or event.

Professional Standards of Care and Scope of Practice

A professional standard of care is based on the standard that would be used by a reasonably **prudent** professional in that line of work. Professional standards of care are specific to professions. For example, a medical assistant is not held to the same standard of care as a physician. Health care workers must always remember, however, that their actions have legal consequences. To that end, there are laws that authorize the **scope of practice**—or scope of care—under which health care workers operate, or function. For example, there are tasks that are within the scope of practice for a registered nurse, such as administering medications, and there are tasks that are *not* within the registered nurse's scope of practice, such as prescribing medications.

In any health care setting, a worker must limit the methods and procedures he or she uses to the appropriate legal scope of practice for his or her health occupation. A health care facility's policies and procedures manual provides further guidelines as to the authority and responsibilities of each type of health care worker in that facility.

Understanding Medical Liabilities

Health care workers are obliged to do everything they can to offer high-quality care to their patients and take steps to reduce errors. If it is determined that a health care worker provides less than the best quality care, he or she may be guilty of committing medical **malpractice**. Malpractice means "bad practice"—care that leads to faulty practice or neglect. Malpractice is a commonly heard term, but actually refers to one type of unintentional tort. For example, suppose a construction worker accidentally pokes his hand on a rusty nail. He goes to the emergency room and the doctor who sees him does not order a tetanus shot or check to see when he last had one. The construction worker is later stricken with lockjaw. This action would be considered malpractice. The doctor could be held legally responsible, or **liable**, for his actions.

In medical malpractice lawsuits, the legal system examines the facts of each case and determines whether or not the health care professional is guilty.

The types of errors that can lead to medical malpractice lawsuits include inaccurate **diagnosis**, failure to diagnose a condition, lack of **informed consent**, and mistakes during surgery.

Just because a mistake was made and a lawsuit was filed, the professional who made the mistake has not necessarily committed medical malpractice. All the facts are presented to the legal system and the decision is made by a jury or judge.

- Discuss ways health care workers other than physicians might be responsible for malpractice.
- Emphasize how understanding one's responsibilities can help stop malpractice before it occurs.
- Point out to students that a facility's policies and procedures manual should reflect federal and state legislation regarding health care professionals' legal responsibilities; staying current with that manual will help them avoid legal difficulties.

Apply It

- Provide enough time to complete this assignment.
- Have students write a description of the scope of practice for the occupation they selected.
- Allow an opportunity for students to review their classmates' findings so that they can compare and contrast.

Language Arts Link

Tort Law

A tort is a wrongful act that results in physical injury, property damages, or damages to a person's reputation. Tort law usually provides the victim with rights to compensation for the damages done.

Using the Internet or a library, research the different types of tort law. Select one that interests you and find a medical case example. In your word processing program, write a report about the case describing each party's claim, how they supported their claims, and the result.

Check the spelling and grammar and correct any errors. Be sure to cite any sources that you use in the format required by your teacher.

Exchange reports with a classmate. Provide feedback and corrections as necessary. Read your classmate's comments and revise your report as necessary.

Other Legal Issues

In addition to medical malpractice, workers in the health care field need to be aware of the following issues that may arise in the workplace:

- *Assault* is a threat or an attempt to injure another person. *Example:* A health care worker threatens to hit a patient/client or co-worker.
- *Battery* is the unlawful touching of another person without his or her consent, with or without **resultant** injury. Assault and battery are often charged together because of the successful attempt to injure. Both assault and battery are violations of criminal law, but they may also be subject to a civil lawsuit filed by a patient to recoup damages. *Example:* A health care worker hits a patient/client or co-worker; or a doctor operates on a patient without obtaining a signed consent form.
- *Felony* is a serious criminal offense that carries a penalty of imprisonment for more than one year and possibly the death penalty. *Example:* A health care worker withholds treatment for a terminally ill patient, which causes the patient's premature death.
- *Harassment* is any verbal or physical abuse of a person because of race, religion, age, gender, or disability. Any conduct that creates significant anguish for another person is harassment. Both state and federal criminal laws apply to harassment, but a civil lawsuit for harassment may also be filed. *Example:* A health care worker makes a joke about the religion of a patient.
- *Libel* is writing untrue matter that is **defamatory** about an individual or group to a third party. Libel is a violation that pertains to civil law. *Example:* A newspaper writes damaging information about a local health care institution. The information is false. The paper is charged with libel. What you write in a patient record could be libelous if you make a

resultant
(ri ZUHL tunt)
Resulting from an action.

defamatory
(dee FAM uh tor ee)
Statement that causes injury to another's reputation.

Health Care Legislation

Federal and state laws regarding health care are continually updated and revised. It is the responsibility of a health care worker to stay up-to-date with legislation that affects the profession in which he or she works.

Information about legislation that specifically applies to health care facilities is presented in policies and procedures manuals. Workers must read their manuals in order to know the laws that apply to the facilities where they work. In addition, they must pay attention to e-mails, memos, and other correspondence about changes to policies and procedures.

Understanding Your Legal Obligations | Chapter 5 113

- Review the types of errors that might lead to malpractice, emphasizing that this is not a complete list.
- Provide examples of malpractice.
- Provide examples of methods for medical error reduction and prevention in various health care settings.
- Emphasize that health care workers must not practice any methods outside the appropriate scope of practice set of methods for their particular occupations.
- Provide examples of situations when a charge of malpractice might be made, but the professional is not found liable.
- Discuss how legislation affects a health care worker's scope of care.

TEAMWORK

Divide the class into two teams. Ask each team to think up illegal scenarios that might occur in a health care facility and write them on separate index cards. Randomly select a scenario and ask team one to identify whether it is criminal or civil. Select a different scenario and ask team two the same question. The team that identifies the most correctly wins.

Language Arts Link—Tort Law

- Review the definition of tort law, and how it applies to clinical negligence.
- Remind students that a thesis statement presents their main idea, and the information in the document should support the thesis.
- Remind students about your school's Internet policy and emphasize that they should use reputable Web resources. Remind them to keep a list of sources.
- If students do not have access to the Internet, be sure to direct them to other resources, such as books and periodicals.
- Evaluate the document based on whether the facts are correct and support the thesis, on its organization, and on spelling and grammatical errors.

Health Care Legislation

- Point out that continuing education and lifelong learning are as beneficial to the health care worker as staying up-to-date with health care legislation.
- Explain that the field of health care is dynamic, with new ideas, products, and treatments being developed and introduced on an almost daily basis.
- Ask students to discuss ways they can keep up-to-date on health care issues. These include attending national and local meetings held by professional organizations; participating in online forums and chats; and subscribing to print, online, and other forms of media that focus on health care issues.

Teaching Tips

- Emphasize that there are many legal problems that might affect a health care worker.
- Discuss why it is important to understand all of the different legal responsibilities.
- Point out that these legal situations are not specific to a health care environment, but can be applied to actions that occur in a health care environment.
- Review the list of legal terms and issues.
- Emphasize invasion of privacy, and discuss how it relates to confidentiality.
- Discuss reasonable care. Note that it may seem like reasonable care is open to interpretation, but that in reality it is based on the standards of practice.

Apply It

- Provide enough time for students to prepare their presentations. Encourage them to research common misdiagnoses of ankle injuries.
- After each team's presentation, have the other class members act as a "jury" and decide if the incident qualifies as malpractice.
- After all the teams have completed their presentation, have a class discussion to determine whether the doctor and hospital are guilty of malpractice.

ACTIVITY

Make a poster or chart listing examples of the different types of errors that might lead to medical malpractice. List the types of errors in one column, and then give examples in another column. Use illustrations to embellish the poster.

misrepresentations
(mis rep ri zen TAY shuns)
Untruths; lies.

Apply It

In groups of six, you will role-play the following scenario in front of the class:

A teenage girl comes into the emergency room with a swollen ankle sustained during a soccer game. The attending doctor misdiagnoses the injury, which results in a long-term injury that later requires surgery. The girl's parents file a lawsuit against the physician and hospital.

Assign one team member to be the girl and another to be the doctor. Assign two members of the group to be the legal representatives of the physician and hospital and two members to be the legal representatives of the patient. Research state and federal laws to determine if the incident qualifies as malpractice.

obligation
(ob li GEY shuhn)
Moral responsibility.

statement such as, "Mr. M is hoarding painkillers," when in reality, Mr. M is only requesting and taking the medication that has been prescribed.

- *Slander* is a spoken statement of false charges or **misrepresentations** that defame or damage another's reputation. Slander is also a violation pertaining to civil law. *Example:* A health care worker tells friends that a patient who is well-known was treated for a drug overdose when in fact she was treated for a serious medical problem.
- *False imprisonment* is a civil tort in which a person is held or retained against his or her will. *Example:* A physician or a health care worker refuses to allow a patient to leave the hospital.
- *Invasion of privacy* is a civil tort that unlawfully makes public knowledge of any private or personal information without the consent of the wronged person. *Example:* A health care worker gives personal information to a newspaper about a patient/client or co-worker, or a health care worker leaves the door open while bathing a patient.
- *Reportable conditions*, such as *abuse*. Abuse is defined as intentionally inflicting injury or damage to another with violence or cruelty. Abuse falls under the heading of intentional torts. There are three types of abuse: physical, verbal, and sexual. The health care worker is obligated to file a confidential report to the county health department when child or adult abuse is suspected. Reports are also required when certain diseases are diagnosed. It is important to check your facility's policy and procedures manual for a current listing of reportable diseases and the procedure for reporting abuse. *Example:* A child is at the doctor's office for a checkup and the doctor sees bruises and burns and suspects child abuse.
- *Negligence* is the failure to perform in a reasonably prudent manner. The legal definition for negligence is when a person "does not do what a reasonable and careful person would do, or does do what a reasonable and careful person would not do." *Example:* A health care worker forgets to lock the brakes on a wheelchair, and the patient/client is injured.
- *Reasonable care* is the legal **obligation** of health care workers. They must perform according to the standards of practice expected in their community for comparable workers. *Example:* Drawing blood, as seen in **Figure 5.3**, takes training and skill. If a laboratory aide draws blood from a patient/client after watching the procedure several times but without proper training in the procedure, then reasonable care was not exercised.
- *Sexual harassment* is defined by federal regulations as "unwelcome sexual advances, requests for sexual favors, and other verbal and physical contact of a sexual nature." Innocent remarks, inappropriate pictures, and written material can be perceived as sexual. You can guard against harassment accusations by not making personal remarks or sexual gestures and by not participating in sexually explicit discussions around co-workers. *Example:* A co-worker gets really close and frequently touches another person when talking. The closeness and physical touch could be interpreted as sexual harassment, even if it is innocent.

CUSTOMIZED INSTRUCTION

Less Advanced Students

Legal terms and definitions may be difficult to understand. Try to provide everyday language explanations of the legal information, or direct students to a Web site such as dictionary.law.com, or nolo.com/glossary.cfm.

At-Risk Students

Make sure students understand the concept of risky behavior, which is an activity that puts your health and wellness in danger. Provide examples of risky behavior for teenagers, such as stealing, vandalism, giving out personal information online, smoking cigarettes, drinking alcohol, abusing drugs, and dropping out of school. Ask students what measures a teen could take to avoid engaging in risky behaviors.

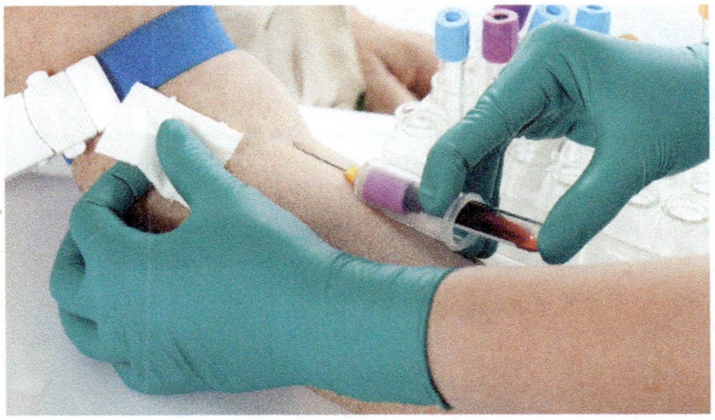

Figure 5.3
This health care professional was trained to draw blood. Why would it be dangerous to try to draw blood without proper training?

Labor Laws

Individuals employed in the health care field have the same workers' rights as those employed in other industries, as mandated by the U.S. Department of Labor (DOL). These laws are applicable to businesses, job seekers, workers, retirees, and contractors. Following is a brief description of some of the major laws:

- Wages and Hours: The Fair Labor Standards Act prescribes standards for wages and overtime pay, and the employment of minors.
- Workplace Safety and Health: The Occupational Safety and Health Act requires employers to provide their employees with work and a workplace free of recognized, serious hazards.
- Workers' Compensation: Requires employers to pay for insurance that provides cash benefits and/or medical care for workers who are injured or become ill as a direct result of their job.
- Employee Benefit Security: Regulates employers that offer pension or welfare benefits to their employees.
- The Family and Medical Leave Act: This law requires employers of 50 or more employees to give up to 12 weeks of unpaid, job-protected leave to eligible employees for the birth or adoption of a child, or for the serious illness of the employee, or a spouse, child, or parent.

- *Social media* policies determine what health care workers can and cannot post to their personal social media. These policies protect patient privacy as well as shield workers from legal troubles. Always remember that what you post online is not as private as you think and far more permanent.

Summary

Health care workers have a responsibility to provide the highest quality care within their scope of practice. A failure to provide the best care can result in lawsuits. Lawsuits are decided by the legal system based on the facts of the case. Health care workers must be aware of other legal responsibilities they face, including neglect, confidentiality and privacy laws, incorrect or missed diagnosis, etc. Being informed and staying up-to-date on the policies and procedures that govern your workplace will help you avoid legal trouble.

Section 5.3 Review Questions

1. What is a health care worker responsible for providing in order to avoid legal repercussions?
2. How can you evaluate yourself effectively?
3. What is medical malpractice?
4. Give some examples of negligence or illegal behavior that could result in legal repercussions.
5. What are the four common errors that could lead to a medical malpractice lawsuit?
6. What is slander?

Understanding Your Legal Obligations | Chapter 5 115

Figure Focus

5.3 This health care professional was trained to draw blood. Why would it be dangerous to try to draw blood without proper training?

Answer: If a person tried to draw blood without the proper training, a patient could be seriously injured.

Labor Laws

- Review the labor laws and discuss how they were enacted to protect workers in all industries.
- Emphasize the importance of understanding your rights and responsibilities as an employee as it will help you make decisions about where to work and whether or not your employer is treating you fairly.
- Discuss the issues of discrimination and harassment in the workplace. While laws are in place to prevent discrimination and harassment, employees can take measures to cope with and overcome it.

Section 5.3 Review Questions

1. Answer: Health care workers are obliged to do everything they can to offer high-quality care to their patients.
2. Answer: You can evaluate yourself effectively by keeping a journal, being honest about how you are doing, being constructive, evaluating how your work decisions affect others, and asking peers for feedback.
3. Answer: Medical malpractice is failure of a professional person, such as a physician, to render proper services through reprehensible ignorance or negligence or through criminal intent, especially when injury or loss follows.
4. Answer: Some example of negligence or illegal behavior that could result in legal repercussions include assault, battery, slander, libel, false imprisonment, invasion of privacy, and sexual harassment.
5. Answer: The errors that could lead to a medical malpractice lawsuit include inaccurate diagnosis, failure to diagnose a condition, lack of informed consent, and mistakes during surgery.
6. Answer: Slander is a spoken statement of false charges or misrepresentations that defame or damage another's reputation.

CHAPTER 5 REVIEW

Chapter Review Questions

1. Answer: The Patient's/Client's Bill of Rights is intended to improve the quality of health care by protecting the patient/client as well as involving the patient/client in health care.
2. Answer: Confidential
3. Answer: HIPAA protects information in medical records; conversations between health care providers about patient care or treatment; health insurance information; patient billing information; and most other information about a patient's health.
4. Answer: Advance directives help patients communicate their wishes about medical treatment before a time in which illness or injury makes them unable to make their wishes known.
5. Answer: An ombudsman is a social worker, nurse, or trained volunteer who makes certain that the patient/client is not abused and that the person's rights are secure.
6. Answer: Licensure is given by a governmental agency when a person meets the qualifications for a particular occupation.
7. Answer: A health care worker tells friends that a famous person was treated for a drug overdose when in fact he or she was treated for a serious medical problem, or a health worker tells a friend that a doctor is infected with AIDS and in fact is not.
8. Answer: A newspaper writes a damaging article about the chief of staff at a local hospital, reporting that he is stealing from the hospital when in fact he is making legal donations.
9. Answer: Assault
10. Answer: A scope of practice is a legal set of directives developed by a state board that governs practice for a health care professional.

CHAPTER 5 REVIEW

Chapter Review Questions

1. Explain the Patient's/Client's Bill of Rights. (5.1)
2. When something is __________, it is held in secret. (5.2)
3. What information is protected by HIPAA? (5.2)
4. Why are advance directives helpful? (5.2)
5. What does an ombudsman do? (5.2)
6. Who grants licensure, and when do they grant it? (5.2)
7. Give an example of slander. (5.3)
8. Give an example of libel. (5.3)
9. What are you guilty of if you hit a client or patient? (5.3)
10. What is a scope of practice? (5.3)

Activities

1. Review the legal issues discussed on pp. 113–114 of Section 5.3 and use the Internet or the library to research articles about these issues. Working in pairs, select three issues and investigate the legal, ethical, and professional ramifications of unacceptable or discriminatory behavior. Create a slide show presentation with at least three slides per issue: one that defines the issue; one that provides at least two examples; and one that summarizes the consequences of such behavior.
2. Working with a partner, do additional research on Health Insurance Portability and Accountability Act (HIPAA) policy standards and why compliance to these standards is so important. When you're done with your research, create a T-chart with medical information that is confidential under HIPAA on the left and information that is exempt from HIPAA on the right. Once you have your chart completed, answer the following question: Does HIPAA allow an employee to decline to disclose their own vaccine status to an employer?
3. Working with a partner, research various professional associations. Using your word processor, create a handbook describing the association and the role that professional associations play in career development. Share your handbook with your classmates.
4. Working with a partner examine various legal and ethical behavior standards. Based on what you learn, create your own set of standards.

116 Chapter 5 | Understanding Your Legal Obligations

Activities

1. Direct students to refer to the list of legal terms and issues in Section 5.3 while compiling their list.
2. Students should be familiar with how to create a T-chart, but if they are not, show them an example.
3. You may wish to compile all of the student handbooks into a master handbook that lists professional organizations.
4. Again, you may wish to compile all of the standards that students come up with into a master list of standards.

CHAPTER 5 REVIEW

Case Studies

1. A surgeon is operating on a patient's liver. While the operation is going on, the patient dies of a heart attack. The patient had a very advanced case of heart disease, but the surgeon was unaware of that problem. Do you think this is malpractice? Explain your answer.
2. A nurses' aide working in a nursing home is caring for a woman who is 95 years old and in reasonably good health. While the aide is bathing the patient, the patient has a heart attack and dies. Do you think this is malpractice? Explain your answer.

Thinking Critically

1. **Legal and Ethical**—One of your patients tells you he is worried about having no will. He has no money to pay for an attorney. How would you advise this patient? What resources are available in your community for such a person? Use this as a research opportunity. Check with the county court and the local bar association. Look for current articles about similar scenarios.
2. **Patient Education**—A patient/client asks about advance directives. Describe how you will respond.
3. **Patient's Rights**—In this chapter, you learned about the Patient's Bill of Rights adopted by the American Hospital Association. What other changes do you feel need to be made in light of recent changes and advances made in the health care field?

Portfolio Connection

Patient advocacy is a practice that defends and promotes issues that help ensure appropriate health care.

With the many challenges that affect health care today, there is a greater awareness of the need to defend patient rights. Think of three ways you can be an advocate for patients' rights. In your word processing program, write a one-page essay that explains your ideas. File it in your career portfolio.

Try to identify three ways in which you can be an advocate for patient's rights. Write a short report explaining the current status of patient's rights and include your ideas on how you can be a patient advocate.

PORTFOLIO TIP

Before you file your document, check that it is free of errors and formatted in an attractive, professional manner. Be sure to follow industry based standards as you create and collect material for your portfolio.

Understanding Your Legal Obligations | Chapter 5 117

Case Studies

1. Students should refer to Section 5.3 for information about what constitutes malpractice.
2. Students should refer to Section 5.3 for information about what constitutes malpractice.

Thinking Critically

1. Direct students to consider the consequences of not having a will. Provide time for students to research his or her response. Students should produce a written response to the patient.
2. Direct students to Section 5.2 for information on advance directives. Students should write their response, but you may also allow them to perform skits.
3. Direct students to create a list of medical advancements since 1992, and use it to guide their response to this question.

Portfolio Connection

- Explain patient advocacy.
- Point out that Patient Advocate is an actual job title, but that all health care workers should be patient advocates.
- Discuss some of the issues that might concern patient advocates.
- Web sites to recommend are patientadvocate.org and npaf.org.
- Remind students of your school's Internet policy and emphasize that they should only use reputable sites.
- Remind them to keep a list of sources for a bibliography or future reference.
- Encourage students to review their own work carefully before adding it to their portfolio, and to use a peer review to improve their work.
- Check to make sure that students have completed the assignment and added it to their portfolio.

ACTIVITY

A patient advocate might be a lawyer, a government official, a volunteer, or health care professional. Research the job to find out if it might be a career that interests you. Use Internet resources, books, and periodicals to learn about patient advocacy, and then contact a patient advocate to discuss the job. Write a job description and a career ladder for a patient advocate, including educational and certification requirements, and average salary range.

6 Medical Ethics

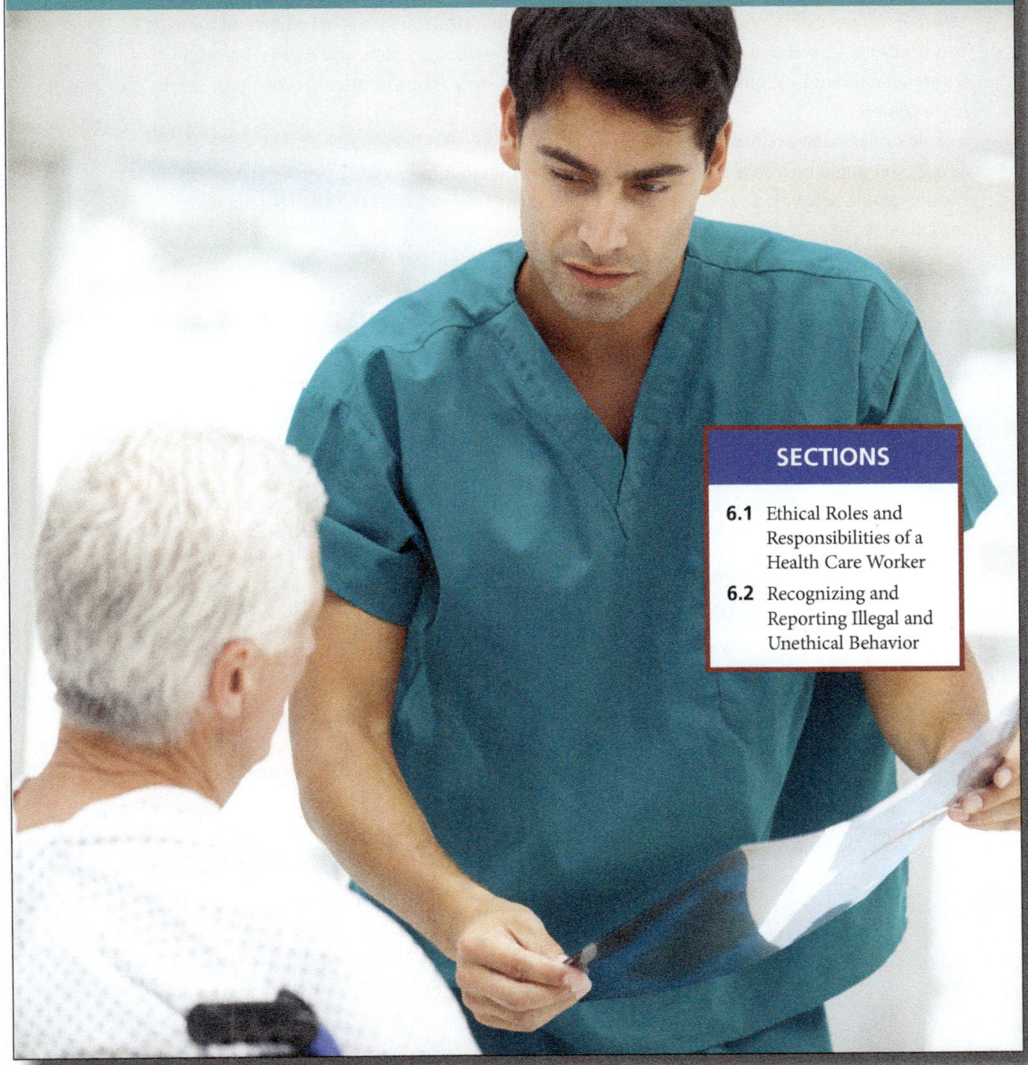

SECTIONS

CHAPTER 6 OVERVIEW

Chapter 6 focuses on the important topic of ethics and how it relates to health care workers. It covers the ethical responsibilities of health care workers and how to recognize and report unethical behavior in others.

Section 6.1: In Section 6.1, students learn how to act ethically as a responsible health care worker. Students learn the importance of the code of ethics. They learn about value indicators, and why each health care worker is responsible to his or her employer, co-workers, and patients.

Section 6.2: Section 6.2 covers how to recognize and report unethical behavior. Students learn the legal implications of unethical behavior and why it is important to report it.

Advance Preparation	
Review	■ Chapter text for Sections 6.1 and 6.2.
Contact	■ Professional organizations, state employment office, and personnel departments to request documents, pamphlets, handouts, or forms detailing their codes of ethics. ■ Guest speakers such as attorneys or health care professionals to discuss the importance of ethical behavior.
Prepare	■ Magazine and newspaper articles on topics such as ethical behavior in health care. ■ A list of Web sites that provide information about ethics in health care—such as healthpronet.org and hosa.org.

FOCUS AND ENGAGE

Getting Started

- This activity encourages students to start thinking about ethical behavior in all walks of life; not just in health care.
- Distribute information such as newspaper and magazine articles about ethics in the classroom.
- If your district offers ethics classes, invite a teacher or administrator to speak, and distribute a syllabus.

Introduce the Section

a. Review the content of the Background paragraph, discussing the role ethics plays in protecting the worker, patient, and employer, and in providing quality care.
b. Ask students if they have ever faced an ethical dilemma, such as whether to tattle on a friend, and how they dealt with it.
c. Introduce the concept of ethical responsibility as different from legal responsibility.
d. Review the objectives for the section.

Vocabulary Review

a. Key terms are defined in the margins of the text on the page where they first appear.
b. Pronounce each word, and have the students repeat the pronunciation out loud.
c. Discuss each definition.

Getting Started

You have learned that to provide the highest quality care to patients/clients, you must communicate in a clear and honest manner, be sensitive to differences, and conduct yourself in a professional and ethical manner. Ethics are a set of beliefs about what is right and what is wrong. Some ethics are established by society. They determine how people are supposed to behave, usually in terms of human rights, responsibilities, and justice. Some ethics are personal and based on what you believe to be positive character traits, such as honesty, compassion, and loyalty. Some ethics are established by groups of people, such as health care workers or members of a professional organization.

Think of examples of organizations to which you belong that have a code of ethics. For example, you might be a member of a student organization that has a code of ethics that outlines the acceptable behavior and responsibilities given to members. As a class, discuss what you think should be included in a code of ethics for your classroom.

SECTION 6.1 Ethical Roles and Responsibilities of a Health Care Worker

Background

Members of the health care team must be aware of their ethical roles and responsibilities. This awareness protects them, the patients, their co-workers, and the facility where they work. Ethical issues differ from legal issues in health care settings. Legal issues protect patients and workers because they are based on laws, which, if not obeyed, will result in legal consequences. Ethical behavior is not based on laws, but ensures quality patient care, positive work relationships, and a well-managed work environment.

Objectives

When you have completed this section, you will be able to do the following:

- Match key terms with their correct meanings.
- Summarize the code of ethics that every health care worker follows.
- Explain why following a code of ethics is important.
- Use the value indicators to explain the employee's responsibilities to his or her employer.
- Explain how each health care worker affects the health care team.
- Demonstrate communication objectives that promote patient satisfaction.

Community

Prepare a chart listing the code of ethics for a local retirement community or senior center. Compare your chart with those prepared by your classmates.

120 Chapter 6 | Medical Ethics

CUSTOMIZED INSTRUCTION
English Language Learners
Have students write each key term and its pronunciation on one side of an index card and its definition on the other side.
More Advanced Students
Instruct students to use the Internet and other resources to research how health care organizations in your area are addressing ethical issues in the workplace. Have them report their results to the class.

CUSTOMIZED INSTRUCTION OVERVIEW	
Less Advanced Students	Pages 123, 128
More Advanced Students	Pages 120, 128
English Language Learners	Pages 120, 125
Special Needs Students	Pages 124, 129
At-Risk Students	Pages 123, 129

Value Indicators

Health care workers are expected to live by values that show others respect. You show respect by treating others with dignity, demonstrating a spirit of service, performing your duties with excellence, and treating others fairly.

Medical **ethics** dates back to the Hippocratic Oath, which is widely believed to have been written by Hippocrates in the 4th century B.C. One of the earliest principles to come from this oath is to "first, do no harm." Western medical ethics have evolved to include values derived from the Muslim, Jewish, and Christian religions, including noted thinkers such as al-Razi, Maimonides, and Thomas Aquinas. In recent times, professional codes of medical ethics have incorporated legal principles to more formally spell out what conduct is expected of health care workers.

Each person determines how values are reflected in his or her day-to-day actions. An employer describes what values are important and how to demonstrate them while working. (Figure 6.1) These descriptions are usually found in an employee handbook or policy and procedure book.

Apply It

Research various codes of medical ethics from different historical periods, or for different health care professions. Choose two codes and compare them, citing differences and similarities. Identify any legal principals addressed by the codes. Prepare a brief speech for the class, explaining what you agree with in each code, and why.

ethics
(ETH iks)
Social values; conduct; description of what is right and wrong.

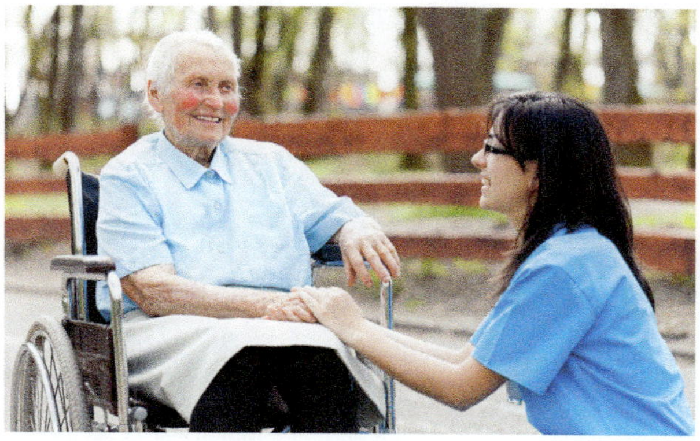

Figure 6.1
Values are reflected in your body language and your verbal responses. What kind of body language shows that you are kind?

Apply It

Invite a representative of the local organ procurement agency or an organ recipient to the classroom to discuss the legal and ethical issues pertaining to organ donation and procurement.

Common values that are emphasized in the workplace are described below:

- **Dignity.** You treat people with dignity when you are honest, truthful, trustworthy, sincere, and respectful. Always do what is needed to the best of your abilities and ask for assistance when tasks are beyond your understanding or ability. Dignity is communicated through active listening, being clean (Figure 6.2), being positive, showing understanding, demonstrating **civility**, and being respectful of all people.
- **Service.** Service means responding to patients/clients and co-workers with an understanding of their unique needs. You show kindness and patience, and make comments that are positive, courteous, and helpful.

civility
(si VIL i tee)
Exhibiting politeness and respect in communication with others.

Medical Ethics | Chapter 6 121

Apply It

- Direct students to Chapter 1 for information on medical history.
- Students should write a speech that lasts between 3 and 5 minutes.
- Encourage them to practice delivering the speech to family, friends, or in front of the mirror.
- Ask each student to prepare one or two questions to ask their classmates.
- Advise students to think about all of the possible questions, and to prepare answers.

Apply It

- If you cannot arrange for a visit from an organ procurement specialist, have the students research the topic using books and the Internet.
- Ask students to create a chart listing the pros and cons of organ donation.

TEACH

Discuss

- Explain that dignity, excellence, service, and justice influence ethical values.
- Ask students to discuss how these values are expressed in their everyday life, including family, school, and work. Prompt them to give specific examples such as how they are treated by store clerks. They may want to discuss fair treatment and respect.
- Keep in mind that some of their opinions may be negative, and that they may disagree with you on certain issues. Do not respond negatively, but use inquiry to bring further discussion. For example, say, "Tell me more."

Teaching Tips

- Explain the use of value indicators:
  - Discuss how the value indicators are expressed verbally and non-verbally.
  - Have students identify, compare, and contrast personal, professional, and organizational ethics.
  - Review the descriptions of dignity, service, excellence, and fairness/justice.
  - Discuss how the value indicators are used to categorize the health care worker's responsibilities.
  - Emphasize that together, they outline a code of ethics.
- Discuss the concept of a code of ethics: guidelines that govern proper and moral behavior.

Figure Focus

6.1 Values are reflected in your body language and your verbal responses. What kind of body language shows that you are kind?

Answer: The responses should include a smile, a gentle touch, and a friendly expression.

Community

- Allow class time for students to prepare the chart.
- Encourage students to use a word processing table to create a professional-looking chart that is easy to read.
- Allow time in class to discuss similarities and differences in students' charts.

Teaching Tips

- Discuss Patient/Customer Satisfaction in the context of excellence and service.
- Call students' attention to Table 6.3 Patient and Customer Satisfaction Guidelines on pp. 122–123.
- Discuss factors that contribute to poor customer relationships.
- Point out that, like any other type of business, health care must meet customer expectations.
- Have students list customer expectations in a health care setting.
- Point out that patients who come to a facility are external customers. Internal customers are employees of a facility involved in the process of providing services to external customers.
- Discuss the consequences of unmet customer expectations.

Figure Focus

6.2 Good grooming is important. What does good grooming tell clients and patients about you?

Answer: It tells clients that you respect them enough to be neat and clean at work.

socioeconomics
(soh see oh ek uh NOM iks)
Related to the cultural or social and financial factors of life.

appropriate
(uh PROH pree it)
Suitable, correct.

Apply It

Bioethics examines moral right and wrong within medicine and health care—organ donation, euthanasia, human cloning, and genetic engineering are just a few of the issues facing health care providers today. Choose an issue of your interest and create a list of pros and cons surrounding that issue. Share your ideas with your class, and justify each of your pros and cons.

- **Excellence.** Performance excellence is taking responsibility for yourself, your team's decisions, and the results. You adapt to changing needs by learning new skills, knowledge, and behaviors that encourage continuous improvement. Accepting and seeking feedback help you improve your performance excellence.
- **Fairness/Justice.** You treat all people with mutual respect and provide the same dignity, service, and performance excellence regardless of the patient's race, beliefs, ethnic background, or **socioeconomics**. You also use supplies and available resources effectively to provide **appropriate** care and a safe environment for everyone.

Health care workers demonstrate their core values and qualities in everything they do. **Tables 6.1** and **6.2** outline your responsibilities within each of the key value indicators for health care.

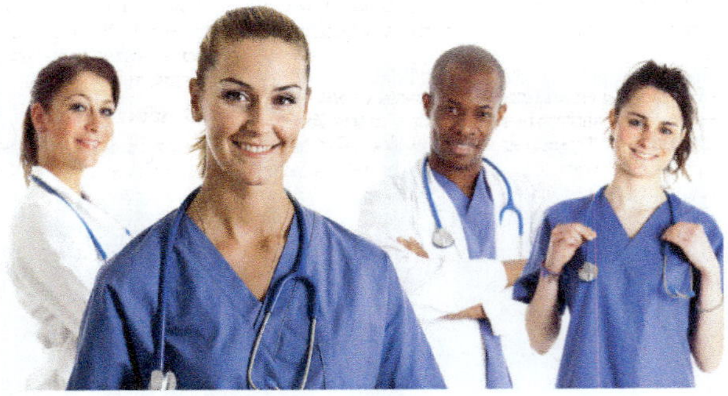

Figure 6.2
Good grooming is important. What does good grooming tell clients and patients about you?

Patient or Customer Satisfaction

Patients and clients are more than citizens with rights. They are also customers buying goods and services. Patient and customer satisfaction is an essential element in providing effective health care. Demonstrating the values of service and excellence helps patients and their families feel satisfied with the care they receive. They are told:

- What is needed
- Why it's needed
- Who will provide the service
- When it will be provided
- How it will be provided

Health care workers who successfully provide patient/client satisfaction practice the service guidelines outlined in **Table 6.3**.

When a patient's expectations are not met, there are consequences. The patient may change doctors or refuse to receive treatment from a particular health care professional in a facility. Changing caregivers can compromise a patient's care.

Career-Ready Practices

You are conducting an orientation session for new health care employees at your hospital. Your topic is the values that you expect your employees to exhibit. Make sure you discuss how an employee's actions and decisions can impact not only the patients, but also other employees and the organization in general.

It is important for career-ready individuals to recognize their roles and responsibilities on the job and consider what they can do and the tools they can use to enhance the workplace, the community, and the environment.

Create a slide show using your presentation software and share it with the class.

122 Chapter 6 | Medical Ethics

Career-Ready Practices

- Direct students to Chapter 3 for information on values.
- Students should create a presentation that lasts between 3 and 5 minutes.
- Encourage them to practice delivering the presentation to family, friends, or in front of the mirror.
- Ask each student to prepare one or two questions to ask their classmates.
- Advise students to think about all of the possible questions, and to prepare answers.
- This activity gives students real-world experience in applying the following Career-Ready Practice: Consider the Environmental, Social, and Economic Impacts of Decisions.
- For more information on the Career-Ready Practices, visit careertech.org/career-ready-practices.

In addition, the loss of a patient—or customer—is detrimental to a health care facility's business. Besides losing that patient's business, he or she may spread negative comments about the unsatisfactory care through word of mouth. To avoid negative consequences, focus on communicating successfully and respecting patients/clients.

project
(pruh JEKT)
To show or reflect.

confidential
(kon fi DEN shuhl)
Private; personal; restricted; secret.

Table 6.1 Code of Ethics

Ethics is a code of conduct representing ideal behavior for a group of people. A health care worker observes the following code of ethics. Often, health care facilities have special committees that develop the code of ethics for that facility. All health care workers at the facility are expected to know, understand, and abide by the facility's code of ethics.

Dignity	Service	Excellence	Fairness/Justice
Know your limitations. Know what you are trained to do and what you are capable of doing. *Be sincere.* Always be honest and trustworthy in the performance of your duties. Expect your salary in return for your work. Do not solicit gifts or additional money. *Be well groomed.* ■ Always clean your uniform, shoes, hair, nails, skin, teeth, and body to prevent the spread of disease-causing bacteria. ■ Be sure your uniform is free of wrinkles, tears, and runs. All buttons must match. Shoes and laces must be clean and bright. ■ Wear a name tag. It is required in most states. ■ Do not wear excessive jewelry. It harbors bacteria and can cause you or your patients injury. Wedding rings and watches are acceptable. ■ Never wear perfume or aftershave lotion. They make some people who are ill feel even worse and may trigger an allergic reaction.	*Be a good citizen.* Respond to the needs of others. Demonstrate concern for meeting those needs. *Be caring.* Try to understand the unique needs of others. Respond quickly and effectively to problems that arise while you are working.	*Be accountable.* Seek out and use feedback from others to learn. Take responsibility for yourself and for your team's actions, decisions, and results. *Be informed.* Learn from your experiences. Seek growth and development opportunities for yourself and others. *Follow the rules and regulations.* ■ Read the policies and procedures manual. ■ Practice Standard Precautions and the Bloodborne Pathogen Rule.	*Be loyal.* This applies to patients/clients, co-workers, and your employer. Always **project** a positive attitude toward the institution where you are employed. *Respect the privacy of others.* Always keep privileged information about any personal or private matter **confidential**.

Medical Ethics | Chapter 6 123

Teaching Tips

- Review Table 6.1, Code of Ethics, with the class.
- Point out that the column headings correspond to the value indicators.
- Suggest students read the table column by column instead of row by row.
- Read and discuss each statement.
- Discuss how different professions might have different codes of ethics. For example, ask students how the code of ethics for a police officer might be different or similar to the code of ethics for a salesperson.
- To reinforce the concept of a code of ethics, have the class discuss and develop a code of ethics for your classroom.
- Discuss why the code of ethics for health care workers might be more stringent than the code of ethics for a different profession.
- Distribute copies of codes of ethics from professional organizations, and have students read them out loud.

ACTIVITY

Write a paragraph about an actual situation when you or someone you know had to make an ethical decision. Alternatively, write a fictitious story about such a situation.

ACTIVITY

After reading and discussing the values listed in the text, think of other values that might be important qualities for health care professionals. List and define at least one, and then share it with the class.

CUSTOMIZED INSTRUCTION

Less Advanced Students

Less advanced students may have trouble reading the tables. Allow adequate time to read and discuss each item.

At-Risk Students

Each of the value indicators is defined in Table 6.1. Ask students to provide examples of how they apply each in their daily activities. For example, if you come to class on time, you demonstrate that you follow the rules, which falls under the Excellence value. Encourage students to think of as many examples as possible. You might want to have them work with a partner to identify in each other how they apply these values on a day-to-day basis.

TEAMWORK

In small groups, role-play a situation that depicts ethical or unethical conduct. Present the simulations to the class.

Teaching Tips

- Review the value indicators.
- Explain that they can also be used to categorize an employee's responsibility to his or her employer.
- Discuss the importance of being a responsible employee.
- Review Table 6.2, Responsibilities of an Employee.
- Again, point out that the column headings correspond to the value indicators.
- Begin a review of Table 6.3, Patient and Customer Satisfaction Guidelines.
- Explain that this table uses the Service/Excellence value indicator as its foundation.
- Discuss the relationship between communication and customer satisfaction.
- Refer students to the information regarding patient/customer satisfaction on pp. 122–123, and to keep it in mind as they review Table 6.3.

Table 6.2 Responsibilities of an Employee

Employees are required to assume certain responsibilities. The responsibilities that are most important to employers include being dependable, honest, and well groomed; displaying a good attitude; and following the rules and regulations of the organization.

Dignity	Service	Excellence	Fairness/Justice
Communicate effectively. ■ Express ideas, information, and viewpoints clearly. ■ Use active listening skills, and seek to understand others. ■ Create and maintain positive working relationships. ■ Understand and respect differences in people. ■ Be supportive of others' success when they do well.	*Have a good attitude.* ■ Be willing to help your co-workers. ■ Be aware of your body language and facial expressions, and reflect a positive outlook. ■ Be respectful by changing your behavior when it appears to irritate others. ■ Work effectively under pressure.	*Be dependable.* ■ Be on time. ■ Report in when you arrive. ■ Report to the person taking care of your assignment prior to leaving your area. ■ Do your job to the best of your ability. ■ Call your supervisor ahead of time on those occasions when you are unable to be at work.	*Be honest.* ■ Never clock in or out for another person. ■ Never take anything from the facility that is not yours. ■ Never say that you have completed a task when you have not. ■ Work with commitment and enthusiasm to improve the care patients/clients receive.

Table 6.3 Patient and Customer Satisfaction Guidelines

Communication Objective	Service/Excellence	Behavior
■ Demonstrate open, honest, and respectful communication. ■ Present ideas, information, and viewpoints clearly, both verbally and in writing. ■ Listen actively and seek to understand others. ■ Anticipate and strive to understand the unique needs of those serving as well as those served. ■ Respond to the needs of those served and demonstrate concern for meeting those needs. ■ Tailor each interaction to the specific needs of the person and/or situation. ■ Seek growth and developmental opportunities for yourself and others. ■ Adapt to changing needs by acquiring new skills, knowledge, and behaviors. ■ Learn from your experiences.	■ Welcome patients, family members, and visitors in a warm, friendly manner. ■ Listen to and communicate with one another and the people you serve. ■ Think before you speak. ■ Have respect for each person's privacy, comfort, and dignity. ■ Use good elevator manners. ■ Provide a safe, clean environment. ■ Anticipate the wants and needs of those served. ■ Strive to do your best.	■ Introduce yourself to the patient and his or her family. ■ Address the patient by Mr. or Ms. unless directed otherwise. ■ Make eye contact and smile. ■ Explain who you are and what you do. ■ Listen attentively. Do not interrupt. ■ Wear your name badge. ■ Adhere to the dress code. ■ Clarify with more questions if necessary. ■ Address the person's needs and take whatever action is necessary. ■ Do not argue. ■ Try to eliminate distractions when communicating with patients and families. ■ Communicate clearly and positively. ■ Make sure patients understand their treatment or procedures. ■ Encourage patients to ask questions. ■ Respect patient confidentiality in all settings. ■ Keep noise and conversation levels low. ■ Interview patients in private.

(continued)

124 Chapter 6 | Medical Ethics

CUSTOMIZED INSTRUCTION

Special Needs Students

Ask students who may have trouble discussing or articulating ethics and values to draw a picture illustrating one code of ethics as presented in Table 6.1.

Table 6.3 Patient and Customer Satisfaction Guidelines (continued)

Communication Objective	Service/Excellence	Behavior
		■ Close curtains and doors during exams and procedures. ■ Remember to care for the whole person—body, mind, and spirit. ■ Use the elevator as an opportunity to make a favorable impression. ■ Be friendly. ■ Remember confidentiality—do not discuss patients, their care, or any business on elevators. ■ Once on an elevator, make room for others and push the door open button for them. ■ Stand aside as others enter or exit. ■ Be alert to unsafe conditions. Correct, warn, and/or report safety hazards for immediate repair. ■ Pick up and dispose of litter. ■ Keep all areas neat, orderly, and clutter-free. ■ Be aware and sensitive to the different cultures and religious beliefs of patients. ■ Communicate any anticipated delays. ■ Be prepared to address special needs, such as hearing impairments, language barriers, and disabilities. ■ Focus on education, comfort, and privacy needs at all times. ■ Anticipate and provide appropriate comfort measures. ■ Identify better ways to serve patients and their families. ■ Be a role model. ■ Promote cooperation and teamwork. ■ Take opportunities to improve your skills. ■ Seek out and constructively use feedback from others. ■ Show appreciation and thank your co-workers.

Apply It

Because there are often difficult ethical decisions that must be made while providing health care, hospitals typically have *ethics committees*. They may be composed of physicians, chaplains, administrators, nurses, and many more. They usually are responsible for helping to guide care givers and families when uncomfortable or difficult decisions must be made. Decisions such as removing a ventilator, withholding care, and transplants are examples of such activities. Specific policies and procedures are established for each committee to follow.

Research ethics committees for your local hospital or other hospitals. Determine who comprises that committee and read about their responsibilities. Consider the pros and cons of the committee.

Why are these committees necessary? What kinds of decisions do they have to make?

Teaching Tips

- Continue reviewing Table 6.3.
- Explain that the Communication Objective column lists goals for the health care provider.
- Explain that the Service/Excellence column lists the value indicator guidelines.
- Explain that the Behavior column lists the ways the health care provider can meet the goals and practice the value of service/excellence.

TEAMWORK

In small groups, brainstorm specific examples of how a patient is a customer, purchasing goods and/or services from the health care provider. Discuss your ideas with the class.

CUSTOMIZED INSTRUCTION

English Language Learners

Ask students to comment on facial and other nonverbal expressions or gestures that provide context in their primary language. Do they provide the same context or meaning to those whose primary language is English or another language?

What's New?—Biotechnology and Ethics

- Discuss the relationship between technology and ethics.
- Explain that health care professionals work together to develop rules and codes for newly emerging technologies.
- Discuss stem cell research, and why it has been controversial.
- Ask students if they have an opinion on stem cell research.
- Ask students if they know of other technologies that might be considered controversial. For example, egg harvesting and freezing, or genetic modification.

What other kinds of diseases might be treated with stem cells?

Answer: In the future, stem cells may be useful in any application for which new tissue is needed, including creating new nerve tissue.

Section 6.1 Review Questions

1. Answer: A code of ethics represents ideal behavior for a group of people.
2. Answer: Dignity, Service, Excellence, Fairness/Justice
3. Answer: Each health care worker assumes certain responsibilities. The responsibilities that are most important to employers include being dependable, honest, and well groomed; displaying a good attitude; and following the rules and regulations of the organization. These responsibilities directly affect the health care team.

What's New?

Biotechnology and Ethics

Sometimes biotechnology allows scientists to study medical treatments that create ethical questions. Other times, it helps alleviate the ethical problems. For example, scientists have known for years that stem cells might be very useful in treating many different diseases, such as Parkinson's disease. Stem cells are very basic, undeveloped cells that can develop into many different kinds of cells. Scientists hope that one day they can grow new tissues and organs using stems cells.

Until recently, however, human stem cells were only available from tissues of human embryos. This created an ethical problem: Is it acceptable to use human embryonic tissue to help fight diseases? Is it ethical not to treat all diseases as effectively as we can? This is a case in which biotechnology presents an ethical problem.

Recently, scientists have discovered how to make human stem cells out of ordinary skin cells. This is helpful, because it's sometimes difficult to use one person's tissue in another person's body. Moreover, the new process eliminates the ethical problems associated with using human embryonic tissue. In this case, biotechnology may help alleviate an ethical dilemma.

What other kinds of diseases might be treated with stem cells?

Summary

As a health care worker, you are part of a very important team. You must demonstrate many qualities both in the care of your patients/clients and in your responsibility to your employer. Health care workers are expected to conduct themselves in an ethical manner. Ethical behavior protects you, your patients/clients, their families, the staff, and your place of employment. Dignity, service, excellence, and fairness/justice are essential for every health care worker.

Section 6.1 Review Questions

1. Explain why following a code of ethics is important.
2. What values are important in health care?
3. Explain how each health care worker affects the health care team.
4. How can good communication promote patient satisfaction?
5. Identify three behaviors from the patient and customer satisfaction guidelines.
6. Quality health care workers show a commitment to certain values, including fairness/justice. Describe some actions that show fairness/justice.

126 Chapter 6 | Medical Ethics

4. Answer: Good communication promotes patient satisfaction by demonstrating the values of service and excellence, and it helps patients, their families, and their friends feel satisfied with their care. Health care is given with respect and with a sincere attitude.
5. Answer: Answers will vary but might include: make eye contact and smile, listen, address the patient's needs, make sure patients understand their treatment and procedures, respect patient confidentiality, and be aware of cultural differences.
6. Answer: Answers will vary but might include: being loyal to patients/clients, co-workers, and your employer, projecting a positive attitude toward the institution of employment, respecting the privacy of others, keeping information confidential, being honest, never taking anything from the facility of employment, never saying a task is completed when it is not, and working with commitment and enthusiasm to improve patient care.

Recognizing and Reporting Illegal and Unethical Behavior

SECTION 6.2

Background

Health care workers must be aware of their ethical responsibilities for the protection of their patients/clients, their co-workers, their employers, and themselves. One of a health care worker's main responsibilities is to recognize and report unsafe, illegal, or unethical behaviors occurring in their work environment.

Objectives

When you have completed this section, you will be able to do the following:

- Match key terms with their correct meanings.
- Explain the importance of reporting illegal and unethical incidents.
- Identify three expectations of every employee regarding the treatment of others.
- Identify three resources that can help you report illegal or unethical behavior.

Career Connect

Research the job of a medical ethicist. What are their typical responsibilities? What are the education and training requirements? What types of facilities or offices do they typically work in? What type of character traits do you think a medical ethicist should possess?

Recognizing Reportable Incidents

Health care workers are responsible for helping to protect everyone in the work environment. If you suspect illegal behavior or unethical conduct, that incident must be reported. A reportable incident is any event that can adversely affect the health, safety, or welfare of patients/clients, co-workers, and others within your place of work. There are many ways a health care worker's behavior can have negative or adverse effects. Here are a few examples:

- A nurse might administer the wrong medicine
- A cleaning person might unplug important equipment
- A doctor might **harass** another employee
- An administrator might misuse hospital funds
- An employee might disclose a patient's condition to a reporter

harass
(huh RASS)
To behave in an offensively annoying or manipulative way.

There is no set list of reportable behaviors. Rather, it is required and expected that every employee will:

- Obey the laws of the city, state, and federal government
- Fulfill his or her job requirements to the best of his or her ability, including following a code of ethics and respecting others
- Treat everyone in the hospital environment with care, dignity and respect

Medical Ethics | Chapter 6 127

FOCUS AND ENGAGE

Introduce the Section

a. Review the content of the Background paragraph, explaining that one of the most important ethical responsibilities of a health care worker is to recognize and report unethical behavior in others.
b. Explain that reporting unethical behavior helps to guarantee a safe, healthy environment for patients, workers, and employers.
c. Discuss the objectives for the section.

Vocabulary Review

a. Key terms are defined in the margins of the text on the page where they first appear.
b. Pronounce each word, and have the students repeat the pronunciation out loud.
c. Discuss each definition.

TEACH

Discuss

- Ask students if they have ever encountered unethical behavior in others, such as lying or cheating.
- Ask students how they feel about reporting unethical behavior in others. Some might have a strong opinion about "ratting" or "tattling."
- Discuss the difference between unethical and illegal behavior, and whether the two ever overlap.
- Discuss how the policies and procedures of an organization can make dealing with unethical behavior easier to handle.

Reinforce and Review

- Review the code of ethics and the value indicators from Section 6.1.
- Review the legal responsibilities of the health care worker covered in Chapter 5.

Teaching Tips

- Define and explain reportable incident.
- Spend as much time as possible covering how to recognize reportable incidents.
- Give specific examples of reportable incidents, at every level at a health care facility.
- Review the examples in the text, explaining what makes them "reportable" and discussing which are illegal and which are unethical.
- If possible, provide newspaper clippings of unethical behavior that made the news nationally, or in your area.
- Discuss the legal, employment and professional consequences of illegal and unethical conduct.

Career Connect

- Ask a medical ethicist or legal representative to visit the class. If this is not possible, have students use the Internet to research the career, including educational requirements and job descriptions.

ACTIVITY

Make a two-column chart. In one column list unethical incidents you might encounter as a health care worker. In the second column, indicate whether you think the incident is reportable or not, and why.

Teaching Tips

- Emphasize that there is no set list of reportable incidents.
- Discuss examples of reporting policies at different types of healthcare facilities.
- Discuss the difference between procedures and policies. You may want to display a policy book and a procedure book for comparison.
- Emphasize that students must follow policies and procedures to protect the patient, their co-workers, the employer, and themselves.

Apply It

- If desired, have teams of three role-play the situation. You may want to have a list of specific scenarios for the role-playing.
- Alternatively, have students develop scenarios on their own.
- If there is disagreement about the reporting, open it up for class discussion.

Apply It

You are an emergency room health care employee who has witnessed another employee take a personal call on her cell phone while questioning a patient who has just come in complaining of stomach pain. You consider this to be a reportable activity. What course of action would you take?

Reporting Illegal, Discriminatory, and Unethical Behavior

Reporting an illegal or unethical incident helps ensure the health, safety, and welfare of everyone in the hospital environment. Follow your employer's policy regarding how you report illegal, discriminatory, or unethical incidents. The policy should be clearly outlined in the employee manual. If your employer does not provide an employee manual, consult with your immediate supervisor or the human resources department.

Consequences of Illegal and Unethical Behavior

Illegal and unethical behaviors may result in an employee being put on probation or fired. Illegal behavior can result in criminal charge or a civil lawsuit. In some cases, an employee who has exhibited unethical behavior will be required to take specialized training to better understand the behavior they are expected to exhibit in the workplace.

Language Arts Link

Ethical and Professional Standards

As a health care worker, it's essential that you maintain a high degree of professional standards and always adhere to a code of ethics that includes providing caring service and treating people fairly and with dignity.

Working with a partner, participate in a collaborative discussion building on each other's ideas regarding what you feel are some of the key qualities that will make a successful health care worker. When you have identified enough ideas, create a document describing your principles, policies, and intentions. This type of policy is called a *manifesto*. Present your information in paragraph form, conveying a clear and distinct perspective and selecting the most significant and relevant facts.

Be sure to proofread your work to see if you can improve it by making it clearer, more concise, or more interesting. Check the spelling and grammar and correct any errors.

Exchange your policy with another team. Provide feedback and corrections as necessary, and then exchange back. Read your classmates' comments and revise your document as necessary.

128 Chapter 6 | Medical Ethics

Language Arts Link—Ethical and Professional Standards

- Define manifesto for the class, and discuss the type of information students should include. If possible, hand out samples of a manifesto.
- Instruct students to include at least five items in their manifesto.
- If students will be using the Internet, remind them about your school's Internet policy, and to use reputable Web resources.
- Remind them to keep a list of sources.
- Evaluate the document based on originality, appropriateness, organization, and on spelling and grammatical errors.

CUSTOMIZED INSTRUCTION

Less Advanced Students

Although there is no set list of reportable incidents, it might help less advanced students grasp the concept if they can see a list of many different types of incidents. You may want to develop such a list, or work with the class to develop a list.

More Advanced Students

Have more advanced students compare a policy manual from two different health care facilities and report to the class on the similarities and differences they find.

Summary

In this section, you learned the importance of recognizing and reporting unethical and illegal behavior. Although illegal behavior may result in legal action, both illegal and unethical behaviors have consequences. When health care workers perform their duties within these boundaries, they help ensure the safety and welfare of everyone around them and help prevent both medical and legal problems. There are resources at your workplace to help you report unethical or illegal incidents.

Section 6.2 Review Questions

1. Explain the importance of reporting illegal and unethical incidents.
2. Identify three expectations of every employee regarding the treatment of others.
3. Identify three resources that can help you report illegal or unethical behavior.
4. Provide three examples of reportable behaviors.
5. What does it mean to harass someone?
6. How do you know that a behavior is unethical?

Medical Ethics | Chapter 6 129

CUSTOMIZED INSTRUCTION

Special Needs Students

It may be difficult for some students to overcome the idea that reporting an incident is tattling. Emphasize that reportable incidents usually result in harm to someone—the patient, worker, or employer—and not only is it okay to report, it is a legal obligation.

At-Risk Students

Many students (and workers) are hesitant to report unethical or illegal behavior because they do not want to be labeled as a "snitch," or they are afraid of retaliation. Discuss measures that are in place at your school (or in the workplace) that allow a student to report an incident either anonymously or that allow them to do so privately and without the fear of others finding out.

Section 6.2 Review Questions

1. Answer: Health care workers are responsible for helping to protect everyone in the work environment.
2. Answer:
   - Obey the laws of the city, state, and federal government.
   - Fulfill his or her job requirements to the best of his or her ability, including following a code of ethics and respecting others.
   - Treat everyone in the hospital environment with care, dignity and respect.
3. Answer:
   - Your employee manual should explain clearly how you should report illegal and unethical conduct.
   - Your manager should be able to help you report illegal and unethical behavior.
   - Your human resources department.
4. Answer:
   - A nurse might administer the wrong medicine.
   - A cleaning person might unplug important equipment.
   - A doctor might harass another employee.
   - An administrator might misuse hospital funds.
   - An employee might disclose a patient's condition to a reporter.
5. Answer: Harass means to behave in an offensively annoying or manipulative way.
6. Answer: When the safety and well-being of someone else is at risk

CHAPTER 6 REVIEW

Chapter Review Questions

1. Answer: The responsibilities that are most important to employers include being dependable, honest, and well groomed; displaying a good attitude; and following the rules and regulations of the organization.
2. Answer: A code of ethics represents ideal behavior for a group of people.
3. Answer: Dignity, Service, Excellence, Fairness/Justice
4. Answer: Ethical
5. Answer: If an incident puts the health, safety, and welfare of a person at risk, it is reportable.
6. Answer: Human resource department
7. Answer: Health care workers are expected to live by values that show others respect, and you show respect by treating others with dignity, demonstrating a spirit of service, performing your duties with excellence, and treating others with fairness/justice.
8. Answer: If someone does not treat another person respectfully or behaves in an offensive way, it can negatively affect people in the hospital. This is also true if a person is dishonest, discourteous, behaves in a harassing manner, or discloses matters of a private nature. Finally, if someone does not perform their job properly, this can also negatively affect patients and other employees.
9. Answer: Reporting an illegal or unethical incident helps ensure the health, safety, and welfare of everyone in the hospital environment.
10. Answer: Obey the laws of the city, state, and federal government. Fulfill his or her job requirements to the best of his or her ability. Treat everyone in the hospital environment with care, dignity, and respect.

Activities

1. Students should include a thesis statement and support their opinion with facts or real-world examples. Point out that the incident does not have to be health care related.
2. Encourage students to be creative with this assignment. They may want to create an actual handbook. Direct them to imagine a fictitious company, including a name and a type of business.
3. As extra credit, students may wish to create a poster illustrating some of the unsafe conditions they encountered.

CHAPTER 6 REVIEW

Chapter Review Questions

1. What four responsibilities are most important to employers? (6.1)
2. Why is the code of ethics important? (6.1)
3. What are the four key value indicators? (6.1)
4. The controversy surrounding the use of human embryonic tissue in research to help fight diseases presents a(n) ________ dilemma. (6.1)
5. How can you determine if an incident is reportable? (6.2)
6. To help you report an illegal or unethical incident, you may refer to your employee manual, your manager, or ________________. (6.2)
7. Why is it important to treat everyone in the hospital environment with respect and dignity? (6.2)
8. Name three ways in which someone's behavior can negatively affect the people in the hospital. (6.2)
9. Why is reporting an illegal or unethical incident important? (6.2)
10. What is expected of every health care employee? (6.2)

Activities

1. Write an essay about how you would report an illegal or unethical incident at your school. Who would you tell? What would you say? Would it matter if you knew the person who did the unethical or illegal activity? In your essay, explain why it is important to report these incidents, and how reporting them helps keep everyone in your school environment safe.
2. Working in pairs, create a section of an employee handbook to address illegal and unethical behavior. Explain what makes a behavior unethical or illegal and provide examples. Remember to include reporting guidelines for the employees.
3. The next time you have a chance to visit your local hospital (for job-shadowing or community service), assess and make note of any possible unsafe conditions. Prepare a brief report for your class as if you were reporting unsafe conditions to a supervisor.

130 Chapter 6 | Medical Ethics

CHAPTER 6 REVIEW

Case Studies

1. While doing your rounds, you find a patient in mild distress. After checking their chart, you realize that the wrong dosage of a medication was administered. You know that this is easily corrected. What do you do?
2. A famous actress is in the hospital under an assumed name for elective surgery. The next day, a tabloid carries the story of her admission for a fatal ailment, citing an "inside" hospital source. You know who was responsible. What do you do?
3. Medical advances in biotechnology are occurring every day. In-vitro fertilization is one of those advances. Research the ethical, moral, and legal issues it raises. Be prepared to discuss these with the class.
4. A health care worker at a hospital is found to have the HIV virus. Should patients at the hospital be informed of this?
5. An organ donor organization has determined that organs will be sold to the highest bidder. Should this be allowed to happen? Should people be allowed to sell their organs for donation?

Thinking Critically

1. **Communication**—Being an effective communicator involves active listening, honesty, and assertiveness. Think about the last time you had to tell another person something unpleasant. Were your comments constructive or destructive? Write a skit explaining how you could change destructive comments into constructive ones; then act it out in class. Use the health care value indicators to help you decide what and how to send your message.
2. **Value Indicators**—It is particularly important to show your employer that you have a good attitude. Give three examples of how you would exhibit this when interacting with co-workers.
3. **Patient Satisfaction**—Patient Satisfaction is an important part of the health care worker's role. Refer to Table 6.3 and select two communication objectives. Write an explanation of how behavior that reflects these objectives benefits patients and, their families and helps provide appropriate medical services.
4. **Biotechnology**—Sometimes biotechnology helps to alleviate ethical problems; other times it can present an ethical dilemma. Provide an example of a situation that reflects each of these scenarios.

Medical Ethics | Chapter 6 131

Case Studies

1. In their responses, students should include a complete explanation for their actions.
2. In their responses, students should include a complete explanation for their actions.
3. Students may write a report or create a chart.
4. Direct students to research the topic before answering.
5. Remind students that this is an opinion piece, with no right or wrong answer. They should include a thesis statement, and support their opinion with facts or real-world examples.

Thinking Critically

1. If students cannot think of an example, ask them to reverse it: When was the last time someone told them something unpleasant? You may want students to work in groups for the second part of this activity.
2. Point out that this refers to interaction with co-workers, not patients. You may want to encourage students to select one of the three examples, and draw a poster to illustrate it.
3. Remind students of the roles that service and excellence play in customer satisfaction. In addition to writing their responses, students may want to perform skits demonstrating the behavior.
4. Direct students to refer to their responses to Case Study 3 for ideas. Point out that they should provide two examples: (1) one of technology that helps alleviate ethical problems; and (2) one that presents an ethical dilemma. The responses might display the student's opinions and attitudes, which may be different from your own.

Portfolio Connection

- This is another opportunity for self-examination.
- Remind students to be honest and sincere when listing their behaviors.
- They may want to discuss the assignment with family members or friends who know them well.
- Encourage students to think about the report carefully, including a complete action plan.
- Check to make sure that students have completed the assignment and added it to the portfolio.

CHAPTER 6 REVIEW

Portfolio Connection

Your values and the way you express them affect your success in your occupation. The values discussed in this chapter provide basic guidelines for working closely with others in health care. Think about your strongest personality traits. List behaviors you exhibit when you are happy and when you are sad. Compare those behaviors with behaviors that reflect the health care values discussed in this chapter. Write a clear explanation of three behaviors you display. Include:

- At least one behavior that best reflects health care values; Describe why the behavior fits the value.
- At least one behavior that does not reflect health care values; Describe why the behavior does not fit the values.

Develop and describe a plan to change this behavior into a positive value-based action. Include the following in your action plan:

- Negative behavior, with an explanation about what makes it negative or outside the health care values discussed in this chapter
- Action that changes the behavior, with an explanation about how it fits the health care values
- Evaluation plan, including a time line to determine the final outcome of the action plan

Write your action plan in your word processor. Proofread your work and format it attractively. Place it in your portfolio in the section for Written Samples.

PORTFOLIO TIP

Before you file your portfolio samples, check that you have followed a step-by-step process in each document. It makes your written or recorded presentations clear and logical.

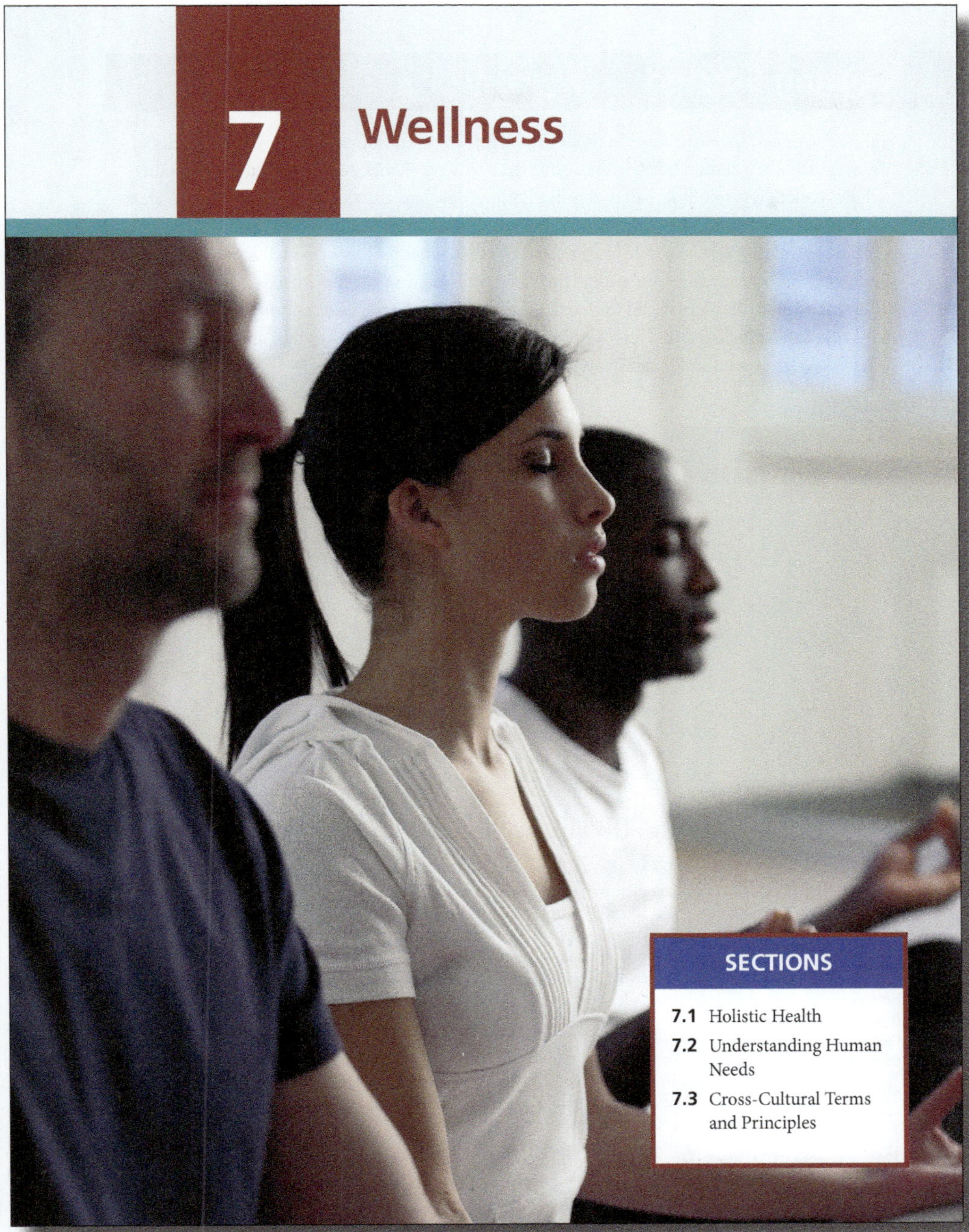
7 Wellness

SECTIONS

7.1 Holistic Health

7.2 Understanding Human Needs

7.3 Cross-Cultural Terms and Principles

CHAPTER 7 OVERVIEW

Chapter 7 introduces the concept of wellness, and how it impacts health and quality of life.

Section 7.1: In Section 7.1, students learn about holistic health. The section focuses on ways the mind, body, spirit, and social involvement can be balanced to affect a person's well-being and health.

Section 7.2: Section 7.2 covers understanding human needs from both a psychological and physiological point of view. It looks at the needs of patients, as well as the needs of workers.

Section 7.3: Section 7.3 introduces students to cross-cultural differences that might affect attitudes and approaches to health care. Specifically, it focuses on communicating among different cultures.

Advance Preparation	
Review	■ Chapter text for Sections 7.1, 7.2, and 7.3.
Contact	■ Organizations and agencies such as the American Heart Association, the American Diabetes Association, the Cancer Society, or the American Holistic Health Association that promote the understanding, screening, and prevention of disease and illness, to request brochures, pamphlets, or handouts. ■ Guest speakers such as holistic health practitioners or cultural liaisons or interpreters to visit the class. ■ A biofeedback professional to visit the class. ■ A pet-therapy administrator who might be willing to visit the class, or allow the class to visit during a session at a long-term care facility.
Prepare	■ Magazine and newspaper articles on topics such as holistic health, wellness, and preventive care. ■ Magazine and newspaper articles on cross-cultural communication. ■ A list of supporting Web sites such as americanheart.org, diabetes.org, cancer.org, and ahha.org.

FOCUS AND ENGAGE

Getting Started

- List items for a comfort kit. You may want students to research catastrophic disasters, such as Super Storm Sandy, or local disasters, such as fires that leave people homeless. Gather newspaper or magazine articles on the topic.
- This activity helps students think about basic human needs in the context of community service.
- Have students work in small groups to develop their lists, and allow them enough class time. Discuss the lists as a class.
- You may want to provide information such as newspaper or magazine articles about local disasters, such as fires or floods, and global disasters, such as Hurricane Katrina.
- You could invite a representative from the Red Cross to speak to the class about the type of disaster relief that they provide.

Introduce the Section

a. Review the content of the Background paragraph, discussing the concept of wellness.
b. Compare the proactive approach to health care that includes wellness and preventive medicine to a more traditional reactive approach, which focuses on healing and curing.
c. Review the objectives for the section.

Vocabulary Review

a. Key terms are defined in the margins of the text on the page where they first appear.
b. Pronounce each word, and have the students repeat the pronunciation out loud.
c. Discuss the definition of each word.

Getting Started

Humans *need* certain basic items in order to survive. We *want* things to improve our quality of life, or to achieve a certain lifestyle. Basic human needs are shelter, food, and water. Our wants include work that is fulfilling, safety, family relationships, and access to health care. The level of access to these wants and needs has a direct effect on our lifestyle and quality of life.

Each community is susceptible to some sort of crisis, whether it is a flood, hurricane, tornado, earthquake, or other unforeseen event. During a crisis, many of the basic needs may be jeopardized. To help with preparation for a crisis that may occur in your community, make a list of items that can be included in a "comfort kit"—a package that can be prepared ahead of time and delivered to those who suffer catastrophic loss.

SECTION 7.1 Holistic Health

Background

Responsible health care promotes lifestyles that encourage wellness. It is important for the health care worker to understand that mind, body, spirit, and social involvement must be balanced. Understanding wellness promotes good health in the health care worker and in the patient/client.

Objectives

When you have completed this section, you will be able to do the following.

- Match key terms with their correct meaning.
- List three parts of holistic health.
- Explain wellness and preventive care.
- Compare holistic health to disease-oriented care.

Health and Wellness

The World Health Organization defines health as follows: "Health is a state of complete physical, mental, and social well-being and not merely the absence of disease or **infirmity**." This definition of health has been expanded with the recent growth and emphasis on **holistic** health. Today we think in terms of the body working as a unit (mental, physical, spiritual) to maintain and promote optimum wellness through daily actions. Wellness is the overall feeling of well-being and the understanding that everything is going right in your life.

infirmity
(in FIR mi tee)
Unsound or unhealthy state of being.

holistic
(hoh LIST tik)
Pertaining to the whole; considering all factors.

In health care, *holistic* refers to the well-being of the whole person. It is important to meet physical needs as well as mental and spiritual needs when giving care. Holistic health care is a part of the wellness approach, which encourages good health and a positive self-image. Understanding these needs helps you care for yourself and for your patients/clients.

134 Chapter 7 | Wellness

TEACH

Discuss

- Display pamphlets from organizations that advocate a holistic approach to health care.
- Discuss the importance of treating the whole patient—mind, body, and spirit.
- Ask students if they have any experience with holistic health care, and to consider how holistic care might impact wellness.

CUSTOMIZED INSTRUCTION OVERVIEW	
Less Advanced Students	Pages 136, 146
More Advanced Students	Pages 135, 145
English Language Learners	Pages 135, 143
Special Needs Students	Pages 135, 147
At-Risk Students	Pages 138, 154

Wellness and Preventive Health Care

Wellness and preventive health care emphasize keeping patients well, and not waiting until they are ill, to provide treatment. The concept of wellness changes throughout the life span, and it is important to identify the concepts of wellness for each stage of the life span. For example, from infancy through early childhood, wellness reflects growth and development. For senior citizens, wellness reflects an ability to live an active and engaged lifestyle. Screenings are tests or examinations that are done to identify a disease or condition before symptoms appear. Age, gender, family history, and genetic risk factors are indicators as to whether or not a person should have particular screenings. This type of preventative care makes it easier to treat most diseases and conditions early: when treatment is often more successful. Health education is vital to helping clients maintain good health. These are examples of community outreach education programs that encourage wellness and prevention of disease. A holistic approach includes all of the following sections.

aerobic
(ai ROH bik)
Requiring oxygen.

elimination
(i lim uh NEY shuhn)
Process of expelling or removing, especially of waste products from the body.

Physical Fitness

Physical fitness keeps us alert and energetic in activities of daily living. It gives us enough energy to enjoy leisure time and to respond when emergencies arise. It can be achieved through:

- Routine physicals
- Adequate rest
- Good nutrition
- Good posture
- Avoiding risky behavior, including the use and abuse of substances such as alcohol and tobacco
- **Aerobic** exercise
- Immunizations
- Well-baby checks
- Weight control
- **Elimination** of body wastes

Physical fitness is the result of regular exercise, proper diet and nutrition, and proper rest for physical recovery.

Physical exercise is bodily activity that develops and maintains physical fitness and overall health. This helps to strengthen muscles and the cardiovascular system, and to boost the immune system. Exercise helps prevent heart disease, cardiovascular disease, diabetes, and obesity. It also improves mental health and helps prevent depression.

Besides exercise, correct posture is a simple but very important way to keep the back and spine healthy. It is more than cosmetic—good posture and back support are critical to reducing the incidence and levels of back pain and neck pain.

Nutrition

A diet is all of the food consumed by a person. Dietary habits are the decisions an individual or culture makes when choosing what foods to eat. Each culture holds some food preferences and some food taboos. Individual dietary choices may be more or less healthy, but proper nutrition requires the appropriate intake and absorption of vitamins, minerals, and fuel in the form of carbohydrates, proteins, and fats. Dietary habits and choices play a significant role in health and mortality, since deficiencies, excesses, and imbalances in diet can produce negative impacts on health, which may lead to diseases such as cardiovascular disease, diabetes, scurvy, obesity, or osteoporosis.

Health Screenings

Many health care organizations offer screenings at low or no cost, and often the services are provided in mobile units to serve patients/clients in remote areas or who may not have a means of transportation for getting to and from a hospital, clinic, or doctor's office. Conditions that are commonly screened for before symptoms occur include: breast cancer in women, colorectal cancer, diabetes, high blood pressure, glaucoma, high cholesterol, osteoporosis, and prostate cancer in men.

Age, gender, family history, and genetic risk factors are indications for whether a person should have particular screenings.

With a partner, identify a health care organization in your community that offers screenings. Research how access to such services promotes wellness and helps prevent disease. Share your findings with the class.

Wellness | Chapter 7 135

CUSTOMIZED INSTRUCTION

English Language Learners

Have students write each key term and its pronunciation on one side of an index card and its definition on the other side.

More Advanced Students

Use the Internet to research the development of holistic medicine. Report your results to the class.

Special Needs Students

There may be students in the class who have chronic health concerns, such as asthma or allergies. They might feel comfortable discussing in class the extra measures they must take to ensure their physical well-being.

Teaching Tips

- Discuss holistic health, emphasizing the importance of understanding that physical, mental, and social well-being must be balanced.
- Point out that mental (mind), physical (body), emotional (spirit), and social interaction as a path to wellness is a relatively new approach.
- Emphasize that holistic health focuses on the way the entire body works as an integrated unit. For example, biofeedback teaches people to change physical symptoms by using the mind.
- Introduce the three categories of holistic health: physical fitness, spiritual fitness, and mental fitness. Mention that financial fitness also plays a role in a person's health and well-being.
- Discuss the factors that contribute to physical fitness.
- Discuss the value of preventative health care and how health screenings can contribute to preventative care.
- Ask students to describe other strategies for prevention of diseases besides health screenings.

Health Screenings

- Explain that health screenings are a preventative measure to help prevent diseases as well as to diagnose them early when they are more treatable.
- Explain that screenings are often offered for free and that many health care providers have mobile units that set up in different locations to offer screenings.

ACTIVITY

Is holistic health care the same as alternative medicine? Research the question using the Internet, the library, or by talking to professionals. Make a decision based on the information you find, and then write your answer in paragraph form. Share your answer with the class.

Teaching Tips

- Discuss proper nutrition.
- Explain how to interpret the MyPlate graphic. Point out that everybody is different, which means everybody has different requirements when it comes to food intake.
- Discuss healthy food choices.
- Discuss the importance of physical activity.
- Discuss moderation, and portion control.

Figure Focus

7.1 The United States Department of Agriculture (USDA) developed MyPlate (choosemyplate.gov) to provide the information you need to choose a healthy diet. Why is it important to have a healthy lifestyle?

Answer: Good health is considered to be a state of physical, mental, and emotional well-being; it is not merely being free from illness. Preventive health care focuses on healthy eating and activity to help us stay physically and mentally fit, and to help us fight off illness or injury.

"Financial Fitness"

- Discuss how financial concerns can contribute to stress.
- Point out that developing and sticking to a personal budget and establishing and working toward financial goals can contribute to financial well-being, which in turn contributes to overall fitness and wellness.

"Financial Fitness"

Finances are assets in the form of money. Your personal finances include the money you earn, spend, and save.

Some people live "paycheck-to-paycheck," meaning they spend all that they earn. They may have trouble paying their bills; they may not put financial needs before wants; or they may not understand planning ahead financially. People who live this way may have stress and worries.

When you take control of your finances, you set financial goals and make healthy financial decisions for both your needs and wants. Managing your money makes you financially "fit" and contributes to your overall well-being. Furthermore, when you understand the differences between financial needs and wants, you can make responsible choices that will have a positive impact on your community and the economy.

Trending in nutrition today is the consumption of supplemental vitamins and minerals in the diet. There are many options available in nutrition stores, as well as grocery stores and online. Alternative diets (liquid, fat-free, vegetarian, vegan, high-protein, etc.) are often marketed as the answer to obesity, Type 2 diabetes, and other health problems. Alternative diets and supplements should be researched thoroughly before initiating them, and you should consult with nutritional health professionals.

To make healthy choices, you need to know what your body needs. Diet is the food you eat. Nutrition is a science that studies the way the food you eat nourishes your body. When you eat a healthy diet and have good nutrition, your body is getting what it needs to work at its best level. Different foods contribute different nutrients—the parts of food that your body requires. Recognizing that food is a resource you can use to stay healthy and happy can help you choose the best foods and food combinations and maintain a healthy diet.

So what is a healthy diet? A healthy diet gives your body balanced nutrition. (**Figure 7.1**) Like a car, if you give your body the right fuel, it will run great and last a long time. If you give it the wrong fuel, it might break down. To achieve a healthy diet, you should eat a balanced variety of foods from different food groups.

Other basic guidelines include:

- Eating a variety of fruits and vegetables, including dark green vegetables, yellow vegetables, and beans
- Eating calcium-rich foods, such as low-fat milk, cheese, and yogurt
- Eating whole grains
- Eating lean meats, fish, poultry, and nuts
- Limiting the amount of fats, salts, and sugars that you eat
- Drinking plenty of water

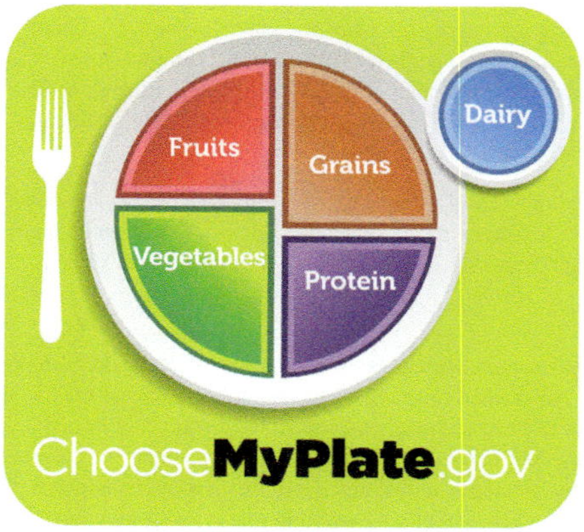

Figure 7.1
The United States Department of Agriculture (USDA) developed MyPlate (choosemyplate.gov) to provide the information you need to choose a healthy diet. Why is it important to have a healthy lifestyle?

136 Chapter 7 | Wellness

ACTIVITY

Access the choosemyplate.gov Web site via the Internet, and explore the site. Use the Daily Food Plans page to create a customized food guide, and print it, or write down the information. Review the Physical Activity links to determine how much physical activity you need to burn the calories you take in. Use the SuperTracker tool to plan, analyze, and track your diet and physical activity.

CUSTOMIZED INSTRUCTION

Less Advanced Students

Give less advanced students ample time to learn their way around the ChooseMyPlate.gov Web site. Make sure they are comfortable using the SuperTracker tool. Encourge them to download the tool on their home computers.

Substance Abuse

The impact of substance abuse, including tobacco, alcohol, and drugs, crosses all societal boundaries and affects both genders, every ethnic group, and people in every tax bracket. Smoking tobacco particularly damages the respiratory and the circulatory systems. Regular use results in diseases that cause death or severe disability. During pregnancy, chemicals from the tobacco smoke pass through the mother's blood to the baby through the placenta and reduce the oxygen and blood flow to the baby.

Excessive alcohol use increases the risk of many harmful health conditions, such as unintentional injuries, including traffic injuries or falls. It is associated with violence, child neglect, and risky sexual behavior. In addition, alcohol poisoning can occur, which is a medical emergency that results from high blood alcohol levels that suppress the central nervous system and can cause loss of consciousness, low blood pressure and body temperature, coma, respiratory depression, and death. Long-term alcohol problems include chronic disease and neurological impairments. During pregnancy, miscarriage, stillbirth, and a combination of physical and mental birth defects that last throughout life can occur.

Drug abuse is defined generally as the use of a psychoactive drug or performance enhancing drug for a non-therapeutic or non-medical effect. Some of the most commonly abused drugs include alcohol, amphetamines, barbiturates, benzodiazepines, cocaine, methaqualone, and opium alkaloids. Use of these drugs may lead to criminal penalties in addition to physical, social, and psychological harm.

Energy and Rest

Physical and mental activities require energy and create waste products. As our energy level goes down and wastes accumulate, we experience fatigue and a need to rest. During rest, energy is restored, and the waste buildup is diminished, allowing for recovery and growth. Rest and sleep are dependent upon our ability to relax. To get a good night's rest, try to sleep in a dark, quiet, cool room.

Mental Fitness

Mental fitness allows us to interact effectively with others and to feel balanced. Mental fitness manifests in a positive self-image. Mentally healthy people:

- Self-direct (being the captain of your own ship)
- Have a sense of belonging
- Trust their own senses and feelings
- Accept themselves
- Have high **self-esteem**
- Practice stress management

Stress is what you feel when you have to handle more than you are used to. Often, your body responds in the same way as it would if you were in danger—hormones speed up your heart, make you breathe faster, and give you a burst of energy. This is sometimes known as the fight-or-flight stress response. Some stress is normal and even useful; for example, it can help you win a race or finish an important job on time. But if stress happens too often or lasts too long, it can have negative

Apply It

According to recent studies, many chronic health conditions are preventable, yet they account for a large percentage of deaths and their treatment has contributed significantly to the rise in health care costs. Working in teams of three to five, identify a chronic health condition (i.e., high blood pressure, back/neck pain, and type 2 diabetes) or environmental health issue, such as (i.e., ebola, measles outbreak, and exposure to mold in older buildings).

Create a presentation that discusses who is affected by the issue, the impact it has had on the economy and society, and how it could have been prevented or should be addressed in the future.

self-esteem
(SELF i STEEM)
Belief in oneself.

Teaching Tips

- Review the problems that arise from excessive alcohol use.
- Review the effects of drug abuse.
- Point out that illegal drugs, prescription, and over-the-counter medications can be abused.
- Discuss the importance of a good night's sleep for renewing the body and the mind.
- Introduce the topic of mental fitness.
- Review the concepts of mental fitness and the factors that contribute to mental fitness.
- Discuss the importance of self-esteem in everyday life.
- Review the symptoms of stress.

Apply It

- Break students into groups as you deem appropriate.
- They may need help identifying some environmental health issues. You might suggest asbestos; lead exposure; water, air, or noise pollution.
- Provide specifics as to the type of presentation you want: hard copy, PowerPoint, etc.

ACTIVITY

Have students create a list of unhealthy lifestyle choices, and then use their lists to identify factors that contribute to good health and a positive self-image.

TEAMWORK

Working in small groups, have students brainstorm ways that people might be able to improve their self-esteem. Create a presentation about one way to improve self-esteem. You might use a slideshow presentation program, or write an inspirational speech illustrated with posters. Deliver your presentation to your class or to a group of people who might benefit, such as a girl scout troop, or a homeless shelter.

Teaching Tips

- Review the list of ways of identifying the cause of stress.
- Discuss the methods students can use to mitigate stress.
- Rest, physical activity, and proper nutrition are all effective methods of mitigating stress.
- Introduce the topic of spiritual fitness.
- Review the factors that contribute to spiritual fitness.

Apply It

- Divide class into teams of two or three.
- Encourage students to brainstorm for stressful situations.
- Allow class time for students to compare and contrast the strategies they suggested.

Apply It

- Pair students to review types of fitness.
- Remind them that overall fitness leads to a positive self-image.
- Allow class time for students to compare and contrast their lists of positive behaviors and traits.

Apply It

In teams of three to four, discuss potentially stressful situations in the workplace, such as having a heavy workload, or not getting along with a co-worker. Then, develop a list of strategies for dealing with stressful situations in the workplace. Share your list with the class to compare and contrast strategies for dealing with stress on the job.

Apply It

With a partner, review the types of fitness discussed in this section. Create a list that identifies behaviors and traits that contribute to overall fitness, or a positive self-image as well as those that can lead to a negative self-image. Compare and contrast your list of positive behaviors and traits with the lists of your classmates.

effects on your well-being. You can experience headaches, an upset stomach, back pain, or trouble sleeping. It can weaken your immune system, making it harder to fight off disease. It can make you moody, tense, or depressed. Relationships may suffer, and you may not do well at work or school.

To identify stressors, you have to know:

- What event caused the stress
- Why you feel stress
- How much stress you are feeling
- If you feel negatively or positively about the situation

Before you can control stress, you must determine what is causing it. So, you should:

- Gather information or data
- Identify the problem
- List possible solutions
- Act on your solution
- Evaluate the results
- Make a plan

In order to cope with stress, look for ways in which to reduce it, and learn healthy ways in which to relieve it. Some methods might include better time management, taking good care of your health, getting plenty of rest, regular exercise, not smoking, limiting alcohol intake, learning to say "no" if you are too busy, and asking for help. You can talk to family, friends, or a counselor. You can write down things that are bothering you, or find other ways to express your feelings. Finally, take time to do something you enjoy or to relax yourself (yoga, massage, aromatherapy, etc.). Also, manage the physical reaction to stress by breathing deeply, reflecting on the cause of stress, and choosing another way to react.

Spiritual Fitness

Spiritual fitness allows us to experience meaning and purpose in life. It provides a sense of comfort with others, creating greater acceptance of behaviors, attitudes, and beliefs. It includes:

- Enjoying companionship
- Sharing ideas and thoughts
- Having a sense of belonging
- Showing enthusiasm for life

Holistic health requires health care workers to promote physical, mental, and spiritual well-being. For example, a patient experiencing stomach pain may be referred to a psychologist if the physician suspects that the patient is under emotional stress. The psychologist may refer him to a biofeedback specialist for stress management. This process continues until the patient's/client's needs are met in all areas.

Relationships

Interpersonal relationships, whether with family, friends, or co-workers, can have important health implications. Positive relationships can boost mental and physical health and provide patients with a support network to help them navigate trying times. Negative relationships, however, can exacerbate declining health

138 Chapter 7 | Wellness

ACTIVITY

Create a chart with three columns. In one column, list ways you meet your physical fitness needs. In the second column, list ways you meet your spiritual or social needs. In the third column, list ways you stay mentally healthy. Examine your chart, and then select one area in which you would like to improve. Create a plan for how you will achieve this goal.

CUSTOMIZED INSTRUCTION

At-Risk Students

Ask students to describe how school contributes to their well-being. Be prepared with prompts, such as: "School is a safe place so it contributes to emotional well-being;" or, "School offers a healthy lunch and opportunities to exercise so it contributes to physical well-being;" and so forth.

Personal Wellness

Time Management

Time management is a critical skill for succeeding in your personal life, at school, and in your career. Employers want you to make the most of your time—to them, time is money. To achieve your personal, academic, and professional goals, you will have to manage your time effectively and set priorities—decide which tasks must be completed first.

Once you have set your priorities, you develop a time frame for completing each task. For example, you have a goal of completing your term paper on April 15, and it is now April 1. Determine which tasks must be completed first and the deadline for completing each. Following is an example:

- On April 1, I will create an outline.
- On April 2, I will review it with my teacher.
- From April 3–April 8, I will research my topic and take notes.
  - On April 3, I will use the school library.
  - On April 4, I will go to the public library.
  - On April 5, I will conduct my interview.
  - On April 6 and 7, I will organize my notes.
  - On April 8, I will review my outline and notes to make sure I have no gaps.
- From April 9–11, I will write the first draft.
- From April 12–14, I will review and revise.

If you avoid distractions and concentrate on following your schedule, your term paper will be done on time—and you'll be able to take credit for a job well done!

and even be the cause of health issues. Health professionals should help identify problematic relationships and provide patients the tools to cope or even eliminate these negative relationships while fostering positive ones.

Alternative Health Care

The National Library of Medicine classifies alternative medicine as a complementary therapy. These therapeutic practices are not currently considered an integral part of conventional medical practice. They do not follow generally accepted medical methods and may not have a scientific explanation for their effectiveness; they are unconventional. Therapies are termed as *complementary* when used in addition to conventional treatments; they are considered *alternative* when used instead of conventional treatment.

Fundamental to alternative medical practice is a strong bond between patient and doctor; the need to work as a team. These doctors do not see themselves as the source of healing; patients must take active responsibility for their health and well-being.

Initially, these therapies were used by individuals who had run out of other options—individuals with immune deficiencies, cancer, chronic back pain, arthritis, and other conditions. Today, more and more people are turning to alternative health care for wellness care. Some examples of alternative medicine include the use of herbal remedies, acupuncture, yoga, massage therapy, and spiritual healing. For example, a woman with breast cancer chooses to treat

Community

Review the activities offered at a local senior center or retirement community. How many of them focus on spiritual fitness? Do they offer complementary or alternative techniques for helping residents achieve well-being?

Community

- Check with the local senior centers and/or retirement communities and get permission for students to conduct this activity. Then, check with a local fitness or spiritual activity center to see who is willing to volunteer their services.
- Ask students to check on the range of activities offered to residents at the senior center or retirement community.
- Once the instructor has conducted the class, ask students to interview the residents to see how they reacted to the class.

Personal Wellness—Time Management

- Time management is something that will help students across all their endeavors.
- Explain what time management is, then ask students for examples of situations in which they either managed their time well or poorly. What were the results? If they did not manage their time well, how would they change what they did?
- Provide a sample project for students—such as creating a term paper, working on a group project, or conducting an Apply It activity.
- Set a deadline and ask students to provide a timeline and "to do" list. Review to see if the students' lists and timelines are reasonable.

Teaching Tips

- Discuss the meaning of generally accepted medical methods as compared to unconventional methods.
- Review the difference between complementary therapy and alternative therapy.
- Discuss alternative medicine without being subjective one way or another.
- Point out that many treatments that were once considered alternative, are now generally accepted, such as physical therapy or diet.
- Conversely, point out that some alternative treatments have been scientifically proven to deliver no benefits to the patient, such as some herbal remedies.
- Ask students to discuss the pros and cons of alternative therapies:
  - May provide relief when conventional treatments fail
  - Not covered by insurance
  - Not regulated
- Discuss the role of a patient as an active partner in holistic and alternative therapy.

Teaching Tips

- Review the jobs and professions available for holistic practitioners.
- Point out that some are outside the medical profession, while others are practiced by medical professionals.
- Discuss education and certification requirements for alternative medicine professions.

Apply It

- Create a list of alternative care options offered in your area.
- Pass this out to students and have them check off any alternative medical professionals with whom they or their family have had experience.
- Make sure you include an "Other" category with a line on which students can note the type of care received (e.g., aromatherapy).
- Chart responses on a computer (or ask for a volunteer who will do this for extra credit). Print out the results in the form of a bar chart.

Apply It

Take a survey of the students in your classroom. How many of them (or their families) have used alternative medical professionals? Create a chart that shows the types of alternative care delivered—for example, chiropractic, acupuncture, aromatherapy, hypnotist, or midwife.

her cancer by eating a special macrobiotic diet instead of having radiation and chemotherapy, which is the standard medical practice. Or, an elderly person with arthritis uses acupuncture to treat arthritis pain instead of taking medications.

The use of alternative medicine, of course, has its drawbacks. Many in the mainstream medical community believe that these alternative therapies, in conjunction with standard treatments, provide comfort for the patient. However, they argue that relying on these therapies alone and without doctor approval is dangerous and can even be fatal. The disease might be getting worse, even if the patient "feels" better, because it is not being adequately treated.

Using herbs that are not FDA approved may cause interactions with other medications or vitamins. It may be easier to overdose on a specific regimen that has not been adequately tested. Just because a product is natural does not mean it is safe. One example of this is foxglove, which is a component of digitalis, used to treat heart conditions. Foxglove, with unsupervised use, can also be a poison.

There are minimal, if any, regulations or federal guidelines associated with alternative medicine. For example, over-the-counter herbs are not regulated and the patient cannot be sure of any standard of preparation in their formulation. This could make the patient a target for unscrupulous activity. Finally, insurance companies may not cover alternative medical treatments unless they are used in conjunction with traditional therapies.

Public Health

As you have seen so far, promoting wellness is an essential part of preventing illness for individual patients and health care professionals have many tools at their disposal to do so. It is important to consider though that promoting wellness can extend well beyond the scope of what individual health care teams can do. This field of health sciences is termed public health, the study and development of policies that promote health and wellness of entire communities.

Public health initiatives come in many different forms. A large part of what these professionals do involves outreach and community education on how to avoid illness, such as telling people how to properly store food, wash their hands frequently, get regular exercise, etc. They also include policy and law changes, such as restricting the sale of certain products to minors, mandatory vaccinations for school children, or even limits on pollutants in drinking water. In some cases, they may also involve control of the organisms that transmit diseases (vectors) like mosquitoes and ticks. All of these strategies can be employed to reduce the load on health care services in a community by promoting wellness. The global impact of disease prevention through public health programs, both financially and in terms of quality of life, cannot be overstated.

With such a large scope of work to be done with the community, public health initiatives require the various health care teams that serve the community to form strong, positive relationships and cooperate extensively. This not only lessens the burden on individual teams, but it allows teams within different areas of health care (nutrition, fitness, etc.) to lend their expertise to an overall holistic approach to public health.

140 Chapter 7 | Wellness

ACTIVITY

Some alternative treatments have been around for centuries, such as acupuncture. Some are relatively new, such as aromatherapy. Select and research one alternative treatment, then create a poster to illustrate it. Display the posters at a health and wellness assembly.

TEAMWORK

Divide the class into two or three teams. Provide a list of qualities or actions such as "enthusiasm for life" or "attending religious services." Have each team identify the appropriate holistic health category—physical, mental, or spiritual—for each item in the list. Have the teams discuss their lists with the class.

Jobs and Professions

There are a wide variety of careers that are outside of the mainstream medical world. There are physicians and nurses who specialize in alternative medical treatments, such as homeopathy and naturopathic medicine. Others focus on breath therapy, environmental medicine, and nutrition. Many who choose a career in alternative health care are entrepreneurs, or those who start their own business.

Following is a description of some of the more widely practiced alternative medical treatments:

- **Acupuncture**. The insertion of thin, stainless steel needles into the skin at specific locations to affect the flow of energy in the body. Making sure energy is not blocked facilitates symptom relief and healing of illness.
- **Homeopathy**. Developed in Germany in the 18th century, homeopathic remedies are created from plant, animal, or mineral products greatly diluted in water or alcohol.
- **Massage therapy**. A wide variety of physical manipulative techniques promote relaxation and treat conditions caused by tension, such as headaches or insomnia.
- **Naturopathic medicine**. Although similar to traditional medicine, naturopathic physicians avoid drugs, major surgery, and cutting-edge technology and rely on treatment designed to strengthen the body's own healing capabilities. For example, preparations such as vitamins, nutritional supplements, and herbs might be used to treat and prevent disease.
- **Prayer and spirituality**. Often considered "alternative" by conventional medical standards, prayer and spirituality help patients maintain a sense of purpose, meaning, and hope in the face of pain, suffering, and uncertainty.
- **Chinese traditional medicine**. Utilizing methods such as herbal remedies, acupuncture, diet, meditation, and exercises such as qigong and tai chi, this therapy seeks to achieve overall balance of health in preventing as well as treating illness. Qigong is an aspect of traditional Chinese medicine that involves the coordination of different breathing patterns with various physical postures and motions of the body. Tai chi is a gentle exercise program derived from martial arts, but composed of slow, deliberate movements, meditation, and deep breathing, which enhance physical health and emotional well-being.

There are a wide range of career choices in alternative medicine. They include:

- **Psychologist**. An expert in the systematic investigation of the human mind, including behavior, cognition, and affect. Psychologists are usually categorized under a number of different fields, the most well-known being clinical and counseling psychologists. Licensed psychologists need an academic doctoral degree.
- **Social worker (rehabilitation worker)**. Concerned with social problems, their causes, their solutions, and their human impacts. Social workers work with individuals, families, groups, organizations and communities.

Career-Ready Practices

The knowledge and skills you obtain through education and experience have a variety of real-world, on-the-job applications. For example, the critical-thinking skills you use to perform an experiment in science class would be valuable when you are diagnosing a patient. The communication skills you use to keep two friends from arguing would be helpful when you are dealing with a patient who is upset about his hospital bill.

Research an alternative medical treatment that interests you. It can be one covered in this section or one you have heard of on your own. What type of education and training does it require? What special skills, knowledge, or personality traits should you possess in order to practice it? What academic and technical skills have you already acquired that would prepare you for a job in this area? Share your findings with the class.

Wellness | Chapter 7 141

ACTIVITY

Holistic health involves preventive care, wellness, and treatment of the entire person, leading to a positive self-image. Traditional disease-oriented care involves diagnoses and treatment of illness, and treatment of the disease, not the total person. In your opinion, what are the benefits and drawbacks to these two approaches? Write a personal essay explaining your opinion. Include a thesis statement, and back it up with supporting facts or real-life examples.

Teaching Tips

- Point out that many of the professions that are listed are common and accepted among the medical community, such as social worker and midwife.
- Also, note that some of the professions may be specialties or areas of interest for traditional medical practitioners. For example, a registered nurse may also be a certified midwife, and a physician might study the effects of herbal remedies.
- Discuss why a career in alternative therapy will probably require entrepreneur skills.

Career-Ready Practices

- Students are to research an alternative medical treatment that interests them.
- They can choose from those discussed in the text, but encourage them to research others if desired.
- You might ask students to create a presentation—oral, written, or slideshow—about the treatment they chose.
- This activity gives students real-world experience in applying the following Career-Ready Practice: Apply Appropriate Academic and Technical Skills.
- For more information on the Career-Ready Practices, visit careertech.org/career-ready-practices.

Teaching Tips

- Provide information about regulations in your state regarding alternative medicine and practitioners.
- Also, provide links to Web sites for more information.
- For the government's take on alternative medicine, refer to the National Institute of Health's Web site: https://nccih.nih.gov/.

Figure Focus

7.2. What are the advantages of using a midwife?

Answer: The presence of a midwife can be a comfort for many women, especially first-time mothers-to-be. They are there from the beginning of the birthing process through and after completion of delivery. While many obstetricians have multiple patients at one time, a midwife can usually devote exclusive attention to a woman during labor. They are there to monitor labor, guide, and support the woman. For many women, this allows them to be more in control of the birthing process.

Figure Focus

7.3 A chiropractor holding a patient's head performing alignment. What benefits can a chiropractor provide patients?

Answer: Many chiropractic treatments deal specifically with the spine and the manipulation of the spine. The chiropractic approach to health care stresses the patient's overall health. Chiropractors provide natural, drugless, non-surgical health treatments, relying on the body's recuperative abilities. They also recognize that many factors affect health, including exercise, diet, rest, environment, and heredity; and they tend to first try to recommend changes in lifestyle, rather than drug therapy.

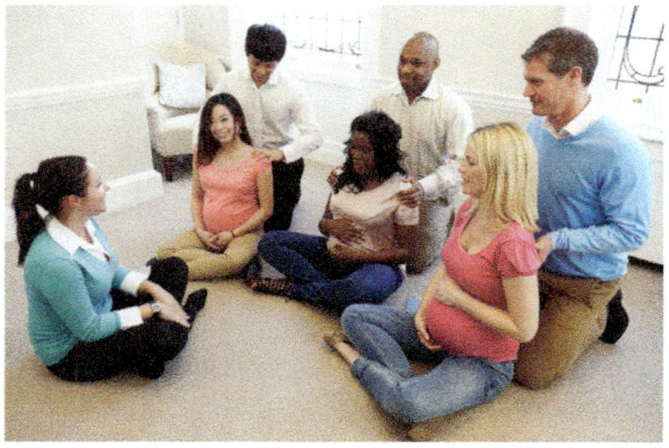

Figure 7.2
What are the advantages of using a midwife?

Generally, social workers need a professional degree in social work; and usually they must obtain a license or be professionally registered.

- **Midwife**. Practitioner who specializes in normal pregnancy, childbirth, and the postpartum. (**Figure 7.2**) They generally strive to help women have a healthy pregnancy and natural birth experience. Midwives also provide general women's health care. Direct-entry midwives learn midwifery through self-study, apprenticeship, a midwifery school, or a college- or university-based program separate from the discipline of nursing.
- **Biofeedback specialist**. Trained to use a form of alternative medicine that involves measuring a patient's bodily processes such as blood pressure, heart rate, skin temperature, galvanic skin response (sweating), and muscle tension, and conveying such information to the patient in real time in order to raise his or her awareness and conscious control of the related physiological activities. Specialists must pass a certification exam.
- **Parish nurse specialist**. Registered nurse who commits to the healing missions of a church. They work to help fellow parishioners find support in crisis or with day-to-day struggles. They also work directly with parish staff to educate on wellness and a better quality of life. Nurses must be registered and meet the standard nursing educational requirements.
- **Acupressurist**. Uses a form of traditional Chinese medicine in which the health care provider stimulates certain pressure points to encourage the flow of vital energy (Qi) along the specific pathways called meridiens. This is often used to control chronic pain such as migraine headaches or backaches. Acupressure is generally classified as massage, and training may be offered through massage schools or independent seminars.
- **Acupuncturist**. Uses a form of traditional Chinese medicine that treats specific health disorders with the insertion of fine needles into the body at specific points where the flow of energy is thought to be blocked. To be certified, an acupuncturist must attend an accredited school of acupuncture and pass a licensing exam.
- **Palliative care specialist**. Palliative care is the active total care of patients whose disease does not respond to curative treatment, including control of pain, of other symptoms, and of psychological, social, and spiritual problems. The goal is to provide the best possible quality of life for patients and their families. Palliative care specialists typically work in teams and usually are needed when the disease is advanced, life expectancy is short, and problems become complex and more urgent. Palliative care specialists are board certified physicians and must meet all of the standard requirements.
- **Ayurvedic practitioner**. Uses a traditional system of Indian medicine, in which the basic texts analyze the human body in terms of earth, water, fire, air, and ether as well as the three bodily humours (wind, bile, and phlegm).

Figure 7.3
A chiropractor holding a patient's head performing alignment. What benefits can a chiropractor provide patients?

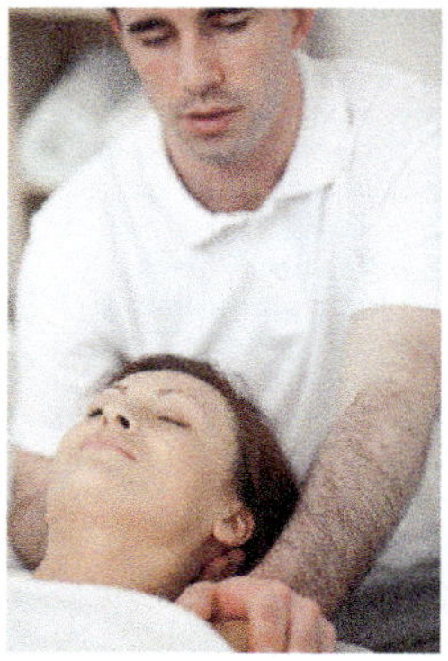

142 Chapter 7 | Wellness

To prevent illness, these practitioners emphasize hygiene, exercise, herbal preparations, and yoga. To cure ailments, they rely on herbal medicines, physiotherapy, and diet. Specialists must take specific courses and pass a certification exam.

- **Chiropractor**. Treats patients whose health problems are associated with the body's muscular, nervous, and skeletal systems, especially the spine. Chiropractors use manipulation and specific adjustment of body structures, such as the spinal column, to rebalance the nervous system and the body. (Figure 7.3) They must be licensed, which requires two to four years of undergraduate education and passing national and state exams.
- **Aromatherapist**. Uses essential oils extracted from plants as therapy to promote health and well-being. These can be inhaled by patients, introduced internally, or applied topically. They must pass a training course and receive a certificate.
- **Hypnotist**. Trained in inducing trance states and therapeutic suggestions to address a wide range of medical and psychological issues, such as fears, phobias, anxiety, sleep disorders, etc. Hypnotists must take a course (about a month long) and pass a test to be certified.

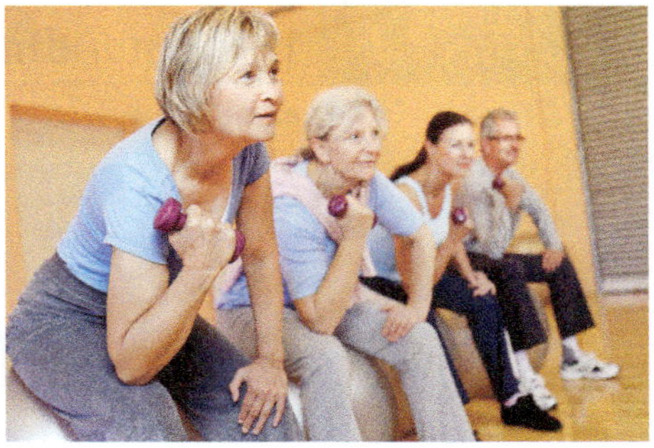

Figure 7.4
Enjoying companionship, sharing ideas, having a sense of belonging, and showing enthusiasm for life are vital to well-being. What is a way that a person might show enthusiasm for life?

Summary

The holistic approach to health is important because it includes all aspects of a person's well-being. When a person is in balance physically, mentally, and spiritually, that person can experience life in a positive way and enjoy a greater sense of well-being. (Figure 7.4) The trend in health care is toward wellness and preventive care. The health care worker has a responsibility to help the patient understand different care choices and the role that each of these therapies may play in seeking a goal of optimal wellness.

Section 7.1 Review Questions

1. How does the definition of health presented by the World Health Organization go beyond physical conditions?
2. What are some habits that can help a person to stay physically fit?
3. In what ways is spiritual fitness related to a person's well being?
4. In a holistic approach to health care, a patient with neck pain might be referred to a psychologist. How might this help the person?
5. Name three professions involved in maintaining the health and wellness of others.
6. Name two conditions and explain how they might be treated using alternative therapies.

Wellness | Chapter 7 143

Teaching Tips

- Remind students that the idea of wellness and preventive care is relatively new.
- In the past, people went for care when ill or injured. The health care provider's role was to "fix" the patient.
- Today, the emphasis is on preventing illness. To encourage wellness, preventive care is important. It includes health education and physical screening tests, such as mammograms and PSA (prostate specific antigen).

Figure Focus

7.4 Enjoying companionship, sharing ideas, having a sense of belonging, and showing enthusiasm for life are vital to well-being. What is a way that a person might show enthusiasm for life?

Answer: A person might smile, take on new tasks, try new activities, or interact with others.

Section 7.1 Review Questions

1. Answer: The definition of health presented by the World Health Organization goes beyond physical conditions by thinking of the body as a unit—mental, physical, and spiritual.
2. Answer: Some habits include: routine physicals, adequate rest, good nutrition, good posture, aerobic exercise, immunizations, well-baby checks, weight control, elimination of body wastes, and avoiding substance abuse.
3. Answer: Spiritual fitness gives us meaning and purpose in life.
4. Answer: Sometimes patients are under emotional stress, which makes them have pain, and that's why a psychologist could be helpful.
5. Answer: Professions are psychologist, social worker, midwife, biofeedback specialist, chiropractor.
6. Answer: Answers will vary but could include:
   - Pregnancy: A woman can choose a midwife as her primary care giver.
   - Migraine headaches: A person experiences migraine headaches can choose acupressure.
   - Anxiety/sleep disorders: A person experiencing anxiety or sleep disorders can choose to see a hypnotist.

CUSTOMIZED INSTRUCTION

English Language Learners

English language learners might come from cultures where practices considered alternative in the U.S. are considered mainstream care. Ask them to share their experiences with these practices.

FOCUS AND ENGAGE

Introduce the Section

a. Review the content of the Background paragraph, emphasizing the importance of stability for complete health.

b. Explain that the section covers both the needs of the patient as well as the needs of the health care worker.

c. Discuss the objectives for the section.

Vocabulary Review

a. Key terms are defined in the margins of the text on the page where they first appear.

b. Pronounce each word, and have the students repeat the pronunciation out loud.

c. Discuss each definition.

TEACH

Discuss

- Emphasize the importance of meeting both the physical and psychological needs of patients and health care workers.
- Ask students to share experiences of when they felt their basic needs were unmet. They may have been thirsty, tired, or hungry.

Teaching Tips

- Discuss Maslow's Hierarchy and the five levels of basic needs.
- If desired, print an image of the hierarchy from a Web site such as simplypsychology.org/maslow.html or edpsycinteractive.org/topics/conation/maslow.html.
- Point out that basic needs include both the physiological and psychological.
- Refer to the tables on pp. 145–148 to discuss each category of physiological and psychological needs.

SECTION 7.2 Understanding Human Needs

Background

Each of us has needs that must be satisfied to maintain stability. Understanding a person's physiological and psychological needs—and helping patients/clients communicate these needs—is essential for every health care worker.

Objectives

When you have completed this section, you will be able to do the following:

- Match vocabulary terms with their correct meanings.
- Name four psychological needs that must be met to maintain stability.
- Name four physiological needs that must be met to maintain stability.
- Explain five benefits of pet-facilitated therapy.
- Recognize the importance of valuing differences in the people with whom you work.
- Match five defense mechanisms with the correct descriptions.
- Explain how you use defense mechanisms daily.

Meeting the Needs of Patients/Clients

For many years, psychologists have studied people to better determine what makes each of us act the way we do. One theory put forth more than 60 years ago by American psychologist Abraham Maslow suggests that our actions are motivated by the desire to fulfill our needs. Maslow developed a hierarchy of five levels of needs, called appropriately Maslow's Hierarchy. Often displayed as a pyramid, the most basic needs are at the bottom levels. These are physiological needs, such as oxygen, food, water, shelter, and the need to feel secure. Once these needs are met, the individual seeks to fulfill more complex needs. These are more psychological and social in nature, such as family, friendship, love, achievement, respect, and esteem. When all of these needs are satisfied, then the need for *self-actualization*, a person's need to be and do what he or she thinks they were born to do, becomes important.

It is important for the health care worker to understand and show sensitivity to the needs of their patients/clients. Physiological needs can be divided into four categories. Biological needs are listed in **Table 7.1a**; safety needs in **Table 7.1b**; sensory needs in **Table 7.1c**; and motor activity needs in **Table 7.1d**.

144 Chapter 7 | Wellness

- Review the four categories of physiological needs. Emphasize that these needs are the foundation of life.
- Discuss how understanding these needs can help a health care worker recognize the reasons for certain behaviors and respond appropriately.
- Point out that it is part of a health care worker's responsibility to identify when these needs are not being met.

TEAMWORK

Have you ever been thirsty, tired, or hungry? Have you choked or had an asthma attack and been unable to breathe? As a group, prepare a skit depicting a situation where one of your biological needs is unmet and present it to the class.

Table 7.1a Biological Needs—Food, Water, Sleep, and Waste Elimination

Threatened by Illness	Communication Needs	Age-Specific and Communication Needs	Cultural Awareness	Reporting and Recording Observations
■ Food and water may be withheld before various procedures or surgery is performed. ■ Sleep may be interrupted because of the environment, noises, or anxiety. ■ Elimination is frequently affected by changes in routine, foods, or medication.	■ Be committed to reflecting the value of dignity. Use effective communication skills that demonstrate holistic care. Be alert to the biological needs and communicate how they will be met during patient care. ■ For new patients explain: • Physician's orders concerning activity, food, use of the bathroom, and any expected special procedures; • Mealtimes; • How to request assistance or ask questions. ■ Always ask patients if they have any special requests or questions. ■ When sleep must be interrupted, inform the patient before he or she goes to sleep.	■ Use words that the patient can understand. Ask a translator to ensure that words and thoughts are fully communicated. ■ Allow decisions concerning food and sleep to be made by the patient when possible. ■ Tell patients what to expect. ■ Reassure children and parents of times they can be together. ■ Address people by their proper names and titles, especially older people. ■ Ask coherent patients if they have any specific fears. Address their fears honestly and with sensitivity, always treating people with dignity. Ask for assistance when necessary. ■ Remember that comments like "don't worry" are never helpful.	■ Many cultures of the world: • Believe that illness is caused by a supernatural power; • Use various herbs to treat illness and may request a specific diet; • Consider the color white to be bad luck. Medical personnel in white may cause an increase in fear; • Believe that hot and cold air currents negatively affect health. Be alert to drafts. ■ See Section 7.3 of this chapter for more information.	■ Report to your supervisor and record in the medical record: • Special requests; • Expressed fears;. • Your instructions about the medical routine; • Your observations of how the patient and family received instructions concerning the routine and potential limitations of food, water, interrupted sleep, and expected preparation for procedures that may affect elimination.

Wellness | Chapter 7 145

Teaching Tips

- Explain biological needs: Biological needs are survival needs. These must be met to maintain life: air, food, water, sleep, and elimination.
- Review Table 7.1a together as a class.
- Emphasize ways of communicating with the patient about his or her needs.

CUSTOMIZED INSTRUCTION

More Advanced Students

Have more advanced students look into the ways depriving people of basic needs affects their physical and psychological well-being. For example, they might research sleep deprivation, fasting, or hunger strikes. Have them present their findings to the class.

Teaching Tips

- Explain safety needs: Safety needs involve feeling secure as well as avoiding bodily harm and injury.
- Review Table 7.1b together as a class.
- Point out that feeling secure is a valid need, and just as important as actually being in a safe environment.
- Remind students that they should never ignore a patient's fears, and should treat all concerns seriously.

Table 7.1b Safety Needs—Needs to Feel Secure and to Avoid Bodily Harm and Injury

Threatened by Illness	Communication Needs	Age-Specific and Communication Needs	Cultural Awareness	Reporting and Recording Observations
■ Patients needing medical procedures and treatments may feel insecure. They may be facing hospitalization for the first time and are afraid they will be hurt or die. They may be entering a long-term care facility where they will live for the rest of their lives. They may wonder: • What will happen to me? • How will I be treated? • Will I be safe? ■ Patients may also be worried about pain or accidents that could occur during procedures.	■ Be sure that the patient fully understands what you are saying. Use pictures, culturally appropriate gestures, writing and/or a translator to ensure understanding. ■ Tell patients what they can expect from you and your team. Introduce yourself and your team. Your reassuring presence and warm touch may be enough to help a patient feel safe. ■ For new hospital patients: • Tell patients how to request assistance or contact you—explain the call system and intercom. ■ Show your commitment to service and treating others with dignity by always doing what you say you're going to do. This helps create trust and builds a sense of security for patients and their families.	■ Think of the patient's age and ability to understand before speaking. Use the patient's words as much as possible. Speak at his or her level. ■ When caring for pediatric patients, ask the family if special words or objects communicate special things. For example, a child may call a special toy or blanket a "binky." ■ When possible, allow family or significant others to be present if the patient requests their presence.	■ Be alert to body language and other forms of communication that may provide clues to the patient's state of mind. ■ See Section 7.3 of this chapter for more information on various cultural beliefs that may affect the way health care is given.	■ Report to your supervisor and record in the medical record: • Special requests; • Expressed fears; • Your instructions about medical routine; • Your observations of how the patient and family received instructions.

146 Chapter 7 | Wellness

CUSTOMIZED INSTRUCTION

Less Advanced Students

Less advanced students may have trouble deciphering the tables. Try pairing them with other students so they can read and interpret the tables as a team.

Table 7.1c Sensory Needs—Stimulation of the Five Senses (Hearing, Seeing, Feeling, Smelling, Tasting) as Well as Intellectual Stimulation

Threatened by Illness	Communication Needs	Age-Specific and Communication Needs	Cultural Awareness	Reporting and Recording Observations
■ When the senses are not stimulated they diminish. For example, when a patient is not able to eat, intravenous fluids may be used. Because the smell and taste sensors are not stimulated, when the patient begins to eat again it will take time for taste and smell to return to normal. ■ The senses are less responsive to stimulation as we age. Geriatric patients may have lost one or more of their senses. They may have difficulty hearing or seeing which may increase their fear and cause anxiety.	■ Communicating with people experiencing a sensory loss takes patience and imagination. Try some of the following to stimulate their senses. • People with hearing loss can experience music by touching a speaker while it plays music. They can feel rhythm vibrate through the speaker. • Patients with touch-impaired senses usually lose feeling in their hands and feet. When it is reasonable, touch their face or arms with things that they want to feel, such as a warm towel. • Sight-, smell-, and taste-impaired patients appreciate your description of colors, smells, or flavors in their environment. For example, you might say, "Remember the smell of turkey roasting and fresh bread baking? That's what it smells like today." ■ When working with people, show your commitment to excellence by being sensitive and remembering to use techniques that help people experience their senses.	■ The loss of senses during the aging process also adds to the loss of well-being. As a health care worker you can help restore a sense of well-being by being aware and using techniques that help people experience or remember the feelings of their five senses. ■ When you are aware of sensory loss, talk to the person and ask what helps him or her experience the lost sense. Try various techniques that will help stimulate the senses, always explaining what you are doing.	■ The various cultures of the world relate differently to touch, gestures, and personal space. As a health care worker it is important that you are mindful of the various cultures and the potential barriers relative to the body senses. ■ See Section 7.3 of this chapter for more details.	■ Report to your supervisor and record in the medical record: • Special requests; • Expressed fears; • Your instructions about medical routine; • Your observations of how the patient and family received instructions.

Wellness | Chapter 7 147

Teaching Tips

- Explain sensory needs: Sensory needs require stimulation of the senses and the mind.
- Remind students of the five senses:
  - Hearing
  - Sight
  - Taste
  - Smell
  - Touch
- Review Table 7.1c together as a class.
- Ask students to share personal stories they might have of relatives or friends who have lost sensory perception.
- For example, they may have a grandparent who has lost hearing or sight.
- Emphasize the importance of compassion.

TEAMWORK

Working in pairs, practice describing objects for visually impaired patients. Have one partner wear a blindfold while the other describes an object without naming the object. When the blindfolded partner identifies the object correctly, switch roles.

CUSTOMIZED INSTRUCTION

Special Needs Students

Be sure to engage students with visual or hearing impairments in the discussion about sensory needs. What tools or devices help them communicate and ensure their needs are met?

Teaching Tips

- Explain motor activity needs: Motor activity needs involve moving or exercising the body.
- Review Table 7.1d together as a class.
- Explain the term *atrophy*.
- Note that safety needs may also be of concern when addressing motor activity needs.
- Point out that patients may not always recognize the benefits of motor activity, and may resist because:
  - It may hurt.
  - It may seem unnecessary.
  - They may be tired.
- Discuss ways a health care provider can overcome a patient's resistance.
- Ask students to share personal stories or experiences they may have had wearing a cast.

TEAMWORK

Imagine you are a health care provider treating a patient who just had surgery. It is vital for him to get out of bed and start walking. In pairs, present a skit demonstrating how you would go about getting the patient up and about.

Table 7.1d Motor Activity—Movement or Exercise of the Body

Threatened by Illness	Communication Needs	Age-Specific and Communication Needs	Cultural Awareness	Reporting and Recording Observations
■ When muscles are not stimulated they atrophy (shrink) and eventually weaken and can even become frozen. The results of a lack of muscle stimulation may or may not be reversible depending on the length of time the muscle was not stimulated. For example, when a cast is removed from an arm or a leg after a long period, the arm or leg is usually much smaller than the one which was not in a cast. The casted limb was not able to stimulate the muscles so they shrank and became weak. Weakened muscles can prevent free and easy movement.	■ Be sure that the patient fully understands what you are saying. Use pictures, culturally appropriate gestures, writing and/or a translator to ensure understanding. ■ People who experience difficulty moving around must be informed about how to reach you and others at all times. ■ Inform the person that you are aware of his or her condition and will take precautions to protect any special needs. ■ Explain the procedures that you will use to ensure the patient's safety as you help him or her move or as you do procedures. ■ Share expected times that procedures and other things will happen, and always follow through with the schedule.	■ Remember to ask patients if they follow a certain procedure that best accommodates their limited or painful movement. Never do anything contradictory to your training or good judgment. ■ When appropriate, encourage people to do as much as possible on their own to promote self-sufficiency.	■ Be alert to your patient's customs concerning personal space. Always tell the patient what you are going to do before you start to move or touch him or her. ■ Be aware of cultural taboos about touching the head and appropriate versus inappropriate hand gestures. ■ See Section 7.3 of this chapter for more details.	■ Report to your supervisor and record in the medical record: • Special requests; • Expressed fears; • Your instructions about medical routine; • Your observations of how the patient and family received instructions.

148 Chapter 7 | Wellness

Psychological needs are divided into four categories. Adequacy and security needs are listed in Table 7.2a; social approval and self-esteem needs in Table 7.2b; order and meaning in life needs in Table 7.2c; and self-growth needs in Table 7.2d.

Understanding their **physiological** and **psychological** needs helps you be a better health care worker. You are able to recognize the reasons for certain behaviors and respond appropriately.

physiological
(fiz ee uh LOJ I kuhl)
Pertaining to normal body functions.

psychological
(sahy kuh LOJ I kuhl)
Pertaining to the mind.

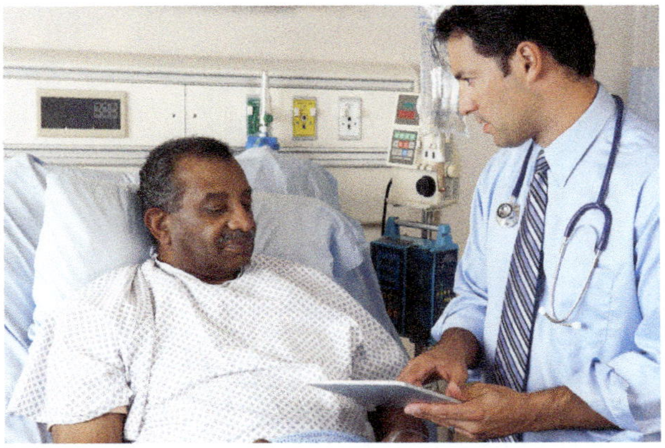

Figure 7.5
Clients worry about many things when hospitalized. How can you help calm a patient?

Pet-Facilitated Therapy

Recent studies have focused on the **value** of the human-pet bond, showing that petting or stroking a pet has an immediate effect on the body. Most people studied showed:

- A slowing heartbeat
- Deeper breaths
- Fewer abnormal heartbeats
- Lowered blood pressure
- An increased sense of well-being

value
(VAL yoo)
Importance, worth.

Over 50 percent of American households have pets, primarily for the companionship that they provide. Research shows that even when people do not respond well to other people, they do respond to pets. They talk to their pets. They care for the needs of their pets. When there is a human–animal bond, people often find new meaning in life. They feel less lonely. They feel needed because their pets are totally dependent on them. They have a reason to get out of the house to buy food for their pets. The pet may be just the friend or responsibility they need to help feel better or to feel good about themselves. Research also shows that fish swimming gracefully in an aquarium with swaying plants creates a relaxing environment that reduces stress.

Wellness | Chapter 7 149

Teaching Tips

- Review the four categories of psychological needs.
- Ask students how they feel these needs are met or unmet in their lives.
- Introduce pet-therapy as an example of an alternative therapy that has shown proven results. The discussion of pet therapy is continued on p. 152.

Figure Focus

7.5 Clients worry about many things when hospitalized. How can you help calm a patient?

Answer: Discuss what must be done to promote good health and to treat specific conditions; encourage the patient to comment and ask questions; provide opportunities for the patient to be involved as much as possible in decision-making.

ACTIVITY

Do you have a pet? Write a personal essay about how your pet helps you physically and/or psychologically. If you do not have a pet, write about how you think a pet might help you. Share your essay with the class.

Teaching Tips

- Explain adequacy and security needs: Need to feel in control and able to cope.
- Review Table 7.2a together as a class.
- Explain social approval and self-esteem needs: Need to be recognized and accepted by others.
- Review Table 7.2b together as a class.

TEAMWORK

Select an illness, disease, or condition. To help patients understand the selected topic, work as a team to develop a brochure, pamphlet, or handout about it. You should try to answer as many questions as possible, including information about symptoms, causes, and treatments, as well as statistical information, if it is available.

Table 7.2a Adequacy and Security—Need to Feel in Control and Capable of Coping

Threatened by Illness	Communication Needs	Age-Specific and Communication Needs	Cultural Awareness	Reporting and Recording Observations
■ When a condition occurs that requires medical treatment, it is easy to feel a loss of control. Medications and various procedures and disease processes can change the way the body feels and what a person is capable of doing. ■ Loss of a sense of control affects physical and emotional well-being.	■ Discuss what must be done to promote good health and to treat specific conditions. Encourage the patient to comment and make decisions as much as possible. ■ Show your commitment to dignity and justice by providing opportunities for patients to be involved as much as possible in decision making.	■ When possible, provide the opportunity for patients to make decisions such as what they will eat or wear.	■ Be aware of cultural customs that show respect or disrespect. For example, making direct eye contact in some cultures is disrespectful. Adapt your behavior and language to show respect for each person.	■ Report to your supervisor and record in the medical record: • Signs of insecurity; • Voiced inadequacies; • Your observations; • Special requests; • Your observations of how the patient and family received instructions.

Table 7.2b Social Approval and Self-Esteem—Recognition and Acceptance by Other People

Threatened by Illness	Communication Needs	Age-Specific and Communication Needs	Cultural Awareness	Reporting and Recording Observations
■ When illness limits what a person is able to do at work, at home, or in social situations, depression can occur. This in turn can affect the success of treatment. The patient's ability to support his family may be taken away by an illness that causes job loss. This causes extreme stress.	■ It is important to spend time with patients who feel isolated. Patients in quarantine or who have visible body changes may feel different and isolated from their friends and family. Spending time with them and learning about their life can help them feel accepted. ■ Encourage family and friends to include them in activities and events when possible. ■ Show your commitment to dignity by practicing active listening skills. Show interest in the patient's concerns and past experiences. ■ Inform the patient and family of available helpful resources (e.g., social services).	■ When caring for children, use terms they can understand. ■ Be positive even when you want to say something negative. ■ As a health care worker, you can help restore a sense of well-being by staying alert to your patient's preferences. Use resources within your facility to encourage and promote socialization with others who may be having similar experiences. ■ Use age-appropriate vocabulary. Do not use childish gestures or language to talk with an elderly person.	■ Use culturally appropriate gestures and words to show respect. Honoring a person's culture is an effective way of reinforcing self-esteem and showing social approval. ■ Be aware of dietary needs or restrictions. ■ Encourage family and friends to display pictures and articles that may bring warm and comforting memories.	■ Report to your supervisor and record in the medical record: • Signs of low self esteem; • Voiced inadequacies; • Your observations concerning any change in behavior; for example, withdrawal, passive behavior, wanting to give things away, refusing to see people; • Special requests; • Your observation of how the patient and family received instructions.

150 Chapter 7 | Wellness

Table 7.2c Order and Meaning in Life—Understanding of What Is Going on in One's Environment

Threatened by Illness	Communication Needs	Age-Specific and Communication Needs	Cultural Awareness	Reporting and Recording Observations
■ When illness occurs, it is difficult to know what to expect or how to plan for the future. ■ Meaning and purpose in life are in question if an illness changes the way we do things. ■ Order that brings a sense of control is lost, leaving a feeling of being out of control and uncertain.	■ Tell patients what to expect before, during, and after procedures to help them psychologically prepare for the experience. ■ Listen to the patient so you will have an understanding of his or her concerns. ■ Respond with understanding. For example, "We will be starting your physical therapy today and I'm bringing you the schedule so you will know when to expect the therapist."	■ Use words that the patient can understand. Ask for a translator to ensure that words and thoughts are fully communicated. ■ Write information and schedules on a paper that the patient and family can refer to. Use pictures for children, like a clock with the hands pointing to a time you will return.	■ Use culturally appropriate gestures and words to show respect. ■ Be aware of routine cultural activities that bring meaning to the patient.	■ Report to your supervisor and record in the medical record: • Signs of low self esteem; • Voiced inadequacies; • Your observations concerning any change; • Special requests.

Table 7.2d Self-Growth—Need for Fulfillment Beyond Basic Needs

Threatened by Illness	Communication Needs	Age-Specific and Communication Needs	Cultural Awareness	Reporting and Recording Observations
■ Illness often consumes our thoughts. Patients who experience a long illness or physical changes that limit their abilities may experience a loss of personal growth.	■ Use active listening skills to identify patients' special interests. Encourage them to share the details of these interests. When appropriate, discuss possible options with the care team that will allow the patient to experience learning. Your commitment to treating others with dignity are a reality when you take action in this way.	■ Use words that the patient can understand. Ask for a translator to ensure that words and thoughts are fully communicated. ■ When caring for children, introduce activities at the child's level of understanding. ■ Be sure enough time is given to teach and not frustrate the patient of any age.	■ Seek culturally appropriate learning for the patient. ■ Some cultures view games as childish; being sensitive to cultural attitudes will help the patient accept new opportunities.	■ Report to your supervisor and record in the medical record: • Voiced discouragement or being bored; • Your observations concerning mood changes; • Special requests; • Involvement of any kind that promotes learning.

Teaching Tips

- Explain order and meaning in life needs: Need to understand what is going on around oneself.
- Review Table 7.2c together as a class.
- Explain self-growth needs: Need to find fulfillment in areas of life beyond the basic needs.
- Review Table 7.2d together as a class.

ACTIVITY

Have students create a poster depicting one way they meet their own psychological need for self-growth and fulfillment. Display the posters in the classroom or on a bulletin board.

Teaching Tips

- Continue the discussion of pet therapy.
- Discuss how research has found that patients respond to pets in many positive ways:
    - Reduced loneliness
    - Increased exercise
    - Added meaning to life
    - Reduced stress
- Discuss the difference between the benefits of pet-ownership and the benefits of pet-therapy (in a long-term care facility, hospital, or nursing home).
- Discuss the characteristics of a healthy relationship. These include respect, honesty, trust, and open communication.
- Stress the importance of effective communication in building workplace relationships:
    - When you listen and respond to someone, you show respect.
    - When you provide objective comments, you show honesty.
    - When you share ideas and opinions, you show trust.
    - When you are willing to discuss differences, you show openness.
- Explain that you are more likely to be a productive and satisfied employee when you are with people you respect and trust, and who respect and trust you.

Figure 7.6
What are some of the benefits of pet therapy?

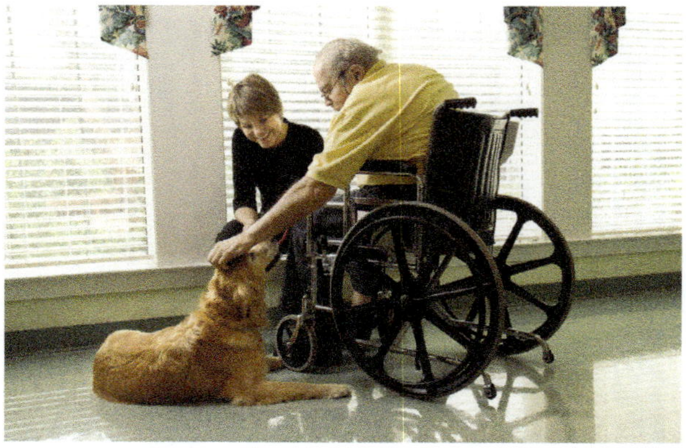

Based on this research, the medical community actively promotes healthier lifestyles through the companionship of pets. People who are experiencing many changes in their lives often find a pet to be the one unchanging element. Some people may be lonely and find that a pet is a good companion, while others simply enjoy the pleasure and presence of a pet.

Pet-facilitated therapy can be used as a treatment. Animals are taken into convalescent homes and children's hospitals. Some hospitals have arranged to have a pet live on the premises. Other programs have been developed with the Humane Society, and pets are brought in to visit on a regular basis. Pet-facilitated therapy is especially effective in the home. An aging person may feel depressed and alone. A pet brings new meaning to life. Now there is something that really needs him or her and is affectionate and loving. The same kind of therapy is effective for a sick child.

Meeting the Needs of Co-Workers

Recognizing how to meet the needs of your patients/clients makes you a better health care worker. Recognizing human needs in the staff you work with helps make you a successful member of the health care team. But you must also understand the importance of healthy relationships with your co-workers.

Like any other relationship, the relationships you build at work can affect your on-the-job success, job satisfaction, physical health, and overall well-being. Building positive working relationships helps you in the following areas:

- **Makes you more productive.** Working well with others helps avoid conflict, which usually leads to work being done faster and better.
- **Gives you additional opportunities to learn.** Your co-workers can be excellent resources for helping you improve your skills.

152 Chapter 7 | Wellness

Figure Focus

7.6 What are some benefits of pet therapy?

Answer: Pets can bring meaning to life, offering affection and devotion. Through pet therapy, a person might feel less lonely.

- **Makes work more enjoyable.** While work isn't meant to be all fun and games, it can be less stressful and more agreeable if you like the people you work with.
- **Makes you feel better.** When the work environment is positive, friendly, and supportive, you will wake up looking forward to the work day. This working environment will promote both your physical and emotional well-being.

On the other hand, negative working relationships can lead to conflicts, which can decrease productivity, increase stress, and even be the cause of dismissal. In addition, a negative work environment can cause physical illness and emotional anxiety that can also lead to illness.

Valuing Differences

You will encounter people with different backgrounds and experiences in your workplace. You are likely to encounter people from different societies with different cultures. Sometimes, these differences can cause conflict:

- You might think the food a co-worker eats in the lunchroom smells bad, even though it is common in his or her native country.
- You might be frustrated trying to understand a co-worker who speaks English as a second language.
- You might become impatient waiting for a disabled co-worker to complete a task you know you could do faster.

Understanding the differences between your co-workers makes it easier to communicate, which, in turn, helps you to find common bonds. Though you may have different cultures, beliefs, backgrounds, or skills, you are all working toward the same goals: to get your work done and help your organization succeed. At work, focusing on the common goals you and your co-workers share will help you see past the differences to resolve conflicts.

Community

Form teams of five. Each member will select a society with a different ethnic group and research practices and beliefs on what causes illness, how it should be treated, and who is involved in the treatment. Use the Internet and library to gather information. If possible, interview members of the ethnic group. In your word processing or desktop publishing program, create a brochure that provides brief demographic information on the ethnic group and describes their beliefs on health care. With permission, share the brochure with local health care providers.

Defense Mechanisms

Defense mechanisms are mental devices that help people cope with various situations. Health care workers who are aware of defense mechanisms better understand themselves, their co-workers, their supervisors, and their patients' behavior. Following are some common defense mechanisms:

- **Rationalization.** Finding good reasons to replace the real reason for behavior in order to maintain self-esteem. *Example:* Mark did poorly on a test and explained it by saying, "I'd rather be popular than smart."
- **Compensation.** Substituting one goal for another. *Example:* Mary really wanted to be on the track team but wasn't good enough. Instead, she joined the choir and became a soloist.
- **Projection.** Placing the blame for your actions on someone or something else because you cannot accept the responsibility. *Example:* "I didn't get a good grade in my health occupations class because the teacher doesn't like me."

TEAMWORK

In small groups or pairs, select one type of need, such as biological or safety. Think of a motivational slogan encouraging co-workers to meet that need in one another. Draw a poster illustrating the slogan.

Teaching Tips

- Ask students to consider the importance of etiquette, manners, and understanding when it comes to dealing with differences among co-workers.
- Explain that cross-cultural communication is a critical skill for all employees, regardless of their job or the industry in which they work.
- As companies continue to expand their international business, employees at all levels must learn to deal with cultural and ethnic differences.
- Also, cultural diversity within the workplace requires employees to be open-minded and flexible.
- Review each of the defense mechanisms.
- Ask students to identify any defense mechanisms that they use, or that they have seen others use.
- Emphasize that everyone uses defense mechanisms every day in order to cope with unexpected or difficult situations.
- Discuss how recognizing defense mechanisms in others will help make a person a more effective health care worker.

Community

- Decide whether you will allow class time for students to research the report, or if it will be a homework assignment.
- You may want to have a list of possible topics and resources they can use.
- Encourage students to use a presentation graphics software program to develop the report.
- Provide class time for students to practice delivering the report.

Science Link—Fight-or-Flight Response

- Review the causes and effects of a fight-or-flight response.
- Discuss the historical importance of the fight-or-flight response in preserving human life.
- Ask students to consider whether such a response still has merit in modern times.

What is a good way to slow your breathing and heart rate after a fight-or-flight response?

Answer: Students may suggest doing five minutes of physical activity, such as jumping jacks, push-ups, or a quick jog to eliminate excess stress hormones.

TEAMWORK

In small groups, randomly select one of the defense mechanisms listed on pp. 153–154 of the section text. Perform a skit depicting someone using the defense mechanism in a health care environment. The class should be able to identify the defense mechanism.

aggressiveness
(uh GRES iv ness)
Tendency to start fights and quarrels or to attack without reason.

hostility
(hos STIL i tee)
Unfriendliness; ill will toward another.

idolizing
(AHYD l ahyz ing)
Loving to excess.

- **Sublimation.** Redirecting feelings toward a constructive objective. *Example:* You enjoy playing tennis and you use the game to work out **aggressiveness** and **hostility** instead of directing those feelings toward others.
- **Identification.** **Idolizing** someone you would like to be like. *Example:* Margaret especially admired her music teacher. She began to walk and dress like her.

When you are aware that everyone uses defense mechanisms, and when you know what they are, you are able to better understand your behavior and the behavior of others.

Science Link

Fight-or-Flight Response

You can probably recall a situation in which you felt threatened or scared. Perhaps your teacher surprised you with an unexpected test or you had an argument with a classmate. In situations like these, your heart pounds, your muscles tighten, and your mind races. You are experiencing a fight-or-flight response.

The fight-or-flight response, also known as the acute stress response, was first described by the American physiologist Walter Cannon in 1927.

He described it as an inborn response that prepares the body to either deal with or flee from a perceived threat in order to survive. In response to the threat, changes occur in the nerve cells of the body, and hormones such as adrenaline and cortisol are released into the blood stream.

The combination of nerve cell and chemical activity causes the rate of respiration to increase. Blood is shunted away from the digestive tract and directed into muscles and limbs, which require extra energy and fuel for running or fighting. The pupils of the eyes dilate as the person's awareness of the surroundings intensifies. At the same time, the perception of pain decreases. Essentially, the fight-or-flight response bypasses your thinking mind and puts your body into an attack mode.

Long ago, the fight-or-flight response often saved people from physical threats, such as saber-toothed tigers and opposing warriors. Today, the threats are different. They might be found on the soccer field, in the classroom, or at the office. The response has also changed. Running and fighting are not always appropriate or feasible options—for example, in the case of an unexpected pop quiz. Nonetheless, the response prepares your body to deal with the situation in order to protect yourself.

The natural conclusion of fight-or-flight is physical activity. Some researchers suggest that without the physical conclusion, people can suffer from the buildup of stress hormones. Some people experience symptoms such as muscle tension, headache, upset stomach, racing heartbeat, deep sighing, or shallow breathing. Others may experience anxiety, poor concentration, depression, hopelessness, frustration, anger, or fear.

Perhaps the easiest way to slow the body's activities after a fight-or-flight response is through physical exercise. Exercise helps the body break down excess stress hormones, thereby restoring both body and mind to a calmer, more relaxed state.

What is a good way to slow your breathing and heart rate after a fight-or-flight response?

Develop a model to illustrate how intake and expulsion of air to and from the lungs is affected in response to physical activity at given intervals; for example, running or skipping in place at three two-minute intervals (breaths per 15 seconds multiplied times four for a one-minute count).

Plan and conduct an investigation to provide evidence that the heart rate increases in response to physical exercise.

154 Chapter 7 | Wellness

CUSTOMIZED INSTRUCTION

At-Risk Students

Explain that conflict can cause stress and fear, and sometimes make you feel threatened. When you feel this way, you may not be reasonable or realistic about the situation. Ask students to create a list of what they do (or could do) to calm down and control their emotions. Some suggestions: taking a deep breath, counting to ten, exercising, identifying your role in the conflict, brainstorming solutions, asking someone for advice, or simply removing yourself from the situation.

Personal Wellness

Depression

Everyone feels sad or blue once in a while when situations go wrong or disappointments arise. For some people, however, sadness is a constant emotion—even when there is no obvious reason for it. This disorder, known as depression, is not a passing mood or a sign of weakness. People who suffer from depression cannot simply "get over it" or assume it will go away.

The symptoms of depression go beyond mere sadness. People who suffer from depression may also experience any or all of the following symptoms:

- A change in sleeping patterns
- A change in eating habits
- An increase in fatigue
- Unexplained aches and pains
- A loss of interest in activities and friends
- Difficulty concentrating
- Feelings of hopelessness, helplessness, and worthlessness

The causes of depression vary from one person to another. Low self-esteem, pessimism, and anxiety are major contributing factors in some types of depression. Physical changes, such as a stroke, heart attack, or hormone disorders can also lead to depression. Stresses at home or school, life and relationship changes, and family history are also important factors.

If you or someone you know displays any symptoms of depression, there are several steps you can take to start the healing process. Begin by identifying any problems that might be causing the symptoms. For example, consider living conditions, relationships, diet, physical fitness, and spiritual beliefs. Regain control of your life by looking for ways to fix problems and eliminate sources of sorrow. Develop a healthier diet, get regular exercise and sleep, and establish a support system of friends and family. Set realistic goals each day, and determine priorities in your life.

If symptoms persist, seek a professional counselor who can help you work through issues and refer you to a physician if medication is required. Health care workers should be aware of the signs and symptoms of depression. Basic tools used to screen the patient for depression should be available for use in the health care setting. Mental health resources for referral should be made available to the patient. This is a part of providing the patient with holistic care.

Treatment for depression can last for months or years, but a combination of psychotherapy and medication can often reduce or even eliminate symptoms of depression.

How might an increase in exercise help defeat mild depression?

Summary

Human beings have physiological needs, which include biological needs, safety needs, sensory needs, and motor activity needs. They also have psychological needs, which include the need to feel adequate and secure, to have social approval and self-esteem, to have order and meaning in life, and to experience self-growth. These needs must be met at all times. It is important to always be aware of these needs in our patients/clients, our co-workers, our supervisors, and ourselves.
All people use defense mechanisms to help them feel comfortable inside. These include rationalization, compensation, projection, sublimation, and identification.

Wellness | Chapter 7 155

Personal Wellness—Depression

- Emphasize that there is a difference between being sad for a short time and being depressed.
- Review some of the causes and symptoms of depression.
- Discuss holistic approaches to treating depression, as well as resources that might be available in your area for someone suffering from depression.
- Discuss medical approaches to treating depression, such as meeting with a psychiatrist, or drug therapy.

How might an increase in exercise help defeat mild depression?

Answer: Exercise, along with a balanced diet, gives the body the energy it needs to conduct normal activities and to respond to unexpected situations as they arise. It helps enable a person to interact successfully with others rather than feeling isolated. Exercise increases the production of natural endorphins, which help a person feel better. When people feel well physically, their thoughts become clearer, positive beliefs are easier to form, and perceptions are more open. People who feel tired and physically run down, on the other hand, tend to focus on the negative aspects of every situation.

Section 7.2 Review Questions

1. Compare and contrast physiological and psychological needs. Give an example of each.
2. What are some physical effects on a person who strokes a pet?
3. Briefly explain the Maslow Hierarchy.
4. List one benefit of building and maintaining positive relationships with your co-workers.
5. What are defense mechanisms, and why do people use them?
6. What causes the fight-or-flight response?
7. Evaluate and describe positive effects of work relationships on physical and emotional health. Give one example of how positive work relationships can affect your physical health. Give one example of how positive work relationships affect your attitude and sense of well-being.
8. Evaluate and describe negative effects of work relationships on physical and emotional health. Give one example of how negative work relationships can affect your physical health. Give one example of how negative work relationships affect your attitude and sense of well-being.

SECTION 7.3 Cross-Cultural Terms and Principles

Background

Health care workers interact with people from many cultural backgrounds. It is important to know culturally acceptable and effective gestures, terms, and behaviors. This knowledge allows the health care worker to adapt his or her care and communication techniques to meet individual needs. The patient/client receives quality care, and the experience is a positive one.

Objectives

When you have completed this section, you will be able to do the following:

- Explain how culture influences behavior.
- Identify culturally acceptable and effective gestures, terms, and behaviors.
- Recognize communication techniques that create a positive exchange of information.
- Identify common folk medicine practices.
- Compare and contrast cultural differences.
- Explain how understanding cultural beliefs affects you as a health care worker.

Society, Culture, and Behavior

Society is referred to as a group of people who share a common area, culture, and behavior patterns. When caring for and working with people from various societies with different cultures, you must understand their cultural background. Understanding allows you to have positive experiences and to communicate effectively. Our understanding and opinions of different societies and other cultures

156 Chapter 7 | Wellness

Section 7.2 Review Questions

1. Answer: Physiological needs pertain to normal body functions and psychological needs pertain to the mind. Examples of physiological needs are food, water, air, and sleep. Examples of psychological needs are safety, self-esteem, and independence.
2. Answer: Physical effects include: slower heartbeat, deeper breaths, few abnormal heartbeats, lowered blood pressure, and increased sense of self-worth.
3. Answer: The Maslow Hierarchy is often displayed as a pyramid in which the most basic needs are at the bottom levels. These are physiological needs, such as oxygen, food, water, shelter, and the need to feel secure. Once these needs are met, the individual seeks to fulfill more complex needs. These are more psychological and social in nature, such as family, friendship, love, achievement, respect, and esteem. When all of these needs are satisfied, then the need for self-actualization—a person's need to be and do what he or she thinks they were born to do—becomes important.
4. Answer: Benefits include making you more productive, giving you additional opportunities to learn, and making work more enjoyable.
5. Answer: Defense mechanisms are mental devices that help people cope with various situations, and people use them to make them feel comfortable and to make their behavior seem reasonable.
6. Answer: Situations in which you feel threatened or scared are causes for the fight-or-flight response.
7. The answers students give will be based on their personal frame of reference including positive experiences they have had that may be limited at this point in their lives. You might let them know that as their world expands these answers may change and how they need to consider ways to repeat and expand on those experiences they see as positive to their personal well-being.
8. The answers students give will be based on their personal frame of reference including negative experiences they have had at this point in their lives. You might let them know that as their world expands they might consider ways to eliminate or influence these negative experiences.

FOCUS AND ENGAGE

Introduce the Section

a. Review the content of the Background paragraph, emphasizing the importance of understanding people from different cultures.

develop through our life experiences. Culture includes a shared background. This means that cultural groups share things such as:

- Language
- Communication style
- Belief system
- Customs
- Attitudes
- Perceptions
- Values

Language and communication styles and some customs are recognizable to people outside of a specific cultural group. But other things, such as belief systems, attitudes, perceptions, and values are less recognizable. Think of a tree. The trunk, branches, and leaves are all visible—like language, communication styles, and some customs are apparent in people. The roots of a tree, however, grow deep underground and nourish it to keep it strong—but they are not visible. So it is with culture: Belief systems, attitudes, perceptions, and values all come together to create a strong foundation that helps form a person.

Taking interest in different cultures broadens your thinking and opens doors to new ideas. When we refuse to be open and accepting of cultural differences, we can easily **prejudge** and form prejudices. Some prejudices include:

prejudge
(pree JUHJ)
To decide or make a decision before having the facts.

- **Agism.** A person is judged to be too old or too young.
- **National.** A person is judged based on his or her country of origin.
- **Physical.** A person is judged based on his or her appearance.
- **Mental.** A person is judged based on his or her intellect, knowledge, and opinions.
- **Religious.** A person is judged based on his or her religious beliefs.
- **Racial.** A person is judged based on his or her race.

You can overcome prejudice by learning about others:

- Keep an open mind.
- Seek out additional information. Why do people think the way they think? For example, why does someone think people of another culture are lazy or not smart?
- Watch documentaries and read books, magazines, and newspapers for information.
- Consider many resources before you form an opinion.
- Evaluate all the information. Ask yourself if it is true or false.

There are some basic points to keep in mind when experiencing aspects of a different culture:

- Values are an important part of every culture. Cultures have values and ideals that they believe, yet individual conduct may not always reflect those values. For example, a culture may value and honor their national flag, but not everyone in the cultural group may have a flag or display it.
- Behavior is influenced by many things, in addition to an individual's culture. Age, financial status, education, gender, experience, relationships, and health are all factors that affect behavior.

Wellness | Chapter 7 157

b. Point out that health care workers frequently come into contact with people from other cultures, both as patients and co-workers.
c. Review the objectives for the section.

Vocabulary Review

a. Key terms are defined in the margins of the text on the page where they first appear.
b. Pronounce each word, and have the students repeat the pronunciation out loud.
c. Discuss the definition of each word.

TEACH

Discuss

- Display magazines about other cultures.
- Ask students if they have preconceived ideas about people from other cultures.
- Discuss the importance of communication and understanding between health care workers and patients in order to facilitate effective care.

Teaching Tips

- Explain that culture is the commonality among individuals and groups:
  - Basic beliefs, moral/ethical codes of behavior, and values
  - Language and communication styles
  - Customs, reflected in feasts and celebrations, clothing, grooming, and other rituals
- Review the list of common things shared by a group and relate them to the classroom as a group, or your school.
- There may be students from different cultures in the class. Ask them to share information about their language and customs.
- Explain that culture influences behavior.
- Discuss preconceived ideas or stereotypes.
- Emphasize that in today's global society, you must be able to work with people from many different cultural backgrounds.
- Point out that understanding cultural differences allows positive interactions.
- Discuss the influences that shape individual prejudices or acceptance of other cultures.

ACTIVITY

Draw a tree diagram depicting your own culture. Include the visible characteristics such as language, dress, and customs on the branches and leaves. Include the less visible characteristics such as values and beliefs on the roots.

ACTIVITY

Prepare a presentation about a culture different from your own. You may use a presentation software program, or write a report supported with a poster. Include information about language, geographic origins, beliefs, customs, celebrations, and other distinguishing facts.

Teaching Tips

- Review some ways of overcoming prejudice.
- Discuss the concept of "finding common ground" with others. For example, many cultures value education, many have common religious beliefs, many have similar attitudes toward family.
- Introduce the concepts of ethnicity, culture, gender, and race.
- Emphasize that they are not the same:
  - Culture: Behaviors, beliefs and actions characteristic of a particular social, ethnic, or age group.
  - Ethnicity: Identity with or membership in a particular racial, national, or cultural group and observance of that group's customs, beliefs, and language.
  - Gender: The differences between men and women and how they are treated and expected to behave may be influenced by culture, but being aware of cultural aspects is only one consideration. Gender equity is a goal for many.
  - Race: A human population that is considered distinct based on physical characteristics.
- Review the difference between assimilation and acculturation.
- Emphasize the importance of tolerance and understanding for all people, and particularly for health care workers.
- Explain objective behavior. Compare it to subjective behavior.
- Discuss how understanding different cultures prepares a health care worker to meet the needs of all patients.

- Look for the common characteristics of different cultures or to seek a common ground. For example, we are all part of the human race so food is common to all of us. We can explore different flavors, which are created by spices, cooking techniques, and so on. We also all have seasons of the year that have special meaning and that are celebrated through traditions.

Ethnicity, Culture, Gender, Age, and Race

Career Connect

Visit your local fire department, Red Cross office, or emergency room and research the problems they face when working in communities of different cultures. How do they address their needs? Do they have specific training? How does it impact their jobs?

We often refer to culture, ethnicity, and race interchangeably. Culture relates to the behaviors, beliefs, and actions characteristic of a particular social, ethnic, or age group. Ethnicity refers to identity with or membership in a particular racial, national, or cultural group and observance of that group's customs, beliefs, and language. Race is a human population that is considered distinct based on physical characteristics, such as skin color. The U.S. Census Bureau collects data on the following racial categories: White American, African American, Asian American, European American, Hispanic American, Middle Eastern/Arab American, and Native American.

Our country is known as the "melting pot" because its population consists of people representing many different cultures. Cultural assimilation—or the integration of members of an ethno-cultural group into an established, generally larger community—has occurred, and often results in the smaller group's characteristics being absorbed into the larger group.

Acculturation, on the other hand, is the exchange of cultural features that results when groups come into continuous firsthand contact. The original cultural patterns of either or both groups may be altered, but the groups remain distinct.

It's important for the health care worker to exhibit sensitivity—understanding the value of cultural differences and treating each person with respect and dignity. For example, a traditional Muslim woman is not allowed to be examined by male members of the medical staff. It is always preferable that a female member of the medical staff is present.

Health care professionals need to be objective and should not be predisposed to a set opinion or idea; for instance, you cannot assume that all elderly patients are incapable of accurately describing their symptoms or making viable decisions about their care. They must also be concerned about ethnocentricity, a belief in the superiority of one ethnic group. Western medicine, for example, is not necessarily superior to alternative Chinese treatments. Finally, health care professionals must avoid stereotyping, which means you express an unfair or untrue belief that all people or things with a particular characteristic are the same; for example, all pregnant women have food cravings.

Being open and willing to learn about others sometimes requires you to choose your words carefully. It is best to avoid saying things like:

- "We're all alike; we're all human." A statement like this ignores the important differences that bring depth and richness to life. A person's dignity could be diminished causing her to feel that she needs to blend in more. People may change their names to fit in or avoid traditions that may draw attention to the differences.

158 Chapter 7 | Wellness

Career Connect

- Contact the agencies well in advance of the class in order to arrange the visit.
- If you cannot arrange a visit, encourage students to contact and visit someone from the agency on their own time.
- Alternatively, ask students to contact and interview someone who works with different cultures to discuss the issues they face.

ACTIVITY

Have students develop a personal philosophy statement regarding gender equity.

- "We should stay with our own culture; we are too different." This statement may cause fear and separation. When fear causes separation, defensive attitudes and behavior often follow. Arguments or fights are often the result of such fear. Learning about other cultures is enriching and broadens our view about life. Understanding other cultures usually brings a more complete understanding of your own culture and helps you communicate better with others.

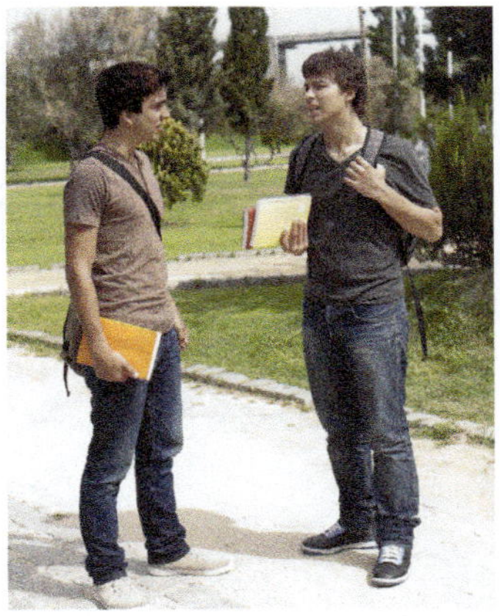

Figure 7.7
Respecting personal distance. What types of actions show that you respect another person's personal distance?

Citizens of the United States represent many societies and cultures. The influence of Asian populations has increased significantly over the current and recent past. This influence has brought ancient medicines and medical techniques such as yoga and treatments using herbal medicines that had not previously been embraced as part of the country's traditional Western medicine. As more citizens have begun to explore the benefits of combining these ancient practices with Western medicine referred to as Complementary and Integrative Medicine (CIM), the diverse influence has had a dramatic impact on contemporary aspects of health care delivery. CIM has become so widely practiced that the National Institutes of Health has created the National Center for Complementary and Integrative Medicine. In addition, the U.S. Food and Drug Administration established an approved list of CIM products used for medicinal purposes.

Gestures and Body Language

Personal Space and Touching

Personal space is the space needed to feel comfortable when we are with other people. (Figure 7.7) Personal space and touching are defined in different societies as close-contact and more-distant contact. (Table 7.3)

People in close-contact societies are comfortable with less space between them. An individual in a close-contact society may be more likely to touch an arm or shoulder of another person while in conversation. It is important to use caution when touching. A touch can be easily misunderstood.

Table 7.3 Close-Contact and Distant-Contact Regions

Close-Contact Regions		Distant-Contact Regions	
Africa	Mediterranean	Canada	Native Americans
Indonesia	Southern Europe	Great Britain	Middle Eastern
Latin America	French	Northern Europe	Arabic Nationalities
Hispanic Americans		United States	Asian Americans
Common Behavior			
■ Men hold hands with men and women hold hands with women.		■ People greet one another with a handshake or hand gesture.	
■ Men and women greet eachother by kissing on both cheeks.		■ Close friends or family members may hug each other.	

Teaching Tips

- Introduce the topic of gestures and body language.
- Explain that these are important means of communication in all cultures, but that they do not always meant the same thing.
- Emphasize that the way a health care worker behaves is as important as how he or she speaks.
- Point out that many health care workers are "touchers," meaning that they frequently reach out physically to touch others around them.
- Note that some cultures find touching offensive. Even in the U.S., many people feel threatened when someone enters their personal space.
- Discuss the difference between close-contact societies and more-distant-contact societies.
- Review Table 7.3 together as a class, identifying the regions on a globe or a map.
- Try to name one or more cultures in each region.
- Note that under the heading Common Behavior, the items in the left column align with the close contact regions and the items in the right column align with the distant-contact regions.

Figure Focus

7.7 Respecting personal distance. What types of actions show that you respect another person's personal distance?

Answer: Not standing too close, not speaking directly into another person's face, and not touching someone without permission.

ACTIVITY

Americans frequently use touching to greet or respond to others, while other cultures do not. Select a culture and then draw a chart or poster illustrating the way people from that culture greet each other.

Teaching Tips

- Review Table 7.4 together as a class.
- Discuss the different cultural attitudes to touching.
- Remind students not to be judgmental.
- Note that there are other Southeast Asian cultures that are not included in the table.
- Review different customs regarding greetings.
- Review Table 7.5 together as a class.
- Identify the close-contact societies and more-distant-contact societies.
- Point out the regions on a map or globe.
- Have students act out the different greetings.

Some Southeast Asian cultures believe that a person's spirit is on the head. Touching the head is often considered an insult. Table 7.4 explains who is permitted to touch or not touch the head.

Table 7.4 Guidelines Restricting Touch and Physical Closeness in Southeast Asian Cultures

Cambodian	Vietnamese	Laotian
■ Only a parent can touch the head of a child. ■ Members of the opposite sex never touch each other in public, not even brothers and sisters.	■ Only elderly people can touch the head of a child.	■ It is necessary to ask permission to move near another person.

Greetings

Greeting another person is important in all cultures. The way a greeting is given and received often determines how positive or negative the meeting is. Table 7.5 describes greetings in various cultures.

Table 7.5 Guidelines for Greeting People

Anglo-American	Latin American	Cambodian, Laotian	Vietnamese	Hmong
Shake hands if desired.	Shake hands or hug.	Do not shake hands. Instead, put hands together at different levels. 1. Equal status—hands must be at chest level. 2. Older person or stranger—hands must be at chin level. 3. Relative or teacher—hands must be at nose level.	Salute by joining both hands and moving them against the chest.	Bow head or shake hands.

Hand Gestures

Hand gestures help communicate many things. It is very important to use correct gestures so that others are not offended. Figure 7.8 illustrates gestures that are offensive in other cultures.

Eye Contact

In some cultures, eye contact may indicate that a person is listening, sincere, or honest. In other cultures, direct eye contact is considered to be hostile or disrespectful. Table 7.6 explains some cultural views about eye contact.

160 Chapter 7 | Wellness

ACTIVITY

Make a two-column chart. In column one, list gestures, facial expressions, or hand signals. In column two, list the way you interpret these nonverbal means of communication. For extra credit, add a third column listing the way a different culture might interpret the same gestures, facial expressions, or hand signals.

TEAMWORK

Divide the class into two or three teams. Have each team create a list of emotions or ideas. Have the other teams try to act out the items on the list using gestures, facial expressions, and body language.

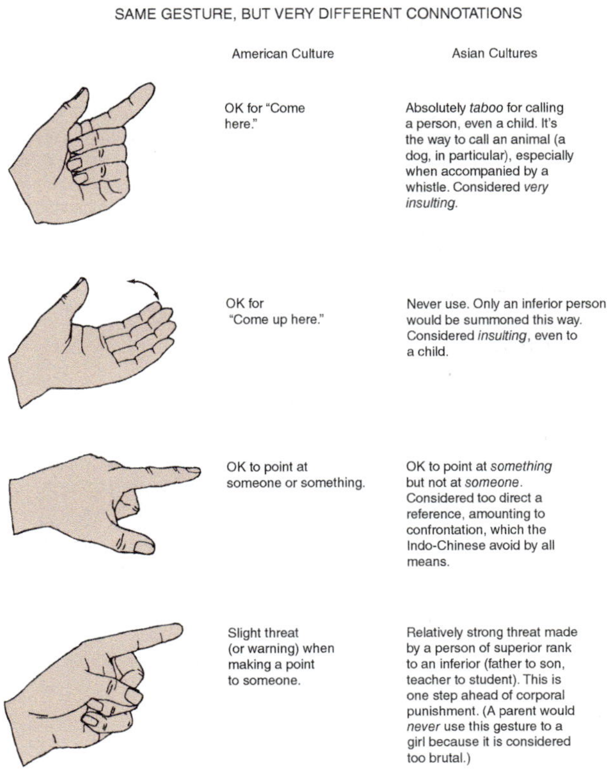

Figure 7.8
Hand gestures. How are the two types of pointing gestures different?

Table 7.6 Eye-Contact Guidelines

Anglo-American	African Americans	Navajo	Japanese, Southeast Asian, Hispanic
■ Eye contact is important; it indicates interest, honesty, and listening.	■ Eye contact may not be important. Being in the same room indicates attentiveness.	■ Direct eye contact is avoided. ■ Peripheral vision is used. ■ Direct stares are considered hostile or a way to scold children.	■ Eye contact is avoided as a form of respect.

Figure Focus

7.8 Hand gestures. How are the two types of pointing gestures different?

Answer: One gesture refers a person's attention to another person or object. The other gesture suggests a strong statement or threat. The two gestures impart very different messages.

Teaching Tips

- Review different customs and responses to greetings, hand gestures, and eye contact.
- Hand gestures are often offensive in one culture but not in another.
- Eye contact may be unacceptable in some cultures, but a lack of eye contact is unacceptable in the United States.
- Review Table 7.6, Eye-Contact Guidelines, together as a class.
- Explain peripheral vision.
- Point out the regions on a map or globe.
- Have students act out the different ways of making and responding to eye contact.

Teaching Tips

- Discuss family organization.
- Emphasize that it is important for health care workers to understand the relationships between family members when interacting and communicating with patients.
- Explain the following family structures:
  - Nuclear: Mother, father, children.
  - Patriarchal: Fathers, husbands, brothers, and sons make decisions.
  - Matriarchal: Mothers, wives, sisters, and daughters make decisions.
  - Extended family: Multi-generational, living together, and making decisions.
- Introduce the topic of verbal communication with people of other cultures.
- Discuss how hard it can be to understand someone who is just learning to speak English. Ask students to imagine how hard it must be for them to understand English-speakers.
- Review the list of ways to ensure effective communication.
- Discuss how medicine practiced in other cultures may seem strange to us.
- Emphasize that it is important to respect the belief and work involved in medicine from other cultures.
- Note that some practices that seemed odd in the past have now become common in the United States, such as acupuncture.

Family Organization

The structure of family is important in all cultures. There are nuclear families, a term developed in Western society referring to the basic family group—usually a mother, father, and children. There are also extended families—kinship groups consisting of a family nucleus and various relatives, such as grandparents, usually living in one household and functioning as a larger unit. In addition, there are patriarchal and matriarchal family structures. In a patriarchal family, the actions and ideas of men and boys are dominant over those of women and girls, while in a matriarchal society, the female (especially the mothers of a community) dominate.

Each culture has its own set of beliefs and values that must be incorporated into any health care interaction.

Apply It

Decorate the outside of a brown paper grocery bag with pictures, symbols, icons, and materials that illustrate who you are. Do not use anything that will easily give away your identity. Things you should try to illustrate include your heritage, gender, languages spoken, age, hobbies, groups to which you belong, interests, and values.

Place the bags around the room and number each one. Create a numbered list and write down who you think each bag belongs to.

Communicating Effectively with People from Other Cultures

When speaking with people from other cultures, the tone of your speaking voice is as important as the gestures you use. The tone of your voice is defined by voice quality, volume, and pitch. Voice tones cause positive or negative reactions from others. Clear pronunciations are more easily understood. When speaking to others who are learning English, communicate accurately and efficiently:

- Speak clearly; do not slur words.
- Speak so that they can hear you easily.
- Do not raise your voice or yell.
- Speak in moderate tones.
- Pronounce the entire word; do not draw it out or shorten sounds.
- Summarize often.
- Confirm their understanding.
- Clarify when necessary.

Folk Medicine

traditional
(truh DISH uh nl)
Customary beliefs passed from generation to generation.

Folk medicine is a collection of **traditional** beliefs and customs for treating pain or illness. Many who practice folk medicine believe that natural materials, such as herbs, spices, and spiritual prayers and rituals keep evil spirits away and allow the body to heal.

As a health care worker, you must take the time to understand common medical practices of patients/clients from other cultures.

Read magazines and books about other cultures. Ask questions. Your interest and understanding will contribute to the patient 's well-being and ensure that the experience is positive for both of you.

162 Chapter 7 | Wellness

Apply It

- Assign students the first part of the project as homework: gather the items and pictures they want to use to create the paper bag.
- You may have them decorate the bags at home or in class.
- Allow time in class to share the bags and discuss them.
- Students should be prepared to explain why they selected included items.

ACTIVITY

Draw a picture of your nuclear family. Then, draw a picture of your extended family. Discuss the difference with the class.

Following is an overview of common folk medicine practices in various cultures. Note that some practices that cause pain or discomfort are not considered abusive because they are based on a belief of the culture.

Armenians

- Give the mother a party one week after a baby is born. The mother is served bread, which she dips into a paste of margarine, sugar, and flour. This is a celebration of the birth of the child.
- Prohibit a menstruating woman from attending church, taking a shower, or eating spicy foods.

Asians

- Think that health is balance of yin and yang.
- Use treatments such as herbal remedies and acupuncture.
- Use cupping with heated bamboo.

Cambodians

- Use herbs as medicine.
- Use cupping for headaches. Cupping leaves a round mark on the forehead. A cotton ball saturated in alcohol is placed in a glass and set on fire. After burning for a few seconds, the cotton is discarded. The heated glass is placed upside down over the painful area.
- Use coining for pain. Oil or ointment is applied to the skin. Then a large coin is used to rub the painful area in one direction until the blood is raised to just below the surface of the skin. This leaves red areas on the skin.
- Consider the color white to be a sign of bad luck. White indicates mourning and death. Think about a Cambodian's first visit to a caregiver. Is it possible that the white uniform might seem frightening?

Central and South Americans

- Use herbal home remedies.
- Discourage a menstruating woman from getting her head wet and from eating cucumbers, oranges, lemons, pork, lard, and deer meat.

Europeans

- Believe that illness is caused by outside sources.
- Focus on treating with medication, surgery, diet, and exercise.

Wellness | Chapter 7 163

Teaching Tips

- Review the information about different cultures that is included in the section text.
- Point out the geographic origins of the cultures on a map or globe.
- If there are students from other cultures in the class, ask them to share information about medical practices that might be different in their native countries.
- When possible, identify similarities between cultures, such as Europeans and Americans, or Koreans and Chinese.

ACTIVITY

Write a folk tale that involves folk medicine. Start by selecting a culture and finding out what types of folk medicine they might use. In the story, include the name of the culture and the geographic location. Make the folk medicine the focus of the story, but include as many details about the culture that you can, such as language and beliefs. Be respectful toward the culture. Share your folk tale with the class.

ACTIVITY

Many cultures—including North Americans—believe that plants and herbs have medicinal power. Select one plant or herb that is thought to be medicinal. Make a poster or presentation that shows the plant or herb and lists the medicinal properties. Include information about the cultures that use it.

Teaching Tips

- Continue reviewing the folk medicine of different cultures as described in the text.

Apply It

- Explain to students that you are looking for a traditional custom or belief held by their ancestors, not necessarily their parents.
- Once students have noted the beliefs on a card (one per parent, should they be of different backgrounds), they should bring the cards to school.
- Mix up the cards and read them aloud to the class. Ask for suggestions as to the culture described.
- Note the cultures on the board with additional check marks next to those cultures mentioned more than once.

Hispanics

- Believe that health is a reward from God.
- Believe in good luck.
- Use heat and cold remedies to restore balance.
- Rely on prayers and massage.

Hmong and Mien Tribes

- Perform spiritual ceremonies to please the spirits that cause illness.
- Use herbal home remedies, including opium.

Apply It

Think of a traditional belief or custom about health care, reflective of your heritage. On an index card, write an example from your paternal family lineage and another from your maternal family lineage. Circulate the cards to other classmates. Can you determine what culture is represented by the belief or custom?

Iranians

- Believe that poor health is predetermined (fatalism).
- Use herbs, foods, rituals, and magic formulas for healing.
- Believe the "Evil Eye" (a person or animal that causes injury through a look) causes sudden illness.
- When of the Islamic faith, require washing of the face and hands before prayer.
- Require periodic baths for cleansing.

Koreans

- Practice alchemy, a medieval practice of magic and natural herbal remedies.
- Use acupuncture.
- Go to hot springs for bath rituals and massage.
- Use energy and brain stimulants.

Middle Easterners

- Believe that health is spiritual and cleanliness essential.
- Believe males dominate and make decisions on health care.
- Believe in spiritual causes of illness, such as the "evil eye."

Native Americans

- Use herbs and spices.
- Use modern medical practices.
- Some rely on a healer/shaman (medicine man or woman) to remove pain and evil spirits.
- Believe that health is harmony with nature.
- Believe that a tolerance of pain signifies power and strength.
- Believe that illness is caused by supernatural forces and evil spirits.

South Africans

- Believe in maintaining harmony of body, mind, and spirit.
- Believe the causes of ill health are spirits, demons, or punishment from God.
- Use prayer or religious rituals as treatment.

Vietnamese

- Commonly use herbal medicine.
- Use cupping for head pain, cough, muscle pain, and motion sickness.
- Use acupuncture for musculoskeletal problems, visual problems, and other ailments.

Table 7.7 lists typical terms used by non-English-speaking Asian cultures to describe health problems.

Table 7.7 Terms That Describe Health Problems

Term	Condition
Weak heart	Palpitations, dizziness, faintness, feeling of panic
Weak kidney	Impotence, sexual dysfunction
Weak nervous system	Headache, malaise, inability to concentrate
Weak stomach or liver	Indigestion
Skinniness	Sickliness
Fire, hot	Dark urine, flatulence, constipation
Air/wind, cold	Illness was caused by too much air

Spiritual Beliefs

When dealing with people from other cultures, it is important to demonstrate respect for a patient's spiritual beliefs and practices. You can uncover these beliefs by talking to the patient. In helping to meet these spiritual and religious needs, the health care professional has to relate to each patient as unique and distinctive. You must be willing to listen, and to respect any symbols or books on which the patient relies. It is important to explore the patient's fears and doubts and help him or her maintain hope. Sometimes, it can help to encourage the patient's religious community or clergy involvement for support. Finally, it is very important to refrain from imposing your own beliefs on to the patient.

There are differences between spirituality and religion. Spirituality refers to matters of the spirit or soul, as distinguished from material things. Religion is a belief in a supernatural power or powers regarded as the creator and governor of the universe; or beliefs based on the teachings of a spiritual leader. Some people are agnostics; they believe that it is impossible to know whether or not there is a God. You may also have patients who are atheists, who deny or do not believe in the existence of any supreme being.

Teaching Tips

- Introduce Table 7.7 by reminding students that even verbal communication methods may vary by culture.
- Review Table 7.7 together as a class.
- Note that these terms may not be used by all Asian cultures.
- Ask students from other cultures if their family members have any specific terms that describe medical conditions.
- Introduce the topic of spiritual beliefs.
- Emphasize the difference between religious beliefs and spiritual beliefs.
- Emphasize that health care workers must respect the spiritual and religious beliefs of all people.

ACTIVITY

Compare the folk medicine traditions of one culture with the folk medicine traditions of a different culture. Depict the differences and similarities in a chart, or write a brief report. Include information about the geographical location of the culture.

Language Arts Link—Cultural and Spiritual Beliefs

- You may want students to write a rough draft, or use a story web to organize their thoughts for the letter.
- Encourage students to use proper letter formatting, such as including a return address.
- Because they are writing to a peer, they can use informal language.
- Evaluate the letters based on the amount of information included, whether the information is accurate, and on spelling and grammatical errors.

Language Arts Link

Cultural and Spiritual Beliefs

A person's cultural and spiritual beliefs may affect how they respond to different situations. Imagine that you have a pen pal in another country. Write a letter to your friend describing how your cultural and spiritual beliefs affect your attitudes towards health care.

Ask your friend to share health care practices that are similar or different than the health care you can receive. Include at least three key points on your beliefs, and ask for a response from your friend for the same points.

Research the different practices. Complete a compare and contrast display (poster, chart, or slide show) of the different health care practices based on the two different sets of cultural and spiritual beliefs as described in each letter. Point out the strengths and limitations of both sets of practices. Consider the possible concerns, biases, and values that might affect health care practices if they were exchanged between the two countries. When comparing the two, would you be willing to try health care practices from a different country?

Health care providers must be careful to be considerate of any patient's beliefs. They can make medical decisions that are consistent with the patient's spiritual and/or religious views. They should support the patient's use of spiritual coping during the illness, encouraging him/her to speak with their clergy or spiritual leader, or referring the patient to a hospital chaplain, appropriate religious leader, or support group that addresses spiritual issues during illness.

Family Traditions

Family support is an important part of patient care. Some family traditions are unique to individual families. Other traditions are a blend of beliefs and traditions from cultures, as well as from spiritual and religious beliefs and practices. As a health care provider, you must make it a priority to relate to family members in a positive and productive manner. Being aware of family traditions that can help nurture a patient will benefit everyone involved with a patient's care.

ACTIVITY

Have students research a tradition modeled by their own families. Suggest that they interview several family members as primary sources.

TEAMWORK

In pairs, discuss your spiritual beliefs, particularly as they relate to health care. Practice listening carefully and respectively to each other.

What's New?

Demographics

Every ten years, the U.S. Census Bureau conducts a survey to learn about the demographics of the country. Demographics are statistical data summarizing the population in terms of such characteristics as age, race, marital status, language spoken at home, location, and income level. The last major census took place in 2010. At that time, the data showed that nearly 13 percent of the population consisted of people born in other countries.

It also showed that more than 20 percent of the population over five years of age spoke a language other than English at home. Varying percentages of those people spoke English at different ability levels outside the home as well.

These statistics showed a continued increase in the everyday use of languages other than English since the 1990 census. In some states, the number of people not speaking English at home has risen even higher—43 percent in California, 36 percent in New Mexico, and 34 percent in Texas.

These data suggest that the American population is continuing to undergo major changes that affect the way people understand and interact with each other. Health care workers need to be especially aware of the evolving population and take cultural differences into account when providing care.

How might the language spoken at home affect a person's health care in this country?

Summary

Cultural beliefs are very important to all societies. You give quality care when you take the time to understand and respect patients of other cultures. Caring about them as individuals will help them improve more quickly. If they are not ill, your caring builds mutual respect for future meetings.

Section 7.3 Review Questions

1. What experiences do members of a cultural group usually share?
2. In what way can culture be compared to the parts of a tree?
3. Give an example of a prejudice.
4. What are two ways of overcoming prejudice?
5. What is a customary method of greeting someone in an Anglo-American culture?
6. Why might it be considered rude to speak loudly when trying to communicate with someone who is learning English?

Wellness | Chapter 7 167

What's New?—Demographics

- Note that the latest census bears out the trends that have been in place for more than 10 years.
- If possible, refer to the statistics for your community or state for demographic information.
- Take this opportunity to discuss how knowing a second language can be a benefit when looking for employment.

How might the language spoken at home affect a person's health care in this country?

Answer: It might mean that the person is not comfortable speaking English. He or she may not present symptoms accurately and completely because of limited English language skills. Also, if health care providers only speak English when prescribing medicine and other treatments, the person may not interpret the information correctly.

Section 7.3 Review Questions

1. Answer: Language, communication style, belief system, customs, attitudes, perceptions, and values
2. Answer: Culture can be compared to the parts of a tree because some cultural characteristics are visible like the trunk, branches, and leaves of tree whereas others are less visible like the root system of a tree which is underground.
3. Answer: Answers will vary. Some examples: A woman is not hired because of her age; a man is not hired because of his race; an overweight woman is not hired because of her physical appearance.
4. Answer: Keep an open mind; look for additional information; watch documentaries, read books, magazines, and newspapers for information; look at many resources before you form an opinion; and evaluate all the information.
5. Answer: Shake hands
6. Answer: Voice tones cause positive and negative reactions from others.

TEAMWORK

In small groups, develop and present a skit showing how emergency medical personnel might respond to a patient with limited or no English-speaking ability. You might develop one skit showing an effective response, and one showing an ineffective response.

CHAPTER 7 REVIEW

Chapter Review Questions

1. Name and describe three types of fitness included in a holistic approach to health. (7.1)
2. What does it mean to describe an activity as aerobic? (7.1)
3. A person needs a bandage to help a wound heal. Classify this as a physiological or a psychological need. Explain your choice. (7.2)
4. What is pet-facilitated therapy? (7.2)
5. Why is it important to establish healthy relationships with other staff members on a health care team? (7.2)
6. Give an example of rationalization as a defense mechanism. (7.2)
7. What does it mean to idolize someone? Why is this a negative behavior? (7.2)
8. What does it mean to exhibit age prejudice in the workplace? (7.3)
9. What is wrong with the statement, "All people are alike; they are human" in terms of cultural awareness? (7.3)
10. How does the use of eye contact vary in different cultures? (7.3)

Activities

1. Check out your physical health by measuring your pulse (which is reflective of your heart rate). Practice measuring your pulse. Count the number of beats in 10 seconds and multiply the number by 6. Record this number as beats per minute (bpm). Throughout a day, measure your pulse in different situations; for example, while rushing to get ready for school, during a test, while listening to a teacher's lecture, while stroking a pet, or resting in bed. Compare the changes throughout the day, and identify any relationship between your pulse and your mood or stress level.
2. Using the Internet for research, select an alternative health practice or therapy, and describe its history and use, including intended benefits.
3. Using the Internet for research, select a complementary and integrative medicine and determine if it is included on the FDA list of approved products.
4. Select an annual event, such as the beginning of a new year or a birthday. Interview five people from different cultures about how they treat this event. Collect the information in a brief report, and present it to the class.
5. Research practices used by three different societies, and describe how those practices are used to solve problems related to health.
6. Compare practices used by the three selected societies to solve problems related to health. Describe your findings.
7. Prepare a timeline with five columns divided into 10 year age spans beginning with age 20. In each column, identify and list three health practices particular to that age group that can lead to the feeling of wellness. In addition to the health practices, identify two concepts of wellness that will result for each age group within the health practices. Include that information on your timeline. Share your timeline with the class.

168 Chapter 7 | Wellness

CHAPTER 7 REVIEW

Chapter Review Questions

1. Answer: Physical fitness makes us alert and energetic in our daily lives; mental fitness allows us to interact effectively with others and to feel balanced; spiritual fitness allows us to experience meaning and purpose in our lives.
2. Answer: An activity that is aerobic requires oxygen.
3. Answer: Answers may vary but should include an appropriate explanation: physiological need, because the wound needs protection from infection; psychological need, because the person believes a bandage will help heal and alleviate pain.
4. Answer: Pet-facilitated therapy can be used as a treatment—animals may be taken into convalescent homes and hospitals. Pet-facilitated therapy helps a person with loneliness and responsibility which can give meaning in life.
5. Answer: Rapport with other staff members makes everyone feel worthwhile and accepted.
6. Answer: Answers will vary. Kathy told a friend about a very confidential secret that her sister told her. She explained it by saying, "Well, if it was a secret, my sister shouldn't have told me to begin with."
7. Answer: Idolize means to care for someone to excess. It is a negative behavior because it takes away a person's own identity.
8. Answer: Exhibiting age prejudice in the workplace might indicate that you: (1) don't hire older people; (2) assume that an older person can't perform certain tasks (like using a new computer program); or (3) don't ask their advice on issues dealing with the current marketplace (thinking that they don't understand the current generation).
9. Answer: A statement like this ignores the important differences that bring depth and richness to life. A person's dignity could be diminished causing her to feel that she needs to blend in more. People may change their names to fit in or avoid traditions that may draw attention to their differences.
10. Answer: In some cultures, eye contact indicates that a person is listening, sincere, and honest, but in other cultures, direct eye contact may be hostile or disrespectful.

Activities

1. Have students prepare for this activity by setting up a table in which they can record the time of day, the pulse rate, and the situation. Specify how many times they should check their pulse rate. Have them write their conclusions below the table.
2. Refer students to the Web site https://nccih.nih.gov/ and have them scroll down to the various lists to make a selection, and complete their activity.
3. Refer students to www.fda.gov/RegulatoryInformation/Guidances/ucm144657.htm for the information needed to complete this activity. The site is dense with information and you may ask the students to just determine which category the Complementary and Integrative (Alternative) Medicine they selected falls into and if that is a regulated category. Categories are: 1. Drug and New Drug; 2. Device; 3. Food; 4. Food Additive; 5. Dietary Supplement; 6. Cosmetic; and 7. Biological Product. The site states which are regulated.
4. Encourage students to be creative with this assignment. They may want to draw a picture, videotape the interviews, or make a booklet.

CHAPTER 7 REVIEW

8. In teams of two, select a "country of origin" based on the predominant immigrants living in the local area. Using Web sites and library sources, research and select one healing practice traditional to the culture of the country of origin selected. Study the history of the practice, and when, where, and how it was introduced. (Some will trace back thousands of years.) Research and describe how migration patterns, cultural beliefs, values, and rituals of the country of origin's society have influenced the practice of Western medicine. Complete a comparison chart that shows the cultural norms, values, and rituals of the country of origin's society and those commonly practiced in the United States.
9. Give an example of a positive work environment (may be a class if you are not yet employed), and describe how it made you feel when it was time to arrive and participate. Were you looking forward to being there?
10. Give an example of a negative work environment (may be a class if you are not yet employed), and describe how it made you feel when it was time to arrive and participate. Did you have any physical discomfort? Did it have an effect on your attitude for the day?
11. Describe how you might evaluate negative relationships at work or in a class and contribute to improving the condition. How can healthy relationships contribute to your success at school or on the job?
12. Evaluate the effects of both physical and emotional health as a result of positive relationships with peers, family, and friends in promoting a healthy community.
13. Evaluate the effects of both physical and emotional health as a result of negative relationships with peers, family, and friends in promoting a healthy community.
14. Choose a health science topic that impacts the health of people in various countries across the globe. Some ideas include selecting a disease such as HIV/AIDS, COVID-19, or malaria. Research the public health initiatives different countries have taken to prevent this disease and the impact these practices have had so far.
15. Talk with your classmates about the role that health care professionals should have in preventing illness in the community and how professionals in various fields can contribute together. Come up with ideas for how the different health care teams can work together to foster positive relationships with both each other and the community.

Case Studies

1. You are assigned a patient from Iran. Her family is concerned about leaving her alone during the day, so they admit her to a long-term care facility. The patient is convinced that she is going to die because her family brought her to the hospital. Explain what basic need is not being met and develop a plan to meet that need for the patient. Strategize ways you could communicate information accurately and efficiently to this patient.
2. Your co-worker is gentle and caring, but he has a loud voice and waves his hands around when he talks. You observe that some of your Cambodian patients seem to be afraid of him and tend to back away or avoid being around him. Explain why the Cambodian patients might respond to your co-worker in this way. What could you do to help your co-worker communicate his gentle, caring nature to the Cambodian patients?

Wellness | Chapter 7 169

5. Refer students to pages 162–165 Folk Medicine (now referred to as Complementary and Integrative or Alternative Medicine) and select one practice from three different countries listed for their research.
6. Use the three selected from the lists for the comparison and findings descriptions.
7. Suggest that the students each interview someone within each of the five age groups, asking each person to name three health practices that lead to the feeling of wellness. Also ask each person to identify two concepts of wellness. After completing the timeline, ask the students to share their findings and determine if there are commonalities across the reports.
8. Note that this is a fairly extensive activity and may take several days to complete. Ask the teams to complete research to find the predominant immigrant groups living in the community. Distribute the groups across the teams so all groups will be represented. Have the students determine the "country of origin" for each immigrant group, for example if they are Spanish speaking they may be from Mexico, Cuba, Central America, or South America. Ask the students to complete the healing practice part of the activity. Next ask the students to trace the information for the remainder of the activity. This may require personal interviews to determine how the immigrants arrived in the community.
9. This is an activity that asks students to be introspective and think about their feelings and reactions. Some of the students may struggle to think of a good experience and may have to be encouraged to come up with something. Suggest that if they can't think of any positive work or school experience they may want to think of a personal or social experience that they enjoyed.
10. Students will likely have an easier time coming up with an experience that left them with negative feelings. You may want to suggest that they either work to improve the situation or find something positive to focus on.
11. You may wish to have students share their findings with the class.
12. This activity might lead to the students creating a community service project based on their positive experiences that could improve the physical and emotional health for a group that may be struggling (homeless children, elderly living in assisted care, young people with injury or illness causing extended medical care, etc.).

ACTIVITY

Have students keep a personal food diary for a week. They should write down everything they eat in the diary. They should include the amount and the number of calories. If possible, they may want to include nutritional values as well. At the end of the week, ask the students to assess whether they made healthy choices or not.

13. Students might be asked to consider negative relationships that may have caused some to have poor attendance at school, failing grades, or little interaction with colleagues. A class discussion might focus on how to assist those in negative environments. This could be part of the community service project suggested for Activity 12.
14. Ask the students to contrast the approaches taken by different countries. Which approaches seem to be most effective? Why?
15. Have the students think about how so many different agencies and teams contributed to the control of COVID-19. Ask them what public health officials did well/poorly and what they would have done if they were health professionals.

Case Studies

1. Students should respond to this case study in writing. Advise them that if they think more than one basic need is not being met, they should address that as well.
2. Students should address the Cambodian culture specifically when responding to this case study.
3. Collect the flyers from the local grocery stores and make them available to students. To help students get organized, show them how to set up a menu. Refer them to the Web site ChooseMyPlate.gov for the nutritional requirements.
4. A sample answer might be: Explain to the couple how you are attempting to help. Then try to determine the types of herbs the father has been using. Discuss these herbs with a pharmacist or complete Internet research to see if there is medication that includes or is closely related to the herbs that can be used to treat the problem. If so, try to locate a health care professional familiar with Thailand beliefs or a respected elder from the Thailand community to inform the father that the herbs are part of the medication but in a different form. If not, share what you have learned with the health care professional and let them determine how to proceed.

CHAPTER 7 REVIEW

3. You will develop a weekly menu with a budget of $110.00 to feed a family of four. Describe the family. Is it a family with a 10-year-old boy and a baby? A couple and their parents? A family with teenagers? You must pick all your food ingredients from local grocery store flyers with food items and prices on them. Menus, including breakfast, lunch, dinner, and snacks for seven full days, must meet the daily nutritional requirements identified in the MyPlate program (see ChooseMyPlate.gov). Menus should also meet the specific needs of individual family members (formula, baby food, etc.).
4. A young couple along with the husband's elderly father has recently moved to the United States from Thailand. The father has taken ill and appears to need medical care. The three arrive at the hospital but the father is refusing any treatment declaring that he has herbs that will take care of the problem. The son is very concerned as the father has tried the herbs but continues to run a high fever and seems disoriented. Demonstrate an understanding of diversity influencing contemporary aspects of health care by describing what action you might take to help provide care for the father.

Thinking Critically

1. **Communication**—You always talk to your adult patients/clients using their title and last name as you have been trained. You cannot help noticing that many of them respond cheerfully to a co-worker who uses first names. You suspect that some of your patients/clients think you are too formal. Write a paragraph describing how you could handle this situation.
2. **Cultural Competency**—Make a list of some of the different reactions to pet therapy that you would expect from different cultures, for example, various Asian groups as well as South American and Mediterranean.
3. **Medical**—Compare and contrast the World Health Organization's definition of health with the meaning of holistic.

Portfolio Connection

Mrs. Summers is an alert, ambulatory, 85-year-old patient. You observe that she argues about everything and with everyone. You cannot remember her ever agreeing to or being willing to do anything. In your word processor, develop a plan to identify why Mrs. Summers is so argumentative. Your plan must clearly identify what you would do to involve other people. In your plan, clearly identify her behavior, what causes it, and what the positive and negative outcomes are for her. Include ...roposed solution, a method of evaluation, and a timeline. When yo... ...pleted your plan and checked the format and gram... ...in the section of your portfoli...

PORTFOLIO TIP

Be aware of the tone and volume of your voice, especially when talking to patients from different cultures, with sensory disabilities, or a language barrier. Find a partner and role-play some situations, using ...

TEAMWORK

On p. 162, there is a list of suggestions for ways you can communicate effectively with people who are not English-proficient. In small groups, work together to think of other methods to add to the list, such as using easy-to-understand terms, or not using distracting hand movements. Compare your list with the lists developed by the other groups.

Thinking Critically

1. Remind students to write complete answers. Also remind them that there may not be a "right" or "wrong" answer.
2. This activity may require research into a culture's attitude toward pets.
3. Remind students how to compare and contrast different concepts. Direct students to the Web site of the World Health Organization for more information: who.int.

Portfolio Connection

- Note that there are two assignments: (1) Developing a plan for Mrs. Summers; and (2) Researching two cultural groups.
- Allow time in class for students to present their oral reports on the cultural groups.
- Check to make sure that students have completed the written assignments and added them to their portfolio.

8 Teamwork

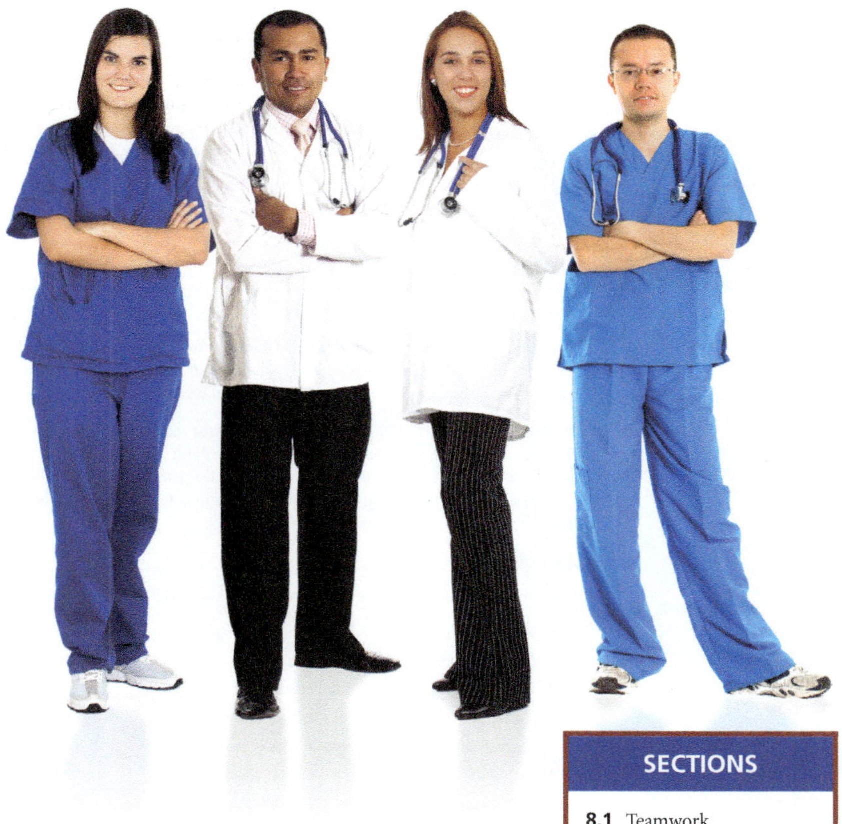

SECTIONS

CHAPTER 8 OVERVIEW

Teamwork is vital to the success of health care professionals. Chapter 8 examines the roles of individuals as part of a team, as well as the importance of a team for providing effective health care.

Section 8.1: Section 8.1 explores all aspects of teamwork, including the components of a team, the concept of working as a team, different types of teams in health care, how to identify and set team goals, and how to resolve conflicts that arise among team members.

Advance Preparation	
Review	■ Chapter text for Section 8.1.
Contact	■ Guest speakers who can speak on the importance of teamwork, such as human resources professionals, team leaders, or coaches.
Prepare	■ Teamwork motivational posters and sayings, available on commercial Web sites such as quotations.about.com and motivational-inspirational-corner.com. ■ Magazine and newspaper articles on teamwork in health care. ■ A list of Web sites that provide information about teamwork in health care—such as ihi.org. (Note that many colleges and universities provide information on effective teamwork on their Web sites.)

FOCUS AND ENGAGE

Getting Started

- This activity is designed to promote effective communication, which is the cornerstone of effective teamwork.
- Provide the scissors and paper for cutting out the shapes.
- Alternatively, if time is an issue, provide the shapes to each pair.
- After the exercise, discuss how speaking and listening are vital to working as a team.

Introduce the Section

a. Review the content of the Background paragraphs, discussing the concept of teamwork.

b. Explain that teams are comprised of individuals who understand their roles as members of the team. Emphasize communication and conflict resolution.

c. Review the objectives for the section.

Vocabulary Review

a. Key terms are defined in the margins of the text on the page where they first appear.

b. Pronounce each word, and have the students repeat the pronunciation out loud.

c. Discuss the definition of each word.

Getting Started

Health care is provided by a team of professionals. A successful team relationship depends on all team members working together. They rely on each other to provide accurate and precise information. They trust one another to fulfill their responsibilities. If one team member does not do his or her share, the entire team suffers as does their employer and, most importantly, the patient/client.

To practice both listening and verbal communication skills, choose a partner and cut out two exact copies of a variety of shapes in different sizes and colors, including rectangles, squares, diamonds, circles, and so forth. Each team member gets one set of the cut outs.

Sitting back to back, one team member should arrange the shapes in a selected design describing the arrangement as it is formed. The other teammate will attempt to replicate the design. When completed, compare your designs. Then switch roles and repeat the exercise. What did you learn about your listening and verbal communication skills?

SECTION 8.1 Teamwork

Background

Managed care organizations and other health care providers have formed health care teams that enable them to provide a higher level of care to the patient/client, and to meet the challenges of economic change and increased competition.

It is vital in today's medical field to know how to work with others on a team. Understanding the responsibilities of team members and how to contribute as part of a team; learning how to cooperate and **collaborate** with team members; and practicing conflict resolution are skills that will help you not only on the job but in all other areas of your life as well.

collaborate
(co LAB er ate)
To work together to achieve a specific goal.

teamwork
(TEEM work)
Cooperative effort from a group of people contributing towards a common goal.

dynamics
(di NAM ic s)
Motivating or driving forces.

conflict
(KON flikt)
A contradiction, fight, or disagreement.

Objectives

When you have completed this section, you will be able to do the following:

- Match key terms with their correct meanings.
- Identify types of health care teams.
- Explain how a team builds cohesiveness and fosters productivity.
- Recognize characteristics of effective teams.
- Explain the roles and responsibilities of team members.
- Recognize underlying factors and situations that may lead to conflict.
- Apply verbal and nonverbal communication skills in a team setting.
- Apply conflict resolution strategies in a team setting.

172 Chapter 8 | Teamwork

CUSTOMIZED INSTRUCTION

English Language Learners

Have students write each key term and its pronunciation on one side of an index card and its definition on the other side.

Special Needs Students

Pair special needs students with regular learners for the Getting Started exercise. Provide extra time, if necessary, so they do not feel rushed while describing their shapes or trying to re-create the pattern described by their partners.

CUSTOMIZED INSTRUCTION OVERVIEW

Less Advanced Students	Pages 175, 179
More Advanced Students	Pages 176, 178
English Language Learners	Pages 172, 178
Special Needs Students	Pages 172, 177
At-Risk Students	Pages 173, 179

The Making of a Team

A team is a group of more than two people who cooperate in order to achieve a specific goal. Teaming is also a word used in health care, defined as coming together as a team to achieve quality health care. When you are part of a team, you have access to all the knowledge, experience, and abilities of your teammates. Through **teamwork,** you have more ideas, achieve more goals, and solve more problems. A healthy relationship as a team member contributes to your well-being and to success on the job. Your teammates respect you and value your contribution to their achievements.

Group **dynamics** are the motivating or driving forces that influence the actions and identity of the team. Some examples include personality styles, team roles, office layout, tools and technology, a company's culture, and procedures. A team's identity is also formed by the nature and purpose of the work to be done by the team. It is important to periodically step back and evaluate the dynamics of your group to see where you can make improvements.

Most teams develop through a series of stages. At first, members of the new team might feel nervous. Individuals might have to interact with other members who they do not know well. They might also begin tasks that are new to them.

As teammates begin to work together, members might misunderstand or misinterpret each others' behaviors. A teammate might disagree with another's opinion.

This kind of **conflict** is natural and can actually strengthen a team as members learn to resolve their differences. Many teams will eventually achieve **cohesiveness.** The team will feel a sense of unity or team identity.

Once groups establish this unity, they are poised to be productive and achieve their goals. This productive period lasts as long as the group dynamics do not change. Some teams might eventually break apart because team members move to new teams or leave a company.

The Team Concept

The challenges of a team relationship come from having different people working together. Even if everyone agrees on a common goal, they may not agree on how to achieve that goal. Your friends might agree to celebrate the end of the school year together, but some of you might want to go to the lake; some might want to play Frisbee in the park; and still others might want to have a picnic.

The same challenges apply in most health care settings. Quality health care depends on every health care worker doing his or her part. Each member is an important part of the **interdisciplinary** team. Professionals with different backgrounds, different education, and different interests all work together to provide appropriate quality care.

The RN collaborates with the members of the interdisciplinary team and coordinates the care delivered to the patient. The RN determines the holistic plan of care and effectively delegates tasks by using the *five rights of* **delegation**:

cohesiveness
(koh HEE siv niss)
State of being well-integrated or unified.

interdisciplinary
(in ter DIS uh pluh ner ee)
Involving two or more disciplines.

delegation
(del i gat shun)
To give another person responsibility for doing a specific task.

Career-Ready Practices

Form teams of four to five. As a group, select a health-related facility in your community where you *all* think you might like to volunteer. Remember, career-ready individuals recognize the importance of engaging all members of the team in the decision-making process. They understand that each member of the team has a responsibility to contribute and help the team work productively to make decisions, solve problems, and adjust plans accordingly.

Then, research volunteer opportunities at the facility. For example, find out what volunteers typically do, how many hours a week they volunteer, and if there are any age restrictions. Explore transportation options for getting to and from the facility. Identify the personal and professional benefits you could gain from volunteering at the facility.

Using your word processor or desktop publishing software, create a one-page flyer that promotes volunteering at the facility. Delegate tasks as appropriate.

Then, get involved and volunteer. It's a great way to give back to your community!

Teamwork | Chapter 8 173

TEACH

Discuss

- Display teamwork motivational posters and read teamwork motivational sayings, such as, "The achievements of an organization are the results of the combined effort of each individual," by Vincent Lombardi.
- Discuss the meaning of the posters and sayings.
- Ask students if they have been part of a team, and to share stories of what made the team successful or unsuccessful.

Teaching Tips

- Introduce the concept of team dynamics.
- Review the factors that determine team dynamics.
- Point out ways that personnel from different departments contribute to a single team. Include departments such as office staff who are responsible for scheduling or recordkeeping, as well as nurses, nutritionists, and physicians.

CUSTOMIZED INSTRUCTION

At-Risk Students

Have students work as a team to develop a list of volunteer opportunities in the classroom and in the school. In the list, they should describe the opportunity, the duties of a volunteer, and how to become involved. For example, does your class need a team of volunteers to handle paper recycling?

Career-Ready Practices

- You might help the groups by suggesting roles for each member, such as a team leader, a project manager, a researcher, and so on.
- Remind students that the goal of this activity is to inspire classmates and other students to get involved and volunteer. They should keep this in mind as they design their flyers.
- Remind them that volunteering can be an effective way to network and develop contacts who can help them with their job search and career pursuits.
- This activity gives students real-world experience in applying the following Career-Ready Practice: Work Productively in Teams while Using Cultural/Global Competence.
- For more information on the Career-Ready Practices, visit careertech.org/career-ready-practices.

Teaching Tips

- Read the five rights of delegation out loud with the class.
- Review the types of health care teams.
- Discuss team identity, and how it is determined by the nature and purpose of the work to be performed. Illustrate this by comparing different teams, such as one working in an emergency room to a team working in a long-term care facility.
- Review pitfalls that may arise when a new team is formed, or when a new member joins an existing team. For example, team members may not know who is responsible for a specific task, or one team member may think he or she knows more than the team leader.
- Review factors that encourage cohesiveness, such as effective communication, trust, and understanding of team roles.
- Emphasize that each individual brings something unique to a team.
- Point out that team members can rely on each other for knowledge and ideas.

Apply It

- Make sure students consider all possibilities for the team experience, whether it's a school group, community group, church group, or social group.
- If necessary, help them determine the team's goal. Again, stress that this doesn't have to be a formal, written goal or plan.

Apply It

An effective team cooperates to achieve a specific goal. Think of a team you are involved with currently, or were involved with in the past. This can be a sports team, a school club, a community organization, or any other organized group that required you to cooperate with others. Describe the group dynamics. What was the team's goal and did the team achieve it?

feedback
(FEED bak)
Information received as a result of something done or said.

discipline
(DIS uh plin)
A branch of instruction or learning, such as cardiology.

collaborate
(kuh LAB uh reyt)
To work together.

interdependent
(in ter di PEN duh nt)
Depending on each other.

Career Connect

Visit the office of a dentist (or other health care professional) who runs a "one man" shop. Then, visit the office of a group of doctors (for example, a group of internists, each with a different specialty). Which environment do you prefer? Think about the pros and cons of each type of operation.

- **Right task.** Identifying an appropriate caregiver-patient relationship.
- **Right circumstances.** Verifying that the correct patient setting and resources are available.
- **Right person.** Identifying who is trained and capable of doing the task.
- **Right direction/communication.** Providing a clear, short description of the task and clarifying limitations and the expected result.
- **Right supervision.** Providing appropriate monitoring, assistance, and **feedback**.

Health care teams can be a combination of nurses, physicians, physician assistants, therapists, laboratory technicians, and many other professionals on staff. All departments are responsible for quality patient care, even if they are not providing hands-on care. For instance, if the medical records department fails to keep correct files of the patient/client chart, the physician will not have the test results and history needed to provide appropriate care. If housekeepers do not clean properly and bacteria are present, patients/clients might contract additional diseases. Each team member is responsible for fulfilling their own roles on the team so that the team works together to meet the needs of their patients.

Remember: It is the team effort of all health care workers that provides the best service to the patient/client!

Types of Health Care Teams

There are many types of health care teams today:

- Ad hoc groups are formed for a limited amount of time to address a specific problem. These can be composed of members from many departments. They might address issues such as redesigning a hospital floor or improving patient check-in procedures.
- A nominal care group includes a physician who refers a patient to different specialists. These specialists provide care independently; however, the physician coordinates the flow of information among the specialists.
- A unidisciplinary group is organized around a single discipline. These are relatively permanent groups, such as nursing units or hospital floors.
- A multidisciplinary team is made up of practitioners from multiple **disciplines** who may work with a patient/client during the same time period; however, the practitioners each have their own goals and recommendations. The practitioners do stay informed about what each other is doing.
- An interdisciplinary team consists of practitioners from two or more disciplines who work in the same setting. (**Figure 8.1**) Members contribute their opinions about treatment plans and then **collaborate** to implement one plan based on one set of goals. Members of an interdisciplinary team communicate often and are **interdependent**.

Team Goals

Once a team is formed, its members must determine the goal and how they will achieve it. Goals might focus on professional needs, patient needs, or team needs.

174 Chapter 8 | Teamwork

Career Connect

- Contact the health care professionals to arrange the visits ahead of time.
- If it is not possible to visit, invite the professional(s) to speak to the class.
- Alternatively, try to set up a telephone or e-mail interview.

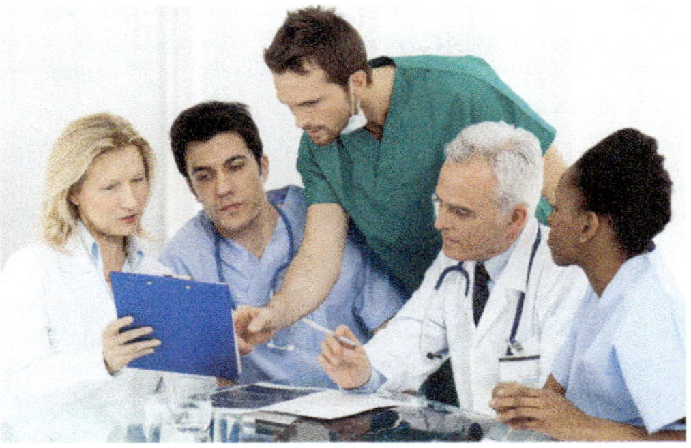

Figure 8.1
An interdisciplinary team works together to achieve common goals. How is an interdisciplinary team different from other types of teams?

They might include ways of exchanging information or evaluating outcomes. To develop meaningful goals, members will need to communicate clearly about individual goals with mutual respect so that these can be incorporated into the shared goals of the group.

In some cases, the team will want to develop a broad **mission statement** that all members can support. Keep in mind that you should set goals that have observable, measurable end points. When you want to achieve something quickly, you set short-term goals. You can accomplish short-term goals in the near future—maybe even today. It is usually easy to define short-term goals because they are specific and not very complicated. For example, you might want an elderly patient recovering from knee surgery to be able to stand up on their own and walk with assistance within two weeks.

mission statement
(MISH uhn STEYT muhnt)
A summary describing the aims, values, and overall plan of an organization or individual.

A long-term goal is something you want to achieve in the more distant future—maybe a year from now or maybe even more distant than that. Defining long-term goals may be more difficult than defining short-term goals. For example, you might want the elderly patient to be able to live on their own in six months.

Prioritizing goals will help members of the team stay focused and promote cohesiveness. In addition, team members may revise or add new goals based on a patient's needs.

prioritizing
(prahy AWR itahyz)
Arranging or dealing with in the order of importance.

Team Roles and Tasks

An interdisciplinary team usually consists of members representing several different professions, such as physicians, social workers, psychiatrists, physical therapists, massage therapists, medical assistants, nursing service workers, radiology workers, dieticians, and even home health care workers.

Often, there is overlap in the skills of the various team members. Several may have expertise in interacting with patients, forming care plans, and educating patients. Others can diagnosis and treat illness. Therefore, health care teams must develop **roles**.

roles
(rol s)
A position, responsibility, or duty.

Figure Focus

8.1 An interdisciplinary team works together to achieve common goals. How is an interdisciplinary team different from other types of teams?

Answer: Remind students of the different types of teams. Their answers to the question should include a definition of interdisciplinary, and that members contribute their opinions about treatment plans and then collaborate to implement one plan based on one set of goals.

Teaching Tips

- Review the three types of team goals:
  - Professional needs, such as a supportive work environment and clearly defined career paths.
  - Patient needs, such as food, medicine, and comfort.
  - Team needs, such as clearly defined roles, goals, and communication.
- Discuss the difference between individual goals and team goals.
- For example, individual goals, such as a promotion or raise, might benefit one person only, while team goals, such as providing patient care, or implementing a new method of organization, might benefit a patient or the entire facility.
- Compare short-term goals with long-term goals.
- Review the definition of an interdisciplinary team.
- Emphasize the importance of understanding one's role within a team.

CUSTOMIZED INSTRUCTION

Less Advanced Students

As a team, have students create a mission statement for the class. The statement should be two to three sentences that summarize the aims, values, and overall plan for the class. If necessary, provide a brief course description to help them get started.

TEAMWORK

As a class, with the teacher acting as a facilitator, work together to define a list of goals for the semester, term, or year. You may want to start by developing a mission statement, or using the mission statement you develop in the Language Arts Link on p. 179. Next, define a list of goals. Finally, prioritize the goals. Post the mission statement and goals on a bulletin board where you can see them every day.

Teaching Tips

- Discuss the ways in which roles are defined. For example, some roles may be self-evident, or defined by a job such as that of a dietician, or physician. Some roles may be defined by the team goals, or task at hand, such as who is responsible for communicating with family members.
- Emphasize the need for strong leadership in order to make the team work well.
- Review the characteristics of a strong, effective leader.
- Discuss the different types of leaders:
  - Democratic: Invites input
  - Autocratic: Absolute power
  - Laissez-faire: Lets team members take charge

Apply It

- Use the same teams from the Career-Ready Practices activity on p. 173.
- Encourage students to refer to the list of characteristics that make a strong leader.
- Limit discussion during the voting, but spend time reviewing the ballots afterward.

tasks
(task)
A function to be performed; job.

Many teams begin by identifying the necessary **tasks** before negotiating the roles. A team's goals help to define these tasks. Tasks might include activities such as ordering diagnostic testing, taking a patient's vital signs, contacting the patient, or writing prescriptions.

Decisions about each team member's role depends on availability, level of training, or a team member's preferences. For example, a nurse's role on the health care team is to coordinate patient care, protect the patient from illness, and teach the patient and/or family members.

Another nursing role might be assisting with mobility—a function evaluated by the physical therapist with specific activities prescribed, such as assisting the patient with transfer using a walker, carried out by the nursing staff. Assigning roles to each team member helps to eliminate conflict and establish expectations.

Commonly, one or more members of the health care team will serve as the leader(s) of the group. In the past, physicians often had the role of team leader in the health care setting. However, today many health care teams promote a more equal participation.

The leadership of a team may shift depending on the nature of the problem to be solved. Emphasis on providing holistic care has increased the roles and responsibilities of non-physician providers.

A good team leader is energetic, organized, reliable, charismatic, intelligent, creative, and often has a sense of humor.

Apply It

Form teams of five or more. By secret ballot, select a team leader for your team. On your ballot, identify the person you're voting for and list three qualities that would make him or her a successful leader.

In addition, a strong professional leader exhibits the following characteristics:

- Respects the rights, dignity, opinions, and abilities of others
- Understands the principles of democracy
- Works with a group and guides the group toward a goal
- Understands his or her own strengths and weaknesses
- Displays self-confidence and willingness to take a stand
- Communicates effectively and states ideas clearly
- Shows self-initiative and a willingness to work
- Completes tasks
- Shows optimism
- Is open-minded and can compromise
- Praises others and gives credit to others
- Is dedicated to meeting high standards

All strong leaders do not operate in the same type of environment. A democratic leader will make the final decision, but invite other members of the team to contribute to the decision-making process. This usually increases job satisfaction, because members of the team feel appreciated and respected. In addition, this leadership style can help to develop skills of team members.

ACTIVITY

Think up a motivational team building quotation or saying of your own and create a poster to illustrate it. Display the posters on a bulletin board.

CUSTOMIZED INSTRUCTION

More Advanced Students

Have more advanced students select one type of health care team and draw a diagram or flow chart illustrating how members of the team interact with each other.

Conversely, an autocratic leader has absolute power over the team. Members have little opportunity to offer suggestions, and often resent being treated in this manner. Sometimes this style of leadership is appropriate for routine and unskilled employees, but in most instances, it results in high turnover and absenteeism.

A leader might take a *"laissez-faire"* approach. This French phrase means "leave it be" and is used to describe a leader who leaves team members alone to get on with their work. This style of leadership works best with an experienced staff.

Skilled leaders recognize and cope with diversity, differing levels of skill, and different personalities. A successful leader has to assume responsibility for:

- Organizing and coordinating the team's activities
- Encouraging everyone to share ideas and give opinions
- Motivating all team members to work toward established goals
- Assisting with problems, decision making, and problem-solving
- Monitoring the progress of the team
- Providing reports and feedback to all team members on the effectiveness of the team

While a strong leader is important to the success of a team, team members must also be committed to the group's **productivity**.

Some important qualities of a good team member include developing good interpersonal relationships, which involves:

- Working for agreement on decisions (i.e., being open-minded and willing to compromise)
- Sharing thoughts and feelings openly and honestly (i.e., being friendly and cooperative)
- Involving others in the decision-making and problem-solving process
- Trusting and supporting other team members (i.e., assisting others when they need help)
- Admitting that problems exist rather than blaming them on others
- Listening carefully when another person is sharing ideas or beliefs
- Influencing others by involving them in the issues
- Encouraging and supporting the development of team members
- Respecting and tolerating individual differences (i.e., respecting opinions even when you don't agree with them)
- Identifying and working through conflict openly
- Considering and using new ideas and suggestions from others
- Encouraging feedback on own behavior
- Understanding and being committed to team goals and objectives
- Maintaining a positive attitude and learning to laugh at yourself
- Avoiding criticism of other team members

Meetings

Meetings are important in the workplace. In a health care setting, where patient care requires teamwork, meetings are an efficient way to communicate among team members.

There are different types of meetings: a team meeting for coworkers to communicate about team duties, such as patient care; a staff meeting for supervisors and managers to communicate information to a group about topics such as policies and schedules; a status meeting for team members to report on how patients are doing, procedures, schedules, and so forth.

productivity
(proh duhk TIV i tee)
The power to reach goals and get results.

Teaching Tips

- Review the responsibilities of a strong leader.
- Explain productivity.
- Discuss how the actions of one team member can enhance or detract from the entire team's productivity.
- Ask students to consider how the actions of one person has affected productivity in their own lives.
- Review the important qualities of a good team member.
- Point out how many of the qualities of a good team member involve effective communication.
- Some examples:
  - Sharing thoughts and feelings
  - Listening carefully
  - Encouraging feedback

Meetings

- Review the additional communication practices, such as meetings and record keeping.
- Discuss advantages and disadvantages of using meetings as a means of communication.

CUSTOMIZED INSTRUCTION

Special Needs Students

Special needs students may have trouble communicating effectively in a group environment. Encourage them to practice one-on-one communication first, then expand to working with two others, and so on until they are comfortable with the entire group.

ACTIVITY

Select one of the important qualities of a good team member. Write, draw, or act out a scenario that demonstrates the quality.

Teaching Tips

- Emphasize the importance of team communication.
- Review the components of effective communication:
  - Active listening
  - Giving and receiving feedback
  - Checking for comprehension
- Emphasize the importance of a communication network.

Apply It

- If necessary, have students review the sample careers discussed in Chapter 3. They should focus on the Therapeutic Services, Diagnostic Services, Health Informatics, and Support Services pathways.
- This will have them better understand the various roles of health care team members.
- They might also want to review the Patient Care Partnership (Patient's Bill of Rights) discussed in Chapter 5.

Figure Focus

8.2 How do strong communication skills help a health care team provide better service to the patient?

Answer: Strong communication skills among team members ensures that ideas, concepts, knowledge, and information regarding a patient's care are shared with the appropriate resources.

TEAMWORK

Divide the class into small groups. Have each person write one positive comment about each of the other members of the group. Share the comments.

- Learning good communication skills so you can share ideas, concepts, and knowledge
- Performing your duties to the best of your abilities

Team Communication

Effective interpersonal communication is vital to the smooth functioning of any team. (**Figure 8.2**) Team members should be skilled in active listening, giving and receiving feedback, and checking for comprehension.

It is also important for a team to develop an effective communication network. For example, team members should establish who relays information to whom within the team. The team must work to share relevant information in the most efficient way possible.

Some other important communication practices for a health care team include the following:

- A clear and effective system of recording patient information
- A regularly scheduled meeting for members to discuss patient's progress
- A regularly scheduled meeting to evaluate the team's function and development
- A procedure for communicating with other groups inside or outside the health facility

As with communication skills for interacting with patients, quality of care is also dependent upon the skills used for team discussions. When preparing for a specific practice or procedure, one member of the team may be called upon to complete research and present the findings, particularly if a new diagnosis has been identified or new practice is being implemented. As the team member doing the research, it is important to plan and prepare an effective presentation for the rest of the team as though it were for a large audience.

Teams can also learn to communicate better and practice dealing with emotional and stressful situations such as trauma and chronic and terminal illness using role play, providing valuable experience in a lower stakes situation.

Apply It

Form teams of five. A new patient has been admitted to your hospital and her care has been assigned to your team. What channels of communication will you follow to provide the best quality care possible? Create a poster that illustrates the tools and resources you will use to communicate information to all those involved in her care.

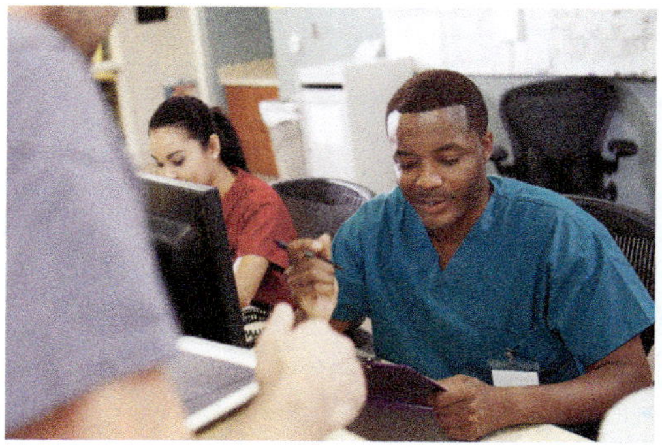

Figure 8.2
How do strong communication skills help a health care team provide better service to the patient?

Conflict Resolution

Health care team members represent a variety of skills, professional backgrounds, and opinions. In addition, interdisciplinary collaboration can be complex. With these types of dynamics, conflict between team members is inevitable.

178 Chapter 8 | Teamwork

CUSTOMIZED INSTRUCTION

More Advanced Students

More advanced students might assume they should always be the team leaders. Create situations where they must be subordinate to others in group activities or class discussions, so that they can understand the dynamics from a team member's point of view.

English Language Learners

As a group, have students discuss what techniques a team might use to overcome language barriers between members. Have students create a list of guidelines for overcoming language barriers that any type of team could follow. Their list should address: making sure all members understand the goal and their individual responsibilities in meeting the goal, speaking clearly (and more slowly), using a translation dictionary or an interpreter, and exercising patience and understanding if something needs to be repeated or explained.

Language Arts Link

Teamwork and Mission Statements

It is vital in the medical field to know how to work with others. When working as a team, it is critical that each member is aware of each individual's role and responsibilities. It is also essential that each team member has the same end goal in mind. A mission statement, which is a brief statement of purpose, can ensure that all team members will work collectively for the same purpose and result.

Work in a team to create a mission statement for this course. Be sure to include your team's responsibilities, values, and main objectives. During discussions in preparing the statement, build on each team member's ideas, respond thoughtfully to diverse perspectives, resolve contradictions, and determine if additional information is needed to complete the task.

Each team should prepare a presentation conveying a clear and distinct perspective on their mission statement. Part of working as a team is determining who is best suited and prepared for each job. Each team member should practice delivering the mission statement; then, as a team, decide who the presenter will be.

Conflict is a disagreement between two or more people who have different ideas. Conflict at work can make you angry and cause you to resent the other people on your team. If it is left unresolved, conflict can make it difficult or even impossible to successfully meet your responsibilities.

Some workplace conflicts are small, such as a disagreement about who gets to use the printer first or who put a file in the wrong drawer. Others are more significant, such as a disagreement over who will be the manager of a new project or who will get a promotion.

You can usually resolve minor conflicts easily by talking about them and coming to a **compromise** or building a consensus. A consensus means to come to an agreement. Managing workplace conflict does not always mean eliminating the conflict completely. It means that you are able to recognize what is causing the conflict and that you can cope with it in an honest and respectful way. All members of a team need to feel comfortable in offering feedback or discussing their ideas.

compromise
(KOM pruh mahyz)
A settlement of differences between parties by each party agreeing to give up something that it wants.

Successful teams often have a procedure or set of guidelines in place for handling conflict. These can be as simple as avoiding name-calling, speaking in a calm manner, or focusing on putting the needs of the patient first. Sometimes a team may want a **facilitator** to help resolve the conflict.

facilitator
(fuh SIL i tey ter)
A person responsible for leading or coordinating a group.

Techniques to resolving a conflict and building a consensus are listed below:

- Give all team members a chance to express their views and listen carefully.
- Be respectful of all team members.
- Set clear expectations and identify the conflict or problem.
- Gather the facts about the problem.
- Agree to work toward a solution.

Teamwork | Chapter 8 179

Language Arts Link—Teamwork and Mission Statements

- You may want to have examples of mission statements available to show to the class.
- Encourage the groups to assign specific roles, such as a team leader, a secretary, and a communicator.
- Teams may prepare an oral presentation, illustrated with a poster or created with a presentation program.
- Evaluate the mission statements based on content and organization, as well as on spelling and grammar. Also evaluate the way the group worked together as a team and presented their project.

Teaching Tips

- Emphasize that conflict in and of itself is not always a problem. It is usually only conflict that goes unrecognized and unresolved that is a problem.
- Point out that conflict resolution can lead to more effective communication, as well as confidence and trust in a team and its members.
- Discuss factors that contribute to conflict, such as personality problems or misunderstandings.
- Discuss factors that contribute to conflict resolution, such as constructive feedback, honesty, and open communication.

CUSTOMIZED INSTRUCTION

Less Advanced Students

Provide enough time for less advanced students to understand the process of conflict resolution. Explain that it is a step-by-step procedure and that the end result should be satisfying to all parties.

At-Risk Students

Working in pairs, have students create a one-page flyer that defines and illustrates the following four conflict resolution concepts: (1) Negotiate: Discuss options that will lead to an agreement that satisfies everyone. (2) Compromise: Settle a conflict by agreeing to accept less than what your originally wanted. (3) Resolve: Find a solution to the conflict. (4) Apologize: Express remorse or acknowledge that you are sorry for something.

TEAMWORK

Form groups of at least eight and stand in a close circle. Create a human knot: Put one hand in the circle and grasp only the hand of someone across from you. Put the other hand in the circle, and grasp the other hand of a different person (not the person next to you). Without releasing either grasp, work to "untie" the human knot. Do not break contact, although you can relax the grip enough to twist or rotate.

Teaching Tips

- Emphasize the importance of compromise and negotiation for conflict resolution.
- Discuss the role of a facilitator.
- Ask students to consider how they resolve conflicts with family members or friends, and to share personal experiences with the class.
- Review the steps for resolving a conflict.
- Emphasize that conflict is not always a bad thing, and that it can help a team grow stronger when it is resolved effectively.

- Deal with one problem at a time.
- Brainstorm possible solutions.
- Focus on common interests (such as patient wellness).
- Mediate disputes and negotiate decisions with the team members.
- Use objective criteria when possible.
- Invent new solutions where all team members gain.
- Implement the plan.
- Evaluate and review the problem-solving process after implementing the plan.

Analyzing Team Performance

A vital feature of a team that works well together is the ability to critically assess team performance and outcomes. Strong teams take time to reflect on how the decisions made by the group led to both positive and negative experiences for the patient without resorting to blame. This process is crucial as it allows the team to improve their tactics and modify their decision making on future cases.

Summary

Most health care organizations need well-functioning teams that understand the all-important end goal of providing quality health care to patients/clients. To be successful in your career and as a member of a team, you need an understanding of group dynamics. You should help to develop team goals and understand your role in achieving these goals.

You will likely experience conflict in your team at some point in your career. That's why it is important to develop strong communication skills and be willing to work with others to resolve the conflict. Each team member is responsible for helping to identify the problem and brainstorm solutions.

Section 8.1 Review Questions

1. How does being part of a team help you do your job better?
2. Explain the difference between a multidisciplinary health care team and an interdisciplinary health care team.
3. What are some things a team should do in order to be one cohesive unit?
4. Name three qualities a good team member should have.
5. List two things a health care team should do to have good communication.
6. What is the role of a facilitator?
7. What is the purpose of teaming?

180 Chapter 8 | Teamwork

Section 8.1 Review Questions

1. Answer: Being part of a team gives you access to all the knowledge, experience, and abilities of your teammates.
2. Answer: A multidisciplinary team is made up of practitioners from multiple disciplines who may work with a patient/client during the same time period. These team members have their own goals and recommendations, but they do stay informed about what each other is doing.
   An interdisciplinary team consists of practitioners from two or more disciplines who work in the same setting. Members contribute their opinions about treatment plans and then collaborate to implement one plan based on one set of goals. Members of interdisciplinary teams communicate often.
3. Answer: To become a cohesive unit, a team should establish goals and a mission statement that all team members agree on. The team should prioritize their goals to help members of the team stay focused and promote cohesiveness
4. Answer: Team members should have good interpersonal relationships including:
   - Working for agreement on decisions
   - Sharing thoughts and feelings openly and honestly
   - Involving others in the decision-making process
   - Trusting and supporting other team members
   - Admitting to problems rather than blaming them on others
   - Listening carefully when another person is sharing ideas or beliefs
   - Influencing others by involving them in the issues
   - Encouraging and supporting the development of team members
   - Respecting and tolerating individual differences
   - Identifying and working through conflict openly
   - Considering and using new ideas and suggestions from others
   - Encouraging feedback on own behavior
   - Understanding and being committed to team goals and objectives
   - Maintaining a positive attitude and learning to laugh at yourself
   - Avoiding criticism of other team members
   - Learning good communication skills so you can share ideas, concepts, and knowledge
   - Performing your duties to the best of your abilities
5. Answer: A health care team should have a clear and effective record system, a regularly scheduled meeting for members to discuss patient's progress, a regularly scheduled meeting to evaluate the team's function and development, and a procedure for communicating with other groups inside or outside the health care facility
6. Answer: A facilitator is responsible for leading or coordinating a group, often in conflict resolution.

7. Answer: A word used in health care defined as coming together as a team to achieve high-quality health care.

CHAPTER 8 REVIEW

Chapter Review Questions

1. Why is teaming important? (8.1)
2. List five examples of group dynamics. (8.1)
3. What is an interdisciplinary team? (8.1)
4. Why is assigning roles and tasks to team members so important? (8.1)
5. Describe the five rights of delegation. (8.1)
6. Compare the five types of health care teams. (8.1)
7. What is a mission statement? (8.1)
8. List five characteristics of a good team leader. (8.1)
9. What are some of the responsibilities a successful leader must assume? (8.1)
10. List five steps to resolving conflict among team members. (8.1)

Activities

1. In order for a team to function well, it is important to build relationships with all of your teammates. One way to develop a relationship is to find common bonds. For example, you and another team member might both enjoy playing soccer. Or, you might both have brothers or sisters. Or, you might both play the guitar. Discovering common bonds helps you understand the other person so you can work together successfully— exhibiting the ability to cooperate, contribute, and collaborate—as a member of a team.

   In teams of four, identify at least five common bonds among you. How would the things you all have in common help you function better as a team? What role does communication play in healthy relationships and team success?
2. In the same group of four you formed in Activity 1, review the definition of group dynamics discussed in this chapter. Working collaboratively, assess your group's dynamics. What are your strengths? What are your weaknesses? Did everyone on your team cooperate on the project and contribute equally?
3. A new treatment for Ebola will be introduced for a patient in the facility recently diagnosed with the condition. Your team will be assisting the physician in charge, and you have been asked by the other team members to complete research on the specifics of the procedures that will be used. Describe your plan for gathering the data and preparing your presentation for the team.
4. Have your instructor assign you a group case study to diagnose a fictional patient and recommend treatment. Afterwards, take the time to come together again as a group and evaluate the group's performance and the health care outcomes for your patient. Think of the impacts of the decisions the group made and suggest modifications for future case studies.
5. In a group, role play how a health care team might deal with telling a patient that they are likely to pass away in the next few days and how you can help the patient through this. You can try again with each person taking on a new role on the team. Make sure you apply critical-thinking, adaptability, and consensus-building techniques to solve this problem.
6. Think about the personal relationships you have with family and friends. Identify the role of communication skills in building and maintaining healthy relationships. Practice your new communication skills with a friend.

Teamwork | Chapter 8 181

CHAPTER 8 REVIEW

Chapter Review Questions

1. Answer: Teaming is important because an individual has only limited knowledge and experience and by bringing together different people with a variety of backgrounds, more ideas are generated and more problems are solved.
2. Answer: Team dynamics are defined by personality styles, team roles, office layout, tools and technology, a company's culture, and procedures.
3. Answer: An interdisciplinary team consists of practitioners from two or more disciplines who work in the same setting. Members contribute their opinions about treatment plans and then collaborate to implement one plan based on one set of goals.
4. Answer: Assigning roles and tasks to team members is important because there may be overlap in roles and defining each team member's tasks will help define their role.
5. Answer:
   - Right task: Identifying an appropriate caregiver-patient relationship.
   - Right circumstances: Verifying that the correct patient setting and resources are available.
   - Right person: Identifying who is trained/capable of doing the task.
   - Right direction/communication: Providing a clear, short description of the task and clarifying limitations and the expected result.
   - Right supervision: Providing appropriate monitoring, assistance, and feedback.
6. Answer:
   - Ad hoc groups: Formed for a limited amount of time to address a specific problem. These may be composed of members from many departments.
   - Nominal care group: Includes a physician who refers a patient to different specialists. These specialists provide care independently; however, the physician may coordinate the flow of information among the specialists.

6. *(continued)*
   - Unidisciplinary group: Organized around a single discipline.
   - Multidisciplinary team: Made up of practitioners from multiple disciplines who may work with a patient/client during the same time period, but these practitioners each have their own goals and recommendations.
   - Interdisciplinary team: Includes practitioners from two or more disciplines who work in the same setting. Members contribute their opinions about treatment plans and then collaborate to implement one plan based on one set of goals.
7. Answer: A mission statement is a summary describing the aims, values, and overall plan of an organization or individual.
8. Answer:
   - Respects the rights, dignity, opinions, and abilities of others.
   - Understands the principles of democracy.
   - Works with a group and guides the group toward a goal.
   - Understands own strengths and weaknesses.
   - Displays self-confidence and willingness to take a stand.

- Communicates effectively and states ideas clearly.
- Shows self-initiative and a willingness to work.
- Completes tasks.
- Shows optimism.
- Open-minded, can compromise.
- Praises others and gives credit to others.
- Dedicated to high standards.

9. Answer:
   - Organizing and coordinating the team's activities, including meetings.
   - Encouraging everyone to share ideas and give opinions.
   - Motivating all team members to work toward established goals.
   - Assisting with problems.
   - Monitoring the progress of the team.
   - Providing reports and feedback to all team members on the effectiveness of the team.
10. Answer:
   - Give all team members a chance to express their views and listen carefully.
   - Be respectful of all team members.
   - Identify the conflict or problem.
   - Agree to work toward a solution.
   - Deal with one problem at a time.
   - Brainstorm possible solutions.
   - Focus on common interests (such as patient wellness), not positions.
   - Use objective criteria when possible.
   - Invent new solutions where all team members gain.
   - Implement the plan.
   - Evaluate and review the problem-solving process after implementing the plan.

CHAPTER 8 REVIEW

Case Studies

1. Your interdisciplinary team consists of a physician, social worker, psychiatrist, and medical assistant. Some of the suggested treatments for a patient appear to be independent of one another, rather than part of a cohesive treatment plan. What is the problem here and how would you resolve it?
2. You and a member of your interdisciplinary team are not getting along because you feel that he is often bossing you around. He tells you to do things that you think he should be doing. In addition, you are sometimes not sure about how to do the things that he asks you to do. He thinks that you are being lazy and not doing your job. How can you use critical-thinking skills to express your needs, wants, and emotions to resolve this conflict?

Thinking Critically

1. **Group Dynamics**—Group dynamics are the motivating or driving forces that influence the actions and identity of the team. Use examples from a recent team project to describe personality styles, team roles, and culture. Working with a small group, role play different situations that demonstrate both good and bad group dynamics. Have another team assess your group's dynamics.
2. **Making a Team**—Most teams go through a series of stages. Initially, new team members may feel nervous. Sometimes they misinterpret others' behaviors. The situation involves new people and new tasks. Describe the process by which a team becomes a cohesive and productive unit.
3. **Conflict**—Conflict may occur in any group because of misunderstandings or strong personalities. How do you resolve conflict successfully and professionally in the workplace? Evaluate the effectiveness of the conflict-resolution techniques you described. Why is it important to maintain healthy relationships with your co-workers? How can this help you succeed on the job?

PORTFOLIO TIP

The manner in which you present your activity to your classmates is very important. Remember that you're building a team. All members of the team must feel that they are working together toward a specific goal.

Portfolio Connection

Health care teams are a critical part of today's health care system. Successful teams help provide a higher level of care to the patient/client, and to meet the challenges of economic change. Therefore, every health care worker needs to do his or her part to contribute to the team's goal.

There are many resources that can help you better understand what it takes to build a team. Use the Internet, library, and other resources to research team-building activities, such as ropes courses, minefield exercises, "mission impossible," or "team survivor" types of assignments.

Design an activity that can be used in a health care setting to build a team. ... strengths into team assets, learning to blend personal goals ... and building effective communication skills ...

Activities

1. You may want to assign teams. Common bonds can be as simple as being in the same class together. Encourage students to explore the common bonds that may not be apparent; for example, maybe they all like the same type of music.
2. Encourage students to think critically about their team dynamics. Students may want to perform a skit demonstrating their team's dynamics.
3. Students should provide a written response for the plan and an outline with the media strategies for the team presentation (PowerPoints, handouts, demonstration, discussion, or other).
4. You can assign specific roles to each member of the group. On subsequent case studies, have them swap roles.
5. This is also an opportunity for students to practice compassion and empathy. You can have a student role play as the patient for added benefit.
6. Have the students report back on how things went with their friend.

Case Studies

1. Student responses should be in writing. Alternatively, encourage students to work in groups and present a skit illustrating the situation and the resolution.
2. Again, students should respond to the case study in writing. You may also allow them to present a skit illustrating the situation and the resolution.

Thinking Critically

1. Alternatively, allow them to use a fictional team situation from a movie or television show.
2. Encourage students to express their responses as a step-by-step list of procedures.
3. Refer students to the section on Conflict Resolution on pp. 178–180.

Portfolio Connection

You may want to provide resources for this assignment—books on team building or links to Web sites such as humanresources.about.com. Remind students that they must write up their activity so they can include it in their portfolio. They may also want to prepare posters illustrating their idea, or create a slide show presentation to use when selling the idea to the class. Encourage them to practice before presenting their activity to the class. You may want to have the class select one or two of the activities and test them out. Check to make sure that students have completed the written assignments and added them to their portfolio.

9 Effective Communication

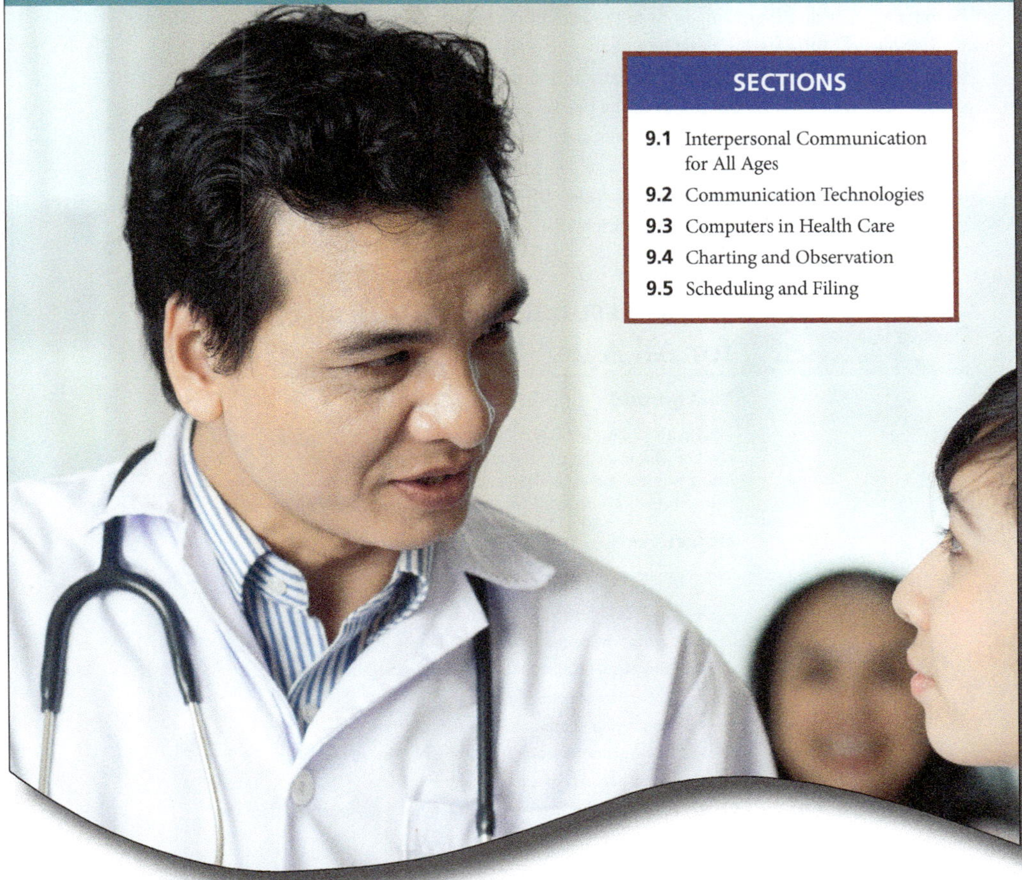

SECTIONS

Advance Preparation

- Review: Chapter text for Sections 9.1, 9.2, 9.3, 9.4, and 9.5; and chapter procedures.

Contact:

- Local health care facilities to request copies of Internet and e-mail policies, as well as blank forms for charting and observation.
- Acute-care facility to request a tour so students can observe computerized procedures in various medical services.
- Local health care facilities to request a tour or job shadow opportunities in the filing and scheduling departments.
- Guest speakers who have experience with scheduling, filing, and recordkeeping.
- A guest speaker to explain computers.

Prepare:

- Have on hand correctly and incorrectly filled out charts and observation forms.
- Magazine and newspaper articles on advances in communications technology and computers in health care.
- Magazine and newspaper articles on verbal and nonverbal communication.
- A list of Web sites that provide information about effective communication—such as hhs.gov/ocr/civilrights/resources/specialtopics/hospitalcommunication/.

CHAPTER 9 OVERVIEW

Communication in health care involves more than just talking and listening. It also includes sharing information such as records and treatment plans. Chapter 9 covers all aspects of communications in health care, including interpersonal communications, charting, and the role of computers and other technology.

Section 9.1: Section 9.1 covers interpersonal communications. The section title refers to "all ages" because communicating with children and seniors may require different techniques.

Section 9.2: In Section 9.2, students are introduced to the role of communications technology, including software programs, telephone systems, facsimile machines, e-mail, and the Internet.

Section 9.3: Section 9.3 looks specifically at how computers are used in health care professions for diagnostics, education, recordkeeping, and more. It also examines issues of confidentiality and ethics, as they relate to the use of computer technology.

Section 9.4: In Section 9.4, Charting and Observation, students learn proper methods for observing patients, and how to record information on health records and charts.

Section 9.5: The final section focuses on how to schedule appointments and tests and standard methods of filing information, such as patient records.

FOCUS AND ENGAGE

Getting Started

- This activity is designed to demonstrate how easily information can be misinterpreted.
- After passing the message around the circle, compare the original message with the final message.
- Discuss the problems that might result if the final message is used in place of the original message.

Introduce the Section

a. Review the content of the Background paragraph, emphasizing that communication is more than just talking.
b. Point out that health care workers must communicate with many different people, in many different roles throughout the course of the day.
c. Review section objectives.
d. Review the different ways people communicate, and the different information they pass from one to another.

Vocabulary Review

a. Key terms are defined in the margins of the text on the page where they first appear.
b. Pronounce each word, and have the students repeat the pronunciation out loud.
c. Discuss each definition.

Getting Started

Effective communications are essential to providing appropriate and quality health care. In one study by a large health care organization, it was determined that on an average two-day stay in an acute care facility, patient information is shared among 47 different health care professionals. Clearly, if communications are not shared with care and accuracy, diagnosis and treatment can be inappropriate and even dangerous to the patient outcome.

To show how information must be shared accurately and appropriately and how very easy it is for mistakes to occur, join your classmates in a circle and with a message from your teacher whisper the information into the ear of the person next to you until the circle is completed. The last person in the circle will share what is heard. The results are then compared to the original message. A discussion led by the teacher will consider the results of treatment if the information is different than the original message. (*Example:* Mr. Johansen in room 222 was admitted this morning and is agitated and appears disoriented.)

SECTION 9.1 Interpersonal Communication for All Ages

Background

The health care worker should understand that there are many factors in communication. A knowledge of these techniques will increase your skills in communicating with co-workers and patients/clients. With this knowledge, you will be able to do a better job and to make good observations about your patients.

Objectives

When you have completed this section, you will be able to do the following:

- Match key terms with their correct meanings.
- Explain why communication is important.
- Name elements that influence our relationship with others.
- List barriers to communication.
- Identify your communication assertiveness level.
- List elements necessary for communication to take place.
- Describe actions of a good listener.
- Differentiate between verbal and nonverbal communication.

184 Chapter 9 | Effective Communication

CUSTOMIZED INSTRUCTION

English Language Learners

Have students write each key term and its pronunciation on one side of an index card and its definition on the other side.

Special Needs Students

Special needs students may take longer learning effective methods for communicating. Allow extra time for pairing special needs and non-special needs students to practice interpreting nonverbal communication.

CUSTOMIZED INSTRUCTION OVERVIEW

Less Advanced Students	Pages 192, 213, 228
More Advanced Students	Pages 187, 200, 202
English Language Learners	Pages 184, 190
Special Needs Students	Pages 184, 196, 206
At-Risk Students	Pages 186, 187

Effective Patient Relations and Communication Skills

Communication is essential in the exchange of ideas, feelings, and thoughts. Communication helps us to understand the needs of others and how best to meet those needs. Developing good communication skills helps to build and maintain healthy relationships. There are several kinds of communication. These include words (either written or spoken), gestures, facial expressions (frowns, smiles), body posture, touch, and listening. The following discussion has important information to help you become a better communicator with patients, families, coworkers, supervisors, and other members of the health care team.

Apply It

Think-Pair-Share: Think about the different ways you would communicate as a health worker in a pediatric office vs. working in a nursing home. Take three minutes to write down the differences. Pair with a classmate and discuss your responses. Share with the class.

Effective patient relations are a necessity. To communicate effectively, we need to work through a process that includes engaging, understanding, educating, and creating a sense of collaboration.

Engagement is a connection between the health care professional and patient that sets the stage for establishing a collaboration. Barriers to engagement by the health care professional might include mistakes like not introducing yourself, asking pointed and critical questions, and interrupting the patient/client.

An understanding health care professional will make patients feel accepted. To exhibit understanding of a patient's needs, you might first make introductions with the patient fully clothed, in a safe environment. You can allow the patient to share thoughts and feelings and respond by repeating them in your own words. Sharing anecdotes—without being too personal—can also help to create a positive bond between the patient and health care professional. (**Figure 9.1**)

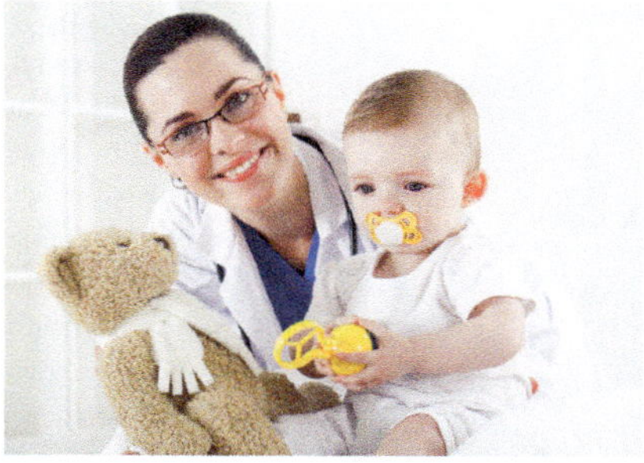

Figure 9.1
A pediatrician gives a toy to a baby. Why is it important to engage patients?

Educating the patient includes helping to increase knowledge and understanding and minimize anxiety. Health care professionals should assume that all patients share many of the same questions, including:

- What is happening to me?
- What will I have to do?
- Will it hurt?
- When will I have the results?

To have good communication, you must be certain to answer all of the patient's questions. If you are unable to answer the questions, assure the patient you will find out from other sources. Avoid using complicated, clinical terms and be clear. Determine if you have answered the patient's questions by using statements such as, "Have I answered your questions?", "Do you have questions about anything I have not covered?", or "Is there anything you want to add to the information I have obtained about you?".

Creating a collaborative relationship occurs with good communication. The health care professional and patient work together regarding the problem and the treatment plan. Many times, a patient may think he or she knows the problem.

Effective Communication | Chapter 9 185

TEACH

Discuss

- Ask students how they communicate with friends and family. Do they use different methods for different people? Do they use verbal or nonverbal communications?
- Discuss ways people communicate without words: storming angrily out of a room, sulking at the dinner table, or smiling at someone.

Reinforce and Review

- Review the concept of teamwork as covered in Chapter 8, and the ways teams identify goals and resolve conflict.
- Review cultural attitudes to body language, such as eye contact and personal space, covered in Chapters 6 and 7.

Teaching Tips

- Review the four components of effective communication between a health care worker and a patient:
  - Engagement
  - Understanding
  - Education
  - Partnership
- Emphasize that communication is a process that allows people to share thoughts, ideas, and feelings.
- Point out that communicating with patients is one of the most important roles for all health care workers, not just those in direct care situations.
- For example, receptionists take phone calls and schedule appointments, housekeeping staff might handle patients' personal belongings, nutritionists might receive menu requests, etc.

Figure Focus

9.1 A pediatrician gives a toy to a baby. Why is it important to engage patients?

Answer: It is important to engage a patient because it creates a connection between the health care professional and patient that sets the stage for establishing a partnership.

Apply It

- While this exercise asks students to identify the differences in communication techniques, you might also prompt them to consider similarities. For example, active listening is an important communication skill when dealing with youngsters as well as older patients.

TEAMWORK

In pairs, randomly select a health care occupation. Have one team member act as the health care worker, and the other act as a patient. Perform a short skit that illustrates communication between the two.

Teaching Tips

- Review the eight components of good communication that allow you to send a clear message:
  - Use active listening skills.
  - Use a positive tone.
  - Watch your body language.
  - Treat patients and co-workers with respect.
  - Be precise and detailed about what you expect.
  - Model the behavior you want others to follow.
  - Explain your reasoning.
  - Discuss any conflicts in a calm and rational way.
- Point out that sending a clear message is not the same thing as sending a positive or "good" message. Even bad news or difficult information must be delivered clearly.
- Explain that prejudice may be a bias about anything—not just race—and that it is not always a negative bias. For example, someone might believe that wealthy people are all smart.

You need to make sure the patient and/or family members understands the diagnosis, plan, and treatment.

Non-effective communications are often due to the health care team member feeling incompetent or lacking confidence, not knowing what to say, or feeling that he or she doesn't have the skills or knowledge needed. It can also be due to fear of saying something wrong or of arousing strong emotions in others and in ourselves. Other barriers to effective communication might include working with patients that speak a language that you are not familiar with or for which you do not have skills. Non-effective communications can have a significant impact on the outcomes of the care to be provided, such as the treatment needed, prescription directions, or patient discomfort. It is important to be well prepared for and confident in your career responsibilities and that you communicate effectively.

Apply It

Bring in two photos, depicting scenes or activities with people, from magazines or newspapers. The scenes should reflect a variety of cultures and countries.

As your teacher shows each photo to the class, write down the first thing you think of on a 3 × 5 card. You do not need to write your name on the cards. Your teacher can read these anonymous note cards. What can you learn about yourself and your classmates from your reactions?

Sending a Clear Message

Good communication means that you are sending a clear message in an effective manner—one that is understood by both your co-workers and your patients. It is especially important that medical information is accurately communicated in a health care setting. Messages are used to convey needs and wants. A need is a something you can't live without. A want is something you desire. Humans need certain basic items in order to survive. We want things to improve our quality of life. It is important that while you are able to express emotions, you do not let your message get overwhelmed by them. In order to convey a clear message that communicates your needs and wants in an effective way, you must:

- Communicate clearly and concisely, both verbally and in writing. Communication is clear when you use words and body language that other people can understand, and concise when you convey information clearly and comprehensively in as few words as possible.
- Use active listening skills.
- Speak in a positive tone.
- Be aware of your body language.
- Be sure to use language and terms that the patient can understand.
- Treat patients and co-workers with respect.
- Be precise and detailed about what you expect.
- Model the behavior you want others to follow.
- Explain your reasoning.
- Discuss any conflicts in a calm and rational way. Don't let your emotions take over.
- Self-advocate by clearly and calmly expressing your needs, wants, and emotions.

Communicating clearly is the key to creating a high quality health care team and establishing a positive relationship with your patients. Developing communication strategies is key to success in the health care setting.

186 Chapter 9 | Effective Communication

Apply It

- You may want to have students work in small groups to select the photos.
- Have magazines available in the classroom for students to use.
- Try not to let the class know the point of the exercise before they write their responses to the photos, or they may not be honest about their feelings and reactions.
- Do not be judgmental, and do not let the class discussion become judgmental.

CUSTOMIZED INSTRUCTION

At-Risk Students

Make sure students understand the definition of prejudice. In most cases, prejudices are negative opinions that are not based on fact. Discuss methods for eliminating prejudices against another. For example, respect what others say; respect what others think is important; and be considerate of the feelings of others.

Elements That Influence Your Relationships with Others

Prejudices

All people form opinions or **biases** as they are growing up. These **prejudices** affect how they feel about other people and how they relate to them. You may have very strong feelings about the backgrounds or the values of your patients or co-workers. Your feelings affect how you communicate. For instance, if you believe that certain people are lazy, overly emotional, or **inferior**, you need to think about your prejudices. When you understand your prejudices and feelings, you have an opportunity to overcome them.

Frustrations

When you care for and work with others, you may experience **impatience**, **annoyance**, and even anger. Perhaps other people do not understand your directions, or they may move too slowly. You feel irritated. These feelings interfere with your ability to communicate. Take time to understand why you feel frustrated. Evaluate the situation, and then try to correct it. It is your responsibility to control your behavior and to understand that patients, families, and co-workers have problems that are the cause of their behavior.

How you act toward others and how they act toward you affect the quality of **communication**. If you are disinterested or bored, if you are in a bad mood, if you wish you were someplace else, communication breaks down. However, if you show interest and concern for others, you will experience worthwhile communication, your job will become easier, and you will be more effective.

Life Experiences

People have new experiences every day. These experiences help us know what to expect in day-to-day living and how to act in certain situations. The most effective communication is based on shared experiences. These may be experiences you went through together or experiences that you both went though individually. Perhaps you grew up in the same community, went to the same school, or even share the same language. It may be as simple as liking the same type of movies, music, or books.

You will usually have more effective communication with someone who has shared some of your experiences. Of course, the reverse can be true as well; less shared experiences can cause communication to be more difficult and frustrating. This is especially true in the area of **slang** and **dialect**.

To be a more effective communicator, look for things that you have in common with the other person. You can do this by listening to what they say and how they say it, and looking for something familiar and then focusing a bit more on that shared experience. As you find more and more areas in common, your communication with that person will become more effective.

biases
(BAHY uhs ez)
Tendencies; prejudices.

prejudices
(PREJ uh dis ez)
Judgments or opinions formed before the facts are known.

inferior
(in FEER ee er)
Lower, second-rate, substandard (e.g., one product is inferior in quality to another product).

impatience
(im PEY shuh ns)
Intolerance, edginess.

annoyance
(uh NOI uhns)
Irritation (e.g., to feel irritated with a co-worker or patient).

communication
(kuh myoo ni KAY shuhn)
Act of exchanging information.

slang
(slanNG)
Language of informal words and phrases; typically restricted to a particular context or group of people.

dialect
(di e lekt)
Language peculiar to a specific region or social group.

Effective Communication | Chapter 9 187

CUSTOMIZED INSTRUCTION

More Advanced Students

You might have more advanced students spend time researching medical technology that helps sensory-impaired people communicate; for example, cochlear implants for the hearing impaired or cornea transplants for the visually impaired. They can report their findings to the class.

At-Risk Students

Have students cut out a picture of a person from a newspaper or magazine and paste it to a sheet of paper. Have them call out facial expressions, gestures, posturing, and clothing and what they think those things communicate about the person. As a group, discuss prejudices or biases that one might form based on another's appearance.

Teaching Tips

- Discuss why certain people or situations make students feel uncomfortable.
- Discuss the impact of frustration and attitude on communication.
- Discuss what "life experience" means.
- Explain shared experience, and discuss why it might be easier to communicate with someone who shares your life experiences.
- For example, students may have an easier time communicating with peers who attend the same school than they do with peers who attend a different school.
- Discuss cross-generational communication: young people communicating with seniors.
- Ask students to share stories of communicating with elderly relatives.

Community

- You may want to have a list of agencies or organizations, which you have already contacted, available for students.
- You may want to invite a representative of one or more organizations to speak to the class.
- You may want to set a timetable for this activity, so you can plan class time for compiling the list of concerns and issues.

Teaching Tips

- Explain what a barrier is. Discuss:
  - Labeling
  - Types of sensory impairment
  - Why talking too fast is a barrier
  - Types of cognitive impairment
- Discuss the four essential elements needed for communication to take place:
  - Message
  - Sender
  - Receiver
  - Feedback
- Ask students to name factors that might interfere with these elements, such as an unclear message, a distracted receiver, no acknowledgement that the message was received, etc.

Career-Ready Practices

- Students may list skills discussed in the text, as well as others they feel are important for communicating on the job.
- Examples of interpersonal communication skills are:
  - Being clear
  - Being personal
  - Being positive
  - Getting to the point
  - Using active listening
  - Thinking before you respond
- This activity gives students real-world experience in applying the following Career-Ready Practice: Communicate Clearly, Effectively and With Reason.
- For more information on the Career-Ready Practices, visit careertech.org/career-ready-practices.

labeling
(LEY buhl ing)
Describing a person with a word that limits them (e.g., lazy, stupid).

courteous
(KUR tee uhs)
Polite; considerate toward others.

Career-Ready Practices

Interpersonal communication is the verbal and nonverbal interaction between two or more people and is one of the primary means of exchanging information in a health care setting. Given the nature of the information—which can sometimes mean life or death for a patient—it is critical for every health care worker to communicate thoughts, ideas, and action plans clearly, concisely, and effectively. Career-ready individuals are skilled at interacting with others; they are active listeners, and speak clearly and with purpose to others. They utilize effective strategies for communicating wants, needs, and emotions.

In your word processor, create a list of ten interpersonal communication skills to practice on the job. Focus on skills that ensure the accuracy of information and eliminate any errors in its exchange. Share your list with the class.

Aging and Communication

What happens when a younger health care professional deals with an older patient, or vice versa? There are, of course, possible physical issues that make communication with the elderly more difficult, such as hearing or vision problems. There may be mental or emotional issues, such as older people who are afraid of losing the ability to think, reason, or explain themselves. Finally, there may be certain cultural issues, such as believing the doctor is always right or being afraid to complain about aches and pains.

There are also fewer shared experiences between younger and older individuals, so it becomes even more important to work on finding some common ground that you may share.

Barriers to Communication

Recognizing barriers to communication—both verbal and nonverbal—allows you to become an understanding health care worker. The following are five major communication barriers:

- **Labeling.** Deciding the other person is mean, lazy, a complainer, or difficult causes a breakdown in communication. You do not pay attention to the message being sent. If you listen, you might find out the reason for the behavior.
- **Language barriers.** When two people who have different native tongues try to communicate in a single language, problems may arise if one person does not understand the language well enough.
- **Sensory impairment.** Deafness or blindness can be a communication barrier. Always evaluate the people you are communicating with to be certain that they do not have a sensory impairment. Sensory impairment is when one of the senses—sight, hearing, smell, touch, taste, and spatial awareness—is no longer normal.
- **Talking too fast.** It is especially important when you are working with elderly people to speak slowly. Communication can break down when the message is delivered too rapidly.
- **Cognitive impairment.** Cognitive impairment includes developmental level, memory, perception, problem solving, emotional reaction, and idea formulation. These types of impairments might result from aphasia (a loss of understanding), autism, brain injury, Parkinson's, Alzheimer's, or old age. Be careful to make sure your patient understands what you are saying. You may want them to tell you, in their own words, what you have just explained to them. Or, you may write down suggestions for them.

Developing skills in communication helps you become a better health care worker. It is important always to be **courteous** and understanding. Take time to evaluate gestures, facial expressions, and tone of voice in order to understand what is really being said. You may feel frustrated, angry, or irritated, but as a health care worker, it is up to you to attempt to understand and to listen. Hearing accurately and then responding appropriately are essential. Remember to communicate your messages so that they can be understood easily.

188 Chapter 9 | Effective Communication

TEAMWORK

Randomly select a topic. In pairs, sit back to back and carry on a conversation about the selected topic. Face each other and carry on a conversation about the same topic. Write or discuss the ways that the two conversations differed, how you felt about them, and why.

Elements of Communication

For communication to take place, there are four essential **elements**:

- **A message.** There must be something that you want to convey to another person. Perhaps the purpose of the message is to give information or to acquire information. Perhaps there is something you want another person to do.
- **A sender.** Unless there is someone who wants to send a message, there cannot be communication.
- **A receiver.** Even if there is a message and a sender, there must be a receiver. If there is no one to receive the message, communication is incomplete.
- **Feedback.** Capturing feedback is of critical importance. If you do not appear to be listening and then act on what you are told, why would people tell you anything?

Interference with any of these elements can disrupt communication. Remember that in order to ensure clear and effective communication:

- The message must be clear.
- The sender must deliver the message in a clear and concise manner.
- The receiver must be able to hear and receive the message.
- The receiver must be able to understand the message.
- Interruptions or distractions must be avoided.

How can we ensure clear and effective communication? We have to remember that communication is a two-way street. You must listen to others to make sure they listen to you. If you're interested in what the other person has to say, that person will more likely be interested in you. Remember to smile and maintain eye contact, so that the other person knows that you are interested in him or her. Use your voice and body language to show your enthusiasm.

On the other hand, there are many elements that can disrupt communication. Don't be competitive or make it seem as if what you have to say is more important than what the other person is saying. Watch your body language. You don't want to appear bored or disinterested. Don't hunch your shoulders, fold your arms across your body, fidget, tap your feet, twiddle your hair, or play on your cell phone. Finally, don't be too aggressive or pushy in your conversation.

Good Listening Skills

When you think of communication, you may not think of listening. However, listening is a very important element in all communication. If you do not receive the message that is being sent, communication has not taken place. Your understanding of how to be a good listener makes you a better health care worker.

- **Show interest.** It is important for you to show interest in the person who is sending you a message. (**Figure 9.2**) If you follow all of the other rules of being a good listener but tune out the message because you are not interested, communication will not take place.

elements
(L uh ment z)
The basic assumptions or principles of a subject.

Community

Visit a local organization dedicated to the culture of a specific group (e.g., Asian Americans or Native Americans). Work with volunteers of that organization to better understand the way their members address health care issues. What problems do they have?

If no local organization exists, visit a senior day care center or nursing home, and interview the patients. Create a list of concerns or issues, compile it across the class and share it with your local hospital, if appropriate.

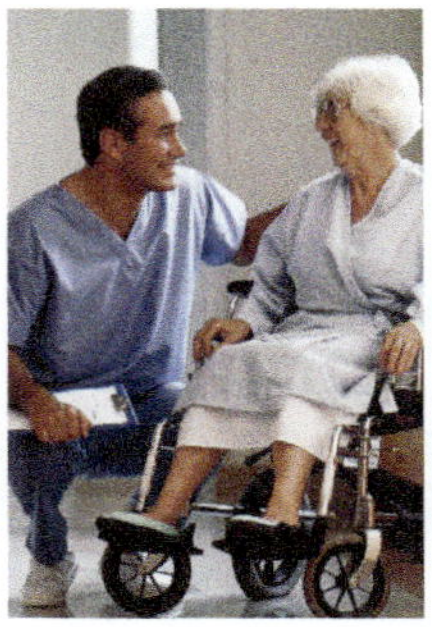

Figure 9.2
Good eye contact, a gentle touch, and your body inflections show that you are interested in what is being said. How is showing interest an important part of listening? What are several observations you can make about this interaction?

Effective Communication | Chapter 9 189

Teaching Tips

- Review the five components of clear communication:
  - Clear message
  - Effective delivery
  - Effective reception
  - Understanding
  - No distractions
- Emphasize the two-way nature of communication.
- Remind students that communication is not just between a health care worker and a patient, but also between health care workers and a patient's family members, employers and employees, co-workers, team members, etc.
- Explain that listening and active listening are not the same, and discuss the difference.
- Ask students how well they listen when they are not interested, and to share stories of problems that may have come from not listening carefully.
- For example, they may have missed a homework assignment, or bought the wrong item at the store.
- During the discussion, interrupt the students frequently, ask questions but ignore the answers, give directions too quickly.
- Afterward, ask students how it feels to be interrupted, ignored, or misunderstood because the other person is not paying attention.
- Review the qualities of a good listener:
  - Show interest
  - Hear the message
  - Do not interrupt
  - Pay attention
  - Maintain a positive attitude

Figure Focus

9.2 Good eye contact, a gentle touch, and your body inflections show that you are interested in what is being said. How is showing interest an important part of listening? What are several observations you can make about this interaction?

Answer: Showing interest allows you to tune in to a message. If you tune out the message because you are not interested, communication will not take place. From this interaction, you can observe that the caregiver and patient have a positive relationship, and that the patient is comfortable with him.

ACTIVITY

Make a poster depicting one element of effective communication, such as active listening, or one barrier to effective communication, such as talking too fast. Display the posters in the classroom or on a bulletin board.

Teaching Tips

- Review the three common styles of communication: assertive, passive, and aggressive.
- Emphasize the difference between assertive and aggressive.
- Discuss examples of all three. For example, ask students which style they might use if they are pulled over for speeding, which style they might use with a sibling, and which style they might use with a friend.
- Encourage students to use the following techniques for assertive behavior:
  - Use a level tone of voice.
  - Use strong "I" statements, which are direct and honest and do not attribute blame to the other person.
  - Repeat your assertion as often as necessary.
  - Find something on which you can agree with the other person.
  - Reach a workable compromise.

Apply It

- Before students begin, have them review good listening skills.
- Time their conversations and cue them when to switch speakers.
- Have students share the strategies they developed to improve their listening skills.

Apply It

- Remind students to consider the issues of cross-generational communication.
- Plan class time to let students discuss what they learned from the activity.

Apply It

With a partner have a conversation about career goals. Each of you should share your thoughts and ideas for two to three minutes. As you listen to your partner, observe your listening skills. Are you showing interest? Do you find yourself interrupting, or wanting to interrupt?

Take a few minutes to write down observations about your listening skills. Note any personal barriers to listening that you notice. Review the guidelines for good listening skills on this page and make a plan for how you can improve your listening skills.

Apply It

Role play with a classmate. You are a nurse and your classmate is an elderly patient who has a hearing impairment and has just been diagnosed with a treatable form of cancer. What steps can you take—verbal and/or nonverbal—to establish successful communication? How can you demonstrate care, empathy, and compassion?

Then, reverse roles. This time, your classmate is a medical assistant, and you are a teenager who is not a native English speaker and is trying to get information on his father who was rushed to the hospital after falling off a ladder. What steps might the health care professional take in this situation in order to communicate effectively?

Have classmates outline the positive and negative aspects of the communication. How could the situation have been improved? Also, discuss the emotion, tone, body language, and volume.

- **Hear the message.** Health care workers frequently think that they understand what is being said to them when sometimes they really do not. It is important to repeat what you believe you heard to be certain you heard correctly. It is not necessary to repeat exactly what was said, but check for understanding of the general message. Watch the speaker closely to observe actions that may contradict what the person is saying. Evaluate how well you listen and if you are using all of the above skills during and after each conversation with patients and health care team members.
- **Do not interrupt.** Have you ever tried to send a message and been frustrated by the receiver's interrupting you? Allow the sender to give you the entire message without interruptions. If you need to ask a question to clarify the meaning, be patient and wait until the sender is finished. She or he may give you the information you need without your questions.
- **Pay close attention.** This is critical. Eliminate distractions by moving to a quiet area for the conversations. Avoid thinking about how you are going to respond. Try to eliminate your own prejudices and see the other person's point of view.
- **Maintain a positive attitude.** Keep your temper under control, even if you become irritated.

Being a good listener takes patience. You need to concentrate on being a good listener until the skills become easy for you. As a health care worker, good listening is an essential skill. Good listening skills also help you follow directions, make good observations of patients, and understand your fellow workers.

Assertive Communication

Communicating assertively is an honest and direct way to say what you feel or think. Being assertive allows you to express your feelings and thoughts. You must believe you have the right to be heard and believed by others. You recognize that it is okay for you and for others to say no when it is appropriate. For example, when you are asked to perform a skill you are not trained to do, it is appropriate for you to refuse. You could then offer to assist as needed to accomplish a goal or task. This type of open, honest communication shows that you are a genuine person with self-respect and confidence. Assertiveness says that you have an awareness of and respect for others. To communicate strong health care values effectively, it is important for you to be an assertive communicator.

There are three common styles of communication:

- *Unassertive*, or *passive*, communication allows others to control the conversation or situation.
- *Assertive* communication does not take power or authority away from others. It empowers individuals to speak up and be heard.
- *Aggressive* communication occurs when power is taken away from others and communication breaks down.

190 Chapter 9 | Effective Communication

CUSTOMIZED INSTRUCTION

English Language Learners

Have students repeat the following sentence to a partner three times, with emphasis on the italicized word. Ask the team how emphasizing the different words in each sentence changes the meaning of what's been said.

- *I* did not tell Mr. Meyer you were late. (Emphasizing the word "I" implies that someone else told Mr. Meyer.)
- I did not tell *Mr. Meyer* you were late. (Emphasizing "Mr. Meyer" implies that you did not tell Mr. Meyer, but you may have told someone else.)
- I did *not* tell Mr. Meyer you were late. (Emphasizing "not" makes it clear that it did not happen.)

Most people communicate in all three of these styles, depending on their feelings or thoughts at the time. Health care workers are more effective when they use assertive communication skills. You can develop your skills over time.

Nonverbal Communication

Communication also takes place in nonverbal ways. It is not necessary to speak in order to send a message. You send messages with your eye contact, facial expressions, **gestures**, and touch.

gestures
(JES cherz)
Motions of a part of the body to express feelings or emotions (e.g., nodding yes or no).

- **Eye contact.** Making eye contact with the person with whom you are communicating is important. Eye contact lets others know that you are paying attention. When you do not make eye contact, you send others a message that you are not interested or that you wish to avoid them.
- **Facial expressions.** A smile sends a different message than a frown does. It is possible to say something very kind and still send a message of anger with your eyes. Try to think of an instance when you knew that what was being said was not what was meant. How did you know? The expression on the sender's face probably sent you a different message.
- **Gestures.** Shrugging your shoulders, turning your back, and leaving the room while someone is talking to you certainly convey a lack of interest in the sender's message. A message of disinterest has been sent through gestures.

Science Link

Communication Differences Between Men and Women

Studies have shown that, in general, men and women vary in the way they use nonverbal communication. Differences between men and women are found in their body movements, eye contact, and use of space.

Women tend to use facial expressions to express more emotion than men. They are more likely to smile and more likely to use facial and body expressions to show friendliness. In contrast, a man does not smile as much and is more likely to interrupt a person who is smiling. While women may show some friendly nonverbal cues, their posture tends to be more tense than men's posture. Men are more relaxed and more likely to use gestures.

While women do not often stare, men use staring to challenge power. This nonverbal cue for power is also seen when observing the behavior of a man during an initial gaze. Men will wait for the other person to turn away, while women are more likely to avert their eyes on initial gaze. Men also use staring to signal interest. Instead of staring, women signal interest by maintaining eye contact.

Investigate and describe the probability as to whether the differences in communication traits between men and women are due to genetic or environmental factors.

Create an in-class simulation with half the group participating in an interaction related to a health care process (patient-professional communication) and the other half making observations as to how the boys and girls in the class communicate.

How might these differences between men and women affect communication in the workplace?

Science Link—Communication Differences Between Men and Women

- Discuss the different communication techniques attributed to men and women.
- Ask the students if they agree, and then ask why, or why not.

How might these differences between men and women affect communication in the workplace?

Answer: This difference may cause more conflict or misunderstandings in the workplace. For example, a man may misinterpret the nonverbal message of a woman who stands close to him. In addition, a smiling woman may have a harder time getting a point across in a meeting without being interrupted.

TEAMWORK

In pairs, practice assertive communication. Have one team member take an aggressive role, such as an uncooperative patient, or a pushy supply sales representative. Have the other team member use assertive communication techniques. Switch roles.

Teaching Tips

- Explain—and demonstrate—types of nonverbal communication:
  - Eye contact
  - Facial expressions
  - Gestures
  - Touch
- Discuss messages sent by these nonverbal actions.
- For example, what is conveyed by taking someone's hand in your own? What is conveyed by rolling your eyes or chewing your fingernails?
- Be sure to reinforce nonverbal communication that makes a positive impression:
  - Standing or sitting up straight with your shoulders squared communicates confidence and attentiveness.
  - Folding your hands in your lap or leaving your arms at your sides indicates open-mindedness.
  - Maintaining eye contact shows you are interested and focused.
  - Smiling indicates confidence and agreement.

Teaching Tips

- Review the two types of verbal communication.
- Discuss the importance of conveying yourself clearly when speaking and writing.
- Explain to students that most employers are looking for job applicants who have some degree of writing skills. A recent survey of companies indicated that 90 percent of them always take writing into account when hiring for any position. Regardless of the job level, you must know how to document, report, and communicate in the written form.

Career Connect

- If possible, provide a list of health care professionals in the area who are willing to communicate with your students.
- Direct students to pay particular attention to the ways in which the health care professionals communicate with others.

Language Arts Link—Human Development and Aging

- You may want to direct students to use the section text as their primary source for this report.
- You may want to have students draft an outline or story web, to organize their ideas for the report.
- Review the purpose of a thesis statement. In this case, it should explain what the student believes is the importance of developing effective communication skills.
- If students will be using the Internet for additional research, remind them about your school's Internet policy.
- Emphasize that they should use reputable Web resources, such as sites sponsored by the government or educational institutions.
- Remind them to keep a list of sources to use for a bibliography, and so they can go back to the sites when they review their career plan in the future.
- Evaluate the document based on how well it addresses the thesis, organization, and spelling and grammar.

- **Touch.** Touch can convey great caring, warmth, concern, and tenderness. It can also convey anger, rejection, and distaste. Touch is a very important part of your communication. It is important that your nonverbal communication be supportive and positive.

Career Connect

What kind of a communicator are you? Do you like to talk? Are you shy? Do people consider you to be a "good" listener?

Interview a health care specialist in a field that appeals to you (for example, a pediatrician, a gerontologist, an insurance specialist). Ask if you can shadow them for a day. Is this the kind of environment in which you are comfortable? Observe effective communication techniques during your shadowing experience.

Verbal Communication

Verbal communication includes spoken and written messages.

- **Spoken messages.** When you speak to someone, you send a message. The tone of your voice, the language you use, and the message you send are interpreted by the receiver. Always speak clearly and concisely. This ensures that your message is understood.
- **Written messages.** You communicate frequently with the written word. You take messages and orders. You may write notes in the patient's/client's chart or enter them in documentation related to health science. You may also need to leave instruction of co-workers. It is important to spell correctly, use proper grammar, and write in a clear and concise manner.

Communicating with a patient can itself be part of the healing process. Therapeutic communication is a set of strategies for communicating with patients that can put them at ease and help them to recover faster by improving their emotional well-being. Some of these strategies include things like active listening, asking the patient questions to help them understand their own feelings and experiences, offering hope to patients that are in despair, and sometimes even sitting silently with a patient to help them feel less alone.

Language Arts Link

Human Development and Aging

Being able to communicate important information to a patient, the patient's family, a colleague, or your supervisor is an essential skill in any health care profession. Communication has many forms: written communication, oral communication, and nonverbal communication using body language.

Write a brief report on the importance of developing effective communication skills. Include the importance of the ability to express your ideas and directives clearly and persuasively. Convey clear and distinct information so the listener can follow what is being said. Consider when a word or phrase is important to comprehension when discussing health care directives, practices, procedures, or documentation. Considering the types of information that might be shared, detail why accurate and appropriate communication skills are essential to anyone who wishes to work in a health care profession.

Be sure to proofread your work to see if you can improve it by making it clearer, more concise, or more interesting to read. Check the spelling and grammar and correct any errors.

Exchange reports with a classmate. Provide feedback and corrections as necessary, and then exchange back. Read your classmate's comments and revise your report as necessary.

CUSTOMIZED INSTRUCTION

Less Advanced Students

Be sure to allow adequate time for less advanced students to complete the Language Arts Link activity. Try to pair less advanced students with average or more advanced students for the peer review.

ACTIVITY

Write a paragraph deliberately using incorrect grammar and spelling, or illegible handwriting. Swap papers with a classmate. Write your interpretation of your classmate's paragraph. Discuss whether you were able to correctly interpret the information.

Professionalism

Professional standards needed by health workers include a model of excellent care and service. Professionalism brings together **soft skills**: **work ethic**, character, relationships, teamwork, communication, honesty, **cultural competence**, personal image, personal health, and wellness.

Health care involves interactions with a variety of people. Etiquette in health care is more than good manners. It includes establishing respectable relationships with patients, colleagues, and supervisors. Health professionals set the tone for interaction with patients and visitors. Workers are assessed by the way they communicate and their body language and appearance.

Everyone from the receptionist to the physician must do their part to convey a sense of courtesy, caring, and helpfulness in a friendly and open way. Smiling and appropriate touch lets patients know they matter. Professionalism encompasses medical knowledge, personality, and the ability to understand patients and communicate concern.

San Diego, California-based medical marketing firm Sullivan Luallin Group created C.L.E.A.R. to provide health professionals with guidance on proper ways to deliver services. C.L.E.A.R. stands for connect, listen, explain, ask, and re-connect. Behaviors outlined are simple, but people do not always follow them because they are bogged down by the routine and repetition of their jobs.

C.L.E.A.R. Health Care Service Model[1]

Connect

- Acknowledge immediately
- Establish eye contact and smile
- Use the patient's name
- Use a friendly, helpful voice tone
- Say "please" and "thank you"

Listen

- Maintain eye contact
- Be relaxed
- Don't interrupt
- Use "active" listening techniques
- Repeat information for accuracy

soft skills
(soft skilz)
Cluster of personality traits—communication, language, personal habits, friendliness, and optimism—that characterize relationships with other people.

work ethic
(werk e-thik)
Values based on hard work and diligence.

cultural competence
(kulch-ral kam-pe-tens)
Ability to interact effectively with people of different cultures and socioeconomic backgrounds.

Apply It

Role-Plays: Working in groups, prepare a role-play of negative and unprofessional health worker behaviors. Other students should put themselves in the position of the patient/client who deserves to be treated with respect and professionally. At the end of each role-play, conduct a discussion of how the health workers might respond more appropriately.

1. Courtesy of Sullivan Luallin Group. Author: Darice Britt. See more at http://source.southuniversity.edu/healthcare-professionalism-how-important-is-proper-bedside-manner-132067.aspx.

Effective Communication | Chapter 9 193

Teaching Tips

- Review the components of professionalism:
  - Work ethic
  - Character
  - Relationships
  - Teamwork
  - Communication
  - Honesty
  - Cultural competence
  - Personal image
  - Personal health
  - Wellness
- Provide examples of the qualities and actions that demonstrate an employee's professionalism. These include:
  - Arriving early to meetings.
  - Using proper language and avoiding slang.
  - Stating your opinions confidently and speaking clearly.
  - Dressing in a professional manner.
  - Avoiding talk about personal matters.
- Introduce the C.L.E.A.R. service model and make sure students understand what each letter stands for.

Apply It

- Allow students class time to prepare their role-plays.
- Students should refer to the C.L.E.A.R. model in order to make suggestions on appropriate behavior.

Teaching Tips

- Continue your review of the C.L.E.A.R. service model.
- Ask students to suggest personal qualities that demonstrate their idea of professionalism. These might include integrity, courtesy, honesty, dependability, and responsibility.

Section 9.1 Review Questions

1. Answer: Communication can be through written or spoken words, gestures, facial expressions, body posture, touch, and listening.
2. Answer: Prejudices, frustrations (annoyance/impatience), and life experiences might influence relationships with others.
3. Answer: Barriers to communication include labeling, sensory impairment, talking too fast, and cognitive impairment.
4. Answer: The four elements are a message, a sender, a receiver, and feedback.
5. Answer: Good listening skills are important because if a message hasn't been received/understood, then communication has not taken place. Good listening skills also help you follow directions, make good observations of patients, and understand your fellow workers.
6. Answer: Assertive communication is an open, honest way to say what you think and feel. Assertive communication does not take power or authority away from others. It empowers individuals to speak up and be heard.

Explain

- Describe what's going to happen
- Answer questions with patience
- Let patients know about expected delays
- Speak slowly; repeat as necessary

Ask

- "Were all your questions answered?"
- "Is there anything else I can do…?"
- "Did you understand…"

Re-connect

- Check back frequently with waiting patients
- Direct patient where to go next
- End with a friendly parting comment

Evaluating Communication Skills

Good communication requires consistent evaluation of the communication methods—both verbal and nonverbal—to ensure healthy relationships with individuals throughout the lifespan. Take the opportunity to use these criteria the next time you communicate, particularly with people who are older, younger, or of a different ethnic background than you.

- Have I considered how this person's age and experience might affect their understanding?
- Have I given appropriate background on the topic?
- Am I aware of my nonverbal body language such as facial expressions and hand gestures?
- Have I solicited feedback in a way that will lead to a more fruitful discussion of the topic?

Summary

Communication requires a sender, a receiver, and a message. The message may be verbal or nonverbal, and many factors influence the effectiveness of communication. These factors include prejudices, frustrations, attitudes, and life experiences. Good listening skills are important to ensure successful communication, and an awareness of barriers to good communication is important.

Section 9.1 Review Questions

1. Identify three types of communication.
2. What elements might influence our relationships with others?
3. Name four barriers to communication.
4. List the four essential elements of communication.
5. Why are good listening skills so important?
6. What is assertive communication?

194 Chapter 9 | Effective Communication

Communication Technologies

SECTION 9.2

Background

Communication between health care providers is vital to patient care. Today's technology has helped to improve the efficiency and the speed at which a message or file can be sent to another person. A worker in the health care environment needs to know how to use common software programs in order to access and record important patient information. In addition, workers need to be well-trained to work with phones, fax machines, e-mail, and the Internet in order to complete daily tasks.

Objectives

When you have completed this section, you will be able to do the following:

- Match key terms with their correct meanings.
- Demonstrate responding, transferring a caller, and taking a message.
- Apply basic listening skills.
- Use communication technology such as a fax machine, e-mail, or Internet to access and distribute data and other information.

Apply It

Play telephone. Pair up with a partner. One should be a caller to a health care professional's office; the other should be the receptionist. See how the receptionist responds, no matter how the patient acts.

Is the patient angry or annoyed? Does the patient keep repeating his or her questions? Is the receptionist clear and understanding? Then, switch roles.

Telephone Communication

The telephone is an important communication tool between you and those you serve. All departments in the health care setting require good telephone communication skills. You may be asked to answer the telephone, take a message, or respond to a request. Always follow good communication standards when answering an incoming or placing an outgoing call. (**Figure 9.3**)

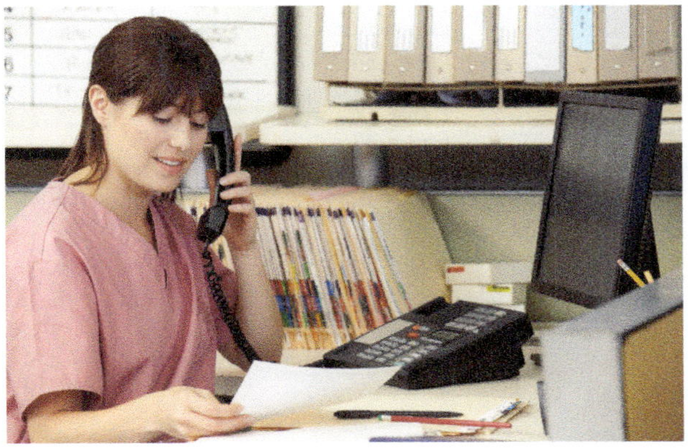

Figure 9.3
Medical professional scheduling an appointment over the phone. Why are telephone communication skills important in health care?

Effective Communication | Chapter 9 195

FOCUS AND ENGAGE

Introduce the Section

a. Review the content of the Background paragraph, emphasizing that technology has made communications for the health care professional more efficient.
b. Point out how important it is that that health care workers understand how to use the available communications technologies.
c. Review the objectives for the section.

Vocabulary Review

a. Key terms are defined in the margins of the text on the page where they first appear.
b. Pronounce each word, and have the students repeat the pronunciation out loud.
c. Discuss the definition of each word.

TEACH

Discuss

- Ask students if they have ever encountered an annoying or frustrating phone call.
- Discuss how the lack of nonverbal communication cues, such as tone and facial expressive might impact telephone, fax, and e-mail correspondence.

Reinforce and Review

- Review the guidelines and techniques of effective communication.
- Reinforce the role of verbal communication in a health care environment.

Teaching Tips

- Introduce the topic of telephone communication.

Apply It

- You may want to assign specific roles for the activity.
- For example, the caller might be a parent calling about a sick child, or someone who recently received a diagnosis that requires surgery.
- The receptionist might be having a bad day, or might be new.
- Plan class time to discuss the activity.

Figure Focus

9.3 Medical professional scheduling an appointment over the phone. Why are telephone communication skills important in health care?

Answer: Telephone communication skills are important in health care because you use the telephone to communicate with patients as well as with co-workers, supervisors, and other health care professionals.

Teaching Tips

- Review the guidelines for taking incoming calls.
- Discuss the information that should always be included when taking a message for someone else.
- Emphasize that if telephones are in public areas, it is important to take measures to ensure confidentiality is not broken.
- Emphasize the risks of making personal calls while at work; it can lead to reprimands or loss of job.
- Review Table 9.1 together as a class.
- Discuss the behaviors associated with each communication objective.
- Point out that the communication objectives are aspects of effective communication.
- Compare the appropriate and inappropriate words and phrases.

pertinent
(PUR tn uh nt)
Relating directly to the matter at hand; relevant.

etiquette
(ek-i-kit)
Rules of acceptable social behaviors.

Telephones at workstations are for communication of health care issues **pertinent** to those you serve. Personal calls and socializing must be done on your break or outside of your assignment or work time. See **Table 9.1** for indicators that promote patient/client satisfaction when talking on the telephone and **Table 9.2** for telephone guidelines.

Table 9.1 Indicators That Promote Patient/Client Satisfaction When Talking on the Telephone

Communication Objective	Service/Excellence	Behavior
■ Demonstrate open, honest, and respectful communication. ■ Present ideas, information, and viewpoints clearly both verbally and in writing. ■ Listen actively and seek to understand others.	■ Use good telephone **etiquette**. ■ If the doctor asks you to screen calls at an office or clinic, answer the phone and identify the caller, or use caller ID. Politely notify the caller that the doctor is unable to speak at the moment. Then, offer to take a message so the doctor can return the call.	■ Answer the telephone cheerfully. ■ Use a pleasant, caring, and sincere tone of voice. ■ Answer the telephone on the first ring if possible. ■ Speak clearly and courteously. ■ Remember to thank the caller when a call is returned. ■ Identify yourself and give your title (e.g., "This is Monica, nurse assistant."). ■ Identify your department or doctor's office (e.g., "Dr. Smith's office"). ■ Thank the caller for calling. ■ Allow the caller to hang up first to ensure that the caller has said everything he or she wanted to say. ■ Use appropriate words and phrases. **Appropriate:** • May I have your name, please? • Would you repeat that, please? • How may I assist you? • I'm sorry; I didn't understand. **Inappropriate:** • What's your name? • What did you say? • What do you want? • Huh?

196 Chapter 9 | Effective Communication

CUSTOMIZED INSTRUCTION

Special Needs Students

If students have speech impairments, you may want to emphasize alternatives to telephones, such as fax machines, e-mail, and text messaging.

Table 9.2 Telephone Guidelines

Being Prepared	Placing a Caller on Hold	Transferring a Caller
■ Have the necessary materials: • Pencil • Message pad • Telephone • Facility and public telephone directory ■ Before placing a call: • Prepare questions to ask. • Gather information to share with the person you are calling. • Determine appropriate action to take. ■ Follow the patient/client satisfaction indicators in Table 9.1.	■ Ask the caller if he or she can hold and wait for the response. ■ Check every 30 seconds to see if the caller wants to continue to hold. ■ Ask if you may take a message. ■ Transfer the call as soon as possible. ■ Follow the patient/client satisfaction indicators in Table 9.1.	■ Explain where you are transferring the caller and to whom. ■ Give the caller the number you are transferring to. ■ If possible, stay on the telephone and introduce the caller to the person receiving the call. ■ Follow the patient/client satisfaction indicators in Table 9.1.

Writing a Message	Leaving a Message
■ Record time and date. ■ Write clearly: • The caller's name—verify spelling. • The telephone number—read back the number. ■ Summarize information with the caller by repeating the message. ■ Sign or initial the message. ■ Record the action you take to deliver the message. ■ Follow the patient/client satisfaction indicators in Table 9.1.	■ State: • Whom you are calling for. • Your name and where you are calling from. • Your message— remembering to follow confidentiality guidelines. • The times that you will be available for a return call. ■ Document date, time, and message left. ■ Follow the patient/client satisfaction indicators in Table 9.1.

Fax Communication

If a health care employee needs to send a patient's record to another provider, the worker may use a **facsimile** or **fax machine**. A fax transmission is a way to send or receive printed pages or images over telephone lines by converting them to and from electronic signals. You may work on a computer, or have access to a printer, that is connected to a phone line so that you can send and receive faxes directly from your computer or printer. In order to send a fax, you must have a telephone number used for faxes by the person to whom you want to send the documents. There are a few things you should remember when sending a fax:

- Use a **cover page**. A cover page is the first page of a fax that gives the receiver important information about the fax. It should include your name, contact number, number of pages being sent, the name of the recipient, and any other important information.
- Confirm that the intended **recipient** received the fax. Since a fax often contains important patient information, call or e-mail the recipient to ensure that he or she has received it.

facsimile/fax machine
(faks muh SHEEN)
A device that sends and receives printed pages or images as electronic signals over telephone lines.

cover page
(KUHV er peyj)
The first page of a fax.

recipient
(ri SIP ee uhnt)
A person or thing that receives.

Effective Communication | Chapter 9 197

Teaching Tips

- Review Table 9.2 together as a class.
- Instruct students to read the table column by column, not row by row.
- Point out the importance of having a writing utensil and paper on hand when on the phone, even when you are the one making the call.
- Discuss "talking points" and why it is a good idea to write down questions or topics you will need to discuss before making a call.
- Ask students to share personal stories of successful or frustrating phone calls.
- For example, they may have been placed on hold for a long time, or transferred to the wrong person. They may have had trouble communicating with someone who spoke a different language.
- Introduce the topic of fax communication.
- Students may be unfamiliar with a fax machine. It may help to have one on hand to use to demonstrate the process.
- Compare a fax machine to a copy machine, explaining that the copy is received at the remote location.
- Display a sample cover page, and review the information that should be included on a cover page.

ACTIVITY

Create and fill out a fax cover sheet for sending a document. You may use a software program, such as Microsoft Word, which includes templates for fax cover sheets, or design and create one by hand.

TEAMWORK

Divide the class into groups of three. One person will be a caller, one will be a receiver, and one will be an evaluator. The caller and receiver should act out a telephone call scenario, while the evaluator determines whether the call is positive or negative. Switch roles so that each student has the opportunity to act as a caller, receiver, and evaluator. Discuss factors that made a call positive or negative.

Teaching Tips

- Introduce the topic of e-mail communication. Most students will be familiar with e-mail.
- Review the guidelines for creating professional e-mail messages.
- Discuss the difference between the shorthand they may be accustomed to using when communicating with friends, and the appropriate language for professional correspondence.
- Emphasize the importance of proofreading messages before sending them, both to check for errors, but also to make sure they convey the information as intended.

Figure Focus

9.4 Health care professional working online. What are the advantages of health care workers using the Internet and e-mail?

Answer: Using the Internet makes it possible for health care workers to access information from a wide range of sources. They can conduct research, and access patient information. Using e-mail provides an additional methods of communicating with patients and co-workers.

- Remember that you may be dealing with confidential information. If you are sending confidential or potentially sensitive information, call ahead and let the recipient know to be ready. Using an online fax may help avoid security issues, as it lets users send and receive faxes from the privacy of their own computers.

E-Mail Communication

E-mail is an important method of communication in the health care business. However, health workers sending e-mails should choose their words carefully. A person cannot hear vocal inflections in an e-mail; therefore, sarcasm and humor should not be used in a business e-mail because they may lead to miscommunication or misunderstandings.

Remember that any message you send is permanent and may be forwarded to others. Do not use a business e-mail address to send trivial or highly sensitive information.

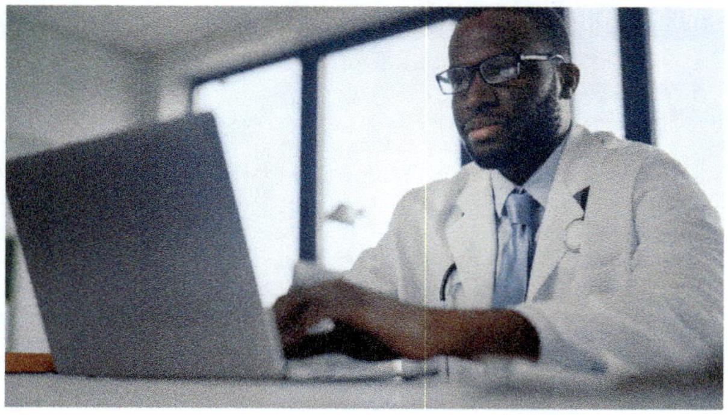

Figure 9.4
Health care professional working online. What are the advantages of health care workers using the Internet and e-mail?

Before you hit send, follow these guidelines to write a professional e-mail:

- Begin with a salutation.
- Include short, simple, and straightforward information. If a message is long, discuss the topic in a short e-mail, and use an **attachment** to provide details. An attachment is a file linked to an e-mail message. You may also break up a longer e-mail that has many topics into multiple, shorter e-mails that discuss each topic separately.
- Read your e-mail aloud to check the tone of your message. Using please and thank you with requests ensures a polite tone.
- Proof the content for spelling and grammar mistakes. Remember that you should use upper and lower case when writing.

attachment
(uh TACH muhnt)
A file linked to an e-mail message.

- Remember to include important contact information at the end of your e-mail. This includes your name, position, company, telephone number, e-mail address, and perhaps fax number.
- Include a subject on the subject line of the e-mail.
- Use features such as **blind carbon copy** and **carbon copy** when appropriate. Carbon copy (Cc) is used to send a copy of your e-mail to another recipient. For example, you may send an e-mail to a patient, but carbon copy a doctor on the e-mail so that he or she knows what was sent to the patient. Blind carbon copy (Bcc) is used when an e-mail is sent to multiple people. Blind carbon copy allows a recipient to read the message; however, the recipient cannot see the other e-mail addresses to which the message was sent. This is beneficial because it protects the recipients' e-mail addresses and eliminates clutter in the e-mail.

Respond to incoming e-mails within 24 hours. If you need more time to respond, call or e-mail that you are looking into the matter and will get back to the person as soon as possible. Also be sure to answer all questions when responding to an e-mail. When sending an e-mail with questions, allow one or two days for a response. If you need an immediate response, you may want to call the person.

In health care, **memorandums** (memos) are used as reminders, to persuade an action, to issue a directive or to provide a report. Memorandums can be delivered via e-mail. When sending a memorandum via e-mail, be sure to:

- Confirm the memorandum looks as intended in print and on the screen.
- Use fonts/graphics that are clear on all recipients' computers.
- Ensure attachments are readable by all recipients.

The Internet

Many health care positions may require a worker to find or access information online. (Figure 9.5) In order to gain access, employees usually need to have a **username**. Usernames are names used to gain access to a computer system.

Once on the computer, employees may research and access information on the **Internet**. The Internet is a worldwide computer network that provides information on many subjects. When researching information, it is important to choose a **Web site** that is **credible**. Not every medical Web site is supported by research or written by experts in the medical field. Some examples of credible sources on the Internet include organizations such as the

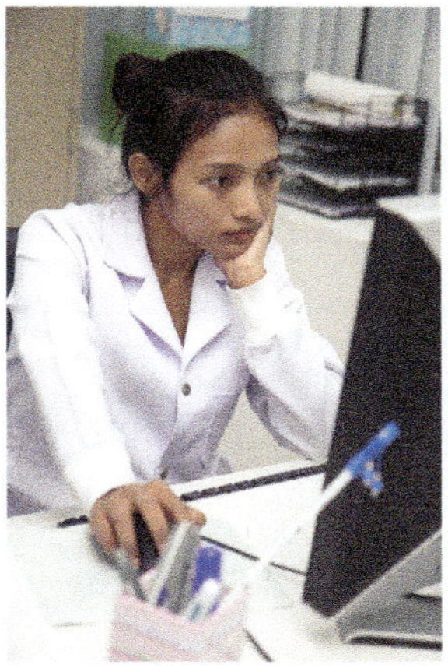

blind carbon copy
(blahynd KAHR buhn KOP ee)
An e-mail feature that allows a person to send an e-mail to multiple people without them seeing the other receivers' e-mail addresses.

carbon copy
(KAHR buhn KOP ee)
An e-mail feature that allows a person to send a copy of an e-mail to another person.

memorandum
(mem e RAN dum)
A short note written to help a person remember something or to remind a person to do something.

username
(YOO zer naym)
A unique identifier composed of alphanumeric characters, used as a means of initial identification to gain access to a computer system or Internet Service Provider.

Figure 9.5
Many health care workers may use the Internet to find information quickly. What should you remember when searching for information on the Internet? What is the function of a Web browsers?

Internet
(IN ter net)
A worldwide computer network with information on many subjects.

Web site
(WEB sahyt)
A group of pages on the Internet developed by a person or organization about a topic.

Teaching Tips

- Review the etiquette of responding to e-mail.
- Discuss memorandums. If possible, display a sample memo.
- Explain that the recipient may want to print the memo, or other message, to keep on file as a record.
- Introduce the topic of the Internet.
- Discuss the risks of assuming all information on the Internet is reliable and factual.
- Point out that one way to determine if information found online is factual is to find the same information at multiple, unrelated sites. It helps if at least one of the sites is known to be credible.
- If you cannot locate the information at multiple sites, you should assume it is unsubstantiated.
- Remind students that they should never use information they find on the Internet in a report or presentation without attributing it to its source.
- If you have Internet access in the classroom, show students examples of credible Web sites, such as redcross.org, or a site associated with a local health care facility.

Figure Focus

9.5 Many health care workers may use the Internet to find information quickly. What should you remember when searching for information on the Internet? What is the function of a Web browser?

Answer: Choose Web sites that are credible and reliable. These may include sites sponsored by organizations, the government, or educational institutions. Remember that not all information online is true or accurate. A Web browser is software designed for locating and viewing information stored on the Web.

ACTIVITY

Select a health-related question. Find at least three credible Web sites that provide the same answer to the question. Record the name and address of each site.

Teaching Tips

- Display and discuss your school's Internet policy.
- Review the type of content that might be considered inappropriate for viewing or sharing in a professional environment.
- Emphasize that information posted online in any forum—including blogs or social networking profiles—should be considered public. Students should never post information they would not want employers to see.
- Explain that employers often implement e-mail and Internet policies for the following reasons:
  - Lower productivity that often results from employees who do personal Web surfing, shopping, blogging, texting, etc., on company time.
  - The loss of confidential information; for example, sensitive data about the organization's internal operations appearing on a social networking page.
  - The increased vulnerability to viruses from employees who are careless about e-mailing and downloads.

Career-Ready Practices

- Students are to research the benefits of using electronic communications and Internet technology to provide care to patients.
- Students may use information from the section text or gather information from other resources.
- Make sure their posters illustrate at least five benefits.
- This activity gives students real-world experience in applying the following Career-Ready Practice: Use Technology to Enhance Productivity.
- For more information on the Career-Ready Practices, visit careertech.org/career-ready-practices.

credible
(KRED uh buhl)
Worthy of belief or confidence; trustworthy.

reliable
(ri LAHY uh buhl)
Dependable, accurate, honest.

Career-Ready Practices

Electronic communications and Internet technology have drastically changed the way patients seek health care services and the way they are delivered. Career-ready individuals recognize how new and existing technologies can improve productivity and enhance the overall patient/client experience. It can help them complete tasks more efficiently and solve workplace problems.

Research the benefits of caring for patients electronically. These might include the "self-documenting" of e-mail correspondence as opposed to unrecorded telephone calls and face-to-face conversations; fewer disruptive telphone calls and unnecessary office visits; and decreased costs for both the caregiver and the patient. Create a poster that illustrates at least five benefits. Present it to your class.

Community

Work with students in the local middle school or junior high school computer classes. Create a poster that lists the dos and don'ts of safe online communication—how to act in blogs, chat rooms, or sites such as Facebook, Instagram, Twitter, etc. Participate in a discussion, outlining different uses of the Internet for students.

American Cancer Society or the Leukemia and Lymphoma Society. Web sites sponsored by the government such as the Food and Drug Administration Web site are also **reliable**. Educational institutions such as John Hopkin's University are also quality sources.

A domain name is used as an Internet address to identify the location of a particular Web page. For example, the URL for the American Cancer Society is *www.cancer.org*. The domain name is *cancer*.

In addition, some health care providers create Web sites that provide important information to patients. These Web sites may include directions to the facility, office hours, contact phone numbers and e-mail addresses, as well as other helpful information.

A Web browser is software designed for locating and viewing information stored on the Web. Although their look is different, most Web browsers, including the popular Mozilla Firefox, Google Chrome, and Microsoft Internet Explorer, share some common features, such as Navigation Buttons, Address Box, and Favorites or Bookmarks.

E-Mail and Internet Policies

With the current use of technology in the workplace, most companies have policies regarding use of the Internet and e-mail for personal business while at work. Employees may be required to read and sign a company's policy concerning Internet and e-mail use.

While some companies allow employees to use the Internet and e-mail for personal use on a limited basis, companies' policies prohibit employees from sending disruptive or offensive e-mail. This may include forwarding jokes or pictures that have been e-mailed to an employee.

In addition, employees may not access Web sites that contain pornographic material or discriminatory messages. E-mail and Internet access should always be used in a manner that is accurate, appropriate, ethical, and lawful.

In order to ensure that workers are following these policies, many companies monitor their employees' e-mail and Internet use. Computer programs today help companies identify e-mails or Web site visits that may be inappropriate. Employees should always remember that any e-mail or file on a company computer is not confidential and may be read by someone in a company's technology department or a manager.

If an employee notices a violation of a company's policy, the company usually asks the employee to notify a supervisor. Often a company policy explains that a violation will result in disciplinary action and may even cause a person to lose his or her job.

200 Chapter 9 | Effective Communication

Community

- Students are to work with middle school/junior high school students to create a poster on the dos and don'ts of online communication.
- This activity might also apply to elementary schools in your area.

CUSTOMIZED INSTRUCTION

More Advanced Students

Challenge more advanced students to write an Internet Usage Policy document for a health care facility. Encourage them to look up a few different policies online, or by contacting local facilities. Then, they can select a type of health care facility, and write a new, thorough policy.

What's New?

Electronics and Health Care

Today's cell phones cause much less interference and modern medical equipment is better shielded. However, the most recent guidance still warns against their use in critical or intensive care units, stating that they could interfere with dialysis machines, defibrillators, ventilators, and monitors. So, with the exception of holding phones next to critical care equipment, there is no convincing evidence for blanket bans on the grounds of electromagnetic interference. But, there might be other reasons why phones are not so desirable in health facilities. Phones are hard to clean. On top of the hygiene problems, there are issues of privacy. Most phones come complete with cameras and sometimes people just can't resist taking pictures. The *LA Times* reported that staff at one hospital even took photos of a 60-year-old man dying from multiple stab wounds and put them up on Facebook. In that case, perhaps phones in health facilities need some monitoring.

Despite the minor problems associated with using cell phones in health care environments, advancing technologies offer beneficial uses for cell phones in regard to health care, such as allowing doctors and health workers to respond faster to emergencies. Twitter, a Web site that offers social networking and microblogging services, enables doctors and other medical personnel to send and receive tweets—text-based posts of up to 140 characters—about health care issues and questions. Health care apps—applications that may be accessed on cell phones—are available, as well. You should keep in mind that patients and clients are finding access to health care information via these technological sources. Remind them that, like medical information they find on the Internet, health care information they receive in a tweet or with an app should be discussed in greater depth with their doctors.

Summary

The telephone, e-mail, fax, and the Internet are four ways that technology helps health care workers send and receive information. Not only do you need to know how to work the technology, you also need to know proper etiquette when using it. In all instances, a health care employee should use technology professionally and responsibly. Telephones are helpful for a more immediate contact with another employee or patient. E-mail and fax machines can be used to send documents. The Internet can help health care worker find information on a topic or allow health care workers to present important information to their patients.

Section 9.2 Review Questions

1. What are two ways you can promote patient/client satisfaction when talking on the phone?
2. Name three guidelines when writing a telephone message.
3. What should you do if you have to send confidential or sensitive information in a fax?
4. Why should you avoid sarcasm and humor in an e-mail?
5. How is the Internet a useful tool in the health care field?
6. Why would you use blind carbon copy (Bcc) rather than carbon copy (Cc) on an e-mail?

Effective Communication | Chapter 9 201

What's New?— Electronics and Health Care

- Discuss why cell phones cause problems in medical facilities.
- Ask students to role-play telling a member of a patient's family to turn off his or her phone.
- Emphasize that information posted via any type of social-networking or microblogging services should be evaluated carefully before passing it along to others.
- Health care apps provide quick and easy access to medical information that might help a patient make a decision to seek medical attention. However, discuss how information received through an app should be discussed with a doctor.

Section 9.2 Review Questions

1. Answer: Answers will vary but could include answer the telephone cheerfully, use a pleasant and clear tone, speak clearly and courteously, thank the caller when a call is returned, identify your department or doctor's office, and identify yourself by name and title.
2. Answer: Record time and date, write clearly (the caller's name, telephone number), summarize information with the caller by repeating the message, sign or initial the message, and record the action you take to deliver the message.
3. Answer: If you are sending confidential or potentially sensitive information, call ahead and let the recipient know to be ready. Using an online fax service may help avoid security issues, as it lets users send and receive faxes from the privacy of their own computers.
4. Answer: A person cannot hear vocal inflections in an e-mail and the use of sarcasm or humor may lead to miscommunication.
5. Answer: The Internet is a useful tool in the health care field because it provides information on many subjects and some health care workers create Web sites that contain information for patients (directions, hours, contact information).
6. Answer: Blind carbon copy allows a recipient to read the message but the recipient cannot see the other e-mail addresses to which the message was sent. This is beneficial because it protects the recipients' e-mail addresses and eliminates clutter in the e-mail.

FOCUS AND ENGAGE

Introduce the Section

a. Review the content of the Background paragraph, pointing out that computers are tools to help health care professional work with information.

b. Emphasize that computer technology allows workers to communicate with each other by sharing information.

c. Point out that knowing how to use computers makes a person more employable.

d. Review the objectives for the section.

Vocabulary Review

a. Key terms are defined in the margins of the text on the page where they first appear.

b. Pronounce each word, and have the students repeat the pronunciation out loud.

c. Discuss the definition of each word.

TEACH

Discuss

- Discuss the ways computers make work easier and more efficient.
- For example, a word processing program makes it easier to write and rewrite a letter or report, a database program makes it possible to save accurate records, and a calendar program simplifies scheduling.

Teaching Tips

- Start by asking students how much experience they have using computers. Almost all students will have experience, but some may have more than others.

SECTION 9.3 Computers in Health Care

Background

Computers are essential in health care. Health care agencies use computers in most departments to help save time and improve accuracy. They are used for record keeping, diagnostic tests, education, research, treatment, patient monitoring, and many other tasks. Health care workers must have a basic understanding of how computers work and how they are used in health care in order to communicate effectively and be employable.

Objectives

When you have completed this section, you will be able to do the following:

- Match key terms with their correct meanings.
- List and explain how computerized diagnostic tests help diagnose disease or illness.
- State how environmental services use computers.
- Describe ways that information services use computers.
- Discuss ethics and confidentiality as they relate to computers.

Computers in General

During the past 50 years, computer technology has grown and changed at an unbelievable rate. The early computers were made of vacuum tubes and required large, environmentally controlled rooms. They often overheated and became inoperable for many hours. Repairing them was time consuming. Large systems were very expensive, and only the largest organizations were able to afford them. Today's computer technology allows computers to be smaller, more powerful, and less expensive. Computer equipment that is used today is the result of a development process. Models and devices continue to change frequently as new technology becomes usable and marketable.

Basic Computer Components and Functions

Computers have basic components and functions that you need to learn about in order to understand computer terminology. All computers allow users to input information, process information, and provide ways to output information.

Inputting

input
(IN poot)
To enter data into a computer for processing.

The most common device used to **input** data into a computer is a keyboard. In addition to alphanumeric keys, a keyboard has function keys, punctuation keys, arrow keys, and conjunction keys. Function keys have different purposes, depending on the software that is running on the computer. Arrow keys, along with a mouse, can be used to move the cursor around on the computer screen so

202 Chapter 9 | Effective Communication

- Explain that as computers advance technologically, they become smaller and smaller. Early computers filled entire rooms. Now, people carry the same amount of information in a handheld device.
- Point out that in the past, it was necessary to cut into a patient to see internally, but now computers offer noninvasive technologies.

CUSTOMIZED INSTRUCTION

More Advanced Students

Provide the opportunity for students that are extremely proficient with computers to share their experience with the class. For example, you might ask them to give a demonstration or presentation about computers in general.

you can control where you input information. Conjunction keys are used in combinations that are specific to the software that is running. For example, in some programs, when the Alt key is pressed in conjunction with the Shift key and the letter t, the current time is entered.

With advances in mobile-device technology, touch screens are becoming a frequently used data input method. Touch screens, or touch pads, are common inputting devices for tablet or handheld computers. They are also used on computers in places where many people can access information, such as at a kiosk that gives directions in a medical facility. Uses for touch-screen technology in health care are growing. For example, touch screens have been developed that allow cancer patients to accurately show where their pain is and how bad the pain is at times when they may have trouble communicating with their caregivers.

For some types of computer systems used in health care facilities, tablet computers that require a stylus for inputting data may be used. (**Figure 9.6**) A stylus looks like a pen or pencil, but using it on a tablet computer that is designed for this type of inputting allows a user to write information that can be digitally interpreted and stored. For example, some hospitals and medical offices may have patients enter their personal information directly into tablet computers; the information is digitally input into the computer system and does not need to be transcribed by a person in order to be added to the patient's medical record.

Other input devices include external hard-disk drives, CD-ROMs, DVD-ROMs, USB flash drives, and optical drives. These devices are used for both inputting and storing data, or information.

File hosting services such as iCloud and Dropbox offer cloud storage for documents, apps, notes, contacts, etc., that can be accessed on whatever computer and most devices a health worker may be using. This allows information to be easily shared and accessed.

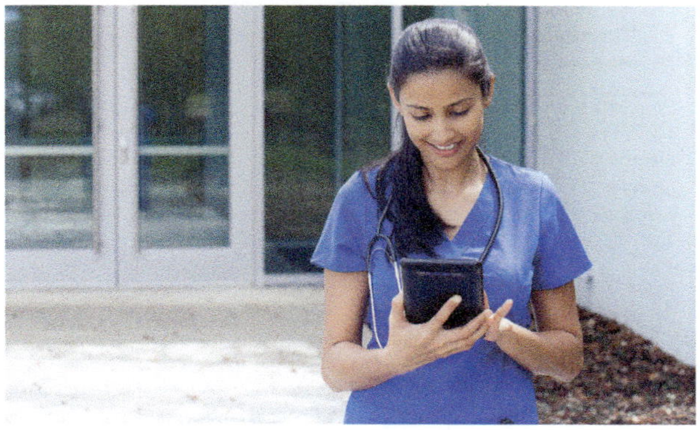

Figure 9.6
Tablets are being used more and more in health care settings. What are some advantages? What are some disadvantages of using a tablet?

Effective Communication | Chapter 9 203

Figure Focus

9.6 Tablets are being used more and more in health care settings. What are some advantages? What are some disadvantages of using a tablet?

Answer: Tablets are small and portable. This is an advantage in that health care workers can always have the tablet with them. This can also be a disadvantage, because tablets can be misplaced or stolen. Students may have other answers.

Teaching Tips

- If possible, display the basic computer components, and demonstrate their usage. If you do not have a computer system in the classroom, provide a handout, or display an image.
- For inputting, display how to use the keyboard and/or mouse.
- If possible, demonstrate touch-screen technology; if not, discuss experiences students have had with touch screens, such as with ATM machines.
- Point out the special keys such as ENTER and ESC.
- Display or describe tablet computers, and discuss why they are beneficial in health care settings.
- Demonstrate inputting by performing a basic calculation in a spreadsheet program, or keying a paragraph in a word processing program.
- Print a page to demonstrate output.

ACTIVITY

Draw a picture of a basic computer system. Label each component, and describe its function.

Teaching Tips

- Emphasize the vast amount of information that is required by health care workers.
- Review the procedures for which computers are frequently used in a health care facility.
- Point out that many systems are linked so that workers can share information. Discuss electronic health record software. For example, a physician in an emergency room might enter an order for a diagnostic test into a computer system. A technician in the radiology department then receives the order.
- Discuss how this type of process helps eliminate errors.
- Discuss collaborative, or groupware applications such as databases and electronic charting applications. Point out that, as their description implies, these types of groupware applications facilitate group work.
- Review the benefits of keeping electronic records. For example, records can be easily accessed by necessary personnel, they can easily be transferred from one office to another, they help eliminate errors, they take up less space than paper records, etc.
- Discuss potential drawbacks, such as unauthorized access to patient records.
- Discuss basic transferrable computer skills. These include:
    - Turn a computer on and start a program.
    - Type on a computer keyboard without making many mistakes.
    - Access the Internet and move from one Web site to another.
    - Use a search engine to do basic Internet research.
    - Write and send e-mail.

Processing

A computer processes the information that is input and returns the information to the person who input it or to someone in another department. The **central processing unit** (CPU) is the working unit of the computer. The CPU consists of many electronic components and microchips. The CPU can process only the information it receives; if it receives incorrect information, it processes incorrect information. This is where the phrase "Garbage in, garbage out" comes from. You must be accurate when you enter information.

central processing unit
(SEN truhl pros es ing yoo nit)
The part of a computer that interprets and carries out instructions.

output
(OUT poot)
To produce information; turn out.

Outputting

Just as there is more than one device for inputting information into a computer, there are several devices for outputting. The two most common items used to **output** are the monitor and the printer. The health care worker uses both.

Monitor

The monitor, or display screen, of a computer allows a user to see what is happening. The computer monitor is a screen that displays peripheral output to the user.

Printer

A printer is used to print the processed information on paper. Information printed on paper is called *hard copy* and can be filed with the patient's records. In most work environments, you will use the same printer as a group of your co-workers. Output can also be stored or transferred to external hard drives, or other input devices.

Use of Computers

Computers are processors of information. They process large amounts of information at incredible speeds, accurately, and consistently. Computers are used to communicate standards of care and to guide the practitioners in making patient care decisions.

System Policies, Procedures, and Regulations

As computers and technology are used in health care, it is critical to remember that policies and procedures for their use are established by health care facilities, accreditation agencies, and government entities. Regulations regarding the use of technology are established to protect patient confidentiality and maintain standards of care, as well as providing methods to analyze patient care data, all of which help to improve the quality of care. All health care providers and employees must follow these policies and procedures so that there are no breaches of security and privacy.

Wherever your career path in the health field takes you, you will do a portion of your work on a computer. Hospitals and medical and dental offices are converting their methods of keeping medical records, as well as accounting and purchasing functions, to storage and processes that use computers. Some health care agencies have computer diagnostic services where a complete physical examination is analyzed by a computer.

In the hospital, a computer performs many functions. The following are some of the procedures computers assist with:

- Recording physicians' notes and orders
- Creating a nursing treatment/work sheet based on physician orders and updating automatically with each additional physician order
- Creating templates for interventional protocols
- Charting at bedside

204 Chapter 9 | Effective Communication

- Patient monitoring (Figure 9.7)
- Ordering or changing diets
- Ordering unit supplies
- Ordering medications and therapies
- Processing charges for nursing care equipment
- Ordering lab work and receiving lab results
- Recording lab results for patient records
- Scheduling x-rays, special tests, and surgeries
- Processing discharges
- Performing diagnostic testing
- Medical billing
- Emergency dispatch
- Researching via the Internet

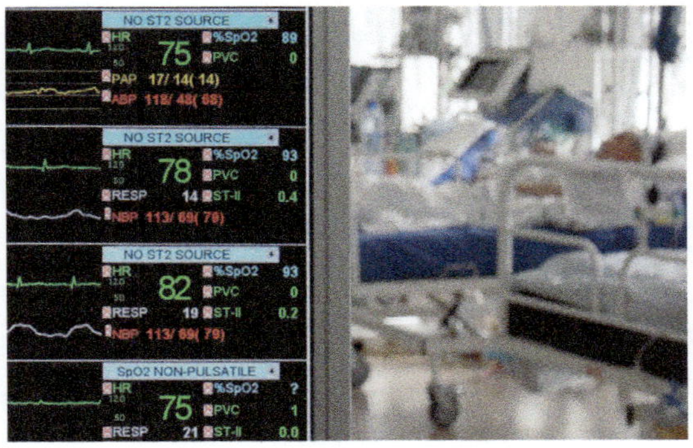

Figure 9.7
Computers help monitor a patient's vital signs.

In medical and dental offices, computers can be used to schedule appointments, set up a recall system, bill patients, schedule lab work, dial the telephone, manage the security system, and keep the inventory. Computers are an important part of the search for correct specific patient/client data that meets the **HEDIS** requirements. HEDIS is a tool used by more than 90 percent of America's health plans to measure performance on important dimensions of care and service. Electronic medical records are a necessary method of monitoring patient/client progress and quality health care; they provide data that allows physicians to provide timely disease management.

HEDIS
Healthcare Effectiveness Data and Information Set; an organization that provides quality care guidelines.

The key benefit to electronic medical record systems is that they make information available to multiple staff at locations hundreds of miles apart at the same time. This also increases flexibility for medical professionals. Web services also play a role in providing data; for example, laboratory results are immediately sent to a Web site, allowing physicians or other professionals to access them. Medical professionals can access complete patient/client data that previously was available only in the paper medical record. Pharmacists can put notes in the system regarding drug interactions. There are medical environments that have a separate department dedicated to the development and use of software specific to their clients. These systems often support research and product development. Not all medical environments have the funds and training available to implement electronic medical data systems; however, the systems will gradually become more affordable and therefore more accessible over time.

An electronic medical record (EMR) is a digital version of a paper chart that contains a patient's **demographics**, medical history, and clinical data from one practice or one provider's office. Electronic health records (EHRs) go beyond the data collected in the provider's office and include a more comprehensive patient history. EHRs are designed to contain and share information from all providers involved in a patient's care. EHR data can be created, managed, and consulted

demographics
(dem uh GRAF iks)
Information in a patient's record that includes such data as age, sex, address, education, family, and other such social or vital information.

Effective Communication | Chapter 9 205

Figure Focus

9.7 Computers help monitor a patient's vital signs.

Point out how computers can store information more efficiently and can record even more details than a person can observe.

Reinforce and Review

- Note that HEDIS was introduced and discussed in Section 2.2 of Chapter 2.
- Under the direction of the National Committee for Quality Assurance (NCQA), the Healthcare Effectiveness Data and Information Set (HEDIS) was developed to establish guidelines on the quality of health care given in this country.
- HEDIS is a tool used by more than 90 percent of the country's health plans to:
  - Measure health plan performance
  - Identify physicians and other providers who give high-quality medical care to their patients/clients
  - Identify physicians and other providers who do not meet the quality care guidelines

ACTIVITY

Ask students to list all their technology skills and experience on paper. For example, they might be experienced in online research, using a word processing program, creating and working with computer graphics and video, and working with digital photographs.

You might encourage them to also consider the skills they have obtained from using video games, computer simulations, and social networking sites. For example:

- Video games provide opportunities to use critical-thinking skills, such as decision making, problem solving, and conflict management. They also require students to understand and follow rules and to devise strategies for achieving goals.
- Computer simulations challenge students to recreate a modeled or modified version of a real-world situation or scenario. Students exercise creativity and also use problem-solving and decision-making skills.
- Social networking sites engage students in topics of conversation with others who have the same interests. They can also help them expand their network of career contacts.

Have students exchange their lists with a partner. They should review their partner's list and then write a paragraph explaining how their partner's skills and experience would be useful on the job.

Teaching Tips

- Review the ways computers are used in therapeutic services.
- For example, discuss inventory systems related to health care and databases of information, such as drugs, symptoms, and diseases. Also, discuss monitors and other machinery.
- Review the ways computers are used in diagnostic services.
- Explain that invasive procedures were common diagnostic tools before computerized diagnostics were available.

APPLY IT

- Encourage students to think about how computers can improve effectiveness and reduce costs.

Apply It

Turn to a classmate for a brief discussion. Envision the role of a medical records or health information manager or health professional such as a physician, nurse, or medical assistant who have responsibilities to document in the health record. Brainstorm and write down as many ideas as the two of can come up on how the use of computers can improve documentation in the health record and ultimately improve patient outcomes. After five minutes, share your thoughts with the class. Reflect on the health care industry without the availability of computers for documentation of patient care.

by authorized providers and staff from across more than one health care organization. Unlike EMRs, EHRs also allow a patient's health record to move with them—to other health care providers, specialists, hospitals, nursing homes, and across states. Providers who use EHRs report improvements in their ability to make better decisions with more comprehensive information. Electronic health record (EHR) adoption requires investment of time and money, but the benefits often outweigh costs, and financial incentives may be available to help providers make the transition.

A Personal Health Record (PHR) is a record controlled by the individual and may include health information from a variety of sources. With a standalone PHR, patients fill in information from their own records, and the information is stored on patients' computers or the Internet. A standalone PHR can also accept data from external sources, including providers, pharmacies and laboratories. With a standalone PHR, patients could add diet or exercise information to track progress over time. Patients can decide whether to share the information with providers, family members, or anyone else involved in their care.

A tethered, or connected, PHR is linked to a specific health care organization's electronic health record (EHR) system or to a health plan's information system. With a tethered PHR, patients can access their own records through a secure portal and see the trend of their lab results over the last year, their immunization history, their medication records, and/or due dates for screenings.

The use of technology for providing health care services from research to diagnosis and treatment; patient and practitioner support; and to recording and reporting of results, new practices, and procedures are constantly being explored, adopted, and incorporated throughout the industry. As the health care industry becomes more dependent on technology, it is important to identify potential malfunctions of technological equipment and the use of other technology and how it might impact the quality of patient outcomes. To ensure a malfunction does not compromise patient care, recording, or reporting, recognize and explain to the staff responsible for equipment repairs or technology malfunctions.

Therapeutic Services

If you choose to enter an occupation in the therapeutic services, you will have opportunities to work with a computer each day. In the pharmacy, drugs are inventoried using a computer. A computer also assists the pharmacist in keeping track of medications that a person receives. The computer can alert the pharmacist when one medication acts as an **antagonist** to another medication or contains a substance that causes an allergic reaction. In physical and occupational therapy, a computer assists paralyzed patients to walk. In respiratory therapy, a computer keeps critically ill patients in **homeostasis**. In emergency services and intensive care areas, computers do direct patient/client monitoring and are programmed to warn health care workers when a potentially dangerous condition occurs.

Diagnostic Services

In diagnostic services, highly sophisticated computers are being used. In the past, surgery and other **invasive** procedures were used to reach a diagnosis.

antagonist
(an TAG uh nist)
Something that works against.

homeostasis
(hoh mee uh STEY sis)
Constant balance within the body. This balance is maintained by the heartbeat, blood-making mechanisms, electrolytes, and hormone secretions.

invasive
(in VEY siv)
Entering the body.

206 Chapter 9 | Effective Communication

CUSTOMIZED INSTRUCTION

Special Needs Students

There are many computer programs, as well as hardware components, that have been developed specifically for special needs students, or customized for use by special needs students. For example, there may be larger font sizes for the visually impaired, or special input devices. If possible, make these options available to students.

Today, computerized diagnostic equipment helps diagnose many illnesses. Using computerized equipment removes the risks of surgery and reduces the pain and discomfort of invasive tests. Computerized tests include the following:

- The *CAT scanner* does computerized axial **tomography**. This test allows an organ to be **transversely** dissected to help find abnormalities (such as tumors) without surgery. A photograph is taken to provide the radiologist and the physician with a permanent record for future use.
- The *Coulter counter* completes multiple examinations of many blood specimens in seconds.
- The *electrocardiogram computer* creates pictures on a computer screen. It prints out the electrical activity of the heart. This helps the physician diagnose heart disease correctly.
- The *magnetic resonance imaging* (MRI) computer scans the body. (**Figure 9.8**) The scanner produces a cross-sectional image of the body. This helps the physician find tumors, see the results of medication and treatment, and diagnose the cause of an illness or disease.
- The *positron emission tomography* (PET) computer is also a scanner. It produces a three-dimensional image that shows an organ or bone from all sides.
- The *ultrasound imager* computer produces a picture of internal organs, tumors, aneurysms, and other abnormalities. It also produces pictures of the fetus developing in the uterus to help with fetal monitoring. These pictures can be seen on the monitor or can be processed on photographic film.
- *Wearable medical devices*, such as portable heart monitors, blood sugar monitors, and pulse oximeters, measure vital signs and levels of chemicals in the body. By monitoring actual, real-time events, these devices assist in providing data that can improve treatment of diseases and disorders.

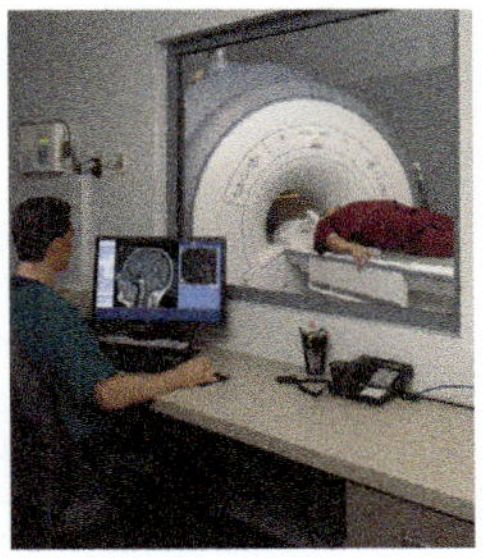

Figure 9.8
A technician uses the computer monitor to see what is happening with the MRI scan taking place.

The latest electronic technology scans an organ and not only provides pictures, but it can also create a three-dimensional object out of plastic. This object is an exact replica of the organ scanned in the patient's body. It allows the physician to practice difficult or experimental surgical procedures on the plastic replica before performing the procedure on the patient.

Support Services

Careers in support services also offer an opportunity to work with computers. Central supply services/central processing services are computerized for reordering inventory and for billing. Supplies are even categorized and identified by bar scanners like those you see in the grocery store.

tomography
(tuh MOG ruh fee)
X-ray technique that produces film of detailed cross sections of tissue.

transversely
(trans VURS lee)
In a cross direction.

Apply It

Technology has myriad applications in the five pathways in the Health Science Career Cluster. While building and developing your computer and technology skills will serve you well in just about any health care profession you choose, understanding what to do in the case of equipment malfunctions or technology glitches are equally important skills. In some cases, it could mean life or death for the patient/client!

Many health care organizations employ a technology or medical equipment manager to monitor and maintain technological equipment. Use the Internet and other resources to research the duties and responsibilities of a worker in the health care technology management field. What is their role in training other care workers on identifying and reporting malfunctions and other issues?

Figure Focus

9.8 A technician uses the computer monitor to see what is happening with the MRI scan taking place.

Explain that an MRI scan displays data, or output, on the computer monitor, so the technician can see what is happening.

Teaching Tips

- Discuss each of the six computer devices that are used for diagnostic testing.
- Ask students to share personal experiences (or experiences of family members) with computerized testing such as x-rays or MRIs, or breath or heart monitors.
- Review the ways computers are used in support services.
- Explain that inventory requests for work, materials, and food can be made on computers instead of through the mail. This makes the process faster, and dependent on fewer people.
- Point out that computerized calculations are more reliable than manual calculations.
- Review the ways computers are used in health informatics.
- Explain that electronic medical records have revolutionized records management:
  - Improved access to patient information
  - Statistics for research are more easily acquired and shared
  - Information required by HEDIS can be more easily identified
  - Diagnoses and treatment plans are determined faster, and are more accessible

Teaching Tips

- Review the ways computers are used in biotechnology research and development.
- Introduce the topic of contingency planning.
- Point out that disasters are not the only reason it is important to have a contingency plan.
- Explain that it is important to save data entered in a computer if you want it to be available for future use.
- Also point out that most health care facilities have contingency plans in place, such as automatically scheduled backups and generators to keep the power running.

Personal Wellness—Computer-Related Repetitive Strain Injury

- Explain ergonomics, which is the design of equipment to minimize physical strain, fatigue, and discomfort.
- Discuss and demonstrate the proper position for sitting and working at a desk and computer.

What other daily activities might be affected by repetitive strain injury?

Answer: Any activity involving repetitive use of a muscle, limb, or joint. That includes playing a musical instrument, sewing, knitting, playing a sport like golf or tennis, or using tools like a saw or hammer.

Apply It

The use of telecommunication and the Internet has resulted in a delivery of health care via computers and telephone systems. Many health care systems, physicians, and insurance companies provide patients with access to medical services via cell phones and video chats. Patients contact the provider via online chats or portals that allow the health care provider to view and discuss the health care issue with the patient without having to leave home.

Use the Internet to research telemedicine practices for Medicare, Medicaid, and other insurance providers. What are some advantages and disadvantages of this health care delivery system?

Health Informatics

Careers in health informatics require the use of computers in a variety of ways. Medical records workers manage and process records on computers. With diagnostic-related groupings, the computer is used to help categorize and track patients in the medical system. Health unit coordinators/unit secretaries use the computer to process many of the orders, transmitting requests to other departments.

The growing need to access medical data from patient/client files quickly requires health care providers to use computerized information systems. This means that to be employable, every health care worker must be comfortable working on computers.

Biotechnology Research and Development

Careers in biotechnology research and development involve high-level research and require workers to have computer technology skills. Computers are used in such areas as clinical trials, development of medicines and treatments, the research of such topics as genetic defects and inherited traits, and investigation of crimes by analyzing data.

Personal Wellness

Computer-Related Repetitive Injury Strain

Repetitive strain injuries happen when repeated physical movements do damage to tendons, nerves, muscles, and other soft body tissues. Nowadays, you may spend hours a day typing or clutching and dragging a mouse. An increase in the amount of time spent at the computer over the years has led to an increase in this type of injury. Some common types of repetitive strain injuries are carpal tunnel syndrome, bursitis, and tendonitis.

Typical symptoms of a repetitive strain injury include a tightness, soreness, or burning in the hands, wrists, fingers, forearms, or elbows. You may also experience tingling or numbness, coldness, or loss of strength or coordination in the hands. While most symptoms occur with the hands and arms, you may also feel pain in the upper back, shoulders, or neck.

While this type of injury can be painful, it can be prevented. You should use correct typing technique and posture, the right equipment setup, and good work habits in order to stay healthy. Be sure to sit up straight when using a computer. In addition, when you are typing, make sure that your wrists are straight and level. Your wrists should not be resting on anything, and your fingers should be in a straight line with your forearm. Also, check your work area to be sure that you do not have to stretch to reach the keys or read the computer screen. Anything that creates awkward reaches or angles in the body will create problems. Other helpful practices include using a light touch on the keyboard or mouse, keeping your arms and hands warm, and taking breaks to stretch and relax.

What other daily activities might be affected by repetitive strain injury?

208 Chapter 9 | Effective Communication

Contingency Planning

Whenever human beings depend on machines, **contingency** plans need to be made just in case the machine stops functioning. When a computer is not functioning, it is said to be down. Downtime can be scheduled to allow a new program to be entered into the computer's memory or to make changes. Downtime can also be unexpected (e.g., due to a power failure or component failure). Hospitals and medical/dental offices have learned that it is important to have an alternative plan if failure occurs.

contingency
(kuhn TIN juhn see)
Event that may occur but is not intended or likely to happen.

Despite modern technology, you still need to know manual methods of entering orders. The use of computers can make you more efficient in your job. With time, you will learn all of the things the computer can do, and you will learn how to do them. Practice is important in learning how to use the computer to its fullest capability.

Personal Information Management (PIM)

Working in a medical setting requires management of a variety of documents and information: reports, forms (paper and digital), e-mails, instruction sheets, Web pages, and so forth. Technology can assist with the tasks of handling information, creating ease and efficiency. The goal of personal information management is for the correct and complete information to be available at the right time and in the right format. Reducing or eliminating errors and saving time with technology tools and software applications that function as personal information managers (PIMs) can make you a better employee.

Ethics and Confidentiality

The health care worker must remember the importance of ethics and confidentiality when using a computer. Computers contain privileged information that must be protected. Keep your identification code or password confidential to protect you and the patient.

Summary

In this section you read that computers are an essential part of health care. All health care services have gained a greater ability to treat, diagnose, and care for patients/clients through computerization. Computers do shut down occasionally, making contingency planning important.

The responsible use of computers means that all users must keep information learned about patients/clients confidential. Keeping your identification code or password a secret is also your responsibility.

Section 9.3 Review Questions

1. Name two devices used for inputting.
2. Which part of the computer processes information?
3. List three procedures in which a computer might be used.
4. Why might a physician use magnetic resonance imaging?
5. How are computers used in support services?
6. Why is a contingency plan important when working with computers?

Effective Communication | Chapter 9 209

Personal Information Management (PIM)

- Discuss how Personal Information Management (PIM) applications can help increase workplace efficiency.
- Introduce the topic of Ethics and Confidentially as it relates to computers in health care.
- Ask students what ethical and legal guidelines they think apply to computers in the health care environment.
- Review guidelines pertaining to computers:
  - Never give your password to anyone.
  - Never reveal patient information.
  - Never look up patient information unless you are authorized to do so.
  - Never look up information about friends or co-workers.

ACTIVITY

Find out the guidelines for creating a "strong" password. Then, create a three-column chart or table that lists sample passwords in one column, a designation as either strong or weak in the second column, and an explanation of why it is either strong or weak in the third column.

Section 9.3 Review Questions

1. Answer: Inputting devices include: keyboards, microphone, touch screen, stylus, external hard-disk drives, CD-ROMs, DVD-ROMSs, USB flash drives, and optical drives.
2. Answer: The central processing unit (CPU) processes information.
3. Answer: Any three of the following:
   - Recording physicians' notes and orders
   - Creating a nursing treatment/work sheet based on physician orders
   - Updating automatically with each additional physician order
   - Creating templates for interventional protocols
   - Charting at bedside
   - Ordering or changing diets
   - Ordering unit supplies
   - Processing charges for nursing care equipment
   - Ordering lab work and receiving lab results
   - Recording lab results for patient records
   - Scheduling x-rays, special tests, and surgeries
   - Processing discharges
   - Performing diagnostic testing
   - Researching via the Internet
4. Answer: A physician would use an MRI to find tumors, see the results of medication and treatment, and diagnose the cause of an illness or disease.

5. Answer: Central supply services/central processing services are computerized for reordering inventory and for billing. Supplies are even categorized and identified by bar scanners like those you see in the grocery store.
6. Answer: Sometimes computers stop functioning or downtime is scheduled, and if this occurs it is important to have a contingency and for health care workers to know how to do things manually.

FOCUS AND ENGAGE

Introduce the Section

a. Review the content of the Background paragraph, pointing out that charting means documenting your observations.
b. Explain that both charting and observation are forms of communication; observing requires communicating with the patient, and charting requires communicating with co-workers.
c. Review the objectives for the section.

Vocabulary Review

a. Key terms are defined in the margins of the text on the page where they first appear.
b. Pronounce each word, and have the students repeat the pronunciation out loud.
c. Discuss each definition.

SECTION 9.4 Charting and Observation

Background

Observation and documentation are key components of health care. Your ability to observe patient/client behavior and symptoms will directly affect their care. Accurate documentation provides information needed to make decisions about their care. It is important that you develop sharp observation, reporting, and documentation skills.

Objectives

When you have completed this section, you will be able to do the following:

- Match key terms with their correct meanings.
- Explain the difference between subjective and objective observations.
- Explain which type of reporting allows immediate feedback and action.
- List information that must be on all health records.
- Apply five general charting guidelines.

Observation

observation
(ob zur VEY shuhns)
Something that is noted or recorded.

Every health care worker is responsible for observing the patient/client. Even if you are not responsible for charting, you must report your **observations** to your supervisor. You are responsible for making observations moment by moment. Your observation skills must be fine-tuned so that you are aware of the patient's mental and physical state. This awareness helps you and your co-workers to be more effective.

When interacting with patients and their families, use all of your tools to evaluate the situation. Your tools are four of your five senses: sight, hearing, touch, and smell:

- *Look* for all visible signs that may indicate a reason for the client's complaint.
- *Listen* carefully. Don't put thoughts or words into others' mouths. Be sure that you understand fully what you are told.
- *Feel* for changes in the skin, body temperature, abnormal structures, and so on.
- *Smell* unusual odors, which are often the first clue to a problem (e.g., fruity breath, foul stools).

subjective
(suhb JEK tiv)
Relating to a symptom or condition perceived by the patient and not by the examiner.

There are two types of observations:

- **Subjective** *observations* cannot be seen. They are ideas, thoughts, or opinions. If you cannot see it, feel it, hear it, or smell it, it is a subjective observation. (The patient complains of pain—you cannot see it, feel it, hear it, or smell it.)

210 Chapter 9 | Effective Communication

TEACH

Discuss

- Explain that observation is more than just looking at someone.
- Ask students to pair up and observe their partner for a set amount of time, such as one minute. Have them turn away, and then write down their observations.
- Discuss the observation experience.

Reinforce and Review

- Review nonverbal communication, such as facial expressions and gestures.
- Review written communication, including the importance of clear, legible handwriting.

Teaching Tips

- Emphasize that the goal of observation is to identify the status of the patient's mental and physical state.
- Discuss how four of five senses help in evaluating a situation.

ACTIVITY

Have students close their eyes. Make a small change somewhere in the room. Ask the students to identify the change.

- **Objective** *observations* can be seen. If you can see it, feel it, hear it, or smell it, it is an objective observation. (The patient has a cut—you can see it.)

The health care worker must report and record all subjective and objective observations. Any unusual event or change in a patient must be reported verbally to the supervisor and then documented on the client's legal record.

objective
(ahb JEK tiv)
Relating to a symptom or condition perceived by someone other than the person affected.

Reporting

Reporting unusual events or any change in behavior or condition is every health care worker's responsibility. Observation of people in a waiting area or a patient care area is important. Verbal reports to a supervisor allow immediate feedback and action when necessary. For example, you must always report changes in blood pressure, breathing, or coloring (e.g., pale, **flushed**) and any indications that a person is in **distress**.

It is also important to report anyone who acts strangely, threateningly, or weakly or appears to be in pain. Do not wait for others to report unusual observations. You may prevent a serious situation by reporting your observation in a timely manner.

Apply It

Create a list of signs and symptoms and patient chief complaints to share with the class. Encourage a discussion to identify each as either subjective or objective observations.

Medical Reporting. There are many kinds of medical reporting. As mentioned above, there are the reports that a health care worker might make to document observations. There are also medical billing reports, insurance reports, code analysis reports, and other administrative reporting functions.

Medical Records. A medical record is a systematic documentation of a person's medical history. It can be the actual physical folder for the patient as well as the body of information that makes up each patient's health history. Medical records are personal documents, and there are many ethical and legal issues surrounding them, such as the degree of third-party access and appropriate storage and disposal.

flushed
(flush d)
Showing reddening of the skin.

distress
(di STRES)
Great pain or suffering.

Documentation

Documentation is required in all medical and dental settings. **Documentation** is a record of the patient's progress throughout treatment. The documentation may either be in print or electronic format. Many people may be responsible for documenting information on a single patient/client. This record provides the information needed to allow each health care provider to give the care that best benefits the patient.

documentation
(dok yuh men TEY shuhn)
A record of something, such as a patient's progress.

notation
(noh TEY shuhn)
The act of noting, marking, or setting down in writing.

All records must contain certain information:

- Client's name
- Client's age
- Client's address
- Identification number
- Diagnosis
- Physician's orders

Depending on the department where the record is kept, other information may be required. Each health care worker who cares for the patient makes a **notation** on the chart. (Your facility policy tells you if you are required to chart. Even if you do not chart, you must always report your observations.) In the past, a health care worker's notations were always handwritten. Now, however, much patient

Apply It

When you go to the doctor, ambulatory care clinic, dental office, etc. what kind of medical records do you observe?

Effective Communication | Chapter 9 211

Teaching Tips

- Explain the difference between subjective and objective observations.
- Ask students to name symptoms they might observe in a patient, and identify whether each symptom is subjective or objective.
- Introduce the topic of reporting.
- Review the difference between medical reporting and medical records.
- Emphasize the importance of reporting all observations.
- Point out that early reporting based on observation can save lives. Examples include:
  - Changes in vital signs
  - Life-threatening problems
  - Anything that changes or is different
- Emphasize that it is better to report an insignificant matter than to fail to report a serious matter.
- Review types of behavior that should be reported, and discuss why.
- Introduce the topic of documentation. Review the information that must be entered on every record.

Apply It

- Have students brainstorm additional signs and symptoms that weren't on the original list.

Apply It

- Ask students to consider physical records, such as printouts and folder/filing systems, as well as electronic records; for example, are they asked to sign in for their appointment using a touch screen?

ACTIVITY

Provide access to one, or more, samples of electronic medical documents. If access is limited at your school, you might contact a sales representative from a company that sells medical applications and/or hardware. Have students access data from these documents and interpret the information.

TEAMWORK

In small groups, plan a skit that demonstrates observation and reporting. Perform the skit for the class. For extra credit, the audience can identify whether the observation in the skit is objective or subjective.

Apply It

- Students are to research instances in which poor charting or incorrect information in medical records resulted in poor patient outcomes or medical malpractice lawsuits.
- Have students share their findings with the class, being sure to point out what mistake was made in the recorded information and the result.

Teaching Tips

- Emphasize that a medical record is both a medical and a legal record.
- Discuss other information that may be entered on the chart.
- Stress that documentation:
  - Is the only record that shows what the health care worker has completed
  - Is a legal record
  - Must be correct
  - Must be concise, clear, and meaningful
- Explain that the chart protects the worker as well as the patient, because it legally indicates the worker's interaction with the patient.
- Point out that each facility has policies about who must chart.
- Emphasize that even if your position is not required to chart, you must still report your observations.
- Display examples of correctly and incorrectly filled out charts.

information is entered directly into computers, including chart notations. If charts are kept electronically in the facility where you work, be sure you know how to properly record and save the notations you make. These notations should contain specific information about the client, including:

- Care or treatment given
- Time of treatment
- How the patient tolerated the care or treatment
- Any observations that would be helpful to other health care workers
- Information that the patient has given that would affect treatment

chart
(CHART)
To write observations or records of patient care.

legible
(LEJ uh buhl)
Capable of being read easily.

This documentation is admissible in a court of law. This means that anything you write is considered to be true. If you do not write down something that you did for the patient, it is assumed that it was not done. As you can see, it is very important to be accurate and careful when you **chart**.

Everyone must follow these general guidelines for charting:

- Use ink for record keeping. In some facilities, different colors are used for different shifts.
- Entries must be **legible**. If your writing is hard to read, you should print.
- If you make an error, do not erase it or scratch it out or cover it up. Draw a single line through the error so that it can still be read. Write "error" next to it, and then place your initials next to the correction (e.g., "error/KG Patient tolerated procedure well"). If you are working with electronic charts, you will need to learn how to correct errors in the system your facility uses.
- Entries should be in short phrases—concise, clear, and meaningful. You do not need to write complete sentences. You do not need to use the patient's name because you are writing in the patient's chart.
- Document in order of occurrence. All entries should be entered in a timely manner, preferably as the care is provided. For example, all medications and treatments must be documented at the time given. Any incidents or patient activities should be documented in the order in which they took place.
- All entries that you make are followed by your signature. You sign with your first initial, your last name, and your title. If you are making entries in an electronic chart, you still must "sign" the entries you make.

Apply It

Internet Search: Emphasize the importance of accuracy in entering correct information in the patient's chart or electronic medical record by researching medical charting mistakes that have resulted in poor patient outcomes and medical malpractice legal battles.

Hospital Chart

The rules listed above apply to all charting. However, additional charting may be required. This is especially true for the nurse assistant. Each facility has its own policy and procedures for charting. Learn what these are. There are some standard types of charting that all nurse assistants are required to do:

- *Nurses' notes* may be in **narrative** or check-off form. These notes state:
  - What personal care was given
  - What activities the client participated in
  - The patient's skin condition

narrative
(NAR uh tiv)
A story or account of events.

212 Chapter 9 | Effective Communication

- Review the general guidelines for charting.
- Discuss the components of a hospital chart.
- Review the components of nurses' notes.

- General observations about the client
- Any unusual occurrences
- Any complaints that the client has
- What treatments were given
- Any information that is important to the patient's well-being

- During your career, you may be asked to document in many different styles. To avoid confusion in this book, we will use the following style:
  - Date
  - Military time
  - A description of the care or treatment given, complaints and problems, all written as ordinary sentences
  - Signature (first initial, full last name) and certification

  Many facilities provide flow sheets with charting examples and when employed you will follow those examples.

- The **graphic chart** is a record of the patient's vital signs. All graphic charts have time blocks and numbers that relate to temperature, pulse, and respiration. On some graphic charts there is also space for blood pressure, intake and output, bowel movements, and weight. (**Figure 9.9**) Graphic charts are useful because they contain like measurements over time. When placed together, the nurse can quickly scan and determine the patient's baseline and any alterations from baseline.

graphic chart
(GRAF ik charct)
A visual record of data in graphic or tabular form.

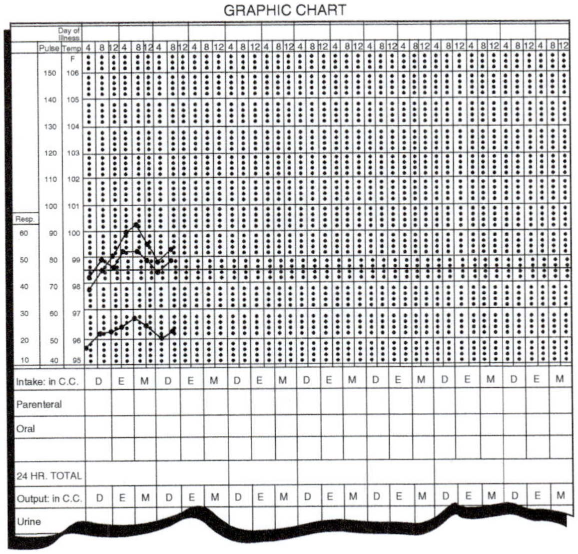

Figure 9.9
Graphic chart with intake and output section. What types of things are included on a graphic chart?

Effective Communication | Chapter 9 213

Teaching Tips

- Emphasize that the procedures and policies for charting vary from facility to facility.
- Discuss the components of a graphic chart.
- Review the importance of tracking a patient's vital signs.
- Emphasize that a graphic chart displays changes over time, which is extremely helpful in monitoring the status of a patient.

Figure Focus

9.9 Graphic chart with intake and output section. What types of things are included on a graphic chart?

Answer: A graphic chart includes a record of a patient's vital signs. Graphic charts have time blocks and numbers that related to temperature, pulse, and respiration. On some graphic charts there is also space for blood pressure, intake and output, bowel movements, and weight.

CUSTOMIZED INSTRUCTION

Less Advanced Students

Have less advanced students copy information from a completed chart to a blank chart, practicing writing or printing neatly.

Teaching Tips

- Review other parts of a chart, such as:
  - Front sheet
  - Medical history
  - Daily progress report
  - Discharge plan
  - Reports from other team members, such as a social worker or nutritionist
  - Treatment records from other departments
- Reinforce the importance of confidentiality as it relates to charts.
  - Never read a chart unless authorized.
  - Never leave a chart in an area where unauthorized personnel may access it.
  - Never write inaccurate or untrue information on a chart.

Section 9.4 Review Questions

1. Answer: Subjective observations cannot be seen; for example, feelings, thoughts, or opinions. Objective observations can be seen. If you can feel it, hear it, see it, or smell it, it is an objective observation.
2. Answer: Information that should be on a patient record includes the client's name, age, address, identification number, diagnosis, and physician's orders.
3. Answer:
   - Make entries legible.
   - Scratch out errors (do not erase) by drawing a single line through the error so that it can still be read and then place your initials next to the correction.
   - Write in short phrases. You do not need to write complete sentences.
   - Make concise, clear, and meaningful entries.
   - Sign each entry.
   - If using an electronic charting system, follow the procedures for the system, including "signing" entries and making corrections properly.

Other parts of the chart include:

- A front sheet with personal information, such as name, address, marital status, place of employment, and admission diagnosis
- A physical examination and a medical history
- The daily progress report written by the physician
- There may be:
  - A discharge plan
  - A social worker's report
  - Treatment records from other departments or from specialists

Documentation is a very important responsibility. Learn how to write good records, and always be responsible and careful when you chart.

Apply It

Imagine that you are taking care of a male patient and a lady calls the hospital stating she is his daughter. She wants to know the patient's diagnosis, what is going on with him, and how is he doing. What do you say? The patient is on a ventilator and unable to communicate verbally. Do you answer her questions? Would it go against HIPAA if you shared information?

Confidentiality

In 1996, the federal government passed the Health Insurance Portability and Accountability Act (HIPAA) to establish strict standards to maintain and protect confidentiality of health care records and information. This act allows patients to control how their medical record information is used. Patients are able to see copies of their records and limit who has access to this information. Every health care worker and provider must be aware of the requirements in this act and be certain to protect the privacy and confidentiality of the patient's medical record.

When communicating any information concerning the client, remember that it is confidential and is not discussed unless it affects the treatment. The physician and patient will decide if family members or others will share the information.

Summary

In the health care field, you will need to record both subjective and objective observations. It is your responsibility to report any unusual events or change in behavior. In addition, you will be required to maintain documentation of a client/patient's care. Accuracy is important in order for health care workers to provide the best care for a client/patient. Always remember that the information in a client/patient's chart is **confidential**.

confidential
(kon fi DEN shuhl)
Limited to persons authorized to use information or documents

Section 9.4 Review Questions

1. Explain the difference between subjective and objective observations.
2. Name three pieces of information that should be on a patient record.
3. List three notations you should include when charting.
4. Why is it important to chart carefully?
5. What is the benefit of verbal reporting?
6. What additional items may a nurse's assistant be required to include as part of a chart?
7. What is a graphic chart?

214 Chapter 9 | Effective Communication

4. Answer: Charting provides accurate details about a patient's actions, reactions, and treatment. These charts can be used in court, so all notations must be true. If something is not noted, then it is assumed that it was not done. Accuracy is important if we are to provide the best care for patients.
5. Answer: Verbal reports to a supervisor allow immediate feedback and action when necessary.
6. Answer: Additional items include a discharge plan, social worker's report, and treatment records.
7. Answer: A graphic chart is a visual record of data in graphic or tabular form. It is a record of the patient's vital signs and all graphic charts have time blocks and numbers that relate to temperature, pulse, and respiration. Graphic charts are useful because they contain like measurements over time.

TEAMWORK

Divide the class into two teams. Read a symptom to each team in turns. For each symptom they correctly identify as objective or subjective, the team receives one point, and extra credit if they can explain why.

Scheduling and Filing

SECTION 9.5

Background

As a health information technician or medical assistant, you will provide essential support for the medical staff and for patients. You will often be the first person the patient/client meets, either on the phone or in person. You may be in charge of gathering important health information from patients and keeping records up to date. You may also schedule office visits and work in bookkeeping and billing. The health information technician or medical assistant works to ensure that health providers have the information they need to provide appropriate care and that the office runs smoothly.

Objectives

When you have completed this section, you will be able to do the following:

- Match key terms with their correct meanings.
- List the guidelines for scheduling clients/patients for appointments.
- Describe a tickler file.
- List five filing systems.
- List two kinds of registration forms.
- Demonstrate how to schedule appointments.
- Demonstrate how to schedule a new client/patient: first time visit.
- Demonstrate how to schedule an outpatient diagnostic test.

Scheduling

For a smooth-running day it is important to know how to schedule clients/patients for office visits, procedures, and surgeries. Scheduling is done in one of two ways: appointments are written manually in an appointment book, or a computer system maintains appointment schedules.

Scheduling Office Visits

When scheduling visits, follow these guidelines:

1. A patient/client visit is scheduled every 15 minutes, 30 minutes, or hourly, depending on your provider's specialty. (**Figures 9.10** and **9.11**)
2. Learn to recognize the patients/clients who require more time with the provider.
3. Always ask the purpose of the appointment (for example, checkup, cold) to allocate enough time for the visit.
4. Ask the patient/client what would be the most convenient time for an appointment.
5. If you are not able to schedule the patient/client at the time and date requested, express regret and ask for a second choice.

Apply It

Pair Compare: Work in pairs to discuss the importance of accurate medical appointment scheduling. Each pair writes down all the negative outcomes from poorly scheduled appointments for 2–3 minutes. Pair forms teams of 4 and summarize all their discussion points. Randomly survey teams for their answers to emphasize one of the most frequent complaints patients voice regarding medical office visits.

Effective Communication | Chapter 9 215

FOCUS AND ENGAGE

Introduce the Section

a. Review the content of the Background paragraph, pointing out that a health information technician is usually responsible for filing and scheduling.
b. Explain that other workers may also file information and schedule appointments.
c. Emphasize that both filing and scheduling require communicating with patients and co-workers, and involve keeping track of important information.
d. Review the objectives for the section.

Vocabulary Review

a. Key terms are defined in the margins of the text on the page where they first appear.
b. Pronounce each word, and have the students repeat the pronunciation out loud.
c. Discuss each definition.

TEACH

Discuss

- Explain that the person responsible for scheduling appointments is often the first contact a patient has with a health care facility.
- Discuss the importance of making a good impression.

Reinforce and Review

- Review telephone communication skills.
- Reinforce the importance of communicating in a clear and effective manner, whether it is on the phone, in writing, or in person.

Teaching Tips

- Review the scheduling guidelines for office visits.

Apply It

- Encourage students to consider any negative outcomes at recent medical appointments of their own.
- Make sure they consider all aspects of the appointment experience, from parking to the waiting room experience to signing out or leaving the appointment.

ACTIVITY

Research the typical or standard interval for scheduling different types of appointments or procedures. For example, find out how long a well-baby appointment with a pediatrician should be, and how long an annual mammogram appointment should be. Create a chart showing the times for each appointment.

Teaching Tips

- Discuss the two methods of scheduling: computerized and manual.
- Discuss reasons why it is important to use the correct scheduling interval.
- Review the information that should always be on an appointment card. If possible, display sample appointment cards.
- Point out that some offices have cancellation policies. If so, be sure to mention the policy and to provide it in writing.
- It may also be necessary to ask the patient to bring certain information to an appointment, such as prior x-rays, MRIs, or health data sheets.

Figure Focus

9.10 Standard appointment sheet. What problems might result if you do not recognize when a particular patient's visit will take longer than that of some other patients?

Answer: If one patient's visit runs longer than you've allotted for an appointment, the visits of the next patients will be delayed. The schedule for the whole day can be thrown off. The provider will be behind all day, and patients will be unhappy when they have to wait for scheduled appointments.

Figure Focus

9.11 Medical appointment schedule for more than one service at a time. One of Dr. Smith's patients is also having back problems that day. She will probably need an ultrasound. What time should you schedule her appointment with Dr. Smith?

Answer: The earliest one could reasonably be scheduled would be at 8:30. That allows time for Mrs. Green's test to be completed before Dr. Smith's patient uses the machine.

Apply It

Research health science careers in information technology (IT). Identify the skills required to be successful in an IT career and the job requirements. What types of technology should an IT worker be familiar with? Create a poster or presentation exhibiting several careers along with examples of the technology these workers would use.

6. Ask for a phone number where the patient/client can be reached during the day in case a cancellation is necessary.
7. Offer to call the client/patient as cancellations occur if the patient/client desires an earlier appointment. Use a tickler file as a reminder. (See the next sections for a description of a tickler file.)
8. Always repeat the appointment time and date to the patient/client to avoid confusion.
9. When a patient/client cancels an appointment, note the date, time, and reason for the cancellation in the chart.
10. Give all patients/clients appointment cards when scheduling a follow-up visit. Put the following information on the appointment card:
    - Provider's name
    - Provider's address and phone number
    - Patient's/client's name
    - Date and time of next appointment

Figure 9.10
Standard appointment sheet. What problems might result if you do not recognize when a particular patient's visit will take longer than that of some other patients?

Date 1-8-16

7	30	IAN GALLAGHER			
	45	DEE ANN SHERMAN			
8	00	//////////////////			
	15	MARY KELHI			
	30				
	45				
9	00				
	15				
	30				
	45				
	00				

Figure 9.11
Medical appointment schedule for more than one service at a time. One of Dr. Smith's patients is also having back problems that day. She will probably need an ultrasound. What time should you schedule her appointment with Dr. Smith?

Month ________
Date ________
Day ________

	Dr. Smith	Dr. Jones	Ultrasound Machine
8:00			
8:15		GREEN, LOIS 412-6190	
8:30		BACK PAIN	DR. JONES: MRS. GREEN
8:45			
9:00			
9:15			
9:30			
9:45			

ACTIVITY

Write a personal essay about an experience scheduling an appointment. It may have been with a health care professional or with someone else. Discuss whether it was a positive or negative experience, and why.

Procedure 9.1 Scheduling Office Visits

BACKGROUND: Careful scheduling is essential for a well-run office. Appointments must be scheduled to prevent long waits for patients while also keeping the staff working at top efficiency. Accommodating the patient as much as possible tells the patient that you are concerned about him or her.

Preprocedure

1. Assemble materials:
   a. Pen or pencil
   b. Appointment book
   c. Appointment reminder cards for tickler file
   d. Appointment cards
   e. Calendar
   f. Procedure list with approximate time allotments for each procedure
   g. Written instructions for patient/client preparation prior to visit
2. Prepare provider schedules for at least three months:
   a. Mark out vacation or holiday times.
   b. Schedule monthly, weekly, or daily meetings.
   c. Mark schedule to identify hours for patient/client appointments.
3. Follow the correct procedure for the type of appointment system in your office.
4. Write clearly and neatly so that names and procedures are easy to read.

Procedure

5. Schedule appointments.
   a. By phone:
      (1) Clarify reason for appointment.
      (2) Discuss most convenient time for client/patient (e.g., a.m., p.m.).
      (3) Offer various times.
      (4) Ask for proper spelling of first and last names once a time is chosen.
      (5) Ask for information, such as birthday or Social Security number, if name is common (e.g., Smith, Jones).
      (6) Write patient's/client's telephone number and where he or she can be reached during the day of appointment.

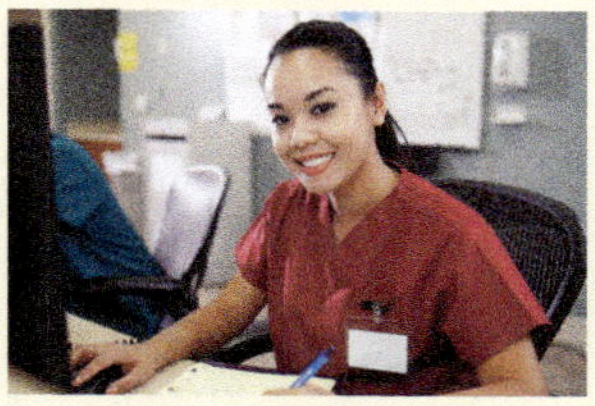

      (7) Allocate **sufficient** time for the visit when scheduling a procedure.
   b. In person:
      (1) Follow steps 1 to 6 of procedure above.
      (2) Give patient/client an appointment card with date and time of appointment.
   c. For appointments more than three months in the future:
      (1) Ask patient/client to address an appointment reminder card.
      (2) Fill in month patient is to return.
      (3) Instruct patient/client that a card will be sent as a reminder to call and make an appointment.
   d. Place appointment reminder card in tickler file so that it is sent at the correct time.

sufficient
(suh FISH suhnt)
Enough.

Procedure Tips

9.1 Scheduling Office Visits

- Review the background information.
- Review the reasons why scheduling is important.
- Discuss why it is important to respect the patient during the scheduling procedure.
- Discuss the preprocedure steps. Point out that the necessary tools should always be available at the workstation or desk.
- Emphasize that it is the technician's responsibility to know and understand the scheduling requirements of the office staff.
- Emphasize the importance of communication with the staff to keep the calendar up-to-date.
- Review the procedure steps.

PROCEDURE PRACTICE

- Demonstrate the steps for Procedure 9.1, Scheduling Office Visits, as many times as necessary, or ask students to demonstrate the steps. Have students practice and perform the procedure until they are competent.

TEAMWORK

In pairs, practice scheduling routine office visits. One student will act as a patient, and the other as the health care worker. Switch positions and repeat the activity.

Teaching Tips

- Review the guidelines for scheduling surgeries and procedures.
- Emphasize that the technician must be knowledgeable about the policies and procedures at the facility where the appointment will take place.
- Explain the importance of giving the patient clear instructions for procedures and surgeries.
- Point out that many patients are nervous when scheduling such appointments, and it is the health care professional's responsibility to be forthright and respectful.
- Review the guidelines for scheduling diagnostic tests.
- Emphasize that diagnostic test—like surgeries and procedures—are likely to be performed at a different facility.
- Note that in some cases, you will schedule the test for the patient, and in other cases, the patient will contact the test facility directly.
- Explain the importance of a tickler file:
  - Helps to keep the office organized and running smoothly
  - Facilitates communication with the patients
- Review the steps for creating a tickler file.

Scheduling Surgeries/Procedures

Learn how your provider wants to schedule surgery and procedures in the hospital or office. Use the following guidelines to help you with this scheduling:

- Determine how long each procedure takes.
- Learn how to schedule patients/clients around these procedures.
- Establish what days and times your provider prefers to do surgeries.
- Learn the admitting procedure for the hospital where your provider performs surgery.
- Provide the patient/client with the following information:
  - Surgery time
  - Time patient/client needs to arrive at the office or hospital
  - Registration instructions (admitting forms) if going to the hospital
  - The hospital's address, telephone, and directions
  - Written instructions to follow prior to surgery (for example, *NPO after midnight*)
- Give the client/patient verbal and written instruction because the person may be nervous or apprehensive and forget what you said.
- Maintain good lines of communication with the office personnel of all referring providers and assisting providers.

Learning how your office functions allows you to schedule a smooth-running day.

Scheduling Diagnostic Tests

Diagnostic procedures are frequently scheduled to be performed in other facilities. The following is basic information necessary to schedule an appointment:

- Patient's/client's name
- Age or date of birth
- Reason for the diagnostic test

Give the client/patient the appointment information and instructions to prepare for the test. When scheduled for a test like an upper gastrointestinal series (UGI), give written guidelines that explain how to prepare for the test.

Tickler File

tickler file
(TIK ler fayhl)
Special file kept to remind you of tasks that need to be done at a certain time.

A **tickler file** reminds you of tasks that need to be done at a certain time (for example, by day, week, or month). When you create a tickler file, arrange 12 file dividers in a file. You need 1 divider for each month and 1 for each day of the month (1 through 31). When a client/patient needs to be seen at a later date:

1. Fill out a reminder card with the patient's/client's name and address.
2. Fill in the blank space with the date of the patient's/client's last visit.
3. Place the card in the file the month prior to the next required visit.

218 Chapter 9 | Effective Communication

4. Each month, take cards from that month's folder, and mail them to the client/patient.

Check the tickler file routinely because this file tells you what to do and when to do it. The card that is in the file reminds you to notify the client/patient to make an appointment. (**Figure 9.12**) There are also tickler file software programs that automatically "pop up" reminders on the screen of your computer monitor without you having to check a file. Even with an electronic tickler file, however, the reminder information must be entered carefully and completely.

> As you requested, Dr. R. C. Smith is reminding you that it has been __________ since your last visit.
>
> Please call (555) 888-0000 to schedule an appointment.
>
> R. C. Smith, M.D.
> 11372 City Drive
> Scottsdale, WA 88888

Figure 9.12
Appointment reminder card to be placed in a tickler file. When should you look through the file to remind yourself to send the reminder card?

Procedure 9.2 Scheduling a New Patient/Client: First-Time Visit

BACKGROUND: Gathering essential information from each new patient provides the information needed for patient care and timely billing for services rendered. The patient feels secure when everything is taken care of efficiently.

Preprocedure

1. Assemble materials:
   a. Appointment book
   b. Scheduling guidelines
   c. Telephone
   d. Pencil

Procedure

2. Ask patient/client for the following:
   a. First, last, and middle names
   b. Birth date
   c. Home address
   d. Telephone number
3. Ask patient/client if this is a referral. If yes:
   a. Determine information you need from the referring provider.
   b. Add this information to the medical chart. (Your provider needs to send a consultation report to the referring provider.)
4. Ask what the chief complaint is and when it started.
5. Find the first appointment that allows the appropriate amount of time.
6. Offer a choice of days and times.
7. Enter the following:
   a. Patient's/client's name NP next to name indicating new patient)
   b. Time and date of appointment
   c. Patient's/Client's day telephone number
8. Explain payment procedure (e.g., patient/client must pay for visit, your office will bill).
9. Give directions to the office.
10. Explain parking arrangements.

Postprocedure

11. Repeat day, date, and time the appointment is scheduled.

Figure Focus

9.12 Appointment reminder card to be placed in a tickler file. When should you look through the file to remind yourself to send the reminder card?

Answer: You should look through the tickler file daily to check for tasks, such as sending reminder cards, that need to be done that day.

Procedure Tips

9.2 Scheduling a New Patient/Client: First-Time Visit

- Ask students why scheduling a first visit may be different from scheduling someone who has been there before.
- Review the background information.
- Review the preprocedure steps.
- Review the procedure steps.
- Review the postprocedure steps.

PROCEDURE PRACTICE

Demonstrate the steps for Procedure 9.2, Scheduling a New Patient/Client: First-Time Visit, as many times as necessary, or ask students to demonstrate the steps. Have students practice and perform the procedure until they are competent.

TEAMWORK

In pairs, practice scheduling a new patient/client first time visit. One student will act as a patient, and the other as the health care worker. Switch positions and repeat the activity.

Procedure Tips

9.3 Scheduling Outpatient Diagnostic Tests

- Review the background information.
- Ask students what signs might indicate that a patient is nervous.
- Discuss why patients may be more nervous about scheduling diagnostic tests than they are for a regular exam.
- Review the preprocedure steps.
- Review the procedure steps.
- Review the postprocedure step.
- Note that it may be necessary to mail instructions to the patient. If so, you must be sure to mail them in plenty of time so they arrive in advance of the scheduled appointment.

PROCEDURE PRACTICE

Demonstrate the steps for Procedure 9.3, Scheduling Outpatient Diagnostic Tests, as many times as necessary, or ask students to demonstrate the steps. Have students practice and perform the procedure until they are competent.

Teaching Tips

- Describe the two types of registration and client information forms.
- Explain that these forms may be sent to patients in advance of the visit, to save time.
- If possible, display a client information form.
- Review the information that should be included on a client information form.

Procedure 9.3 **Scheduling Outpatient Diagnostic Tests**

BACKGROUND: Patients are often fearful about diagnostic tests. Scheduling the diagnostic tests as soon as possible and when it is most convenient for the patients gives them confidence that they are cared for in a timely and caring way.

Preprocedure

1. Assemble materials:
   a. Written order from provider
   b. Patient's chart
   c. Test preparation instructions for client/patient
   d. Name, address, and phone number of laboratory
   e. Telephone

Procedure

2. Read provider's order.
3. Ask patient/client when he or she is available.
4. Call test lab.
5. Order test:
   a. Set up time and date
   b. Give name, age, address, and telephone number of patient/client
   c. Ask if there are special instructions for patient/client prior to the test
6. Provide patient/client with the following:
   a. Name, address, and telephone number of laboratory
   b. Date and time
   c. Instructions (in writing) for preparation prior to test
7. Verify instructions with patient/client.

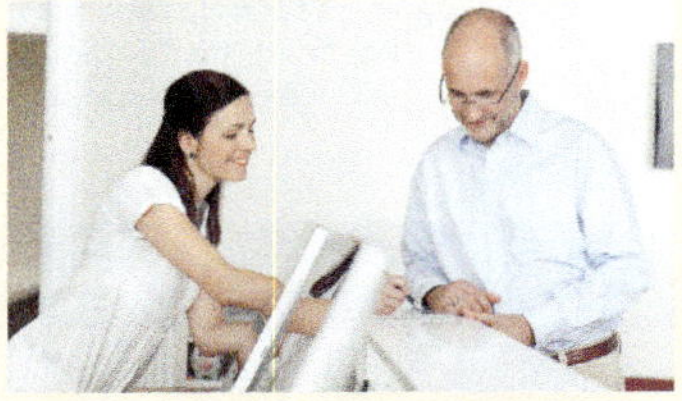

8. Record test time in patient's/client's chart.

Postprocedure

9. Put a reminder in the tickler file or on a calendar to check for results.

Registration

New patients/clients must complete two basic forms when registering:

1. Client/patient information forms
2. Medical history forms

Client/Patient Information Forms

The client/patient information form gives the following information:

- Patient's/client's name, address, and phone number
- Birth date, sex, marital status, and Social Security number
- Patient's/client's employer name, address, and phone number
- Insurance company's name, address, and phone number
- Insured's employer name, address, and phone number
- If the patient/client is a minor, name of the responsible party

ACTIVITY

Fill out a client information form.

TEAMWORK

In pairs, practice scheduling an outpatient diagnostic test. One student will act as a patient, and the other as the health care worker. Switch positions and repeat the activity.

Personal Wellness

Health Risks

As a health information technician, your contact with patients will be casual. You will be talking to them, getting and giving information, but you will have little if any physical contact. Nonetheless, anyone working in a health care environment is at some risk of infection. So, how much at risk of infection are you and what can you do to reduce your risk?

Hepatitis B Virus (HBV) is one of the most serious infections. It is typically spread through sexual contact, by sharing needles among drug users, and by accidental needle sticks, which represent the greatest risk to health care workers. HBV cannot be contracted by casual contact with infected patients. Check with your supervisor. You may be entitled to an inoculation against HBV at no cost.

Human immunodeficiency virus (HIV) is primarily transmitted by sexual contact and intravenous drug use. It is not transmitted by casual contact, through contaminated food or water, or through the air.

Influenza is a common illness that often brings patients into the medical facility. To protect yourself from infection and to avoid spreading the flu to other patients, you should consider getting an annual flu vaccination. Check with your supervisor about the provider's policy.

The health information technician may be exposed to other microorganisms that can be spread through casual contact in the medical facility. The best precaution against infection is to regularly and frequently wash your hands. Keep your hands away from your mouth. If you develop any signs or symptoms of illness, report them immediately.

How does your health affect the health of patients? How can you protect them?

Medical History Forms

The medical history form gives the provider the necessary information to evaluate the patient's/client's physical condition. The patient/client must give you the following information (Figure 9.13 and Figure 9.14):

- Previous surgeries
- Allergies
- Chronic illness
- Medications taken
- General medical history
- Childhood diseases

Both forms must be completed accurately to serve the needs of both the client/patient and the provider.

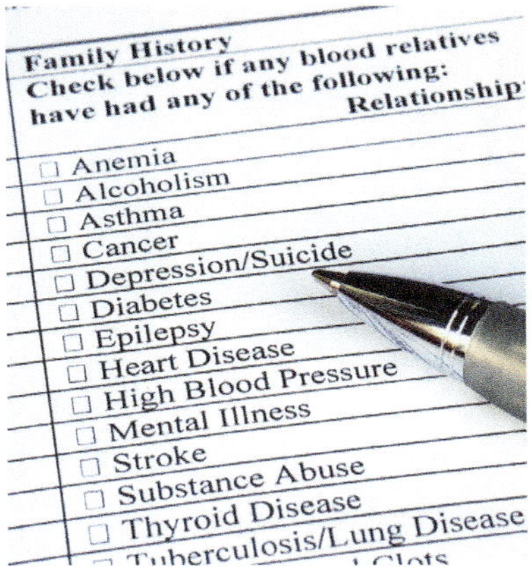

Figure 9.13
A patient must complete a handwritten or electronic medical history form. Why is this information necessary?

Personal Wellness—Health Risks

- Review the types of illnesses which are easily transmitted in an office environment.
- Discuss the importance of hand washing.
- Introduce hand sanitizers.

How does your health affect the health of patients? How can you protect them?

Answer: Whenever you are sick, you bring pathogens and the risk of infection to patients you come in contact with. You can protect patients by staying healthy yourself, by managing rather than ignoring signs of illness, and staying home if you have a contagious illness that can infect patients.

Teaching Tips

- If possible, display an actual medical history form. (Alternatively, refer to Figure 9.14 on the next page.)
- Review the information that should be included on a medical information form.
- Discuss why it is important to collect this information from all patients.

Figure Focus

9.13 A patient must complete a handwritten or electronic medical history form. What information does a medical history form provide?

Answer: Previous surgeries, allergies, chronic illness, medications taken, general medical history, childhood diseases.

Teaching Tips

- Discuss problems that might arise if a health care professional does not have access to a patient's medical history form:
    - The patient might be allergic to prescribed medication.
    - The patient might already by taking a medication that conflicts with a prescribed medication.
    - A symptom might be part of a pre-existing condition.
- Review confidentiality as it pertains to a medical history form.

Figure Focus

9.14 Medical history form. Under Marital Status, what do the initials S M D W stand for?

Answer: Single, married, divorced, widowed

Figure 9.14
Medical history form. Under Marital Status, what do the initials S M D W stand for?

GREEN VALLEY MEDICAL GROUP, INC.
MEDICAL HISTORY

NAME ____________ DATE OF BIRTH ____________
OCCUPATION ____________ MARITAL STATUS: S M D W

ALLERGIES:
Are you allergic to:

Penicillin	Yes ___	No ___
Sulfa	Yes ___	No ___
Aspirin	Yes ___	No ___
Codeine	Yes ___	No ___
Tetanus Injections	Yes ___	No ___
Iodine	Yes ___	No ___
Foods	Yes ___	No ___
Tape	Yes ___	No ___

Other ____________

MEDICATIONS:
List all medications, including over the counter, you are currently taking:

____

HABITS:
Do you:

Smoke? Yes ___ No ___ How Much ___
Drink Alcohol? Yes ___ No ___ How Much ___
Drink Beverages That Contain Caffeine?
Yes ___ No ___ How Much ___
Limit Cholesterol Yes ___ No ___
Use Other Substances Yes ___ No ___
What? ____________

EXERCISE:
Do you on a regular basis:

Walk	Yes ___	No ___
Run	Yes ___	No ___
Bike	Yes ___	No ___
Swim	Yes ___	No ___
Aerobic Exercise	Yes ___	No ___
Other	Yes ___	No ___

MENSTRUAL HISTORY (FEMALES):
Date of last PAP & results ____________
Date of last normal period ____________
Date of last mammogram & results ____________
Length of cycle (days) ____________
Usual duration (days) ____________
Number of pregnancies ____________
Number of children ____________

PRESENT COMPLAINTS:
Do you have:

Headaches	Yes ___	No ___
Fever	Yes ___	No ___
Cough	Yes ___	No ___
Chest Pains	Yes ___	No ___
Nausea	Yes ___	No ___
Vomiting	Yes ___	No ___
Diarrhea	Yes ___	No ___
Constipation	Yes ___	No ___
Black Stools	Yes ___	No ___
Bloody Stools	Yes ___	No ___
Painful Urination	Yes ___	No ___
Recent Weight Gain or Loss	Yes ___	No ___

Other Complaints ____________

PAST ILLNESS:
Have you ever had:

High Blood Pressure	Yes ___	No ___
Heart Trouble	Yes ___	No ___
Pneumonia	Yes ___	No ___
Hepatitis	Yes ___	No ___
Cancer	Yes ___	No ___
Diabetes	Yes ___	No ___
Tuberculosis	Yes ___	No ___
Asthma	Yes ___	No ___
Ulcers	Yes ___	No ___
Seizures	Yes ___	No ___
Sexually Transmitted Disease	Yes ___	No ___
Blood Disorder	Yes ___	No ___

Other ____________

OPERATIONS:
Have you had any surgery:

Appendix	Yes ___	No ___
Tonsils	Yes ___	No ___
Gallbladder	Yes ___	No ___
Stomach	Yes ___	No ___
Hemorrhoids	Yes ___	No ___
Female Organs	Yes ___	No ___
Thyroid	Yes ___	No ___
Hernia	Yes ___	No ___
Heart	Yes ___	No ___

Other ____________

222 Chapter 9 | Effective Communication

ACTIVITY

Attempt to participate in class or everyday activities while using one or more of the following to experience sensory deprivation or loss:

- Wear glasses that are coated with a lubricating jelly.
- Put cotton in ears.
- Wear heavy gloves or mittens.

At the conclusion, write or discuss how the experience affected you.

What's New?

Digital Paperwork

Health care providers rely upon information from admittance forms, patient histories, lab forms, insurance forms, and much more to make the medical and business parts of the organization successful. Currently most of these forms are completed by using a paper form and pen. Information on paper forms has limited usefulness, however, so, in many cases, someone transcribes, or copies, the written information to a computer.

Periodically, new forms are completed on patients, and that information must also be entered into the computer system. Transcribing all this information represents an enormous amount of staff time that might be better spent on patient care. It also increases the possibility of errors being introduced as the information is copied.

New digitalized systems are emerging to simplify and streamline the process. Some of it is already being seen in many facilities.

Tablet PCs, for example, have special light-weight and portable slate display screens. The forms appear on the screens and can be written on with a special pen, or stylus. Handwriting recognition software reads the handwriting. Information is instantly digitalized and can be transferred to the computer system without the need for separate transcribing.

Another new technology even eliminates the display screen with special paper and digital pens. Patients simply fill out the medical forms as they normally do. The digital pens record the information as patients write. Again, the laborious manual transcription from paper forms to computer is eliminated.

How can a digitalized system like one of these improve the quality of patient care?

Filing

Filing Systems

Proper filing helps ensure you can find information when you need it. (Figure 9.15) The filing system serves to:

- Store information and records safely
- Keep related materials together
- Retrieve files quickly when needed

The following are the five most common systems:

1. Alphabetical
2. Numerical
3. Color coding
4. Chronological
5. Geographic

Apply It

Make three copies of the medical history form shown in Figure 9.14. Gather information for the form from three family members or close friends. After you have completed the forms, discuss as a class what information was most difficult to obtain. As a class, create a filing system for all the completed forms.

What's New?—Digital Paperwork

- Discuss the types of technology that make electronic recordkeeping possible.

How can a digitalized system like one of these improve the quality of patient care?

Answer: A digitalized system will improve patient care in several ways. First, it will help eliminate errors in records that will result from mistakes in transcribing the information. As a result, treatment will be more accurate. Secondly, because so much time will be saved from transcribing and updating records, more staff hours can be devoted to other areas of patient care.

Teaching Tips

- Ask students if they have any experience with filing systems. At first they may say no. Point out that they might store phone numbers or e-mail addresses, they might keep their class notes organized in a notebook, or they might have a recipe file.
- Review the three main purposes of a filing system.
- Review the five most common filing systems.

Apply It

- Allow students time in class to create the filing system, and discuss the different ways that the files could be organized.

TEAMWORK

Work in groups of five or six. Distribute copies of different client information forms obtained from different health care facilities. Ask each group to compare the forms, noting similarities and differences. Then, have each group design their own form, and create a presentation marketing the new form. Deliver the presentations to the class.

Figure Focus

9.15 A filing system must be followed carefully so that the correct files can be retrieved when needed. Barcodes can help make retrieval more efficient.

Point out how the filing system uses visual and sorting cues so that specific files can be identified.

Teaching Tips

- Review the four basic filing procedures:
  - Sorting, which may be alphabetical, numerical, color-coded, or geographic.
  - Coding, which identifies items belonging to a certain category, such as surgery or laboratory.
  - Indexing, which places items in the order in which they are filed.
  - Storing or filing, which places a large number of items in a system that allows for easy retrieval.
- Introduce the Alphabetical Filing System.

Figure 9.15
A filing system must be followed carefully so that the correct files can be retrieved when needed. Barcodes can help make retrieval more efficient. How?

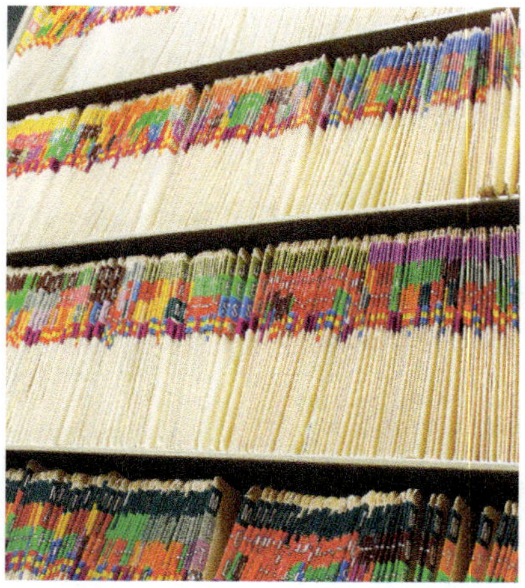

Each filing system involves the same basic procedures:

- Sorting
- Coding
- Indexing
- Storing or filing

sorting
(SAWR ting)
Separating items to be filed according to the filing system being used, such as alphabetical, numerical, color, chronological, and geographical.

coding
(KOH ding)
Identifying items to be filed according to particular categories, such as surgical or laboratory.

indexing
(IN deks sing)
Organizing items in the order they are to be filed.

Sorting is the placement of each item according to the particular filing system you are using. Alphabetical sorting requires placing all items with the same letters together. Numerical sorting requires placing all items with the same numbers together. Color sorting requires placing all items with the same colors together. Chronological sorting requires placing all items with the same dates together. Geographical sorting requires placing all items from the same region together.

Coding identifies items that belong to a certain category. For example, surgical files may be assigned a number or letter to identify them as separate from laboratory files.

Indexing organizes items in the order in which they are filed. The American Medical Records Management Association has established rules that provide guidelines for indexing items.

Alphabetical System

The alphabetical system is simple and economical, and it is the most common method for filing records. This system follows the order of the alphabet.

224 Chapter 9 | Effective Communication

TEAMWORK

Play charades. After the game, discuss how being unable to communicate verbally makes it harder to get your message across. Discuss methods you used to communicate, such as hand signals and facial expressions. Discuss feelings of frustration and annoyance when you could not understand, or be understood.

Sorting

To set up an alphabetical filing system, place all charts with the same first letter of the last name together (all *As*, all *Bs*, and so on):

Cruz
Culver
Masters
Mendoza
Puertas
Putnam
Samuelsen
Samuelson

When there is more than one chart that begins with the same letter, alphabetize by the second, third, fourth letters (or as many as necessary). The boldface letters in the following list determine the file's placement in an alphabetical listing:

Cruz
Culver
Masters
Mendoza
Puertas
Putnam
Samuelsen
Samuelson

Coding

If your files are separated by a code, place all As with the same code together, all Bs with the same code together, and so on. Some systems do not separate coded files. In files that are not separated, the codes identify specific things. For example, an office may have several doctors, and each doctor may be identified by a different color. All charts can be filed together, or they can be separated, depending on the office procedure.

Indexing

Make three columns on a page and label the columns 1, 2, and 3. When filing by name, place the last name in the column labeled 1, the first name in the column labeled 2, and the middle name or initial in the column labeled 3. For example, if the name is Alec Monroe Goldman, it is indexed as:

1	2	3
Goldman	Alec	Monroe

It is important to label charts by this indexing method. This makes placing them in order a simple task.

Effective Communication | Chapter 9 225

Teaching Tips

- Explain the alphabetical filing system.
- Use the telephone book as an example.
- Make sure students understand how to use the second, third, and even fourth letter in the sort.
- Display short lists of words or names and work together as a class to put them in alphabetical order.
- Review the concepts of coding and indexing to differentiate them from basic sorting.
- Make sure students understand what is meant by coding. Explain that many facilities add a code to the patient's name for organizational purposes.
- Make sure students understand why they might index a filing system.
- Have students practice indexing different names, including some with abbreviations, initials, apostrophes, and titles.

ACTIVITY

Provide a random list of names for students to alphabetize. For extra credit, ask students to index the names as well.

Teaching Tips

- Review the different indexing rules.
- Emphasize that these rules are designed to cover all potential situations.
- Discussing methods of storing and filing.
- Review the explanation of using the first letter of the first name to indicate the sequence for filing.

TEAMWORK

Split the class into groups of five or six. Have the students in each group stand and arrange themselves in alphabetical order. Have all the students merge into one group, and arrange themselves into alphabetical order.

Charts with initials instead of a first name are placed before spelled-out names. C. Todd Sherman is indexed as:

1	2	3
Sherman	C.	Todd

Names that are hyphenated are considered one name, as if the hyphen were not there. For example, Kellie Bell-White is indexed as:

1	2	3
Bell-White	Kellie	

Apostrophes are ignored when indexing, so Timothy Gallagher O'Bannon is indexed as:

1	2	3
OBannon	Timothy	Gallagher

Last names with prefixes are joined as one name, so Carlos A. De Leon is indexed as:

1	2	3
DeLeon	Carlos	A.

Abbreviated names are indexed as if they were spelled out in full. For example, St. Gustov Edward is indexed as Gustov Saint Edward, or:

1	2	3
Edward	Gustov	(Saint)

If a title precedes one name or a given name and a middle name, the title is the first indexing number. Father Gerald Rahn, Queen Erin, and Princess Monica are indexed as:

1	2	3
Gerald	Rahn	(Father)
Erin	(Queen)	
Monica	(Princess)	

Titles and degrees before or after a complete name are placed in parentheses after the name for identification. For example, Dr. DeeAnn Marie Sherman or DeeAnn Marie Sherman, M.D., is indexed as:

1	2	3
Sherman	DeeAnn	Marie (Dr.)
Sherman	DeeAnn	Marie (M.D.)

Store or File

Place files in alphabetical order for easy retrieval. Place the names in order by looking for the first letter that is different, indicating the sequence. For example, Gallagher, Kevin DeWayne, is filed before Gallagher, Shaun Patrick Michael, because the *K* in Kevin comes before the *S* in Shaun.

Numerical System

The numerical system is another simple way of maintaining client/patient charts. Use a notebook or computer to record the number assigned to each client/patient.

This allows you to find the client/patient name by the assigned number. The assigned number is often referred to as a medical record number or patient/client number.

- Assigned numbers are placed in numerical order.
- Assign each new patient/client a number (for example, 001, 002, 003).

Keep a log in a notebook or computer of the client/patient name and number as you assign them. This record must be **accessible** to all staff. For example, assign numbers as follows:

accessible
(ak SES uh buhl)
Available to obtain.

File Number	Client/Patient Name
001	Mendoza
002	Samuelsen
003	Putnam
004	Puertas
005	Masters
006	Culver
007	Cruz
008	Samuelson

Terminal Digits

Numbers can indicate many different things. Grouping by **terminal** digits means that you group items according to the last few digits of their assigned number (for example, 432.80, 321.80 or 879.90, 320.90). The terminal digits in these examples are 80 and 90, so all the 80s are filed in order by the first three digits, and all the 90s are filed in the same fashion (for example, 321.80, 432.80 and 320.90, 879.90). Let's pretend that you have items that need to be filed according to their assigned number. First sort these items by grouping all the same number of digits together (for example, all two-digit numbers together, all three-digit numbers together). These are basic rules to follow:

terminal
(TUR muh nl)
Last or ending.

- When zeros precede numbers, ignore them. Zeros are often added to numbers because computers call for a specific number of digits in a space. For example, the sequence 0001, 0935, 0087 is filed 0001, 0087, 0935. Because you ignore zeros before numbers when filing, you sort 0001 as a one-digit number, 0087 as having two digits, and 0935 as having three digits.

Effective Communication | Chapter 9 227

Teaching Tips

- Explain the numerical filing system.
- Point out that the numbers should always be assigned in order, and that skipping a number may lead to confusion.
- Ask students why a numerical system might start with 001, and not just 1.
- Emphasize that using a numerical system may be more reliable than using an alphabetical system, because names may be the same, but each assigned number will be unique.
- Explain terminal digits.
- Review the basic rules for using terminal digits.

ACTIVITY

Provide a random list of names that have been assigned numbers. Ask students to arrange them numerically for filing.

Teaching Tips

- Explain the color coding filing system.
- Explain the chronological filing system.
- Explain the geographical filing system.

ACTIVITY

Provide a random list of names and addresses. Ask students to arrange them geographically for filing.

- Coding is often done by the terminal-digit method. Take the last digits of the assigned numbers and group together all those that are the same. File in ascending order within these groupings. For example, 546.10, 386.30, 957.10, and 752.30 are grouped with all numbers ending with 10 together and all numbers ending with 30 together (546.10, 957.10, 386.30, 752.30).
- Indexing places items in ascending numerical order within their groups. For example, 546.10 and 957.10 are in one group, and 386.30 and 752.30 form another group.
- Place files according to their numerical order.

Color-Coding System

Color coding helps reduce the chance of filing errors. The following are guidelines for using this method:

1. Assign a color sticker to each letter of the alphabet (for example, blue is *A*, yellow is *B*, green is *C*).
2. Determine how many stickers to apply on a patient's/client's chart (depending on chart size). *Example:* If you use three colors on the chart and the client's/patient's name is Mr. Gates, place the stickers in the order that corresponds to the first three letters of the patient's/client's last name (for example, *G* is yellow, *A* is blue, and *T* is purple).
3. Place the color stickers on the side of the chart that faces out when filed.

Chronological System

Chronological filing arranges files in the order of their occurrence, usually by day. This method is most often used in storing research items. Because each day, month, and year can be referred to by number, it is easy to follow the basic numerical system:

1. Sort by placing all items of the same year together.
2. Code each item as in any filing system.
3. Index by placing all files of the same month and year together.
4. File each item by date within the appropriate month and year grouping.

Geographical System

Geographical filing is done according to location. This method is often used for storing records of research studies in specific geographical areas. File alphabetically according to the name of the state, then alphabetically according to the city. File in the following manner:

- Alphabetically according to the state name
- Alphabetically according to the city name
- Alphabetically according to the names of companies

228 Chapter 9 | Effective Communication

CUSTOMIZED INSTRUCTION

Less Advanced Students

Less advanced students may need to spend additional time becoming comfortable with the different types of filing systems. Provide lists or folders that they can use to practice all of the systems.

Whichever filing method you use, follow the basic rules for filing under the appropriate system. The following is an example of filing by company name:

Company Name	City	State
A.G. Corporation	Mills	Illinois
Blosson Inc.	Lakewood	California
Gamble Corporation	Reno	Nevada
General Corporation	Redlands	California
K.G. Inc.	Lakes	Utah
K.M.B. Corp.	Mills	Illinois
M.M. General	Lakewood	California
M.W.G. Corporation	Great Lakes	Florida
Water Inc.	Silverton	Illinois\

The following items are alphabetized by state and city:

State	City	Company Name
California	Lakewood	Blosson Inc.
California	Lakewood	M.M. General
California	Redlands	General Corp.
Florida	Great Lakes	M.W.G. Corp.
Illinois	Mills	A.G. Corp.
Illinois	Mills	K.M.B. Corp.
Illinois	Silverton	Water Inc.
Nevada	Reno	Gamble Corp.
Utah	Lakes	K.G. Inc.

Summary

Scheduling patients is an important part of a well-run medical facility. Appointments for office visits, procedures, and diagnostic tests may be scheduled manually in an appointment book, or on a computer system. When a patient arrives for an appointment, information must be gathered and recorded on client/patient information forms and medical history forms. Follow up appointments by scheduling future appointments and placing appropriate information in a tickler file for further follow-up. Medical records are kept according to a specific filing systems that may be alphabetic, numerical, color coding, chronological, or geographic. Proper filing ensures that patient information can be found when it is needed.

Section 9.5 Review Questions

1. List the ten guidelines for scheduling office visits.
2. Explain what a tickler file is and how it is used.
3. Name the two forms that new patients/clients must complete upon registering.
4. What are the five most common filing systems?
5. List the guidelines for scheduling surgeries/procedures.
6. What are the functions of a filing system?

Effective Communication | Chapter 9 229

Teaching Tips

- Review the list of filing by company name.
- Point out that even though the first record is from Illinois, it is filed ahead of the records from California and Florida because the sort is based on the company name.
- Review the list of items files by state and city.
- Note that the record from Lakewood, California is filed ahead of the one from Redlands, California.
- Ask students why a geographical filing system might not be efficient for filing patient records in a dentist's office. (Most people who use the dentist live nearby.)
- Make sure students understand the review questions, and know where to look for more information.

Section 9.5 Review Questions

1. Answer:
   - A patient/client visit is scheduled every 15 minutes, 30 minutes, or hourly, depending on your provider's specialty.
   - Learn to recognize the patients/clients who require more time with the provider.
   - Always ask the purpose of the appointment to allocate enough time for the visit.
   - Ask the patient/client what would be the most convenient time for an appointment.
   - If you are not able to schedule the patient/client at the time and date requested, express regret and ask for a second choice.
   - Ask for a phone number where the patient/client can be reached during the day in case a cancellation is necessary.

1. *(continued)*
   - Offer to call the client/patient as cancellations occur if the patient/client desires an earlier appointment. Use a tickler file as a reminder.
   - Always repeat the appointment time and date to the patient/client to avoid confusion.
   - When a patient/client cancels an appointment, note the date, time, and reason for the cancellation in the chart.
   - Give all patients/clients appointment cards when scheduling a follow-up visit.
2. Answer: A tickler file is a special file kept to remind you of tasks that need to be done at a certain time by day, by week, or by month. A tickler file is used to send out appointment reminder cards to patients.
3. Answer: The two forms are the client/patient information form and medical history form.
4. Answer: The most common filing systems are alphabetical, numerical, color coding, chronological, and geographic.

5. Answer:
   - Determine how long each procedure takes.
   - Learn how to schedule patients/clients around these procedures.
   - Establish what days and times your provider prefers to do surgeries.
   - Learn the admitting procedure for the hospital where your provider performs surgery.
   - Provide the patient/client with the surgery time, when the patient needs to arrive at the office/hospital, registration instructions, direction to the hospital, written instructions to follow prior to surgery, and maintain good lines of communication with the office personnel.
6. Answer: Store information and records safely, keep related materials together, and retrieve files quickly when needed.

CHAPTER 9 REVIEW

Chapter Review Questions

1. Why is it important to recognize prejudices and biases? (9.1)
2. What are some ways you can exhibit good listening skills? (9.1)
3. Name three communication objectives you should have when talking on the telephone with a client. (9.2)
4. List three items you should include when writing a professional e-mail. (9.2)
5. How might a computer be used in a medical or dental office? (9.3)
6. How can you protect you and your patient when working with computers? (9.3)
7. Name the senses you should use when observing a patient. (9.4)
8. Explain why documentation of a client's/patient's care is needed. (9.4)
9. What information should be included on a medical history form? (9.5)
10. What are the four basic procedures common to each filing system? (9.5)
11. Identify components of non-effective communications and list three possible corrections. (9.1)
12. List three effective skills to use when communicating with a child, a peer, and an older person. List the skills in order of importance, and then evaluate and analyze how each communication skill contributes to maintaining a healthy relationship at each stage of the life span. (9.1)

Activities

1. How would you explain to a new employee the legal importance of clear, concise, and complete documentation? Create a bulleted list of points to be made. Present your points to the class, making sure you clearly articulate your understanding and comprehension of written documentation and how it is used in the medical community as well as in a court of law.
2. Select one of the career pathways. Use the Internet to research the pathway. Once you are done with your research, write a brief report on what you have learned, including required skills, certification, licensure, academic requirements, and continuing education requirements. Research starting salaries for careers in this pathway. If you have e-mail access, send an e-mail to your instructor with the report as an attachment. Remember to follow guidelines for writing a professional e-mail.
3. Identify one technological equipment and research its use for each of the following health care systems. Briefly describe the purpose of the equipment:

   a. Diagnostic systems
   Name of Equipment________________
   Use and Purpose________________
   ____

   b. Therapeutic systems
   Name of Equipment________________
   Use and Purpose________________
   ____

   c. Health Informatics systems
   Name of Equipment________________
   Use and Purpose________________
   ____

   d. Support Services systems
   Name of Equipment________________
   Use and Purpose________________
   ____

   e. Biotech Research and Development systems
   Name of Equipment________________
   Use and Purpose________________
   ____

230 Chapter 9 | Effective Communication

CHAPTER 9 REVIEW

Chapter Review Questions

1. Answer: It is important to recognize prejudices and biases because your feelings affect how you communicate.
2. Answer: Show interest, hear the message, don't interrupt, pay attention, and maintain a positive attitude.
3. Answer:
   - Demonstrate open, honest, and respectful communication.
   - Present ideas, information, and viewpoints clearly both verbally and in writing.
   - Listen actively and seek to understand others.
4. Answer:
   - Begin with a salutation.
   - Include short, simple, and straightforward information. If a message is really long, discuss the topic in a short e-mail, and use an attachment to provide details.
   - Read your e-mail aloud to check the tone of your message.
   - Proof the content for spelling and grammar mistakes.
   - Remember to include important contact information at the end of your e-mail.
   - Insert a subject into the subject line of the e-mail.
   - Use features such as blind carbon copy (bcc) and carbon copy (cc) when appropriate.
5. Answer: Computers can be used to schedule appointments, set up a recall system, bill patients, schedule lab work, dial the telephone, manage the security system, and keep the inventory.
6. Answer: Keep your identification code or password confidential to protect you and the patient.
7. Answer: You use the senses of sight, hearing, touch, and smell.
8. Answer: This record provides the information needed to allow each health care provider to give the care that best benefits the patient. Each health care worker who cares for the patient makes a notation on the chart. This documentation is admissible in a court of law.
9. Answer: Information that should be included on a medical history form includes previous surgeries, allergies, chronic illness, medications taken, general medical history, and childhood diseases.

CHAPTER 9 REVIEW

4. You are working as a medical assistant in a medical office that is located in an area where many of the patients do not have English as their primary language. To ensure a clear understanding of the processes and procedures that will be provided, it will be helpful to formulate a list of questions in the language native to the patients and formulate responses using precise language to communicate directions that are common at the close of the appointment. Create a list of 10 questions and 10 possible responses that will follow the appointment. The class may select to prepare a booklet for use by local health care professionals with the primary language native to the community. Working with a partner, role play how you would communicate medical information accurately and efficiently to a patient whose primary language is not English. Practice expressing ideas in a clear, concise, and effective manner.
5. Research common document formats, both paper and electronic, for taking a patient's medical or dental history. Using industry-based standards, choose one and record your own history.
6. Practice therapeutic communication with a classmate by having them pretend to be a patient in despair. Use the communication strategies you have learned in this chapter—both verbal and nonverbal—to help them through their circumstances. Once you feel comfortable with these techniques, imagine how you would change your strategy if you had a patient dealing with sensory loss.
7. Imagine that you are a nurse reaching the end of your shift. You are excited to go home and get ready for a dinner you had planned with your friends weeks ago. Your supervisor has just asked you to stay another four hours. Practice communicating your needs, wants, and emotions to your supervisor by role-playing different strategies with a classmate.

Case Studies

1. There are many ways in which technology helps health care workers in a clinical setting send and receive information. You are describing the functions of the telephone, fax, e-mail system, and the Internet to a new employee. How would you illustrate the proper use and appropriate etiquette of each of these tools? How would you explain the protocol for identifying and reporting equipment or technology failures?
2. You are in the process of completing your internship as a paramedic, and during your ride-along the unit has been called to a school site accident. It has been raining for a number of days and the roof of the gymnasium has collapsed, trapping students under the stands and injuring several that were in the top row. You are asked to assist with triage but find as you try to determine types and levels of injuries that many of the students only speak Spanish and you do not understand what they are trying to tell you. You are very concerned about non-effective communications leading to potential harm to the students. How should you react?
3. The health care facility where you are employed uses a Personal Health Record (PHR) system for making appointments, reporting test results, and sending appointment reminders. As the Electronic Health Records Specialist you are responsible for distributing this information. Several patients have called asking for the date of their next appointment. Since the information is not appearing on the PHR you consider the possibility of a technology or equipment malfunction. Recognize and explain the process for reporting the technology malfunction. If it should be the equipment rather than the technology, recognize and explain the process for reporting the equipment malfunction.

Effective Communication | Chapter 9 231

10. Answer:
    - Sorting
    - Coding
    - Indexing
    - Storing or filing
11. Refer students to the paragraph on page 186 to locate the three components to select for corrections. Answers will vary.
12. Student answers will vary.

Activities

1. Direct students to write an introductory paragraph explaining what they plan to do, and then write the bulleted list.
2. If you do not have access to e-mail, have the students handwrite the message as they would if they were typing it on a computer.
3. Student research will vary. Students will need to choose technological equipment for each health care system listed. Once the equipment item is selected the students can go online to find the use and purpose, contact the manufacturer, or interview a health care professional that uses the equipment.
4. Ask the students as a class to brainstorm questions they may have been asked when going to a medical or dental appointment, e.g., are you in pain? Or contact a medical/clinical assistant to visit the class and share the typical questions asked of new patients. Also make a list of the types of instructions given following the appointment. Ask students to locate someone either at the school (maybe a student in the class) or at the local hospital that speaks the native language common to the community to review the corresponding language the students generated.
5. Caution students on privacy and what information they should not include for this assignment. You can then have them compare different formats.
6. Ask the students how sensory loss made this more challenging. What other conditions could impair communication? Have the students discuss strategies for dealing with patients with dementia or mental health issues.
7. This is also a good opportunity to discuss work-life balance and have them reflect on their personal priorities.

Case Studies

1. Refer students to Table 9.2 on p. 197 for information specific to this situation.
2. The student answers may vary but should include at least requesting assistance from someone that is fluent in Spanish to interpret, preferably on the medical team members. You might also suggest as an extra credit assignment that students prepare a language guide for emergency use with questions in both English and Spanish.
3. Suggest students interview a department representative at the local hospital for computer set-up and maintenance or a local medical or dental office to determine the process they use for reporting both technology and equipment malfunctions.

Thinking Critically

1. Students should write a personal essay for this, including a thesis statement supported by facts or real-life examples.
2. Direct students to create a table for listing the pluses and minuses. They should write an explanation of the problems in paragraph form. Note that this assignment could be added to the student's portfolio.
3. Refer students to the section on Effective Patient Relations and Communication Skills starting on p. 185 for related information.

ACTIVITY

Create a two-column chart or table. In column one, list health care occupations. In column two, list all of the people that each worker must communicate with in a single day.

Portfolio Connection

- You may want to build a library of books related to communications and assertiveness to have available in the classroom.
- This activity requires self-analysis and evaluation. Direct students to be honest and sincere when identifying the way they communicate.
- Point out that most people use all types of communication methods at one point or another.
- If they struggle to think of experiences that demonstrate different methods of communicating, suggest that the way they communicate might depend on who they are communicating with, and how.

CHAPTER 9 REVIEW

Thinking Critically

1. **Communication**—Describe a recent event in which you or someone else did not use good listening skills. Explain what you or the person you observed could have done differently to demonstrate good listening skills in that situation.
2. **Time Management**—Have you ever thought of good communication as a time saver? Write down the pluses and minuses of taking time to communicate properly. Describe in writing some problems that are caused by failure to communicate properly. Put this list in the personal section of your portfolio to remind you why you should speak with care.
3. **Patient Education**—Explain how you know when patients/clients understand and can do what you have instructed them to do.

Portfolio Connection

The ability to communicate effectively is essential to successful interactions with others. Your decision to develop effective communication skills directly affects your success or failure in the work world. Your experience in a health science education program is the perfect place to focus on developing assertive communication skills.

There are many easy-to-read books on assertiveness training that are helpful in learning about and practicing assertiveness. Go to your local library or resource center, and select and read a book that teaches assertive communication skills.

Identify your most common and least common communication type (unassertive, assertive, aggressive). Think of three recent experiences that demonstrate your use of unassertive or aggressive communication. What caused you to respond the way you did? What could you have done or said that would have made your responses assertive? What was the outcome of the unassertive or aggressive communication?

PORTFOLIO TIP

How you deliver your message in both words and body language may be more important than the message itself: it may decide whether your audience is willing to listen. Think before you speak.

Values can be reflected in your body language and your verbal responses. What kind of body language shows that you are kind?

Explain your answer for all three experiences by writing a short paper. Your explanation must clearly identify the unassertive or aggressive statements or actions, indicate what you would change to create an assertive, effective communication, and compare the expected results with those of the unassertive or aggressive communication.

This assignment helps you evaluate the effectiveness of your most frequently used communication skill and allows you to express it in writing. Assertive written communication skills reflect your ability to communicate effectively in the health care environment. Your ability to demonstrate this skill in your portfolio presents you as an appropriate candidate for higher education or job opportunities. Place this assignment in the "Written Samples" section of your portfolio.

232 Chapter 9 | Effective Communication

- For example, they might be more aggressive with a sibling, more assertive with a peer, and more unassertive with a parent or teacher.
- Check to make sure that students have completed the written assignments and added them to their portfolio.

ACTIVITY

Write a personal essay about a negative attitude that has affected you in your life. It may be an attitude you have directed at someone, or one directed at you. Include ways you could have turned the negative experience into a positive one.

PART II Health Care Knowledge and Skills

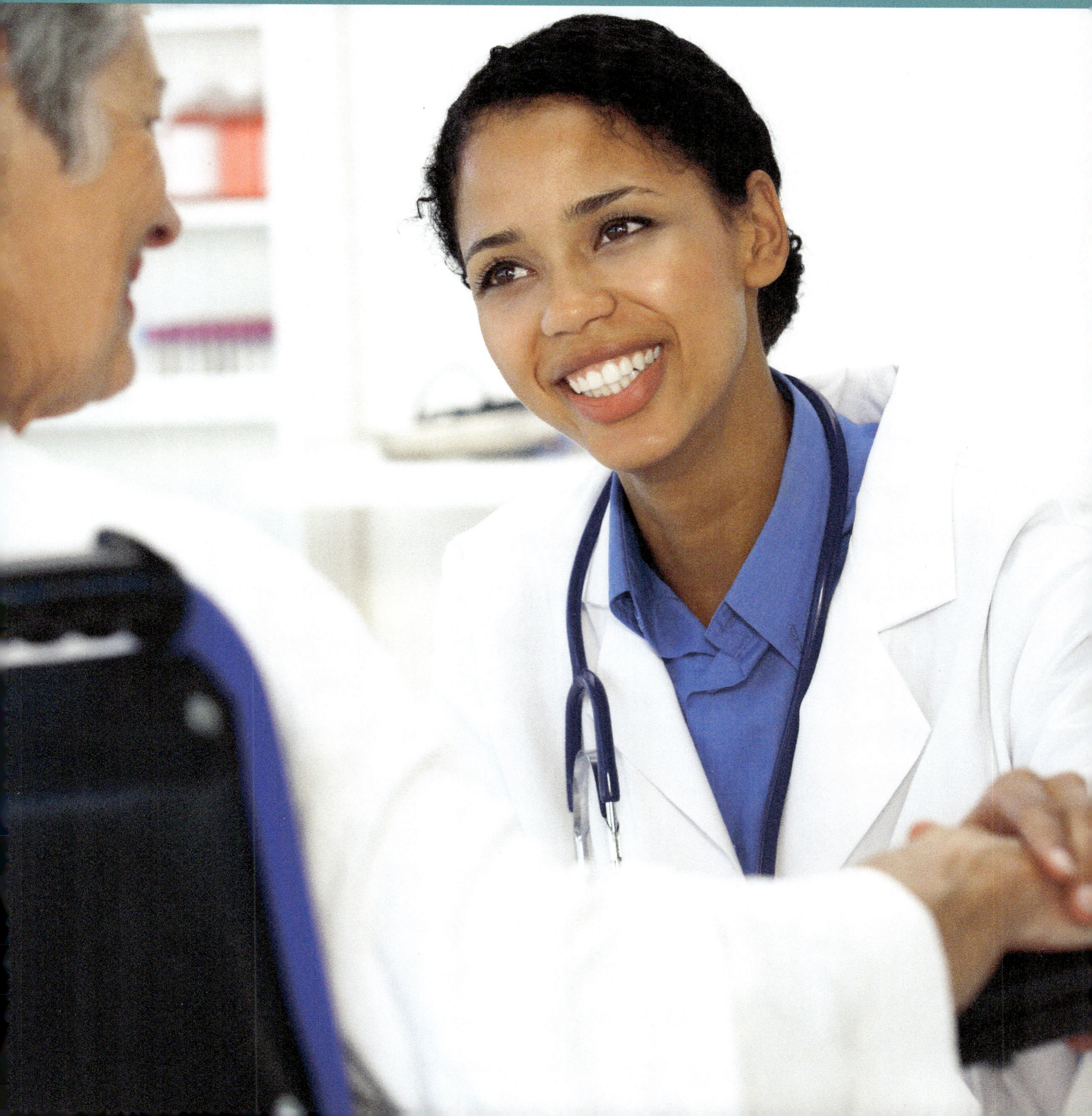

10 Medical Terminology

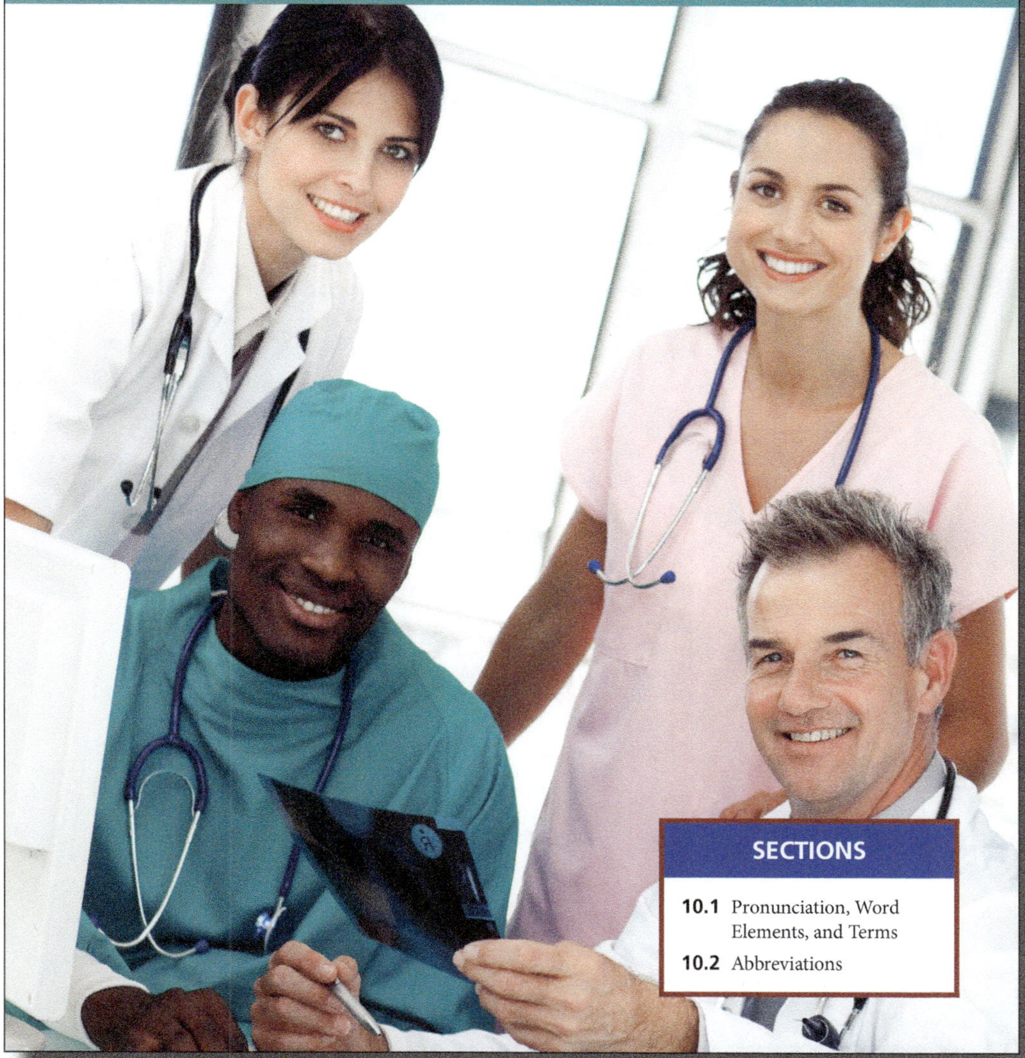

SECTIONS

10.1 Pronunciation, Word Elements, and Terms

10.2 Abbreviations

CHAPTER 10 OVERVIEW

Health care professionals really do have a language all their own. Recognizing and understanding medical terminology is a must for anyone working in a health care facility. Chapter 10 teaches students how to pronounce, identify word elements, and define medical terms and abbreviations.

Section 10.1: Section 10.1 introduces the roots, prefixes, and suffixes used to build medical terms. It covers correct pronunciation and provides definitions for numerous medical terms. It also provides the tools students will need to decipher unfamiliar terms.

Section 10.2: Section 10.2 lists common medical abbreviations.

Advance Preparation	
Review	■ Chapter text for Sections 10.1 and 10.2.
Contact	■ Health care facilities to request materials that include health care terminology, such as care plans or charts.
Prepare	■ Index cards for use as flashcards. ■ Medical dictionaries for use in the classroom. ■ A list of Web sites that provide definitions of medical terms—such as fda.com, dana-faber.org/can/dictionary, and medterms.com. ■ Web sites that list common English language word elements—such as PrefixSuffix.com and betterendings.org.

FOCUS AND ENGAGE

Getting Started

- This activity is designed to help students identify and interpret medical terminology used in context.
- You may want to use the activity before starting the chapter, and then repeat it at the end of the chapter so students can see how much they have learned.

Introduce the Section

a. Review the content of the Background paragraph, explaining that medical terminology is the language used by health care professionals.
b. Emphasize the importance of understanding medical terms, and knowing how to decipher unfamiliar terms.
c. Review the section objectives.

Vocabulary Review

a. Direct students to the key terms.
b. Pronounce each word, and have the students repeat the pronunciation out loud.
c. Discuss each definition.

TEACH

Discuss

- Explain that learning medical terminology is similar to learning a new language.
- Discuss that medical terminology is the language health care workers use to communicate about their work.

Reinforce and Review

- Review the importance of communication for health care professionals.

Teaching Tips

- Introduce the topic of medical terminology.

Getting Started

Health care practices and procedures require a special vocabulary that could be considered a second language. Using a list of common medical terms provided by the teacher, watch a health-care related television program and circle all of the words that are used by the actors. Define the words that you circled and share with the class in a discussion following the activity. Also discuss whether the medical terms in the program were used accurately.

SECTION 10.1 Pronunciation, Word Elements, and Terms

Background

Health care workers use medical terminology in their work every day. It is the professional language that helps them communicate effectively and quickly. All caregivers use medical terminology to record orders, write instructions, take notes, and to chart. Health care workers are unable to perform their job if they cannot use and understand medical terminology.

Objectives

When you have completed this section, you will be able to do the following:

- Match key terms with their correct meanings.
- Define roots, prefixes, and suffixes.
- Define the word elements listed.
- Divide medical terms into elements.
- Combine word elements to form medical terms.

Introduction to Medical Terminology

terminology
(ter muh NOL uh jee)
Specialized terms used in any occupation.

Medical **terminology** can be fun, interesting, and challenging. At first medical terminology may seem hard to learn—it's like learning a new language. However, with practice it becomes easier and easier. You need to learn how to build a medical term, how to pronounce it, and what it means. This section gives you the tools that you need to learn and understand medical terms.

236 Chapter 10 | Medical Terminology

CUSTOMIZED INSTRUCTION
Special Needs Students
Students who have speech disabilities may have trouble pronouncing medical terms and abbreviations. Send a list of terms to their speech therapists so they can practice with proper supervision.

CUSTOMIZED INSTRUCTION OVERVIEW	
Less Advanced Students	Pages 238, 245
More Advanced Students	Pages 245, 249
English Language Learners	Pages 237, 247
Special Needs Students	Pages 236, 246
At-Risk Students	Pages 240, 251

Pronunciation

If you have never heard medical terms pronounced, they may seem very difficult. To make it easier for you, the following are some hints to help you pronounce the terms correctly:

- **ch** sounds like *k*
  Examples: chyme (kīm), cholecystectomy (kō-lə-sis-tek′-tō-mē), chronic (kro-nic), chondroid (kon′-droyd)
- **ps** sounds like *s*
  Examples: psychiatric (sī-kē-a′-trik), pseudomonas (sū-dō-mō′-nas), psychology (sī-kol′-ō-ji), psoriasis (sō-rī′-a-sis)
- **pn** sounds like *n*
  Examples: pneumonia (nū-mō′-ni-a), pneumatic (nū-mat′-ik)
- **c** sounds like a soft *s* when it comes before *e*, *i*, and *y*
  Examples: cycle (sī-kl), cytoplasm (sī′-tō-plazm), cisternal (sis-ter′-nal), centrifuge (sen′-tri-fūj)
- **g** sounds like *j* when it comes before *e*, *i*, and *y*
  Examples: giant (jī′-ent), gestation (jes-tā′-shun), generic (jen-er′-ik), gyration (jī-rā′-shun)
- **i** sounds like *eye* when added to the end of the word to form a plural
  Examples: glomeruli (glō-mer′-ū-lī), villi (vil′-lī), alveoli (al-vē′-ō-lī), bacilli (ba-sil′-lī)

Forming Medical Terms from Word Elements

Medical terms are words that consist of several parts. All medical terms have a word root. Most medical terms have the word root and a prefix, a combining vowel, and a suffix. In some cases, the word has only a prefix or suffix added to the root. When you add different prefixes and suffixes to the word root, you change the meaning of the medical term. The combining vowel makes the word easier to pronounce. You build a large medical term vocabulary when you learn the meanings of word parts and how to combine them. (**Figure 10.1**)

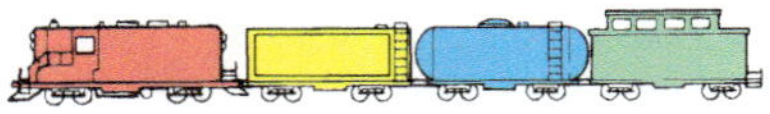

Figure 10.1 Prefix–Root–Root–Suffix. How is a prefix different from a suffix?

- The *word root* is the main part of the word and tells what the word is about. For instance, *cardio* is the root word that means "heart." This is the subject of the word you are going to build.
- The *prefix* is a word element added to the beginning of a word root. The prefix is added to the root to change the meaning or to make it more specific. The prefix *electro* means "pertaining to electricity."

Medical Terminology | Chapter 10 237

Teaching Tips

- Ask students why they think medical terminology is important.
- Point out that medical terminology is concise and exacting. It is vital to be able to distinguish between closely related words.
- Review the pronunciation of the letter sounds.
- Pronounce each sound, and ask the students to repeat the sound out loud.
- Explain word elements, and the basics of word construction:
  - Prefix
  - Root
  - Suffix

Figure Focus

10.1 Prefix–Root–Root–Suffix. How is a prefix different from a suffix?

Answer: A prefix is added to the beginning of a root while a suffix is added to the end of a root. Both prefixes and suffixes change the meaning of the root word.

ACTIVITY

Medical terms are not the only words comprised of word elements. Find ten regular English words that use word elements. Create a chart or table listing the word, its individual elements, and their meanings. Examples include words based on the root *arch*, meaning "chief" or "leader," such as *archangel*, *monarch*, and *archaic*; or *bio*, meaning "life," such as *biography*, *antibiotic*, and *autobiography*.

CUSTOMIZED INSTRUCTION

English Language Learners

Allow students extra time to read through and review Section 10.1. Have students work with a partner to pronounce each of the sounds and examples listed in the "Pronunciation" section.

Figure Focus

10.2 Prefix—Root–Combining vowel–Suffix. What is the role of the combining vowel in the word shown?

Answer: The combining vowel makes it possible to combine several word roots and makes it easier to pronounce the word.

Teaching Tips

- Ask students why they think medical terminology is important.
- Point out that medical terminology is concise and exacting. It is vital to be able to distinguish between closely related words.
- Point out that word elements are like pieces of a puzzle that fit together to create a complete word.
- Emphasize that if students understand the word elements they can decode the terms.
- Emphasize that knowing the rules for combining word elements makes it easier to decode the meaning of the medical terms quickly and accurately.
- Explain that the combining vowels separate the word elements, and help make the terms easier to pronounce.
- Review the rules for combining vowels, emphasizing the examples.
- If students have not yet learned the meaning of the elements used in the examples, ask them to try to decipher the meanings based on the definition of the entire term.
- For example, using the term aden/o/pathy (disease of the glands) they should be able to determine that *aden* means glands, that *o* is the combining vowel, and that *pathy* means disease.

- The *suffix* is an element added to the end of the word root that changes or adds to the meaning of the root. The suffix *gram* means "record."
- The *combining vowel* makes it possible to combine several word roots. It also makes the word easier to pronounce. (Figure 10.2)

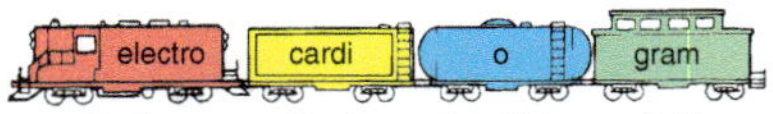

Figure 10.2
Prefix—Root–Combining vowel–Suffix. What is the role of the combining vowel in the word shown?

When all the previous word elements are combined, the word is *electrocardiogram* (electro/cardi/o/gram). It means "an electrical record of the heart."

The following are some examples of (common) English words (Figure 10.3):

Combining Word Elements

Prefix	Root	Suffix	Word
pre	heat	ing	preheating
	gentle	ness	gentleness
	speed	o/meter	speedometer

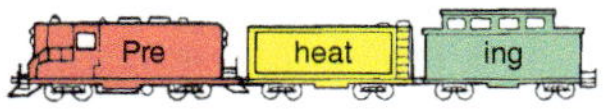

Figure 10.3
Prefix–Root–Suffix. What is the prefix and suffix in the word "Preheating"?

Rules for Combining Word Elements

Rules help make medical terminology easier to learn. When everyone uses the rules, there are fewer mistakes. A mistake in combining a word can change its meaning and cause confusion.

Combining Vowels

- The combining vowel is usually an *o*, for example, *oste/o*. Oste means "bone," and the *o* is the combining vowel. The *o* can be added to join a word root with another word root or a suffix. Sometimes an *i*, *y*, or *u* is used. Combining vowels make it easier to pronounce the term. For example, *osteomyelitis* is easier to pronounce than *ostemyelitis*.
- When the suffix begins with one of the vowels (*a*, *e*, *i*, *o*, *u*), the *o* on the root word is not used. Since *oste/o* ends in *o* and the suffix *-itis* begins with a vowel, the *o* is dropped. The word is *osteitis*, which means "inflammation of the bone."
- The combining vowel is placed between root words, for example, *osteoporosis* (oste/o/por/osis). Pronounce the word with the combining vowel, and you can tell that it is easier to say than *osteporosis*.

238 Chapter 10 | Medical Terminology

Figure Focus

10.3 Prefix–Root–Suffix. What is the prefix and suffix in the word "Preheating"?

Answer: The prefix is *pre-*, which means "before" or "in front of" and the suffix is *-ing*, which means to create an action or process out of preheat.

CUSTOMIZED INSTRUCTION

Less Advanced Students

To help less advanced students grasp the concept of word elements, have them draw posters illustrating medical terms. They should include the term and its word elements on the posters. Display the posters in the classroom or on a bulletin board.

The following words are examples of word elements that have been combined to form a medical term:

aden/o/pathy	disease of the glands
hepat/o/rrhagia	hemorrhage of the liver
poly/arthr/it is	inflammation of many joints
hyster/ectomy	surgical removal of the uterus
hyster/o/salping/ectomy	surgical removal of the uterus and fallopian tubes
oste/o/por/osis	condition of pores in the bone

After you learn the roots, prefixes, and suffixes, you can combine many word parts to form medical terminology. There is always at least one root word, and there may be more than one root word. When you add a prefix or a suffix you create a new word.

Changing Words from Singular to Plural

- Use the rule for changing words from singular to plural that applies to the language the word comes from; for example, the English word *wavelength* adds an *-s* to become *wavelengths*.
- Since many medical terms come from Greek or Latin, use the following rules for Greek or Latin words:
  - Add an *-e* to a word ending in *-a*—for example, *axilla* to *axillae*.
  - Drop the *-ax* at the end of a word and add *-aces*—for example, *thorax* to *thoraces*.
  - Change the *-x* to *-g* in a word that ends in *-nx* and add *-es*—for example, *phalanx* to *phalanges*.
  - Drop *-ix* or *-ex* at the end of the word and add *-ices*—for example, *appendix* to *appendices*.
  - Drop the *-y* at the end of a word and add *-ies*—for example, *myringotomy* to *myringotomies*.
  - Drop the *-us* at the end of a word and add an *-i*—for example, *alveolus* to *alveoli*.
  - Drop the *-on* at the end of a word and add an *-a*—for example, *ganglion* to *ganglia*.
  - Drop the *-is* at the end of a word and add *-es*—for example, *metastasis* to *metastases*.
  - Drop the *-um* at the end of a word and add *-a*—for example, *ischium* to *ischia*.
  - Drop the *-ma* at the end of the word and add *-mata*—for example, *stoma* to *stomata*.

Apply It

Your teacher will set up two or four teams in class. Organize a word game in which one team creates a medical term, using a prefix, root and suffix. The other team has to guess what the word means, identify the prefix and suffix, and determine if it is a real medical term. Then, reverse roles.

Medical Terminology | Chapter 10 239

Teaching Tips

- Review the rules for changing a term from singular to plural.
- Advise students that the only way to effectively learn the elements is to memorize them.
- Explain that you will be assigning them to memorize 12 elements and their meanings each day.
- Follow through by quizzing the students on the 12 elements the following day.
- Introduce the topic of understanding medical terminology.
- Reiterate that once students know the common prefixes, roots, and suffixes, they will have the tools they need for recognizing and understanding medical terminology.
- Go through the examples in the text together.
- Break down a few common terms that they might already be familiar with.

Apply It

- You may want to provide the elements the students should use.
- For example, you could have cards with prefixes written on them, cards with roots written on them, and cards with suffixes written on them. Then, students can line up the card to create words.
- To determine if the term is real, have students use a medical dictionary.

Teaching Tips

- Take the time to review the word elements.
- Show students how to read the table:
  - Point out that every two columns make a set of elements (left column) and meanings (right column).
  - Point out that there are three sets in the table.
  - The prefixes and their meanings are listed first, with a blue background.
  - The roots and their meanings are listed next, with a purple background (p. 241).
  - The suffixes and their meaning are listed last, with a gold background (p. 242).

TEAMWORK

In groups of three, use index cards to create flashcards to use to learn the word elements. One person should be responsible for creating prefix cards, one for root cards, and one for suffix cards. Use the cards to quiz each other on the element meanings.

Understanding Medical Terminology

Knowing prefixes, roots, and suffixes makes it possible to write and decipher common medical and dental terms. For example, if you come across the term *tendonitis*, you can identify the root as *tendon* and the suffix *-itis*. Because this suffix means inflammation, *tendonitis* must describe an inflammation of a tendon.

Now consider the term *arthroscope*. The root is *arthro*, meaning "joint" and the suffix is *-scope*, meaning "picture." An arthroscope is a diagnostic tool that gives physicians a way to take a picture, or form an image, of a structure inside the body, such as a knee.

A related term, *osteoarthritis*, can be interpreted in a similar way. To break this term into parts, find the prefix, root, and suffix. The root is *arthro*, meaning "joint." The prefix is *osteo-*, meaning "bone," and the suffix is *-itis*, meaning "inflammation." By putting the parts of the term together, you can figure out that *osteoarthritis* is an inflammation of the bone's joint.

Prefix	Meaning	Prefix	Meaning	Prefix	Meaning
a, an	without	ecto	outside	ortho	straight
ab	away from	endo	inside, within	pan	all
acr, acro	extremities (arms & legs)	epi	upper, above	para	beside, beyond
ad	toward	ex	out from	peri	around
ambi	both, both sides	hemi	half	poly	many
ante	before	hyper	excessive, above, more than	post	behind, after
anti	against	hypo	deficient, below, less than	pre	before, in front of
aut	self	inter	between	pro	forward
bi	both, two	intra	inside, within	pseudo	false
brady	slow	macro	large	retro	backward
circum	around	mal	bad	semi	half
con	with	mega	large	sub	below
contra	against	meta	between	super	above
di	two	micro	small	supra	above
diplo	double	mono	one, single	tachy	rapid
dors	back	neo	new	tele	distant, far
dys	painful, difficult			trans	across
				ultra	beyond, excess

240 Chapter 10 | Medical Terminology

CUSTOMIZED INSTRUCTION

At-Risk Students

Provide a copy of the Prefix table on this page and the Root and Suffix tables on pp. 241–242 for each student. Encourage them to keep the copies handy as they read through the remainder of this text.

Root	Meaning	Root	Meaning	Root	Meaning
Albino	white	dent	tooth	leuko	white
acro	extremities	derma	skin	lingua	tongue
aden	gland	dextr	right	lip	fat
angio	vessel (blood)	duoden	duodenum	lith	stone
ankyl	crooked, looped	echo	sound	lymph	fluid
arterio	artery	edema	swelling	mamm, mast	breast
arthro	joint	electr	electric	melan	black
aud, aur	ear, hearing	embry	fertilized ovum/ embryo	mening	membrane (pertaining to the covering of the brain or spinal cord)
bio	life	emesis	vomit	meno, mens	menstruate
blepharo	eyelid	enter	intestine	myelo	bone marrow
brachi	arm	epidemic	among the people	myo	muscle
bronchi	bronchial	erythro	red	nares	nose, nostrils
bucca	cheek	esophag	esophagus	necr	death
carcin	cancer	esthesi	feeling	nephro/ren	kidney
cardio	heart	faci	face	neuro	nerve
caud	tail	fascia	band, fibrous	ocul	eye
cephal	head	gastro	stomach	odont	tooth
cerebro	brain	genit	related to birth	onc	tumor
cervic	neck	gingiva	gum	oo	egg
cheil	lip	gloss	tongue	oophoro	ovary
chem.	chemistry, drug	gyne	woman	ophthal	eye
chole	bile	hemo	blood	orchis	testes
cholecyst	gallbladder	hepat	liver	osteo	bone
(c)hondro	cartilage	holo	all	oto	ear, hearing
chrom	color	hom	same, alike	ovario	ovary
coccus	round	hydro	water	ovi	egg
col/colo	colon	hygien	healthful	part	birth, labor
colp	vagina	hystero	uterus, womb	ped, pod	foot
costo	ribs	iri	iris (eye)	ped	child
cranio	skull	kerat	cornea, scaly	phagia	swallow
cut	skin	labia	lip	pharyng	pharynx
cyan	blue	lacrim	tear	phasia	speak
cysto	bladder, sac	lacto	milk	phleb	vein
cyt, cyte	cell	lapar	abdomen		
dacry	Tear duct	laryng	larynx		
dactyl	fingers, toes				

Medical Terminology | Chapter 10 241

Teaching Tips

- You do not have to read each element, but select a few to go over as a class.
- You may want to focus on the twelve you assign for memorization each day.
- Pronounce the selected element out loud, read its definition, and give examples of medical terms that use each element.
- For example, *gastr-* means "stomach" and *-otomy* means "opening into." Combining the two results in *gastrotomy*, which means "an opening into the stomach."
- For a touch of humor, compare the word *gastrotomy* to *gastronomy*, which means "the art and science of fine dining." Use this example to show how precise and exacting medical terminology must be.

ACTIVITY

Select a word element. Define it. Find as many medical terms as you can that use that element.

Teaching Tips

- Remind students that the meaning of most medical terms can be deciphered from the definitions of their word elements.
- Emphasize that students should never assume they know what a term means. If they are not sure, they should look it up.
- Review the medical terms that are listed on this page.
- You may want to have students cover the meanings with a piece of paper.
- Pronounce each term and identify the elements, or ask students to take turns pronouncing the terms and identifying the elements.
- Ask students to try to decipher the meanings based on the word elements.
- Point out that not all terms have all word elements.
- Assign the terms for memorization.

ACTIVITY

Create flashcards for each of the terms in the table, being sure to break each term into its elements—prefix, root, suffix, and combining vowel. Write the definition on the back of the card. Use the cards to memorize the meanings of the terms.

Root	Meaning	Root	Meaning	Root	Meaning
pleur	pleura of the lung	rhin	nose	stric	narrowing
pneumo	lung	salpingo	tube	therm	heat
procto	rectum	semin	seed	thorac	thorax
psycho	mind, soul	sept	infection	thrombo	clot
pulm	lung	soma	body	trachi	trachea
pyelo	pelvis of the kidney	splen	spleen	vas	vessel
pyo	pus	spondyl	spine	vesic	bladder, sac
ren	kidney	squam	scaly	viscera	organ
		stoma	mouth	vit	life

Suffix	Meaning	Suffix	Meaning	Root	Meaning
a, ac	pertaining to	iasis	abnormal condition	penia	deficiency
able	capable of	ic, ical, is	pertaining to	pexy	fixation
al	like, similar, pertaining to	ism	state of	phobia	fear
algia	pain	itis	inflammation	plasty	surgical repair
ase	enzyme	lysis	destruction	plegia	paralysis
cele	hernia	malacia	softening	ptosis	drooping down
cente	puncture	megaly	enlarged	rhagia	bursting forth
cide	causing death	oid	like, similar	sarcoma	tumor, cancer
crine	secrete	ologist	person who studies	sclerosis	hardening
desis	surgical fixation	ology	study of	scope	picture, inspection
ectomy	surgical removal	oma	tumor	spasm	contraction
emesis	vomit	orrhagia	hemorrhage	stasis	stoppage
emia	blood	orrhaphy	suture	trophy	development growth
esthesis	sensation	orrhea	flow	um	pertaining to
genesis, genic	source, origin	osis	condition of	uria	urine
gram, graph	pictures	ostomy	surgical opening	y	the act of or result of an action
ia	a disease; an unhealthy state or condition	otomy	incision into		
		pathy	disease		

242 Chapter 10 | Medical Terminology

Look at the following terms, their parts, and their meanings.

Term	Prefix	Root	Suffix	Meaning
arteriosclerosis		*arterio*, meaning artery	*-sclerosis*, meaning hardening	Condition in which deposits on the artery walls cause them to harden
bicuspid	*bi-*, meaning two	*cuspid*, meaning sharp point		Having two points or cusps
bronchitis		*bronchi*, meaning bronchial tubes leading into the lungs	*-itis*, meaning inflammation	Inflammation of the bronchial tubes
fibromyalgia	*fibro-*, meaning fiber	*myo*, meaning muscle	*-algia*, meaning pain	A condition involving pain in the muscle fibers
hyperventilation	*hyper-*, meaning excessive or above	*ventilation*, meaning breathing		An excessive rate of breathing
hypothyroidism	*hypo-*, meaning below or less than	*thyroid*, relating to the thyroid gland	*-ism*, meaning pertaining to	Pertaining to an underactive thyroid gland
mammogram		*mamm*, meaning breast	*-gram*, meaning picture	Image formed to examine breast tissue
ophthalmology		*opthal*, meaning eye	*-ology*, meaning study of	Study of the eye
otosclerosis	*oto-*, meaning ear or hearing		*-sclerosis*, meaning hardening	A progressive condition that can result in hearing loss
postpartum	*post-*, meaning after	*part*, meaning birth or labor	*-um*, meaning pertaining to	Pertaining to the period after giving birth

How to Use Medical Terminology

Medical terminology provides a system for health workers to communicate with each other. When a patient complains to the doctor about a "pain in the stomach," it can mean many different things. Often the patient is referring to pain in the lower abdominal cavity and not the stomach. For instance, the patient may be assuming that "the stomach" is the entire area between the ribs and the pelvis.

The doctor must ask exactly where the pain is, how it feels, how long it has been a problem, and other questions. After making a diagnosis the primary case provider must be able to tell the health care workers exactly what the problem is. When the entire health care team understands the problem they can treat the patient in the most effective way.

The patient in the above situation could have any of the following or any number of other problems:

- Gastritis
- Hepatitis
- Appendicitis
- Pancreatitis
- Gastralgia
- Ileitis
- Colitis
- Diverticulitis

Medical Terminology | Chapter 10 243

Teaching Tips

- Discuss ways that health care professionals use medical terminology. For example:
  - Providing a precise diagnosis
  - Charting a condition
  - Ordering a test
  - Discussing symptoms with colleague
- Review the eight terms that could describe "a pain in the stomach."
- Ask students to break them into their word elements to decode their meanings.
- Look them up in a medical dictionary for a precise and accurate definition.

Language Arts Link—Health Terms Dictionary

- You may want to assign a specific number of terms for students to add to their dictionary.
- You may allow students to work in groups or teams.
- If students create their dictionary electronically, you may ask them to print it and keep it in a binder.
- Remind students to check their spelling and definitions.
- In addition to including the term and the definition, you may ask the student to identify the word elements and meanings.

Section 10.1 Review Questions

1. Answer: To enunciate or articulate (sounds, words, sentences, etc.).
2. Answer: The prefix is a word element added to the beginning of a word root. The prefix is added to the root to change the meaning or to make it more specific. The suffix is an element added to the end of the word root that changes or adds to the meaning of the root.
3. Answer: The *o* is called the combining vowel and can be added to join a word root with another word root or a suffix
4. Answer: Add an *-e* to a word ending in *-a*; for example, change *axilla* to *axillae.*
5. Answer: Cerebro
6. Answer: The suffix is *ology* and means "the study of."

Language Arts Link

Health Terms Dictionary

Sometimes a step towards learning a new vocabulary term is to actually write it out yourself, rather than just reading it in a textbook or looking it up in the dictionary or on the Internet. To help determine the meaning of unknown or multiple-meaning words or phrases, it may be beneficial to create your own medical dictionary. As you create your medical dictionary, be sure to verify the preliminary determination of the meaning of the word or phrase. It might also be helpful to include the phonetic pronunciation for words that may not sound as they appear.

If you have access to a computer to create your dictionary, you can easily sort the words alphabetically as you enter them. This will make looking up terms easier. If you do not have computer access, you can use a small notebook to make your dictionary.

Go back through the first nine chapters in this text and enter the key terms and definitions in your dictionary. Continue making entries as you complete the course. After you've completed your dictionary, it can serve as an easy reference as you continue your health care preparation or entry level employment.

Summary

Medical terminology is formed by using three components: prefixes, roots, and suffixes. To make the words easier to pronounce, a combining vowel such as *i*, *o*, *y*, or *u* may be used. In this section, you learned many word elements to help you be a better prepared health care worker.

Section 10.1 Review Questions

1. What does it mean to pronounce a medical term?
2. How are prefixes and suffixes used to build medical terms?
3. What is the *o* called in the word adenopathy? Why is it used?
4. How can you change a term ending in *-a* to make it plural?
5. What root word relates to the brain?
6. What is the suffix in the term *endocrinology*? What does it mean?

Language Arts Link

Digital Flashcards

Using your computer or your cell phone, create digital flashcards of various medical vocabulary. In creating the flashcards, include cards that list only a suffix, only a root, and only a prefix. As you master the medical vocabulary, create a dictionary on your computer of common ailments, such as tendonitis, appendicitis, and arthritis. Break the medical vocabulary down into its component parts and accurately interpret what each ailment means.

What's New?

Over-the-Counter Drug Labels

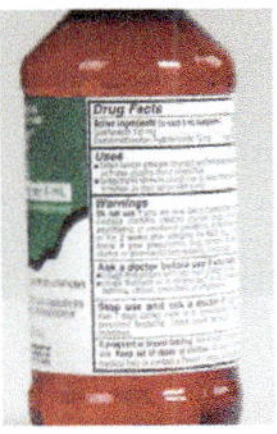

Many drugs are available without a prescription. Labels on these drugs, known as over-the-counter drugs (OTCs), are regulated by the U.S. Food and Drug Administration. Their goal is to make sure that the information on the label clearly states the directions so that a person can choose the right medication to treat symptoms and use the medication correctly.

At one time, labels varied greatly among manufacturers and medications, and label information was often difficult to understand for people not in the medical profession. In 1999, a new regulation required OTC drug manufacturers to use a new, standardized label on all products.

Along with a standardized format, the new drug label uses common terms instead of confusing medical terminology to describe each OTC drug. The new label also requires a type size that is large enough to be easily read, along with added spacing between lines and clearly marked sections to make the label clearer.

Thanks to this law, Drug Facts labels must now list information in the same order, as outlined below. A person should always read every section carefully before taking, or giving, a medicine as each section contains valuable information.

Active Ingredients—This section lists the ingredient or ingredients that make the product work. It is especially important for people taking more than one medicine to make sure that they are not taking too much of the same active ingredient.

Purpose—This section describes the type, or category, of medicine. For example, it might be an antacid or antihistamine.

Uses—This section outlines the symptoms or illnesses for which the product should be used.

Warnings—This section points out situations in which the medicine should not be used. It also indicates when a doctor or other health care professional needs to be consulted, any possible side effects, and when to stop using the product.

Directions—This section describes exactly how and when to use the product. It might also provide amounts to be taken depending on weight or age.

Other Information—This section contains information about how to store the product along with additional information about certain ingredients. This information includes the amount of calcium, potassium, or sodium the product contains.

Inactive Ingredients—This section lists ingredients that are in the product but do not treat the symptoms. This information is particularly important to people with known allergies.

The label of an OTC drug should be checked each time the drug is purchased and used, as manufacturers sometimes change their products and/or labeling. If there is change in a product, a flag or banner is often placed on the front of the package to alert you.

What section of a drug label should you read if you want to know how often to take a medicine?

Medical Terminology | Chapter 10 245

What's New?—Over-the-Counter Drug Labels

- Display examples of over-the-counter drug labels.
- Review the information that is listed on the labels.
- Provide the Web site address for the U.S. Food and Drug Administration (fda.gov) for more information.

What section of a drug label should you read if you want to know how often to take a medicine?

Answer: You should look at the Directions section of the label.

CUSTOMIZED INSTRUCTION

More Advanced Students

Have more advanced students research the risks of drug interactions, and present a report to the class.

Less Advanced Students

Have less advanced students compare the active ingredients in different over-the-counter analgesics, such as Advil, Bayer Aspirin, Tylenol, and Aleve, and then create a chart or poster illustrating the difference.

FOCUS AND ENGAGE

Introduce the Section

a. Review the Background paragraph, explaining that medical abbreviations are used frequently for written communications on documents such as charts and prescriptions.
b. Emphasize that knowing the meaning of an abbreviation is as important as knowing the meaning of a full medical term.
c. Review the objectives for the section.

Vocabulary Review

a. Direct students to the key terms.
b. Pronounce each word, and have the students repeat the pronunciation out loud.
c. Discuss the definition of each word.

TEACH

Discuss

- Ask students if there are any abbreviations they use in everyday life.
- For example, they might use abbreviations when communicating online, such as *LOL* for "laughing out loud," or *TTFN* for "ta ta for now."
- They also might use abbreviations when addressing an envelope.
- Discuss what might happen if they used an incorrect abbreviation, such as a bill payment being delivered to the wrong address.
- Discuss the role of abbreviations in saving time and space on written documents.

SECTION 10.2 Abbreviations

Background

Health care workers use abbreviations to convey information about their patients/clients. Abbreviations help save time and save space on medical documents.

Objectives

When you have completed this section, you will be able to do the following:

- Match key terms with their correct meanings.
- Replace terms with abbreviations.
- Recognize and define abbreviations that are commonly used by health care workers.

Introduction to Abbreviations

abbreviations
(uh bree vee AY shun)
Words that have been shortened.

concisely
(kuhn SICE lee)
In a brief manner; to express in a few words.

Abbreviations are the shortened form of words. They are an efficient way of communicating quickly and **concisely** with other health care workers. You must be very careful when you use abbreviations.

Always use standard medical abbreviations, which have been agreed to by the medical and scientific communities. Additionally, be sure to know the "do not use" list of abbreviations developed by the Joint Commission and can be seen on their Web site: www.jointcommission.org. Never make up an abbreviation. Doing so is confusing and will be a problem if a record is used in a legal action, because no one will understand what you wrote. Never use an abbreviation if you are unsure about its meaning. It is better to write out the word so that it is easily understood.

Be considerate about when you use an abbreviation. Your patients/clients do not know what the abbreviations mean. For instance, *NPO* posted over the bed means "nothing per oral," meaning nothing by mouth. You know what it means, but you should always explain it to your patient/client. The following abbreviations are the most common abbreviations that health care workers use.

Abbreviation	Meaning
@	at
abd.	Abdomen
ABG	Arterial Blood Gas
a.c.	before meals
ADL	activities of daily living
ad lib	as desired
adm	admission
am/AM	morning (midnight to noon)

Abbreviation	Meaning
amb	ambulate/walk
amt.	amount
approx.	approximately
AIDS	acquired immune deficiency syndrome
ASA	aspirin
ASAP	as soon as possible
ASHD	Arteriosclerotic Heart Disease

CUSTOMIZED INSTRUCTION

Special Needs Students

Create lists of terms and abbreviations using a large type font to make it easier for visually impaired students to read.

Abbreviation	Meaning	Abbreviation	Meaning
AU	both ears	DOB	date of birth
ax	axillary, armpit	DON	director of nursing
BE	barium enema	Dr.	doctor
bid/BID	twice a day	dsg	dressing
bm/BM	bowel movement	dx	diagnosis
B/P/BP	blood pressure	D/W	dextrose in water
BR, br	bed rest	ECG/EKG	electrocardiogram
BRP	bathroom privileges	EEG	electroencephalogram
BS	blood sugar	EENT	eye, ear, nose, and throat
bx	biopsy	ER	emergency room
°C	Celsius degree, centigrade	Exc	excision
$\bar{c}$	with	Exp	exploratory
CA	cancer	°F	Fahrenheit degree
Ca	calcium	FBS	fasting blood sugar
CAT	Computerized Axial Tomography	Fe	iron
cath.	catheter	FF	force fluid
CBC	complete blood count	Fl or fl	fluid
CC	chief complaint	ft	foot
cc	cubic centimeters	FUO	fever of unknown origin
CCU	coronary care unit	fx	fracture
CHF	Congestive Heart Failure	GB	gallbladder
Cl	chloride	Gm	gram
cl liq	clear liquids	g	gram
cm	centimeters	GI	gastrointestinal
c/o	complains of	gr	grain
CO_2	carbon dioxide	gtt	drop
COPD	Chronic Obstructive Pulmonary Disease	GU	genitourinary
CPR	cardiopulmonary resuscitation	Gyn	gynecology
CS	central supply	H	Hydrogen
CVA	cerebrovascular accident/stroke	H_2O	water, aqua
D&C	dilatation and curettage	HA	headache
dc, d/c	discontinue	HBV	hepatitis B virus
Del. Rm.	delivery room	Hct	hematocrit
Diff	differential white count	Hg	mercury
DNR	do not resuscitate	Hgb	hemoglobin
DOA	dead on arrival	HOB	head of bed

Medical Terminology | Chapter 10 247

Reinforce and Review

- Review the different word elements.
- Reinforce the importance of clear, concise written communications on charts and other documents.

Teaching Tips

- Emphasize the need for standard abbreviations in health care documentation.
- Explain that an abbreviation is not just the first few letters of a word. Use a common abbreviation such as *Rd.*, or *Ave.*, as an example.
- Emphasize that students should never assume they know an abbreviation. If they are not sure, they should use the full term.
- If they are not sure of the meaning of a written abbreviation, they should look it up, or ask the person who wrote the abbreviation in the first place.
- Once again, tell students that the best way to learn abbreviations is to memorize them.

CUSTOMIZED INSTRUCTION

English Language Learners

Working in pairs, have students quiz each other on the abbreviations and their meanings. One student should say aloud the abbreviation and the other student should answer with the meaning.

Teaching Tips

- Take the time to review the abbreviations on pp. 246–249.
- Show students how to read the table:
  - Point out that every two columns make a set, with the abbreviations in the left column and the full term or meaning in the right column.
  - Point out that some abbreviations use symbols, such as greater than >.
  - Point out that some abbreviations are for complete phrases, not just a single term, such as *DOB* for "date of birth."
- You do not have to read each abbreviation, but select a few to go over as a class.
- You may want to focus on the twelve you assign for memorization each day.

ACTIVITY

Gather the flashcards you created to learn medical terminology. On the front of each card write the correct abbreviation for the term. If necessary, create new cards for new abbreviations.

Abbreviation	Meaning	Abbreviation	Meaning
hr	hour	ML	milliliter
hs	bedtime, hour of sleep	mm	millimeter
ht	height	MRI	magnetic resonance Imaging
hyper	above, high	min.	minute
hypo	below, low	Na	sodium
ICU	intensive care unit	NA	nurse aide/nursing assistant
I & D	incision and drainage	NaCl	sodium chloride
I & O	intake and output	ng	nasogastric tube
IM	intramuscular	noct, noc.	night
inj	injection	NPO	nothing by mouth
int	internal, interior	N/S	normal saline
irrig	irrigation	N&V	nausea and vomiting
IV	intravenous	O_2	oxygen
IVP	intravenous pyelogram	O&P	ova and parasites
K	potassium	Ob	obstetrics
KCL	potassium chloride	Od	overdose
Kg or kg	kilogram	OD	right eye
KUB	kidney, ureter and bladder x-ray	OOB/oob	out of bed
L & D	labor and delivery	OPD	outpatient department
Ⓛ	left	OR	operating room
L	left/liter	OS	left eye
lab	laboratory	ord.	orderly
Lap	laparotomy	ORTH	orthopedics
lb	pound	O.T.	occupational therapy
liq.	Liquid	OU	both eyes
LLQ	left lower quadrant	oz	ounce
LP	lumbar puncture	PAP	Papanicolaou smear
LPN	licensed practical nurse	Path	pathology
LUQ	left upper quadrant	pc	after meals
LVN	licensed vocational nurse	PDR	Physician's Desk Reference
M	minim	PEDS	pediatrics
M.D.	medical doctor	per	by, through
med.	Medicine	pH	measure of acidity/alkalinity
mEq	millequivalent	PID	pelvic inflammatory disease
mg	milligram	pm/PM	afternoon (noon to midnight)
MI	Myocardial Infarction	po	by mouth

248 Chapter 10 | Medical Terminology

Abbreviation	Meaning
post	after
postop, PostOp	postoperative
pre	before
preop, PreOp	before surgery
prn	whenever necessary, when required
Pt, pt	patient
P.T.	physical therapy
$\bar{q}$	every
qd	every day
qh	every hour
q2h	every 2 hours
q3h	every 3 hours
q4h	every 4 hours
qhs	every night at bedtime
qid, QID	four times a day
qod/QOD	every other day
qs	quantity sufficient
qt	quart
R	respiration or rectal
r	rectal
Ⓡ	right
RBC	red blood cell
RLQ	right lower quadrant
RN	registered nurse
R/O	rule out
ROM	range of motion
R.R.	recovery room
RT	respiratory therapy
RUQ	right upper quadrant
R_x	prescription or treatment ordered by a physician
$\bar{s}$	without
SIDS	sudden infant death syndrome
sob	short of breath
spec.	specimen

Abbreviation	Meaning
sp gr	specific gravity
$\overline{ss}$	one half
SSE	soap solution enema
stat	at once, immediately
surg.	surgery
T&A	tonsils and adenoids
TB	tuberculosis
tbsp	tablespoon
TIA	transient ischemic attack
TID/tid	three times a day
TLC	tender loving care
TPR	temperature, pulse, and respiration
tsp	teaspoon
tx	traction
UA or U/A	urinalysis
URI	upper respiratory infection
UTI	urinary tract infection
VS	vital signs
WBC	white blood count
w/c	wheelchair
wt	weight
x	times (2x is 2 times)
x-match	cross match
>	greater than
<	less than
□	increase, elevate, higher
↓	decrease, lower
#	number or pound sign
I	one
V	five
X	ten
L	fifty
C	one hundred
D	five hundred
M	one thousand

Medical Terminology | Chapter 10 249

Teaching Tips

- For selected abbreviations, read its meaning, and give examples of how it might be used in a chart or in a conversation.
- Identify the most common abbreviations.
- Point out that some medical abbreviations might be similar to or the same as other common abbreviations. For example:
  - The medical abbreviation *c/o* means "complains of," while on an envelope *c/o* means "care of."
  - The medical abbreviation *R.R.* means "recovery room," not "railroad."
  - The medical abbreviation *ROM* means "range of motion," not "read-only memory."

CUSTOMIZED INSTRUCTION

More Advanced Students

Have more advanced students look up the difference between an acronym and an abbreviation and then identify which of the common medical abbreviations listed are which.

Teaching Tips

- Remind students to interpret all abbreviations in a medical context.
- Remind students of the importance of communicating with patients. In this case, they should always explain the meaning of abbreviations regarding the patient's care.

ACTIVITY

Make a chart or table listing similar abbreviations that might be easily confused, such as *EEG* and *EKG*, or *B/P* and *BRP*. Include the correct meaning for each abbreviation.

Community

- If it is not possible to visit a pharmacy, perhaps a pharmacist could visit the class.
- Students might ask the pharmacy workers what abbreviations they use most often.
- Direct students to create a professional-looking document for the list of abbreviations.
- Encourage them to use a desktop publishing or word processing program for the activity.
- They might also be able to hand out the list at a local senior center.
- If students are bilingual, ask them to provide translations for the meaning of the abbreviations in the list.

Community

Plan an afternoon at a local pharmacy. See how the pharmacist or pharmacist's assistant explains prescription instructions to people picking them up. Offer to hand out a patient-friendly form that explains the meaning of the abbreviations used on the prescription label.

Summary

Health care workers use abbreviations to help communicate quickly and effectively. Abbreviations are the shortened form of words and help reduce the time needed to chart important information. You have learned the most commonly used abbreviations; however, in your work experience you may find other abbreviations that are not listed here. Never assume that any of the above abbreviations are acceptable in your place of employment. A list of acceptable abbreviations for the organization will be provided for you during the job orientation process.

Section 10.2 Review Questions

1. What is an abbreviation?
2. Why are abbreviations used in medical professions?
3. A doctor writes the following order for a patient: BR. What should the patient do?
4. What abbreviation might indicate that a patient should take in liquids only?
5. If a patient is in the R.R., in what part of the hospital is the patient located?
6. What does TID/tid stand for on a prescription bottle?

250 Chapter 10 | Medical Terminology

Section 10.2 Review Questions

1. Answer: Abbreviations are shortened forms of words.
2. Answer: They are an efficient way of communicating quickly and concisely with other health care workers.
3. Answer: Bed rest
4. Answer: FF (force fluid)
5. Answer: Recovery Room
6. Answer: Three times a day

Personal Wellness

Understanding Medical Prescriptions

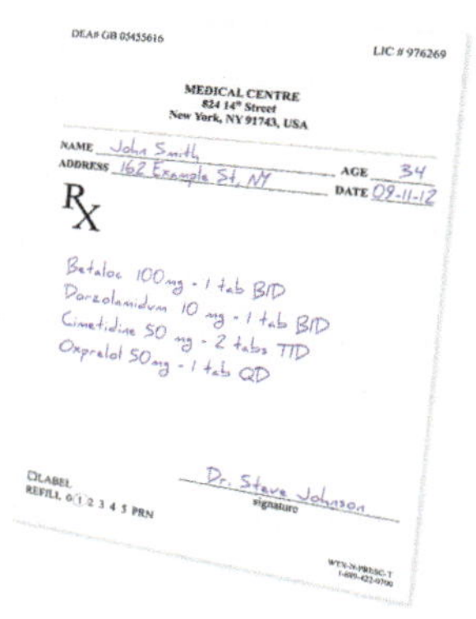

As part of medical treatment, a health care provider may need to write a prescription for a patient. A prescription is a physician's order for the preparation and administration of a drug or device for a patient.

The word *prescription* comes from the Latin *praescriptus*, which is made up of the prefix *prae-*, meaning "before," and the root *scribere*, meaning "to write." A prescription must be written before certain drugs can be prepared and administered to patients.

Some health care providers write prescriptions on paper. Others input information into a computer template. Regardless of the format, all prescriptions have several basic parts:

- The *superscription* (or heading) with the symbol R or Rx, which stands for the Latin word *recipe*, meaning "to take"
- The *inscription*, which contains the names and quantities of the substances to be taken
- The *subscription*, which gives directions for compounding the drug
- The *signature*, which is often preceded by the letter *s*

Health care providers use many abbreviations when writing prescriptions. These abbreviations are translated into common English by pharmacists when the prescription is filled.

However, it is important to understand the prescription as it is written in order to confirm that it has been filled correctly and that the directions have been translated properly. In some cases, it could mean the difference between life and death.

In addition to the abbreviations listed in this section, several additional common abbreviations found on prescriptions and their meanings are listed below:

caps = capsules
da or daw = dispense as written
g (or gm or GM) = gram
gtt. = drops (from "guttae," drops)
h = hour
mg = milligram
ml = milliliter
tabs = tablets
ut dict. = as directed (from "ut dictum," as directed)

What does it mean if a prescription says 2 tabs q4h?

Medical Terminology | Chapter 10 251

Personal Wellness—Understanding Medical Prescriptions

- Use the word elements to break down the word prescription.
- Review the difference between over-the-counter and prescription medications.
- Review the components of a prescription.
- Discuss health care professions that might need to know how to write and interpret a prescription.
- Review the listed abbreviations.

What does it mean if a prescription says 2 tabs q.4h?

Answer: It means to take two tablets every four hours.

ACTIVITY

The instructor should write explicit, complete prescription instructions on slips of paper, using no abbreviations. Students randomly select a slip, and then write the prescription using abbreviations. Students may then swap prescriptions and interpret them.

CUSTOMIZED INSTRUCTION

At-Risk Students

Provide students with various samples of packaging for commonly used over-the-counter medications, such as cough or allergy medicine, anti-itch cream, or pain relievers. Review the directions for use as well as any warnings about the medication. Ask them to comment on any information they find confusing or unclear, and how it could be worded differently.

CHAPTER 10 REVIEW

Chapter Review Questions

1. Answer: Terminology is specialized terms used in any occupation, so medical terminology is specialized terms used in medical occupations.
2. Answer: o
3. Answers may vary: Anti-inflammatory, antibody, antigen
4. Answer: The end
5. Answer: o, i, y, u; o is the most commonly used.
6. Answer: Thinning of the bones with reduction in bone mass due to depletion of calcium and bone protein. Predisposes a person to fractures, which are often slow to heal and heal poorly.
7. Answer: Ganglia (delete the *on* and add *a*)
8. Answer: Tooth
9. Answer: am/AM or pm/PM
10. Answer: Twice a day

Activities

1. Direct students to set up the table before beginning the activity.
2. Direct students to set up a table for this activity as well. They should include three columns: one for the abbreviation, one for the meaning, and one for notes on how the abbreviation is useful.
3. This activity may be more difficult than it sounds at first. Direct students to select a song or poem that includes anatomical terms.

CHAPTER 10 REVIEW

Chapter Review Questions

1. What is medical terminology? (10.1)
2. Identify the combining vowel in the term *osteoporosis.* (10.1)
3. Write a word with the prefix *anti-*. (10.1)
4. To what part of a root word is the suffix added? (10.1)
5. Which letters can be used as combining vowels? Which letter is most commonly used? (10.1)
6. What is *osteoporosis*? (10.1)
7. How do you make the word *ganglion* plural? (10.1)
8. What is the meaning of the root *dent*? (10.1)
9. What abbreviation might you use when telling time? (10.2)
10. What does the abbreviation *bid* mean when written on a prescription? (10.2)

Activities

1. Using appropriate, credible Web sites, find five medical terms used in a health care setting not presented in this chapter. Using a word processor, transcribe the medical vocabulary by creating and filling in the table below, identifying any prefixes, roots, and suffixes. Give the meaning of each part of the word and combine the parts to define the term. Fill in a table like the one below with the information you gather.

Term	Prefix	Root	Suffix	Meaning
1.				
2.				
3.				
4.				
5.				

2. As you go through a day, pay attention to any abbreviations you encounter. Keep a record of as many as you can. Define each abbreviation and think about how using the abbreviation is useful.
3. Rewrite the words to a favorite song or poem, such as the camp song Dry Bones or Hokey Pokey, using medical terminology used in a health care setting.

Case Studies

1. It has been a long day and your shift is almost over. You are in a hurry to finish your charting and cannot remember some of the abbreviations you are expected to use. You can think of several ways to shorten words that you are using. Is it a good idea to use abbreviations that you make up? Explain what you should do and why.
2. You have several co-workers who have English as their second language. They are having problems learning and understanding medical terminology. They cannot interpret certain terms and are unfamiliar with some common abbreviations. How should you go about helping your co-workers to be more productive?

252 Chapter 10 | Medical Terminology

Case Studies

1. Refer students to p. 246 for information specific to this situation.
2. Encourage students to be creative when responding to this situation. In addition to writing their responses, they may want to create a bilingual dictionary of terms and abbreviations, or bilingual flashcards for use in studying.

ACTIVITY

Select and copy 10 random terms and definitions from a medical dictionary. Using the definitions, decipher the meanings of the word elements that comprise each term. If available, include the correct abbreviation for each term.

CHAPTER 10 REVIEW

Thinking Critically

1. **Communication**—You have a patient who is complaining of multiple symptoms. Write a description of these symptoms using medical terminology so that your supervisor understands what the patient is experiencing. The symptoms include headache, vomiting, stomach pain, and excessive perspiration.
2. **Computers**—Be aware that clients may research their diagnosis on the Internet. Make a list of both the helpful and challenging outcomes of this possibility. Think of some examples of how this could affect a health occupation aide and write them down for your portfolio.
3. **Patient Education**—Take a medical condition, such as osteoporosis or polyarthritis, and write an explanation of the disease assuming that the client you are helping has a limited understanding of English.

Portfolio Connections

Imagine that you are the instructor of a medical occupation class. You want your students to learn to communicate effectively in the health care environment. Create five assignments for your students to complete. Use the information in the medical terminology and abbreviation sections. Look at the objectives in your textbook to guide you in developing what you want your students to accomplish in the assignment. Develop worksheets and evaluations. Provide clear directions for the student. An employer is interested in your ability to use in a meaningful way the new information you have learned. Add this to your portfolio. This exercise demonstrates your skills in organizing and articulating what you are learning.

PORTFOLIO TIP

Remember that your clients are not experts in medical terminology and may not understand the abbreviations that you and your colleagues use. Try to use everyday language when talking to clients and getting feedback from them. If you are giving an important instruction or explanation, check to be sure they have understood your comments.

Medical Terminology | Chapter 10 253

Thinking Critically

1. Direct the student to be as thorough as possible. Remind the student that many medical terms are similar but have very different meanings, so they should be careful and accurate.
2. Encourage students to try looking up different medical terms online to see what a patient might find when researching a diagnosis on the Internet. Suggest a site such as webmd.com as a reference. Note that students could add their response to this problem to their portfolio.
3. Advise students to refer back to Chapter 7, Wellness, for information on cross-cultural communications, and Chapter 9, Effective Communication, for information on communicating in general.

Portfolio Connection

- Direct students to use the worksheets and evaluations for this chapter as a template or guide for their original work.
- Remind students that they should include all five assignments, plus supporting material, in their portfolio.
- Check to make sure that students have completed the written assignments and added them to their portfolio.

TEAMWORK

In small groups, prepare a skit demonstrating a problem that might arise from misinterpreting an abbreviation on a patient's chart. Present the skit to the class.

11 Medical Math

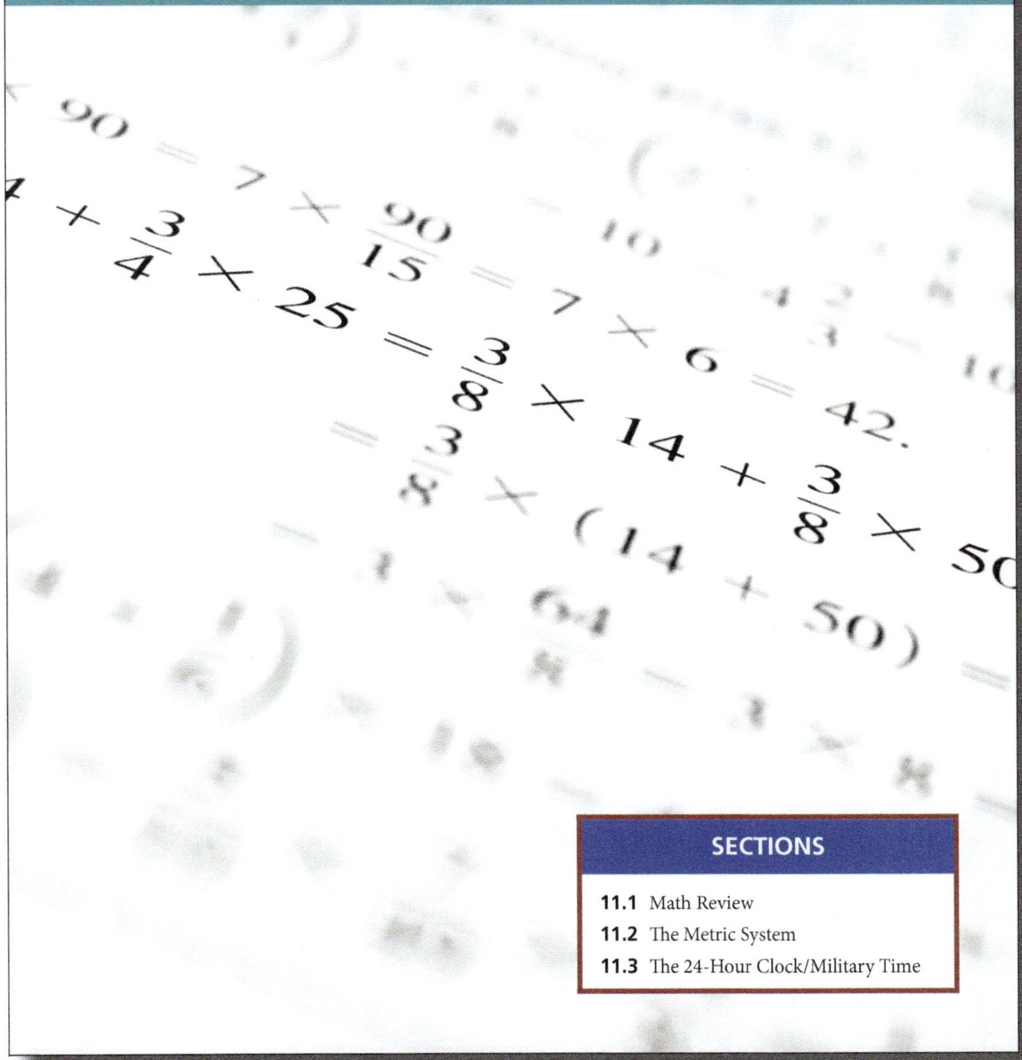

SECTIONS

CHAPTER 11 OVERVIEW

Knowledge of basic mathematics is a must for most health care occupations. In Chapter 11, students review basic math skills, study the metric system, and learn how to use a 24-hour military clock.

Section 11.1: Section 11.1 is a review of basic math skills, including addition, subtraction, multiplication, and division of whole numbers, decimals, fractions, and percentages.

Section 11.2: Section 11.2 introduces the metric system. Students learn the basic units of measurement and how to convert standard units to metric units.

Section 11.3: In Section 11.3 students learn how to use 24-hour clock to tell time.

Advance Preparation	
Review	■ Chapter text for Sections 11.1, 11.2, and 11.3.
Contact	■ A local pharmacy to request a tour, or to invite a pharmacist to speak to the class about the importance of math.
Prepare	■ Index cards for use as flashcards. ■ A list of Web sites that provide support for basic math—such as math.about.com and math.com.

FOCUS AND ENGAGE

Getting Started

- This activity is suitable for small groups.
- You may want them to measure items using standard measures at the beginning of the chapter, and then using metric measures after completing the chapter.
- Or, have the students convert the measurements after completing the chapter.

Introduce the Section

a. Review the content of the Background paragraph, providing specific examples of how math is used in health care occupations.

b. Explain that direct care providers such as nurses and physicians are not the only ones who must know math. It may be even more important for inventory planning, billing, and housekeeping.

c. Review the section objectives.

Vocabulary Review

a. Direct students to the key terms.

b. Pronounce each word, and have the students repeat the pronunciation out loud.

c. Discuss each definition.

TEACH

Discuss

- Ask students their attitudes and feelings toward math. Many may have negative feelings.
- Explain that math has real-world implications in the health care environment.
- Discuss problems that can arise from incorrect calculations or poor measurements.

Teaching Tips

- Introduce the math review section.

Getting Started

Measure the length or width of a variety of different items in and around the classroom. You can include the height of the desk, the width of a chair, the height of a doorway, the length of the chalkboard, the width of a textbook, etc. Then, convert these measurements to the metric system.

Next, identify items by their metric measurements; for example, find something that is 32 cm long or find something that is 1m high. Convert these measurements to the customary U.S. units.

SECTION 11.1 Math Review

Background

Health care workers are required to solve mathematical calculations when doing various tasks, such as dosage calculation and unit conversions for patient weight and height. Knowing basic math concepts and knowing when to apply them are essential skills for all health care workers. To be a successful health care worker, you should know how to add, subtract, convert standard figures into metric figures, calculate percentages, and manipulate fractions. Because math skills are critical to success in all health care jobs, this chapter begins with a math skills review.

Objectives

When you have completed this section, you will be able to do the following:

- Match key terms with their correct meanings.
- Add and subtract whole numbers, decimals, and percentages.
- Multiply and divide whole numbers, fractions, mixed numbers, decimals, and percentages.
- Convert decimals to percentages and percentages to decimals.

256 Chapter 11 | Medical Math

CUSTOMIZED INSTRUCTION

Special Needs Students

You may need to allow special needs students to use assistive tools, such as a calculator, as necessary.

CUSTOMIZED INSTRUCTION OVERVIEW

Less Advanced Students	Pages 258, 272
More Advanced Students	Pages 257, 269
English Language Learners	Pages 257, 260, 277
Special Needs Students	Pages 256, 276
At-Risk Students	Pages 267, 274

Numbers

Numbers are expressed in different forms:

- Whole numbers
- Nonwhole numbers
- Mixed numbers
- Percentages

Numbers that have more than one digit are defined by their place value. For example, the number 7777 is given the following values:

	7	7	7	7
Place value →	*thousands*	*hundreds*	*tens*	*ones*

This number is described by saying "seven thousand, seven hundred seventy-seven." Numbers are written with a comma placed to the left of every third digit. The number 7777 is properly written "7,777." The number 22222 is given the following place values:

	2	2	2	2
Place value →	*ten thousands*	*thousands*	*hundreds*	*tens*

It is written "22,222" and described as "twenty-two thousand, two hundred twenty-two."

Numbers indicating less than a whole number are placed to the right of a decimal. The number 7777.255 is given the following place values:

	7	7	7	7	2	5	5
Place value →	*thousands*	*hundreds*	*tens*	*ones*	*tenths*	*hundredths*	*thousandth*

It is written "7,777.255" and described as "seven thousand, seven hundred seventy-seven and two hundred and fifty-five thousandths."

Roman Numerals

You often find Roman numerals on clock faces; in numbered lists, such as are used in an outline; and as numbering for annual events. Roman numerals also are used in writing prescriptions, so a pharmacist must interpret "III tabs t.i.d." as "take three tablets a day." The Roman numeral system is decimal, which means it is based on the number 10, but the system does not use place value and does not include a zero.

Roman numeral values:

I = 1	VI = 6
II = 2	VII = 7
III = 3	VIII = 8
IV = 4	IX = 9
V = 5	X = 10
L = 50	D = 500
C = 100	M = 1,000

Roman numerals may be written with uppercase or lowercase letters.

Whole Numbers

Whole numbers are the counting numbers and zero. Whole numbers do not contain decimals or fractions. *Examples:* 1, 2, 3, 10, 15, 18, 0. Ignore zeros before whole numbers. *Example:* 025 → Ø25 and is written "25."

Nonwhole Numbers

Nonwhole numbers are numbers that have decimals. *Examples:* 7,777.255, 12.25, 5.9.

Mixed Numbers

Mixed numbers are whole numbers and a fraction. *Examples:* $12^{1}/_{4}$ or $45^{3}/_{4}$.

whole numbers
(HOHL NUHM bers)
Numbers that do not contain decimals or fractions (e.g., 1, 2, 3).

nonwhole numbers
(non HOHL NUHM bers)
Numbers with decimals (e.g., 6.25, 9.85).

mixed numbers
(mikst NUHM bers)
Numbers with whole numbers and a fraction (e.g., 6¼, 7½).

Medical Math | Chapter 11 257

Teaching Tips

- You should administer a pretest before beginning this section to identify the math skills of each student.
- Students should complete the test in class without the use of a calculator or reference material.
- Students who pass the pretest with 100% may be excused from the rest of the section.
- Other students should continue with the section.
- Review the ways numbers can be expressed:
  - Whole numbers: Counting numbers that do not contain decimals or fractions
  - Nonwhole numbers: Contain decimals
  - Mixed numbers: Whole numbers with fractions
  - Percentages: Indicate a part of a whole, where the whole is one hundred
- Percentages are described with a % sign. For example, 7% means seven for every one hundred, or seven per hundred.
- Review place values.
- Explain the place value of numbers from ones to ten thousands, and tenths to thousandths.
- Have students write Roman numerals for numbers that you give them. Have volunteers write the correct Roman numerals on the board so the class can check their accuracy in using Roman numerals.

CUSTOMIZED INSTRUCTION

More Advanced Students

Ask more advanced students to act as tutors or mentors to other students in the class.

English Language Learners

Have students write each key term and its pronunciation on one side of an index card and its definition on the other side. Have them read each term and definition aloud to a partner.

Teaching Tips

- Spend adequate time on percentages.
- Emphasize that 100% is the whole of something, and parts of the whole are represented as percentages.
- Use a visual example, such as four quarters, which are each 25% of a dollar; a pizza; or a slice of bread.

Figure Focus

11.1 Percentages. If there were five bananas in the figure, what percentage would one banana represent?

Answer: 20%

Teaching Tips

- Review the concepts of adding whole numbers:
  - Finding the total of two or more numbers
  - Keeping numbers in the appropriate column
  - Adding numbers in the right column first and then each column to the left

percentages
(per SEN tij es)
Portions in relation to a whole (e.g., 65%, 22%).

Percentages and Ratios

The word *percent* means "by the hundred"; 100 percent = the whole or all of something. The symbol for percent is %. (**Figure 11.1**) *Example:* Four bananas = 100% or all of the bananas present. When one banana is sold, 1/4 (one-fourth) or 25% of them are gone and ¾ (three-fourths) or 75% are left.

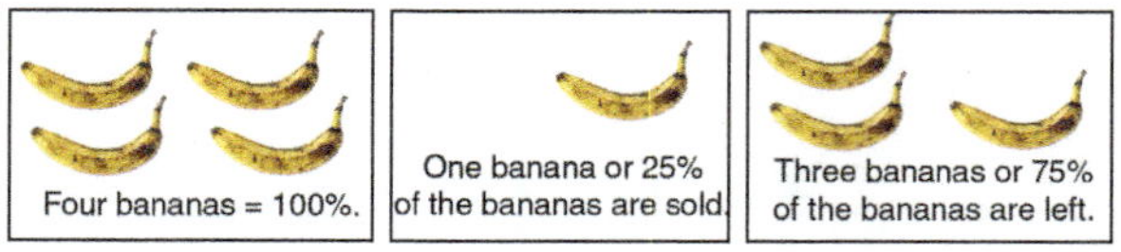

Figure 11.1
Percentages. If there were five bananas in the figure, what percentage would one banana represent?

Addition

Addition is the totaling of two or more numbers. For example, 2 computers in the reception area + 3 computers in accounting = a total of 5 computers in the office. To add, place numbers in columns. Put a line under the last number in the column. Add all the numbers above the line and write the total or sum of the numbers below the line.

Examples:

	2	34
	+ 3	+ 4
Total	5	38

When adding more than one column of numbers, always keep the numbers in each column in a line under each other. This helps you add the correct numbers together. Always start adding numbers in the right column first.

Example:

11 + 234 + 10 + 4 is written like this:

```
  11
 234
  10
+  4
 ---
 259
```

When figuring numbers that total more than 10 in a column, it is necessary to carry numbers to the left of the column being added. In the next example, the first column of 1 + 4 + 0 + 9 = 14. In the total, the number to the left of the 4 is 1. Move or carry the 1 to the column at the left and add it to the top number of that column (8), then add the remaining numbers in the column, 1 + 8 + 8 + 1 = 18. The number to the left of the 8 is 1. Move or carry the 1 to the column at the left and add it to the top number of that column (3), then add the remaining numbers in the column, 1 + 3 = 4. The total is 484. (See the examples that follow.)

CUSTOMIZED INSTRUCTION

Less Advanced Students

Set up specific times outside of class to provide extra help to less advanced students. The math department may already have a system in place for after school help, or you may be able to arrange for accomplished students to provide tutoring.

Example 1:

		$^{1}8$	1
	$^{1}3$	8	4
		1	0
+			9
Total	4	8	4

(carry 1) 81
(carry 1) 384
10
+ 9
484

= 14; leave the 4 in the total row and carry the 1 to the top of column at the left.
= 18; leave the 8 in the total row and carry the 1 to top of the column at the left.
= 4; place the 4 in the total row of the column added.

Example 2:

			$^{1}8$	1
		$^{3}9$	8	4
			9	0
+			9	9
Total	1	2	5	4

(carry 1) 81
(carry 3) 984
90
+ 99
1,254

= 14; leave the 4 in the total row and carry the 1 to the top of column at the left.
= 35; leave the 5 in the total row, carry the 3 to top of the column at the left.
= 12; leave the 2 in the column you're working in at the total row, carry the 1 to the column at the left. (Since there is no number above the total line, write the 1 in the total column.)

Subtraction

Subtraction is the opposite of addition. Subtracting numbers means taking a number away from another number. Simple subtraction problems are written in the following way:

subtraction
(suhb TRAK shuhn)
Taking a number away from another number; the operation opposite of addition.

84
− 23
61

or 84 − 23 = 61

136
− 12
124

or 136 − 12 = 124

Check your answer by adding the answer to the number subtracted. If your answer is correct, your total will equal the number at the top of your problem.

Examples:

84 check
− 23
+ 61 = 84

or 23 + 61 = 84

136 check
− 12
+ 124 = 136

or 12 + 124 = 136

Medical Math | Chapter 11 259

Teaching Tips

- Demonstrate how to carry numbers from one column to the next.
- Work through Example 1 with the class.
- Invite volunteers to work through Example 2 with the class.
- Spend adequate time to be certain students understand the concept of carrying numbers.
- Review concepts of subtracting whole numbers:
  - Keeping numbers in the appropriate column
  - Subtracting numbers in the right column first, and then each column to the left
- Review ways to check answers.

ACTIVITY

Use subtraction to figure out how much food you can purchase for $25.00. Determine how much certain items cost, such as a bottle of water, an apple, a hamburger, etc. Start with the $25.00, and subtract the cost of the first item. From the result, subtract the cost of the second item. Continue until you have no money left. Try the activity again with different items.

Teaching Tips

- Explain and demonstrate the procedure for subtracting by borrowing.
- Explain the different ways multiplication problems can be written.
- Emphasize the value of knowing the multiplication tables:
  - Quick way to add numbers
  - When memorized, it makes it easy to quickly know the answer to basic problems
- Remind students that they are not to use calculators while working through this chapter.
- Refer students to Table 11.1, Multiplication Table, and explain how to read the multiplication table.
- Test their ability to read the table by asking them to find the answer to basic problems, such as: What is 6 × 4?
- Share any tips or shortcuts you might know, such as multiplying by 5 is like counting by fives, anything times 1 is itself, anything times 0 is zero, anything times 10 ends in a zero, and the rule of nines.
- Explain how to multiply fractions and mixed numbers.
- Emphasize that for multiplication, the fractions do not have to have the same denominator.
- Review how to simplify fractions after multiplication.
- Introduce long multiplication.
- Explain that it is a multi-step process, but that if they take it one step at a time, it is not difficult.

Subtracting by Borrowing Numbers

Borrow a number from the column to the left. This allows a larger number, such as 8, to be subtracted from 5. See the following examples to help you understand.

Examples:

```
 ²3̸ ¹5     5 becomes 15 when 1 is borrowed from the 3
− 1  8     3 becomes 2
 [1  7]
```

```
 ¹2̸ ¹⁶7̸ ¹2̸   2 becomes 12 when 1 is borrowed from the 7
− 1   9   5   7 becomes 6 because you borrowed 1; 6 becomes 16
 [0̸   7   7]  when 1 is borrowed from the 2; 2 becomes 1
```

Multiplication

multiplication
(muhl tuh pli KEY shuhn)
Finding the product of two numbers.

Multiplication is a quick, easy way to add. For example, $9 + 9 + 9 = 27$, but an easier process is $3 \times 9 = 27$. Adding large numbers is bulky and takes a lot of time. Multiplication is much easier.

To multiply numbers easily, memorize the multiplication table. (**Table 11.1**) Memorizing this table allows you to calculate numbers quickly and without difficulty. You probably already know the basics of multiplication.

The following symbols are used to indicate multiplication: ×, ()(), ·, or *. These symbols are used in writing problems. Examples:

$\begin{array}{r} 8 \\ \times 9 \\ \hline 72 \end{array}$ or $8 \times 9 = 72$ or $8 \cdot 9 = 72$ or $(8)(9) = 72$ or $8 * 9 = 72$

Using calculators is helpful when figuring complicated calculations; however, you are responsible for knowing how to calculate numbers without a calculator. Most of the calculations in your work are simple and easy to figure without the use of a calculator.

Table 11.1 Multiplication Table

	1	2	3	4	5	6	7	8	9	10
1	1	2	3	4	5	6	7	8	9	10
2	2	4	6	8	10	12	14	16	18	20
3	3	6	9	12	15	18	21	24	27	30
4	4	8	12	16	20	24	28	32	36	40
5	5	10	15	20	25	30	35	40	45	50
6	6	12	18	24	30	36	42	48	54	60
7	7	14	21	28	35	42	49	56	63	70
8	8	16	24	32	40	48	56	64	72	80
9	9	18	27	36	45	54	63	72	81	90
10	10	20	30	40	50	60	70	80	90	100

260 Chapter 11 | Medical Math

CUSTOMIZED INSTRUCTION

English Language Learners

On a sheet of paper, have students write five multiplication problems and their answers using Table 11.1 as a reference, if necessary. Have them orally quiz a partner on their five problems.

Math Link

Adding and Subtracting Decimals and Fractions

Decimals

For decimals, the process of adding and subtracting numbers is similar to the process for adding and subtracting whole numbers. The only difference is how the numbers are aligned in the column. Numbers should be aligned by the decimal point as in the following examples:

$$\begin{array}{r} 12.136 \\ +\ 10.246 \\ \hline 22.382 \end{array}$$

$$\begin{array}{r} 23.453 \\ -\ 10.37 \\ \hline 13.083 \end{array}$$

Fractions

A fraction is made up of two parts: a numerator, which is the number on top, and a denominator, or the number on the bottom. To add or subtract a fraction, the denominator must be the same. Consider the following examples:

Example 1:

$$\frac{1}{4}+\frac{3}{4}=\frac{1+3}{4}=\frac{4}{4}=\frac{1}{1}=1$$

Example 2:

$$\frac{1}{5}+\frac{2}{5}+12\frac{4}{5}=\frac{1}{5}+\frac{2}{5}+\frac{64}{5}=\frac{1+2+64}{5}=\frac{67}{5}=\frac{133}{5}$$

Example 3:

$$\frac{2}{3}-\frac{1}{3}=\frac{2-1}{3}=\frac{1}{3}$$

Note that Example 1 shows a simplified fraction, or a fraction that does not have any common factors (other than 1) for the numerator and denominator. Example 2 shows a mixed number, which is converted to a fraction to be added or subtracted.

In some cases, fractions will need to be converted so each fraction being added has a common denominator. Consider the following example:

$$\frac{1}{3}+\frac{1}{2}=?$$

Step 1: Convert each fraction so they have a common denominator.

The denominators, 2 and 3, are factors of 6, so multiply both the nominator and the denominator of each fraction by the number that makes the denominator equal to 6.

$$\frac{1}{3}\times\frac{2}{2}=\frac{2}{6}$$

$$\frac{1}{2}\times\frac{3}{3}=\frac{3}{6}$$

Step 2: Add fractions.

$$\frac{2}{6}+\frac{3}{6}=\frac{5}{6}$$

For subtraction, follow the same process to make fractions that have the same denominator. Simplify fractions after adding and subtracting as needed.

Step 1: Convert each fraction so they have a common denominator.

$$\frac{3}{4}\times\frac{1}{3}=\frac{3}{12}$$

$$\frac{1}{4}\times\frac{1}{3}=\frac{1}{12}$$

Step 2: Subtract fractions.

$$\frac{3}{12}-\frac{1}{12}=\frac{2}{12}$$

(continued)

Math Link—Adding and Subtracting Decimals and Fractions

- Review the methods for adding and subtracting decimals.
- Provide examples for the students to use as practice.
- Review the terminology of fractions:
  - Numerator
  - Denominator
  - Factor
  - Common factor
  - Simplified fraction
- Review the methods for adding and subtracting fractions.
- Make sure students understand the difference between the numerator and the denominator.
- Emphasize the importance of the denominator being the same in order to add or subtract fractions.
- Review the process of converting fractions to a common denominator.
- The answers to the four problems are: 11.39; $5\,^{13}/_{60}$; 2.12; $1\,^{5}/_{12}$

What will happen if you don't convert fractions to a common denominator before adding or subtracting them?

Answer: If you don't convert the fractions so they have the same denominator, you will get the wrong answer. You cannot add or subtract fractions that have different denominators.

ACTIVITY

Tell students that they probably use math more often than they realize. For example, you use it when you shop and when you cook. You might use it to figure out how many pages of homework you must read, or how many hours you spent at work. Have students keep track of how many times each day they use math. Record the information in a chart or table. Have students compare their results.

TEAMWORK

In small groups, use index cards to create flashcards to use to learn the multiplication table. Write the problem on one side of the card, and the result on the back. Use the cards to quiz each other.

Teaching Tips

- Explain how to multiply fractions and mixed numbers.
- Emphasize that for multiplication, the fractions do not have to have the same denominator.
- Review how to simplify fractions after multiplication.
- Introduce long multiplication.
- Explain that it is a multi-step process, but that if they take it one step at a time, it is not difficult.

TEAMWORK

In small groups, use index cards to create flashcards to use to learn the multiplication table. Write the problem on one side of the card, and the result on the back. Use the cards to quiz each other.

Math Link (cont)

Add or subtract the following:

$3.45 + 2.34 + 5.6$

$3\frac{3}{4} + \frac{2}{3} + \frac{4}{5}$

$3.4 - 1.28$

$2\frac{3}{4} - \frac{11}{3}$

What will happen if you don't convert fractions to a common denominator before adding or subtracting them?

Describe how fractions and decimals are used for medical processes and procedures. Solve a real medical problem involving multiplication of fractions and mixed numbers. Compare a medical process or procedure measurement, using decimals to hundredths, by reasoning about the size to be recorded.

Multiplying Fractions

numerators
(NOO muh rey ters)
The top numbers of fractions.

denominators
(di NOM uh ney ters)
The bottom numbers of fractions.

Like a whole or nonwhole number, fractions can be multiplied. The **numerators**, or top numbers of the fractions, are multiplied; and the **denominators**, or bottom numbers of the fractions, are multiplied. For example:

$$\frac{3}{4} \times \frac{12}{15} = \frac{3 \times 12}{4 \times 15} = \frac{36}{60} = \frac{3}{5}$$

Note that the final answer for the example above is simplified, or reduced. To reduce the fraction, you must divide the numerator and denominator by the largest number that goes into both—in this case, 12.

To multiply mixed numbers, convert the number to a fraction first. For example:

$$1\frac{3}{4} \times 2\frac{2}{3} = \frac{7}{4} \times \frac{8}{3} = \frac{56}{12} = 4\frac{8}{12} = 4\frac{2}{3}$$

Long Multiplication

When you are multiplying numbers that have more than one digit, it is sometimes necessary to carry and add. See the following examples to review these steps.

The next problem does not require carrying numbers. It does require multiplying and adding.

A.

		5	2
	×	3	2
	1	0	4

2 × 2 = 4; place 4 in the first column, below 2 and 2.
2 × 5 = 10; place 0 in column under the 5 and 3 and place 1 in column at left.

B.

		5	2
	×	3	2
	1	0	4
+ 1	5	6	

3 × 2 = 6; place 6 in column under the 5, 3, and 0.
3 × 5 = 15; place 5 in column under 1 and place 1 in column at left.

C.

		5	2
	×	3	2
	1	0	4
+ 1	5	6	
1	6	6	4

Add together, keeping each number in the correct column.
Answer

This problem requires carrying, adding, and multiplying:

A.

	$^{1}8$	$^{1}9$	8
×	5	6	2
1	7	9	6

2 × 8 = 16; place 6 in first column and carry 1 to top of column at left. 2 × 9 = 18 + 1 [that was carried] = 19; place 9 in column under 9 and 6 and carry 1 to top of column at left. 2 × 8 = 16 + 1 [that was carried] = 17; place 7 in column under 8 and 5 and place 1 in column at left of 7.

B.

		$^{5}8$	$^{4}9$	8
	×	5	6	2
	1	7	9	6
5	3	8	8	

6 × 8 = 48; place 8 in column under 9, 6, and 9 and carry 4 to the top of column at left. 6 × 9 = 54 +4 [that was carried] = 58; place 8 in column under 8, 5, 7 and carry 5 to top of column at left. 6 × 8 = 48 + 5 [that was carried] = 53; place 3 in column under 1 and place 5 in column at left next to 3.

C.

			$^{4}8$	$^{4}9$	8
		×	5	6	2
		1	7	9	6
	5	3	8	8	
4	4	9	0		

5 × 8 = 40; place 0 in column under 8, 5, 7 and 8 and carry 4 to the top of column at left. 5 × 9 = 45 +4 [that was carried] = 49; place 9 below 1 and 3. Carry 4 to top of column at left. 5 × 8 = 40 + 4 [that was carried] = 44; place 4 below 5 and place 4 next to 4 in column at left.

D.

			8	9	8
		×	5	6	2
		$^{1}1$	$^{1}7$	9	6
	$^{1}5$	3	8	8	
+ $^{1}4$	4	9	0		
5	0	4	6	7	6

Add together, keeping each number in the correct column.
Answer

Teaching Tips

- Explain the steps of long multiplication.
- Work through steps A, B, and C of the first example.
- Point out that the problem requires you to multiply, line up the numbers correctly, and add the results.
- Work through steps A, B, C, and D of the second example.
- Explain why carrying the numbers to the next column is necessary (place value).
- Go over the examples again, if necessary, or provide additional examples.
- Have students volunteer to demonstrate one of the math problems for the class.

Teaching Tips

- Emphasize that knowing the multiplication table aids in division as well.
- Explain the ways in which division problems may be written.
- Explain how to divide numbers.
- Explain remainders.
- Point out that remainders can be expressed as decimals or fractions.
- Carefully step through the sample division problems for dividing by a one-digit number.

Division

division
(di VIZH uhn)
The process of separating into parts; the operation opposite of multiplication.

Division is the opposite of multiplication. Knowing the multiplication table is essential when dividing. As a health care worker, you may divide to determine costs per item or to determine the amount of items used daily. Here is a simple example: A medical office budget allows $600 a year for magazines. You are responsible for selecting and ordering the magazines. As you survey appropriate magazine subscriptions, you determine that the average annual cost is $35 per magazine. To determine how many subscriptions you can purchase, you divide $35 into $600. This problem is written as follows:

600 ÷ 35, or 35)600

```
    17  magazine subscription
35)600
```

To understand how 17 magazine subscriptions can be purchased for $600, review the following division skills:

Dividing three-digit numbers by one-digit numbers:

812 ÷ 4 — Divide hundreds — Divide tens — Divide ones

```
Divide hundreds     Divide tens                    Divide ones
   [2]                [20]                           [203]
 4)812              4)812                          4)812
   8                  8↓                             8
   0                  01} 4 does not divide          01
                      00  into 1. Place a 0          00↓
                       1  next to the 2 in            12
                          the answer.                 12} Divide 4 into 12.
```

Community

Volunteer in an elementary school class or after-school program. Use your time to work with students who are having trouble with math. You can use either paper and pencil practice or math tutorial programs to help them.

Dividing four-digit numbers by one-digit numbers:

7,216 ÷ 9

```
   [8]        [80]        [801]        [801 R or 7/9 or 0.8]
9)7,216    9)7,216     9)7,216      9)7,216.0    Add 0s to carry answer.
  7 2        7 2↓        7 2 ↓        7 2
               1            16           16
               0             9            9↓
               1             7            7 0
                                          6 3
                                            7
```

Answer is $801\frac{7}{9}$ or 801.8

remainder
(ri MEYN der)
The amount left over after division that is less than a whole number.

As shown in the example, "R" stands for **remainder**. The remainder is what is left over that is less than a whole number. A remainder is usually expressed as a fraction or a decimal.

Dividing Fractions

To divide fractions, you will need to invert, or turn over, the divisor (dividing number) in the calculation. So, the denominator will be on top and the numerator will be on bottom. Then, you multiply the fractions to find the answer. For example:

Step 1: Invert the divisor.

$$\frac{7}{10} \div \frac{2}{9}$$

So, $^{2}/_{9}$ is converted to $^{9}/_{2}$.

Step 2: Multiply the fractions.

$$\frac{7}{10} \times \frac{9}{2} = \frac{7 \times 9}{10 \times 2} = \frac{63}{20} = 3\frac{3}{20}$$

Note that the answer was converted from a fraction to a mixed number. When dividing mixed numbers, you will need to convert them to fractions first.

So, for example:

$$3\frac{7}{8} \div \frac{21}{4}$$

would convert to

$$\frac{31}{8} \div \frac{9}{4}$$

before you can divide the numbers.

Language Arts Link

Using Word Problems to Help Home Health Care Workers' Math Skills

As a health care worker, you must be able to use mathematical calculations that are appropriate and accurate for a given medical task, process, or procedure. In teams of three or four, in a word problem format, create a series of equations and inequities in one or more variables that will be used to solve real medical problems. For example:

- A weight measurement is taken for a mother and baby at 147 pounds. The mother weighs 133 pounds. How much does the baby weigh? (Answer: 14 pounds)
- A patient is allowed 2.5 quarts of fluid intake each day. There are 32 ounces in a quart. How many ounces of fluid will the patient receive at each of 3 meals? (Answer 26.7 ounces)
- There are 10 3" × 3" triple-layer gauze pads in a box, and your department uses an average of 5 boxes each week for general wound care. There are 25 2" × 2" specially treated pressure ulcer gauze pads in a box, and an average of 3 boxes are used each week. To monitor expenses, your supervisor wants to know what percentage of the total gauze pads used are 2" × 2" pads. (Answer: 60%)

Using these examples, create a workbook for the class. Be sure to proofread your work to see if you can improve it by making it clearer, more concise, or more interesting to read.

Check the spelling and grammar and correct any errors. Exchange your workbook with another team. Provide feedback and corrections as necessary, and then exchange back. Read your classmates' comments and revise your document as necessary.

ACTIVITY

Make a poster illustrating fractions. For example, use a clock to illustrate halves, a pizza to illustrate eighths, or a pie to illustrate thirds. Display the posters in the classroom or on a bulletin board.

Teaching Tips

- Explain how to divide fractions.
- Point out that it is simply a matter of flipping the fraction upside down, and then multiplying.
- Remind students that division is the opposite of multiplication, which will help them understand why it is necessary to flip the fraction and then multiply it.
- Explain that mixed numbers should be converted to fractions before flipping and multiplying.
- Review the procedure for converting mixed numbers to fractions.
- Review the procedure for simplifying fractions.

Language Arts Link—Using Word Problems to Help Home Health Care Workers' Math Skill

- Make sure students understand what a word problem is.
- You may want to assign a specific number of word problems to each group or team.
- Alternatively, you may want to assign a specific level of difficulty to each group or team. For example, one team might be responsible for easy problems, one for intermediate, and one for advanced.
- Remind students that they must be clear and concise so that others will understand what the problem is asking.
- Also, remind students that the problems should involve a situation that a health care professional would encounter in the workplace.
- You may want to share finished projects with another class.

Teaching Tips

- Review the rules for decimals:
  - Numbers to the left of the point are whole numbers.
  - Numbers to the right of the point are less than one.
- Review the steps for dividing decimals by a whole number.
- Review the table that provides the decimal and percentage equivalents of fractions:
  - .10 = $^1/_{10}$ = 10%
  - .25 = $^1/_4$ = 25%
  - 6.25 = 6 $^1/_4$ = 625%
- Review other decimal and percentage equivalents of common fractions:
  - .5 = $^1/_2$ = 50%
  - .33 = $^1/_3$ = 33%
  - .75 = $^3/_4$ = 75%
- Suggest students memorize these equivalents.
- Explain the procedure for converting decimals to percentages:
  - Move the decimal two spaces to the right.
  - Replace the decimal point with a % sign.

ACTIVITY

Randomly select a percentage. Create a poster that illustrates the selected percentage. For example, you might draw half a sandwich to illustrate 50%, or three quarters to illustrate 75%. Display the posters in the classroom or on a bulletin board.

Decimals, Percentages, and Fractions

Numbers to the left of a decimal are whole numbers. Numbers to the right of a decimal are less than one.

Dividing *decimals* by whole numbers:

$24.5 \div 4 = 4\overline{)24.5}$ Place the decimal point in the answer directly above the decimal point in the dividend.

$$\begin{array}{r} 6.\\ 4\overline{)24.5}\\ \underline{24} \end{array} \qquad \begin{array}{r} 6.1\\ 4\overline{)24.5}\\ \underline{24}\downarrow\\ 5\\ \underline{4}\\ 1 \end{array} \qquad \begin{array}{r} 6.125\\ 4\overline{)24.500}\\ \underline{24}\\ 5\\ \underline{4}\downarrow\\ 10\\ \underline{8}\downarrow\\ 20\\ \underline{20} \end{array}$$

Add 0s to carry answer.

Numbers to the right of a decimal point indicate less than one whole. For example, 1.5 is the same as $1^1/_2$.

Examples:

Decimal		Percentage		Fraction(s)
0.10	=	10%	=	$^{10}/_{100}$ or $^1/_{10}$
0.25	=	25%	=	$^{25}/_{100}$ or $^1/_4$
6.25	=	625%	=	$6^{25}/_{100}$ or $6^1/_4$

Change a decimal number into a percentage by moving the decimal two places to the right.

Examples:

0.5 = 0.5 0. = 50%

30.0 = 30.0 0. = 3000%

0.04 = .0 4. = 4%

Apply It

Pick out 10 items in your refrigerator or kitchen cabinet, such as cereal, juice, or household cleaners. Create a chart and convert all of the ingredient measurements on the label to decimals.

To change a percentage into a decimal number, replace the percent sign with a decimal and move the decimal two spaces to the left.

To find the percentage of a number, first change the percentage to a decimal. Then multiply that decimal by the number.

Examples:

15% of 63 change 15% to 0.15 then multiply 0.15 × 63 = 9.45

9.45 is 15% of 63

20% of 100 change 20% to 0.20 then multiply 0.20 × 100 = 20

20 is 20% of 100

266 Chapter 11 | Medical Math

Apply It

- Show an example of the label measurement in class.
- For example, point out the volume of a soda bottle, or the weight of a box of cereal.
- Alternatively, have students convert the percentages of vitamins, sodium, protein, sugars, etc.
- Suggest they set up a table for entering the values: in column 1 they list the ingredient, in column 2 the percentage, and in column 3 the decimal.

Math Link

Ratios and Proportions

Ratios and proportions are used in health care to calculate medication dosages and convert measurements. A *ratio* is a comparative relationship between two or more things. An example of a ratio is 30 ml to 1 ounce, written as:

30 ml:1 oz *or* 30 ml/1 oz *or* 30 ml to 1 oz

Always include the named units of the items you are comparing (e.g., ml and oz); otherwise, the two items are merely numbers, and could easily be misinterpreted.

A *proportion* is a relationship of one part to another, or the whole, with respect to size, quantity, or amount. Proportions can use ratios to solve problems such as medication dosages, measurements, and other calculations required in health care. Think of a proportion as an analogy in English.

Example: A physician orders an antibiotic to be given to the patient in the amount of 500 mg every 12 hours. The medication label reads: 250 mg/5 cc. How many cc units are given with each dose every 12 hours?

First, state the analogy:

250 mg is to 5 cc as 500 mg is to *X* cc

Next, set up the equation:

$$\frac{250 \text{ mg}}{5 \text{ cc}} = \frac{500 \text{ mg}}{X \text{ cc}}$$

Next, cross multiply, and divide to solve for *X*:

$250 \text{ mg} \times X \text{ cc} = 500 \text{ mg} \times 5 \text{ cc}$

$250X = 2500$

$X = 10$

So, 10 cc are given with each dose every 12 hours.

Summary

In this section, you reviewed the skills for adding, subtracting, multiplying, and dividing whole numbers, nonwhole numbers, mixed numbers, fractions, and percentages. You also practiced converting percentages, decimals, and fractions.

Section 11.1 Review Questions

1. For each of the following pairs of numbers, add and subtract the numbers:
   a. 178, 23
   b. 56.78, 12.2
   c. 56%, 34%
2. Find the answer for each of the following:
   a. 2×9
   b. $^{1}/_{4} \times {}^{15}/_{16}$
   c. $13^{3}/_{4} \times 7^{8}/_{9}$
   d. 45.67×3.45
   e. 33% of 60
3. Find the answer to each of the following:
   a. $56 \div 8$
   b. $^{5}/_{6} \div {}^{1}/_{3}$
   c. $12^{1}/_{2} \div 5^{2}/_{3}$
   d. $23.43 \div 2.3$
   e. Identify the number for which 27 is 60% of the number.
4. Convert the following decimals to percentages:
   a. 0.0033
   b. 0.789
   c. 1.001
5. Convert the following percentages to decimals:
   a. 45%
   b. 23.5%
   c. 0.45%
6. For each of the following pairs of decimals, add and subtract the numbers:
   a. 2.567, 1.382
   b. 0.789, 0.294
   c. 1.934, 0.536

Medical Math | Chapter 11 267

CUSTOMIZED INSTRUCTION

At-Risk Students

Pair students with more advanced learners to work through the Review Questions. Make sure they set up each problem correctly and show their work.

Section 11.1 Review Questions

1. Answers:
   a. $178 + 23 = 201$
      $178 - 23 = 155$
   b. $56.78 + 12.2 = 68.98$
      $56.78 - 12.2 = 44.58$
   c. $56\% + 34\% = 90\%$
      $56\% - 34\% = 22\%$
2. Answers:
   a. 18
   b. $^{15}/_{64}$
   c. $288\,^{1}/_{6}$
   d. 157.5615
   e. 19.8
3. Answers:
   a. 7
   b. $2\,^{1}/_{2}$
   c. $2\,^{7}/_{34}$
   d. 10.18696
   e. 45
4. Answers:
   a. 0.33%
   b. 78.9%
   c. 100.1%
5. Answers:
   a. .45
   b. .235
   c. .0045
6. Answers:
   a. $2.567 + 1.382 = 3.949$
      $2.567 - 1.382 = 1.185$
   b. $0.789 + 0.294 = 1.083$
      $0.789 - 0.294 = 0.495$
   c. $1.934 + 0.536 = 2.47$
      $1.934 - 0.536 = 1.398$

FOCUS AND ENGAGE

Introduce the Section

a. Review the content of the Background paragraph, explaining that the metric system is an alternative method of measurement.

b. Emphasize that all health care professionals must be able to use the metric system.

c. Review the objectives for the section.

Vocabulary Review

a. Direct students to the key terms.

b. Pronounce each word, and have the students repeat the pronunciation out loud.

c. Discuss the definition of each word.

TEACH

Discuss

- Ask students if they have any experience using the metric system. For example, what sizes do soda bottles come in? Has anyone ever run in a 10 K race?
- Explain that all metric units are based on 10.
- Discuss why it might be easier to work with units based on 10 than to work with the standard measurement units.

Reinforce and Review

- Review basic math skills.
- Reinforce the importance of knowing how to compute and measure precisely in a health care environment.

SECTION 11.2 The Metric System

Background

The health care worker is expected to measure and calculate weights, heights, and volume in metric units of measure. Understanding how to convert standard and metric units of measure is an essential requirement of all health care professionals.

Objectives

When you have completed this section, you will be able to do the following:

- Match key terms with their correct meanings.
- State the metric unit of measure used to determine length, distance, weight, and volume.
- Use metric terms to express 100 and 1,000 units of measure.
- Use metric terms to express 0.1, 0.01, and 0.001 units of measure.
- List four basic rules to follow when using the metric system.
- Identify metric measures of length and volume.
- Convert ounces to cubic centimeters/milliliters, pounds to kilograms, and ounces to grams.

Apply It

A popular metric mnemonic is "King Henry Died Drinking Chocolate Milk." This can help you keep the prefixes straight: kilo, hecto, deca, deci, centi, and milli. Working with a partner, come up with your own mnemonic device.

Using the Metric System

The health care industry uses the metric system for measuring. The metric system is used by 90 percent of the world and is known as the International System of Units. Table 11.2 will help you learn the metric terms, their abbreviations, and what they measure. Each metric unit in this table is a single unit of measure. Table 11.3 explains terms used when more than one unit of measure (meter, gram, liter) is being measured. Following are examples of more than one unit:

- Measures of weight:

  1 hectogram = 100 grams

  1.5 hectograms = 150 grams

  1 kilogram = 1,000 grams

  1.5 kilograms = 1,500 grams

length
(LENGTH)
The measure of something from end to end.

- Measures of **length**:

  1 hectometer = 100 meters

  1.5 hectometers = 150 meters

  1 kilometer = 1,000 meters

  1.5 kilometers = 1,500 meters

Table 11.4 explains terms used when *less than one unit* of measure is being measured. Following are examples of less than one unit:

268 Chapter 11 | Medical Math

ACTIVITY

Research what countries other than the United States use the standard system of measurement.

Apply It

- Encourage students to have fun with this activity.
- Students should share their mnemonic devices with the class.

- Measures of length:
  1 decimeter (dm) = 1/10 or 0.1 of a meter
  1 centimeter (cm) = 1/100 or 0.01 of a meter
  1 millimeter (mm) = 1/1000 or 0.001 of a meter
- Measures of volume:
  1 deciliter (dL) = 1/10 or 0.1 of a liter
  1 milliliter (mL) = 1/1000 or 0.001 of a liter

Table 11.2 Metric Terms, Their Abbreviations, and What They Measure

Term	Abbreviation	Measures	In Place of
meter	m	Length	inch, foot, yard, mile
gram	g	Weight	ounce, pound
liter	L*	Volume	fluid ounce, cup, pint, quart, gallon

*Capital *L* is commonly used to prevent confusion of lowercase letter *l* and the number *1*.

Table 11.3 Metric Terms, Their Abbreviations, and What They Measure

Term	Abbreviation	What It Measures
kilo	k	1,000 units
hecto	h	100 units

Table 11.4 Metric Terms, Their Abbreviations, and What They Measure

Term	Abbreviation	What It Measures
deci	d	1/10 or 0.1 unit
centi	c	1/100 or 0.01 unit
milli	m	1/1000 or 0.001 unit
micro	μ	1/1000000 or 0.000001 unit

There are four basic rules to follow when using the metric system:

- Numbers indicating less than one unit are always written in **decimal** form, not as fractions. *Example:* 1/10 = 0.1 or 1/100 = 0.01 or 1/1000 = 0.001.
- When writing decimals, if there is no number before the decimal, always write a 0. *Example:* .1 is 0.1, .5 is 0.5, .75 is 0.75.
- Abbreviations for metric terms are never plural; they are always written in singular form. *Examples:* grams is *g*, not *gs*, and liters is *L*, not *Ls*. Always capitalize the abbreviation L for liter to reduce confusing the lowercase l with the number 1.
- Leave a space between the number and the abbreviation, as shown in the following examples: 8 g or 0.1 dm.

decimal
(DEH sim uhl)
A number containing a decimal point.

Medical Math | Chapter 11 269

Teaching Tips

- Review the main metric units:
  - A meter, which measures length
  - A gram, which measures weight
  - A liter, which measures volume
- Discuss the value of the metric system:
  - Used frequently in health care
  - Very precise
  - Used by 90% of the world
- Explain that certain prefixes are added to the three main terms to indicate multiples, or more than one:
  - A *kilo-* means 1,000 units.
  - A *hector-* means 100 units.
- Explain that other prefixes are added to the three main terms to indicate percentages, or less than one:
  - A *deci-* means 1/10 or 0.1 unit.
  - A *centi-* means 1/100 or 0.01 unit.
  - A *milli-* means 1/1000 or 0.001 unit.

CUSTOMIZED INSTRUCTION

More Advanced Students

Ask more advanced students to plan, create, and deliver a marketing presentation to convince the United States to switch to the metric system.

Teaching Tips

- Review the four basic rules to follow when writing metric units:
  - Write numbers less than one as a decimal, not a fraction.
  - Include a leading 0 to the left of the decimal point if there is no other number in that place.
  - Write abbreviations in the singular, not plural.
  - Always leave a space between the number and the abbreviation.
- Distribute container and rulers marked in both standard and metric units.
- Compare the standard units of measure and the metric units:
  - Yard vs. meter
  - Ounce vs. cubic centimeter
  - Quart vs. liter
- Review the Celsius or Centigrade scale for measuring temperature.

Figure Focus

11.2 Comparison of standard and metric units of length. About how many centimeters are in one inch?

Answer: About 2.5 cm per inch.

Using the Metric System to Measure

Meters, Centimeters, and Millimeters

meterstick
(MEE ter STIK)
A measuring stick one meter long that is marked off in centimeters and usually millimeters.

A **meterstick** can be used to measure length in the following units:

- Centimeters (cm) (**Figure 11.2**)
- Millimeters (mm)
- Meters (m)

One meter is slightly more than 3 feet.

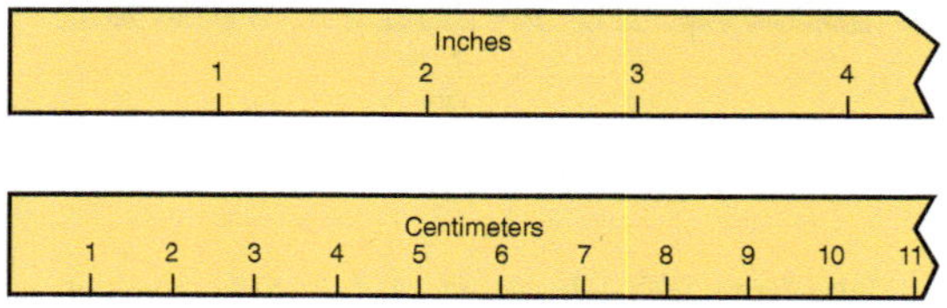

Figure 11.2
Comparison of standard and metric units of length. About how many centimeters are in one inch?

Liters, Milliliters, and Cubic Centimeters

- A liter (L) is slightly larger than a quart.
- A milliliter (mL) is 1/1000 of a liter.
- Cubic centimeters (cc) are interchangeable with mL.

scales
(SKEYLZ)
Instruments with marks that help to determine weight or mass.

Scales can be used to measure weight in grams, hectograms, and kilograms.

Celsius (C) and Centigrade

The metric measure of heat is Celsius or centigrade, which are the same. Boiling water (at normal pressure) measures 100° in Celsius, but 212° in Fahrenheit, and as water freezes it measures 0° in Celsius, but 32° in Fahrenheit. Most people think of a "normal" body temperature as an oral temperature of 37° Celsius (98.6° Fahrenheit).

ACTIVITY

Create a four-column chart or table. In the first column, list specific items you can measure, such as how far away you live from school, how much water you drank at lunch, or how heavy your backpack is. In the second column, write the type of measurement, such as length, volume, or weight. In the third column, write the metric unit you should use for the measurement. In the fourth column, write the standard unit you should use for the measurement.

Changing Standard Measures to Metric Measures

It is easy to change liquid or volume measurement by multiplying 30 cc/mL times the number of ounces. (Table 11.5)

Table 11.5 Changing Ounces to Milliliters and Cubic Centimeters

1 oz medicine	1 oz × 30 cc/mL = 30 cc = 30 mL
8 oz water	8 oz × 30 cc/mL = 240 cc = 240 mL
6 oz soup	6 oz × 30 cc/mL = 180 cc = 180 mL
4 oz juice	4 oz × 30 cc/mL = 120 cc = 120 mL
12 oz soda	12 oz × 30 cc/mL = 360 cc = 360 mL

Health care workers use various types of measuring devices to measure liquid.

To change measurements of **mass** or weight, compare pounds with kilograms and grams with ounces. One pound equals 0.45 kg; 1 kilogram equals 2.2 lb. (Table 11.6)

Table 11.6 Changing Pounds to Kilograms and Kilograms to Pounds

110 lb changed to kilograms: 110 lb × 0.45 kg/lb = 49.5 kg
200 lb changed to kg: 200 lb × 0.45 kg/lb = 91 kg
50 kg changed to lb: 50 kg × 2.2 lb/kg = 110 lb
91 kg changed to lb: 91 kg × 2.2 lb/kg = 200 lb

- To change pounds to kilograms, multiply the number of pounds by 0.45 lb/kg.
- To change kilograms to pounds, multiply the number of kilograms by 2.2 lb/kg.

One ounce (oz) equals 30 grams (g). To change ounces to grams, multiply 30 g/oz by the number of ounces. To change grams to ounces, divide 30 g/oz into the number of grams. (Table 11.7)

Table 11.7 Changing Ounces to Grams

1 oz changed to grams: 1 oz × 30 g/oz = 30 g
8 oz changed to grams: 8 oz × 30 g/oz = 240 g

Apply It

Use the chart created in the Apply It earlier in this chapter. Take the same 10 and convert all of the measurements to metric units. If you did not do that exercise, then select 10 items in your refrigerator or kitchen cabinet, such as cereal, juice, or household cleaners. Create a chart and convert all of the ingredient measurements on the label to the metric scale.

mass
(MASS)
The amount of matter.

Career Connect

Complete a job shadow experience at a hospital or retail pharmacy. List the various mathematical calculations that are used in the processing/filling of prescriptions. Determine the different careers represented by those that are working in the pharmacy and the education preparation required for each.

Teaching Tips

- Review the metric terms, their abbreviations, and what they are used to measure.
- Advise students to memorize the conversion equivalents:
  - One ounce (oz) equals 30 grams (g).
  - One pound (lb) equals .45 kilograms (kg) or one kilogram equals 2.2 pounds.
- Explain how to convert liquid or volume measurements from standard to metric:
  - Multiply the standard measurement in ounces by 30 cc/ml.
- Remind students that cc and ml are the same.

Apply It

- The previous Apply It activity can be found on p. 266.
- Students can simply add a column to the existing table for the metric measurement.

Career Connect

- If students are not able to arrange a job shadow, they may be able to interview a worker.
- Alternatively, you may be able to arrange for a worker to visit the class and discuss his or her job, and the math skills that are required.

Math Link—Metric Prefixes

- You may want to display a measuring device that has both metric and standard measurements, such as a ruler or beaker.
- Review the metric prefixes.
- Review the process for converting milliliters to liters.

How many milliliters are in 25 liters?

Answer: There are 25,000 milliliters (mL) in 25 liters (L).

Teaching Tips

- Explain how to convert mass or weight measurements from standard to metric, or from metric to standard:
  - Multiply the standard measurement in pounds by .45 kilograms.
  - Multiply the metric measurement in kilograms by 2.2 pounds.

ACTIVITY

Convert your current weight from pounds to grams, or kilograms. Convert your current height from inches to meters.

ACTIVITY

Do you ever prepare instant foods such as hot chocolate, oatmeal, or macaroni and cheese by adding water? In this activity, select an instant food item, and calculate how much water you must add in metric measurements. Then, measure the correct amount.

CUSTOMIZED INSTRUCTION

Less Advanced Students

You may need to spend time reinforcing memorization of the multiplication table to help less advanced students with the process of converting from standard to metric measurements.

Math Link

Metric Prefixes

In the United States, most everyday measurements are made using standard units such as ounces, pounds, and feet. In the medical industry, however, many measurements are made using metric units, examples include measuring and weighing medications, physical therapy angles, and intake and output recording. The meter (m), gram (g), and liter (L) are basic metric units. The metric system is a system of measurement that is based on 10, which greatly simplifies calculations. By multiplying or dividing by 10, a new metric unit can be reached.

Different metric units can be identified by their prefixes. If you recognize the prefix, you immediately know information about the given measurement. For example, 1 *kilo*meter equals 1,000 meters, while 1 *milli*meter equals 1/1000 of a meter.

You may often need to convert from one unit to another. Converting between units is accomplished by moving the decimal point. Look at the decimal relationships in the chart. For example, suppose you are given a measurement of 1.5 kilograms, but you need the measurement in grams.

To convert from kilograms to grams, move the decimal three places to the right. So 1.5 kilograms is equal to 1,500 grams.

Prefix	Symbol	Exponent Form	Decimal Equivalent
kilo-	k	103	1000
hecto-	h	102	100
deka-	da	10	10
—	—	—	—
deci-	d	10^{-1}	0.1
centi-	c	10^{-2}	0.01
milli-	m	10^{-3}	0.001

How many milliliters are in 25 liters?

Determine a medical process or procedure that uses metric measures. Choose a level of accuracy appropriate for the selected process or procedure measurement.

Summary

We have discussed the basic units of measure in the metric system. These include meters, grams, and liters. When the prefix *kilo* is used before a basic unit of measure, it multiplies the unit 1,000 times. When *hecto* is used, it increases the basic unit by 100 times. We have also discussed how less than one unit is expressed by using prefixes of *deci*, 1/10 of a unit; *centi*, 1/100 of a unit; and *milli*, 1/1000 of a unit. You have learned four basic rules to follow when using the metric system, methods of converting standard units to metric units, and various ways to measure.

Section 11.2 Review Questions

1. What is a metric unit for each of the following measurements: length, distance, weight, and volume?
2. For a metric unit, what prefixes denote 100 units, 1000 units, 1/10 unit, 1/100 unit, and 1/1000 unit?
3. List four basic rules to follow when using the metric system.
4. What is the relationship between ounces, cubic centimeters, and milliliters?
5. Convert the following values as indicated:
   a. 3 lb to kg b. 50 oz to g c. 5 kg to lb d. 100 g to oz
6. How do you change pounds to kilograms?

272 Chapter 11 | Medical Math

Section 11.2 Review Questions

1. Answer: Length: centimeters, millimeters, meters, and others; Distance: meters, kilometers, hectometers, and others; Weight: grams, kilograms, hectograms, and others; Volume: liter, milliliter, cubic centimeters, and others
2. Answer: 100 units = hector; 1,000 units = kilo; 1/10 unit = deci; 1/100 unit = centi; 1/1000 unit = milli
3. Answer: Numbers indicating less than one unit are always written in decimal form, not as fractions. When writing decimals, if there is no number before the decimal, always write a 0. Abbreviations for metric terms are never plural; they are always written in singular form. Always capitalize the abbreviation L for liter to reduce confusing the lowercase l with the number 1. Leave a space between the number and the abbreviation.

The 24-Hour Clock/Military Time

SECTION 11.3

Background

Medical facilities frequently use the 24-hour clock system. The 24-hour clock clearly states time and eliminates confusion when documenting information. A health care worker is required to understand and interpret time in every health care setting.

Objectives

When you have completed this section, you will be able to do the following:

- Match key terms with their correct meanings.
- Recognize time on a 24-hour clock.
- Express 24-hour time/military time verbally and in writing.
- Convert Greenwich time to 24-hour time.

Introduction to the 24-Hour Clock/ Military Time

In the health care setting, it is important that time be stated in a clear, concise manner. All medical records are legal documents. Time indicates when treatment, medication, and other activities are done and how long procedures or incidents last. A 24-hour clock eliminates the confusion between A.M. (12 midnight to 12 noon) and P.M. (12 noon to 12 midnight) hours. It provides a clear, concise record for recording medical services. The military services were the first to use a 24-hour clock; therefore, the 24-hour system is often referred to as **24-hour time/military time**. Table 11.8 shows you the difference in expressing **Greenwich** and military time. (Figure 11.3)

Military time is always expressed in four digits, and no colons are used to separate hours and minutes. Always use a 0 to complete the four-digit number (for example, for 1:00 A.M., use 0100 instead of 100). When expressing military time, remember to state it in hundreds: for example, zero one hundred hours (0100) is 1:00 A.M.; eleven hundred hours (1100) is 11:00 A.M.; twenty-three hundred hours (2300) is 11:00 P.M.

It is easy to remember that morning hours are 0100 to 1200 hours. The afternoon and nighttime hours can be added to the 1200 hours of noon. For example:

- To determine how 5:00 P.M. is expressed in military time, add 1200 and 0500 (1200 + 0500 = 1700 hours).
- To determine how 12 midnight is expressed in military time, add 1200 and 1200 = 2400 hours.

24-hour time/military time
(MIL i ter ee TIEM)
Method of telling time by counting each hour consecutively for 24 hours (i.e., . . . 11, 12, 13, . . .).

Greenwich time
(GREN ich TIEM)
Standard time, a 12-hour clock.

Apply It

Create a poster board comparing Greenwich Time and 24-Hour/ Military Time. Research who uses each type of time and why we use two different accountings for time.

Present this information to 4th and 5th grade classes. Then, create a short 20 question flashcard game for the class. Hold up a card with a question on it, such as "What time do you start school?" or "What time do you eat dinner?" and ask who can tell you what that is in Military time.

Medical Math | Chapter 11 273

4. Answer: They measure liquids. An ounce is equal to 30 cc (cubic centimeters) or 30 mL (milliliters); a milliliter is $^{1}/_{1000}$th of a liter; cubic centimeters are interchangeable with milliliters.
5. Answers: a. 1.35 kg; b. 1,500 g; c. 11 lb; d. 3.33 oz
6. Answer: To change pounds to kilograms, multiply the number of pounds by 0.45 lb/kg.

FOCUS AND ENGAGE

Introduce the Section

a. Review the content of the Background paragraph, explaining that the Greenwich clock uses only 12 hours.
b. Emphasize that the 24-hour clock is more precise because you do not have to differentiate between A.M. and P.M.
c. Review the section objectives.

Vocabulary Review

a. Direct students to the key terms.
b. Pronounce each word, and have the students repeat the pronunciation out loud.
c. Discuss each definition.

TEACH

Discuss

- Ask students if they have any experience using a 24-hour clock. If not, they may have heard it used in military movies.
- Discuss ways time is referenced in health care, such as when a patient is checked, when medications are administered, when surgery is scheduled, etc.
- Discuss problems that might arise if incorrect or imprecise times are referenced.

Reinforce and Review

- Review the importance of clear, concise communication.
- Reinforce the importance of accuracy when charting.

Apply It

- You may want to break this activity into four parts: Part 1: Research the two different types of time. Part 2: Create a poster and presentation about your research. Part 3: Create flashcards. Part 4: Deliver the presentation.
- You may want students to work in small groups.
- You may want to allow class time for students to practice delivering the presentation.

Teaching Tips

- Introduce the topic of the 24-hour clock.

ACTIVITY

Write your daily schedule using the Military/24-hour clock instead of the Greenwich clock.

Teaching Tips

- Explain Greenwich time using A.M. and P.M. times:
  - Most of us use Greenwich time.
  - If A.M. or P.M. are not indicated, it can be confusing.
- Explain Military time:
  - 24-hour clock
  - Fewer mistakes
  - Clearer
- Explain how Greenwich time and 24-hour time relate.

Figure Focus

11.3 24-hour clock: military time. What is the military time for the following: 8:30 A.M., 7:45 P.M., 3:15 P.M., and 12:10 A.M.?

Answers: 0830 hours; 1945 hours; 1515 hours; 0010 hours.

Table 11.8 will help you understand the relationship between Greenwich time and military time.

Table 11.8 Comparison of Greenwich and 24-Hour/Military Time

Greenwich	Military	Greenwich	Military
1:00 A.M.	0100	1:00 P.M.	1300
2:00 A.M.	0200	2:00 P.M.	1400
3:00 A.M.	0300	3:00 P.M.	1500
4:00 A.M.	0400	4:00 P.M.	1600
5:00 A.M.	0500	5:00 P.M.	1700
6:00 A.M.	0600	6:00 P.M.	1800
7:00 A.M.	0700	7:00 P.M.	1900
8:00 A.M.	0800	8:00 P.M.	2000
9:00 A.M.	0900	9:00 P.M.	2100
10:00 A.M.	1000	10:00 P.M.	2200
11:00 A.M.	1100	11:00 P.M.	2300
12:00 noon	1200	12:00 P.M./midnight	2400/0000

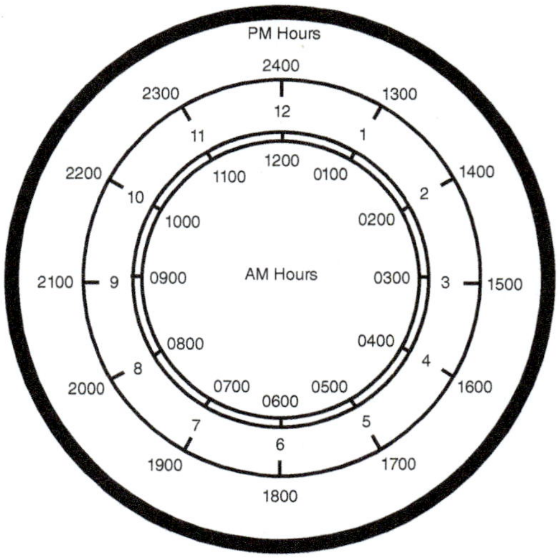

Figure 11.3
24-hour clock: military time. What is the military time for the following: 8:30 A.M., 7:45 P.M., 3:15 P.M., and 12:10 A.M.?

274 Chapter 11 | Medical Math

CUSTOMIZED INSTRUCTION

At-Risk Students

On a sheet of plain paper, have students create their own 24-hour clock, using the one shown in Figure 11.3 as an example. Encourage them to be creative in the design and colors used. Display the clocks around the room.

Summary

In this section, you learned the relationship between Greenwich time and military time and how to determine the time of day using a 24-hour clock. You also learned that the 24-hour clock eliminates confusion between A.M. and P.M. hours.

Section 11.3 Review Questions

1. Describe the 24-hour clock.
2. Why should you use the 24-hour clock to record time?
3. Express the following times numerically in military time: 11:00 A.M., 4:50 P.M., and 11:45 P.M.
4. Express the following times verbally in military time: 3:20 A.M., noon, and 6:15 P.M.
5. Convert the following Greenwich times to 24-hour time: midnight, 5:35 A.M., 8:56 P.M., and 9:34 P.M.
6. What is Greenwich time?

Medical Math | Chapter 11 275

ACTIVITY

Use the Internet to access the Web site of a major airport and find the page that lists arrival or departure times. If the times are listed using the Greenwich clock, convert them to 24-hour time If the times are listed using the 24-hour clock, convert them to Greenwich time.

Teaching Tips

- Emphasize the importance of accurate timing in a health care environment.
- Review the rules for expressing military time:
  - Always use four digits; That means you must always use a leading zero for digits less than 10.
  - Do not use colons to separate hours from minutes.
  - When speaking out loud, state the time in hundreds.
- Practice expressing military time by pointing to time on a Greenwich clock and asking for the Military time.
- Remind students that Greenwich time is based on a 12-hour clock, with A.M. used to indicate the first 12 hours, and P.M. used to indicate the second 12 hours.

Section 11.3 Review Questions

1. Answer: The 24-hour clock clearly states time and eliminates confusion when documenting information.
2. Answer: A 24-hour clock eliminates the confusion between A.M. (12 midnight to 12 noon) and P.M. (12 noon to 12 midnight) hours.
3. Answer: 1100 hours, 1650 hours, 2345 hours
4. Answer: (Students will say times verbally) 0320 hours, 1200 hours, 1815 hours
5. Answer: 2400/0000, 0535, 2056, 2134
6. Answer: Greenwich time is the standard time, 12-hour clock.

CHAPTER 11 REVIEW

Chapter Review Questions

1. Answer: $634\,{}^{4}/_{15}$, $1\,{}^{47}/_{355}$
2. Answer: 1.283, 0.0046, 0.32
3. Answer: m = meter measures length, mL = milliliter measures ${}^{1}/_{1000}$ of a liter for volume, cm = centimeter measures ${}^{1}/_{100}$ of a meter for length, kg = kilogram measures 1000 grams for weight, cc = cubic centimeters measures volume
4. Answer: These measure length. deci = 0.1 or ${}^{1}/_{10}$ unit, centi = 0.01 or ${}^{1}/_{100}$ unit, milli = 0.001 or ${}^{1}/_{1000}$ unit
5. Answer: 120 mL, 300 mL, 960 mL
6. Answer: 2.2 lb, 110 lb, 165 lb
7. Answer: To change pounds to kilograms, multiply the number of pounds by 0.45 lb/kg.
8. Answer: The 24-hour clock uses 4-digit numbers to identify the time of day.
9. Answer: 1300 hours
10. Answer: 4 P.M.

Activities

1. Emphasize that this activity challenges the students' abilities to convert fractions and to use a clock. You might direct students to set up the schedule as a table, with the activity in column 1, the Greenwich time in column 2, and the Military time in column 3.
2. Point out that household measurements refers to standard measures. Point out that the conversions shown are not between standard and metric. They are from one standard measure to another. Explain that students may have to convert to a different standard measure in order to use the formulas they have memorized to convert to metric. For example, they know how to convert from ounces to cc/ml but not from cups to cc/ml. If a measurement is in cups, they can convert cups to ounces and then convert ounces to cc/ml. You may want to demonstrate one or two of the conversions.

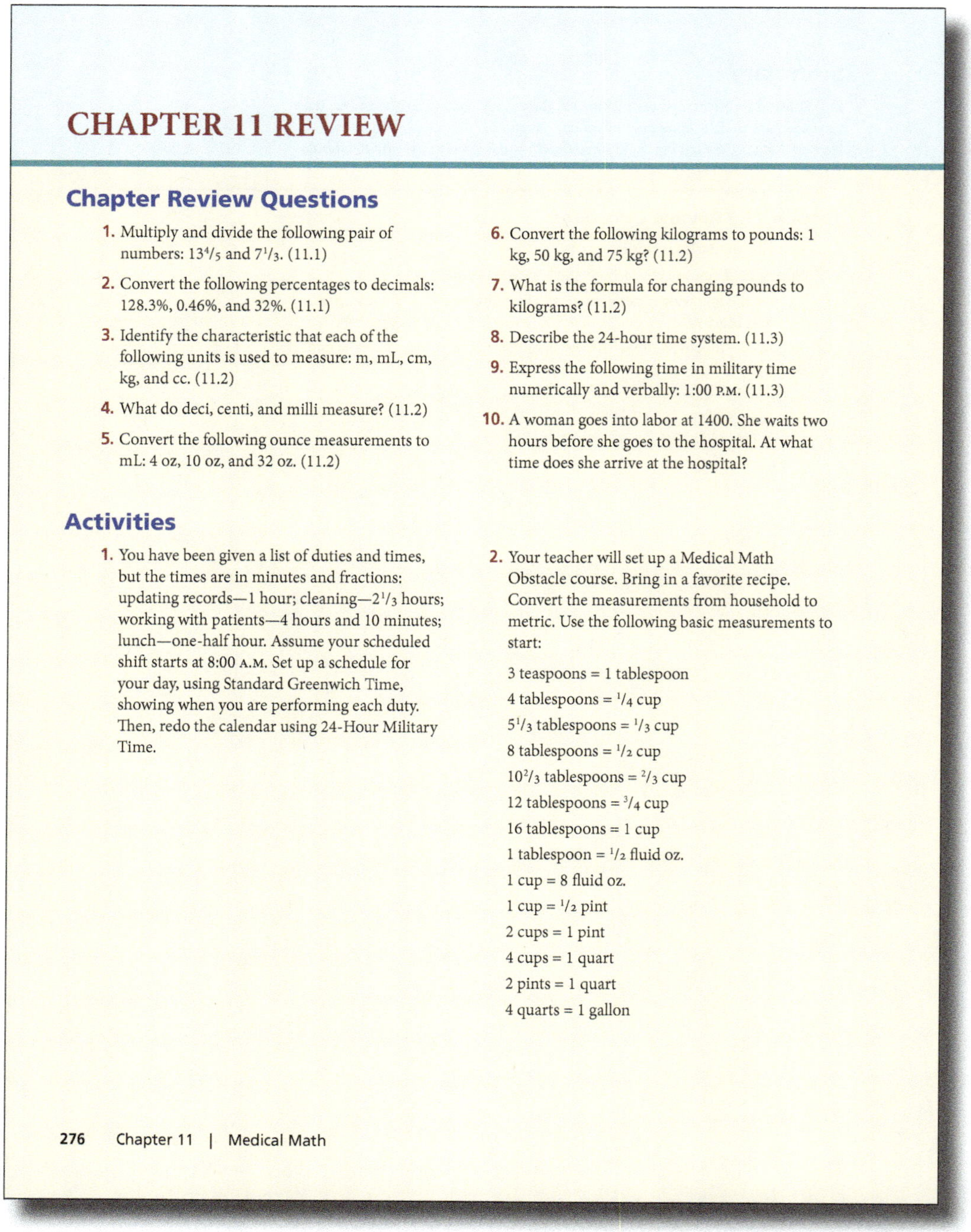

CHAPTER 11 REVIEW

Chapter Review Questions

1. Multiply and divide the following pair of numbers: $13\,{}^{4}/_{5}$ and $7\,{}^{1}/_{3}$. (11.1)
2. Convert the following percentages to decimals: 128.3%, 0.46%, and 32%. (11.1)
3. Identify the characteristic that each of the following units is used to measure: m, mL, cm, kg, and cc. (11.2)
4. What do deci, centi, and milli measure? (11.2)
5. Convert the following ounce measurements to mL: 4 oz, 10 oz, and 32 oz. (11.2)
6. Convert the following kilograms to pounds: 1 kg, 50 kg, and 75 kg? (11.2)
7. What is the formula for changing pounds to kilograms? (11.2)
8. Describe the 24-hour time system. (11.3)
9. Express the following time in military time numerically and verbally: 1:00 P.M. (11.3)
10. A woman goes into labor at 1400. She waits two hours before she goes to the hospital. At what time does she arrive at the hospital?

Activities

1. You have been given a list of duties and times, but the times are in minutes and fractions: updating records—1 hour; cleaning—$2\,{}^{1}/_{3}$ hours; working with patients—4 hours and 10 minutes; lunch—one-half hour. Assume your scheduled shift starts at 8:00 A.M. Set up a schedule for your day, using Standard Greenwich Time, showing when you are performing each duty. Then, redo the calendar using 24-Hour Military Time.
2. Your teacher will set up a Medical Math Obstacle course. Bring in a favorite recipe. Convert the measurements from household to metric. Use the following basic measurements to start:

3 teaspoons = 1 tablespoon
4 tablespoons = ${}^{1}/_{4}$ cup
$5\,{}^{1}/_{3}$ tablespoons = ${}^{1}/_{3}$ cup
8 tablespoons = ${}^{1}/_{2}$ cup
$10\,{}^{2}/_{3}$ tablespoons = ${}^{2}/_{3}$ cup
12 tablespoons = ${}^{3}/_{4}$ cup
16 tablespoons = 1 cup
1 tablespoon = ${}^{1}/_{2}$ fluid oz.
1 cup = 8 fluid oz.
1 cup = ${}^{1}/_{2}$ pint
2 cups = 1 pint
4 cups = 1 quart
2 pints = 1 quart
4 quarts = 1 gallon

276 Chapter 11 | Medical Math

CUSTOMIZED INSTRUCTION

Special Needs Students

Have students write each key term and its pronunciation. There is a lot of memorization in this chapter. Special needs students might benefit from study aids such as large print flashcards for memorizing the multiplication table, metric units, and metric/standard equivalents on one side of an index card and its definition on the other side.

CHAPTER 11 REVIEW

Case Studies

1. A new mother arrives for the baby's first well-baby checkup at 1:00 P.M. You know that she should be taken to an examination room within 5 minutes. Your employer uses military time. Explain how 1:05 P.M. is written in military time. You call the patient's name and ask her to follow you to the scales. You weigh the baby and find she weighs 3.84 kilograms. What will you tell the mother her baby's weight is in pounds and ounces?

2. Health care workers are expected to communicate effectively with co-workers, patients, and their families. In the United States, standard units of measure are common, and metric units of measure are less common. Patients or their families may be expected to measure their medicine and fluid intake and convert these measurements to metric units. It is essential to explain how to do this in terms a patient will understand. Write instructions to a 75-year-old patient explaining the difference between ounces and cubic centimeters. Your instructions must describe how to measure and calculate the patient's 24-hour fluid intake.

Thinking Critically

1. **Safety Alert**—Describe two scenarios in which instructions given to patients using a 12-hour clock may be confusing and put patients at risk. Explain how instructions given using a 24-hour clock can prevent problems.

2. **Medical Math**—A mother gets a prescription for her child. The instructions say to give the child 15mL of antibiotic tid. The mother only has teaspoons at home and does not know how much medicine to give her child. Can you help her?

3. **Math Facts**—Use filling prescriptions as the example for determining accurate measures. In a team of three, complete the following exercise. Fill four simulated prescriptions. Each prescription will require mathematical calculations.

   Medication A is a liquid to be taken as 2 fl. oz., four times a day, until gone. The bottle has 96 oz. How long will it last?

   Give Medication B as 10mg/kg body weight, 2 times per day for 10 days. The patient weighs 79 lbs. Each pill cannot contain more than 200 mg. of Medication B. How many mg. per day would the patient require, and how many pills per day would that be? What would be the mg. dosage of each pill?

   The patient requires 50 mg. of medication C every morning, via teaspoon. The medication solution contains 25 mg. /teaspoon. How many teaspoons must your patient take per day?

   The patient requires 1.25 mg. of Medication D. Medication D comes in a solution of 5 mg. per 5 ml. How many ml of Medication D will the patient receive?

   Teams report on their conclusions and their process for finding the answers.

Medical Math | Chapter 11 277

Case Studies

1. Point out that this activity has two parts: First, students must convert 1:05 to military time. Next, students must convert kilograms to pounds and ounces.
2. You may want to provide the amount of the patient's 24-hour fluid intake. Remind students that they should write concisely and clearly, and to use step-by-step procedures when appropriate. Also, remind students that they are writing instructions for a senior citizen.

Thinking Critically

1. Direct the student to write a complete answer in paragraph form. They should provide specific examples of situations that might be encountered in real life.
2. Point out that students will need to call on their knowledge of medical abbreviations for this problem. Direct the students to provide clear, concise written instructions for the parent. Students may also want to perform a skit in which they help the parent.
3. Note that this activity should be performed in small groups or pharmacy teams. Direct students to show their calculations.

CUSTOMIZED INSTRUCTION

English Language Learners

For Case Study 2, have students read their instructions aloud to a partner. The partner should note any parts of the instruction he or she does not understand and suggest ways to reword it. Students should make revisions as necessary.

TEAMWORK

In small groups, prepare a skit demonstrating a problem that might arise from using standard units of measure instead of metric units in a health care environment.

Portfolio Connection

- If possible students should use a computer spreadsheet program to record the information about the public and private institutions.
- Alternatively, they can set up a table to display the information.
- Check to make sure that students have completed the written assignments and added them to their portfolio.

ACTIVITY

Write a letter to a friend, teacher, or family member about an upcoming event. Mention at least four different times, using only the 24-hour/Military clock.

CHAPTER 11 REVIEW

Portfolio Connections

Research private and public schools for higher education in your career choice. Create a spreadsheet that clearly compares costs for each school, using the following criteria:

- Entrance requirements
- Tuition (costs must be compared equally, that is, semester to semester, quarter to quarter, or hours to hours)
- Books (number of books and the cost for new and used books)
- Supplies and materials (list and compare like items)
- Uniforms (identify all required uniform parts, e.g., shoes, name tag)
- Housing
- Transportation (type of transportation, round-trip miles)
- Miscellaneous
- Financial aid resources (eligibility criteria, amount of dollars available, repayment requirements, and interest rates)

PORTFOLIO TIP

Be sure to visit several facilities of the type in which you hope to work. Remember that one facility alone may not be typical. Keep a dated record of each visit with your reactions noted. Place this in the Personal Tips and Reminders section of your portfolio. This is an important step in your career planning: deciding where you will be happiest working.

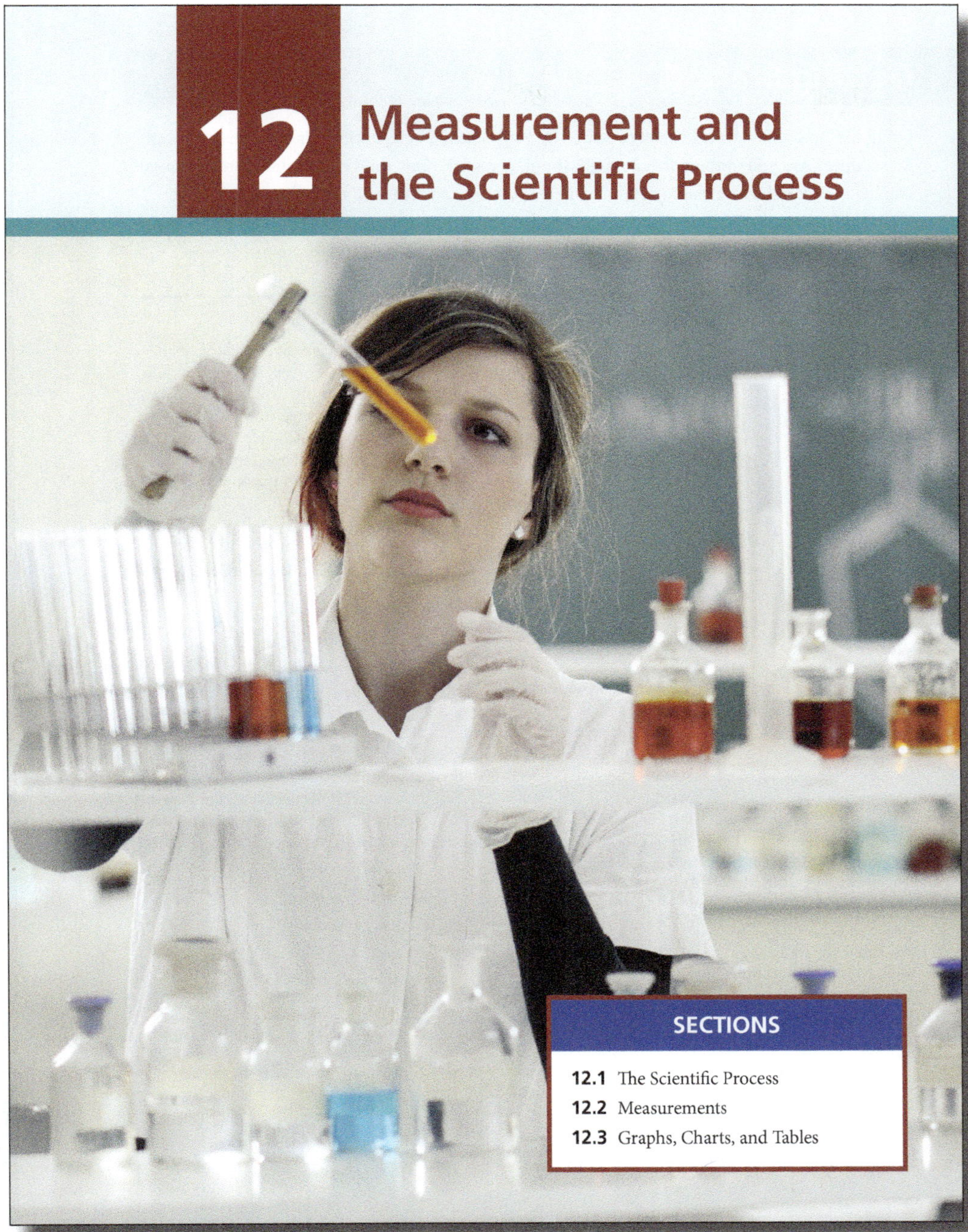

CHAPTER 12 OVERVIEW

In Chapter 12, students learn how to use measurement and the scientific process, as well as how to create and read charts, tables, and graphs. This information helps health care professionals interpret information and communicate with co-workers and patients.

Section 12.1: Section 12.1 introduces the eight steps in the scientific process that scientists use to conduct experiments.

Section 12.2: Section 12.2 follows up the metric system content covered in Chapter 11. It provides more in-depth information about units and tools used to measure. It also discusses the importance of accuracy and precision.

Section 12.3: In Section 12.3, students learn about common charts and graphs used to present data in a health care environment.

Advance Preparation	
Review	■ Review Chapter text for Sections 12.1, 12.2, and 12.3.
Contact	■ A scientist, teacher, or researcher willing to visit the class to discuss the scientific process. ■ A lab at a health care facility, research facility, or school to arrange a tour.
Prepare	■ Samples of medical or scientific journals showing published reports of scientific experiments. ■ Measuring devices such as meter sticks, liters, thermometers, and scales. ■ Samples of different types of charts, graphs, and tables. ■ A list of Web sites that provide information about scientific methods—such as sciencebuddies.org.

FOCUS AND ENGAGE

Getting Started

- Make copies of a Body Mass Index chart and distribute them to the class.
- You can find one—along with a body mass index calculator—at Web sites such as cdc.gov/healthyweight/assessing/bmi.
- Show students how to locate their height in column 1, read across to find their weight, and then identify their BMI.

Introduce the Section

a. Review the Background paragraph, explaining that even workers who do not conduct experiments should understand the scientific process.
b. Emphasize the importance of following the steps in order to insure accuracy of the results.
c. Review the section objectives.

Vocabulary Review

a. Direct students to the key terms.
b. Pronounce each word, and have the students repeat the pronunciation out loud.
c. Discuss each definition.

TEACH

Discuss

- Ask students if any of them have experience with the scientific process in science class, or at a science fair.
- Discuss the importance of following the process, and some of the problems that might arise from not following the process, such as incorrect results.

Reinforce and Review

- Review the importance of observation.

Teaching Tips

- Review the eight steps of the scientific method:
  - Make observations.
  - Ask a question.
  - Develop a hypothesis.
  - Make a prediction.
  - Test the hypothesis.
  - Analyze the results.
  - Draw conclusions.
  - Communicate results.

Getting Started

Using the Body Mass Index Chart provided by your teacher, determine your own personal Body Mass Index. Are you in the normal range? If not, consider a nutrition and exercise program that will help you reach a normal range. You will learn more about nutrition in Chapter 16.

SECTION 12.1 The Scientific Process

Background

Scientists, including medical professionals and biotechnical researchers, often perform experiments to answer the questions they have about the world around them. As a health care professional, it is important for you to understand the scientific method and how the research results are reported. This knowledge is essential to your ability to communicate clinical information to patients and your team. Understanding and using the scientific process also promotes the use of proven and effective methods of health care and the promotion of higher standards of care for all patients.

Objectives

When you have completed this section, you will be able to do the following:

- Match key terms with their correct meanings.
- List eight basic steps of scientific methods.
- Describe a controlled experiment.
- Explain the importance of communication in scientific methods.

Scientific Methods

Scientists, including scientists working in health care, are always asking questions: What medicine will work best to treat this disease? Is the medicine safe? How does the medicine affect people? To answer these questions, scientists use **scientific methods**. The basic steps of scientific methods, which are described in this section, include the following:

- Make observations.
- Ask a question.
- Develop a hypothesis.
- Make a prediction.
- Test the hypothesis.
- Analyze the results.
- Draw conclusions.
- Communicate results.

scientific methods
(SIE uhn tif ik METH uhds)
Processes scientists use to answer questions.

observations
(AHBS uhr vay shuhns)
Using the senses and other means to get information about surroundings.

Making Observations and Asking Questions

How scientists use scientific methods varies depending on what they are trying to find out and what happens during their research. However, all scientific processes start with **observations**.

280 Chapter 12 | Measurement and the Scientific Process

CUSTOMIZED INSTRUCTION
More Advanced Students
Allow more advanced students to look up why knowing one's Body Mass Index (BMI) is important, and report their findings to the class.

CUSTOMIZED INSTRUCTION OVERVIEW	
Less Advanced Students	Page 286
More Advanced Students	Pages 280, 290, 294
English Language Learners	Pages 281, 290
Special Needs Students	Page 284
At-Risk Students	Page 281

Observations

To make observations, a scientist gathers information. He or she may watch, listen, touch, or even smell to gather information. Based on what the scientist observes, he or she asks a question. For example, a scientist observes that some people don't get sick when exposed to a disease, so the scientist might ask why this is happening. He or she might also ask how this information can be used to benefit other people.

Questions

There are many scientific questions that have yet to be answered. Most of those questions are quite big, and it is rarely possible for one scientist, or even one team of scientists, to find answers to big questions. Groups of scientists may work together, or separately, on smaller questions related to the big question and eventually their results provide answers to the big question. A scientific question often begins with the word "why." A why question usually stems from creatively wondering why something is the way it is, or why it isn't another way. Why questions tend to be "big" questions and, as such, are often untestable. Rephrasing a question so that it describes something specific, or asks about a cause, breaks big questions down into testable questions. For example, instead of asking "Why do microorganisms multiply?" the scientist can ask, "Do microorganisms multiply when the temperature is below freezing?" or "Do warm, moist conditions cause microorganisms to multiply." The creativity that sparked the question about why microorganisms multiply is channeled into testable questions.

Community

Take copies of the BMI Chart to students at the elementary or middle school or to another class at the high school you attend and show them how to determine their individual BMI and rate their own results.

Hypotheses

After a testable question has been determined, the scientist will make more observations based on the question. After further observation, the scientist develops one or more **hypotheses**. A hypothesis can be tested. For example, a hypothesis might be that people who run two to three miles daily will not catch bronchitis if exposed to it. Not just an educated guess, a hypothesis is intended to answer the scientific question that was asked. A hypothesis is about causes that lead to effects.

hypothesis
(HIE poth uh sis)
An explanation for an observation that is based on scientific research and that can be tested.

Predicting Results and Testing Predictions

After a scientist has a hypothesis, he or she will design an experiment to test the hypothesis. (Figure 12.1) The scientist makes a prediction about what will happen during the experiment. All of the experiments that the scientist performs must be recorded and well documented. Accurate record keeping helps the scientist draw conclusions, identify possible errors, and develop new ideas. It also helps other scientists repeat the experiment.

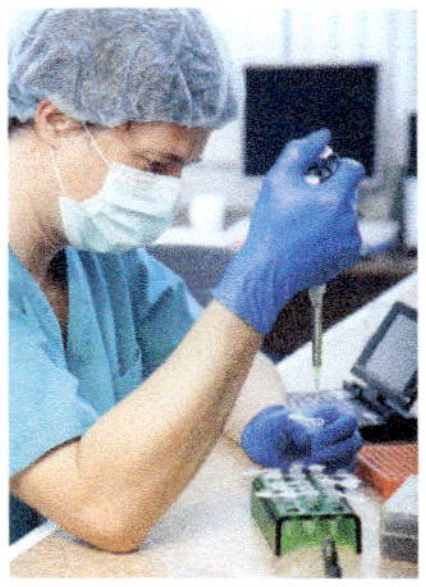

Figure 12.1
A scientist tests his hypothesis. Why do scientists perform controlled experiments?

It is important for any scientist to use **controlled experiments.** In these experiments, all variables except the one being tested are the same and do not change. If more than one variable is changed, it is hard to identify what caused the results of the experiment.

controlled experiments
(kuhn TRULD eks PEER uh muhnts)
Experiments in which only one factor, or variable, is changed.

Teaching Tips

- Review ways to form a hypothesis using a conditional, or if-then, statement: "If I do this, then this will happen."
- Explain that in addition to observation, scientists use research to help develop a hypothesis.
- Emphasize that the purpose of an experiment is to prove whether a hypothesis is right or wrong.
- Ask students to think of ways they might design an experiment to test a hypothesis. For example ask them how they might test the hypothesis that "If I drop an egg from a higher point, it will splatter farther."
- Explain what is meant by a variable. Provide an example, such as for the egg splatter experiment, where the variable would be the height from which the egg is dropped.
- Explain what is meant by a constant. For example, in the egg splatter experiment, use only large eggs, drop all eggs on to the same surface, perform the experiment in the same room, etc.
- Discuss how multiple variables might change the result of the experiment.

Figure Focus

12.1 A scientist tests his hypothesis. Why do scientists perform controlled experiments?

Answer: If an experiment is not controlled, it is difficult to identify what caused the result.

CUSTOMIZED INSTRUCTION

English Language Learners

Have students write each key term and its pronunciation on one side of an index card and its definition on the other side. Have them read each term and definition aloud to a partner.

At-Risk Students

For the Community activity, students are instructed to show other students how to determine their BMI. Some students may be sensitive about their weight and physical attributes. Propose an alternative activity, such as discussing school and community programs that promote health and fitness.

Community

- Make arrangements in advance for your students to visit an elementary school, after school program, or a different class in your school.
- Emphasize to students that they must use positive language when discussing weight and body mass, and that they should focus on lifestyle choices and movement.

Teaching Tips

- Discuss methods of record keeping during an experiment.
- Point out that it is important to document errors or unexpected results, as well as all observations.
- Review how scientists interpret results:
  - Read the data
  - Determine if the hypothesis is supported
- Discuss peer review of scientific results.
- Review ways of communicating results:
  - Publishing
  - Presenting

Section 12.1 Review Questions

1. Answer: Scientific methods are processes scientists use to answer questions. Observations use the senses and other means to get information about surroundings.
2. Answer: Make observations. Ask a question. Develop a hypothesis. Make a prediction. Test the hypothesis. Analyze the results. Draw conclusions. Communicate results.
3. Answer: Developing a hypothesis
4. Answer: It is important for scientists to use controlled experiments. In these experiments, all variables except the one being tested are the same and do not change. If more than one variable is changed, it is hard to identify what caused the results of the experiment.

Career Connect

Are you the type of person who is always asking questions? Do you need to understand the "why" behind every decision? You might want to consider a career in health care research. Study the types of entry level positions available in this field.

Drawing Conclusions and Communicating Results

After a scientist finishes an experiment, he or she analyzes the results to see if the hypothesis is supported. If it is, the scientist will communicate the results. He or she may perform additional research. Sometimes the hypothesis is not supported. This is not a bad thing—the scientist can still use the information. Based on the data, the scientist might run the experiment again to see if there was an error. He or she can use the information to come up with a new hypothesis to test.

After the scientist has analyzed the results and drawn a conclusion, he or she needs to communicate the results to other scientists so other scientists can develop their own hypotheses. This is often done by publishing reports in scientific and medical journals. These reports should clearly describe the experimental process so other scientists can perform the same experiment.

Because math is the language of science, the outcomes of experiments are often reported as numbers. When the results are very small or very large, scientists use "scientific notation" to report their findings. See the following example.

Standard Scientific Notation: $a \times 10^b$ Example: $5{,}400{,}000 = 5.4 \times 10^6$

To write a number using scientific notation, simply move the decimal point from the very end of the number to right behind the first number. Then, count the number of places you moved the decimal and record it as a power of 10.

The ability to replicate an experiment and duplicate the results supports the validity of the hypotheses. Communication also helps scientists compare hypotheses and verify the accuracy of experiments. Finally, clear communication helps scientists trust each other.

Summary

Scientific methods start with observations. Then, scientists ask questions about their observations. They develop a hypothesis, which they test. After analyzing the results, scientists draw conclusions about their experiments and communicate the results to other scientists.

Section 12.1 Review Questions

1. Define the terms scientific methods and observations.
2. What are the eight steps of the scientific method?
3. During which step of the scientific method do scientists propose a possible explanation of their observations?
4. Why is it important to use controlled experiments?
5. Why should scientists communicate their results even if the results don't support their hypotheses?
6. What is a hypothesis?
7. Why do scientist use scientific notation?

282 Chapter 12 | Measurement and the Scientific Process

5. Answer: Scientists should communicate their results even if the results don't support their hypotheses because, based on the data, the scientist might run the experiment again to see if there was an error. He or she can use the information to come up with a new hypothesis to test. The scientist can also communicate the results so other scientists can develop their own hypotheses.
6. Answer: A hypothesis is an explanation for an observation that is based on scientific research and can be tested.
7. Answer: Scientists use scientific notation because it is a convenient way of expressing very large or very small numbers.

Career Connect

- Ask the students to look up the types of careers available in health care research.
- Have them note the education requirements and the entry-level opportunities.

Personal Wellness

Lab Safety

Laboratories pose many safety risks. When working in a lab, you need to consider the following:

1. Follow all safety rules. Your teacher or facility has rules about how you should dress and behave in a lab. Follow these rules to avoid injury.
2. Know your safety symbols. Labs have standard symbols that indicate safety hazards. For example, a bottle of chemicals may have a warning symbol that indicates it is flammable. Work with your teacher or facility to recognize these symbols.
3. Read and follow directions. Anytime you work in a lab, carefully read through the procedure instructions. If you don't understand a step, be sure to clear up any confusion before you start.
4. Use safety equipment. Goggles, gloves, and aprons protect you from injury. Use them anytime you are directed to do so. If you are uncertain whether you need the equipment, ask your supervisor.
5. Keep your workspace clean and neat. Avoid clutter, and clean up your workspace according to your teacher's or facility's instructions.
6. Know emergency procedures. Work with your teacher or facility to understand what you need to do if you are injured or if another person is injured. Certain emergencies, such as eye injuries, need special equipment. Make sure you know where this equipment is located and how it is used.
7. Report all accidents immediately. Even if an accident is minor, tell your teacher or supervisor.

A bottle has a symbol showing goggles on it. What should you do?

Science Link

Using the Scientific Method

The scientific method is a good way to organize your thoughts and elicit the types of information needed. A health care professional can use the scientific method to help him or her interact with patients and co-workers about treatments, potential pharmaceutical interactions, and possible side effects.

The scientific method has eight distinct steps:

1. Make observations.
2. Ask a question.
3. Develop a hypothesis.
4. Make a prediction.
5. Test the hypothesis.
6. Draw conclusions.
7. Analyze the results.
8. Communicate results.

Construct an explanation for a simple chemical reaction experiment using the scientific method to determine the results. Working in teams of two, construct a six-column table, labeling each column beginning on the left: Powder, Appearance, Reaction with Water, Reaction with Iodine, Reaction with Rubbing Alcohol, and Reaction with Vinegar. Add four rows to your table for each of four unknown powders. Your teacher will provide you with several unknown powders. Identify the appearance of each of the powders (fine, gritty, smooth, and lumpy). Wear goggles to protect your eyes and mix each powder with each chemical. Record the reaction of each in the appropriate column.

Hypothesize the identity of each mystery powder. Locate a chart with the accurate powder identity. Compare your results to determine if your hypothesis is accurate. Report the results by documenting each step in the scientific method. Match the results with each team in the class to determine which teams' hypothesis was most accurate.

Identify a simulated patient diagnosis and describe how the outcome would benefit from using the scientific method to determine treatment.

Measurement and the Scientific Process | Chapter 12 283

Personal Wellness—Lab Safety

- Review the risks of working in a lab.
- Review the steps to insure safety.
- Review emergency procedures.

A bottle has a symbol showing goggles on it. What should you do?

Answer: You should wear goggles to protect your eyes.

Science Link—Using the Scientific Method

- Decide whether you will have the students perform the experiment in class or out.
- You may want to do the experiment together as a class.
- Before beginning, review the scientific method with the class:
  - What is the control?
  - What are the variables?
  - What is the research?
  - What is the hypothesis?
- Explain how you want students to document the experiment.
- Display a sample lab notebook.
- Allow time for peer review and discussion of the results.
- You may want to develop a rubric for evaluating the activity that includes points for how well the students complete each of the steps.

ACTIVITY

If any students have participated in a science fair, ask them to bring in their project and present it to the class.

FOCUS AND ENGAGE

Introduce the Section

a. Review the content of the Background paragraph, discussing the types of measurements that may be required.

b. Explain that workers must know when to make measurements, what tools to use, and how to record the information.

c. Review the objectives for the section.

Vocabulary Review

a. Direct students to the key terms.

b. Pronounce each word, and have the students repeat the pronunciation out loud.

c. Discuss the definition of each word.

TEACH

Discuss

- Ask students if they know the difference between an estimate and an actual measurement.
- Ask if they have ever relied on an estimate. For example, they might estimate an amount for a recipe, or estimate the length of time it might take to travel somewhere.
- Discuss when it might be appropriate to estimate, when only a precise measurement will do, and the problems that might arise from using an estimate.

Reinforce and Review

- Review the metric system.
- Review basic math skills.

SECTION 12.2 Measurements

Background

Health care workers often need to make measurements. They may need to record temperature, the size of a wound, or the weight of a patient. Health care workers must understand what devices and units are used to make each of these measurements. They also need to understand the importance of estimating, accuracy, and precision in making measurements.

Objectives

When you have completed this section, you will be able to do the following:

- Match the key terms with their correct meanings
- Identify tools used to measure length, time, temperature, volume, and mass/weight.
- Identify units used to measure length, time, temperature, volume, and mass/weight.
- Describe the process of estimating.
- Round various numbers.
- Relate accuracy and precision to the validity of results.
- Explain how estimating may affect accuracy and precision.

Tools for Making Measurements

Scientists use many different tools to make measurements. As a health care worker, you may need to use some of these tools. It is important to understand which tool is used to make a measurement.

Length

The standard units for length are inches (in), feet (f), and miles (mi). The metric units for length include the millimeter (mm), centimeter (cm), meter (m), and kilometer (km). For most of the measurements you will need to make, you will likely use a ruler or meterstick. Sometimes, you may use a flexible measuring tape.

The basic unit of length measurement is the meter. A meter is close to a yard in length (1 meter = 1.093 yard). In addition, there are:

- 2.54 centimeters in 1 inch
- About 1.6 kilometers in 1 mile
- 1,000 meters in 1 kilometer
- 1,000 millimeters in 1 meter

Temperature

Two scales that are used to measure temperature are the Celsius (°C) scale and the Fahrenheit scale (°F). You will most likely use the Fahrenheit scale. You will likely

Teaching Tips

- Display tools for measuring, such as meter sticks, thermometers, beakers, and scales.
- Review the units and tools for measuring length.

CUSTOMIZED INSTRUCTION

Special Needs Students

Special needs students may benefit from customized measuring devices, such as those with units marked in a larger size, raised, or in Braille. If you cannot obtain such devices for your classroom, you may be able to make some.

use electronic thermometers to measure temperature. The following formula can be used to covert between °C and °F:

$°C = \frac{5}{9} \times (°F - 32)$ $°F = \frac{9}{5} \times (°C + 32)$

Time

Time is measured in minutes and seconds. A stopwatch is used to measure time. You may need to record fractions of a second.

Volume

Volume measures the amount of space that something takes up. For solid objects that have measurable sides, volume is calculated by multiplying width by length by height. For liquids, instruments such as graduates and measuring cups are used to measure volume. The metric units used to measure volume include cubic centimeters (cc), milliliters (mL), and liters (L). The standard measurements include teaspoons (tsp), tablespoons (T), cups (C), pints (pt), quarts (Qt), and gallons (G). Some standard conversions are:

- 1/5 teaspoon = 1 milliliter
- 1 teaspoon = 5 milliliters
- 1 tablespoon = 15 milliliters; 1 fluid ounce = 30 milliliters
- 1/5 cup = 50 milliliters
- 1 cup = 240 milliliters
- 2 cups (1 pint) = 470 milliliters
- 4 cups (1 quart) = .95 liter
- 4 quarts (1 gallon) = 3.8 liters

volume
(VAHWL yoom)
The amount of space that an object or liquid takes up.

Apply It

Divide into small groups. Each group will start at one of four measuring stations. Each station will have a specific measuring tool (either a ruler or a cylinder) and an item which can be measured with that tool, as appropriate.

To record accurate measurements, find the smallest division on the instrument. Measure the items and record the length or volume you feel is accurate (with no direction from the teacher). Then, move to the next station. After all of your classmates have been to all stations, compare findings and discuss correct or incorrect answers.

Mass and Weight

Everything around you, including air, is made up of matter. **Mass** measures the amount of matter in an object. Mass is something that everything has no matter where it is. So something's mass will be the same wherever it is located—on Earth or on the moon. The metric measurement units for mass are grams (g) and kilograms (kg). We use a balance (a special kind of weighing machine) to measure mass. (Figure 12.2a)

In physical science, mass differs from **weight**. Weight measures the force of gravity on an object. So, your weight is different on the Earth than it would be on the moon, because there is more gravity on the Earth than on the moon. The standard units for weight include pounds (lb) and ounces (oz). Scales, including electronic scales, are used to determine weight. (Figures 12.2b and 12.2c)

In the health care setting, the term you will use is *weight*, but it sometimes describes mass rather than weight. That is because the two are connected. Something with a bigger mass will weigh more than something with a smaller mass (assuming they're in the same place).

mass
(MAS)
The amount of matter in an object.

weight
(WAIT)
Measures the force of gravity on an object; varies due to distance between objects and mass.

Measurement and the Scientific Process | Chapter 12 285

Teaching Tips

- Explain the units and tools for measuring temperature.
- Demonstrate how to read a thermometer.
- Discuss when you would measure temperature.
- Explain "normal" body temperature.
- Review the formulas for converting between Celsius (centigrade) and Fahrenheit:
  - °C = 5 / (°F – 32) 9
  - °F = 9 / (°C + 32) 5
- Explain the units and tools for measuring time:
  - 60 seconds in a minute
  - 60 minutes in an hour
  - 24 hours in a day
- Demonstrate how to write time: hh:mm:ss.
- Discuss how to measure and write time that is less than one second:
  - Fractions of a second are usually measured in tenths or hundredths.
  - They can be written by placing a decimal point after the seconds value.
- Demonstrate how to use a stopwatch.
- Demonstrate how to use a second hand on a clock or watch.
- Review the units and tools for measuring volume.
- Review the tools and units for measuring mass and weight.
- Review the difference between mass and weight.
- Demonstrate how to use a balance or scale.

Apply It

- Have the items to measure ready.
- Try to involve different types of measurement, such as length, volume, and temperature.
- Emphasize precision; remind students to be as accurate as possible.
- Limit discussion between groups during the activity.
- Allow time for comparing the results and discussing different results.

Figure Focus

12.2 (a) A balance measures mass. (b) Scales measure weight. (c) An electronic, or digital, scale provides precise weight measurement. There are many different kinds of scales, such as the spring scale and digital scale shown here (b, c), or the common bathroom scale. If you wanted to find out how many ounces of food a person is going to eat, which tool would you use?

Answer: Scale

Math Link—Converting Between Units of Volume in the Metric System

- Review the conversion information.
- Step through the example problems with the class.

Why types of things might be measured in volume in a dental office?

Answer: Things that might be measured in volume in a dental office include materials for creating study models.

Figure12.2
(a) A balance measures mass. (b) Scales measure weight. (c) An electronic, or digital, scale provides precise weight measurement. There are many different kinds of scales, such as the spring scale and digital scale shown here (b, c), or the common bathroom scale. If you wanted to find out how many ounces of food a person is going to eat, which tool would you use?

(a) (b) (c)

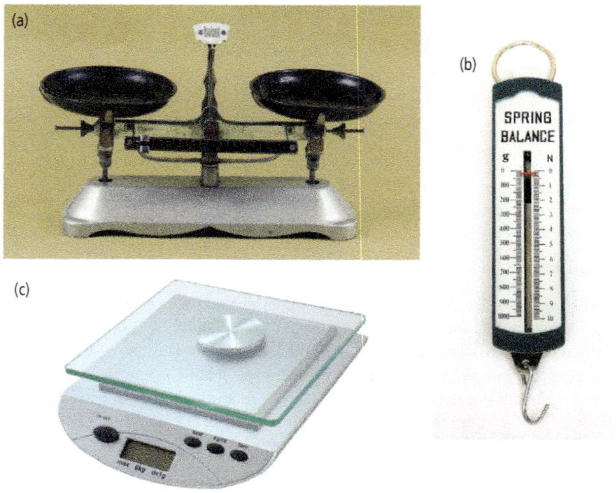

Math Link

Converting Between Units of Volume in the Metric System

All health care workers need a basic understanding of the metric system in order to complete daily duties. For example, a dental assistant may be asked to measure and mix materials when completing such tasks as creating study models. In order to measure volume, a dental assistant may use units such as milliliters, cubic centimeters, liters, and cubic liters.

Volume is the amount of space in a three-dimensional object. Volume can be measured with things such as beakers, measuring cups, measuring spoons, and graduated cylinders.

The following lists conversion information to change to different units of volume:

- 1,000 milliliters (mL) = 1 liter (L)
- 1 cubic centimeter (cm^3) = 1 milliliter (mL)
- 1,000 liters (1 L) = 1 cubic meter (m^3)

Example 1: Convert 3000 milliliters to liters.

1,000 mL = 1 L

1,000 × 3 = 1 L × 3

3,000 mL = 3 L

Example 2: Convert 500 cubic centimeters into liters.

Since 1 cm^3 = 1 mL then 500 cm^3 = 500 mL

You can use this information to help you figure out the answer.

1,000 mL = 1 L

1,000 / 2 = 1 / 2

500 mL = .5 L

If 500 mL equal .5 L then 500 cm^3 also equals .5 L.

a. Convert 10 cubic centimeters to milliliters.

b. Convert 2 cubic meters to liters.

c. Convert .25 liter to cubic centimeters.

What types of things might be measured in volume in a dental office?

List the materials used to create study models. What are the appropriate quantities for each material? Why is it important that the quantities are exact?

286 Chapter 12 | Measurement and the Scientific Process

CUSTOMIZED INSTRUCTION

Less Advanced Students

Allow less advanced students to spend extra time reading and recording measurements. Provide the formulas for converting between different scales.

What's New?

Metric Units in the United States

Most nations around the world use metric units every day. In these countries, distances are measured in kilometers, lengths are measured in centimeters and millimeters, and volumes are measured in liters and milliliters. In the United States, we use standard units, such as miles, feet, inches, and ounces. If the metric system is so widely used, why doesn't the U.S. use it?

In fact, in the 1970s, there was a large push in the U.S. to use metric measurements. The government sponsored research studies that indicated the U.S. would eventually join the rest of the world in using metric measurements. However, this change still hasn't occurred, and fewer people are interested in making it happen. The metric system is only regularly used by people in science and medicine, mathematics, industry, and the military.

Part of the reason the U.S. has not converted to the metric system is that the public simply doesn't use these measurements regularly. Also, the transition would be expensive. For example, any sign indicating distance in miles along a highway would need to be replaced.

Because the U.S. has not converted to the metric system, we have occasionally run into problems. For example, the Mars Climate Orbiter project failed because one of the contractors on the project used standard measurements. Everyone else working on the project used metric measurements. Because of the error, the orbiter burned up in the atmosphere of Mars.

Even though metric measurements are not always used in the U.S., they can still be found on everyday items such as food labels. Many cosmetics, drinks, and nutritional supplements rely on the metric system. Several sports events, such as track and field, are measured in kilometers and meters rather than miles and feet.

Some organizations are still lobbying for the U.S. to use the metric system. It remains to be seen if we will ever make the transition.

What is a benefit of using the metric system?

Estimating

When making measurements or recording numerical data, you may need to **estimate**. Estimates can be used to quickly find approximate values. Estimating may involve rounding numbers.

estimate
(EH stuh muhnt)
Determine approximate value of a number.

To round, identify the place value that will be rounded. Then, identify the digit to the right of it. If the digit to the right is less than five, drop the digit and all numbers to the right of it. For example, the value 6.743 would be rounded to 6.74 in the hundredths place, 6.4 in the tenths place, and 7 in the ones place. If the digit is equal to or greater than five, round the place value up to the next number and drop the digits. For example, the value 23.565 would be rounded to 23.57 in the hundredths place, 23.6 in the tenths place, and 24 in the ones place.

What's New?—Metric Units in the United States

- Review the difference between the metric system and the standard system used in the United States.
- Discuss reasons why the U.S. uses the standard system.
- Remind students that the metric system was discussed in Chapter 11.

What is a benefit of using the metric system?

Answer: Because most other countries use the metric system, a benefit of using the system in the U.S. would be that it is easier to communicate data with people in other countries.

Teaching Tips

- Discuss reasons for estimating.
- Review the steps for rounding a number:
  - Identify the place value to round.
  - Identify the digit to the right.
  - If the digit is equal to or less than 5, round down.
  - If the digit is equal to or greater than 5, round up.
- Explain that rounding may be used to make fractions or decimals into a whole number.
- Review the process of rounding large numbers.

TEAMWORK

In small groups, list five cities in your state in a table. Look up the actual population of each of the cities and record it in the table. Round the population numbers to the nearest 100. How about to the nearest 1,000?

Teaching Tips

- Discuss why it is important to use accuracy and precision when measuring.
- Review methods for insuring accuracy and precision:
  - Measure more than once.
  - Use the proper tools and units.
  - Be sure tools are calibrated correctly.
- Review the steps for calculating an average:
  - Add all values.
  - Divide by the total number of values.

ACTIVITY

Use a thermometer to register the temperature of water at different stages: straight from the tap, with ice, and at "room temperature." Record the results in a table or graph. For extra credit, record the results in both Celsius and Fahrenheit.

Section 12.2 Review Questions

1. Answer: A measuring cup or a graduate is used to measure volume.
2. Answer: Metric units to measure length include millimeter, centimeter, meter, and kilometer. Metric units to measure volume include cubic centimeters, milliliters, and liters. Metric units to measure mass include grams and kilograms.
3. Answer: To convert kilograms to pounds multiple the kilograms by 2.2. 4.54 kg × 2.2 = 9.988 lbs, or about 10 lbs. You are carrying the heavier container.
4. Answer: A mile is approximately 1.6 kilometers. Your sister is walking father (3 miles × 1.6 = 4.8 kilometers).
5. Answer: Accuracy is how close a measurement is to the actual value. Precision is how the close the values of the measurement are to each other. For data to be valid, they must be both accurate and precise. Otherwise, there is an error.
6. Answer: Sometimes estimating involves identifying numbers in the tens, hundreds, or thousands place. In this case, the value 3,456 would be rounded to 3,000. Notice that the rounded numbers in these cases differ more greatly from the actual value, so the estimate may cause errors.

Sometimes estimating involves identifying numbers in the tens, hundreds, or thousands place. In this case, the value 2,345 would be rounded to 2,350, 2,300, or 2,000. Notice that the rounded numbers in these cases differ more greatly from the actual value, so the estimate may cause errors.

accuracy
(AK yuhr uh see)
How close a measurement is to the actual value.

precision
(PREE si shuhn)
For multiple measurements of the same thing, how close the values of the measurements are to each other.

Accuracy and Precision

When making measurements, it is important to maintain both **accuracy** and **precision**. Accurate measurements are close to the actual value of the thing being measured. Measurements are often repeated to ensure accuracy.

You may be asked to make a measurement three times. If the measurements are precise, they will not differ much from each other. Then, you will average the measurements. Doing so increases the likelihood that your final value is accurate, especially if the three measurements are precise, or near each other in value.

For data to be valid, they must be both accurate and precise. Otherwise, there is an error in the data. Estimating can decrease the accuracy and precision of measurements, so it should be used carefully.

Apply It

Practice estimating quantities and then taking the precise measurements. Set up a box filled with soil, a beaker filled with water, a jar filled with M&Ms, etc. Estimate the weight of each sample and note it on a card. Take the actual weight and see who is closest.

Summary

Many tools are used to make measurements—rulers, metersticks, stopwatches, thermometers, graduates, balances, and scales to name a few. The tool used depends on the characteristic being measured. Some tools measure length; other tools measure temperature. To be valid, measurements must be both accurate and precise. Estimating is a useful tool to identify approximate values, but it can introduce errors because it reduces accuracy and/or precision.

Section 12.2 Review Questions

1. If you wanted to measure the volume of liquid a patient drinks, what tool would you use?
2. What metric units are used to measure length, volume, and mass?
3. You and your friend are stacking the supply cabinet in the school nurse's office. You pick up a container that weighs 12 pounds, and he picks up one that weighs 4.54 kilograms. Who is carrying the heavier container?
4. As part of your health class, you are told to walk 3.22 (rounded) kilometers three times a week. Your sister claims to walk 3 miles three times a week. Who is walking farther?
5. What is the relationship between accuracy and precision?
6. How does estimating the number 3,456 to the nearest thousand affect accuracy?

288 Chapter 12 | Measurement and the Scientific Process

Apply It

- Have the items to measure ready.
- You might use the same items as in the Apply It activity on p. 285. You may even combine the two activities.
- Try to involve different types of measurement, such as length, volume, and temperature.
- You could make the activity a contest, and award extra credit or a prize to whoever comes closest.
- Complete the activity by reviewing when it is appropriate to estimate and when an accurate measurement is necessary, and discussing problems that might arise from estimating.

Tables, Graphs, and Charts

SECTION 12.3

Background

A health care worker will need to keep careful records in the course of care for a patient. Sometimes, complex information will need to be interpreted and organized into a table, graph, or chart. A health care worker will need to know how to read technical materials and data in a table, graph or chart. Sometimes, a caregiver will need to organize data in such ways.

Objectives

When you have completed this section, you will be able to do the following:

- Match key terms with their correct meanings.
- Describe three types of graphs.
- Explain what kind of data is represented by tables and each type of graph.
- Draw three types of graphs.

Data Tables

As a health care worker, you are going to need to read or make tables. Tables are used to organize **data** and to help record information. For example, a patient's temperature needs to be recorded every hour for a 24-hour period. A table can be used to organize this data. Tables can also be used to record observations and other verbal data.

data
(DA tuh)
Information.

The first feature of a table is column labels, located at the top of each column in the table. In the example described above, the column labels would most likely be "Time of Day" and "Patient's Temperature." The column labels should be clear and concise. The columns of a table often show the relationship between **variables**. In the example, time and temperature are the variables. **Table 12.1** shows part of a sample table based on the example.

variables
(VAR ee uh buhls)
Any factor that can change or be present in varying amounts.

Table 12.1 Sample Table—Temperature Change over Time

Time of Day	Patient's Temperature
0800	102.3°F
0900	103.1°F
1000	103.0°F
1100	102.9°F
1200	102.3°F
1300	101.0°F
1400	99.5°F
1500	98.9°F

Measurement and the Scientific Process | Chapter 12 289

Teaching Tips

- Explain how data tables are used in health care.
- Demonstrate how to set up a data table and how to label columns and rows.
- Point out that information other than numerical data, such as observation, may be entered in a tables.
- Look at Table 12.1 together as a class.
- Ask students to identify the highest temperature of the day, and at what time it occurred.
- Ask students to identify the lowest temperature of the day, and at what time it occurred.
- Ask if they can identify a trend or pattern from the information in the table.

FOCUS AND ENGAGE

Introduce the Section

a. Review the content of the Background paragraph, explaining that tables, graphs, and charts are used to present data so it can be easily read and understood.

b. Emphasize that students have already been using tables, graphs, and charts to communicate written information.

c. Review the objectives for the section.

Vocabulary Review

a. Direct students to the key terms.

b. Pronounce each word, and have the students repeat the pronunciation out loud.

c. Discuss the definition of each word.

TEACH

Discuss

- Ask students if they have experience using graphs or charts. For example, they may have read a timetable, such as a bus schedule.
- Explain that all three display information so it can be read and understood.
- Discuss the type of information you might display in a table, graph, or chart.

Reinforce and Review

- Review the importance of recording information.
- Review the importance of using clear, concise communication skills.

Teaching Tips

- Explain that the terms chart and graph are often synonymous.
- Review the three common types of graphs:
  - Bar graph to compare data sets
  - Line graph to show trends over time
  - Circle graph/pie chart to show percentages or proportions
- Display examples of different types of charts and graphs.

Figure Focus

12.3 (a) Bar graph; (b) Line graph; (c) Circle graph. If you wanted to compare the number of people in a hospital who are nurses' aides, registered nurses, physical therapists, counselors, and doctors, what kind of graph would you use?

Answer: Use a bar graph to show the total number of each occupation. A circle graph could be used to display the percentage of each occupation in relation to the total number of workers in the hospital.

ACTIVITY

Write your daily schedule as a table.

Graphs and Charts

Several types of graphs and charts are used to visually organize data. Usually, they show numerical data. A health care worker may not need to create these graphs and charts, but he or she will need to understand how to read them. There are several types of graphs and charts, but the most common are the following:

axes
(AKS ees)
Reference lines that mark the borders of a graph; graphs may have two or more axes (singular, axis).

- **Bar graph:** Uses vertical or horizontal bars to represent numerical data. Bar graphs have vertical and horizontal **axes**. Bars are proportional to the numerical value they represent. (See Figure 12.3a for an example of a bar graph.)
- **Line graph:** Uses a line drawn through plotted points to show how one variable is affected by another. These graphs are often used to show time relationships and trends. Like bar graphs, line graphs have axes. (Figure 12.3b is an example of a line graph.)
- **Circle graph:** Also called a pie chart, circle graphs are circles that are divided into sections, similar to the way a pie might be sliced. However, the "pieces" in a circle graph are not usually even. Circle graphs are used to show **proportions** and percentages. (Figure 12.3c is an example of a pie graph.)

proportions
(pruh POR shuhns)
Parts of a whole.

Figure12.3
(a) Bar graph; (b) Line graph; (c) Circle graph. If you wanted to compare the number of people in a hospital who are nurses' aides, registered nurses, physical therapists, counselors, and doctors, what kind of graph would you use?

(a)
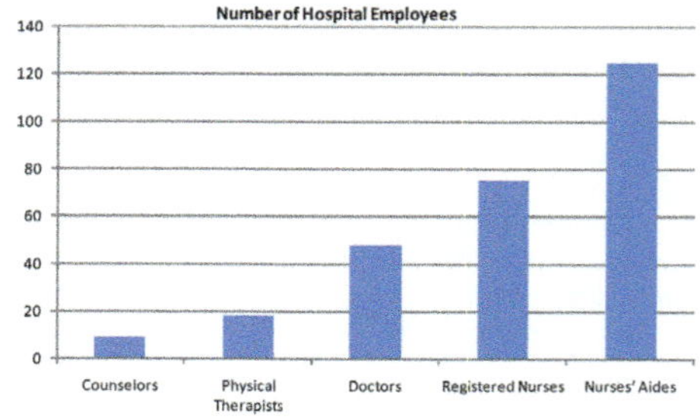

(b)
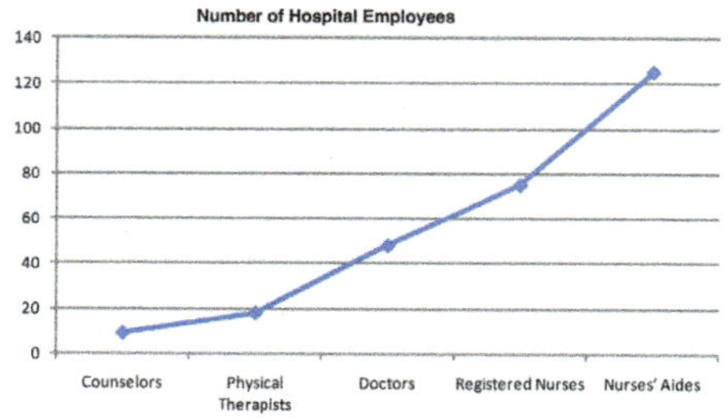

(c)
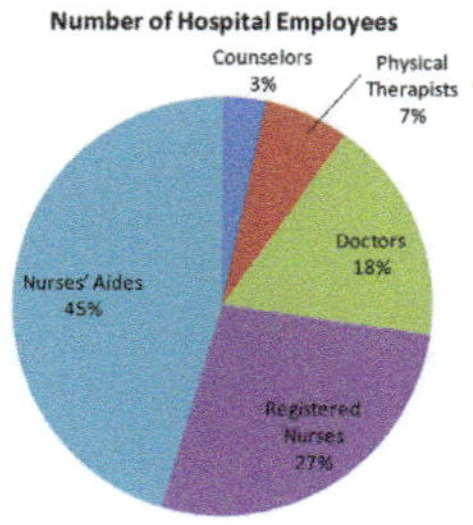

CUSTOMIZED INSTRUCTION

More Advanced Students

Allow advanced students to use a spreadsheet program such as Microsoft Excel to create charts and graphs.

English Language Learners

Have students look through newspapers, magazines, or online for an example of a bar graph, line graph, or circle graph. They should write a sentence that explains what the selected graph illustrates and share it with a classmate.

Summary

Tables, graphs, and charts are important tools for organizing data. Data are often numerical, but can also be verbal. Tables are used to record both numerical and verbal data. Graphs and charts are used for numerical data. Three types of graphs and charts include bar graphs, line graphs, and circle graphs.

Section 12.3 Review Questions

1. Define the terms *data* and *variables*.
2. How do tables differ from graphs and charts?
3. List and describe three types of graphs.
4. Should a bar graph be used to show temperature changes over time? Explain your reasoning.
5. If you wanted to show percentages from a survey, which type of graph would you use? Why?
6. What type of chart best shows time relationships and trends?

Measurement and the Scientific Process | Chapter 12 291

Section 12.3 Review Questions

1. Answer: Data is information and variables are any factor that can change or be present in varying amounts.
2. Answer: Tables are used to record both numerical and verbal data. Graphs and charts are used for numerical data.
3. Answer: Bar graphs use vertical or horizontal bars to represent numerical data. Bar graphs have vertical and horizontal axes. Bars are proportional to the numerical value they represent. Line graphs use a line drawn through plotted points to show how one variable is affected by another. These graphs are often used to show time relationships and trends. Like bar graphs, line graphs have axes. Circle graphs are circles that are divided into sections, similar to the way a pie might be sliced. The "pieces" in a circle graph are not usually even. Circle graphs are used to show proportions and percentages.
4. Answer: A bar graph is used to show numerical data, but use a line graph to show the time relationship of temperature readings that are taken over time.
5. Answer: To show percentages, a circle graph should be used because it shows the pieces in relationship to the whole.
6. Answer: A line chart uses a line drawn through plotted points to show how one variable is affected by another and is used to show time relationships and trends.

CHAPTER 12 REVIEW

Chapter Review Questions

1. Answer: Make observations. Ask a question. Develop a hypothesis. Make a prediction. Test the hypothesis. Analyze the results. Draw conclusions. Communicate results.
2. Answer: Observations
3. Answers will vary, but should indicate an experiment where only the variable changes.
4. Answer: Accuracy
5. Answer will vary but could include the following: temperature, fluid intake, urine output, patient's weight, size of a wound, etc.
6. Answer: For solid objects that have measurable sides, volume is calculated by multiplying width by length by height. For liquids, instruments such as graduates and measuring cups are used to measure volume.
7. Answer: For data to be valid, they must be both accurate and precise. Otherwise, there is an error in the data.
8. Answers will vary.
9. Answer: Circle
10. Answer: Tables are used to organize data and to help record information. Tables can also be used to record observations and other verbal data.
11. Answer: 17.98 liters
12. Answer: 110 lbs

CHAPTER 12 REVIEW

Chapter Review Questions

1. What are the eight steps of scientific methods? (12.1)
2. Before starting an experiment, scientists make ______, which help them ask questions. (12.1)
3. Give an example of a controlled experiment. (12.1)
4. In measurements, ______ describes how close a measurement is to the actual value of the thing being measured. (12.2)
5. Give three examples that show when health care workers might take measurements. (12.2)
6. How is volume calculated? (12.2)
7. Why is precision and accuracy important when making measurements? (12.2)
8. Give examples of when a bar, line, and circle graph would be used in health care. (12.3)
9. Sheila wants to show proportions in a graph. She should use a ______ graph. (12.3)
10. Why would a health care worker need to create a table? (12.3)
11. Mr. Smith, who was raised in Europe, has come in for a consultation before his physical. He is told that he has 19 quarts of salt water in his body. He wants to know how many liters that is. What is your response (rounded to two decimals)? (12.2)
12. At your school physical, you are told that you weigh 49.9 kilograms. You get concerned until your friend explains that you actually weigh ________ pounds (rounded to the nearest pound). (12.2)

Activities

1. Draw a circle graph to show the percentage of the day a worker spends on each of his or her duties. Remember that a circle graph, also known as a pie chart, is a circular chart divided into triangular areas proportional to the percentages of the whole pie. Think about an apple pie. If someone eats half of it and someone else eats a third, each of those pie sizes will be different.
2. Interpret the technical data in the table below and use it to draw a line graph. Remember that a line graph is a graph in which line segments join points representing different values. Describe any trends that are shown in the graph. Are there other types of graphs that you can use to show the data? Explain your reasoning.

Time of Day	Heart Rate (beats per minute)	Time of Day	Heart Rate (beats per minute)	Time of Day	Heart Rate (beats per minute)
0100	46 bpm	0900	63 bpm	1700	66 bpm
0200	45 bpm	1000	64 bpm	1800	65 bpm
0300	47 bpm	1100	65 bpm	1900	64 bpm
0400	47 bpm	1200	65 bpm	2000	63 bpm
0500	48 bpm	1300	66 bpm	2100	63 bpm
0600	47 bpm	1400	65 bpm	2200	60 bpm
0700	50 bpm	1500	65 bpm	2300	56 bpm
0800	60 bpm	1600	67 bpm	2400	50 bpm

Activities

1. Point out that this activity is similar to Activity 1 in the review for Chapter 11. Emphasize that this activity challenges the students' abilities to convert fractions and to use a clock as well as create a pie chart. You might choose to allow students to use a spreadsheet program to enter the data and create the chart.
2. Remind students that a line graph shows trends over time. You might choose to allow students to use a spreadsheet program to enter the data and create the graph. Emphasize that they should write the answers in complete paragraph form.

CHAPTER 12 REVIEW

Case Studies

1. Health care researchers are tracking the early development of children who show definitive signs of allergies by age 5. They need to take 25 subjects and track their development by charting their weight, height, and instances of illness. How would they do this? Would they start with a table? What type of graphs or technical materials might they use? How could they present the information so that it could be easily interpreted? Create a data set and set up a test model.
2. Create a hypothesis based on your work in this course or another science class, such as biology. Design an experiment that will test the hypothesis. What kind of documentation will you need to develop?

Thinking Critically

1. **Presenting Data**—Describe two scenarios, based on your present classes, in which it would be better to present data in tables or graphically. How would you present the information?
2. **Medical Math**—There are two scales that are used to measure temperature—Celsius (°C) scale and the Fahrenheit scale (°F). You will most likely use the Fahrenheit scale, but in many other areas of the world Celsius is more common. Why is this?
3. **Scientific Processes**—During an experiment, a scientist gets results that do not support her hypothesis. She communicates her results to other scientists. What else can she do?

Portfolio Connection

Transferable skills can be used on almost any job, and employers are always looking for employees who possess them. They are called transferable skills because you can transfer them from one situation or career to another. Being able to communicate effectively with other people is a transferable skill. So is being proficient in math and science as well as in the use of basic computer applications. Problem-solving and time management are also transferable skills.

Your portfolio is a place to showcase the basic, transferable skills that you possess. For instance, have you used spreadsheet software to create charts and graphs for analyzing numerical information or completed labs in science class that illustrate your understanding of the scientific process? Make a list of transferable skills for your portfolio. Briefly describe your familiarity with each as "Basic," "Intermediate," or "Expert." Gather at least one sample that shows your successful application of the skill.

PORTFOLIO TIP

Use your word processing or spreadsheet software to create your list of transferable skills in a neatly formatted table. Be sure to label your samples as "Exhibit A," "Exhibit B," and so forth. Your samples can be copies of your original work. Place the list and samples in the "Written Reports and Assignments" section of your portfolio.

Measurement and the Scientific Process | Chapter 12 293

ACTIVITY

Draw posters depicting the steps of the scientific method. Display the posters in the classroom.

ACTIVITY

Find the published results of a scientific experiment in a printed publication or online. Identify the hypothesis, experiment used to test the hypothesis (including variable and controls), prediction, and results. Write a report explaining the experiment, and present it to the class.

Case Studies

1. Encourage students to put some thought into how the researchers would go about setting up this study, and to document their thoughts in writing. Explain that they should fabricate the data set information, and enter it into a table. Remind them to select the appropriate graph type(s) for displaying the data. You might choose to allow students to use a spreadsheet program to enter the data and create the graph(s).
2. Remind students to use the scientific methods when developing their hypothesis and experiment. Point out that it is not necessary to perform the experiment, only to design it.

Thinking Critically

1. Direct the student to write a complete answer in paragraph form. They might illustrate their answers by creating the tables and/or graphs.
2. Students should research the Celsius scale to find out where and why it is used. They should answer in essay form, with a thesis and supporting statements. Remind them to include source information, if necessary.
3. Refer students to Section 12.1 for information specific to this situation. Remind them to provide a complete answer with specific suggestions of what the scientist should do.

Portfolio Connection

- Stress the importance of transferable skills.
- Students may be surprised by all of the transferable skills that they already have.
- Have students work with a partner to brainstorm skills that they may have.
- Check to make sure that students have completed the written assignments and added them to their portfolio.

TEAMWORK

In small groups, think of a hypothesis you would like to test and design a controlled experiment for it. Write a proposal for the experiment, including what you would use as a variable and what would be the constants. Make a prediction as to what you think the results will be. If the group does not agree on the prediction, include all predictions.

CUSTOMIZED INSTRUCTION

More Advanced Students

Have more advanced students research other temperature scales, and report their findings to the class.

13 Your Body and How It Functions

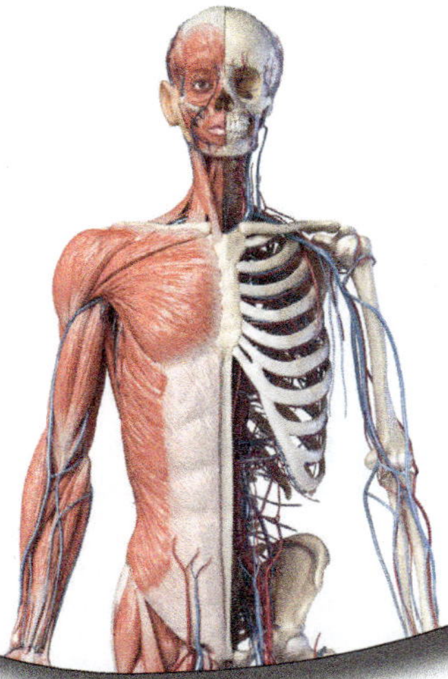

CHAPTER 13 OVERVIEW

Chapter 13, Your Body and How It Functions, provides an overview of the structure and major systems of the human body. It is designed to introduce the student to basic anatomy, human biology, and some of the problems and diseases they might encounter as health care workers. It also lists related jobs and professions.

Section 13.1: Section 13.1 is an introduction to the body, including the overall structure, and the relationships between cells, tissues, organs, and the major body systems.

Section 13.2: Section 13.2 covers the skeletal system, including the names, locations, and functions of bones and joints.

Section 13.3: In Section 13.3, students learn the purpose of the muscular system, including the names and locations of muscles and how they control movement.

Section 13.4: Section 13.4 introduces the circulatory system. It covers the functions of arteries, veins, and the heart, as well as blood.

Section 13.5: In Section 13.5, students learn how the lymphatic system helps the body fight disease and build immunity.

Section 13.6: Section 13.6 covers the respiratory system, the lungs, and how they function to provide oxygen and remove carbon dioxide and water vapor.

Section 13.7: Section 13.7 provides an overview of the digestive system, explaining how the body breaks down food into nutrients, and how it eliminates waste.

Advance Preparation	
Review	■ Chapter text for Sections 13.1 through 13.13.
Contact	■ Medical professionals to visit the class to discuss their professions, and why understanding the human body and its systems is important for all health care professionals.
Prepare	■ Anatomy and physiology charts. ■ Posters or pictures of human anatomy and systems. ■ Videos of the human body and the different systems covered in the chapter. ■ Halloween skeletons for activities. ■ Sticky notes for activities. ■ A list of Web sites that provide information about anatomy and the human body—such as getbodysmart.com.

Section 13.8: In Section 13.8, students learn how the urinary system maintains the water balance within the body.

Section 13.9: Section 13.9 covers the endocrine systems. Students learn the names and locations of the glands and how they function.

Section 13.10: Section 13.10 introduces the nervous system. It includes coverage of the senses, the ear, and the eye.

Section 13.11: In Section 13.11, students are introduced to both the male and female reproductive systems.

Section 13.12: Section 13.12 covers the integumentary system. Students learn the composition of the skin and how it protects the body.

Section 13.13: In Section 13.13, students are introduced to DNA and how genetics impact the body and disease.

FOCUS AND ENGAGE

Getting Started

- Define *forensic*. Explain that the detectives on television shows such as *CSI* are forensic detectives.
- Review the formulas in the activity, explaining what the letters *r*, *t*, *h*, and *H* stand for. Point out that *h* and *H* are not the same.
- Review methods of measuring length.
- Discuss the results of the activity as a class.

Introduce the Section

a. Review the Background paragraph, explaining that in order to help people, health care workers must have a basic understanding of the body and how it works.
b. Review the objectives for the section.

Vocabulary Review

a. Direct students to the key terms.
b. Pronounce each word, and have the students repeat the pronunciation out loud.
c. Discuss each definition.

TEACH

Discuss

- Ask students if any of them have studied biology in science class.
- Discuss how complex and remarkable the human body is, and how we take things, like breathing and moving, for granted.
- Share amazing facts about the body. (Refer to a Web site such as https://sciencebob.com/research-help/the-body-zone/amazing-body-facts/.)

Reinforce and Review

- Review medical terminology.

Getting Started

Your bones tell a lot about your body. Archaeologists and forensic scientists study bones to estimate a person's height, build, and age. This data is helpful in learning about ancient people and in solving crimes. The lengths of major bones such as the humerus, radius, or tibia can be substituted into formulas to find a person's height.

Measure the length of your radius (r), tibia (t), and humerus (h) bones to the nearest half-inch. Using the following formulas, approximate your height (H) in inches. Are the calculated heights close to your actual height?

Male	Female
$H = 32.2 + 2.4t$	$H = 28.6 + 2.5t$
$H = 29.0 + 3.0h$	$H = 25.6 + 3.1h$
$H = 31.7 + 3.7r$	$H = 28.9 + 3.9r$

Imagine that an archaeologist found an 18-inch tibia on the site of an American colonial farm. Do you think it belonged to a man or a woman? Why?

SECTION 13.1 Overview of the Body

Background

The health care worker assists people who are ill, injured, or seeking a healthy lifestyle. Understanding the body's structure and functions provides the health care worker with the basic knowledge necessary to help each person reach his or her goal. When you understand normal body functions you will recognize disease processes.

Objectives

When you have completed this section, you will be able to do the following:

- Match key terms with their correct meanings.
- List cell functions.
- Identify main parts of the cell and explain their functions.
- Describe the relationship between cells, tissues, organs, and systems of the body.
- Identify terms relating to the body.
- Label a diagram of the body cavities.
- Explain why health care workers must have a basic knowledge of body structures and how they function.

296 Chapter 13 | Your Body and How It Functions

CUSTOMIZED INSTRUCTION

Less Advanced Students

This chapter includes many new vocabulary words and medical terminology. Provide less advanced students with a list of terms and definitions at the beginning of the chapter so they can get a head start on learning them.

CUSTOMIZED INSTRUCTION OVERVIEW

Less Advanced Students	Pages 296, 342
More Advanced Students	Pages 297, 309, 372
English Language Learners	Pages 297, 377
Special Needs Students	Pages 302, 326
At-Risk Students	Pages 301, 391

Introduction to The Body

The Cell

The **cell** is the smallest structural unit of the human body. Cells are **microscopic**. This means that they are so small they can be seen only with the aid of a microscope. The body is made up of millions of cells, each programmed to do a specific job that allows the body to **function**. Each cell reproduces, grows, uses oxygen and **nutrients**, digests food for energy, eliminates waste, produces heat and energy, and is able to move. Many cells can repair themselves. The structure of the cell includes (Figure 13.1):

- Golgi apparatus: Packages and transports substances around the cell.
- Secretory vesicles: Structures that fuse with the cell membrane and releases substance from the cell.
- Lysosomes: Responsible for destroying toxins and debris.
- **Cytoplasm**: A jellylike substance that house or contains all of the organelles.
- Rough endoplasmic reticulum: Tubular structure containing ribosomes, which are responsible for producing proteins.
- Peroxisome: Responsible for breakdown of fatty acids.
- **Nucleus**: The control center of the cell and contains the DNA.
- Centriole: Cylindrical cell structure composed mainly of a protein called tubulin.
- Mitochondria: Sausage-shaped structures that produces energy for the cell.
- Ribosomes: Round structures located on endoplasmic reticulum and makes proteins.

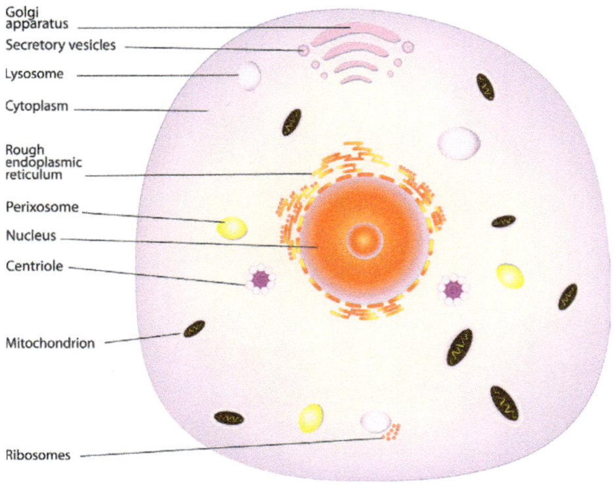

Figure 13.1
Where is the nucleus located in a cell?

cell
(SELL)
Smallest structural unit of the body that is capable of independent functioning.

microscopic
(mahy kruh SKOP ik)
Too small to be seen by the eye but large enough to be seen through a microscope.

function
(FUHNGK shuhn)
Action or work of tissues, organs, or body parts (e.g., the heart's function is to pump blood).

nutrients
(NOO tree ent)
Substances that the cell needs in order to function.

cytoplasm
(SIGH toe plaz um)
The liquid within the cell that surrounds the nucleus and other parts of the cell.

nucleus
(NEW klee iss)
The part of a cell that is vital for its growth, metabolism, reproduction, and transmitted characteristics.

Your Body and How It Functions | Chapter 13 297

Teaching Tips

- Explain that each cell reproduces, grows, repairs itself, uses oxygen and nutrients, digests food, eliminates waste, and is able to move.
- Describe the main parts of the cell and their functions.
- Explain and describe the primary kinds of body tissue:
  - Nerve
  - Epithelial
  - Connective
  - Muscle (skeletal, cardiac, and smooth)
- Explain that blood is also a type of body tissue.
- Discuss disease: any change in the normal structure or function of the body.
- Point out that disease can affect the body at the level of a cell, tissue, an organ, or a system.
- Explain the difference between chronic and acute disease: acute diseases occur suddenly and last a short time; chronic diseases last for a longer period of time—as long as months or years.

Figure Focus

13.1 Where is the nucleus located in a cell?

Answer: Within the cell, surrounded by cytoplasm

CUSTOMIZED INSTRUCTION

More Advanced Students

Assign more advanced students a project in which they research cells and create a presentation, which includes text and graphics, to deliver to the class.

English Language Learners

This chapter includes many new vocabulary words and medical terms. Provide students with a list of terms and definitions at the beginning of the chapter. Before starting each section of the chapter, have students highlight the terms introduced in that section, and then read each term and definition aloud to a partner.

Teaching Tips

- Review Table 13.1 together as a class.
- Review the types of tissue.
- Review the location of the different types of tissue.
- Discuss the function of each type of tissue.
- Describe the relationship between cells, tissues, organs, and systems:
  - Cells make specialized tissues.
  - Tissues combine to form organs.
  - Organs combine to form systems.
  - Systems combine to form the body.
- Spend time on vocabulary as necessary.

Figure Focus

13.2 What are the three types of muscle tissue?

Answer: Striated, smooth, and cardiac muscle tissue

ACTIVITY

Draw a poster or flowchart depicting the relationship between cells, tissues, organs, and systems.

tissues
(TISH yews)
Groups of cells of the same type that act together to perform a specific function.

Tissues

The body is made up of specialized groups of cells. These groups of cells form tissues. These **tissues** have a specific job. There are four primary kinds of tissue in the body: nerve, **epithelial**, connective, and muscle. (Figure 13.2) Table 13.1 describes the locations and functions of each type of tissue.

Table 13.1 Tissues of the Body

Type of Tissue	Location in the Body	Function
Nerve tissue	Throughout the body	Sends impulses to/from the central nervous system and to/from the body systems
Epithelial tissue	Forms the outer skin and lines body cavities and passages to the outside of the body	Protects, secretes, absorbs,and receives sensations (e.g., hot, cold, pressure)
Connective tissue	Bones, tendons, fat tissue	Binds, supports, and connects body tissues
Muscle tissue: 1. Cardiac 2. Smooth 3. Striated	1. Heart muscle 2. Internal organs (e.g., stomach, diaphragm) 3. Throughout the body for movement	1. Contracts heart 2. Contracts internal organs 3. Contracts and flexes to allow movement

epithelial
(e pi THEE lee uhl)
Pertaining to tissue that covers the internal and external organs of the body.

connective tissue
(cuh NEK tiv TISH yew)
Tissue specialized to bind together and support other tissues.

Organs

Groups of tissues make up organs such as the heart, lungs, stomach, and liver. Each organ carries out specific functions for the body. (Figure 13.2) For example, the heart is an organ made up of cardiac muscle tissue, **connective tissue**, and nerve tissue. All three work together to cause our hearts to beat and pump blood throughout our bodies. Figures 13.3a and 13.3b show the organs of the body and their locations.

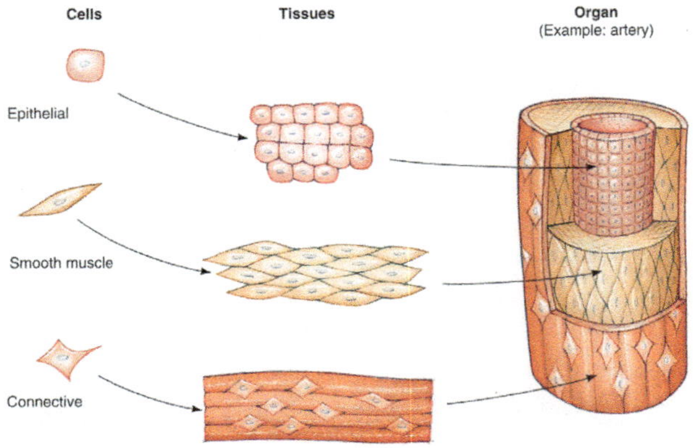

Figure 13.2
What are the three types of muscle tissue?

Figure 13.3a
Organs of the body. Which organ would hepatitis affect?

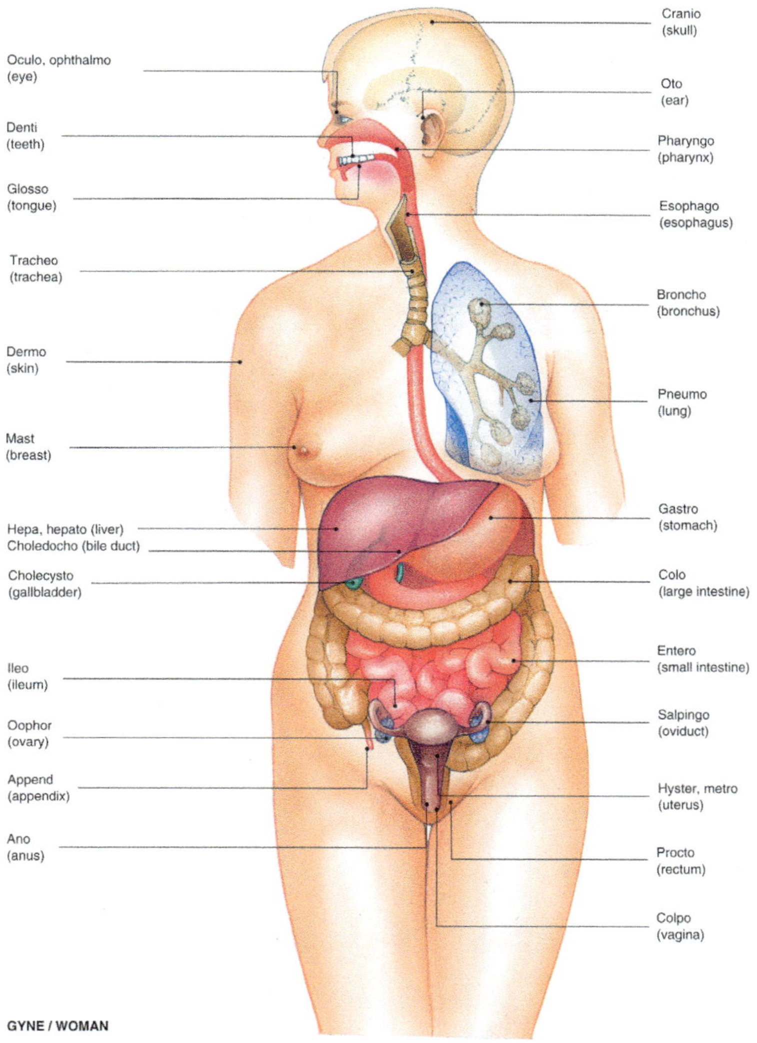

Your Body and How It Functions | Chapter 13 299

Teaching Tips

- Identify the major organs of the body.
- Remind students that tissues combine to form organs.
- Point out that males and females have most of the same organs, but some different organs as well.
- Ask if the class knows why.
- Remind students to use their knowledge of medical terminology when identifying organs.
- Assign students to memorize the names and types of tissue and organs.

Figure Focus

13.3a Organs of the body. What organ would hepatitis affect?

Answer: The liver

TEAMWORK

Working in pairs, sitting facing each other. Write down any tissue that you can see, specifying the type of tissue, where it is located, and what its purpose is. At the end of the exercise, discuss your findings with the class.

Figure Focus

13.3b Organs of the body. What organ would rhinitis affect?

Answer: The nose

Figure 13.3b
Organs of the body. What organ would rhinitis affect?

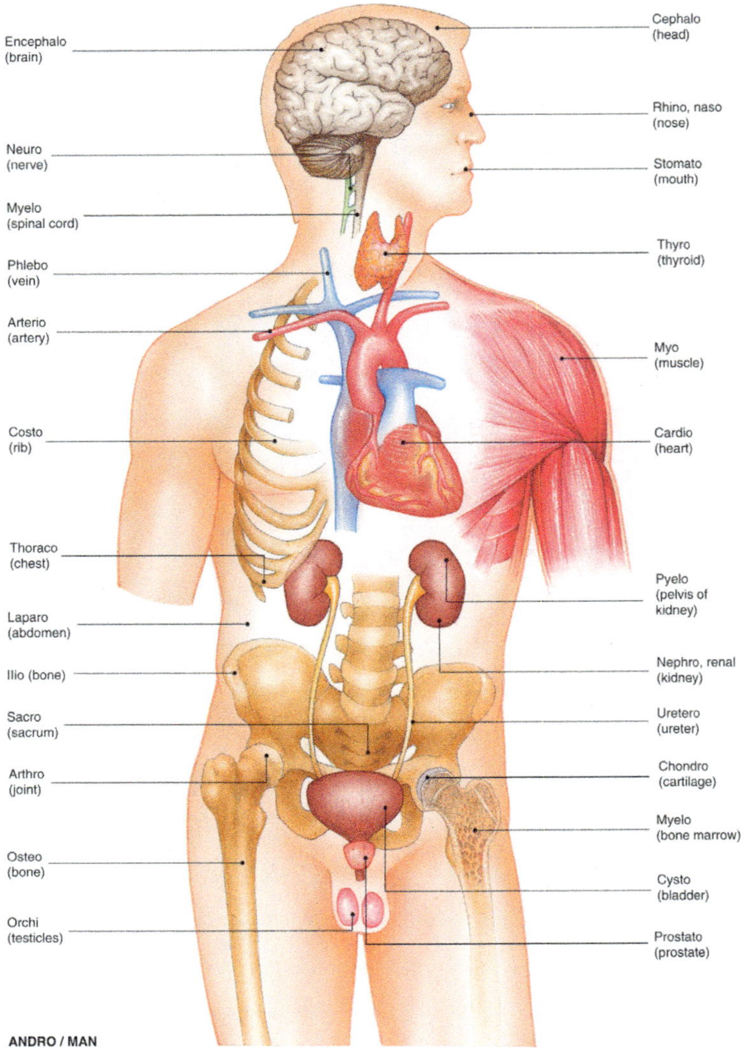

300 Chapter 13 | Your Body and How It Functions

Disease

A change in the normal structure or function of the body is disease. A characteristic set of signs and symptoms is the indication that the normal structure or function has been interrupted. Reasons for such changes in the structure or function of a cell, tissue, organ, or system in the body may or may not be known.

Systems

A system is a group of organs working together to perform a certain function. The body is **composed** of several systems. In the next sections of this chapter, we discuss the following:

- Skeletal system
- Muscular system
- Circulatory system
- Lymphatic system
- Respiratory system
- Digestive system
- Urinary system
- Endocrine system
- Nervous system
- Reproductive system
- Integumentary system

composed
(kuhm POHZD)
Formed by putting many parts together.

structure
(STRUHK cher)
The way that parts of the body are put together.

It is important to understand the unique **structure** and functioning of the body. You need to learn that *cells* combine to form tissues, *tissues* combine to form organs, *organs* combine to form systems, and *systems* combine to form the human body. (**Figure 13.4**)

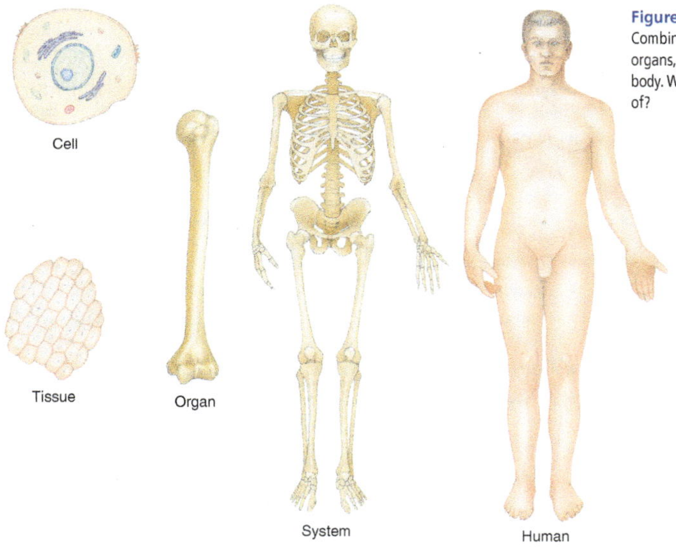

Figure 13.4
Combination of cells, tissues, organs, and systems forms the body. What is an organ made of?

Teaching Tips

- Introduce the systems of the body.
- Remind students that organs combine to form systems.
- Name the eleven systems that are covered in this chapter.
- Select one or two of the systems and use them as examples to summarize how cells, tissues, organs, and systems make up the body.
- Emphasize the importance of understanding the structure of the body.
- Reiterate the relationship between cells, tissue, organs, and systems.

Figure Focus

13.4 Combination of cells, tissues, organs, and systems forms the body. What is an organ made of?

Answer: Tissues

ACTIVITY

Create a table or chart listing the eleven systems that are covered in this chapter. For each system, include an explanation of its function, information about its components (such as organs, tissue, etc.) and one reason why it is important that a health care worker have basic knowledge of this system.

CUSTOMIZED INSTRUCTION

At-Risk Students

Some students may be intimidated by the length of this chapter and the many new vocabulary terms introduced. Explain that 11 of the 13 sections in the chapter cover the 11 systems listed on this page. It might help students to create an index card for each system listed and then add notes and/or pictures as they review the section on that system.

Teaching Tips

- Introduce the topic of directions of the body. Emphasize that the directions of the body are used to communicate information about the patient.
- Discuss problems that might arise from misidentifying a direction of the body.
- Explain the anatomical planes of the body.
- Emphasize that the planes are sections of the body that help identify the location of a specific body part.
- Tell students to think of the midline as dividing the body in half with a left and a right side.
- Point out the most common body directions:
  - Cranial: Near the head
  - Superior: Above or higher
  - Inferior: Below or lower
  - Ventral or anterior: Located near the surface, or in front of coronal plane
  - Dorsal or posterior: Located to the back of the coronal plane
  - Medial: Near the center or midline of the saggital plane
  - Lateral: Away from the midline of the saggital plane
  - Proximal: Nearest the point of attachment
  - Distal: Farthest from the point of attachment or the midline
  - Caudal: Near the sacral region

anterior
(ann TEER ee uhr)
Located in the front; opposite of posterior (e.g., the abdominal wall is anterior to the back).

distal
(DISS tuhl)
Farthest from the point of attachment.

anatomical position
(ann e TOM ik el pozi shun)
The position with the body erect with the arms at the sides and the palms forward.

Organism

An organism is a complex group of systems that work together to serve a particular function. The human body is an organism because all the body systems work together to function as a life.

Chemistry of the Body

Body processes occur effectively because of chemical activities taking place at all times. Elements such as oxygen, hydrogen, carbon, nitrogen, potassium, and many more are responsible for various chemical reactions that keep the body functioning at its optimum. For example, hyperkalemia, or too much potassium, can result in an irregular heart rhythm. Deficiencies and over-abundance of the elements can result in diseases and disorders. Keeping the chemicals in balance (homeostasis) is critical to proper functioning.

Directions of the Body

To document information about patients, use terms that specify regions or directions of the body; for example, to identify locations of pain or injury, write: 1 cm laceration on the right **anterior** forearm, **distal** to the elbow. (Figure 13.5) We normally identify these locations based on the **anatomical position**. The anatomical position is of importance in anatomy because it is the position of reference for anatomical nomenclature. Anatomic terms such as anterior and posterior, medial and lateral, abduction and adduction, and so on apply to the body when it is in the anatomical position.

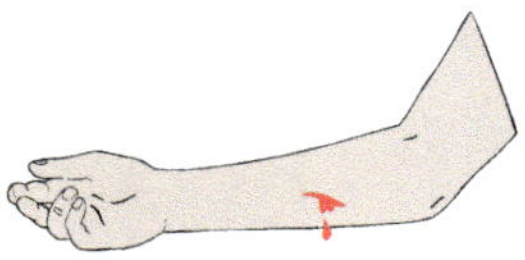

Figure 13.5
To identify the location of this laceration, write: 1 cm laceration on the right anterior forearm, distal to the elbow. What does "the right anterior forearm" mean, in common language?

The body directions are shown in Figure 13.6. Medical professionals often refer to sections of the body in terms of anatomical **planes** (flat surfaces). These planes are imaginary lines—vertical or horizontal—drawn through the upright body. The terms are used to describe a specific body part.

Here are the most common body directions:

- **Cranial:** Located near the head.
- **Superior:** Above or in a higher position. The head is superior to the torso.
- **Inferior:** Below, lower. The knee is inferior to the thigh.
- **Ventral** or **anterior:** Located near the surface or in front of coronal (frontal) plane.
- **Dorsal** or **posterior:** Located to the back of the coronal plane.
- **Medial:** Near the center or midline of the **sagittal** plane. Think of the midline as dividing the body in half with a left and a right side.
- **Lateral:** Away from the midline of the sagittal plane.
- **Proximal:** Nearest the point of attachment.
- **Distal:** Farthest from the point of attachment or the midline.
- **Caudal:** Located near the **sacral region**.

plane
(PLAYN)
A flat surface determined by the position of three points in space.

posterior
(poss TEER ee uhr)
Behind, to the rear, toward the back (e.g., the heel is posterior to the toes).

sagittal
(SAJ i tl)
Body plane that divides the body into right and left parts.

sacral region
(SAY chruhl ree jun)
The area where the sacrum is located; forms the tail end of the spinal column.

302 Chapter 13 | Your Body and How It Functions

Figure Focus

13.5 To identify the location of this laceration, write: 1 cm laceration on the right anterior forearm, distal to the elbow. What does "the right anterior forearm" mean, in common language?

Answer: The front of the right forearm

CUSTOMIZED INSTRUCTION

Special Needs Students

If special needs students have difficulty viewing the figures in the book and reading the callouts, make use of large posters, charts, and anatomical sculptures to help them identify part of the human anatomy.

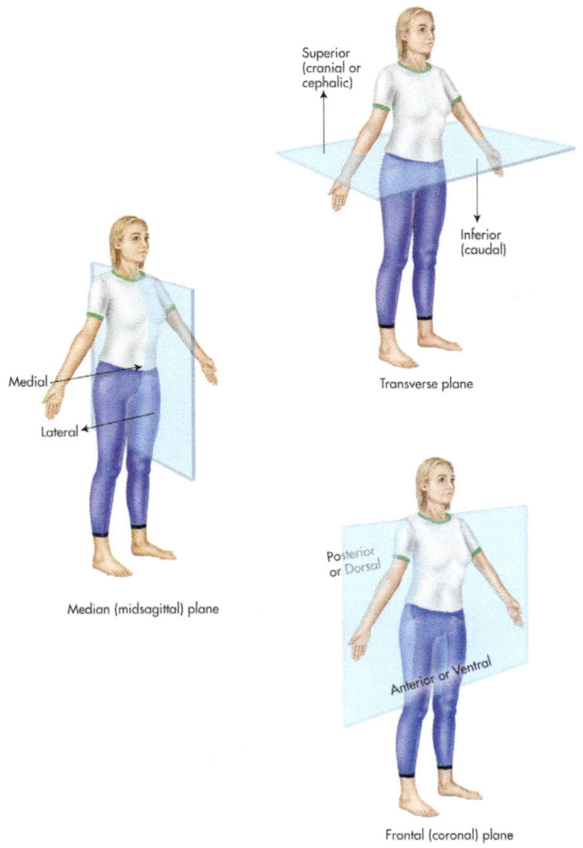

Figure 13.6
Directions of the human body. If an injury were described as a "posterior cranial laceration," where would the injury be?

- **Superficial:** Closer to the outside of the body.
- **Deep:** Further away from the outside of the body; closer to the core.

In addition, health care workers identify the human abdominal region in four quadrants. One horizontal line and one vertical line is passed through the umbilicus, or belly button, which divides the area into upper and lower and left and right, resulting in four quadrants. The Right Upper Quadrant, Left Upper Quadrant, Right Lower Quadrant, and Left Lower Quadrant each house specific organs. It is important that the health care worker knows in which quadrant an organ is located.

Your Body and How It Functions | Chapter 13 303

Teaching Tips

- Explain the directions of the body.

Figure Focus

13.6 Directions of the human body. If an injury were described as a "posterior cranial laceration," where would the injury be?

Answer: On the back of the head

ACTIVITY

Create flashcards for the directions, planes, and cavities of the body. Use the flashcards to study and memorize the information. Play "Simon Says" using the directions and planes of the body. For example, call out, "Simon Says put your hand on your left anterior forearm."

Teaching Tips

- Review Table 13.2 together as a class, identifying and locating the cavities.
- Explain which organs are in each cavity.

Figure Focus

13.7 Body cavities. What is the chest cavity called?

Answer: Thoracic cavity

Apply It

- This is a good activity for small groups or teams.
- You may want to specify the type of materials students should use to create the "anatomy man," keeping in mind that the finished product should be able to stand upright and be large enough that it can easily be labeled with the directions, planes, abdominal regions, and cavities.
- You may choose to have the students label the locations of the organs, rather than trying to make them fit inside the cavities.

MEDICAL TERMINOLOGY

Review the terminology:

- Pronounce each word element, and have students repeat.
- Pronounce each medical term, and have students repeat.
- Allow time for students to write down definitions.
- Select a student to read each definition.
- Assign students to memorize the terms and their definitions.

Cavities of the Body

The cavities of the body are another way to identify location of pain or injury. (**Figure 13.7**) (**Table 13.2**)

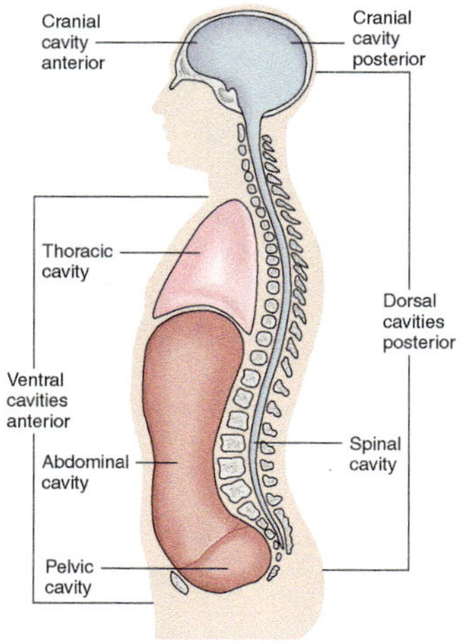

FIGURE 13.7
Body cavities. What is the chest cavity called?

Apply It

Bring in supplies and create an anatomy man, which has to stand up. Then, label the cavities, directions, planes, and abdominal regions. Make organs and then put them in the correct cavity.

vessels
(VES el)
Tubes that carry blood in the body.

tone
(TOHN)
Firmness or tightness.

Table 13.2 Cavities of the Body (see Figure 13.7)

Dorsal Cavities Located Toward the Back of the Body	Ventral Cavity Located Toward the Front of the Body
Cranial cavity—houses the brain; includes the orbit, nasal, and oral cavities	Thoracic cavity—houses the heart, lungs, large blood **vessels**
Spinal cavity—houses the spinal cord	Abdominal cavity—houses the stomach, most of intestines, kidney, liver, gallbladder, pancreas, spleen
	Pelvic Cavity—houses the urinary bladder, part of intestine, rectum, parts of the reproductive system

MEDICAL TERMINOLOGY

aplasia:	failure of any part of the body to develop naturally
endogenous:	anything occurring within the body
exogenous:	anything occurring outside the body
induration:	hardened tissue
infarct:	tissue that has lost blood supply and died
interlobar:	between lobes
intervisceral:	between two organs
intralobar:	within a lobe
necrosis:	condition of dead or decaying tissue
peristalsis:	progressive wavelike movement that occurs in some of the tubes of the body (e.g., intestines, esophagus)
plasma:	liquid part of the blood and lymph
symptom:	any noticeable change in the body or its function
visceratonic:	lack of normal **tone** in an organ

Abdominal Quadrants

To better understand and diagnose issues with the reproductive, digestive, and urinary systems, health care professionals divide the abdomen into four sections, or quadrants. These quadrants and the organs or structures that fall within them are shown in Figure 13.8. These four quadrants are marked by a pair of perpendicular lines: the vertical line separates the left and right sides of the body, while the horizontal line divides the upper and lower half of the abdomen. The intersection of the two lines is located at the navel, making visualizing these quadrants very straightforward.

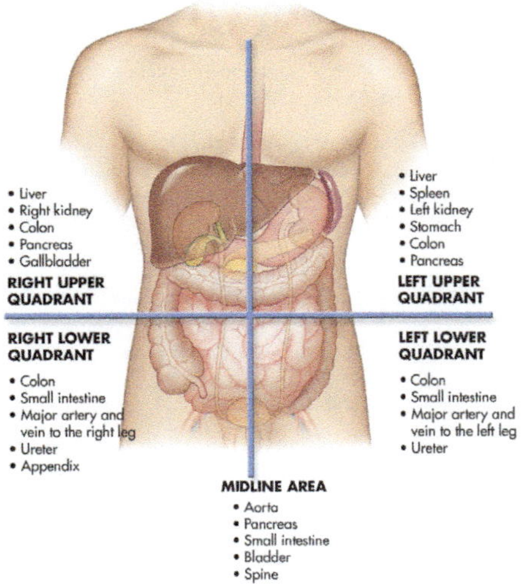

FIGURE 13.8
What are the four quadrants and related organs and structures?

Related Jobs and Professions

Medical Doctor (M.D.)

A medical doctor (M.D.) is a licensed physician who is responsible for comprehensive patient care. An M.D. promotes and maintains health, and treats both injuries and disease. Duties include, but are not limited to: examining patients; obtaining medical histories; ordering, performing, and interpreting diagnostic tests; counseling patients on health-related issues; and prescribing medicines. Many physicians with an M.D. go on to specialize in other areas.

It is not uncommon for an M.D. to work 60 or more hours a week. Most M.D.s work in small, private offices or clinics. Some practice in large health-care organizations, an arrangement that may allow for a less demanding work schedule.

Teaching Tips

- Begin a discussion about the jobs and professions that would be suitable for someone interested in the human body.
- Remind students to refer to Chapter 3 for more information on occupations.
- Discuss the skills and requirements for becoming a medical doctor.
- If possible, invite a doctor in to the class to discuss his or her job.
- Discuss the skills and requirements for becoming a microbiologist.
- Compare a microbiologist with a medical doctor. Which one spends more time with patients and which one spends more time in a lab?
- Discuss the skills and requirements for becoming a pathologist.
- Discuss some of the tests that a pathologist might perform.

TEAMWORK

Divide the class into teams of 8 to 12 students. Hold a "definition bee" in which you read a term and ask one team to define it. If they succeed, they get one point; if not, the other team has a chance. The team with the most points at the end of the competition wins.

Figure Focus

13.8 What are the four quadrants and related organs and structures?

Answer: The four quadrants are the right and left upper quadrants, and the right and left lower quadrants.

Figure Focus

13.9 What skills and interests do you think might be necessary to become a pathologist?

Student answers will vary.

Teaching Tips

- Discuss the skills and requirements for becoming a registered nurse.
- Emphasize the important role that a registered nurse plays in providing direct care and in managing the health care team.
- Discuss the growth prospects of nursing as an industry.
- You may want to refer students to the Web site for the department of labor and statistics (bls.gov) for more information.
- As students proceed through Chapter 13, have them pay attention to the major illnesses and conditions that affect the functioning of the body.
- As students proceed through Chapter 13, have them note diagnostic procedures.

ACTIVITY

Create a table comparing the skills and requirements of each of the nursing professions listed in this chapter.

The education and training for an M.D. are among the most strenuous of any profession. In general, M.D.s complete four years of undergraduate school, four years of medical school, and three to eight years of internship and residency, depending upon the specialty pursued. All candidates must also pass a licensing exam, and they must continue to study throughout their careers to keep up with advances in medical technology.

Microbiologist

A microbiologist is a scientist who studies microbes, or living organisms and infectious agents that are too small to be seen with the naked eye. Because there are so many different species of microbes, microbiologists usually select one type of microbe to study. They focus their research and build their careers in that area.

A small sampling of specialties includes: bacteriologists, who study bacteria; virologists, who study viruses; and immunologists, who study the human body and how it defends itself against disease.

Microbiologists work in almost every industry, and careers in this field are quite varied. At the lowest level are laboratory assistants, who generally have a two-year technical training degree. Those with a four-year degree in biology or microbiology work as research assistants and medical technologists.

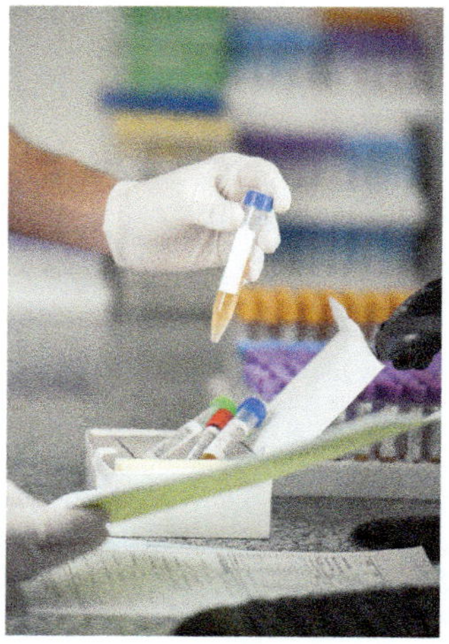

Figure 13.9
What skills and interests do you think might be necessary to become a pathologist?

A master's degree is required for supervisory, technical support, and teaching positions. Microbiologists who perform independent research, teach at the university level, or hold executive-level positions have doctoral degrees.

Pathologist

A pathologist is a medical doctor who examines tissue specimens, cells, and bodily fluids through laboratory tests and then interprets the results to gain an accurate diagnosis. An accurate diagnosis is necessary if the patient is to receive proper treatment. Currently, more than 2,000 different tests can be performed on blood and bodily fluids.

Many times, a pathologist helps a patient's team of doctors select the most appropriate test to gain a complete diagnosis. A pathologist is a critical member of a patient's core medical team.

To become a pathologist, one must complete medical school, a residency program, and an approved residency in pathology. Medical school generally takes four years. Residency training for pathologists lasts anywhere from three to six years, depending upon the specialty. Pathologists work in hospitals, clinics and independent laboratories.

Registered Nurse

Registered nurses (RNs) are involved in every aspect of patient care. Some RNs treat patients. They perform diagnostic tests and analyze the results. They give treatment and medication, and they closely observe patients and record their progress as well as any reactions. Other medical professionals use this detailed record as a basis for proper patient care. RNs also help with patient follow-up and rehabilitation.

Some RNs work with the public rather than individual patients. They educate the public on warning signs and symptoms of various conditions and tell them where to get help. Some RNs run immunization clinics and blood drives. Some are trained in grief counseling. RNs account for the largest health-care occupation. Although they may work in a variety of settings, roughly three out of every five RNs works in a hospital.

To become an RN, one must graduate from an approved nursing program and pass a national licensing exam. There are three main ways to become an RN. One option is to get a bachelor's of science degree in nursing (BSN) through a four-year program at a college or university. A second option is an associate degree in nursing (ADN) through a two- or three-year program at a community or junior college. The third option is to go through a three-year diploma program at a hospital. Advancement opportunities are usually broader for those who complete a BSN program. A master's degree is required to work in administration, teaching or any nursing specialty.

Nurse Practitioner

A nurse practitioner (NP) is a registered nurse who has received additional education and clinical training in the diagnosis and treatment of illness. Most NPs have completed a two- or three-year master's degree program. Some have a doctorate degree in their specialty. These specialties include acute care; adult or family health; gerontology health; neonatal health; oncology; pediatric/child health; psychiatric/mental health; and women's health. NPs may further specialize in everything from allergy and immunology to urology.

Nurse practitioners work in a variety of settings. They can be found everywhere from clinics, hospitals, and private practices to nursing homes, schools, and public health departments. On the job, they order, perform, and interpret diagnostic tests, diagnose and treat common acute illnesses and injuries, prescribe medications and therapies, perform procedures, and educate patients and their families on living a healthy lifestyle.

Licensed Practical and Licensed Vocational Nurse

A licensed practical nurse (LPN), or licensed vocational nurse (LVN) as they are called in Texas and California, provides basic bedside care for patients. Responsibilities are limited as all duties are conducted under the direct supervision of a physician or registered nurse.

A common task for an LPN/LVN is to take a patient's vital signs, which includes temperature, blood pressure, pulse, and respiration. LPN/LVNs also give injections and enemas, monitor catheters, collect samples, and conduct routine laboratory tests. LPN/LVNs also apply dressings, treat bedsores, and give alcohol rubs and massages. They observe patients and report any adverse reactions to medications or treatment. They also help patients with personal hygiene and ensure that patients are comfortable.

Your Body and How It Functions | Chapter 13 307

Teaching Tips

- Discuss the skills and requirements for becoming a nurse practitioner.
- Point out that in many health care facilities, nurse practitioners perform many of the same duties as medical doctors, including seeing patients, diagnosing illness and disease, providing referrals, and more.
- Discuss the skills and requirements for becoming a licensed practical or licensed vocational nurse.
- Discuss the skills and requirements for becoming a nursing assistant.
- Remind students of the nursing career ladder.
- Emphasize that they can start in an entry-level position, and then move up the ladder by continuing their education and gaining professional experience.

ACTIVITY

Select one of the jobs or professions listed in Section 13.1. Create a brochure or pamphlet explaining why the health care worker you selected needs a basic knowledge of body structure and functions in order to perform his or her job effectively.

Section 13.1 Review Questions

1. Answer: Connective tissue is tissue specialized to bind together and support other tissue.
2. Answer: Alimentary canal, liver, pancreas, spleen, kidney, adrenal glands
3. Answer: Heart
4. Answer: Anterior, left medial
5. Answer: Cranial and spinal cavities
6. Answer: Epithelial tissue
7. Answer:
   - Nucleus: regulates the activity of the cell and has an important role in the reproduction of the cell.
   - Cytoplasm: a jellylike liquid where the activities of the cell occur.
   - Cell membrane: outer covering of the cell that keeps the cytoplasm contained. The cell membrane also allows matter to flow in and out of the cell.
8. Answer: Microbiologist
9. Answer:
   - RNs perform diagnostic tests and analyze results and provide treatment and medication. RNs must graduate from an approved nursing program and pass a national licensing exam.
   - LPN/LVNs provide basic bedside care and are under direct supervision of a physician or RN. LPN/LVNs must attend a one-year program at a vocational or technical school. They then must pass a licensing examination.

People wishing to become a LPN/LVN can attend a one-year program at a technical school. They then must pass a licensing examination. Many LPN/LVNs work in hospitals and nursing-care facilities. Others work in physicians' offices, outpatient-care facilities, or for pubic health care agencies.

Nursing Assistant

Nursing assistants (NAs) work under the direct supervision of a nurse. They have extensive daily contact with patients and are the caregivers who help patients perform day-to-day tasks, such as bathing, feeding, and dressing. They help patients walk and go to the bathroom. They transport patients, take vital signs, make beds, and set up equipment. NAs assist patients with activities of daily living and works as part of a collaborative team in the delivery of health care. Because of the physical requirements of the jobs, good physical conditioning is a plus.

NAs work in hospitals, physicians' offices, home health agencies, nursing homes, private homes, and mental health institutions. To become a NA, you need at least a high school diploma followed by 120 hours of training. Some employers offer on-site training. Courses are also offered through high school health science programs, community and state colleges Once training is complete, the NA may have the opportunity to be certified as a nursing assistant.

Summary

In the human body, cells form tissues and tissues form organs. Organs form the organ systems that are part of every individual. As a health care professional, it is important to understand how organs work together within organ systems. A good understanding of these systems can help you to correctly treat disease. It is also important to understand the language that is used to describe the positions of structures within the human body. This will help you to accurately report injury or discomfort in a patient.

Section 13.1 Review Questions

1. What is connective tissue?
2. What organs does the abdominal cavity contain?
3. What organ would arteriosclerosis mainly affect?
4. How would you describe a wound that is on the left front chest, close to the shoulder socket?
5. Which cavities are located in the dorsal region of the body?
6. Which type of tissue protects the outer body and the organs and also receives sensations?
7. Name three major parts of the cell and describe their functions.
8. A ____________ is a scientist who studies living organisms and infectious agents that are too small to be seen with the naked eye.
9. Name two differences between a registered nurse (RN) and a licensed practical nurse/licensed vocational nurse (LPN/LVN).

The Skeletal System

SECTION 13.2

Background

The skeletal system is made of tough bone tissue that supports the body and allows it to move. Some bones cover and protect vital organs, such as the heart and brain. Marrow within bones produces white and red blood cells. As a health care professional, it is important to know the parts of the skeleton, as well as diseases that may affect bone.

Objectives

When you have completed this section, you will be able to do the following:

- Match key terms with their correct meanings.
- Label a diagram of major bones in the body.
- Understand the functions of bones.
- Name the long, short, flat, and irregular bones of the body.
- Identify immovable, slightly movable, and freely movable joints of the body.
- Identify common disorders of the skeletal system.
- Label a diagram of four types of bone fractures.
- Explain why a health care worker must have a basic knowledge of the skeletal system and how it functions.

Introduction to the Skeletal System

Structure of the Bone

The skeletal system is made up of bone and other connective tissues, such as ligaments and cartilage. Bones have their own system of blood vessels and nerves, which allows **circulation** to occur within the bone. (**Figure 13.10**)

The **components** of bone change from conception to old age. In the first month after **conception**, an **embryo**'s skeletal framework is made up of **cartilage**. In the second and third months after conception, you can see calcium deposits in the bone.

Throughout life, calcium continues to form in the bone structure, causing the bone to become hard. This is called ossification. For example, a small child's bone is more **flexible** than the bone of a 30-year-old. The added calcium makes the bones of the 30-year-old harder, less flexible, and more **brittle**. A 60-year-old may lose calcium from the bone. This makes the bone **porous** so that it breaks easily.

circulation
(sur kyuh LEY shuhn)
Continuous one-way movement of blood through the heart and blood vessels to all parts of the body.

components
(kom PO nent s)
Parts or elements of a whole; an ingredient.

conception
(kuhn SEP shuhn)
Occurs when the male sperm fertilizes the female ovum and a new organism begins to develop.

embryo
(EM bree oh)
Living human being during the first eight weeks of development in the uterus.

cartilage
(CAR tuh lij)
Tough connective tissue; forms pads at end of bones, is found in the nasal septum and external ear, and forms the major portion of the embryonic skeleton.

flexible
(FLEK suh buhl)
Able to bend easily.

brittle
(BRIT uhl)
Fragile, easy to break.

porous
(POUR iss)
Filled with tiny holes.

Your Body and How It Functions | Chapter 13 309

FOCUS AND ENGAGE

Introduce the Section

a. Review the content of the Background paragraph, discussing the functions of the skeletal system.

b. Explain that understanding the skeletal system helps health care workers identify and diagnose diseases and illnesses.

c. Review the objectives for the section.

Vocabulary Review

a. Direct students to the key terms.

b. Pronounce each word, and have the students repeat the pronunciation out loud.

c. Discuss the definition of each word.

TEACH

Discuss

- Ask students what they know about bones. Some may have had broken bones.
- Discuss what the body would be like if it had no skeleton. Point out that some animals have exoskeletons—shells or skeletons on the outside.

Reinforce and Review

- Review the information in Section 13.1: cells, tissues, organs, cavities, and body directions.

CUSTOMIZED INSTRUCTION

More Advanced Students

Assign more advanced students a project on the importance of calcium. They should research the role calcium plays in the function of the skeleton system, and prepare a presentation to deliver to the class.

Teaching Tips

- Explain the structure of bones:
  - System of blood vessels and nerves
  - Development from embryonic stage
  - Cartilage is softer
  - Ossification adds calcium, making bones harder
  - Loss of calcium makes bones brittle

Teaching Tips

- Review the skeleton together, identifying the bones.
- Emphasize that students must learn the medical term for the bones. For example, the skull is called the cranium.
- Emphasize that learning the names of the bones will require memorization.

Figure Focus

13.10 The cranium is composed of bones and joints. What types of joints are found in the cranium?

Answer: Immovable

13.11 The vertebrae are composed of 33 bones: cervical (7), thoracic (12), lumbar (5), sacral (5), and coccygeal (4). What type of bones are these?

Answer: Irregular bones

Teaching Tips

- Explain the main functions of bones:
  - Provide framework
  - Protect internal organs
  - Store calcium
  - Produce red blood cells
  - Allow flexibility
- Explain the two groups of bones:
  - Axial—80 bones in the skull, vertebrae, ribs, and sternum
  - Perpendicular—126 bones in the arms, hands, legs, feet, and pelvis

axial
(AX ee uhl)
Pertaining to the central structures of the body (e.g., vertebrae, skull, ribs, and sternum).

Groups of Bones

The human skeleton is divided into two groups of bones. The **axial** skeleton includes 80 bones. (Figure 13.12) These are found in the:

- Skull, made up of bones of the cranium and mandible (Figure 13.10)
- Vertebrae (Figure 13.11)
- Ribs and sternum

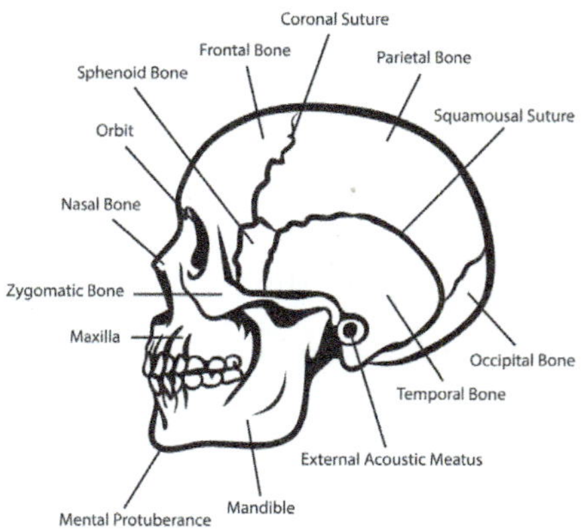

Figure 13.10
The cranium is composed of bones and joints. What types of joints are found in the cranium?

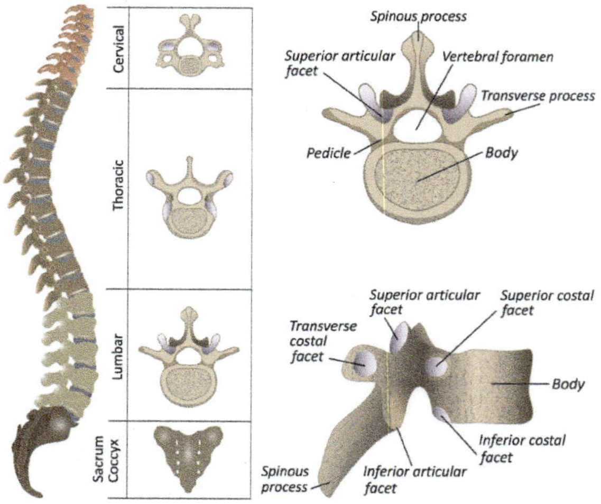

Figure 13.11
The vertebrae are composed of 33 bones: cervical (7), thoracic (12), lumbar (5), sacral (5), and coccygeal (4). What type of bones are these?

310 Chapter 13 | Your Body and How It Functions

TEAMWORK

Divide the class into teams of 8 to 12 students. In turn, name a bone and ask the team to identify it on an unlabeled skeleton or poster. Allow the teams to confer before sending one team member to make the identification. The team is awarded one point for each correct answer. The team with the most points at the end of the activity wins.

The **appendicular** skeleton involves the appendages and includes 126 bones. (**Figure 13.12**) These bones are found in the:

- Arms
- Hands
- Legs
- Feet
- Pelvis

appendicular
(ap pen DIK you ler)
Pertaining to any body part added to the axis (e.g., arms and legs are attached to the axis of the body).

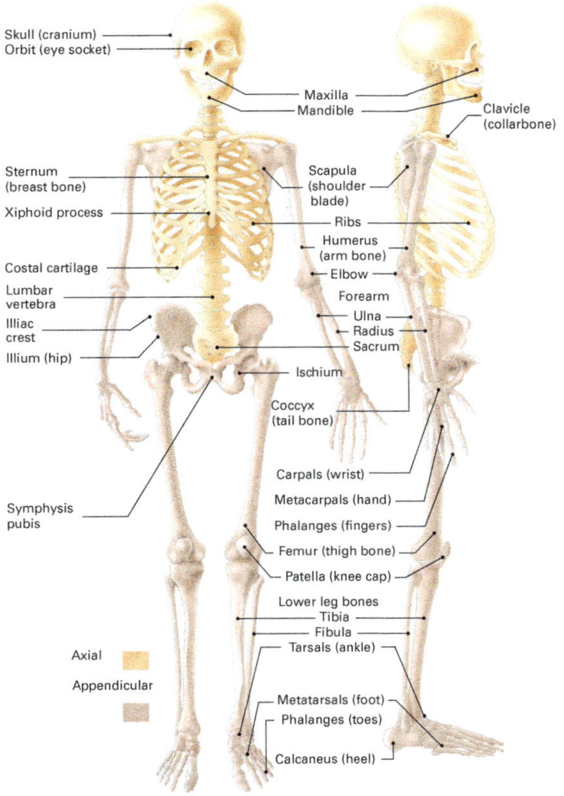

Figure 13.12
The human skeleton is made of bone tissue. There are 206 bones in the body. Where are the tibia and fibula?

Functions of the Bone

Bones perform many functions. Some of these are:

- To serve as a framework for the body, giving the body structure and support.
- To protect internal structures, such as the brain and spinal cord.

Your Body and How It Functions | Chapter 13 311

Teaching Tips

- Review the different types of bones:
  - Long bones are longer than they are wide.
  - Short bones have nearly the same length as width.
  - Flat bones have two layers.
  - Irregular bones do not fit into any of the other three categories.

Figure Focus

13.12 The human skeleton is made of bone tissue. There are 206 bones in the body. Where are the tibia and fibula?

Answer: In the lower leg

ACTIVITY

Create flashcards for identifying bones. On the front side of the flashcard, write the name of the bone. On the back, write the type of bone, which group it belongs to, where it is located, and its function. Use the flashcards to study and memorize the information.

Teaching Tips

- Introduce the topic of joints: the location where bones meet.
- Explain the three groups:
    - Immovable, like the cranium
    - Slightly movable, like vertebral discs
    - Freely movable, like the shoulder
- Describe all of the joints, classifying them:
    - Hinge joint (knee)
    - Ball-and-socket joint (hip)
    - Pivot joint (wrist)
    - Gliding join (lower spine)
- Introduce the topic of ligaments: tissue that holds the bones together.
- Explain that they are part of the skeletal system, even though they are not bones.

ACTIVITY

Lead the class through a series of slow movements. For each movement, students should write down the joint in use, and classify the joint as slightly movable or freely movable.

- To act as a storage area for calcium. This calcium is used in the blood if the diet does not provide enough calcium.
- To produce blood cells (hematopoesis). The red bone marrow produces most of the red blood cells.
- To allow flexibility when muscles move them.

Types of Bones

There are four types of bones:

- *Long bones* (bones that are longer than their width):
    - Humerus
    - Tibia
    - Radius
    - Fibula
    - Ulna
- *Short bones* (length and width are nearly equal):
    - Wrist and hand
    - Ankle and feet
- *Flat bones* (two layers of bone divided by a narrow span):
    - Skull
    - Ribs
    - Sternum
    - Shoulder blade
- *Irregular bones* (bones that do not fit into the shapes of the other three groups):
    - Face
    - Hip
    - Spine

Joints

The point where two bones meet is a joint. Joints are divided into three main groups, depending on the amount of movement permitted. These groups are:

- *Immovable joints:*
    - Cranium (suture joints)
- *Slightly movable joints:*
    - Vertebral discs
    - Sacroiliac joints
    - Symphysis pubis
- *Freely movable joints:*
    - Shoulder and hip joints
    - Elbow, wrist, and finger joints
    - Knee and ankle joints

Ligaments

Ligaments connect to bone and hold bones together. Joints are formed where the bones meet.

penetrates
(PEN i trayts)
Enters or passes through (e.g., a fractured bone passes through the skin).

calcify
(CAL si fy)
To harden by forming calcium deposits.

sedentary
(SED n ter ee)
Immobilized; does not move around very much.

spontaneous
(spon TEY nee uhs)
Occurring naturally without apparent cause.

Common Disorders of the Skeletal System

Table 13.3 Common Disorders, Symptoms, and Preventive Measures/Treatment of the Skeletal System

Condition	Disorder	Symptoms	Preventive Measures/ Treatment
Arthritis	Inflammation of the joints. Can be caused when a joint is damaged, causing the edges of bones in the joint to rub against each other and become irritated.	Pain and swelling in the joints.	Preventing damaging joints by using good body mechanics and limiting continuous repetitive movements that overuse specific joints. Treatments include: pain and anti-inflammatory medications; injections of steroids or gel-like substances to supplement the viscous properties of synovial fluid directly into the joint; non-traditional treatments, such as acupuncture; and, as a last resort, surgery.
Degenerative joint diseases—osteoarthritis	Inflammation of the membrane of the joint. Cause unknown, but changes in the structure of joints occur due to the inflammatory process.	Pain, stiffness, tenderness to the touch, deformity of joint regions.	Treating with anti-inflammatory medication. Surgery is sometimes indicated.
Fracture: ■ Simple ■ Compound ■ Comminuted ■ Greenstick	Broken bone: ■ The bone is broken, but the skin remains intact. ■ The bone is broken and **penetrates** the skin. ■ The bone breaks into many pieces and there are bone fragments in the tissue. ■ The bone is bent and splits, causing an incomplete fracture. (This is most common in children.)	Pain, swelling, and abnormal shape. (Figure 13.13)	Avoiding falls and situations that may put abnormal stress on bones. Treatments include: initially splinting, elevation, and ice; immobilization to help pain; then treatment by reduction (manipulation) to align the broken ends of the bone with or without some form of traction; or open reduction, an internal fixation to surgically repair a fractured bone, usually involving either the use of plates and screws or an intra-medullary (IM) rod to stabilize the bone.
Kyphosis	Abnormal outward curvature of the thoracic vertebrae (hunchback). This condition can be caused from a variety of conditions. (Figure 13.13)	Appearance is the main symptom. In advanced conditions, pain may occur. Early medical care can identify the cause of this condition and early treatment may prevent progression.	Spine-stretching exercises and sleeping without a pillow. Sleeping on a firm mattress that keeps the back as straight as possible may be helpful.

(continued)

Your Body and How It Functions | Chapter 13 313

Teaching Tips

- Review the first part of Table 13.3 together.
- Point out that the table includes the condition, the disorder, the symptoms, and treatments.
- Pronounce the name of the condition for the first four disorders out loud:
  - Arthritis
  - Degenerative joint disease
  - Fracture
  - Kyphosis
- Ask a student to read the description of each disorder.
- Discuss the symptoms of each.
- Discuss the preventive measures and/or treatments of each.
- Differentiate between the four common bone fractures:
  - Simple
  - Compound
  - Comminuted
  - Greenstick

TEAMWORK

In small groups, prepare a skit demonstrating a common disorder of the skeletal system. One student should be a patient, describing symptoms to a health care worker or a team of health care workers. The health care workers should diagnose the disorder, explain it, and prescribe a treatment.

Teaching Tips

- Pronounce the name of the condition for the next six disorders out loud:
  - Lordosis
  - Osteoarthritis
  - Osteomalacia
  - Osteomyelitis
  - Osteoporosis
  - Rickets
- Ask a student to read the description of each disorder.
- Discuss the symptoms of each.
- Discuss the preventive measures and/or treatments of each.

ACTIVITY

Ask students to consider why so many of the common skeletal condition names include the prefix *osteo-*. Have them select one of the terms and draw a poster identifying and defining the word elements.

Table 13.3 Common Disorders, Symptoms, and Preventive Measures/Treatment of the Skeletal System (continued)

Condition	Disorder	Symptoms	Preventive Measures/ Treatment
Lordosis	An inward curvature of the lumbar spine (swayback). This condition can be caused from a variety of conditions. (Figure 13.14)	Appearance is the main symptom; patients have an exaggerated posture. In advanced conditions, pain may occur. Early medical treatment can prevent progression.	Medication (if pain), physical therapy, and use of a brace. In severe cases, with pain and limited range of motion, surgery may be an option.
Osteoarthritis	Also known as degenerative arthritis, a condition in which low-grade inflammation results in pain in the joints, caused by abnormal wearing of the cartilage that covers and acts as a cushion inside joints, and destruction or decrease of synovial fluid that lubricates those joints.	Pain, inflammation, limiting of range of motion. Symptoms may occur in any joint, most commonly knees, hips, hands, and spine.	Relieve pain. Preserve or improve joint function. Reduce physical disability. Treatment can include pain medications, localized steroid injections, topical creams, and—as a last resort—joint surgery.
Osteomalacia	The bones do not **calcify** sufficiently, remaining soft. This is the milder, adult form of the disease. In children, this is called rickets. (See further down on chart.) Related to a lack of vitamin D.	Aches and pains in the lumbar (lower back) region and thighs, spreading later to the arms and ribs. Pain accompanied by tenderness in the involved bones. Difficulty in climbing up stairs and getting up from a squatting position.	Administration of heavy doses of vitamin D. Eating a balanced diet, especially foods with calcium, phosphorus, and vitamin D. Increased exposure to sunshine will result in the production of more vitamin D in the skin.
Osteomyelitis	Infection of the bone that is usually caused by bacteria (often staphylococci) that infects the bone and/or the bone marrow, usually introduced by trauma, or surgery. Number one complication of compound fractures.	Persistent, increasing bone pain with tenderness spreading into muscles, along with a fever.	See a physician early for treatment of infections and avoid accidents that may allow the introduction of bacteria into the body. Treatment includes strong IV antibiotics and, on occasion—in adults—surgery.
Osteoporosis	The bone becomes porous, causing it to break easily. Occurs more frequently in women after menopause, or in people who are **sedentary** or on steroid therapy for a long time.	Pain, especially in the lower back. Fractures that occur easily or with little trauma associated. Often it is the cause of **spontaneous** fractures in elderly women.	Following a proper diet, doing routine moderate exercise, and employing balanced hormone therapy as aging occurs.
Rickets	The bones do not calcify sufficiently, remaining soft. Related to a lack of vitamin D.	Bowlegs and knock-knees enlarged. Knoblike enlargement at ends and sides of bones. Muscle pain, enlarged skull, chest deformities, spinal curvature, enlargement of the liver and spleen, increased sweating, and general body tenderness.	Eating a balanced diet, especially foods with calcium, phosphorus, and vitamin D. Increased exposure to sunshine will result in the production of more vitamin D in the skin.

(continued)

Table 13.3 Common Disorders, Symptoms, and Preventive Measures/Treatment of the Skeletal System (continued)

Condition	Disorder	Symptoms	Preventive Measures/ Treatment
Rheumatoid arthritis	An autoimmune disease that causes chronic inflammation of arthritis in the joints. (Figure 13.15)	Fatigue, lack of appetite, low-grade fever, muscle and joint aches, and stiffness. Joints frequently become red, swollen, painful, and tender. Multiple joints are usually inflamed in a symmetrical pattern (both sides of the body affected).	No cure. Work to reduce joint inflammation and pain, maximize joint function, and prevent joint destruction and deformity. Use a combination of medications, rest, joint strengthening exercises, joint protection, and patient (and family) education.
Scoliosis	A **lateral** (to the side) curvature of the spine. (Figure 13.14)	Congenital malformation of the spine, poliomyelitis, unequal length of legs, and other physical conditions.	Seeking early recognition and treatment may prevent progression of the curvature. Treatments include: exercise, using a brace, and possibly surgically implanting rods.

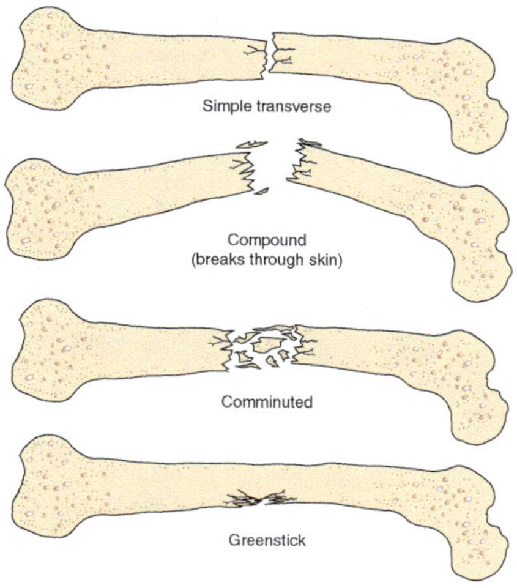

FIGURE 13.13
Common types of bone fractures. Which type of fracture produces many bone fragments?

lateral
(LAT ur uhl)
Relating to the sides or side of.

Apply It

Survey all of your classmates. Ask if they have ever broken a bone, and, if so, which one.

Create a graph—the x-axis should be labeled with the different bones that students broke; the y-axis should be labeled "number of people who have broken this bone."

Analyze the graph. Which bones were broken most? Why might that have happened?

Your Body and How It Functions | Chapter 13 315

Teaching Tips

- Pronounce the name of the condition for the last two disorders out loud:
  - Rheumatoid arthritis
  - Scoliosis
- Ask a student to read the description of each disorder.
- Discuss the symptoms of each.
- Discuss the preventive measures and/or treatments of each.

Figure Focus

13.13 Common types of bone fractures. Which type of fracture produces many bone fragments?

Answer: Comminuted

Apply It

- You may conduct this activity together as a class, or have the students work in small groups.
- You might have them create a form for gathering the data.
- You might have them use a spreadsheet program to enter the data and create the graph.
- Discuss what they can learn from this data.

Figure Focus

13.14 How is the spine of a person with scoliosis different from a normal spine?

Answer: The spine of a person with scoliosis is curved to the side, not straight like a normal spine.

Figure Focus

13.15 Stages of rheumatoid arthritis. What are the characteristics of an arthritic joint?

Answer: Damaged articular cartilage and eroded bone

TEAMWORK

Divide the class into teams of 8 to 12 students. Play a game of Hangman, using the terms covered in Section 13.2.

FIGURE 13.14
How is the spine of a person with scoliosis different from a normal spine?

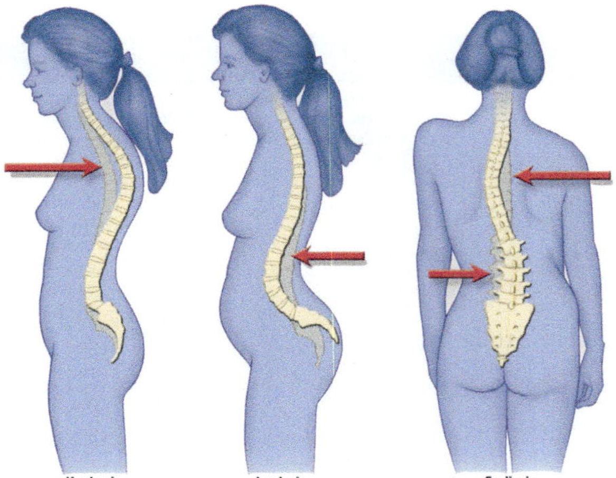

Figure 13.15
Stages of rheumatoid arthritis. What are the characteristics of an arthritic joint?

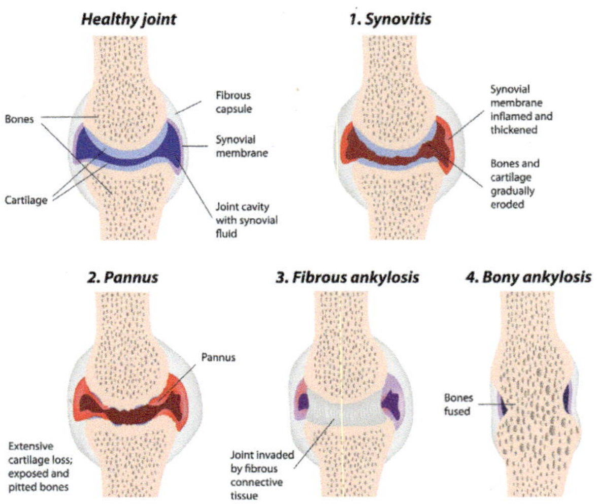

316 Chapter 13 | Your Body and How It Functions

MEDICAL TERMINOLOGY			
arthrodesis:	surgical fixation of a joint	**dactylus:**	toe or finger
caudocephalad:	from tail or coccyx to head	**ilio:**	pertaining to the ilium and femur
cephalalgia:	pain in the head, headache	**lumbosacral:**	pertaining to the lumbar vertebrae and the sacrum
cephalocentesis:	surgical puncture of the head		
cerebrotomy:	incision into the brain	**myelitis:**	inflammation of the spinal cord
chondroma:	tumor consisting of cartilage	**osteomalacia:**	softening of the bone
costochondral:	pertaining to a rib and its cartilage	**osteoplasty:**	plastic repair of the bone
craniomalacia:	softening of the skull bones	**osteosarcoma:**	malignant tumor of the bone
craniosclerosis:	thickening of the skull bones	**osteotomy:**	incision into a bone
dactyledema:	excess fluid in the fingers and toes	**phalanx:**	finger or toe bone
dactylology:	representing words by signs made with the fingers (sign language)	**prosthesis:**	artificial organ or part of the body

Related Jobs and Professions

Orthopedist

An orthopedist, also called an orthopedic surgeon, is a physician who specializes in treating disorders of the musculoskeletal system. The musculoskeletal system is comprised of bones, joints, muscles, tendons, ligaments, nerves, skin, and any of the structures related to these body parts.

fixation
(fik SEY shuhn)
Repair or fix.

Orthopedists use casts to repair broken bones; they prescribe exercise and medication for musculoskeletal injury or disease; and they perform surgeries such as implanting artificial joints or reconstructing damaged limbs. Although historically orthopedists primarily worked with children, modern orthopedists have patients of all ages. Some orthopedists specialize in one area, such as sports injuries, but most treat a wide variety of conditions.

Figure 13.16
What skills and interests do you think might be necessary to become an orthopedist?

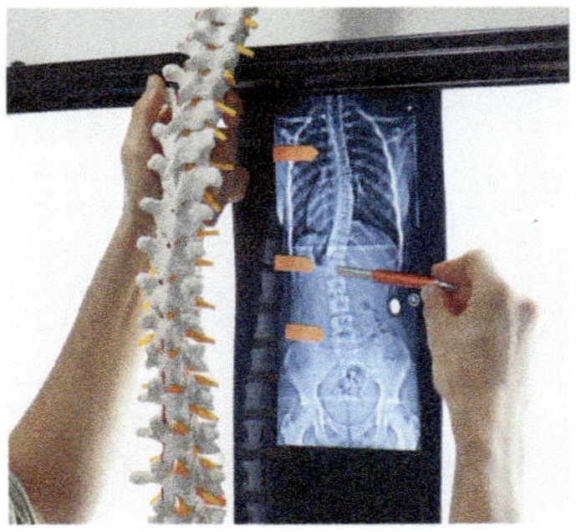

To become an orthopedist, you must first become a physician. That means four years of medical school and passing a medical licensing exam. You then complete one year of general surgery training followed by four years of orthopedic surgery training and two years in clinical practice. At this point, you must take an certification exam. Another year of training is needed to practice in a subspecialty area such as pediatric orthopedics or orthopedic sports medicine. Once certified, orthopedic surgeons must continue to take courses to keep their skills up to date.

Orthopedic Technician

An orthopedic technician, also known as an orthopedic technologist or cast technician, helps physicians and orthopedic surgeons care for and treat patients with orthopedic needs. This work is generally done in a hospital, clinic, or private practice.

The duties of an orthopedic technician are three-fold. First, there is work directly related to patient care. Orthopedic technicians help with such things as the application, adjustment, and removal of casts, splints, and braces. They also help set up,

Your Body and How It Functions | Chapter 13 317

MEDICAL TERMINOLOGY

Review the terminology:

- Pronounce each word element, and have students repeat.
- Pronounce each medical term, and have students repeat.
- Allow time for students to write down definitions.
- Select a student to read each definition.
- Assign students to memorize the terms and their definitions.

Teaching Tips

- Begin a discussion about the jobs and professions that would be suitable for someone interested in the skeletal system.
- Remind students to refer to Chapter 3 for more information on occupations.
- Discuss the skills and requirements for becoming an orthopedist.
- Discuss the skills and requirements for becoming an orthopedic technician.

Figure Focus

13.16 What skills and interests do you think might be necessary to become an orthopedist?

Student answers will vary.

ACTIVITY

Select one of the jobs or professions listed in Section 13.2. Create a brochure or pamphlet explaining why the health care worker you selected needs a basic knowledge of skeletal system in order to perform his or her job effectively.

Teaching Tips

- Discuss the skills and requirements for becoming a prosthetist.
- Review the bones of the body.
- Have the students pronounce aloud the name of each bone as you point to it on a skeleton, or an unlabeled poster or chart.
- Discuss reasons why it is important for all health care workers to have a basic knowledge of the skeletal system and how it functions.
- Students may find it easy to understand why orthopedists must have this knowledge, but you should try to make it relevant for other types of care givers as well.
- For example:
  - A nursing assistant must be able to observe and communicate information about pain in bones or joints.
  - Radiology workers must be able to take x-rays as ordered.
  - A nutritionist must be able to create menus that address skeletal disorders.

adjust, and maintain traction devices. Another aspect to the job is organizational. Orthopedic technicians are responsible for maintaining the cast room as well as orthopedic equipment and devices. The third prong is clerical. Orthopedic technicians manage insurance, medical billing, and coding for orthopedic procedures.

There are three different career levels for orthopedic technicians. Level I, or entry-level positions, requires a high school diploma and at least one year of full-time, on-the-job experience working with orthopedic patients. Level II requires certification from the National Board of Certification for Orthopaedic Technologists (NBCOT) plus either two years of experience, completion of an orthopedic technology training program, or completion of a related program and one year of full-time experience. Level III requires certification, completion of a training program, and up to eight years of experience.

Prosthetist

A prosthetist is a medical professional who evaluates, designs, and creates artificial limbs, or prostheses, for patients who have lost all or part of a limb due to disease or injury.

A prosthetist works with a team comprised of physicians, nurses, and physical and occupational therapists. Once the prosthesis is created, the prosthetist periodically evaluates the device and makes adjustments as needed.

To become a prosthetist, you must earn a B.S. degree and then complete a certificate program in prosthetics. It typically takes four years to earn a B.S. Certificate programs, which include both coursework and clinical experience, take between six months and one year to complete.

Summary

The axial and appendicular skeletons, joints, ligaments, and associated blood vessels and nerves make up the skeletal system. Skeletal system disease or fracture can make movement painful or difficult. In this section, you have learned to recognize skeletal system disorders. You have also learned preventative measures to recommend to patients, so they can avoid skeletal system disorders. A strong and healthy skeletal system is essential to good overall health.

Section 13.2 Review Questions

1. How can a person treat rickets?
2. Which type of bone fracture results in a broken bone that penetrates the skin?
3. What are the three main groups of joints?
4. Contrast the axial skeleton with the appendicular skeleton.
5. Where are the long bones in the body found?
6. Are the maxilla and mandible found in the axial or appendicular skeleton?
7. What is arthritis and what are the symptoms?
8. Identify three duties of an orthopedic technician.

318 Chapter 13 | Your Body and How It Functions

Section 13.2 Review Questions

1. Answer: Eat a balanced diet especially foods with calcium, phosphorus, and Vitamin D, and increase exposure to sunlight.
2. Answer: Compound fracture
3. Answer: Immovable, slightly movable, and freely movable joints
4. Answer: The axial skeleton includes 80 bones found in the skull, vertebrae, ribs, and sternum. The appendicular skeleton involves the skeleton involves the appendages of 120 bones found in the arms, hands, legs, feet, and pelvis.
5. Answer: Humerus, radius, ulna, tibia, fibula
6. Answer: Axial
7. Answer: Arthritis is inflammation of the joints and can be caused when a joint is damaged, causing the edges of bone to rub against each other and become irritated. Symptoms include pain and swelling.
8. Answer: Apply, adjust, remove cast, splints, and braces; Set up, adjust, maintain traction devices; Maintain the cast room, equipment, and devices

TEAMWORK

Divide the class into teams of four to six students. Distribute an unlabeled, large, paper skeleton to each group. For example, use Halloween skeletons. Also distribute a pad of sticky notes. With a time limit, have students label the bones and joints on the skeleton by writing the name on a sticky note and attaching it to the correct location. The team that correctly labels the most parts of the skeleton wins. If a label is misspelled, it does not count.

The Muscular System

SECTION 13.3

Background

The muscles in your body help you to move your arms and legs. They also help to move food, blood, and other materials around your body. In this section, you will learn about types of muscle, their functions, and their movements. You will review the different muscles of the muscular system and learn disorders related to muscles. The muscular system plays a primary role is the principles of body movement. As you study this section, identify and analyze the principles of body movement, such as forces and effects of movement, torque (rotatory force), tension, and elasticity on the human body.

Objectives

When you have completed this section, you will be able to do the following:

- Match key terms with their correct meanings.
- Explain the difference between muscle and bone functions.
- List three major functions of the muscles.
- Match common disorders of the muscular system with their descriptions.
- Match basic muscle movements to their correct names.
- Label a diagram of the muscular system.
- Describe how muscles provide support and movement.
- Explain why the health care worker's understanding of the muscular system is important.

Introduction to The Muscular System

The muscles of the body make all movement possible. Muscles move body parts, allowing for proper functioning, such as heartbeat, breathing, **digestion** of food, and movement of the body from place to place. The next sections help you understand how muscles work.

Muscle Function

Skeletal muscles comprise about 40% of the mass of the average human body. Muscles are the "engine" that your body uses to propel itself. They turn energy into motion. They are efficient at turning fuel into motion; they are long-lasting, self-healing, and can grow stronger with practice.

Muscles are made up of **elastic** fibers. These fibers are like a rubber band that lengthens and shortens. The thick and thin filaments do the actual work of a muscle. Thick filaments are made of a protein called **myosin**. Thin filaments are made of another protein called **actin**.

A muscle **contraction** occurs when these fibers generate tension through the action of actin and myosin cross-bridging—the process that describes the sliding of myosin and actin filaments (a sliding filament mechanism) over each other.

digestion
(dye JES chun)
Process of breaking down food mechanically and chemically.

elastic
(ee LAS tik)
Easily stretched.

myosin
(MI essin)
A protein in muscles that helps them contract.

actin
(AK tin)
A protein present in all cells and in muscle tissue; plays a role in contraction.

contraction
(ken TRAK shun)
A tightening or narrowing of a muscle, organ, or other body part.

Your Body and How It Functions | Chapter 13 319

FOCUS AND ENGAGE

Introduce the Section

a. Review the content of the Background paragraph, explaining that muscles help move your body, and move material around inside your body.

b. Emphasize that health care workers should know basic information about the muscular system to help them better understand and communicate with patients and co-workers.

c. Review the objectives for the section.

Vocabulary Review

a. Direct students to the key terms.

b. Pronounce each word, and have the students repeat the pronunciation out loud.

c. Discuss the definition of each word.

TEACH

Discuss

- Ask students to discuss how they use their muscles.
- Explain that even when they are sitting still or sleeping, they are using muscles.
- Discuss what the body would be like if it had no muscles.

Reinforce and Review

- Review the information in Section 13.1: cells, tissues, organs, cavities, and body directions.
- Review the information in Section 13.2, The Skeletal System.

ACTIVITY

Select one muscle or group of muscles. Draw a poster demonstrating the muscle in action. Label the muscle correctly. Display the posters in the classroom or on a bulletin board.

Teaching Tips

- Introduce the muscular system by explaining that muscles make all movement possible.

Teaching Tips

- Emphasize that movement includes breathing, digestion, and blood flow, as well as walking, waving, running, jumping, etc.
- Discuss muscle function, emphasizing the "engine" comparison.
- Differentiate between the functions of muscles and bones.
- Muscles:
  - Produce heat
  - Produce movement
  - Maintain posture
- Bones:
  - Provide a framework to give structure
  - Protect internal structures
  - Store calcium
  - Produce blood cells in the bone marrow
  - Allow flexibility when muscles move them
- Discuss unique characteristics of muscles:
  - Turn fuel into motion
  - Long-lasting
  - Self-healing
  - Grow stronger with practice
- Discuss the composition of muscle:
  - Elastic fibers like a rubber band
  - Thick and thin filaments

Muscles cannot push; they can only pull. Even when you push against a wall, each muscle in your body is working by pulling. When the muscles relax, they stop pulling.

The main functions of muscles are to:

- Produce heat (**thermogenesis**)
- Produce movement
- Maintain posture
- Protect internal organs

thermogenesis (thur moh JEN uh sis) The production of heat.

Types of Muscle

There are two classifications of muscle:

- **Voluntary** *muscles* that you **contract** when you want to move (e.g., skeletal muscles). (Figure 13.17) You control these muscles; the movement is not automatic.
- **Involuntary** *muscles*, which contract automatically (e.g., stomach, intestine, and heart). The heart pumps blood automatically. The stomach digests food automatically. You cannot tell the heart or stomach to start or stop.

voluntary (VOL en tar ee) Under the control of the person (e.g., you voluntarily raise your arm; it does not rise automatically).

contract (con TRAKT) To shorten, to draw together; muscles shorten when you flex a body part.

involuntary (IN vol en tar ee) Not under control (e.g., muscle twitching).

Tendons

Tendons connect muscles to bones. When the muscle moves, it moves the tendon and bone. The longest tendon is called the Achilles tendon. This is a tendon of the posterior leg; it attaches the calf muscle to the heel bone.

Types of Muscle Tissue

Muscle tissue is classified into three categories:

- *Skeletal muscles* or *striated muscles* are voluntary muscles. These muscles provide movement of the body.
- *Visceral muscles* or *smooth muscles* form the walls of the internal organs of the body (e.g., digestive tract, respiratory passage, and walls of blood vessels). They are involuntary muscles.
- The *cardiac muscle* forms the wall of the heart. This muscle circulates the blood.

320 Chapter 13 | Your Body and How It Functions

ACTIVITY

Hand out two 3 × 5 index cards to each student. On one card, students should write the word "BONES." On the other card, students should write the word "MUSCLES." As you announce a specific function, each student should hold up the appropriate card.

Figure 13.17
Skeletal muscular system. Where is the lattisimus dorsi muscle?

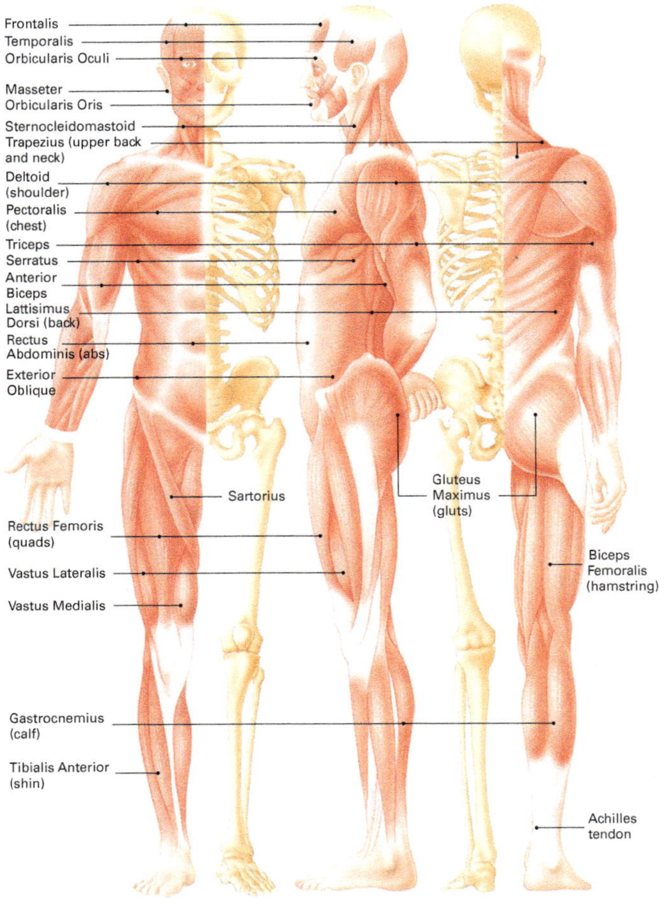

Your Body and How It Functions | Chapter 13 321

Teaching Tips

- Point to each muscle and pronounce the name.
- Ask students to repeat the name.
- Discuss the types of muscles:
  - Voluntary muscles that you control: skeletal muscles
  - Involuntary muscles that contract automatically: visceral muscles
- Explain that tendons connect the muscle to the bone. When the muscle moves, the tendon moves, which in turn causes the bone to move.
- Discuss the types of muscle tissue (refer back to Figure 13.2 on p. 298):
  - Skeletal or striated
  - Visceral or smooth
  - Cardiac, which is found only in the heart

Figure Focus

13.17 Skeletal muscle system. Where is the lattisimus dorsi muscle?

Answer: In the lower back

ACTIVITY

Think about the difference between voluntary and involuntary muscles. For example, can you tell your stomach to digest food? Can you tell your heart to beat? Can you tell your fingers to write the letter A? Make a table that identifies and compares actions based on whether they are the result of involuntary or voluntary muscles.

Teaching Tips

- Review the six basic movements performed by the muscles:
    - Adduct: move a body part toward the midline
    - Abduct: move a body part away from the midline
    - Extend: increase the angle of the muscle
    - Flex: decrease the angle of the muscle
    - Rotate: turn a body part on its axis
    - Supination and pronation: supination is when the ankle appears to be "tipped" to the outside so you are standing on the outside border of the foot; pronation is the flattening out of the arch when the foot strikes the ground.
- Ask for volunteers to demonstrate each type of movement.

Figure Focus

13.18 How is adduction different from abduction?

Answer: Adduction moves a body part toward the midline; abduction moves a body part away from the midline.

Basic Movements of the Skeletal Muscle

There are several basic movements of skeletal muscles (Figure 13.18):

- **Adduct:** moving a body part toward the midline.
- **Abduct:** moving a body part away from the midline.
- **Extend:** increases the angle of the muscle.
- **Flex:** decreases the angle of the muscle.
- **Rotate:** turning a body part on its **axis**.
- **Supination and pronation:** a rotation movement. For example, supination is when the ankle appears to be "tipped" to the outside so you are standing on the outside border of the foot; conversely, pronation is the flattening out of the arch when the foot strikes the ground.

axis
(AX iss)
A center point that can be rotated around.

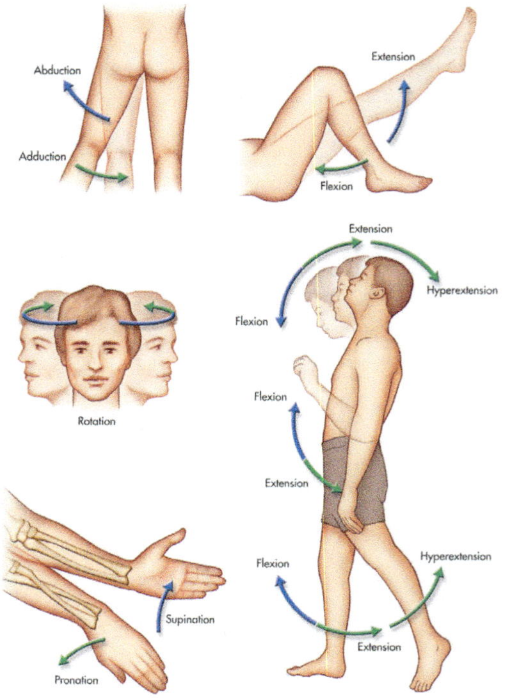

Figure 13.18
How is adduction different from abduction?

322 Chapter 13 | Your Body and How It Functions

TEAMWORK

Divide the class into teams of 8 to 12 students. In turn, name a muscle and ask the team to identify it on an unlabeled poster or chart. Allow the teams to confer before sending one team member to make the identification. The team is awarded one point for each correct answer. The team with the most points at the end of the activity wins.

Common Disorders of the Muscular System

Table 13.4 Common Disorders, Symptoms, and Preventive Measures/ Treatment of the Muscular System

Condition	Disorder	Symptoms	Preventive Measures/ Treatment
Atrophy	The wasting or loss of muscle tissue resulting from disease or lack of use.	Loss of mass and strength; some loss of mobility.	Application of moist heat, whirl-pool baths, and resistive exercises; more active exercises as mobility increases.
Fibromyalgia	Inflammation of the muscle tissues and the fibrous connective tissues.	A chronic stiffness and joint or muscle pain in eight or more specific muscle sites.	Using rest, heat, massage, and medication to relieve inflammation and swelling.
Hypertrophy	Abnormal growth and increase of the size of muscle cells caused by strength training, high-intensity anaerobic exercises, and use of anabolic steroids.	Enlarged muscles, as shown by bodybuilders.	Use lower intensity, longer duration aerobic exercise for health benefits without hypertrophy.
Muscle spasm	Involuntary contractions of the muscle, typically in the calf, thigh, foot, hand, arm, or abdomen.	Severe pain, twitching, tightness of the muscle affected.	Preparing muscles for activity; stretching of the muscle; non-steroidal anti-inflammatory medications.
Muscle strain (also called a torn muscle)	A muscle tear caused by a violent contraction.	Pain, swelling, warmth, and muscle weakness at the site.	Warming up muscles prior to exercise or strenuous activity. Not overextending muscles by trying to lift or pull objects that are beyond your capacity. Treatment includes rest and ice; then, as the pain decreases, use heat, stretch and light exercise to bring blood to the injured area.
Muscular dystrophy	A group of genetically transmitted diseases that progressively **deteriorate** muscle tissue.	Loss of strength with increased disability and deformity.	Using supportive treatment such as physical therapy and orthopedic procedures to minimize deformity. Genetic screening recommended for all family members who might be carriers.
Myalgia	Muscle pain.	Muscle pain and malaise; occurs in many infectious diseases.	Resting, taking medication, and identifying the original cause.
Tendonitis	A painful inflammation of a tendon.	Pain, swelling, stiffness in the local area of the tendon to burning sensation around the whole joint. Slow to heal and rarely regain original strength. Recurrence of injury is common.	Use of anti-inflammatory drugs (not steroids), rest and gradual return to exercise

deteriorate
(dee TEER ee or ate)
Break down.

Your Body and How It Functions | Chapter 13 323

Teaching Tips

- Review Table 13.4 together.
- Point out that the table includes the condition, the disorder, the symptoms, and treatments.
- Pronounce the name of each condition out loud:
  - Atrophy
  - Fibromyalgia
  - Hypertrophy
  - Muscle strain
  - Muscular dystrophy
  - Myalgia
  - Tendonitis
- Ask a student to read the description of each disorder.
- Discuss the symptoms of each.
- Discuss the preventive measures and/or treatments of each.

TEAMWORK

In small groups, prepare a skit demonstrating a common disorder of the muscular system. One student should be a patient, describing symptoms to a health care worker or a team of health care workers. The health care workers should diagnose the disorder, explain it, and prescribe a treatment.

MEDICAL TERMINOLOGY

Review the terminology:

- Pronounce each word element, and have students repeat.
- Pronounce each medical term, and have students repeat.
- Allow time for students to write down definitions.
- Select a student to read each definition.
- Assign students to memorize the terms and their definitions.

Teaching Tips

- Begin a discussion about the jobs and professions that would be suitable for someone interested in the muscular system.
- Remind students to refer to Chapter 3 for more information on occupations.
- Discuss the skills and requirements for becoming a myologist.
- Point out that a mycologist works with disorders affecting the mouth and face.
- Discuss the skills and requirements for becoming a physical therapist.

MEDICAL TERMINOLOGY

myasthenia:	muscle weakness	**myomelanosis:**	abnormal darkening of muscle tissue
myocardium:	heart muscle or cardiac muscle	**myoparesis:**	weakness or partial paralysis of a muscle
myocele:	muscular protrusion (bulging or sticking out through a muscle)	**myosclerosis:**	hardening of a muscle
myocelialgia:	pain of the abdominal muscle	**myothermic:**	pertaining to a rise in muscle temperature
myogenic:	beginning in the muscle	**tenorrhaphy:**	suturing of a tendon
myography:	record of muscle contractions	**tenositis:**	inflammation of a tendon
myoid:	resembling muscle		
myoma:	tumor containing muscle tissue		

Related Jobs and Professions

Myologist

An orofacial myologist diagnoses and treats abnormal patterns of the mouth and face caused by things such as thumb sucking, tongue thrusting, nail biting, and jaw clenching. Left untreated, these habits lead to problems with teeth alignment, speech, chewing, swallowing, and breathing.

The myologist works in conjunction with physicians and dentists to help patients develop new habits that lead to the proper usage and placement of the tongue, lips, and jaw. Myologists consist of professionals such as speech pathologists, physicians, dentists, and dental hygienists who have sought further training in this area.

To become certified by the International Association of Orofacial Myology, candidates, who are already practicing professionals in another area, must complete an approved 28-hour introductory course or internship, be a member in good standing for one year, and pass a take-home proficiency exam and an on-site evaluation.

Physical Therapist

Physical therapists (PTs) work with accident victims and people who suffer from disabling conditions such as lower back pain, fractures, heart disease, and cerebral palsy. They help these patients restore function, improve mobility, relieve pain, and prevent or limit permanent physical disabilities.

PTs test and measure everything from a patient's strength and range of motion to their balance and coordination. They develop individualized treatment plans that may include things such as electrical stimulation, hot packs and cold compresses, ultrasound, traction, or deep-tissue massage.

Physical therapists typically work a 40-hour week. Most PTs work in hospitals, clinics, and private offices. To become a physical therapist, you must graduate from an accredited physical therapy program. The minimum requirement is a B.S. degree. Many have a master's or doctoral degree.

324 Chapter 13 | Your Body and How It Functions

ACTIVITY

Select one of the jobs or professions listed in Section 13.3. Create a brochure or pamphlet explaining why the health care worker you selected needs a basic knowledge of the muscular system in order to perform his or her job effectively.

Sports Medicine Assistant

Working directly under the supervision of a physician, a sports medicine assistant works specifically with athletes. (Figure 13.19) Duties include helping diagnose, treat, and prevent injuries, as well as assisting athletes with their nutrition, training, and conditioning. A sports medicine assistant might recommend protective gear, supervise trainers, or develop training or rehabilitation programs.

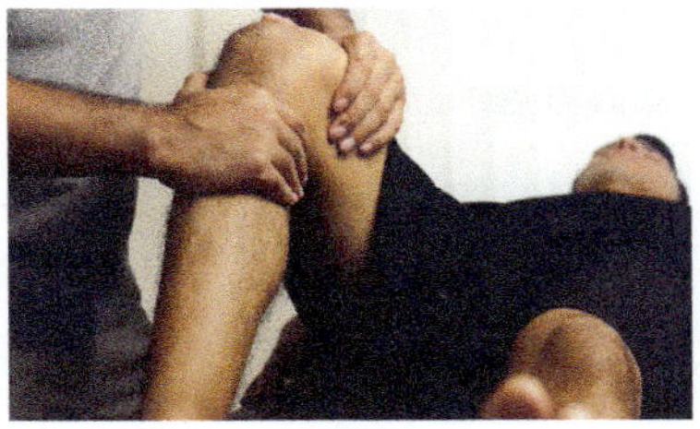

Figure 13.19
What skills and interests do you think might be necessary to work in sports medicine?

Sports medicine assistants can be found in school athletic departments, community recreation programs, health and fitness clubs, sports centers, resorts, clinics specializing in sports medicine, or even in a private practice. To become a sports medicine assistant, you need a four-year degree. This is a growing profession, and the qualifications required are rapidly evolving.

Tenotomist

A tenotomist is surgeon who specializes in tenotomies, or procedures in which tendons are cut. A tenotomy is performed when a muscle has developed improperly, as in the case of a club foot. It is also performed if a muscle becomes shortened and is unable to stretch to its full range of motion. The tenotomist who performs the surgery is a licensed orthopedic surgeon.

Apply It

Working with a frozen piece of licorice and a regular piece of licorice, bend both pieces. The frozen one will snap and break. Discuss why you need to warm up muscles and how muscle tears or strains occur.

Summary

Muscle tissue is made of elastic fibers that lengthen and shorten, helping the body to move, produce heat, and maintain posture. Skeletal muscles allow you to flex and extend your arms and legs. Smooth muscles move food, air, and blood throughout your body. The cardiac muscle pumps blood through your body. In this section, you have learned how muscle disorders can cause pain and inhibit movement. You have also learned that muscle disorders such as muscle strain and torn muscle can be avoided by stretching and avoiding strenuous activity.

Section 13.3 Review Questions

1. How can a person avoid muscle strain?
2. What position is the leg in when you are sitting normally in a chair?
3. Describe the three types of muscle tissue and what they do.
4. What are the three functions of muscles?
5. What does *contract* mean?
6. What is tendonitis and how do you treat it?
7. Describe the different roles of a physical therapist and a sports medicine assistant.

Your Body and How It Functions | Chapter 13 325

Teaching Tips

- Discuss the skills and requirements for becoming a sports medicine assistant.
- Discuss the differences between a physical therapist and a sports medicine aide.
- Discuss the types of injuries someone who specialized in sports medicine might encounter, and why.
- Refer students to Chapter 21 for more information about physical therapy and sports medicine aides.
- Discuss the skills and requirements for becoming a tenotomist.
- Have the students pronounce aloud the name of each muscle as you point to it on an unlabeled poster or chart.
- Review how muscles provide support and allow movement.
- Discuss reasons why it is important for all health care workers to have a basic knowledge of the muscular system and how it functions.
- Students may find it easy to understand why a physical therapist must have this knowledge, but you should try to make it relevant for other types of care givers as well.
- For example:
  - An emergency medical technician must be able to identify and diagnose an injury.
  - A medical educator must be able to explain the need for proper ergonomics.

Section 13.3 Review Questions

1. Answer: Warm up muscles prior to exercise or strenuous activity, not overextending muscles by trying to lift or pull objects that are beyond your capacity.
2. Answer: Flexion
3. Answer: Skeletal muscles or striated muscles are voluntary muscles. These muscles provide movement of the body. Visceral muscles or smooth muscles form the walls of the internal organs of the body (e.g., digestive tract, respiratory passage, and walls of blood vessels). They are involuntary muscles. The cardiac muscle forms the wall of the heart. This muscle circulates the blood.
4. Answer: Produce heat, produce movement, and maintain posture
5. Answer: Contract means to shorten or to draw together. Muscles shorten when you flex a body part.
6. Answer: Tendonitis is a painful inflammation of a tendon. Anti-inflammatory drugs, rest, and a gradual return to exercise are the treatment for tendonitis.

Apply It

- This activity uses licorice to simulate a muscle. The frozen licorice acts like a cold muscle; the warm licorice like a warm muscle.
- You can perform this activity as a class, as individuals, or in small groups.
- During the discussion, ask students to share personal stories of how they warm up before exercising.

7. Answer: Physical therapists help these patients restore function, improve mobility, relieve pain, and prevent or limit permanent physical disabilities. PTs test and measure everything from a patient's strength and range of motion to their balance and coordination. They develop individualized treatment plans for patients. Sports medicine assistants work directly under the supervision of a physician. They work specifically with athletes. Duties include helping diagnose, treat, and prevent injuries, as well as assisting athletes with their nutrition, training, and conditioning.

FOCUS AND ENGAGE

Introduce the Section

a. Review the content of the Background paragraph, explaining that the circulatory system is responsible for moving blood through the body.
b. Emphasize that the circulatory system is one of the most important systems in the body.
c. Review the objectives for the section.

Vocabulary Review

a. Direct students to the key terms.
b. Pronounce each word, and have the students repeat the pronunciation out loud.
c. Discuss each definition.

SECTION 13.4 The Circulatory System

Background

Arteries, veins, and the heart are the main organs of the circulatory system. Blood in the circulatory system delivers oxygen and nutrients to cells and removes waste materials. In this section, you will learn that the circulatory system is one of the most important systems of the body. Any disorder that disrupts the flow of blood can cause brain damage or death. For this reason, health care workers should be familiar with the treatment and prevention of circulatory system disorders.

Objectives

When you have completed this section, you will be able to do the following:

- Match key terms with their correct meanings.
- Name the major organs of the circulatory system.
- Label a diagram of the heart and blood vessels.
- Recognize functions of the circulatory system.
- Identify the common disorders of the circulatory system.
- List the parts of the circulatory system through which blood flows.
- Describe how the circulatory system supports life.
- Explain why the health care worker's understanding of the circulatory system is important.

oxygen
(OX uh jin)
Element in the atmosphere that is essential for maintaining life in most organisms.

waste products
(WAYST praw dukts)
Elements that are unfit for the body's use and are eliminated from the body.

adequate
(AD uh kwit)
Enough, sufficient.

oxygenated
(OX uh jin ate ed)
Containing oxygen.

unoxygenated
(UN ox uh jin ate ed)
Lacking oxygen.

carbon dioxide
(car buhn die OX eyed)
A gas, heavier than air; a waste product from the body.

Introduction to the Circulatory System

Circulation is the continuous one-way movement of blood throughout the body. All of the systems and organs depend on the circulatory system. Arteries carry blood with **oxygen** and nutrients to each cell, and veins carry away the cell's **waste products**. If the circulation is not **adequate**, cells die. When the cells die, tissues begin to die, and the organs stop working properly. This may cause an entire system to stop functioning.

Functions of the Circulatory System

- Carries oxygen and carbon dioxide
- Carries nutrients and wastes
- Circulates hormones and antibodies
- Maintains body temperature and transports heat

Kinds of Blood Vessels

- *Arteries* carry blood from the lower chambers of the heart (ventricles) to all parts of the body. Arteries carry **oxygenated** blood, with the exception of the pulmonary artery. The *pulmonary artery* carries **unoxygenated** blood.
- *Arterioles* are small arteries that connect arteries with capillaries.
- *Capillaries* have very thin walls that allow nutrients, oxygen, and **carbon dioxide** to move in and out of the blood. (Figure 13.20)
- *Venules* are small veins that connect veins with capillaries.

326 Chapter 13 | Your Body and How It Functions

TEACH

Discuss

- Reiterate the importance of the circulatory system.
- Discuss what makes it so important: the lack of blood can lead to severe brain damage or death.
- Emphasize that all systems and organs depend on the circulator system.

Reinforce and Review

- Review the information in Section 13.1: cells, tissues, organs, cavities, and body directions.

Teaching Tips

- Describe the major organs of the circulator system:
  - Heart
  - Arteries
  - Veins

CUSTOMIZED INSTRUCTION

Special Needs Students

To help special needs students identify parts of the heart (as well as other body parts covered in this chapter) try providing pictures or models that include color-coding to differentiate between parts and sections.

- *Veins* carry blood from all the different parts of the body and return it to the heart. Veins carry unoxygenated blood, with the exception of the pulmonary vein. The pulmonary vein carries oxygenated blood. Veins have valves that aid in returning blood to the heart.

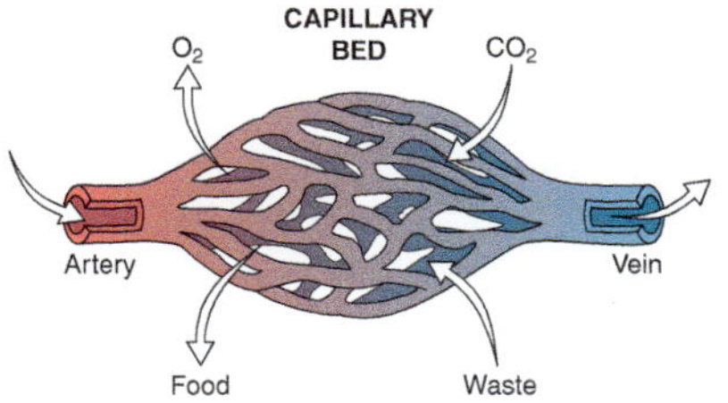

Figure 13.20
Blood vessels and capillary bed of the body. How are gases and other substances exchanged in the capillary bed?

primarily
(pry MARE uh lee)
For the most part; chiefly.

Components of Blood

The blood is a specialized fluid made of solid and liquid components.

- Plasma—liquid component of the blood; contains water, proteins, sugar, and salt that carry hormones, nutrients, and chemicals to the body to maintain homeostasis
- Erythrocytes—red blood cells; contains hemoglobin, which is responsible for carrying oxygen
- Leukocytes—white blood cells; protect the body from infection with antibodies
- Thrombocytes—platelets; responsible for clotting of blood

The Heart

The heart is the pump that forces blood throughout the body. (**Table 13.5**) The outside of the heart is made **primarily** of muscle, and the inside is divided into four hollow chambers. (**Figure 13.21**)

Figure 13.21
Cross section of the heart. What structure separates the two ventricles from each other?

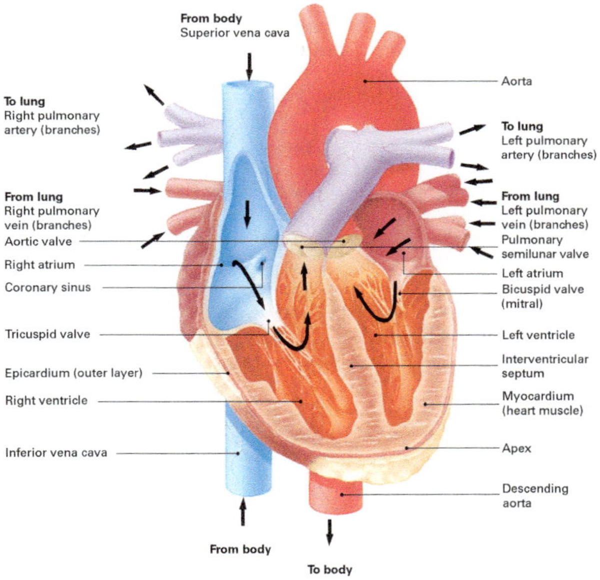

Teaching Tips

- Review the kinds of blood vessels:
  - Arteries
  - Arterioles
  - Capillaries
  - Venules
  - Veins
- Point to and pronounce the parts of the heart, and explain their function.

Figure Focus

13.20 Blood vessels and capillary bed of the body. How are gases and other substances exchanged in the capillary bed?

Answer: Cells take in oxygen from the capillaries and release carbon dioxide to the capillaries. Cells take in food from the capillaries and release waste to the capillaries.

Figure Focus

13.21 Cross section of the heart. What structure separates the two ventricles from each other?

Answer: The interventricular septum

ACTIVITY

Make a chart or table describing and differentiating between the different types of blood vessels.

Teaching Tips

- Review Table 13.5 together as a class.
- Describe the flow of blood through the heart.
- Describe the anatomy of the heart and blood vessels:
  - Outside of heart made of muscles
  - Four chambers
- Describe the composition of the heart wall. Three layers of tissue:
  - Endocardium: smooth inside lining of the heart
  - Myocardium: thickest layer; made of muscle
  - Pericardium: double membrane lining outside of heart
- Describe the four chambers of the heart:
  - Right atrium: receives unoxygenated blood from veins.
  - Right ventricle: receives blood from right atrium and pumps it to lungs through the pulmonary artery.
  - Left atrium: receives oxygenated blood from lungs and pumps it into left ventricle.
  - Left ventricle: pumps blood into aorta, the largest artery in the body.

The heart wall is made of three different layers of tissue:

- *Endocardium* is the smooth inside lining of the heart.
- *Myocardium* is the thickest layer and is made up of muscle.
- *Pericardium* is a double membrane that lines the outside of the heart.

The inside of the heart is divided into four parts or chambers:

- The *right atrium* receives unoxygenated blood from the veins.
- The *right ventricle* receives blood from the right atrium and pumps it to the lungs through the pulmonary artery.
- The *left atrium* receives oxygenated blood from the lungs and pumps it into the left ventricle.
- The *left ventricle* pumps blood into the aorta, which is the largest artery in the body. The aorta delivers the blood throughout the body.

Valves separate the chambers in the heart from the vessels leaving the heart:

- The *tricuspid* valve is between the right atrium and right ventricle. It closes when the right ventricle pumps blood out of the heart. This keeps the blood from flowing back into the right atrium.
- The *pulmonary semilunar* valve lies between the right ventricle and the pulmonary artery. It closes after all the blood from the right ventricle has been pushed into the pulmonary artery. When the valve closes, it stops blood from flowing back into the ventricle.
- The *mitral (bicuspid)* valve is found between the left atrium and the left ventricle. It closes to prevent blood from flowing back into the left atrium when the left ventricle contracts.
- The *aortic semilunar* valve is located between the left ventricle and the aorta. It stops blood from returning to the left ventricle after it has been forced into the aorta.

Table 13.5 Flow of Blood Through the Body

Starts in the right atrium
↓
Through the tricuspid valve
↓
Right ventricle
↓
Through the pulmonary valve
↓
Pulmonary artery
↓
Lungs (oxygen and carbon dioxide exchange)
↓
Pulmonary veins
↓
Left atrium
↓
Mitral valve
↓
Left ventricle
↓
Aortic valve
↓
Aorta ("out to the body")
↓
Arteries
↓
Arterioles
↓
Capillaries (oxygen and carbon dioxide exchange)
↓
Venules
↓
Veins
↓
Superior or inferior vena cava
↓
Right atrium

328 Chapter 13 | Your Body and How It Functions

ACTIVITY

Draw a poster or flowchart depicting the flow of blood through the circulatory system.

Electrical Conduction of the Heart

The electrical conduction process in the heart is responsible for creating the heart beat. As the heart beats, it forces blood through the chambers of the heart to the body and the lungs. Specialized nerve structures allow for the electrical conduction.

The electrical conduction starts in the sinoatrial node, located in the atria of the heart muscle. Once it is stimulated, the signal is passed down through the conduction pathways to the atrioventricular node (located between the atria and ventricles), and the atria contracts. From there, the electrical signal travels to the bundle of His and out to the ventricles from the branches of the right and left bundle branches. This stimulation results in the contraction of the ventricles.

This process normally occurs 60–100 times per minutes, depending on the age.

MEDICAL TERMINOLOGY	
angiocele:	hernia of a blood vessel
arteriosclerosis:	abnormal narrowing of arteries
atherosclerosis:	abnormal hardening and narrowing of arteries due to fatty plague build-up within the walls
bradycardia:	abnormally slow heart rate
cardiogenic:	beginning within the heart
cardiopulmonary:	pertaining to the heart and lungs
cardioscope:	instrument used to examine the inside of the heart
cardiovascular:	pertaining to the heart and blood vessels
carditis:	inflammation of the heart muscle
cyanosis:	bluish discoloration of the skin
ecchymosis:	bruised condition
electrocardiogram:	ECG/EKG, a tracing of heart activity
embolus:	a mass (i.e., blood clot, air) that travels through blood vessels often becoming lodged in a small blood vessel and obstructs it
endocarditis:	inflammation of the inside of the heart
erythrocytosis:	disease of red blood cells
hemostasis:	stoppage of blood flow
hyperemia:	excess of blood in any part of the body
hypertension:	high blood pressure
hypotension:	unusually low blood pressure
intravenous:	IV, within a vein
leukocyte:	white blood cell
leukopenia:	deficiency of white blood cells
tachycardia:	excessively rapid heart rate
thrombus:	stationary blood clot that obstructs circulation

Your Body and How It Functions | Chapter 13 329

Teaching Tips

- Explain that the aorta delivers the blood throughout the body.
- Describe the four valves that separate the chambers from the vessels:
  - Tricuspid valve: between right atrium and right ventricle
  - Pulmonary semilunar valve: between right ventricle and pulmonary artery
  - Mitral (bicuspid) valve: between left atrium and left ventricle
  - Aortic semilunar valve: between left ventricle and aorta
- Differentiate between the function of arteries and veins:
  - Arteries carry oxygenated blood.
  - Veins carry unoxygenated blood.
- Explain the difference between the oxygenation of blood in the pulmonary arteries and all other arteries of the body.
- Describe the flow of blood through the circulatory system.
- Discuss how the circulatory system supports life.
- Emphasize that if there is not adequate circulation, cells die, then tissues die, and organs fail.

MEDICAL TERMINOLOGY

Review the terminology:

- Pronounce each word element, and have students repeat.
- Pronounce each medical term, and have students repeat.
- Allow time for students to write down definitions.
- Select a student to read each definition.
- Assign students to memorize the terms and their definitions.

Teaching Tips

- Review the first part of Table 13.6 together.
- Point out that the table includes the condition, the disorder, the symptoms, and treatments.
- Pronounce the name of each condition out loud:
  - Aneurysm
  - Arteriosclerosis
  - Endocarditis
  - Heart murmur
  - Hypertension
- Ask a student to read the description of each disorder.
- Discuss the symptoms of each.
- Discuss the preventive measures and/or treatments of each.

TEAMWORK

In small groups, prepare a skit demonstrating a common disorder of the circulatory system. One student should be a patient, describing symptoms to a health care worker or a team of health care workers. The health care workers should diagnose the disorder, explain it, and prescribe a treatment.

Common Disorders of the Circulatory System

Table 13.6 Common Disorders, Symptoms, and Preventive Measures/ Treatment of the Circulatory System

Condition	Disorder	Symptoms	Preventive Measures/ Treatment
Aneurysm	An aneurysm is present when the wall of a blood vessel is weakened. Aneurysms may be found in any part of the circulatory system. Among the most serious are those that occur in the head, heart, and aorta. An aortic aneurysm that ruptures usually causes immediate death. A ruptured cerebral aneurysm can cause paralysis, speech and vision disturbances, and death.	Pulsating swelling that produces a blowing sound through a stethoscope. Pain may or may not be present.	Maintaining healthy living can be helpful in keeping blood pressure within normal range. Exercise and diet may also be a factor, but will not ensure the prevention of aneurysms. Treatment depends on where they are located and how big they are; surgery would be used to prevent rupture or to stop bleeding (if rupture has occurred).
Arteriosclerosis	Arteriosclerosis is present when the walls of the arteries become thick and harden, causing vessels to be less elastic. Less blood is able to flow through the arteries because the arteries are narrowed.	Changes in skin temperature and color, changes in peripheral pulses, headache, dizziness, and memory changes. Common in geriatric patients.	Continuing activity throughout aging, getting adequate rest, and avoiding stress.
Endocarditis	An inflammation of the inside lining of the heart that may affect the heart valves. This condition can be caused by a variety of diseases. Survival rate is 65 to 85%.	Chest pain, shortness of breath, and elevated body temperature.	Maintaining good health habits, including good dental care, may help resist this condition. Early diagnosis helps promote successful treatment, which consists of rest and IV antibiotics
Heart murmur	The valve does not close completely, allowing blood to flow back into the chamber it just left. It is most often present in the tricuspid and mitral valves.	Heart sounds that create a blowing sound between heartbeats, which indicate faulty heart valves.	Maintaining a healthy lifestyle may be helpful in preventing murmurs in later life. Some murmurs are present at birth.
Hypertension (also called the "silent killer")	A blood pressure greater than 140/90 places increased strain on the entire circulatory system. Risk of hypertension is increased due to obesity, hereditary factors race (African Americans run greater risk), gender (men run greater risk) and older age. Other factors associated with higher risk include heavy alcohol consumption, diabetes, use of oral contraceptives and lack of exercise.	In some cases, there are no symptoms. In others, anxiety, heart palpitations, profuse sweating, pallor, nausea, and in some cases the lungs collect fluid. May also experience headaches and blurred vision.	Maintaining good health habits may help resist this condition. Early diagnosis helps promote successful treatment. Treatment includes lifestyle changes to minimize risk factors (such as exercise and diet), monitoring blood pressure regularly and taking antihypertensive medication, if necessary.

(continued)

330 Chapter 13 | Your Body and How It Functions

Table 13.6 **Common Disorders, Symptoms, and Preventive Measures/ Treatment of the Circulatory System (continued)**

Condition	Disorder	Symptoms	Preventive Measures/ Treatment
Myocardial infarction (MI) or heart attack	Occurs when the coronary arteries (the muscular blood vessels that carry blood away from the heart) are blocked. This blockage can be due to atherosclerosis, or a blood clot, which is called coronary thrombosis.	Crushing chest pain that may radiate to the left arm, neck, or stomach. The patient may complain of severe heartburn or a gallbladder attack. The patient may look ashen in color and skin may feel clammy. May experience shortness of breath, may feel faint and anxious, and may fear that they are going to die.	Not smoking, maintaining a healthy body weight, eating a balanced diet low in saturated fats, and exercising regularly. Controlling stress is also helpful. Treatment includes opening the blocked artery and restoring blood flow to the affected area of heart muscle (surgery). Treatment is also aimed at preventing further damage and the chance of repeat heart attacks in the future (changes in diet, not smoking, exercise and medication).
Myocarditis	An inflammation of the heart muscle caused by viral, bacterial, or fungal infection, serum sickness, rheumatic fever, chemical agents, or complications from a collagen disease.	Chest pain, shortness of breath, and elevated body temperature.	Maintaining good health habits may help resist this condition. Early diagnosis helps promote successful treatment.
Pericarditis	An inflammation of the outer lining of the heart caused by trauma, malignancy, infection, uremia, myocardial infarction, collagen disease, and other nonspecific conditions.	Chest pain, shortness of breath, nonproductive cough, and rapid pulse. A friction rub can be heard over the heart with a stethoscope.	Maintaining good health habits may help resist this condition. Early diagnosis helps promote successful treatment.
Varicose veins	Enlarged veins that are not efficient in returning blood to the heart. They can occur anywhere in the body but are most often found in the lower **extremities.**	Pain and muscle cramps with a feeling of fullness and heaviness in the legs. Some veins near the skin may look enlarged. May be caused by congenital defects of the veins or by congestion and increased pressure.	Minimizing prolonged times of standing and maintaining good posture can reduce the risk of varicose veins in people without congenital defects.

Related Jobs and Professions

Internist

An internist is a physician who may provide either primary or long-term comprehensive care. They also may specialize in fields such as cardiology, critical care, infectious disease, or pulmonology.

Internists, as the name implies, focus on the health of internal organs. They generally treat illnesses such as high blood pressure or diabetes, which do not require surgery. The majority of an internist's patients are adults.

Internists must complete medical school followed by a three-year residency in which they receive training focused on internal medicine. In order to specialize in a particular area, internists must complete another one to three years of training. Between 20 and 25 percent of all physicians are internists.

extremities
(ex TREM uh tees)
Arms, legs, hands, and feet.

Apply It

Construct a matching game. Create a series of cards naming circulatory disorders or other related medical terminology. Then, create a set of cards with the definition/description of each term. Divide in small groups and play the matching game.

Your Body and How It Functions | Chapter 13 331

TEAMWORK

In small groups, prepare a presentation explaining or demonstrating ways people can behave in order to maintain a healthy circulatory system.

Teaching Tips

- Review the second part of Table 13.6 together.
- Pronounce the name of each condition out loud:
  - Myocardial infarction (MI) or heart attack
  - Myocarditis
  - Pericarditis
  - Varicose veins
- Ask a student to read the description of each disorder.
- Discuss the symptoms of each.
- Discuss the preventive measures and/or treatments of each.
- Begin a discussion about the jobs and professions that would be suitable for someone interested in the circulatory system.
- Remind students to refer to Chapter 3 for more information on occupations.
- Discuss the skills and requirements for becoming an internist.

Apply It

- Start this activity by having each student create a pair of cards: on one card, write a circulatory disorder or other circulatory terminology. On the second card, write the definition or description of the term.
- Distribute the pairs to small groups of students to use for the activity.
- You might choose to collect the cards at the end to use for future activities, or allow students to use them as a study tool.

Teaching Tips

- Discuss the skills and requirements for becoming a cardiologist.
- Review what it means to be a "specialist," such as a cardiologist.
- Explain that a cardiologist sees patients who are referred by another medical professional, usually because of symptoms or the results of diagnostic testing.
- Discuss the skills and requirements for becoming a cardiopulmonary technician.
- Discuss the purpose of a heart and lung machine.
- You may choose to discuss ethical implications of such a machine.
- Discuss the skills and requirements for becoming an ECG/EKG technician.

Figure Focus

13.22 What skills and interests do you think might be necessary to become an ECG/EKG technician?

Student answers will vary.

TEAMWORK

Divide the class into teams of 8 to 12 students. Play a game of Hangman, using the terms covered in Section 13.4.

Cardiologist

Cardiologists are medical doctors who diagnose, treat, and try to prevent problems in the cardiovascular system. The cardiovascular system includes the heart and blood vessels.

Patients are usually referred to a cardiologist by their primary care physicians. If a problem is suspected, the cardiologist checks the medical records, discusses signs and symptoms, conducts tests, and recommends a course of treatment. This may involve medication, lifestyle changes, or surgery. In the case of surgery, patients are sent to a cardiovascular surgeon.

Cardiologists typically work in clinics and hospitals. Some choose to specialize their practice, such as pediatric or adult cardiology. To become a cardiologist, you must graduate from college and then medical school. You must complete a residency and become certified in internal medicine. Then, you must complete another residency and become certified in cardiology. Further specialization requires another residency and certification.

Cardiopulmonary Technician

A cardiopulmonary technician, also called a perfusionist, is someone who operates a heart-and-lung machine. This life-supporting equipment replaces the function of the heart and lungs when they must be temporarily stopped, such as during cardiac surgery.

Cardiopulmonary technicians must pay extremely close attention to detail. They must notice even the slightest change in heart or lung function during surgery as any change could indicate a problem.

Cardiopulmonary technicians may work for hospitals, surgeons, or in a group practice. Some are independent contractors who work for one or more different employers. There are several different routes to this profession.

In general, though, you must have a four-year college degree with an emphasis on medical terminology, respiratory therapy, or nursing. You must then complete a training program that can last anywhere from one to four years. This will result in either a certificate or a master's degree, depending upon the type of program completed. Finally, you pass a test to become certified by the American Board of Cardiovascular Perfusion.

Figure 13.22
What skills and interests do you think might be necessary to become an ECG/EKG technician?

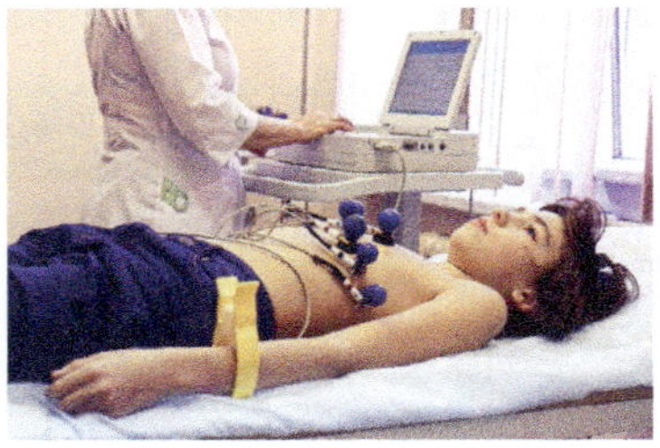

ECG/EKG Technician

ECG/EKG technicians perform tests such as electrocardiograms (EKGs) and stress tests, which help physicians diagnose and treat problems with the heart and blood vessels. (Figure 13.22) These tests record and monitor the electrical impulses transmitted by the heart. Tracking these impulses can identify any irregularities and potential problems.

ECG/EKG technicians work in hospitals and physicians' offices. Community colleges and technical schools offer training in this area, but most ECG/EKG technicians are trained on the job by an EKG supervisor or a cardiologist. Not all ECG/EGK technicians are certified, but there is a growing trend in that direction.

Echocardiogram Technician

Echocardiogram technicians use ultrasound equipment to perform specialized tests called echocardiograms. During these tests, high-frequency sounds waves are transmitted into the heart chambers, valves, and blood vessels to create an image. The technician checks the image on screen for any abnormalities, photographs or videotapes the image, and sends the images and a report to the patient's physician for evaluation.

Nearly three-fourths of all echocardiogram technicians work in cardiology departments in hospitals. Others are employed in physicians' offices or diagnostic laboratories. Although some are trained on the job, most have completed a two- or four-year program in this specialty. Professional certification is available.

Summary

In this section, you have learned that diseases of the circulatory system affect blood vessels or the heart. Heart disease may weaken the muscles of the heart, causing it to pump less effectively. Diseases of the blood vessels may slow or block the delivery of oxygen to cells, causing organs to fail. You have learned the signs of and some treatments for circulatory diseases. You have also learned some ways to prevent circulatory diseases. This knowledge can help you to suggest lifestyle changes to patients to help them avoid circulatory diseases.

Section 13.4 Review Questions

1. What are the major organs of the circulatory system?
2. What is the function of the capillaries?
3. Describe the path that blood takes as it moves from the lungs through the heart and out to the rest of the body.
4. Describe the three layers of tissue that make up the heart.
5. What is an aneurysm?
6. What are actions that people can take to prevent myocardial infarction?
7. What are the differences between an ECG/EKG technician and an echocardiogram technician?

Your Body and How It Functions | Chapter 13 333

Section 13.4 Review Questions

1. Answer: The heart, including blood and blood vessels
2. Answer: Capillaries have very thin walls that allow nutrients, oxygen, and carbon dioxide to move in and out of the blood.
3. Answer: Starts in the right atrium; Through the tricuspid valve; Right ventricle; Through the pulmonary valve; Pulmonary artery; Lungs (oxygen and carbon dioxide exchange); Pulmonary veins; Left atrium; Mitral valve; Left ventricle; Aortic valve; Aorta ("out to the body"); Arteries; Arterioles; Capillaries (oxygen and carbon dioxide exchange); Venules; Veins; Superior or inferior vena cava; Right atrium
4. Answer: Endocardium is the smooth inside lining of the heart. Myocardium is the thickest layer and is made up of muscle. Pericardium is a double membrane that lines the outside of the heart.
5. Answer: An aneurysm is present when the wall of a blood vessel is weakened. Aneurysms may be found in any part of the circulatory system.

Teaching Tips

- Discuss the skills and requirements for becoming an echocardiogram technician.
- Remind students that these technicians perform diagnostic testing using specialized equipment.
- You may want to discuss some of the symptoms that might call for such testing.
- You may also want to discuss results that might come from such testing, and what the next course of action might be (refer to Table 13.6).
- Discuss reasons why it is important for all health care workers to have a basic knowledge of the circulatory system and how it functions.
- Ask students to consider how different types of medical professionals use an understanding of the circulatory system.
- Discuss the expectation that everyone working in a health care environment will understand patient conditions.
- Also, discuss the importance of using correct medical terminology when communicating within a health care environment.
- Finally, discuss the importance of responding appropriately when a medical emergency occurs.

ACTIVITY

Select one of the jobs or professions listed in Section 13.4. Create a brochure or pamphlet explaining why the health care worker you selected needs a basic knowledge of the circulatory system in order to perform his or her job effectively.

6. Answer: Don't smoke, maintain a healthy weight, eat a balanced diet low in saturated fats, exercise regularly, and control stress.
7. Answer: An ECG/EKG technician performs tests such as electrocardiograms (EKGs) and stress tests, which help physicians diagnose and treat problems with the heart and blood vessels. An echocardiogram technician uses ultrasound equipment to perform specialized tests called echocardiograms. The technician checks the image on screen for any abnormalities, photographs or videotapes the image, and sends the images and a report to the patient's physician for evaluation.

FOCUS AND ENGAGE

Introduce the Section

a. Review the Background paragraph, explaining that homeostasis is balance or equilibrium for the body.
b. Emphasize that the lymphatic system helps bodies fight off disease and build immunity.
c. Review the section objectives.

Vocabulary Review

a. Direct students to the key terms.
b. Pronounce each word, and have the students repeat the pronunciation out loud.
c. Discuss each definition.

SECTION 13.5 The Lymphatic System

Background

The lymphatic system allows the body to maintain homeostasis. This system helps the body to fight disease and build immunity. It also prevents the buildup of fluids in tissues. In this section, you will study the structure and functions of the lymphatic system. You will also learn about disorders that affect this system. Disorders that affect the lymphatic system can weaken the body's immune response. Patients who have weakened immunity are less able to fight off disease.

Objectives

When you have completed this section, you will be able to do the following:

- Match key terms with their correct meanings.
- Describe the general functions of the lymphatic system.
- Describe what lymph is.
- Match lymph vessels and organs to their function.
- Explain the difference between an antigen and an antibody.
- Identify common disorders of the lymphatic system.
- Describe how the lymphatic system helps provide immunity and maintain homeostasis.

homeostasis
(hoh mee uh STEY sis)
Constant balance within the body. This balance is maintained by the heartbeat, blood-making mechanisms, electrolytes, and hormone secretions.

interstitial
(in tur STISH uhl)
Space between tissues.

Introduction to the Lymphatic System

The lymphatic system is an important part of the body's defense against disease. (Figure 13.23) It filters out organisms that cause disease, produces white blood cells, and makes antibodies. It also drains excess fluids and protein so that tissues do not swell up. All of these biological and chemical processes contribute to **homeostasis**. Maintaining good health depends on maintaining homeostasis. The body must constantly receive feedback from the body's regulatory mechanisms. For example, when the body's temperature rises, sweating provides feedback. There is a delicate balance between fluid, electrolytes, and pH—illness almost always threatens that balance. Medical interventions, such as intravenous fluids, can also cause imbalances.

Apply It

Create a wound somewhere on your body, using vaseline, cocoa, and tissues. Using yarn, trace the lymphatic path an infection would follow and to determine which lymph nodes would swell. Trace the path from the wound until it empties into the thoracic duct or right lymphatic duct. Determine which it would empty into based on wound location.

The lymphatic system and the circulatory system have structures that are joined together by a capillary system. The lymphatic system is made up of the lymph capillaries, lymph vessels, lymph nodes, spleen, tonsils, thymus, lacteals, thoracic duct, right lymphatic duct, and the cisterna chyli.

Kinds of Lymphatic System Vessels and Organs

- *Lymph capillaries* are tubes that reach into the **interstitial** spaces of most body tissues. The capillaries have very thin walls that allow tissue fluids to move into them. When the fluid moves into the capillary, it is called lymph. The lymph contains waste products and foreign bodies from the cells. The lymph passes from the capillaries to the lymph vessels.

334 Chapter 13 | Your Body and How It Functions

TEACH

Discuss

- Ask students if they have ever had a fever, a bruise that became swollen, or a cut that oozed pus.
- Explain that these are symptoms that show the body is fighting an infection.
- Discuss why the body fights infection.
- Discuss the role of homeostasis and its mechanisms as these relate to the body as a whole.

Reinforce and Review

- Review the information in Section 13.1: cells, tissues, organs, cavities, and body directions.
- Review the information in Section 13.4, The Circulatory System.

Teaching Tips

- Point out that the lymphatic system plays a major role in homeostasis.
- Ask students to predict the consequences of the failure to maintain homeostasis.
- Explain the general function of the lymphatic system is to carry excess tissue fluid to the bloodstream and to protect the body from foreign bodies that cause infection.

ACTIVITY

Imagine that the lymphatic system is a superhero that protects the body the way Superman protects Lois Lane. Draw a comic strip about the lymphatic system, or a poster advertising a new action movie about the lymphatic system.

- *Lymph vessels* are similar to veins. Muscle contractions help move the lymph from the tissues to the lymphatic trunks. Valves prevent backflow of the lymph. The lymphatic trunks receive the lymph from the body. The lymph from the lymphatic trunks empties into the veins and becomes part of the blood **plasma**.
- *Lymph nodes* lie along the lymph vessels. They are located in the neck, armpit, chest, abdomen, elbows, groin, and knees. They filter out bacteria and other waste products from the lymph as it moves toward the lymphatic trunks. They also produce **lymphocytes**, which help the body defend itself against microorganisms.
- *Tonsils* are masses of lymph tissue that are exposed to the outside. They filter tissue fluid, not lymph. They may filter so many bacteria that the pathogens overwhelm the tonsil. The tonsils then become infected, and may have to be removed.
- The *spleen* is behind the stomach. It filters microorganisms and waste products from the blood. The spleen makes lymphocytes and **monocytes** to help the body defend itself against microorganisms. The spleen also stores red blood cells and destroys worn-out red blood cells.
- The *thymus* is in front of the aorta and behind the upper part of the sternum. It is lymphatic tissue that stores lymphocytes that work with the lymphatic system to defend the body. Most of this work is done during childhood; later, it is replaced by fat. The *lacteals* pick up digested fats from the small intestine.
- The *cisterna chyli* stores purified lymph before it empties into the bloodstream.
- *Thoracic* duct is the common trunk of all lymphatic vessels in the body except those on the upper-right side of the body.
- *Right lymphatic* duct is the vessel that carries lymph from the right side of the head, neck, thorax, lung, upper-right limb, right side of the heart, and the diaphragmatic surface of the liver.

plasma
(PLAZ muh)
Watery, colorless fluid containing leukocytes, erythrocytes, and platelets.

lymphocyte
(LIM fo sites)
Type of white blood cell.

monocytes
(MAWN o sites)
Large single-nucleus white blood cells.

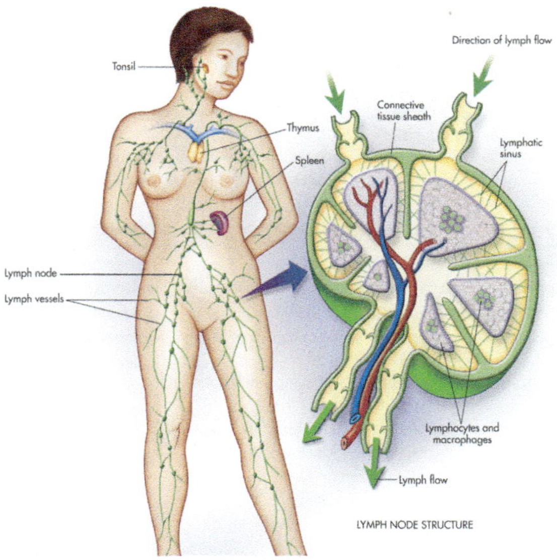

Figure 13.23
What do lymph nodes do?

Your Body and How It Functions | Chapter 13 335

Teaching Tips

- Explain the function of the lymphatic system vessels and organs:
  - Lymph capillaries: tubes that reach into spaces between tissues to remove lymph
  - Lymph vessels: move lymph from tissues to the lymphatic trunks
  - Lymph nodes: filter bacteria and waste from lymph; produce lymphocytes
  - Spleen: filters microorganisms and waste products from blood; makes lymphocytes and monocytes; stores red blood cells; destroys worn-out red blood cells
  - Tonsils: lymph tissues; filter tissue fluid, not lymph
  - Thymus: lymphatic tissue stores lymphocytes
  - Thoracic duct: common duct for all lymphatic vessels except those on the upper-right side of the body
  - Right lymphatic duct: carries lymph from right side of head, neck, thorax, lung, upper-right limb, right side of heart, and diaphragmatic surface of liver
  - Cisterna chili: stores purified lymph
- Explain that the lymphatic system helps the body remove potentially harmful substances, such as microorganisms and other foreign bodies.
- Emphasize that the lymphatic system would not be able to do this on its own; that the immune system is a complicated process that uses chemicals and proteins from other systems.
- Explain the difference between an antigen and an antibody:
  - Antigen: foreign body that causes the immune system to produce antibodies
  - Antibody: substance made by the human body to produce immunity to an antigen
- Have students list the types of immunity and give examples of each type.
- Discuss and differentiate between the types of immunity.

Figure Focus

13.23 What do lymph nodes do?

Answer: Lymph nodes filter out bacteria and other waste products from lymph. They also produce lymphocytes.

Apply It

- This activity is appropriate for small groups, with one student acting as the patient, and two or three others as a health care team tracking the infection.
- You may want to assign each team a particular location for the wound.
- Emphasize that the goal is to track the infection from the wound to either the thoracic duct or the right lymphatic duct.

Teaching Tips

- Discuss types of immunity.
- Differentiate between specific and nonspecific immunity.
- Differentiate between active and passive immunity.
- Explain immune response, and discuss symptoms that indicate the immune response system is working:
  - Fever
  - Pus
  - Inflammation

TEAMWORK

In small groups, prepare a skit demonstrating a common disorder of the lymphatic system. One student should be a patient, describing symptoms to a health care worker or a team of health care workers. The health care workers should diagnose the disorder, explain it, and prescribe a treatment.

ACTIVITY

Divide the class into four immunity groups: nonspecific, specific, active, and passive. Have each group create a detailed list of aspects of their type of immunity. Then, as a class, have the groups take turns explaining various aspects of their types of immunity so that everyone can compare and contrast the types of immunity.

antigen
(ANN tuh jin)
Foreign matter that causes the body to produce antibodies.

antibodies
(ANN tuh bah dees)
Substances made by the body to produce immunity to an antigen.

phagocytes
(FAY go sites)
Cells that surround, ingest, and digest microorganisms and cellular waste.

active immunity
(AK tiv im YOO ni tee)
Protection that occurs when a body produces its own antibodies.

passive immunity
(PASS iv im YOO ni tee)
Protection that occurs when a body receives antibodies from another source.

parasitic
(pare uh SIT ik)
Pertaining to an organism that lives in or on another organism, taking nourishment from it.

The Lymphatic System and Immunity

The lymphatic system helps the body remove substances that are harmful. These substances may be microorganisms or other foreign bodies. The foreign body is called an **antigen**. Examples of antigens are poisons, splinters, and microorganisms. When these enter the body, the body responds by producing **antibodies**. The antibodies attack the antigen. This process is called the *immune response*.

Immune Response

The immune system has many specialized cells. Two types of white blood cells are lymphocytes and **phagocytes**. Phagocytes circulate through the body and ingest diseased and dead cells. Other types of white cells surround foreign bodies and destroy them. All of the white blood cells are important in protecting the body. Some things that tell you that the immune system is working are fever, inflammation, and pus. When these are present, you know that the immune system is responding to protect the body.

Types of Immunity

Nonspecific immunity protects the body, in general, against antigens that can cause infection. The body's nonspecific defenses include intact skin, moist mucous membranes, cilia, saliva, tears, and stomach acids. These defenses work to protect the body against a range of antigens. Specific immunity, however, protects the body against specifically identified antigens, including bacteria, fungi, and viruses.

There are two types of immunity: active and passive. When the body produces its own antibodies, **active immunity** occurs. The first time there is contact with an antigen, the slow process of antibody formation begins. Then, when exposure to the antigen happens again, the combination of antibodies and memory cells specific to that antibody quickly produce even more antibodies. This is natural active immunity. Vaccinations are an artificial means of producing active immunity. When the body receives antibodies from a source outside of itself, **passive immunity** occurs. Antibodies that a baby receives from its mother's breast milk is an example of passive immunity.

MEDICAL TERMINOLOGY

asplenia:	absence of a spleen	**splenectomy:**	surgical removal of the spleen
lymphadenectomy:	surgical removal of the lymph nodes	**splenitis:**	inflammation of the spleen
lymphadenopathy:	enlargement of the lymph nodes	**splenomegaly:**	abnormal enlargement of the spleen
lymphocytopenia:	an abnormally low number of lymphocytes in the blood	**splenorrhexis:**	rupture of the spleen
		splenotomy:	incision into the spleen
lymphocytosis:	abnormally high number of lymphocytes in the blood	**thymectomy:**	surgical removal of the thymus gland
		thymitis:	inflammation of the thymus gland
lymphoma:	tumor made up of lymphatic tissue		
lymphosarcoma:	cancer in the lymphatic tissue		

336 Chapter 13 | Your Body and How It Functions

MEDICAL TERMINOLOGY

Review the terminology:

- Pronounce each word element, and have students repeat.
- Pronounce each medical term, and have students repeat.
- Allow time for students to write down definitions.
- Select a student to read each definition.
- Assign students to memorize the terms and their definitions.

Common Disorders of the Lymphatic System

Table 13.7 Common Disorders, Symptoms, and Preventive Measures/Treatment of the Lymphatic System

Condition	Disorder	Symptoms	Preventive Measures/ Treatment
AIDS (Acquired Immune Deficiency Syndrome)	A collection of symptoms and infections resulting from specific damage to the immune system caused by the human immunodeficiency virus (HIV).	Conditions that do not normally develop in individuals with healthy immune systems, such as infections caused by bacteria, viruses, fungi and parasites. Includes infections, fevers, swollen glands, weakness, chills and weight loss. Affects nearly every organ.	No vaccine or cure for AIDS or HIV. Prevention based on avoiding exposure to the virus. Highly active antiretroviral therapy (HAART) can minimize some symptoms for a while.
Allergies	A misguided reaction by the immune system in response to bodily contact with certain foreign substances, called allergens. These substances are usually harmless and remain so to nonallergic people.	Symptoms vary; can be irritation of the eyes or nose, rash, sneezing, redness, or abdominal pain, diarrhea, or vomiting. Can be as severe as asthma. Insect stings, antibiotics, and certain medicines produce a systemic allergic response that is also called anaphylaxis, a system-wide reaction. (See below.)	Allergy tests to identify allergens. Avoidance or reducing exposure to allergen. Desensitization treatments can reduce reactions. Several antagonistic drugs are used to block the action of allergens or to prevent activation of cells processes, including antihistamines, cortisone, adrenaline, etc.
Anaphylactic Shock	Widespread and very serious allergic reaction.	Dizziness, loss of consciousness, labored breathing, swelling of the tongue and breathing tubes, blueness of the skin, low blood pressure, heart failure, and death.	Immediate emergency treatment is required, usually dose of epinephrine; administration of antivenom in the case of bee or wasp stings.
Elephantiasis	Caused by a **parasitic** thread-like worm, common in tropical and subtropical regions. The worm enters the body from a host bite, usually a mosquito or other insect.	Worm blocks the lymphatic vessels and causes edema and swelling.	Employing mosquito control is the most effective prevention. Treat following infection with medication.
Hodgkin's Disease: Classical cases (95%) Nodular cases (5%)	A malignant disorder characterized by painless, progressive enlargement of lymph nodes. The nodular lymphocyte is most common in young men.	Enlarged lymph nodes, weight loss, low-grade fever, night sweats, anemia, lekocytosis, and skin irritation.	Employing radiation and drug therapy treatments. Cause unknown.
Lupus	Autoimmune disorder that results when the body's own system attacks its tissues and systems; most often affects joints, skin, kidneys, blood cells, brain, heart, and lungs.	Facial rash shaped like a butterfly across the cheeks, fatigue, fever, skin lesions, whiteness or blueness of fingers and toes when exposed to cold or stress, shortness of breath; symptoms vary for every person; difficult to diagnose.	Treatment depends on the symptoms; flare-ups may occur and then subside; nonsteroidal anti-inflammatory drugs; steroids; biologic medications; regular exercise and healthy diet; avoid sun and cold exposure.
Lymphadenitis	Inflammation of the lymph nodes, which may be caused from a variety sources.	Lymph nodes become enlarged, hard, smooth or irregular, red, and may feel hot to the touch.	Using drug therapy treatment.
Mononucleosis/ Epstein-Barr Syndrome (Mono)	Contagious viral infection common in teenagers and young adults caused by the Epstein-Barr virus.	Extreme fatigue, fever, sore throat, head and body aches, swollen lymph nodes, swollen liver and spleen, rash.	Do not share drinks, food, or personal items (e.g., toothbrushes) with infected people; drink fluids, rest, use over-the-counter pain and fever medications; avoid contact sports until fully recovered to protect the enlarged spleen.
Tonsillitis	Infection of the tonsils, frequently caused by streptococcus.	Severe sore throat, fever, headache, malaise, difficulty in swallowing, earache, and enlarged, tender lymph nodes in the neck.	Treating with antibiotics and surgery if infections frequently reoccur.

Your Body and How It Functions | Chapter 13 337

Teaching Tips

- Review Table 13.7 together.
- Pronounce the name of each condition out loud:
  - AIDS—Acquired Immune Deficiency Syndrome
  - Allergies
  - Anaphylactic shock
  - Elephantiasis
  - Hodgkin's Disease (Classical and Nodular)
  - Lymphadenitis
  - Tonsillitis
- Ask a student to read the description of each disorder.
- Discuss the symptoms of each.
- Discuss the preventive measures and/or treatments of each.

ACTIVITY

Make flashcards for the terms associated with the lymphatic system. Use the flashcards to study and memorize the terms and their definitions.

Teaching Tips

- Begin a discussion about the jobs and professions that would be suitable for someone interested in the lymphatic system.
- Remind students to refer to Chapter 3 for more information on occupations.
- Discuss the skills and requirements for becoming an immunologist.
- You may want to point out the difference between an M.D. and a Ph.D. degree.
- Discuss the skills and requirements for becoming an immunology technologist.
- Point out that the aging process affects immunity.
- Discuss immune-related disorders that may affect older people, including slower wound healing, decreased ability to fight disease, autoimmune disorders, and cancer.
- You may want to discuss current research in immunology, and what scientists and researchers are working on the field.

Immunity and Aging

As the body ages, the function of its immune cells decreases. The effect is decreased ability to fight off infection, so the risk of sickness is greater. Immunizations, such as flu shots, may not be as effective, and the protection that is received may not last as long as expected. There also is an increase in some types of cancers because the immune system gradually loses its ability to detect cell defects, as well as correct those defects.

Another area of immunity affected by aging is the body's tolerance of its own cells—an autoimmune disorder occurs when immune cells mistakenly attack organs or tissues when nothing is wrong with them. Often a sign of infection, inflammation can also be an autoimmune response.

Immunotherapy

Immunotherapy is a group of related treatments that use the body's natural immune responses to target and destroy cancer. Patients can be given antibodies that bind the tumor and help the immune system recognize it, enhanced levels of their own white blood cells that have been selected for their ability to attack the tumor and cloned, and even specially engineered white blood cells. These new techniques are creating breakthroughs in cancer treatment and sparing patients from the debilitating side of effects of older chemotherapeutics.

Related Jobs and Professions

Immunologist

An immunologist is someone who studies and/or treats the immune system. An immunologist may be a research scientist who works in a laboratory. The scientist investigates the components needed for a healthy immune system or the diseases that disrupt the immune system.

An immunologist can also be a doctor who treats people with immune system disorders including allergies or autoimmune disease. Some immunologists perform both duties and combine research with patient care.

Immunologists who conduct independent research usually have an advanced degree such as a Ph.D. or M.D., although some jobs only require a master's degree. Training must include a combination of coursework, laboratory research, and a thesis or dissertation, followed by two to four years in a postdoctoral training fellowship. Physicians who work as immunologists typically go to medical school, complete a residency in internal medicine, pediatrics, or a medicine-pediatrics program, and then spend two more years specializing in allergies/immunology.

Immunology Technologist

Immunology technologists study the human immune system and how it responds to foreign invaders. They strive to diagnose, treat, and prevent infections by studying the organisms that cause disease and how they attack the immune system. This work is done under the supervision of an immunologist or a physician. Because of the nature of their work, they often work with other scientists, including chemists, pathologists, geologists, and civil engineers.

Immunology technologists work in a variety of academic and health-related centers. Some work for hospitals; others are employed by research facilities or diagnostic laboratories. People can enter this profession with a B.S. degree in immunology or by completing an immunology technology program at a college or technical institute. Some states require immunology technologists to be licensed.

Summary

The lymphatic system consists of organs and vessels that filter out or destroy antigens and drain excess fluids. In this section, you have learned about disorders of the lymphatic system. These disorders often result in swollen tissues or organs. Therapy with antibiotics or other drugs is often prescribed for lymphatic diseases.

Section 13.5 Review Questions

1. What is the difference between an antigen and an antibody?
2. Which lymph organ filters microorganisms and waste products from the blood?
3. How is the lymphatic system like the circulatory system?
4. What are the symptoms that signal an immune response?
5. What is the cause of AIDS?
6. What is lymphadenitis and what are its symptoms?
7. What does an immunologist do?

338 Chapter 13 | Your Body and How It Functions

ACTIVITY

Select one of the jobs or professions listed in Section 13.5. Create a brochure or pamphlet explaining why the health care worker you selected needs a basic knowledge of the lymphatic system in order to perform his or her job effectively.

Section 13.5 Review Questions

1. Answer: An antigen is foreign matter that causes the body to produce antibodies. Antibodies are substances made by the body to produce immunity to an antigen.
2. Answer: Spleen
3. Answer: The lymphatic system and the circulatory system have structures that are joined together by a capillary system.
4. Answer: Some things that tell you that the immune system is working are fever, inflammation, and pus. When these are present, you know that the immune system is responding to protect the body.
5. Answer: Collection of symptoms and infections resulting from specific damage to the immune system caused by HIV.
6. Answer: Inflammation of the lymph nodes, which may be caused from a variety of sources. Lymph nodes become enlarged, smooth or irregular, red, and may feel hot to the touch.
7. Answer: An immunologist studies and treats the immune system, investigates the components needed for a healthy immune system or the diseases that disrupt the immune system.

The Respiratory System

SECTION 13.6

Background

The respiratory system takes in the oxygen that cells need to remain alive. It also releases waste carbon dioxide and water vapor from the body into the atmosphere. The main organs of the respiratory system are the lungs. Lungs can be damaged by pollutants, such as soot and cigarette smoke. In this section, you will study structures within the lungs and how they function. You will also learn about lifestyle choices that can affect respiratory health.

Objectives

When you have completed this section, you will be able to do the following:

- Match key terms with their correct meanings.
- Label major organs of the respiratory system on a diagram.
- Describe the flow of oxygen through the body.
- Identify common disorders of the respiratory system.
- Describe how the respiratory system supports life.
- Explain why the health care worker's understanding of the respiratory system is important.

Introduction to the Respiratory System

Respiration is breathing. Breathing is necessary to supply life-giving oxygen to each cell in the body and to remove the waste products of each cell. The cell's gaseous waste product is called *carbon dioxide*.

Oxygen enters the body when air is pulled in through the mouth and nose. This process is called **inspiration/inhalation**. **Expiration/exhalation** occurs when the body forces air out of the lungs. This is the body's way of eliminating the cells' gaseous waste (carbon dioxide).

inspiration/inhalation
(in spur AY shun)/
(in hull AY shun)
Process of breathing in air during respiration.

expiration/exhalation
(ex pur AY shun)/
(ex hull AY shun)
Process of forcing air out of the body during respiration.

resonance
(REZ uh nuhns)
The quality of the sound (deep, full, vibrant, etc.).

Structure of the Respiratory System

See Figure 13.24 and Table 13.8.

- The *nasal cavity* (nose) is where air enters the body. The nasal cavity is the preferred passage for air to enter the body. The nasal lining helps stop dust particles and pathogens. If dust and pathogens enter the lungs, the chance for infection is increased.
- *Paranasal sinuses* are mucus-lined cavities in the bones of the face, connected by passageways to the nose, which help to warm and moisten inhaled air. The sinuses also provide **resonance** to the voice. When drainage from the sinuses is blocked, as after a cold, they can become infected (a condition called sinusitis).

Your Body and How It Functions | Chapter 13 339

FOCUS AND ENGAGE

Introduce the Section

a. Review the content of the Background paragraph, explaining that the main organs of the respiratory system are the lungs.

b. Emphasize that the respiratory system enables the body to take in oxygen, which is vital for keeping cells alive.

c. Review the objectives for the section.

Vocabulary Review

a. Direct students to the key terms.

b. Pronounce each word, and have the students repeat the pronunciation out loud.

c. Discuss the definition of each word.

TEACH

Discuss

- Ask students to take a deep breath in, and then let it out.
- Explain that breathing takes in oxygen and gives off carbon dioxide and other waste products.
- Remind students that breathing is vital to life.
- Discuss what happens to the body when it cannot take in oxygen.

Reinforce and Review

- Review the information in Section 13.1: cells, tissues, organs, cavities, and body directions.

Teaching Tips

- Review the process of inspiration/inhalation and expiration/exhalation.

TEAMWORK

In groups of three, use a stopwatch to time how many breaths per minute your partners take at different stages of exercise. One person is the breather, one the timer, and one the counter. Make a table to record the results. For example, time each other when sitting still, after walking around the room, and after walking up two flights of stairs. After collecting the data, display it in a graph or chart. Discuss the results with the class.

Teaching Tips

- Describe the major organs of the respiratory system:
  - Nasal cavity (nose): where air enters
  - Paranasal sinuses: mucus-lined cavities connected to nose
  - Oral cavity (mouth): alternative to nasal cavity where air enters
  - Pharynx (throat): passageway from nose and mouth
  - Epiglottis: flap that closes when food or water is swallowed
  - Larynx (voice box): pouch that creates voice sounds
  - Trachea (windpipe): passageway between pharynx and lungs
  - Bronchi: air passageways connected to the trachea
  - Bronchioles: smallest subdivisions of the bronchi
  - Alveoli: air sacs at the end of each bronchiole
  - Diaphragm: muscular wall divides chest cavity from abdominal cavity

Figure Focus

13.24 Respiratory system. What is the main function of the trachea?

Answer: The trachea is the passageway between the pharynx and lungs.

Figure 13.24
Respiratory system. What is the main function of the trachea?

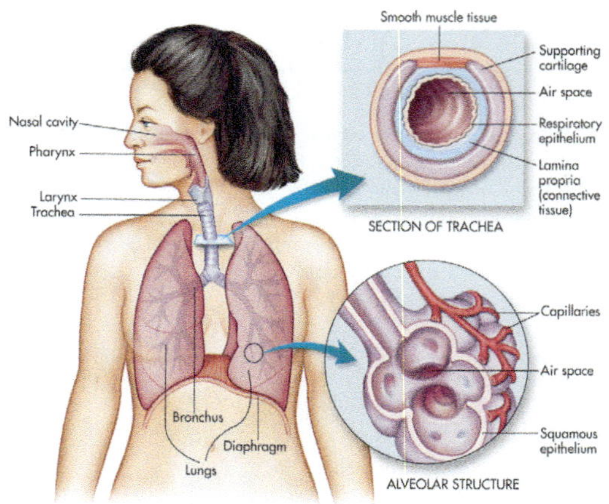

- The *oral cavity* (mouth) is where air enters the body when the nasal passage is blocked or when a person breathes through the mouth.
- The *pharynx* (throat) is the passageway that air enters after leaving the nose and mouth.
- The *epiglottis* is a flap that closes when food or water is swallowed. When it closes, it covers the opening of the trachea that leads to the lungs. This prevents food and water from entering the lungs.
- The *larynx* (voice box) is located just below the epiglottis. It is a **pouch** containing a cordlike framework that creates voice sounds. As air crosses the larynx, sound is created.
- The *trachea* (windpipe) is the passageway between the pharynx and lungs.
- The *bronchi* are air passageways that connect to the trachea. The trachea divides into two main branches, the bronchial tubes that lead into the right and left lungs. The bronchial tubes are lined with hairlike objects called **cilia**. The cilia help move mucus, which catches dust and pathogens, up and out of the lungs.
- The *bronchioles* are the smallest subdivisions of the bronchi.
- The *alveoli* (air sacs) are at the end of each bronchiole. The alveoli are covered with capillaries that absorb oxygen into the blood. Carbon dioxide is forced out of the blood into the alveoli (carbon dioxide and oxygen exchange). Once the carbon dioxide has been released into the alveoli, it can be exhaled from the body.
- The *diaphragm* is the muscular wall that divides the chest cavity from the abdominal cavity. To begin inspiration, the diaphragm moves down, creating a vacuum that pulls air into the lungs. When the diaphragm relaxes and moves upward again, air is exhaled (forced out) from the lungs.

pouch
(POWCH)
Small bag or sac.

cilia
(SYL ee ah)
Hairlike projections that move rhythmically.

340 Chapter 13 | Your Body and How It Functions

TEAMWORK

In groups of 11, prepare 11 cards by writing one stage of the flow of air through the body on each card (refer to Table 13.8 on the next page). Shuffle the cards and then distribute them face down to the team members. At the instructor's command, look at the cards and then arrange the team members into the correct order of the flow of air. The first team to be correctly aligned wins.

Table 13.8 Flow of Oxygen Through the Body

Oxygen enters the body
↓
Nose or mouth
↓
Pharynx
↓
Epiglottis
↓
Larynx
↓
Trachea
↓
Bronchi
↓
Bronchioles
↓
Alveoli (oxygen and carbon dioxide exchange)
↓
Circulatory system
↓
Cell (oxygen and carbon dioxide exchange)

Community

In a team of four, prepare a clinic on how smoking affects the different body systems and present the clinic to a class of middle school students.

Common Disorders of the Respiratory System

Table 13.9 Common Disorders, Symptoms, and Preventive Measures/Treatment of the Respiratory System

Condition	Disorder	Symptoms	Preventive Measures/ Treatment
Asthma	The bronchial tube walls spasm, narrowing the passageways. With the passageways narrowed, it is difficult to exhale.	A suffocating feeling, breathing is difficult, anxiety can easily occur.	Treating with medication helps reduce the swelling in the bronchial tubes and allows air to move easily through the respiratory system. People with asthma should carry their medication with them at all times.
COPD (Chronic obstructive pulmonary disease)	Refers to any of several pulmonary diseases, especially emphysema, in which chronic airway obstruction causes respiratory abnormalities, including shortness of breath.	Shortness of breath, wheezing, decreased exercise tolerance, cough.	Stop smoking. Treatment includes use of inhalers, antibiotic drugs or steroids, and oxygen. Surgery to remove parts of the diseased lung, lung rehabilitation programs, or lung transplants.
Common cold (also known as a viral respiratory tract infection)	A contagious illness that can be caused by a number of different types of viruses.	May feel tired and achy. Nasal stuffiness and drainage, sore throat, hoarseness, cough, and sometimes fever and headache.	Hand washing minimizes spread of colds. No cure. Treatments to minimize specific symptoms include antihistamines, decongestants, and acetaminophen or ibuprofen.

(continued)

Teaching Tips

- Review Table 13.8 together as a class.
- Review the flow of air through the respiratory system.
- Review the first part of Table 13.9 together.
- Pronounce the name of each condition out loud:
  - Asthma
  - COPD (Chronic obstructive pulmonary disease)
  - Common cold
- Ask a student to read the description of each disorder.
- Discuss the symptoms of each.

Community

- This activity is appropriate for small groups.
- You may want to provide class time for students to research and organize the project, or assign it as homework.
- Remind students that the presentation should be appropriate for a middle school class.
- Contact middle school teachers to arrange for your students to visit and present the project.
- They may also be able to present to an after-school program.

TEAMWORK

In small groups, prepare a skit demonstrating a common disorder of the respiratory system. One student should be a patient, describing symptoms to a health care worker or a team of health care workers. The health care workers should diagnose the disorder, explain it, and prescribe a treatment.

Teaching Tips

- Review the second part of Table 13.9 together.
- Pronounce the name of each condition out loud:
  - Emphysema
  - Lung cancer
  - Pneumonia
  - Tuberculosis
  - Upper respiratory infection (URI)
- Ask a student to read the description of each disorder.
- Discuss the symptoms of each.

ACTIVITY

The common disorders of the respiratory system in Table 13.9 are listed in alphabetical order. Create a table that lists them in order of risk. Put the most life-threatening at the top, and the least life-threatening at the bottom. Include the reason you placed the condition where you did.

Table 13.9 Common Disorders, Symptoms, and Preventive Measures/Treatment of the Respiratory System (continued)

Condition	Disorder	Symptoms	Preventive Measures/ Treatment
Emphysema	Progressive disease can result in disability, and, in severe cases, heart or respiratory failure and death. The alveoli become stretched out and are not able to push the carbon dioxide and other **pollutants** out of the lungs. Can be caused from smoking, frequent, untreated respiratory infections, asthma, or abnormal stress on the lungs.	Anxiety, shortness of breath, difficulty breathing, cough, cyanosis, unequal chest expansion, rapid heartbeat, and elevated body temperature.	Achieving a balanced lifestyle that includes adequate rest, a balanced diet, and not smoking helps keep the lungs clean and able to function normally. Treatments include: use of medications, use of oxygen, possible lung transplant.
Influenza	Viral infection of the respiratory system; commonly called "the flu."	Aching muscles and joints, fever, chills, headache, cough, fatigue, and nasal congestion.	Annual influenza vaccination; rest, fluids, fever-reducing medications; antiviral medications may be prescribed.
Lung cancer	**Malignant** tissue in the lungs that destroy tissue. Approximately 75% of cases are due to smoking.	Persistent cough, difficulty breathing, purulent or blood-streaked sputum, chest pain, frequent bronchitis and/or pneumonia.	Treating with radiation and chemical therapy. Surgery may also be an option.
Pneumonia	Inflammation of the lungs, usually caused by bacteria, viruses, or an irritation by chemicals.	Chills and fever, headache, cough, and chest pain.	Treating with antibiotic (if bacterial) and respiratory therapies.
Tuberculosis	Infectious disease caused by the tubercle bacillus. This bacillus is difficult to destroy. The tubercle bacillus can be carried on air currents and dust particles for a long time. When they are inhaled into the respiratory system, the bacillus may become active and destroy tissue.	Listlessness, vague chest pain, decreased appetite, fever, night sweats, and weight loss are early symptoms. Tubercle bacillus most often infects the lungs, but it can also infect other organs of the body.	Treating the bacillus to become inactive keeps it from multiplying and from doing more damage to tissue. It is important for people with tuberculosis to always take their medication. If they stop taking it the bacillus may become active again. A major health risk today is a resistant strain of tuberculosis that does not become inactive with current treatments.
Upper respiratory infection (URI)	Infection of the trachea, larynx, throat, or nose.	Sore throat, congestion of the sinuses, nose, and eye with a fever and tiredness.	Getting adequate rest and eating a balanced diet help prevent infections. Handwashing and covering mouth with sleeved arm when coughing or sneezing can help prevent spread of infection. Infections caused by a virus usually improve after 10–12 days. Bacterial infections may require antibiotics.

pollutants
(puh LEW tents)
Things that contaminate (e.g., smoke, smog).

malignant
(mah LIG nent)
Cancerous.

342 Chapter 13 | Your Body and How It Functions

CUSTOMIZED INSTRUCTION

Less Advanced Students

Try different activities to help less advanced students learn the stages of the flow of air through the body. They might benefit from drawing a flowchart or poster. They might have an easier time remembering more common terms, such as throat for pharynx, voice box for larynx, and wind pipe for trachea. They might benefit from flashcards to use as study aids.

Personal Wellness

The Dangers of Smoking

One of the best ways to protect your health and prevent disease is not to smoke. According to the Centers for Disease Control, smoking causes harm to almost every organ in the body. One out of every five deaths in the U.S. each year is related to smoking.

You might know that smoking causes lung cancer, emphysema, and other respiratory diseases. You might not know that smoking can also cause many other cancers, including cancers of the mouth, larynx, pharynx, esophagus, bladder, kidney, pancreas, cervix, and stomach. Smoking also puts people at a higher risk for coronary heart disease and stroke.

Women who smoke when they are pregnant can damage the health of their fetus. Older women who smoke are more at risk for osteoporosis.

If you don't smoke, you should never start. Cigarettes are highly addictive, so it is difficult to quit smoking. If you smoke now, you should quit. Many health insurance companies have programs that can help smokers to quit. There are also many resources on the Internet to help smokers to become nonsmokers.

What diseases can be caused by smoking?

MEDICAL TERMINOLOGY

apnea:	absence of breathing	**pneumonolysis:**	breakdown of lung tissue
bronchiectasis:	dilation of the bronchi	**pneumothoracic:**	pertaining to the lungs and chest
bronchitis:	inflammation of the bronchial tubes	**pulmonary edema:**	fluid, swelling of the lungs
dyspnea:	difficult or painful breathing	**rales:**	rattling or bubbling sounds in the chest
EENT:	abbreviation for "eyes, ears, nose, throat"	**rhinoplasty:**	plastic repair of the nose
epistaxis:	nosebleed	**rhinorrhea:**	running nose
hypoxia:	lack of oxygen	**sublingual:**	beneath the tongue
intercostal:	between the ribs	**tachypnea:**	rapid breathing
laryngitis:	inflammation of the larynx	**thoracotomy:**	incision into the chest
nares:	nostrils	**trachelosis:**	any condition of the neck
pharyngospasm:	spasmodic contraction of the pharynx	**tracheostomy:**	opening into the trachea
pleurocentesis:	surgical puncture of the pleura	**URI:**	abbreviation for upper respiratory infection

Your Body and How It Functions | Chapter 13 343

Personal Wellness—The Dangers of Smoking

- Review the reasons for not smoking.
- It is likely some students in the class do smoke.
- It is also likely that they know it is not good for them.
- You may want to ask if any are willing to discuss why they started smoking, and why they do not quit.
- Try not to be judgmental. Present the information in a non-confrontational way, so they do not feel that they must be on the defensive.
- Provide links to Web sites with more information such as kidshealth.org, youngwomenshealth.org, or cancer.org.

What diseases can be caused by smoking?

Answer: Lung cancer and many other cancers, emphysema and other respiratory diseases, coronary heart disease, stroke, osteoporosis, and diseases that affect newborns

MEDICAL TERMINOLOGY

Review the terminology:

- Pronounce each word element, and have students repeat.
- Pronounce each term, and have students repeat.
- Allow time for students to write down definitions.
- Select a student to read each definition.
- Assign students to memorize the terms and their definitions.

ACTIVITY

Create an antismoking poster. Display the posters in an area of your school where most students will see it, such as the cafeteria or entry way.

Figure Focus

13.25 What skills and interests do you think might be necessary to become a pulmonologist?

Student answers will vary.

Teaching Tips

- Begin a discussion about the jobs and professions that would be suitable for someone interested in the respiratory system.
- Remind students to refer to Chapter 3 for more information on occupations.
- Discuss the skills and requirements for becoming a pulmonologist.
- Remind students of what a subspecialty is.
- Discuss the skills and requirements for becoming a respiratory therapist.
- You may want to discuss some of the types of respiratory therapy, such as:
  - Administration of oxygen
  - Cardiopulmonary resuscitation (CPR)
  - Management of mechanical ventilators
  - Administering drugs to the lungs
  - Monitoring cardiopulmonary systems
  - Measuring lung function
- Discuss the skills and requirements for becoming a thoracic surgeon.

Related Jobs and Professions

Pulmonologist

Figure 13.25
What skills and interests do you think might be necessary to become a pulmonologist?

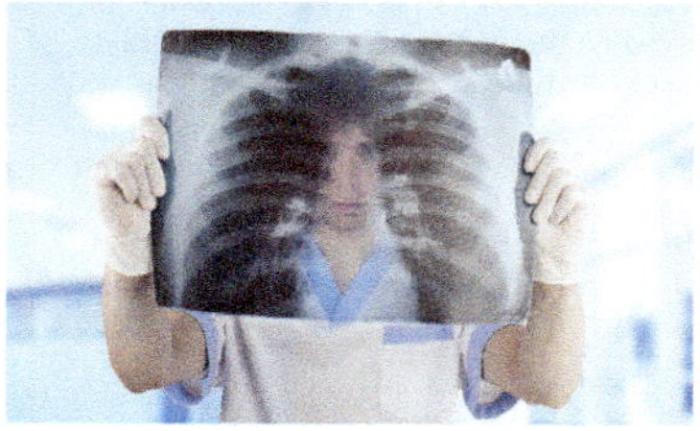

Pulmonologists are physicians who are specially trained to treat diseases and conditions of the chest. (Figure 13.25) These conditions, which affect the lungs and bronchial tubes, include such things as pneumonia, asthma, tuberculosis, and emphysema. Pulmonologists do not perform major surgical procedures, but they do often obtain samples from the lining of a lung or the chest wall for diagnostic testing.

Pulmonology is a subspecialty of internal medicine. This means that in order to become a pulmonologist, you must first become certified in internal medicine. It takes at least seven years to accomplish this. Once this is completed, you must continue your studies for two or three more years focusing on conditions specifically related to the respiratory system.

Respiratory Therapist

Respiratory therapists work with patients who have breathing or other cardiopulmonary disorders. Working under the direction of a physician, these specialists evaluate, treat, and care for patients and are primarily responsible for all respiratory care therapeutic treatments and diagnostic procedures. They also supervise respiratory care technicians, who perform many of these same functions.

Respiratory therapists work with a variety of patients. They may work with premature babies whose lungs are not fully developed. They may also work with elderly patients whose lungs are diseased.

Many respiratory therapists work in hospitals. Some work for home health care agencies and travel to patients' homes. Many programs at colleges, universities, medical schools, and vocational/technical schools offer programs in respiratory therapy.

Some programs offer associate's degrees, which would prepare you for an entry-level position. Others offer bachelor's degrees, which would prepare you for an advanced position in this field. Graduates must then pass a test and become either a Registered Respiratory Therapist or a Certified Respiratory Therapist.

Thoracic Surgeon

A thoracic surgeon is a surgeon who specializes in conditions affecting organs in the chest. Some surgeons specialize in the lungs and esophagus. They are general thoracic surgeons. Others also care for the heart and major blood vessels. They are known as cardiothoracic surgeons. Using minimally invasive procedures, thoracic surgeons perform heart bypass operations and heart and lung transplants. They also remove cancerous tumors. Thoracic surgeons treat patients during and after surgery, as well as while they are in critical care.

Thoracic surgeons attend medical school and then complete five years in a general surgery residency and at least two years in a residency focusing on thoracic surgery.

344 Chapter 13 | Your Body and How It Functions

Pulmonary Technician

Pulmonary technicians care for patients with lung-related problems. These technicians conduct pulmonary function tests, provide respiratory-related care, and treat patients as per a physician's orders. Specific duties include educating patients on medications and the use of oxygen, compiling test results and reviewing those results with physicians, helping physicians change tracheostomy tubing, and maintaining pulmonary function equipment and supplies.

Pulmonary technicians report to a nurse manager, physician, or other appropriate personnel. They typically work in a clinic, hospital, or other facility. This position requires an associate's degree from an accredited respiratory therapy program and certification from the National Board for Respiratory Care.

Oxygen Technician

Oxygen technicians are responsible for understanding the use of the hyperbaric oxygen chamber, used in hyperbaric oxygen therapy (HBOT) programs. They have to check and control the chamber, pneumatic circuits, gas or compressed air reserves, air-compressors, and the rest of the technical parts of the facility. This is a specialized medical treatment in which the patient breathes 100 percent oxygen inside a pressurized chamber.

Commonly known for its use in treating scuba diving complications, modern hyperbaric therapy is also used to treat stubborn non-healing wounds. The therapy quickly delivers high concentrations of oxygen to the bloodstream, which assists in the healing process of wounds and is effective in fighting certain types of infections. These technicians are high-level specialists, needing an official degree with a specialty in Pneumatic Systems, Hyperbaric Technology, or the like.

Otorhinolaryngologist

An otorhinolaryngologist is a physician/surgeon who specializes in head and neck surgery. Common ailments addressed include: head and neck cancer; tumors; sinus and allergic disease; thyroid and parathyroid problems; snoring and sleep apnea; and pediatric ear, nose, and throat issues.

An otorhinolaryngologist might perform open surgery on the salivary or thyroid glands or reconstructive surgery of the head or neck. Other possibilities include microsurgery of the middle ear, sinus surgery, or surgery at the base of the skull. To become an otorhinolaryngologist, you must complete medical school, one year of general surgery residency, and four years of otorhinolaryngology training.

Otologist

An otologist, also known as a neurotologist, is a physician who specializes in conditions affecting the ears. These conditions include problems with balance and dizziness, all types of hearing loss, noises in the ear, facial nerve disorders, persistent infections, congenital malformations of the ear, and tumors of the ear. Trained as a surgeon, an otologist performs surgical procedures such as the repair of eardrum perforations, hearing reconstruction, and tumor removal.

Apply It

Make a lung model using a small plastic cup, a small balloon, a regular size balloon, a straw, and a little play dough.

First puncture a small slit in the bottom of the cup. Insert one piece of a straw cut in half to represent the trachea. Half of the straw piece should be inside the cup, the other half outside the cup.

Put the small balloon around the end of the straw in the cup and secure with a rubber band (represents the lung).

Put play-dough around the slit where you inserted the straw, so no air can escape.

Take the larger balloon and stretch it across the top of the cup to represent the diaphragm.

Gently pull the diaphragm balloon and the lung balloon will inflate. Relax the diaphragm balloon and the lung balloon will deflate. This represents inspiration and expiration.

Your Body and How It Functions | Chapter 13 345

Teaching Tips

- Discuss the skills and requirements for becoming a pulmonary technician.
- Discuss the skills and requirements for becoming an oxygen technician.
- You may want to discuss a hyperbaric chamber. For more information refer to a Web site such as https://www.mayoclinic.org/tests-procedures/hyperbaric-oxygen-therapy/about/pac-20394380.
- Discuss the skills and requirements for becoming an otorhinolaryngologist.
- You might want to discuss why cancers or tumors in the head and neck would fall into the category of respiratory ailments.
- Discuss the skills and requirements for becoming an otologist.

Apply It

- If you choose to conduct this activity in class, have the material ready, or instruct the students to bring them in ahead of time.
- You may want students to work in small groups, or make this a class activity that you do all together.
- Point out that the model will demonstrate inspiration and exhalation.
- After the exercise, discuss whether the model is accurate.

ACTIVITY

Select one of the jobs or professions listed in Section 13.6. Create a brochure or pamphlet explaining why the health care worker you selected needs a basic knowledge of the respiratory system in order to perform his or her job effectively.

To become an otologist, you must attend medical school and then become a trained otorhinolaryngologist. An otorhinolaryngologist, commonly known as an ENT, specializes in problems associated with the ear, nose, throat, and neck. To become an otorhinolaryngologist, you must complete medical school, one year of general surgery residency, and four years of otorhinolaryngology training. To specialize as an otologist, you must complete another residency in that area. All otologists must pass an exam in order to become board certified before practicing medicine.

Summary

In this section, you reviewed the structure and functions of the respiratory system. You learned that the lungs contain a system of branching tubes that get progressively smaller as they get farther away from the trachea. These tubes end in alveoli, or air sacs, that are covered with capillaries. As air flows into the alveoli, the capillaries absorb oxygen and release carbon dioxide.

Oxygen in the capillaries travels to the rest of the body in order to keep cells alive. Some disorders that affect the respiratory system make breathing difficult. This can reduce the amount of oxygen that gets to cells and may cause weakness or death. As a health care worker, you should be familiar with the causes and treatments of respiratory diseases. You should also be aware of the lifestyle choices that can prevent respiratory diseases.

Section 13.6 Review Questions

1. What structure keeps food and water from entering the lungs?
2. Describe the path that air takes as it enters the body.
3. How does the diaphragm help you to breathe?
4. What is asthma and what are the treatments for asthma?
5. Which two respiratory disorders are often caused by smoking?
6. Why would health care professionals need to wear face masks or respirators when treating a patient who has tuberculosis?
7. What are the differences between an otologist and a trained otorhinolaryngologist?

346 Chapter 13 | Your Body and How It Functions

Teaching Tips

- Review the flow of air through the respiratory system.
- Review how the respiratory system supports life:
  - Provide oxygen to cells
  - Provide nutrients and oxygen to tissue of the lungs
- Discuss problems that might arise if the respiratory system cannot function:
  - What if a pulmonary embolism—blood clot—blocks the flow of blood to lung tissue?
  - How might smoking harm the respiratory system?
- Discuss reasons why it is important for all health care workers to have a basic knowledge of the respiratory system and how it functions.
- Ask students to consider why a health care worker should be concerned about the respiratory health of others.
- Discuss the need for health care workers in all positions to use proper medical terminology to communicate with others.
- Discuss the importance of responding appropriately when a medical emergency occurs.

Section 13.6 Review Questions

1. Answer: Epiglottis
2. Answer: Oxygen enters the body; Nose or mouth; Pharynx; Epiglottis; Larynx; Trachea; Bronchi; Bronchioles; Alveoli (oxygen and carbon dioxide exchange); Circulatory system; Cell (oxygen and carbon dioxide exchange)
3. Answer: To begin inspiration, the diaphragm moves down, creating a vacuum that pulls air into the lungs. When the diaphragm relaxes and moves upward again, air is exhaled (forced out) from the lungs.
4. Answer: Asthma occurs when the bronchial tube walls spasm narrowing the passageway, making it difficult to breathe. Medication helps reduce the swelling of the bronchial tubes and allows air to flow easily through the respiratory system.
5. Answer: Emphysema and lung cancer
6. Answer: Tuberculosis is carried through the air currents and dust particles and when they are inhaled they may become active and destroy tissue.
7. Answer: An otologist specialized in conditions affecting the ears. An otologist performs surgical procedures such as the repair of eardrum perforations, hearing reconstruction, and tumor removal. To become an otologist, you must attend medical school and then become a trained otorhinolaryngologist. An otorhinolaryngologist, commonly known as an ENT, specializes in problems associated with the ear, nose, throat, and neck. To become an

otorhinolaryngologist, you must complete medical school, one year of general surgery residency, and four years of otorhinolaryngology training. To specialize as an otologist, you must complete another residency in that area. All otologists must pass an exam in order to become board certified before practicing medicine.

The Digestive System

SECTION 13.7

Background

The digestive system breaks down food into nutrients that can be absorbed by the body. It also passes solid wastes out of the body. In this section, you will learn the organs of the digestive system and the diseases that may affect those organs. You will also learn how lifestyle choices can affect digestive system function.

Objectives

When you have completed this section, you will be able to do the following:

- Match key terms with their correct meanings.
- Label a diagram of the digestive system and its accessory organs.
- Explain the functions of the digestive system.
- Recognize the function of organs associated with the digestive system.
- Match common disorders of the digestive system with their descriptions.
- Describe how the digestive system absorbs nutrients.
- Explain why the health care worker's understanding of the digestive system is important.

Introduction to the Digestive System

In this section, we discuss the body's processing of food. This process prepares nutrients so that they can be used by each cell. Body cells cannot absorb nutrients from food. Food must be changed into a substance that the body cells can use. This process of changing food into a usable substance is known as digestion. Once digestion occurs, nutrients move into the bloodstream and waste moves out. This transfer of nutrients into the blood is called **absorption**. Digestion and absorption are the two main functions of the digestive system.

Digestive Organs

The digestive system is a very long muscular tube that begins at the mouth and ends at the **anus**. This tube, called the **alimentary canal**, is made up of many parts (Figure 13.26):

- The *mouth* (oral cavity) is where food enters the body. The digestive process begins with the mechanical breakdown (the chewing, mashing, and grinding of food by the teeth).
- The *salivary glands* are located under the tongue, near the jawbone, and at the back of the throat. The purpose of the salivary glands is to produce a **secretion** that dissolves food and coats food with a mucus that allows it to pass through the esophagus more easily. **Amylase** from salivary glands also breaks down carbohydrates so that chemical digestion can start in the mouth. By the time food leaves the mouth, it is in the form of **bolus**.

absorption
(ab SAWRP shuhn)
Passage of a substance through a body surface into body fluids and tissues (e.g., nutrients from digested food pass through the wall of the small intestine into the blood).

anus
(EY nuhs)
Outlet from which the body expels solid waste.

alimentary canal
(al uh MEN tuh-ree kuh NAL)
Long muscular tube beginning at the mouth and ending at the anus.

secretion
(si KREE shuhn)
Producing and expelling a special substance (e.g., sebaceous glands secrete oil; salivary glands secrete saliva).

amylase
(AM me layz)
An enzyme in saliva and pancreatic juice that breaks down starch into simple sugars.

bolus
(BOW less)
A soft rounded ball, especially of chewed food.

Your Body and How It Functions | Chapter 13 347

Reinforce and Review

- Review the information in Section 13.1: cells, tissues, organs, cavities, and body directions.

ACTIVITY

Have students create a poster or chart that identifies the parts of the digestive system that are also part of the respiratory system. Include the name of the part, its location, and descriptions of the function it serves in each system.

Teaching Tips

- Introduce the digestive system. Explain that:
  - The digestive system begins at the mouth and ends at the anus.
  - The alimentary canal has many parts.
  - Foods must be processed so that nutrients can be used for energy and growth.

FOCUS AND ENGAGE

Introduce the Section

a. Review the content of the Background paragraph, explaining that the digestive system processes nutrients.

b. Emphasize that digestion makes it possible for the body to absorb nutrients and expel waste.

c. Review the objectives for the section.

Vocabulary Review

a. Direct students to the key terms.

b. Pronounce each word, and have the students repeat the pronunciation out loud.

c. Discuss the definition of each word.

TEACH

Discuss

- Point out that food is used to make energy, and ask if students know how food is absorbed into the body.
- Discuss what life would be like if food could be absorbed through the skin.

Teaching Tips

- Discuss the abdominal regions. Refer students to p. 304 to clarify the abdominal cavity in relation to other cavities of the body.
- Describe the organs of the digestive system:
  - Mouth (oral cavity): where food enters the body
  - Salivary glands: produce a secretion that dissolves food
  - Pharynx (throat): passageway for food
  - Epiglottis: flap that covers the trachea when food or water is swallowed
  - Esophagus: receives food and water from pharynx
  - Cardiac sphincter: ring of muscle fibers where the esophagus and stomach join
  - Stomach: enlarged part of alimentary canal that receives food and water from esophagus
  - Pyloric sphincter: ring-like muscle at the far end of the stomach

Figure Focus

13.26 The digestive system is also called the alimentary canal. Where is the gallbladder located?

Answer: Under the ribs on the right-front side of the body

Figure 13.26
The digestive system is also called the alimentary canal. Where is the gallbladder located?

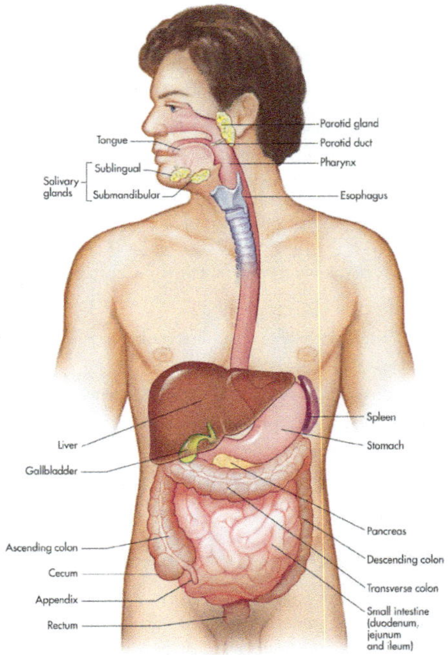

peristalsis
(pear is STALL sus)
Progressive, wavelike motion that occurs involuntarily in hollow tubes of the body.

sphincter
(SVING ter)
Circular muscle that allows the opening and closing of a body part (e.g., anus, pylorus).

chyme
(KIME)
Creamy semifluid mixture of food and digestive juices.

- The *pharynx* (throat) is located at the back of the oral cavity and is a passageway for food.
- The *epiglottis* is a flap that covers the trachea when food or water is swallowed. By covering the trachea, the epiglottis keeps food and water out of the lungs.
- The *esophagus* receives food and water from the pharynx. Food is moved through the esophagus by a rhythmic wavelike motion called **peristalsis**.
- The *cardiac* **sphincter** is a ring of muscle fibers located where the esophagus and stomach join. This muscle keeps stomach contents from moving up into the esophagus.
- The *stomach* is an enlarged part of the alimentary canal that receives food and water from the esophagus. The stomach produces the enzyme, pepsin, which breaks down proteins. The stomach holds food until digestive juices have chemically broken down the food particles into **chyme**. Chyme is a creamy semifluid mixture of food and digestive juices.
- The *pyloric sphincter* is a ringlike muscle found at the far end of the stomach. Its main purpose is to keep food in the stomach long enough to become chyme.

348 Chapter 13 | Your Body and How It Functions

ACTIVITY

Draw a poster illustrating and labeling the parts of the digestive system through which food passes on its way to the stomach.

- The *small intestine* is attached to the stomach at the pyloric sphincter. The small intestine is about 20 feet long. The first 10 to 12 inches of the small intestine are called the *duodenum*. The duodenum receives juices from the pancreas, liver, and gallbladder, which aid in further chemical breakdown of the chyme. This final chemical breakdown is the completion of digestion.
- The small intestine is the portion of the alimentary canal where most absorption takes place. The lining of the small intestine contains many **minute** projections called **villi**. Each villus contains capillaries that absorb nutrients from the food we eat. (**Figure 13.27**) Those food substances that are not absorbed are moved through the 20 feet of the small intestine by peristalsis to the large intestine.
- The *large intestine* is attached to the small intestine and receives food substances that are of little value to the body. The large intestine absorbs water, mineral salts, and vitamins. It secretes (discharges) mucus to aid in the movement of **feces** through the intestine.
- The *rectum*, part of the large intestine, is the last 6 to 8 inches of the alimentary canal. It serves as a storage area for feces.
- The *anus*, also part of the large intestine, is the end of the alimentary canal. It is where fecal material is **evacuated** from the body. Closure of the anus is controlled by the sphincter muscle, a circular muscle that normally maintains constriction of the orifice and which relaxes as required by normal body functioning.

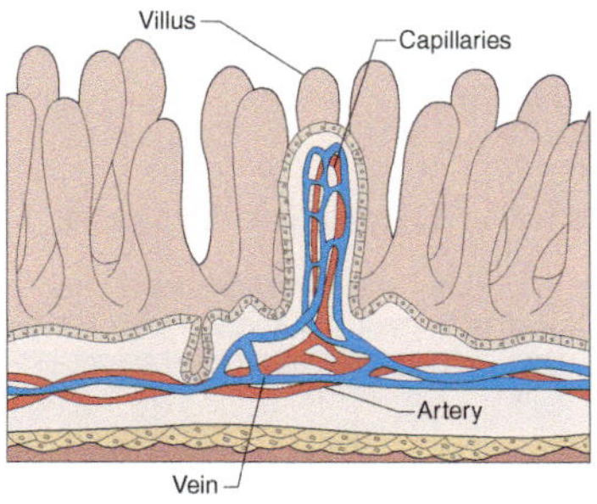

Figure 13.27
Villi in the lining of the small intestine. What function do the capillaries serve in the villi of the small intestine?

minute
(my NEWT)
Exceptionally small.

villi
(VIL eye)
Tiny projections.

feces
(FEE sees)
Solid waste that is evacuated from the body through the anus.

evacuated
(i VAK yoo yet)
Emptied out.

The Accessory Structures

The accessory structures of the digestive system assist in the process of digestion. These structures are the liver, the gallbladder, and the pancreas:

- The *liver*, the largest gland in the body, has many functions. Some of these functions are:
  - Production of bile
  - Removal of poisons that have been absorbed in the small intestines
  - Storage of vitamins
  - Production of heparin, which prevents blood from clotting
  - Production of antibodies, which act against infection and foreign matter

Apply It

Describe what happens after you eat your lunch.

You put food in your mouth. What happens to the food here? Is this chemical or mechanical digestion? Then, what happens in the esophagus? In the stomach? In the small intestine? In the large intestine? Work through each step in the digestive process.

Your Body and How It Functions | Chapter 13 349

Teaching Tips

- Continue reviewing the parts of the alimentary canal:
  - Small intestine: attached to the stomach at the pyloric sphincter
  - Large intestine: receives food substance of little value from the small intestine
  - Rectum: last six to eight inches of the alimentary canal
  - Anus: end of the alimentary canal
- Discuss the accessory structures that are part of the digestive system:
  - Liver
  - Gallbladder
  - Pancreas
- Note that the liver is the largest gland in the body.
- Explain that the liver:
  - Produces bile
  - Removes poisons absorbed by the small intestine
  - Stores vitamins
  - Produces heparin
  - Produces antibodies

Figure Focus

13.27 Villi in the lining of the small intestine. What function do the capillaries serve in the villi of the small intestine?

Answer: They allow the absorption of nutrients from the small intestine into the bloodstream.

Apply It

- This exercise should be done individually.
- You may ask students to write the information in a step-by-step procedure.
- Alternatively, students may create a drawing or presentation that illustrates and explains the process.

Teaching Tips

- Explain the function of organs associated with the digestive system.
- Discuss how the digestive system absorbs nutrients:
  - Food is broken down
  - Nutrients are absorbed
  - Waste is eliminated

MEDICAL TERMINOLOGY

Review the terminology:

- Pronounce each word element, and have students repeat.
- Pronounce each term, and have students repeat.
- Allow time for students to write down definitions.
- Select a student to read each definition.
- Assign students to memorize the terms and their definitions.

Teaching Tips

- Review the first part of Table 13.10 together.
- Pronounce the name of each condition out loud:
  - Cholelithiasis
  - Cirrhosis
  - Colon cancer
- Ask a student to read the description of each disorder.
- Discuss the symptoms of each.

insulin
(IN sel in)
Hormone secreted by the pancreas; essential for maintaining the correct blood sugar level.

- The *gallbladder*, a muscular sac, stores the bile that the liver produces. When chyme reaches the duodenum, the gallbladder squeezes bile into the duodenum to aid in chemical breakdown of the chyme.
- The *pancreas* produces pancreatic juices that also aid in the chemical breakdown of food. It also manufactures **insulin**, which regulates the amount of sugar used by the tissues.

MEDICAL TERMINOLOGY

anorexia:	lack of appetite
antacid:	without acid
buccolingual:	pertaining to the cheek and tongue
cholecyst:	gallbladder
cholelithotomy:	incision for the removal of a gallstone
colitis:	inflammation of the colon
colostomy:	opening into the colon
dysphagia:	difficult or painful swallowing
emesis:	vomiting
emetic:	substance that induces vomiting
enterocele:	hernia involving the intestine
enterocyst:	cyst of the intestinal wall
enterohepatic:	pertaining to the intestines and the liver
gastrointestinal:	GI, pertaining to the stomach and intestines
gastrophrenic:	pertaining to the stomach and diaphragm
gastrosis:	condition affecting the stomach
hepatopathy:	any disease of the liver
hepatoptosis:	liver dropping downward
metabolism:	process by which food is changed into energy for the body's use

Common Disorders of the Digestive System

Table 13.10 Common Disorders, Symptoms, and Preventive Measures/Treatment of the Digestive System and Accessory Structures

Condition	Disorder	Symptoms	Preventive Measures/ Treatment
Appendicitis	Inflammation of the appendix.	Pain in the lower-right abdomen, fever, elevated white blood cell count, nausea/vomiting, abdominal bloating.	Requires immediate medical care; often requires surgical removal of appendix; antibiotics.
Celiac disease	Immune reaction to eating the gluten protein in wheat, rye, and barley; eventually causes damage to the intestine.	Diarrhea, bloating, weight loss, anemia, fatigue, abdominal pain.	Avoidance of any wheat, rye, or barley food products (gluten-free diet); vitamin and mineral supplements; medications to treat intestinal inflammation.
Cholelithiasis *(Accessory Structure)*	Stones in the gallbladder.	Abdominal pain that may radiate toward the back, and heartburn especially after eating.	Eating a low-fat diet. Surgical removal of stones and/or the gallbladder may be necessary.
Cirrhosis *(Accessory Structure)*	Liver cells become damaged, and scarring prevents the liver and other systems from functioning.	Nausea, **flatulence**, decreased appetite, weight loss, clay-colored stools, weakness, and abdominal pain.	Eating a balanced diet rich in protein and vitamins (especially folic acid), getting plenty of rest, and abstaining from alcohol. The liver does have the capacity to regenerate given time and the proper diet.

(continued)

350 Chapter 13 | Your Body and How It Functions

TEAMWORK

Divide the class into teams of 7 to 10. Describe the symptoms of a disorder of the digestive system. Award a point to the first team that can identify the disorder. Award a point to the team that can identify whether it is a disease of the digestive system or the accessory structure. Award a point to the team that can identify the appropriate treatment. The team with the most points at the end of the game wins.

Table 13.10 Common Disorders, Symptoms, and Preventive Measures/Treatment of the Digestive System and Accessory Structures (continued)

Condition	Disorder	Symptoms	Preventive Measures/ Treatment
Colon cancer	Cancer that forms in the tissues of the colon (longest part of the large intestine). Most colon cancers begin in cells that make and release mucus and other fluids.	A change in bowel habits. Rectal bleeding, including bright red or dark blood in your stools or stools that look black. Constant or frequent diarrhea or constipation. Abdominal pain, gas, or bloating. Weight loss and fatigue.	Hard to detect. Use screening tests, such as stool analysis, fecal occult blood tests, or colonoscopy. Treatment includes surgery, chemotherapy, radiation or biotherapy. There are also clinical trials in which a patient can participate.
Constipation *(Digestive System)*	Infrequent, difficult **defecation** of fecal material.	Abdominal pain and cramping, inability to defecate.	Eating a balanced diet with adequate amounts of fruits and vegetables, exercising regularly, and drinking adequate amounts of water help to keep elimination of waste regular. When constipation occurs, medication and/or enemas may be needed.
Crohn's disease	Chronic inflammatory disease of the intestinal tract.	Severe diarrhea, abdominal pain, weight loss, malnutrition, fatigue, blood in the stool.	Medications to manage symptoms; antibiotics; anti-inflammatory medications.
Diarrhea *(Digestive System)*	Abnormal frequent watery stool, usually the symptom of some underlying disorders.	Abdominal cramping that forces frequent defecation and generalized weakness.	Using medication and identifying the condition. It is important to carefully monitor people with diarrhea so they don't become dehydrated, which may cause other serious conditions.
Diverticulitis	Small pouches that bulge outward through the colon, or large intestine, and become inflamed or infected.	Abdominal pain, usually on the left side. If infected, you may also have fever, nausea, vomiting, chills, cramping, and constipation. In serious cases, can lead to bleeding, tears, or blockages.	Treatment focuses on clearing up the infection with antibiotics, resting the colon and preventing future problems, by eating more fiber, drinking lots of fluids, and exercising. Serious cases may require a hospital stay.
Enteritis	Inflammation of the intestines.	Abdominal cramping, **diarrhea**.	See treatment under diarrhea.
Gastric reflux	The backward flow of stomach acid contents into the esophagus.	Heartburn, difficulty swallowing, chest pain.	Lifestyle changes: losing weight, elevating your head, dietary restrictions (avoiding coffee, alcohol, fatty foods, chocolate, and acidic foods). Drug treatment includes antacids, H2 blockers (like Pepcid AC), or proton pump inhibitors (like Prilosec).
Gastric ulcer *(Digestive System)*	Open sore in the stomach.	Pain and sometimes internal bleeding.	Eating a soft bland diet, reducing stress, using medication. When symptoms are not relieved, surgery may be necessary.
Gastritis *(Digestive System)*	Inflammation of the stomach lining. If untreated, it could develop a gastric ulcer.	**Epigastric** pain, indigestion, and burning in the stomach area.	See treatment under gastric ulcer.
Gastroenteritis *(Digestive System)*	Inflammation of the stomach lining and intestines.	Vomiting, abdominal cramping, and diarrhea.	Taking lots of fluids (may be necessary to start an IV to administer fluids if vomiting is excessive) and medication.

(continued)

Your Body and How It Functions | Chapter 13 351

Teaching Tips

- Review the second part of Table 13.10 together.
- Pronounce the name of each condition out loud:
  - Constipation
  - Diarrhea
  - Diverticulitis
  - Enteritis
  - Gastric reflux
  - Gastric ulcer
  - Gastritis
  - Gastroenteritis
  - Hepatitis (accessory structure)
  - Pancreatitis
- Ask a student to read the description of each disorder.
- Discuss the symptoms of each.
- You may want to discuss the types of health care workers who might treat patients with these types of diseases.
- You may want to discuss some of the lifestyle choices that affect the digestive system:
  - Diet
  - Exercise
  - Alcohol consumption

TEAMWORK

In small groups, prepare a skit demonstrating a common disorder of the digestive system. One student should be a patient, describing symptoms to a health care worker or a team of health care workers. The health care workers should diagnose the disorder, explain it, and prescribe a treatment.

Teaching Tips

- Begin a discussion about the jobs and professions that would be suitable for someone interested in the digestive system.
- Remind students to refer to Chapter 3 for more information on occupations.
- Discuss the skills and requirements for becoming a gastroenterologist.
- You may want to discuss endoscopy, and what types of conditions it is used to detect and diagnose.
- Discuss the skills and requirements for becoming a hepatologist.
- Ask students to break the term hepatologist into is word elements.
- Discuss the skills and requirements for becoming a dietician.
- Point out that nutrition is covered in detail in Chapter 16.

ACTIVITY

Write a help wanted ad for one of the jobs or professions listed in Section 13.7. Include the skill and educational requirements, the type of facility where the professional will work, the salary range, and other relevant information.

Table 13.10 Common Disorders, Symptoms, and Preventive Measures/ Treatment of the Digestive System and Accessory Structures (continued)

Condition	Disorder	Symptoms	Preventive Measures/ Treatment
Hepatitis *(Accessory Structure)*	Inflammation of the liver caused by a virus or a poison.	Jaundice, enlarged liver, decreased appetite, abdominal and gastric pain, clay-colored stools, and dark-colored urine.	Eating a balanced diet rich in protein and vitamins (especially folic acid), getting plenty of rest, and abstaining from alcohol. The liver does have the capacity to regenerate given time and the proper diet.
Inguinal hernia	Protrusion of tissue, such as the intestine, through a weak spot in the abdominal muscles, resulting in a bulging when coughing, bending, or heavy lifting.	Bulging in the area of protrusion, burning at the sight of the hernia, pain, heaviness in the groin, swelling.	May require immediate medical attention; wearing a supportive garment (truss) may help; may require surgery to repair weakened abdominal wall and replace protruding tissue into its appropriate location.
Pancreatitis *(Accessory Structure)*	Inflammation of the pancreas caused by an overproduction of its own pancreatic juices.	Severe abdominal pain radiating to the back, fever, loss of appetite, nausea, and vomiting.	Removing any stimulation of the pancreas by removing all stomach contents, IV medication and fluids. Surgery may be necessary.

flatulence
(FLA chu lens)
Excessive gas in the stomach and intestines that causes discomfort.

defecation
(deaf uh KAY shun)
The pushing of solid material from the bowel.

diarrhea
(dahy uh REE uh)
Passage of watery stool at frequent intervals.

epigastric
(ep uh GAS trik)
Pertaining to the area over the pit of the stomach.

jaundice
(JAWN dis)
Yellowing of the whites of the eyes, skin, and mucous membranes.

Related Jobs and Professions

Gastroenterologist

A gastroenterologist is a physician who specializes in the digestive system. A gastroenterologist treats diseases of the gastrointestinal tract, which includes the esophagus, stomach, small intestine, colon and rectum, pancreas, gallbladder, bile ducts, and liver. A gastroenterologist treats conditions including colon polyps, cancer, hepatitis, gastroesophageal reflux (heartburn), and Irritable Bowel Syndrome.

Gastroenterologists are trained in endoscopy, which is the use of narrow, lighted tubes with built-in cameras. By utilizing these instruments, one can see the inside of the intestinal tract.

To become a gastroenterologist, you must complete medical school followed by a three-year residency in internal medicine. Then, you must complete additional specialized training in gastroenterology, which lasts two to three years.

Hepatologist

A hepatologist is a physician who specializes in treatment of the liver. As a hepatologist, you might deal with hepatitis, cirrhosis, genetic or metabolic liver diseases, liver cancer, liver transplants, or metabolic or immunologic issues related to the liver. To become a hepatologist, you must first be trained as a gastroenterologist.

To become a certified gastroenterologist, you must complete college, medical school, a three-year residency in internal medicine, and a two- to three-year fellowship in gastroenterology. To become a hepatologist, you must complete another one-year fellowship in which you will receive both clinical and research training specific to hepatology. Once this training is complete, you must pass an exam to become certified in this field.

Dietician

Dieticians plan food and nutrition programs that help treat or prevent disease. They are often part of a medical team in a hospital, private practice, or other health care facility. Dieticians promote healthy eating habits, evaluate clients' diets, and suggest modifications. Some dieticians specialize in the management of overweight or critically ill patients. (**Figure 13.28**)

Because they help identify and treat health ailments, a detailed knowledge of growth and development, metabolism, and biochemistry of nutrients and food components is required.

To become a registered dietician, you must have at least a bachelor's degree in nutrition or dietetics and complete a 6- to 12-month internship at a health care facility, food service company, or nonprofit agency. You must also pass an exam given by the Commission on Dietetic Registration.

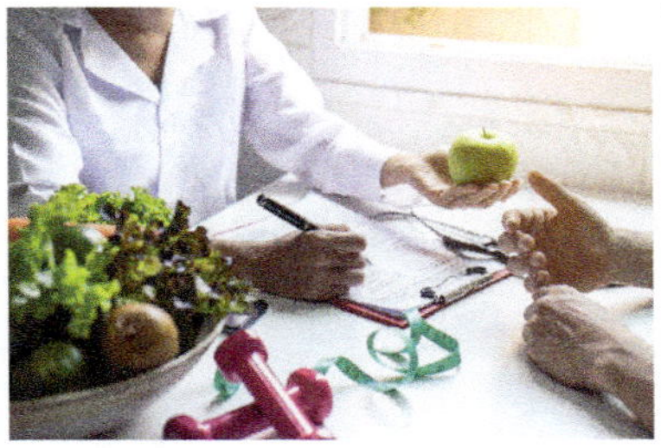

Figure 13.28
What skills and interests do you think might be necessary to become a dietician?

Dietary Aide

A dietary aide prepares and delivers food trays to patients in hospitals or facilities such as nursing homes. Duties may include: reading menu cards to determine which items to place on a tray; placing items on trays; helping the cook prepare food items; preparing foods for soft or liquid diets; pushing a food cart; serving meals to patients; collecting dirty dishes; washing dishes; and recording the amount and type of special foods served to patients. To become a dietary aide, you must have a high school diploma.

Summary

As food travels through the alimentary canal, mechanical and chemical digestion break down the food into nutrients. These nutrients are absorbed by the small intestine. Solid waste materials are excreted through the anus. In this section, you learned about the structure and function of the digestive system. You also learned ways to recognize and treat digestive system disorders. Digestive system disorders often cause abdominal pain. You can often treat these disorders with a low fat or balanced diet or medications.

Section 13.7 Review Questions

1. What is the alimentary canal?
2. What are five functions of the liver?
3. What are the differences in function between the small intestine and the large intestine?
4. What are the accessory structures of the digestive system?
5. What causes hepatitis and what are its symptoms?
6. What does a hepatologist do and what education/training is required?

Section 13.7 Review Questions

1. Answer: The alimentary canal is a long muscular tube beginning at the mouth and ending at the anus.
2. Answer: Production of bile. Removal of poisons that have been absorbed in the small intestines. Storage of vitamins. Production of heparin, which prevents blood from clotting. Production of antibodies, which act against infection and foreign matter.
3. Answer: The small intestine is attached to the stomach at the pyloric sphincter. The first 10 to 12 inches of the small intestine are called the duodenum. The duodenum receives juices from the pancreas, liver, and gallbladder, which aid in further chemical breakdown of the chyme. This final chemical breakdown is the completion of digestion. The large intestine is attached to the small intestine and receives food substances that are of little value to the body. The large intestine absorbs water, mineral salts, and vitamins. It secretes (discharges) mucus to aid in the movement of feces through the intestine.

Teaching Tips

- Discuss the skills and requirements for becoming a dietary aide.
- Review the digestive process and the functions of the digestive organs and accessory structures.
- Discuss reasons why it is important for all health care workers to have a basic knowledge of the digestive system and how it functions.
- Explain that understanding the digestive system alerts you to health problems related to digestion and digestive disease.
- For example, vomit that looks like coffee grinds can indicate internal bleeding.
- Discuss the importance of responding appropriately when a medical emergency occurs.
- Ask students to consider what they would do if a patient were vomiting, depending on the health care position they hold:
  - What if they are a registered nurse?
  - What if they are a nutritionist?
  - What if they are a member of the housekeeping staff?
  - What if they are a receptionist?
  - Does the content of the vomit make a difference in their actions?
  - Does the odor of vomit or feces make a difference?

Figure Focus

13.28 What skills and interests do you think might be necessary to become a dietician?

Student answers will vary.

4. Answers: Liver, gallbladder, and pancreas
5. Answer: Hepatitis is inflammation of the liver caused by a virus or poison. Symptoms include jaundice, enlarged liver, decreased appetite, abdominal pain, clay-colored stool, dark-colored urine.
6. Answer: A hepatologist specializes in the treatment of the liver. To become a hepatologist, you must first be trained as a gastroenterologist. To become a certified gastroenterologist, you must complete college, medical school, a three-year residency in internal medicine, and a two- to three-year fellowship in gastroenterology. To become a hepatologist, you must complete another one-year fellowship in which you will receive both clinical and research training specific to hepatology. Once this training is complete, you must pass an exam to become certified in this field.

TEAMWORK

Divide the class into groups of 7 to 10. Ask each student to write one question about the digestive system on a slip of paper and hand it to you. Ask each group a question, awarding a point for a correct answer and subtracting a point for an incorrect answer. The team with the most points at the end of the game wins.

SECTION 13.8 The Urinary System

Background

The urinary system maintains water balance and flushes liquid wastes out of the body. Urinary system disorders may cause inflammation or obstruction of the organs within the system. As a health care worker, it is important for you to understand the urinary system and to recognize symptoms of urinary system disorders in order to protect patients from organ damage.

Objectives

When you have completed this section, you will be able to do the following:

- Match key terms with their correct meanings.
- Label a diagram of the urinary system.
- Identify the function of organs in the urinary system.
- Match common disorders of the urinary system with their descriptions.
- Describe how the urinary system removes liquid waste and eliminates it from the body.
- Explain why the health care worker's understanding of the urinary system is important.

Introduction to the Urinary System

The urinary system rids the body of liquid waste and assists in the regulation of water and chemical balance. Its functions include:

- The excretion of urine, a liquid waste produced in the body.
- The maintenance of water balance; water balance occurs when the intake of water equals the output of water.
- Regulation of the chemical balance or acid-base balance of the body; the body must maintain a balance of acids and bases in order to function properly.
- Controls blood volume and maintains blood pressure.

These functions are accomplished by the organs of the urinary system. (Figure 13.29)

Structure of the Urinary System

Two kidneys are located at the back of the upper abdomen. Their primary function is to filter (remove) waste products from the blood. Each kidney has the following structure (Figure 13.30):

- The *capsule* is the sac surrounding the kidney.
- The *cortex* is the outer part of the kidney.

354 Chapter 13 | Your Body and How It Functions

FOCUS AND ENGAGE

Introduce the Section

a. Review the Background paragraph, explaining that like some other systems, the urinary system works to eliminate waste from the body.
b. Emphasize that flushing waste via urine is vital to maintaining the balance of water in the body and working to prevent organ damage.
c. Review the objectives for the section.

Vocabulary Review

a. Direct students to the key terms.
b. Pronounce each word, and have the students repeat the pronunciation out loud.
c. Discuss the definition of each word.

TEACH

Discuss

- Discuss how much of the body is composed of water (about 65%).
- Point out that an imbalance of water can result in life-threatening illness.
- Ask students to think of ways the body eliminates water.

Reinforce and Review

- Review the information in Section 13.1: cells, tissues, organs, cavities, and body directions.

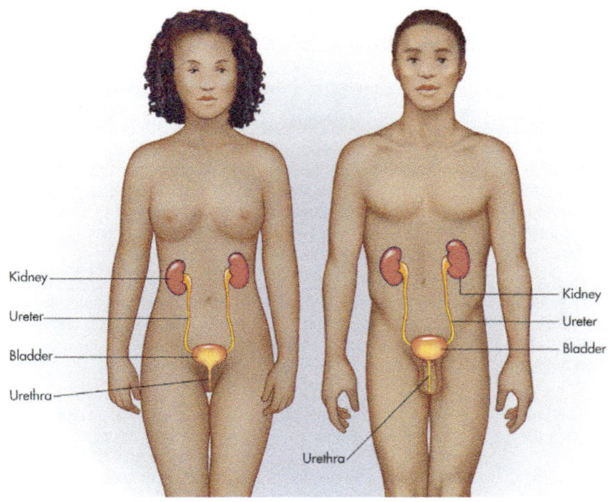

Figure 13.29
The urinary system removes liquid waste from the body. What are the tubes called that move waste from the kidneys to the urinary bladder?

- The *medullais* the inner part of the kidney.
- The **nephron** is the chief filtering **mechanism** of the kidney. Part of the nephron is in the cortex, and part of it is in the medulla. The nephron is made up of:
  - A tiny twisted tube called the *convoluted tubule*.
  - A cuplike capsule called *Bowman's capsule*.
  - A cluster of capillaries in Bowman's capsule called the *glomerulus*.
- The *ureters* are tubes that carry urine (liquid waste) from the kidneys to the urinary bladder.
- The *urinary bladder* is a muscular sac that expands to hold urine received from the kidneys.
- The *urethra* is a tube extending from the urinary bladder to the outside of the body. This allows for the excretion of urine.

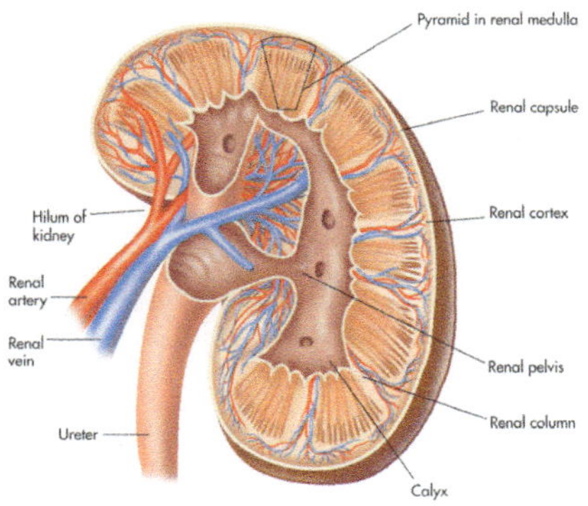

Figure 13.30
Cross section of a kidney. Where is the renal capsule located?

nephron
(NEF rawn)
Functional part of the kidney that filters liquid waste.

mechanism
(MEK uh niz uhm)
Process or a series of steps that achieve a result.

obstruction
(ub STRUK shun)
Blockage or clogging.

dialysis
(die AL iss sus)
Process of removing waste from body fluids.

infuses
(in FYOO z)
Flows into the body by gravity (e.g., IV drips through a tube into the body).

peritoneal cavity
(pear it tun EEL kav it ee)
Area of the body containing the liver, stomach, intestines, kidneys, urinary bladder, and reproductive organs.

edema
(eh DEE muh)
Swelling; abnormal or excessive collection of fluid in the tissues. Usually, the swelling is in the hands, ankles, legs, or abdomen.

Your Body and How It Functions | Chapter 13 355

Figure Focus

13.29 The urinary system removes liquid waste from the body. What are the tubes called that move waste from the kidneys to the urinary bladder?

Answer: Ureters

Figure Focus

13.30 Cross section of a kidney. Where is the renal capsule located?

Answer: The renal capsule surrounds the kidney.

ACTIVITY

Draw a poster illustrating and labeling the parts of the urinary system through which liquid waste passes on its way to leaving the body.

Teaching Tips

- Explain that functions of the urinary system:
  - Excrete urine
  - Maintain water balance in the body
  - Regulate the chemical balance, or acid-base balance
  - Controls blood volume and maintains blood pressure

TEAMWORK

In small groups, look up the scientific definitions of acids and bases. Explain the difference to the class, using at least one specific example of each. Use an encyclopedia or Web site to find information.

Teaching Tips

- Describe the organs and other parts of the urinary system:
  - Kidneys: Filter waste products from blood
  - Renal capsule: Sac surrounding the kidney
  - Cortex: Outer part of the kidney
  - Medullais: Inner part of the kidney
  - Nephron: Chief filtering mechanism
  - Ureters: Tubes that carry urine from kidneys to urinary bladder
  - Urinary bladder: Muscular sac that holds urine
  - Urethra: Tube extending from urinary bladder to the outside of body

Teaching Tips

- Explain how common disorders of the urinary system affect the body.
- Review Table 13.11 together.
- Pronounce the name of each condition out loud:
  - Cystitis
  - Hydronephrosis
  - Kidney or renal failure
  - Nephritis
  - Renal calculi
  - Uremia
- Ask a student to read the description of each disorder.
- Discuss the symptoms of each.

TEAMWORK

Divide the class into teams of 7 to 10. Describe the symptoms of a disorder of the urinary system. Award a point to the first team that can identify the disorder. Award a point to the team that can identify the appropriate treatment. The team with the most points at the end of the game wins.

Common Disorders of the Urinary System

Table 13.11 Common Disorders, Symptoms, and Preventive Measures/ Treatment of the Urinary System

Condition	Disorder	Symptoms	Preventive Measures/ Treatment
Cystitis	Inflammation of the urinary bladder due to infection. The bladder is susceptible to infection because bacteria can easily travel up the urethra to infect the bladder.	Frequent, painful urination, possible blood in urine, fever and chills. More likely to occur in women because of their relatively shorter urethra—bacteria do not have to travel as far to enter the bladder.	Depending on the diagnosis, treating with antibiotics, increased fluid intake, bed rest, medication to control bladder wall spasms, and, when necessary, surgery.
Hydronephrosis	Expanded renal pelvis. Normally caused by an **obstruction** (kidney stone or tumor) that keeps urine from flowing down the ureter.	May experience fever and pain on the side (flank), and, in some cases, urine may contain blood and/or pus.	Removing the obstruction surgically or placement of stints to provide for urinary excretion.
Kidney or renal failure	Nephron of the kidney is unable to filter liquid waste from the blood.	Early signs include fatigue and mental dullness. Later signs include absences of urination, convulsions, GI bleeding, malnutrition, and jaundiced (yellowed) skin that may be covered with a frostlike substance (uremic frost).	Treating with a renal diet and **dialysis**, which is a way to filter waste products from the blood. There are two methods of dialysis: ▪ Hemodialysis, which circulates the body's blood through a machine that filters out the waste and returns the clean blood to the body. ▪ Peritoneal dialysis, which **infuses** sterile fluids into the **peritoneal cavity** and then drains the fluid from the cavity. While the fluid is in the abdomen, waste products are chemically drawn out of tissues and into the fluid. When the fluid drains from the abdomen, the waste is also removed.
Nephritis	Inflammation of the kidney due to infection or arteriosclerosis.	**Edema**, a collection of fluid in the tissues that causes swelling.	Treating with medication or surgery to remove a kidney may be indicated, depending on the cause.
Renal calculi	Kidney stones that develop when the liquid waste from the blood becomes solid.	Sharp, severe pain in the lower back over the kidney, radiating into the groin.	Surgically removing the stones if they do not pass through the ureter and urethra normally.
Uremia	An accumulation of urine substances in the blood occurs when the nephron is unable to completely filter out waste from the blood.	Nausea, vomiting, headache, dizziness, coma, or convulsions; breath and perspiration may smell like urine.	Early diagnosis of kidney dysfunction. Treatment is dialysis.

356 Chapter 13 | Your Body and How It Functions

MEDICAL TERMINOLOGY	
calculi:	stones
cystitis:	inflammation of the bladder
cystoscopy:	inspection of the bladder
diuresis:	passage of abnormally large amounts
glycouria:	sugar in the urine
hematuria:	blood in the urine
nephralgia:	renal pain
nephric:	pertaining to the kidney
nephroid:	resembling a kidney
nephrolithotripsy:	crushing of kidney stones
nephropexy:	surgical attachment of a floating kidney
nephrorrhagia:	renal hemorrhage
nephrostomy:	artificial opening into the kidney
pyelectasis:	dilation of the renal pelvis
pyelitis:	inflammation of the pelvis of the kidney of urine
pyelolithotomy:	removal of kidney stone
pyelometry:	measurement of the kidney's pelvis
renal:	pertaining to the kidney
renal colic:	severe pain in the kidney
uremia:	condition in which blood contains toxins usually excreted from the kidneys
ureteropyelitis:	inflammation of the kidney pelvis and the ureter
urethrism:	irritability or spasm of the urethra

Related Jobs and Professions

Urologist

Urologists specialize in issues related to the male and female urinary tracts and the male reproductive organs. People see urologists for issues ranging from discomfort while urinating to male infertility. Urologists look for such things as signs of infection, blood in the urine, or excess sugars or protein, which could indicate diabetes or other kidney problems.

Because urologists encounter such a wide variety of issues, they must have a broad knowledge of internal medicine, pediatrics, gynecology, and other specialties. Urologists must graduate from medical school and then complete an accredited urology residency program. This program can last up to five years and involves a combination of surgical and clinical training.

Urologists can specialize in a variety of areas, including urologic oncology, male infertility, female urology, or pediatric urology. To practice as a pediatric urologist, one more year of training is required. All urologists must also pass an exam to become certified in this field.

Nephrologist

A nephrologist, also called a renal physician, is someone who specializes in the treatment of patients with kidney diseases. This includes patients with diabetes, polycystic kidney disease, and chronic kidney failure. Many patients must receive dialysis therapy and some will require kidney transplants.

Nephrologists are trained in internal medicine. They do not perform surgery. However, they may do a kidney biopsy in order to obtain a sample of kidney tissue. Their goal is to find ways to preserve patients' remaining kidney function. To become a nephrologist, you must graduate from medical school, complete an internal medicine residency program, and complete a two- to three-year fellowship in nephrology. You must also take an exam to become certified in this field.

Apply It

Form teams of four. Each team should create a model of a functioning urinary system from materials found in their homes (balloons, straws, etc.).

The system should show (1) kidneys that have produced urine, (2) ureters that transport the urine to the (3) bladder that can store the urine, to the (4) urethra, which passes urine out of the body. Conduct an in-class science fair.

Your Body and How It Functions | Chapter 13 357

MEDICAL TERMINOLOGY

Review the terminology:

- Pronounce each word element, and have students repeat.
- Pronounce each term, and have students repeat.
- Allow time for students to write down definitions.
- Select a student to read each definition.
- Assign students to memorize the terms and their definitions.

Teaching Tips

- Begin a discussion about the jobs and professions that would be suitable for someone interested in the urinary system.
- Remind students to refer to Chapter 3 for more information on occupations.
- Discuss the skills and requirements for becoming an urologist and a nephrologist.

Apply It

- You may want to assign this activity well in advance so that students have time to work on their projects.
- If possible, display a sample model that you or a student from a previous class has created.
- Alternatively, you may want to make this a class project, and work on one model together.
- If students cannot create a working model, you may want to offer them an alternative activity, such as creating a presentation with a presentation graphics program.

Figure Focus

13.31 What skills and interests do you think might be necessary to become a dialysis technician?

Student answers will vary.

Teaching Tips

- Discuss the skills and requirements for becoming a dialysis technician.
- You may want to discuss dialysis, and how it works.
- There may be students in the class who have a relative or friend who must undergo dialysis. Ask if they are willing to discuss the process.
- Review the urinary system and how it removes liquid waste and eliminates it from the body.
- Discuss how the body knows what to discard and what to keep.
- Identify the part of the urinary system responsible for filtering water.
- Discuss why a kidney infection is more serious than a bladder infection.
- Discuss what might happen to the body if a kidney fails.
- Discuss reasons why it is important for all health care workers to have a basic knowledge of the urinary system and how it functions.
- Remind students of the importance of responding appropriately when a medical emergency occurs.
- Review the need for health care workers in all positions to use proper medical terminology to communicate with others.
- Look at the following situation from a variety of health care worker perspectives:
  - A patient complains of blood in the urine.
  - What should a physician do?
  - What should a nurse's aide do?
  - What should a front office medical assistant do?

Dialysis Technician

A dialysis technician is the primary caregiver for patients who are undergoing dialysis, which is a process through which waste products are filtered from the blood when the kidneys are not functioning properly. (**Figure 13.31**) Although the dialysis technician performs the actual dialysis treatment, a nurse is responsible for overall patient care. The dialysis technician works under the supervision of that nurse.

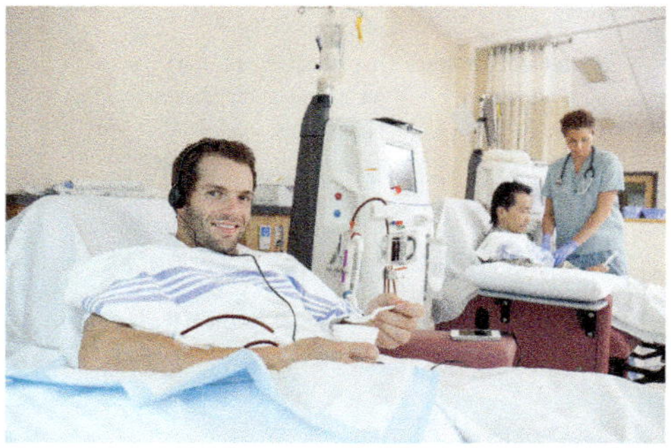

Figure 13.31
What skills and interests do you think might be necessary to become a dialysis technician?

On-the-job duties include assembling supplies, preparing the machine for use, obtaining patient vital signs, administering local anesthetics and drugs under supervision, and closely monitoring the patient before, during, and after dialysis treatment.

Dialysis technicians work in hospitals, outpatient facilities, and home dialysis programs. To become a dialysis technician, you must have a high school diploma. A dialysis technician may be trained on the job, through an employer-sponsored training program, or at a vocational school or community college.

Summary

In this section, you learned that the kidneys are the main organs of the urinary system. Each kidney contains filtering mechanisms called nephrons. Nephrons filter the blood and move excess fluids (urine) into the kidney pelvis. Urine travels from the kidneys to the bladder through tubes called ureters, and out of the body through a tube called the urethra. Kidney diseases can cause fluid buildup or prevent adequate filtering of the blood. Patients may need dialysis or surgery if one or both kidneys stop functioning.

Section 13.8 Review Questions

1. What are the primary functions of the urinary system?
2. What is dialysis and when is it used?
3. What is the purpose of the nephron?
4. What are the symptoms of renal calculi (kidney stones)?
5. Why is kidney failure dangerous to a patient's health?
6. A(n)____________, also called a renal physician, specializes in the treatment of patients with kidney diseases.

358 Chapter 13 | Your Body and How It Functions

ACTIVITY

Select one of the jobs or professions listed in Section 13.8. Create a brochure or pamphlet explaining why the health care worker you selected needs a basic knowledge of the urinary system in order to perform his or her job effectively.

Section 13.8 Review Questions

1. Answer: The excretion of urine; Maintenance of water balance; Regulation of the chemical balance or acid-base balance of the body; and Controls blood volume and maintains blood pressure.
2. Answer: Dialysis is the process of removing waste from body fluids, which is used for kidney or renal failure.

The Endocrine Systems

SECTION 13.9

Background

Glands are small organs that are positioned throughout the body. Some glands release substances, such as tears and sweat, to the outside of the body. Other glands release substances directly into the bloodstream. Many glands produce hormones. Hormones help to regulate many body functions. As a health care worker, you should know the structure, functions, and disorders of the glandular system.

Objectives

When you have completed this section, you will be able to do the following:

- Match key terms with their correct meanings.
- Label endocrine glands on a diagram.
- Identify functions of the endocrine glands.
- Identify common disorders of the endocrine glands.
- Explain the difference between the endocrine and exocrine glands.
- Describe the effects of the endocrine glands on the body.
- Explain why the health care worker's understanding of the glandular systems is important.

Introduction to the Glandular Systems

The glands of the body make substances that help regulate the body processes of growth, **metabolism**, muscle contraction, and many other processes. (Figure 13.32) Glands are divided into two categories. These are the exocrine and endocrine glands:

- *Exocrine glands* have ducts that carry substances to organs, body parts, or the outside of the body. The substance made by the gland is **excreted** and is deposited in the organ or body part. *Examples:*
  - Digestive juices from the salivary glands, pancreas, and gallbladder
  - Milk from the female mammary glands
  - Moisture from the sweat glands
  - Sebum (oil) from the **sebaceous** glands
  - Tears from the **lacrimal** glands
- *Endocrine glands* are glands without ducts. They secrete **hormones** directly into the bloodstream. The secretions from these glands are separated into two main groups:
  - *External secretions* (excretions) are fluids that are carried to a nearby organ or to the outside of the body.
  - *Internal secretions* are hormones that are carried to all parts of the body through the blood and lymph systems. The endocrine glands that secrete hormones are included in Table 13.12.

metabolism
(meh TAB uh liz um)
The body's process of using food to make energy and use nutrients.

excreted
(ex KREET ed)
Thrown off or eliminated as waste material.

sebaceous
(seh BAY shus)
Pertaining to fatty secretions.

lacrimal
(LAK rim uhl)
Pertaining to tears.

hormones
(HOR moans)
Protein substances secreted by an endocrine gland directly into the blood.

Your Body and How It Functions | Chapter 13 359

3. Answer: Nephron is the chief filtering mechanism of the kidney. Part of the nephron is in the cortex, and part of it is in the medulla. The nephron is made up of: a tiny twisted tube called the convoluted tubule; a cuplike capsule called Bowman's capsule; a cluster of capillaries in Bowman's capsule called the glomerulus.
4. Answer: Sharp, sever pain in the lower back over the kidney radiating to the groin
5. Answer: Renal failure is dangerous because it means waste is not being removed from the body.
6. Answer: Nephrologist

FOCUS AND ENGAGE

Introduce the Section

a. Review the content of the Background paragraph, explaining that the endocrine system is made up of glands.
b. Emphasize that there are many different glands located throughout the body.
c. Review the objectives for the section.

Vocabulary Review

a. Direct students to the key terms.
b. Pronounce each word, and have the students repeat the pronunciation out loud.
c. Discuss each definition.

TEACH

Discuss

- Explain that among other substances, tears and sweat are produced by glands in the endocrine system.
- Ask students if they know the purpose of sweat.
- Discuss the importance of keeping the body cool.

ACTIVITY

Draw a poster illustrating and labeling the parts of the endocrine system. Use one color to identify endocrine glands and a different color to identify exocrine glands.

Reinforce and Review

- Review the information in Section 13.1: cells, tissues, organs, cavities, and body directions.

Teaching Tips

- Explain that the endocrine system produces substances that help control bodily functions such as:
  - Growth
  - Metabolism
  - Muscle contraction
- Describe the organs of the endocrine systems.

Teaching Tips

- Differentiate between the two types of glands:
  - Exocrine glands have ducts that carry excreted substances to organs, body parts, or outside the body.
  - Endocrine glands have no ducts. They secrete hormones into the bloodstream.
- Review examples of exocrine glands:
  - Salivary glands produce digestive juices.
  - Female mammary glands produce milk.
  - Sweat glands produce moisture.
  - Sebaceous glands produce sebum.
  - Lacrimal glands produce tears.
- Discuss the two types of secretions produced by endocrine glands:
  - External secretions (excretions) are fluids that are carried to a nearby organ or to the outside of the body.
  - Internal secretions are hormones that are carried to all parts of the body through the blood and lymph systems.
- Review Table 13.12 together as a class.

Figure Focus

13.32 The glandular systems provide substances that help regulate body processes. Which glands are found in the head and the throat?

Answer: Pineal, pituitary, parathyroid, and thyroid glands

Figure 13.32
The glandular systems provide substances that help regulate body processes. Which glands are found in the head and the throat?

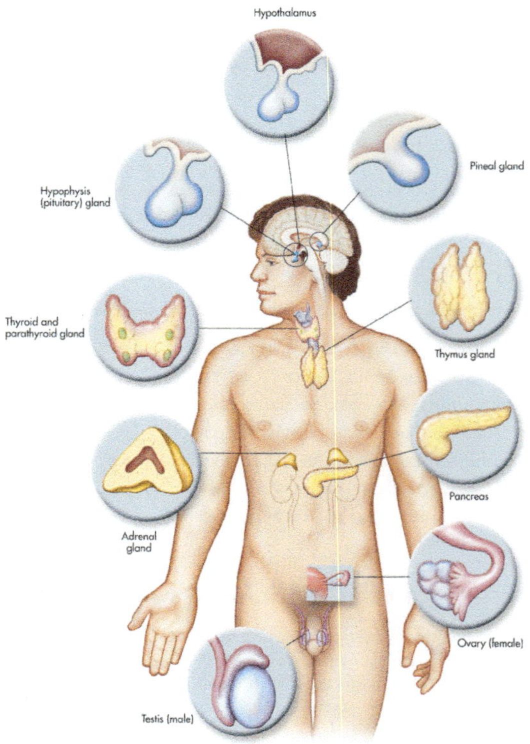

pigmentation
(pig men TAY shun
Natural color of the skin.

Table 13.12 Endocrine Glands, Hormones, and Their Functions

Gland	Hormone	Function
Pituitary	TSH (thyrotropic hormone), ACTH (adreno-corticotrophic hormone), FSH (follicle-stimulating hormone), LH (luteinizing hormone), ADH (antidi-uretic hormone), oxytocin, oytocin, prolactin, and somatotropic hormone	Controls other glands; stimulates growth
Thyroid	Thyroxin	Controls rate of metabolism
Parathyroid	Parathyroid hormone	Regulates calcium and phosphorus metabolism
Pancreas	Insulin from islands of Langerhans	Enables utilization of glucose
Ovaries	Estrogen and progesterone	Develop and maintain female reproductive organs
Testes	Testosterone	Develop and maintain male reproductive organs
Adrenal medulla	Adrenalin	Prepares the body for fight or flight
Adrenal cortex	Corticoids	Aids body in coping with stress or infection
Pineal	Melatonin	May help modulate wake/sleep patterns

360 Chapter 13 | Your Body and How It Functions

ACTIVITY

Make flashcards to use for studying the functions of the endocrine glands in Table 13.12. Write the name of the gland on the front of the card and the hormone and function on the back of the card.

Common Disorders of the Glandular Systems

Table 13.13 Common Disorders, Symptoms, and Preventive Measures/Treatment of the Glandular System

Condition	Disorder	Symptoms	Preventive Measures/ Treatment
Addison's disease	A life-threatening disease caused by insufficient amount of hormones from the adrenal glands.	Weakness, decreased endurance, increased **pigmentation** of the skin and mucous membranes, anorexia, dehydration, weight loss, GI disturbances, anxiety, depression, and decreased tolerance to cold.	Treating with medication, maintaining an adequate intake of fluids, eating a diet high in carbohydrates and protein and low in sodium and potassium.
Diabetes mellitus	Too much sugar (glucose) in the blood, usually the result of the pancreas failing to produce insulin. There are the following types of diabetes: ■ IDDM: insulin-dependent diabetes mellitus. ■ NIDDM: noninsulin-dependent diabetes mellitus. ■ GDM: gestational diabetes mellitus (during pregnancy). ■ Types of diabetes usually associated with pancreatic disease, hormonal changes, adverse effects of drugs, or genetic abnormalities. ■ IGT: impaired glucose tolerance.	Increased thirst (polydipsia) and urination (polyuria), and weight loss. Periods of excessive hunger (polyphagia), and low blood sugar levels (hypoglycemia). The eyes, kidneys, nervous system, skin, and circulatory system may be affected, and infections are common. Atherosclerosis often develops.	Maintaining insulin and glucose levels within normal values through diet, exercise, and medication.
Hyperthyroidism	Increased production of the thyroid secretion.	Excessive sweating, heat intolerance, increased bowel movements; tremors, nervousness, agitation, rapid heart rate. Weight loss, fatigue, decreased concentration. Irregular and scant menstrual flow. In older patients, irregular heart rhythms and heart failure can occur.	Treating the symptoms with antithyroid drugs; radioactive iodine. Surgery to partially remove thyroid gland.
Hypoglycemia	Too little sugar in the blood, usually caused by the excessive production of insulin in the pancreas.	Weakness, headache, hunger, visual disturbances, ataxia, anxiety, personality changes, and, if untreated, delirium, coma, and death.	Taking glucose in orange juice by mouth if the person is conscious, followed by protein,or administering intravenously if the person is unconscious.
Hypothyroidism	Decreased production of the thyroid secretion.	Fatigue, depression, modest weight gain, intolerance of cold, excessive sleepiness, dry or coarse hair, constipation, dry skin, muscle cramps, increased cholesterol levels, decreased concentration, aches and pains, swelling of legs.	Life-long treatment with T-4 form of thyroid hormone. Pill taken once a day, preferably in the morning.

Your Body and How It Functions | Chapter 13 361

Teaching Tips

- Review the Table 13.13 together as a class.
- Pronounce the name of each condition out loud:
  - Addison's disease
  - Diabetes mellitus
  - Hyperthyroidism
  - Hypoglycemia
  - Hypothyroidism
- Ask a student to read the description of each disorder.
- Discuss the symptoms of each.

TEAMWORK

In small groups, prepare a skit demonstrating a common disorder of the endocrine system. One student should be a patient, describing symptoms to a health care worker or a team of health care workers. The health care workers should diagnose the disorder, explain it, and prescribe a treatment.

MEDICAL TERMINOLOGY

Review the terminology:

- Pronounce each word element, and have students repeat.
- Pronounce each term, and have students repeat.
- Allow time for students to write down definitions.
- Select a student to read each definition.
- Assign students to memorize the terms and their definitions.

Teaching Tips

- Begin a discussion about the jobs and professions that would be suitable for someone interested in the endocrine system.
- Remind students to refer to Chapter 3 for more information on occupations.
- Discuss the skills and requirements for becoming an endocrinologist.
- Discuss reasons why it is important for all health care workers to have a basic knowledge of the endocrine system and how it functions.
- Remind students of the importance of responding appropriately when a medical emergency occurs.
- Review the need for health care workers in all positions to use proper medical terminology to communicate with others.

MEDICAL TERMINOLOGY

acromegaly:	enlargement of bones of the extremities	**hyperthyroidism:**	increased production of the thyroid secretion
adenectomy:	removal of any gland	**hypothyroidism:**	decreased production of the thyroid secretion
adenoidectomy:	removal of the adenoids	**lymphocytopenia:**	deficiency of lymph cells
adrenogenic:	originating in the adrenals	**pancreatolysis:**	breakdown of the pancreas
dwarfism:	condition of being abnormally small	**parathyrotoxicosis:**	poisonous condition of the parathyroid
endocrine:	ductless; to secrete within	**pinealoma:**	tumor of the pineal gland
endocrinotherapy:	treatment with endocrine preparation	**pituitarigenic:**	originating in the pituitary
exocrine:	to secrete through a duct	**pituitarism:**	any disorder of the pituitary gland
goiter:	enlarged thyroid gland	**thyroadenitis:**	inflammation of the thyroid gland
goitrogen:	any substance that causes a goiter		

Related Jobs and Professions

Endocrinologist

An endocrinologist is a physician who specializes in the endocrine system. (Figure 13.33) These doctors treat conditions that affect your glands. This may include diabetes, thyroid diseases, metabolic disorders, osteoporosis, hypertension, lack of growth, infertility, or cancer.

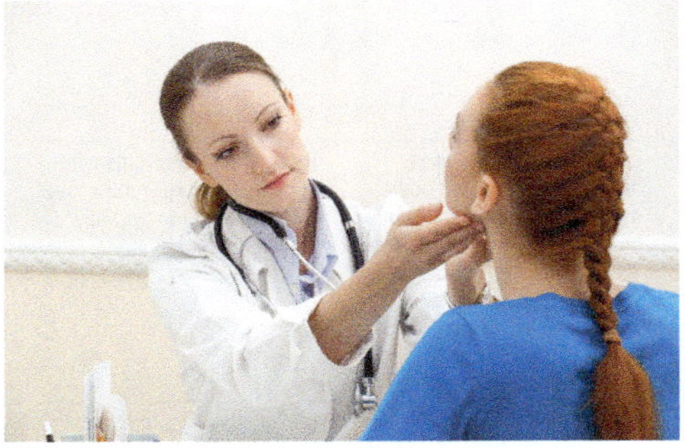

Figure 13.33
What skills and interests do you think might be necessary to become an endocrinologist?

Endocrinologists treat these hormone problems and try to restore a normal balance of hormones in their patients. Endocrinologists also do research to learn how glands work and to find the best treatments for patients with glandular problems.

Like many other specialties, to become an endocrinologist you must first complete medical school and then complete a two- to three-year residency to become certified in internal medicine. Following that, you must then spend two or three more years studying the endocrine system. It takes more than 10 years to become trained as an endocrinologist.

Summary

In this section, you learned that glands produce hormones that help to regulate growth, metabolism, reproduction, and other body processes. Examples of glands include the thyroid, pancreas, ovaries, and testes. Disorders of the glandular system occur when a gland overproduces or underproduces hormones. These disorders may cause illness or death. Some glandular system disorders can be controlled by diet and medications.

362 Chapter 13 | Your Body and How It Functions

Figure Focus

13.33 What skills and interests do you think might be necessary to become an endocrinologist?

Student answers will vary.

ACTIVITY

Create a resume for an endocrinologist looking for a new position. Create a job history, educational credentials, and other relevant information. Refer back to Chapter 4 for information on what to include in a resume.

Section 13.9 Review Questions

1. What substance is produced by the adrenal cortex and what function does this substance have in the body?
2. What is the difference between endocrine and exocrine glands?
3. What do sebaceous glands produce?
4. What is diabetes mellitus and what causes this disorder?
5. Where are the adrenal glands located?
6. What are the symptoms and treatment for hypoglycemia?
7. A(n) __________ is a physician who specializes conditions that affect your glands.

The Nervous System

SECTION 13.10

Background

The nervous system receives, sends, and coordinates internal and external messages. This system helps us to sense and react to things that are happening outside of the body. It also controls automatic internal body functions, such as heartbeat and breathing. In this section, you will learn the structure and functions of the nervous system. You will also learn how diseases of the sensory organs or nerves can affect patients.

Objectives

When you have completed this section, you will be able to do the following:

- Match key terms with their correct meanings.
- Match and select the functions of various parts of the nervous system.
- Label diagrams of the eye and ear.
- Describe the influence of the nervous system on the body.
- Match common disorders of the nervous system with their correct names.
- Explain why the health care worker's understanding of the nervous system is important.

Introduction to the Nervous System

The nervous system is a delicate system of nerve cells (or neurons) linked together to receive **stimuli** and to respond to stimuli. (**Figure 13.34**) Stimuli are anything that cause a reaction or response (e.g., when your hand touches a hot object or when something flies into your eye). Response is the reaction to the stimuli (e.g., moving your hand when it touches something hot or tears in the eye when something flies into it).

stimuli
(STIM you lie)
Elements in the external or internal environment that are strong enough to set up a nervous impulse.

Your Body and How It Functions | Chapter 13 363

Section 13.9 Review Questions

1. Answer: Corticoids are produced by the adrenal cortex and they aid the body in coping with stress or infection.
2. Answer: Exocrine glands have ducts that carry substances to organs, body parts, or the outside of the body. The substance made by the gland is excreted and is deposited in the organ or body part. Endocrine glands are glands without ducts. They secrete hormones directly into the bloodstream.
3. Answer: Fatty secretions
4. Answer: Diabetes mellitus occurs when too much sugar is in the blood usually the result of the pancreas failing to produce insulin.
5. Answer: Adrenal glands are located on top of the kidneys.
6. Answer: Symptoms of hypoglycemia include weakness, headache, hunger, visual disturbances, ataxia, anxiety, and personality changes. If untreated, delirium, coma, and even death can occur. To treat hypoglycemia, drink orange juice followed by protein.
7. Answer: Endocrinologist

FOCUS AND ENGAGE

Introduce the Section

a. Review the content of the Background paragraph, explaining that the nervous system controls our senses.
b. Emphasize that nervous system reacts and responds to internal and external messages.
c. Review the section objectives.

Vocabulary Review

a. Direct students to the key terms.
b. Pronounce each word, and have the students repeat the pronunciation aloud.
c. Discuss each definition.

TEACH

Discuss

- Ask students to name the five senses.
- Discuss the organs responsible for these senses: the eye, ear, nose, tongue, and skin.
- Discuss involuntary reactions to stimuli, such as blinking in bright light, or shivering in the cold.

Reinforce and Review

- Review the information in Section 13.1: cells, tissues, organs, cavities, and body directions.

Teaching Tips

- Show a video on the nervous system, if available.

ACTIVITY

Draw a poster or create a presentation or flowchart that illustrates the path a sensory message takes to reach the brain. For example, illustrate the smell of a fresh-baked pie traveling through the nose to the brain. Label the parts of the nervous system that are involved in receiving, transmitting, and responding to the message.

Teaching Tips

- Explain the function of nerve cells and their role in receiving and responding to stimuli.
- Provide examples of stimuli and the body's response to each:
  - Touching a hot stove—pulling back
  - A car heading toward you—jumping out of the way
  - Dust in the nose—sneezing
  - Dust in the eye—blinking
- Describe and differentiate between the central and peripheral nervous systems.
- Explain that the central nervous system includes the brain and the spinal cord.
- Identify the three main parts of the brain:
  - Cerebrum
  - Cerebellum
  - Medulla

Figure 13.34
Central and peripheral nervous systems. What does the brain do?

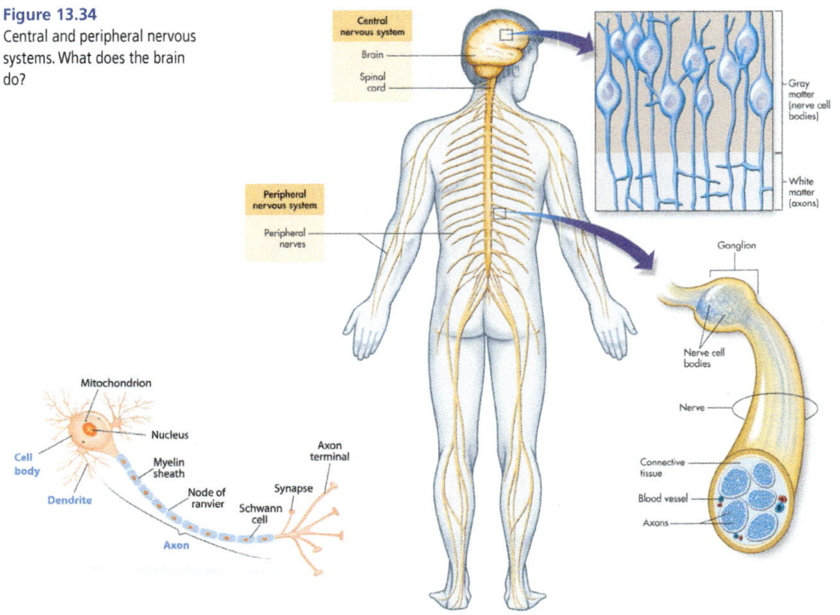

peripheral
(per IF er uhl)
Situated away from a central structure.

The nervous system is divided into two parts: the central nervous system and the **peripheral** nervous system.

The *central nervous system (CNS)* includes the brain and the spinal cord. Nerves of the spinal cord carry messages to and from the brain. The brain has three main parts:

- The *cerebrum* processes thought having to do with memory and learning. It controls voluntary movements and sense interpretation.
- The *cerebellum* coordinates muscle activity and balance so that muscles function smoothly.
- The *medulla*, a part of the brainstem, controls breathing, heartbeat, circulatory action, and digestive movements.

ganglia
(GANG glee ah)
Mass of nerve tissue composed of nerve cell bodies. Ganglia lie outside the brain and spinal cord.

The *peripheral nervous system* includes the nerves and **ganglia** outside the brain and spinal cord. There are:

- Twelve pairs of cranial nerves
- Thirty-one pairs of spinal nerves
- Various nerve branches in body organs
- Divided into the sensory (afferent) and motor (efferent) divisions
- Motor is then divided into somatic (controls skeletal muscle) and autonomic, which regulates sympathetic responses (fight or flight) and parasympathetic responses (rest and digest)

364 Chapter 13 | Your Body and How It Functions

Figure Focus

13.34 Central and peripheral nervous systems. What does the brain do?

Answer: The brain serves as the center of the nervous system.

TEAMWORK

Divide the class into teams of three to five students. Give them a set amount of time to write down specific examples of how the nervous system responds to external and internal stimuli. Compare examples as a class, awarding points for each original example. The team with the most points wins.

All parts of the central and peripheral nervous systems work together to relay messages to the brain. Each message is carried to the correct area of the brain by its specialized neuron or nerve cell.

Each specialized **neuron** leads into a passage that delivers the message or stimuli to the brain or the spinal cord. The areas in the spinal cord that can receive messages cause an action or response to stimuli that does not require interpretation. The stimuli that are received by the brain are interpreted and cause a response.

neuron
(NUR awn)
Nerve; includes the cell and the long fiber coming from the cell.

This response can occur anyplace in the body but is most easily recognized in the sense organs. For example, sound waves are received by the ears; light rays are received by the eyes; the nose and tongue respond to smell and taste; and the nerve endings throughout the body respond to pressure, heat, cold, pain, and touch.

The following are the sensory organs of the body.

The Eye

The eye provides vision. (**Figure 13.35**) It is a ball-shaped organ located in the eye orbit of the skull.

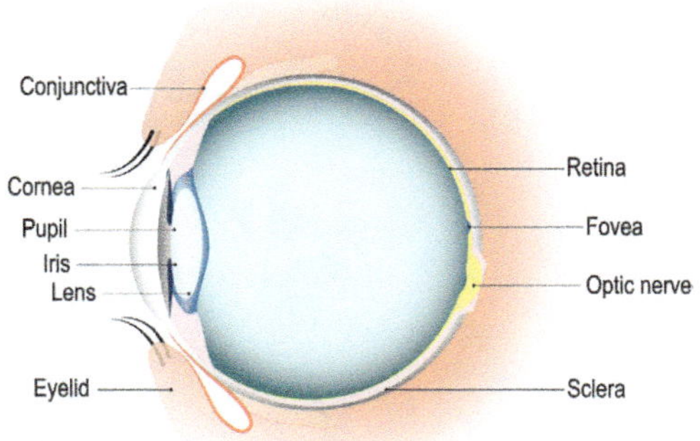

Figure 13.35
The human eye. Where is the cornea of the eye in relation to the lens and iris?

Protection for the Eye

- The lids and eyelashes aid in protecting the eye.
- Tears from the lacrimal **duct** help wash away foreign matter.

Coats of the Eye

- The *sclera*, or the white of the eye, is the outer lining. The front portion of the sclera is clear and is called the *cornea*, or the "window of the eye."
- The *choroid*, the second coating, is heavily **pigmented** to keep light rays from **scattering**.

duct
(DUHKT)
Narrow, round tube that carries secretions from a gland.

pigmented
(PIG men ted)
Colored; relating to various parts of the body (e.g., iris of the eye, lips, moles, freckles).

scattering
(SKAT e ring)
Spreading in many directions, dispersing.

Your Body and How It Functions | Chapter 13 365

Teaching Tips

- Explain that the peripheral nervous system includes the nerves and ganglia outside the brain and spinal cord.
- It includes:
  - Twelve pairs of cranial nerves
  - Thirty-one pairs of spinal nerves
  - Various nerve branches in body organs
- Explain that the central and peripheral nervous systems work together to send messages to the brain.
- Discuss the role of neurons as messengers.
- Discuss the role of the sensory organs:
  - Eyes respond to light.
  - Ears respond to sound.
  - Nose and tongue respond to smell and taste.
  - Nerve endings respond to pressure, heat, cold, pain, and touch.
- Describe the parts of the eye.

Figure Focus

13.35 The human eye. Where is the cornea of the eye in relation to the lens and iris?

Answer: The cornea is on the outside of the eye, covering the lens and iris.

TEAMWORK

Divide the class into teams of 7 to 10. Have each team create two cards. On one, write "Central Nervous System." On the other, write "Peripheral Nervous System." You name a response, such as breathing, heartbeat, pain in a body part, digestion, muscle cramps, balance, blinking, coughing, sneezing, pressure, etc. Each team has 30 seconds to decide which part of the nervous system controls the response, and hold up the appropriate care. Points are awarded for correct answers. The team with the most points at the end of the game wins.

Teaching Tips

- Discuss the function of each part of the eye:
  - Lids and eyelashes protect the eye.
  - Tears from lacrimal ducts wash the eye.
- Discuss the coats of the eye:
  - Sclera, or white of the eye: outer lining
  - Cornea: clear, front portion of the sclera
  - Choroid: second coat heavily pigmented to keep light rays from scattering
  - Retina: innermost coat houses the mechanisms that sense vision
- Discuss the role of the optic nerve.
- Describe the three parts of the ear:
  - External ear has the auricle, external auditory canal, tympanic membrane, or eardrum.
  - Middle ear has three bones—ossicles—that amplify sound.
  - Inner ear has semi-circular canals that transmit sound.

Figure Focus

13.36 Cross section of the ear. Which part of the ear looks like a snail shell?

Answer: The cochlea or inner ear

equilibrium
(ee kwah LIB ree um)
State of balance.

ossicles
(OSS ik uhls)
Three small bones in the middle ear: incus, stapes, and malleus.

amplify
(AM pluh feye)
To increase or elevate a sound (e.g., the ossicles of the ear amplify sound waves).

translate
(trans LEYT)
To make understandable.

- The *retina*, the innermost coating of the eye, houses the mechanisms that sense vision.
- The *optic nerve*, located at the back of the eye, receives a picture and sends it to the brain for interpretation.

The Ear

The ear provides hearing and **equilibrium**. (**Figure 13.36**) The ear can be divided into three main parts:

- The *external ear* includes the following:
  - *Auricle*, or outside projection
  - *External auditory canal*
  - *Tympanic membrane* or eardrum, which separates the external and middle ear
- The *middle ear* is an air space that contains three bones or **ossicles**. These bones **amplify** sound waves received by the tympanic membrane.
- The *inner ear* contains the semicircular canals, which transmit sound waves received from the middle ear to the nerves that allow us to **translate** sound. The inner ear is also responsible for equilibrium.

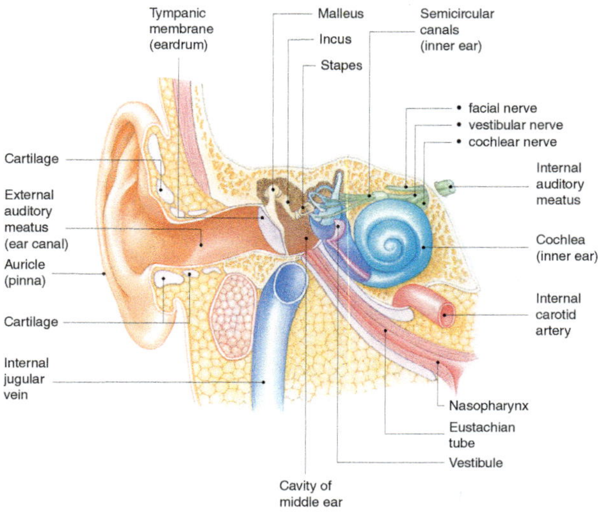

Figure 13.36
Cross section of the ear. Which part of the ear looks like a snail shell?

366 Chapter 13 | Your Body and How It Functions

ACTIVITY

Create a poster or diagram of either the eye or the ear. Label each part correctly.

Organs of Taste and Smell

Sense of Taste

Taste is sensed by receptors in the tongue called taste buds. The taste buds sense four main tastes:

- Sweet
- Salty
- Sour
- Bitter

Sense of Smell

Receptors that receive smells are located high in the upper part of the nasal cavity called the olfactory epithelium. The olfactory nerve sends the smell to the brain for interpretation.

General Senses

General senses are found throughout the body. These general senses are different from the special senses of sight, hearing, taste, and smell; they are not limited to specific areas of the body.

Pressure Sense

Pressure is sensed by the pressure receptors in the **subcutaneous** tissue layer beneath the skin.

Temperature Sense

Heat and cold are sensed by **receptors** that respond only to heat or cold and send messages through nerves to the brain.

Sense of Touch

Touch is sensed by receptors called *tactile corpuscles*. These receptors are found in the dermis layer of skin. They are very close together in the fingertips and the toes and also in the tip of the tongue.

Sense of Pain

Pain is the most important protective sense because it tells us that something is wrong in the body. Pain receptors are found in the:

- Skin
- Muscles
- Joints
- Internal organs

These receptors are nerve fibers that send messages of pain to the brain when parts of the body are injured.

Apply It

Play a game of Mystery Smells. List ten items belonging to a specific place/activity—a school, a ball game, the beach, a specific holiday, etc. that have an odor associated with them. List each item on one side of a 3 × 5 card.

On the opposite side, write a description of the smell. For instance, you might say "dessert" as the word, and "fruity" as the smell. Once the cards are made, try to have your fellow classmates guess the item by the smell and location.

subcutaneous
(sub kyu TAIN ee us)
Beneath the skin.

receptors
(ree SEP torz)
Nerves that respond to stimuli.

Your Body and How It Functions | Chapter 13 367

Teaching Tips

- Discuss the organs of taste and smell.
- Taste:
    - Taste buds in the tongue
    - Four main tastes
- Smell:
    - Receptors in the olfactory epithelium
    - Olfactory nerve sends the smell to the brain for interpretation
- Explain the general senses:
    - Pressure: sensed by pressure receptors in the skin
    - Temperature: sensed by temperature receptors
    - Touch: sensed by tactile corpuscles
    - Pain: sensed by pain receptors in the skin, muscles, joints, and internal organs

Apply It

- Provide 3 × 5 index cards to use in this activity.
- Students may work individually or in small groups.
- Examples of a place that might have an odor associated with it is a movie theater, which might smell like popcorn. An event might be Thanksgiving dinner, which might smell like turkey.

Teaching Tips

- Explain that the general senses are not limited to specific areas of the body.
- Discuss the importance of pain.
- Emphasize that pain informs your brain that something is wrong with your body.
- Explain how common disorders of the nervous system affect the body.
- Review the first part of Table 13.14 together.
- Pronounce the name of each condition out loud:
  - Alzheimer's disease
  - Cataract
  - Conjunctivitis
  - Glaucoma
  - Neuritis
  - Otosclerosis
- Ask a student to read the description of each disorder.
- Discuss the symptoms of each.

TEAMWORK

Divide the class into teams of three to five students. Give them a set amount of time to write down specific examples of how the nervous system responds to external and internal stimuli. Compare examples as a class, awarding points for each original example. The team with the most points wins.

Common Disorders of the Nervous System

Table 13.14 Common Disorders, Symptoms, and Preventive Measures/Treatment of the Nervous System

Condition	Disorder	Symptoms	Preventive Measures/ Treatment
Alzheimer's Disease	A progressive, degenerative disease of the brain that results in dementia.	Personality and behavior changes. Decline in memory. Reduced awareness of one's surroundings and of recent events. Repetitive behavior. Increased restlessness and agitation in late afternoon and evening; wandering. Bowel and bladder incontinence. Suspicion.	No current cure or way to stop the progression of the disease. Medications can improve symptom management; for example, cholinesterase inhibitors help memory and learning.
Cataract	Formation occurs when the lens of the eye loses its transparency. Light is less able to reach the inner eye. Cataracts are the most common cause of blindness and a very common ailment in the geriatric patient.	At first vision is blurred, then distortion and double vision may develop. If not treated, blindness can occur.	For cataracts that have developed through the aging process, treating with removal of the lens and then prescribing contacts or glasses.
Cerebrovascular Accident (stroke)	Interruption to the blood supply in the brain from an obstruction or rupture of the vessel.	Facial drooping, slurred speech, arm weakness, sudden confusion, difficulty walking, blurred vision; symptoms may depend on the location of the interrupted blood supply in the brain.	Prompt emergency medical care when signs of stroke appear that may include clot-busting drugs, surgical removal of the clot, or other surgical procedures.
Concussion/ traumatic brain injury	Violent injury to the head, such as in athletics, auto accidents, falls, etc.	Headache, memory loss, confusion, dizziness, nausea, slurred speech.	Protective helmet; rest; treatment may require diagnostic evaluation such as X-rays, MRI, CT scans.
Conjunctivitis or "pink eye"	Inflammation of the eyelid lining caused from bacteria or irritation from dirt in the eye. Highly contagious.	Red eyes, thick discharge, sticky eyelids in the morning, usually occurring without pain.	Wearing goggles to protect eyes from dirt and debris when possible. For example, when mowing the lawn, sawing wood, etc. Wash hands frequently to prevent transmission. Treatment for infected eyes is usually with antibiotics.
Glaucoma	Caused by increased intraocular pressure (IOP) due to a malformation or malfunction of the eye's drainage structures. Pressure causes the optic nerve and retinal fibers to deteriorate resulting in a progressive, permanent loss of vision. It often appears as a person ages.	*Acute glaucoma*—extreme pain, blurred vision, a red eye and dilated pupil. Nausea and vomiting may also occur. *Chronic glaucoma*—there may be no symptoms except a gradual loss of peripheral vision over time and perhaps a dull pain.	Treating with eye drops; surgery may also be helpful.
Meningitis	Inflammation of the membranes surrounding the brain and spinal cord (meninges).	Sudden high fever, stiff neck, severe headache, confusion, no appetite, nausea/vomiting.	Vaccinations for infants and children according to age schedule; repeat vaccination for teenagers and young adults, particularly living in close quarters such as a dormitory; requires immediate medical care with intravenous antibiotics or antivirals as appropriate; rest, fluids, over-the-counter pain and fever medications.
Myopia/ Presbyopia	Nearsightedness/far-sightedness caused by variations in the shape of the eyeball.	Inability to see at a distance/inability to see up close.	Corrective lenses prescribed by an optometrist or ophthalmologist.

(continued)

368 Chapter 13 | Your Body and How It Functions

Table 13.14 Common Disorders, Symptoms, and Preventive Measures/ Treatment of the Nervous System (continued)

Condition	Disorder	Symptoms	Preventive Measures/ Treatment
Neuritis	Inflammation of a nerve caused by injury, malnutrition, alcoholism, or toxic poison.	Pain, numbness, muscle atrophy, change in reflexes.	Eliminating the cause of irritation if possible. Treatment may consist of pain medication, nerve block procedure, and physical therapy to maintain muscle.
Otitis media	Middle ear infection usually due to bacteria; occurs behind the eardrum.	Ear pain, tugging/pulling at an ear, loss of balance, fever, drainage from the ear, trouble hearing.	May require antibiotics, pain and fever medications; possible ear tube insertions with repeated infections.
Otosclerosis	Hereditary condition in which the bones in the ear change and sounds are not transmitted properly.	Tinnitus (ringing in the ear), then loss of hearing.	No known prevention; treating surgically may be helpful.
Parkinson's	A degenerative disorder of the central nervous system that often impairs the sufferer's motor skills and speech.	Affects movement (tremors, rigidity, instability, shuffling walk), mood, behavior, thinking, and sensation.	No cure at this time. Patient and family education, support group services, general wellness maintenance, physio-therapy, exercise, and nutrition. Medications (most commonly L-dopa) or surgery can provide relief from the symptoms.
Prebyopia	A vision condition in which the crystalline lens of your eye loses its flexibility, which makes it difficult for you to focus on close objects.	Difficulty reading fine print, particularly in low light conditions, eyestrain when reading for long periods, momentarily blurred vision when transitioning between viewing distances.	Not curable, but can be treated with corrective eyeglasses or contacts. New surgical procedures may also provide solutions for those who do not want to wear glasses or contacts, including implanting accommodative intraocular lenses (IOLs).
Presbycusis (deafness)	Loss of hearing that gradually occurs in most individuals as they grow older (usually greater for high-pitched sounds).	Sounds often seem less clear and lower in volume. The speech of others seems mumbled or slurred. High-pitched sounds such as "s" and "th" are difficult to hear and tell apart. Tinnitus (a ringing, roaring, or hissing sound in one or both ears) may occur.	Avoid damaging noises (firearms, lawnmowers, etc.). Use of earplugs or earmuffs can help prevent damage when using machinery. Hearing aids or assistive listening devices can provide further improvement. Training in speechreading can help.
Shingles or herpes zoster	Caused by a virus that can affect any sensory nerve but tends to invade nerves in the chest and head near the temple most often.	Many blisters appear on the skin over nerve routes and cause a great deal of pain. The blisters usually disappear in about a week, but the pain may recur for years afterward.	Treating with soothing creams to elieve itching, topical medications, and pain medications when necessary.

MEDICAL TERMINOLOGY

audiometer:	instrument to measure hearing	**lacrimal:**	pertaining to tear ducts
blepharitis:	inflammation of the eyelid	**ophthalmologist:**	specialist in the study of the eye
blepharorrhaphy:	suturing the eyelid	**otitismedia:**	inflammation of the middle ear
cerebrocular:	pertaining to the brain and eyes	**otoneurology:**	study of the ear and neural disorders
dacryadenitis:	inflammation of a tear duct	**otoplasty:**	plastic repair of cartilage of the ear
gustation:	sense of taste	**otorrhea:**	purulent discharge from the ear
iridocele:	hernia of the iris of the eye		
iridoplegia:	paralysis of the iris of the eye		

Your Body and How It Functions | Chapter 13 369

Teaching Tips

- Review the second part of Table 13.14 together.
- Pronounce the name of each condition out loud:
  - Parkinson's
  - Prebyopia
  - Presbycusis
  - Shingles, or herpes zoster
- Ask a student to read the description of each disorder.
- Discuss the symptoms of each.
- You may want to discuss why conditions of the inner ear affect balance.

MEDICAL TERMINOLOGY

Review the terminology:

- Pronounce each word element, and have students repeat.
- Pronounce each term, and have students repeat.
- Allow time for students to write down definitions.
- Select a student to read each definition.
- Assign students to memorize the terms and their definitions.

TEAMWORK

In small groups, prepare a skit demonstrating a common disorder of the nervous system. One student should be a patient, describing symptoms to a health care worker or a team of health care workers. The health care workers should diagnose the disorder, explain it, and prescribe a treatment.

Teaching Tips

- Begin a discussion about the jobs and professions that would be suitable for someone interested in the nervous system.
- Remind students to refer to Chapter 3 for more information on occupations.
- Discuss the skills and requirements for becoming a neurologist.
- Discuss neurological examinations. Have students identify procedures used for neuro exams.
- Discuss the skills and requirements for becoming an ophthalmologist.
- Discuss the skills and requirements for becoming an otologist.

Figure Focus

13.37 (on the next page) What skills and interests do you think might be necessary to become an otologist?

Student answers will vary.

Related Jobs and Professions

Neurologist

A neurologist is a physician who specializes in nervous system disorders. This includes diseases of the brain, spinal cord, nerves, muscles, and the blood vessels that relate to these structures. Neurologists examine the nerves of the head or neck and test muscle strength and movement. They see how well you move and balance. They test your reflexes. They also examine your sense of sensation, your memory, speech, language, and other cognitive abilities. They do many tests to complete these assessments, including CAT scans, MRIs, and spinal taps.

To become a neurologist, you must complete medical school followed by a one-year internship. At least eight months of that internship must be spent in internal medicine. Then, you must complete a three-year residency in neurology and pass an exam to become a certified neurologist. If you choose to pursue a specialty area, such as child neurology, clinical neurophysiology, or pain medicine, you must complete one to three years of additional training.

> **Neurological Examination**
> More than imaging technology and laboratory tests are needed to determine whether nerves are, or are not, functioning. A neurological examination makes that determination. A neuro exam is a noninvasive series of questions and tests. The exam is divided into sections: mental status; cranial nerves; motor system; sensory system; deep tendon reflexes, coordination, and gait.

Optical Professions

An opthalmologist is a medical doctor who specializes in the eye and the visual system. Their job is to diagnose and treat eye disease. They also treat eye injuries.

This may entail routine eye exams, diagnosis and treatment of eye disorders or diseases, prescribing eyeglasses or contact lenses, surgery, or managing problems caused by systemic illness.

To become an opthalmologist, you must complete college and medical school. That is followed by a one-year clinical internship and at least three years as a hospital resident in opthalmology. To specialize in a specific area, such as a disease, an eye part, or pediatrics, you must complete one or two years of additional training. Once training is complete, opthalmologists must pass an exam to become certified in this profession.

An optometrist examines the eyes and prescribes corrective lenses, such as glasses and contact lenses. They also diagnose and manage eye disease, disorders, and injuries. To become an optometrist, a college degree is required. In addition, a four-year doctor of optometry program of study must be completed. Each state requires that optometrists be licensed.

An opthalmic technologist or assistant may also be employed in an optometrist or ophthalmologist practice. The technician or assistant provides initial eye exams, such as glaucoma testing, and Snellen eye screening tests.

An optician helps to fit glasses and contact lens prescribed by the optometrist or ophthalmologist.

Otologist

An otologist, also known as a neurotologist, is a physician who specializes in conditions affecting the ears. (Figure 13.37) These conditions include problems with balance and dizziness, all types of hearing loss, noises in the ear, facial nerve disorders, persistent infections, congenital malformations of the ear, and tumors

370 Chapter 13 | Your Body and How It Functions

ACTIVITY

Make flashcards to use to learn the medical vocabulary associated with the nervous system.

TEAMWORK

Have students work in pairs to research the procedures of a neurological exam and practice performing neurological exams.

of the ear. Trained as a surgeon, an otologist performs surgical procedures such as the repair of eardrum perforations, hearing reconstruction, and tumor removal.

To become an otologist, you must attend medical school and then become a trained otorhinolaryngologist. An otorhinolaryngologist, commonly known as an ENT, specializes in problems associated with the ear, nose, throat, and neck.

To become an otorhinolaryngologist, you must complete medical school, one year of general surgery residency, and four years of otorhinolaryngology training. To specialize as an otologist, you must complete another residency in that area. All otologists must pass an exam in order to become board certified before practicing medicine.

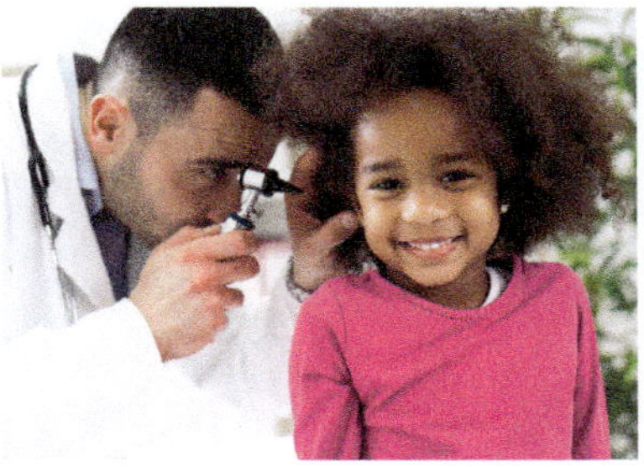

Figure 13.37 What skills and interests do you think might be necessary to become an otologist?

Otorhinolaryngologist

An otorhinolaryngologist is a physician/surgeon who specializes in head and neck surgery. Common ailments addressed include: head and neck cancer; tumors; sinus and allergic disease; thyroid and parathyroid problems; snoring and sleep apnea; and pediatric ear, nose, and throat issues.

An otorhinolaryngologist might perform open surgery on the salivary or thyroid glands or reconstructive surgery of the head or neck. Other possibilities include microsurgery of the middle ear, sinus surgery, or surgery at the base of the skull. To become an otorhinolaryngologist, you must complete medical school, one year of general surgery residency, and four years of otorhinolaryngology training.

Summary

In this section, you learned that the nervous system consists of two parts: the central nervous system and the peripheral nervous system. The central nervous system includes the brain and the spinal cord. The peripheral nervous system is made up of nerves that are outside of the brain and spinal cord.

Sensory organs allow you to detect outside stimuli. Sensory organs include the eyes, ears, nose, and tongue. General sense receptors are found throughout the body. Nervous system disorders can damage nerves or sensory organs. These disorders often interfere with the patient's ability to sense and react to outside stimuli.

Section 13.10 Review Questions

1. List and describe three disorders of the eye.
2. Which tactile corpuscles sense touch and pressure?
3. What four main tastes are detected by the taste buds?
4. Name the ossicles of the middle ear.
5. What structures are part of the peripheral nervous system?
6. Which part of the brain controls breathing and heartbeat?
7. What causes "Pink Eye" and how do you treat it?
8. What does a neurologist do and what education or training is required for this career?

Your Body and How It Functions | Chapter 13 371

Teaching Tips

- Discuss the skills and requirements for becoming an otorhinolaryngologist.
- Have the students break the word *otorhinolaryngologist* into its word elements.
- Review the parts of the nervous system.
- Review the influence of the nervous system on the body.
- Discuss the protective mechanisms that are built into the nervous system.
- Discuss how problems with the protective mechanisms can lead to illness, injury, or disease:
  - If the nerves of the central nervous system in the neck did not exist, would you feel something burning your leg?
  - If there was no blood flow to the medulla, how would the body respond to sensory messages?
  - If there was no blood flow to the optic nerve, would you be able to see?
  - If the ossicle of the middle ear were scarred by infection, would you be able to hear?
- Discuss reasons why it is important for all health care workers to have a basic knowledge of the nervous system and how it functions.
- Remind students of the importance of responding appropriately when a medical emergency occurs.
- For example, who might need to recognize and respond to the symptoms of a stroke?

Section 13.10 Review Questions

1. Answer: Cataract: occurs when the lens of the eye loses its transparency; Conjuntivitis/pink eye: inflammation of the eyelid lining caused from bacteria or irritation from dirt in the eye; Glaucoma: caused by intraocular pressure resulting either from a malformation or malfunction of the eye's drainage structures.
2. Answer: Pressure is sensed by the pressure receptors in the subcutaneous tissue layer beneath the skin. Touch is sense by receptors called tactile corpuscles and they are found in the dermis of the skin.
3. Answer: Sweet, salty, sour, and bitter
4. Answer: Malleus, incus, stapes
5. Answer: The peripheral nervous system includes the nerves and ganglia outside the brain and spinal cord. There are 12 pairs of cranial nerves, 31 pairs of spinal nerves, and various nerve branches in body organs.
6. Answer: Medulla
7. Answer: Inflammation of the eyelid lining caused from bacteria or irritation from dirt in the eye. Treated with antibiotics.

ACTIVITY

Select one of the jobs or professions listed in Section 13.10. Create a brochure or pamphlet explaining why the health care worker you selected needs a basic knowledge of the nervous system in order to perform his or her job effectively.

8. Answer: A neurologist is a physician who specializes in nervous system disorders. This includes diseases of the brain, spinal cord, nerves, muscles, and the blood vessels that relate to these structures. To become a neurologist, you must complete medical school followed by a one-year internship. At least eight months of that internship must be spent in internal medicine. Then, you must complete a three-year residency in neurology and pass an exam to become a certified neurologist.

FOCUS AND ENGAGE

Introduce the Section

a. Review the content of the Background paragraph, explaining that reproduction is the way that animals, plants, and other organisms make offsprings or new versions of themselves.
b. Emphasize that reproduction is controlled by hormones and remind students that the endocrine system controls hormones.
c. Review the objectives for the section.

Vocabulary Review

a. Direct students to the key terms.
b. Pronounce each word, and have the students repeat the pronunciation out loud.
c. Discuss the definition of each word.

TEACH

Discuss

- Ask students to share stories about family members, friends, or even pets, reproducing—having babies.

SECTION 13.11 The Reproductive System

Background

The reproductive system allows humans to reproduce. This system produces sex cells that unite to form a fertilized egg that can develop into offspring. The reproductive system is controlled by hormones. This system usually becomes active during the teenage years. As a health care worker, you should be familiar with this system in order to monitor pregnant patients and prevent or treat reproductive disorders.

Objectives

When you have completed this section, you will be able to do the following:

- Match key terms with their correct meanings.
- Label a diagram of the male and female reproductive systems.
- Match the various organs in the reproductive systems with their functions.
- Match common disorders of the reproductive system with their descriptions.
- Describe how the reproductive system affects the body.
- Explain why the health care worker's understanding of the reproductive system is important.

Introduction to the Reproductive System

Reproduction occurs in all species. Tiny one-celled organisms divide or separate by themselves to reproduce. Most animals require a male and female, each with their own special cells that unite to reproduce. The male and female reproductive systems have several characteristics in common. They are gonads, tubes that carry secretions, and exocrine glands.

- *Gonads* (endocrine glands) or sex glands in the male are called *testes*, and they produce sperm (male gamete). In the female they are called *ovaries*, and they produce ova (female gamete).
- The *tubes* form passageways for the **sex cells**, sperm and ova.

sex cells
(SEX sel)
Cells that allow reproduction to occur; also called gamete.

fetus
(FEE tus)
Infant developing in the uterus after the first three months until birth.

The Female Reproductive System

The main function of the female reproductive system is to produce the ovum for fertilization and to house a developing **fetus**. Reproduction occurs when the male and female sex cells unite within the female. After the union of these cells, the fertilized egg divides and grows for 9 months or 40 weeks and develops into a new individual. Look at Figure 13.38 to identify parts of the female reproductive system.

372 Chapter 13 | Your Body and How It Functions

- Explain that without reproduction, species would cease to exist.
- Emphasize that reproduction occurs in all life, not just humans or animals.
- Discuss different types of reproduction, such as budding on plants, fission in bacteria, and regeneration in starfish.

Reinforce and Review

- Review the information in Section 13.1: cells, tissues, organs, cavities, and body directions.
- Review the information in Section 13.9, The Endocrine Systems.

CUSTOMIZED INSTRUCTION

More Advanced Students

Assign more advanced students a research project comparing different types of reproduction. They might write a report or create a presentation that they can deliver to the class.

- *Female gonads*, the ovaries, are small oval-shaped structures that produce the female sex cells or *ova* and the hormone called **estrogen**. Approximately every 28 days an ovum **matures** and is forced from the ovary and received by the fallopian tube.
- *Fallopian tubes* are muscular tubes about five inches long. The tubes do not connect to the ovaries. When the **ovum** is forced from the ovary into the peritoneal cavity, it floats in the peritoneal fluid. At the end of each fallopian tube, fingerlike projections called fimbriae create a current that sweeps the ovum into the tube.
- Once inside the tube, the ovum is swept forward by small cilia and by peristalsis. The ovum takes about five days to move through the fallopian tube and is then deposited into the uterus.
- The *uterus*, a pear-shaped organ, is attached to the fallopian tubes. While the ovum is maturing, the uterus begins to build an interlining called the **endometrium**. If the ovum is not fertilized in the fallopian tube, it deteriorates shortly after entering the uterus. The endometrium then deteriorates, causing bleeding or **menstruation**. The main function of the uterus is to house and nourish the fertilized ovum until delivery of a fully developed fetus.
- The *vagina* is a muscular tube that houses the neck of the uterus or *cervix*. This tube extends approximately three inches to the outside of the body. The vagina is also known as the birth canal.

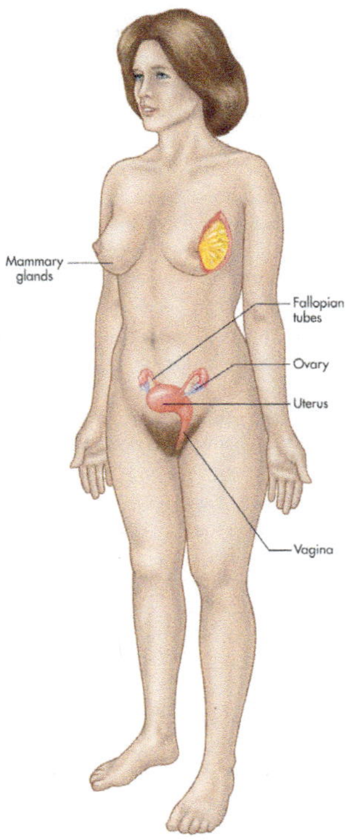

Figure 13.38
Where are the female sex cells (ova) produced?

estrogen
(ESS tro jen)
Female hormone.

matures
(me TCHOOR)
Becomes fully developed.

ovum
(OH vum)
Female reproductive cell that when fertilized by the male develops into a new organism.

endometrium
(en doh MEE tree um)
Interlining of the uterus.

menstruation
(men stroo AY shun)
Cyclic deterioration of the endometrium.

Apply It

Divide into small groups. Each group will create a set of game cards that include answers to specific categories and questions (like on "Jeopardy"), such as female reproductive organs, male reproductive organs, diseases, etc. One student on each team will be the category giver and will read the category to their team. The team can answer as many questions as they can in an allotted time period (i.e., one minute). Teams will get one point for each correct answer. The team with the most points wins.

Your Body and How It Functions | Chapter 13 373

Teaching Tips

- Emphasize that all organisms must reproduce, or they will cease to exist.
- Explain that most animals require a male and a female to reproduce.
- Point out that, for the most part, males and females have different reproductive systems, but that they do share some common characteristics:
  - Gonads (endocrine glands): testes in males and ovaries in females
  - Tubes: passageways for the ova in females and sperm in males
  - Exocrine glands
- Describe the organs of the female reproductive system:
  - Female gonads: ovaries produce female sex cells, called ova
  - Fallopian tubes: help guide ova to uterus
  - Uterus: organ that houses and nourishes fertilized ovum
  - Vagina: muscular tube also called birth canal

Figure Focus

13.38 Where are the female sex cells (ova) produced?

Answer: In the ovaries

Apply It

- Divide the class into two or three teams for this activity.
- You might want to provide the categories, and allow each team to think up five or six questions for each category.
- Set up the game like the game show "Jeopardy." Students pick a category, and the other team reads one of its questions from that category. If the first team answers correctly, they continue. If not, the other team has a turn.

Teaching Tips

- Describe the organs of the male reproductive system:
  - Male gonads: testes produce male sex cells, called sperm
  - Penis: primary male sex organ
  - Epididymis: tube where sperm are stored
  - Vas deferens: passageway for sperm
  - Seminal vesicles: pouches produce secretion to protect and nourish sperm
  - Prostate gland: produce secretion to maintain mobility of sperm
  - Ejaculatory duct: carries sperm through the prostate gland to the urethra
  - Urethra: passage for urine and sperm, through the prostate gland and the penis to the outside of the body

Figure Focus

13.39 Which tube connects to the epididymis and provides a passageway for sperm?

Answer: The vas deferens

The Male Reproductive System

spermatozoa
(spur mat uh ZOH uh)
Male sex cells.

testosterone
(tess TOSS ter own)
Male hormone.

semen
(SEE mun)
Fluid from the testes, seminal vesicles, prostate gland, and bulbourethral glands. Contains water, mucin, proteins, salts, and sperm.

- *Male gonads* or testes are found outside the body, between the legs, in a sac called the *scrotum*. The testes produce the male sex cells or **spermatozoa** (or *sperm*) and the hormone **testosterone**. The *penis* is the primary male sex organ. It lies anterior to the testes. (**Figure 13.39**)
- The *epididymis* is a 20-foot-long tube that is coiled inside the scrotal sac. Sperm are stored here until they mature and are able to move by themselves. As the epididymis extends upward, it becomes the vas deferens.
- The *vas deferens*, the spermatic cord, extends through the abdominal wall and curves over and behind the urinary bladder. It functions as a passageway for sperm.
- *Seminal vesicles* are outpouchings at the end of the vas deferens. They produce a thick yellow secretion that adds to the volume of **semen** and nourishes the sperm.
- The *prostate gland*, located just below the urinary bladder, produces a secretion that maintains mobility of sperm. The *ejaculatory duct* carries sperm from the junction of the vas deferens and the seminal vesicles through the prostate gland and connects to the urethra.

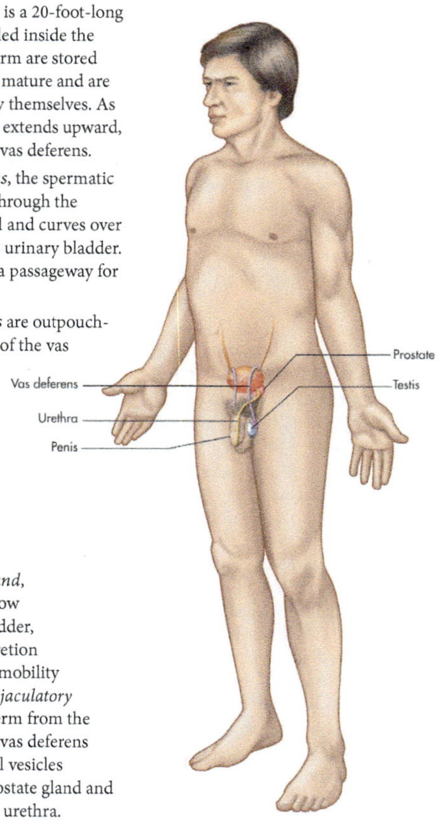

Figure 13.39
Which tube connects to the epididymis and provides a passageway for sperm?

- The *urethra* is a small passage for urine and sperm, and leads from the urinary bladder through the prostate gland and the penis to the outside of the body.

Common Disorders of the Reproductive System

Table 13.15 Common Disorders, Symptoms, and Preventive Measures/ Treatment of the Reproductive System

Condition	Disorder	Symptoms	Preventive Measures/ Treatment
Benign prostatic hyperplasia	Enlarged prostate that is non-cancerous.	Frequent urination, enlarged prostate, difficulty starting urination, urinary dribbling.	Monitoring of the condition, medications, laser surgeries.
Breast cancer	Cancer of the glandular breast tissue. Fifth most common cause of cancer death worldwide. Can occur in men (but rarely) as well as women.	Breast cancer symptoms vary widely—from lumps to swelling to skin changes. Many breast cancers have no obvious symptoms at all. Symptoms that are similar to those of breast cancer may be the result of non-cancerous conditions like infection or a cyst.	Monthly self exams and annual mammograms help early detection. Biopsies are used to confirm the diagnosis. Once detected, may be treated with surgery (lumpectomy, mastectomy, and lymph node dissection), then perhaps radiation, hormonal (anti-estrogen) therapy, and/or chemotherapy.
Cervical cancer	Cancer of the bottom portion of the uterus, the cervix.	Vaginal bleeding and/or discharge, pelvic pain during intercourse.	Regular PAP smears; surgery to remove cancer and/or cervix.
Cryptorchidism	Means "hidden testes." Also called undescended testes.	One or both testes fail to descend into the scrotum.	Administering hormone injections if the testicle does not descend into the scrotum by the age of one year. If this treatment is unsuccessful by the age of five years, surgery is performed to locate the testicle and place it in the scrotum or remove it.
Endometriosis	Painful disorder resulting from overgrowth of the lining of the uterus.	Cramps, painful intercourse, excessive vaginal bleeding, painful periods.	Pain medications, hormone therapy, surgery.
Fibroid tumors	Common in women over the age of 50. They are usually benign.	There may be breakthrough bleeding between menstrual cycles and pressure from the tumor may cause frequent urination. There are often no symptoms.	Physician will monitor size and growth and determine if surgical removal is necessary.
Impotence (Erectile Dysfunction)	The consistent inability to obtain or maintain an erection of sufficient quality for satisfactory sexual intercourse.	Risk increases with age. Can range from a total inability to achieve an erection or ejaculation, an inconsistent ability to do so, or a tendency to sustain only brief erections.	Healthier lifestyle, healthy diet, drink less and exercise more. Oral medications are available. In severe cases, patient may consider penile injections, or implants.
Premenstrual syndrome	Collection of symptoms preceding the onset of menstruation.	Cramps, joint pain, headache, tension, anxiety, insomnia, mood swings	Nonsteroidal anti-inflammatory drugs, diuretics, hormones.

(continued)

Your Body and How It Functions | Chapter 13 375

Teaching Tips

- Compare the organs of the male and female reproductive systems:
  - Point out common characteristics.
  - Point out differences.
- Explain how common disorders of the reproductive system affect the body.
- Review the first part of Table 13.15 together.
- Pronounce the name of each condition out loud:
  - Breast cancer
  - Cryptorchidism
  - Fibroid tumors
  - Impotence (erectile dysfunction)
  - Prostate cancer
  - Sexually transmitted disease (STD)
- Ask a student to read the description of each disorder.
- Discuss the symptoms of each.

TEAMWORK

In small groups, prepare a skit demonstrating a common disorder of the reproductive system. One student should be a patient, describing symptoms to a health care worker or a team of health care workers. The health care workers should diagnose the disorder, explain it, and prescribe a treatment.

Teaching Tips

- Review the second part of Table 13.15 and the end of the table on p. 377 together.
- Pronounce the name of each condition out loud:
  - Acquired Immune deficiency syndrome (AIDS)
  - Chlamydia
  - Gonorrhea
  - Human Papilloma Virus (HPV)
  - Syphilis
  - Testicular cancer
- Ask a student to read the description of each disorder.
- Discuss the symptoms of each.
- Note that the conditions following the item Sexually transmitted diseases (STDs) are examples of specific STDs.
- Describe how the reproductive system affects the body.
- Discuss how hormones affect the body:
  - Appearance
  - Stages of life, such as puberty and menopause
  - Pregnancy
- Discuss organs that are part of different systems that might be affected by the reproductive system:
  - The urinary system
  - The endocrine system
- Remind students that preventative care is part of a healthy lifestyle. Screenings for diseases, such as breast cancer and testicular cancer, can improve the success of treatment and recovery. Discuss the procedures of a breast exam and a testicular exam.

Table 13.15 Common Disorders, Symptoms, and Preventive Measures/Treatment of the Reproductive System (continued)

Condition	Disorder	Symptoms	Preventive Measures/ Treatment
Prostate cancer	Cancer that forms in tissues of the prostate; usually occurs in older men.	May have little or no symptoms in early stages. Trouble passing urine; may gradually lose control of bladder function. A weak or interrupted stream of urine, an urgency to urinate, leaking or dribbling, and more often needing to urinate during the night. Difficulty in having an erection; painful ejaculation; blood in urine or semen.	Annual physical; physical (with attention to any enlargement of prostate); DRE and PSA tests can signal problems; biopsy to confirm. Slow growing so may watch and moniter at first. Treatment may include surgery, radiation therapy, hormone therapy, chemotherapy and other emerging treatments.
Sexually transmitted diseases/ infections (STDs/STIs)	Affect both male and female. The most common sexually transmitted diseases are acquired immune deficiency syndrome (AIDS), chlamydia, gonorrhea, and syphilis (see each that follow).	Symptoms vary as noted below.	For prevention, practice abstinence or use a protective barrier such as a condom during sex, and maintain **monogamous** relationships with uninfected partners. Some treatment options are listed below.
	Acquired immune deficiency syndrome (AIDS): AIDS is most commonly transmitted by sexual contact. It is a contagious disease that causes severe illness and often results in death. The AIDS virus enters the blood of a person from the blood or body fluids of a carrier.	Symptoms include swollen lymph glands, diarrhea, night sweats, abnormal or unusual bleeding, fungal infection of the mouth and throat, loss of memory, fatigue, extreme weight loss, and constant cough. All or some of these symptoms may be present.	Although research is making great strides toward finding a cure, there is no successful treatment that cures AIDS. There are some medications and lifestyle changes that help individuals maintain a fairly healthy state for long periods.
	Chlamydia: A contagious bacterium, Chlamydia trachomatis, that lives in the conjunctiva of the eye and in the urethra and cervix of the uterus.	Purulent discharge from the urethra in the male or the vagina in the female.	Treating with antibiotics.
	Gonorrhea: A contagious bacterium, Neisseria gonorrhoeae, that affects the genitourinary tract and occasionally the pharynx, conjunctiva, or rectum.	Urethritis, dysuria, purulent greenish-yellow urethral or vaginal discharge, red or swollen urethral meatus, itching, burning or pain around the vaginal or urethral opening.	Treating with antibiotics.
	Human Papilloma Virus (HPV): Transmitted through direct contact and causes genital warts and cervical cancer.	Cervical cancer symptoms include abnormal vaginal bleeding, pain in the pelvis or lower abdomen.	Vaccination is strongly recommended in addition to abstinence, decreased number of sexual partners, and protective barriers. Pap smears and pelvic exams are recommended for detection and treatment which includes cryotherapy, LEEP (Loop Electrosurgical Excision Procedure), and hysterectomies.

(continued)

376 Chapter 13 | Your Body and How It Functions

ACTIVITY

Use models in a lab to have students perform a testicular exam and a breast exam.

Table 13.15 Common Disorders, Symptoms, and Preventive Measures/Treatment of the Reproductive System (continued)

Condition	Disorder	Symptoms	Preventive Measures/ Treatment
STDs/STIs *(cont)*	*Syphilis:* Caused by a spirochete transmitted through sexual contact. It can affect any organ or system of the body. The spirochete is able to pass through the human placenta causing congenital syphilis in a newborn infant.	First stage—small, painless red pustule on the skin or mucous membrane (is contagious). Second stage—approximately two months later, generalized malaise, anorexia, nausea, fever, headache, loss of hair, bone and joint pain, skin rash that does not itch, sores in the mouth (remains contagious). Third stage—may not develop for many years. Appearance of soft, rubbery tumors that may cause a deep burrowing pain. Tumors may appear in any organ or system in the body.	Treating with antibiotics.
Testicular cancer	Cancer that occurs in the testes, located inside the scrotum. Compared with other cancers, relatively rare, but the most common cancer in younger males between the ages of 15 and 35.	There may be no symptoms. Discomfort or pain in the testicle or a feeling of heaviness in the scrotum. Enlargement of a testicle or a change in how it feels. Excess development of breast tissue (this may be normal in adolescent boys who do not have testicular cancer). Lump or swelling in either testicle.	Monthly self exams (there is no known effective screening technique, so none is recommended). Once detected, may be treated with surgery to remove the testicle, radiation, or chemotherapy; one of the most treatable and curable cancers.

monogamous
(mun OG ah mus)
Having a sexual relationship with only one partner during a period of time.

MEDICAL TERMINOLOGY

amenorrhea:	scant or no menstruation	**mammectomy:**	surgical removal of breast (or mastectomy) tissue
cervicitis:	inflammation of the cervix	**mastalgia:**	pain in the breast
colpectasis:	dilation of the vagina	**menorrhagia:**	excessive menstrual flow
colpoplasty:	plastic surgery on the vagina	**metrorrhexis:**	rupture of the uterus
dysmenorrhea:	painful or difficult menstruation	**oophorocystectomy:**	removal of an ovarian cyst
ectopic pregnancy:	pregnancy outside the uterus	**orchiopexy:**	fixation of the testes in the scrotum
gonorrhea:	flow from the genitals caused by infection	**orchioplasty:**	plastic surgery of the testes
gynecomastia:	abnormal enlargement of one or both breasts in men	**orchitis:**	inflammation of the testes
hysterectomy:	removal of uterus	**phimosis:**	refers to a tightness of the foreskin over the end of the penis
hystersalping oophorectomy:	removal of the uterus, fallopian tubes, and ovaries	**prenatal:**	occurring before birth
insemination:	injection of semen into the female reproductive system	**postnatal:**	occurring after birth
lactation:	secretion of milk from the breast	**sterile:**	unable to produce young
leukorrhea:	whitish vaginal discharge	**tubal ligation:**	procedure in which fallopian tubes are blocked
		vasectomy:	procedure for male sterilization

Language Arts Link—Career Study

- You may want to provide a list of resources such as Web sites or local facilities that students can use to research information about the career path they select.
- Also, remind them that the information in Chapter 3 is a good place to start.
- Remind students about your school's Internet policy and emphasize that they should use reputable Web resources.
- Remind them to keep a list of sources to use for a bibliography.
- If students do not have access to the Internet, be sure to direct them to other resources.
- For evaluation, you should verify that the information is correct, and you should mark spelling and grammatical errors.

MEDICAL TERMINOLOGY

Review the terminology:

- Pronounce each word element, and have students repeat.
- Pronounce each term, and have students repeat.
- Allow time for students to write down definitions.
- Select a student to read each definition.
- Assign students to memorize the terms and their definitions.

CUSTOMIZED INSTRUCTION

English Language Learners

Some English Language Learners may be uncomfortable presenting their report to the entire class. Allow them the option to share it with a small group or a partner.

ACTIVITY

Make flashcards for the terms associated with the reproductive system. Use the flashcards to study and memorize the terms and their definitions.

Teaching Tips

- Begin a discussion about the jobs and professions that would be suitable for someone interested in the reproductive system.
- Remind students to refer to Chapter 3 for more information on occupations.
- Discuss the skills and requirements for becoming an embryologist.
- You may want to introduce a discussion of the ethical questions involved with embryonic medicine.
- You may want to discuss infertility, and some of the treatments or measures available.
- Discuss the skills and requirements for becoming a gynecologist.
- Discuss the skills and requirements for becoming an obstetrician.
- Emphasize that many obstetricians are also gynecologists—called OB/GYN.

Related Jobs and Professions

Embryologist

Embryologists study the early growth and formation of life. Clinical embryologists work with human embryos. They study the stages of pregnancy and watch how embryos grow and change day by day. Many embryologists work in infertility clinics. They help infertile couples have children. To do this, they collect eggs and sperm from patients for examination and they check fertility levels. Sometimes, they prepare egg and sperm samples for in vitro fertilization.

Other times, an embryologist will combine the egg and sperm so that it grows into an embryo, which can be preserved and implanted at a later date. Embryologists may also study abnormalities in embryos. Their goal is to discover why abnormalities occur and how they may be prevented.

Embryologists are highly trained in advanced laboratory techniques. They may work in hospitals, clinics, laboratories, or for a government agency, pharmaceutical company or biotechnology firm.

The minimum requirement for this position is a four-year bachelor's degree in embryology, microbiology, or biochemistry. You must also have a background in genetics. This will qualify you to be a laboratory assistant or technician. To become a senior researcher, you must have a master's degree or a Ph.D.

Gynecologist

Gynecologists are physicians who specialize in the female organs and reproductive system. They manage hormonal disorders, treat infections, perform pap smears, diagnose cancers of the reproductive system, and perform operations such as hysterectomies. Much of a gynecologist's work is to perform routine check-ups so that serious problems do not occur. Some gynecologists specialize in a specific area such as critical care medicine, gynecologic oncology, or reproductive endocrinology.

To become a gynecologist, you must graduate from college and medical school. You must then complete a four-year gynecology residency and two years of clinical practice. One to three additional years of training is required if you decide to pursue a specialty area. All gynecologists must pass an exam to become certified before practicing medicine.

Obstetrician

An obstetrician is a physician who cares for women throughout childbirth. Some of their patients are women who are having complications during pregnancy. Obstetricians closely monitor the mother's health and diagnose any abnormalities or health issues in the developing fetus. If an issue does arise, the obstetrician may refer the mother to a specialist for treatment.

Many doctors who become obstetricians also train as gynecologists. To become an obstetrician, you must complete college and medical school. You must also complete a four-year residency specializing in obstetrics and gynecology and two

378 Chapter 13 | Your Body and How It Functions

ACTIVITY

Select one of the jobs or professions listed in Section 13.11. Create a brochure or pamphlet explaining why the health care worker you selected needs a basic knowledge of the reproductive system in order to perform his or her job effectively.

more years of clinical practice. One to three more years of training is required for those who pursue an area of specialization. All obstetricians must also pass a national examination to become certified to practice in this field.

Midwife

Midwives are trained medical professionals who care for and support women throughout normal pregnancies. (Figure 13.40) This care extends from the onset of pregnancy to just after delivery. Midwives stress communication with the mother and provide individualized health care information, emotional and social support, and continuous hands-on assistance during labor and delivery. If any problems arise, the midwife does not deliver the baby but calls for an obstetrician.

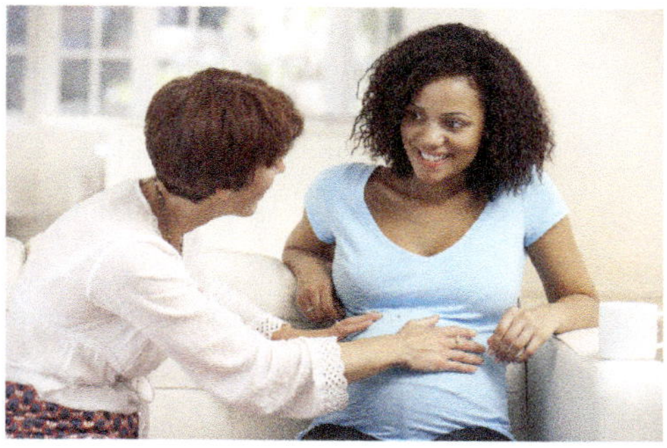

Figure 13.40
What skills and interests do you think might be necessary to become a midwife?

There are two types of midwives in the United States: direct-entry midwives and nurse-midwives. Direct-entry midwives are not nurses. However, they have at least a bachelor's degree, have completed specific health science courses, graduated from an accredited midwifery education program, and have passed a national exam to become certified. Nurse-midwives are registered nurses who have completed an accredited midwifery program and passed an exam to become certified.

Summary

In this section, you learned that male and female reproductive systems have different structures and produce different hormones. However, both systems produce sex cells. You also learned about disorders of the reproductive system. These disorders include cryptorchidism, fibroid tumors, and sexually transmitted diseases, such as AIDS and syphilis. As a health care worker, you can help patients to avoid sexually transmitted diseases by suggesting lifestyle and behavioral changes.

Section 13.11 Review Questions

1. How are the male testes similar to the female ovaries?
2. Describe how a mature egg gets to the uterus.
3. What do the seminal vesicles do?
4. Which sexually transmitted diseases can be treated with antibiotics?
5. What are the symptoms of fibroid tumors?
6. What two professions deal with childbirth and how do these professions differ?

Teaching Tips

- Discuss the skills and requirements for becoming a midwife.
- Point out that midwives are sometimes considered part of alternative medicine (refer to Chapter 7).
- Review the function of each organ in the reproductive system.
- Discuss outside influences that might affect the reproductive system, such as smoking, nutrition, and environmental factors.
- Review problems that might arise in the reproductive system cannot function.
- Discuss reasons why it is important for all health care workers to have a basic knowledge of the reproductive system and how it functions.
- Review the need for health care workers in all positions to use proper medical terminology to communicate with others.
- For example, ask students to consider what it means when a person says "I'm having a hot flash."
- Review the importance of responding appropriately when a medical emergency occurs.

Figure Focus

13.40 What skills and interests do you think might be necessary to become a midwife?

Student answers will vary.

Section 13.11 Review Questions

1. Answer: The male and female reproductive systems have several characteristics in common. They are gonads, tubes that carry secretions, and exocrine glands.
2. Answer: A mature egg (ovum) is received by the fallopian tubes. When the ovum is forced from the ovary into the peritoneal cavity, it floats in the peritoneal fluid. At the end of each fallopian tube, fingerlike projections called fimbriae create a current that sweeps the ovum into the tube. Once inside the tube, the ovum is swept forward by small cilia and by peristalsis. The ovum takes about five days to move through the fallopian tube and is then deposited into the uterus.
3. Answer: Seminal vesicles are outpouchings at the end of the vas deferens. They produce a thick yellow secretion that adds to the volume of semen and nourishes the sperm.
4. Answer: Chlamydia, gonorrhea, and syphilis can be treated with antibiotics.

5. Answer: Breakthrough bleeding between menstrual cycles and pressure from the tumor may cause increased urination.
6. Answer: An obstetrician is a physician who cares for women throughout childbirth. Some of their patients are women who are having complications during pregnancy. Obstetricians closely monitor the mother's health and diagnose any abnormalities or health issues in the developing fetus. Midwives are trained medical professionals who care for and support women throughout normal pregnancies. This care extends from the onset of pregnancy to just after delivery. Midwives stress communication with the mother and provide individualized health care information, emotional and social support, and continuous hands-on assistance during labor and delivery. If any problems arise, the midwife does not deliver the baby but calls for an obstetrician.

TEAMWORK

Divide the class into teams of 8 to 12 students. Play a game of Hangman, using the terms covered in Section 13.11.

SECTION 13.12 The Integumentary System

Background

In this section, you will learn about the integumentary system, which is commonly known as the skin. This system forms a protective barrier around the organs of the body. It keeps out pathogens and prevents injury to internal organs. It helps to regulate body temperature and eliminates wastes through sweat glands.

The integumentary system also senses stimuli, which allows the body to react to changing environmental conditions. As a health care worker, you should know the structure and functions of the integumentary system in order to treat disorders that may damage skin and make the body more vulnerable to injury or disease.

Objectives

When you have completed this section, you will be able to do the following:

- Match key terms with their correct meanings.
- Label a diagram of a cross section of skin.
- List the five main functions of skin.
- Identify three main layers of the skin.
- Match common disorders of the integumentary system with their descriptions.
- Describe how the integumentary system protects the body.
- Explain why the health care worker's understanding of the integumentary system is important.

Introduction to the Integumentary System

The skin is the body's largest organ and is the first line of defense against infection. It contains several kinds of tissue, including epithelial, connective, and nerve tissues. This comprises skin, hair, and nails. It also contains sweat and oil glands. The combination of these tissues and glands works together as the integumentary system. (**Figure 13.41**) The main functions of the skin are to:

- Protect the underlying body parts from injury and the invasion of pathogens and UV light
- Regulate body temperature by controlling the loss of body heat
- Eliminate wastes through perspiration
- Store energy in the form of fat and vitamins
- Sense touch, heat, cold, pain, and pressure through receptors
- Produce vitamin D

380 Chapter 13 | Your Body and How It Functions

FOCUS AND ENGAGE

Introduce the Section

a. Review the Background paragraphs, emphasizing that the integumentary system is the skin.
b. Explain that the skin is a protective barrier for the body.
c. Review the objectives for the section.

Vocabulary Review

a. Direct students to the key terms.
b. Pronounce each word, and have the students repeat the pronunciation aloud.
c. Discuss the definition of each word.

TEACH

Discuss

- Students are likely to not consider the skin a "system" or an organ.
- Explain that it is both.
- Discuss the purpose of the skin, and what the body would be like without skin.

Reinforce and Review

- Review the information in Section 13.1: cells, tissues, organs, cavities, and body directions.

ACTIVITY

The skin has some unique features, such as the ability to regenerate and to change color. Use reference books and the Internet to learn interesting and unusual facts about the skin and other parts of the integumentary system. Make a list and share it with the class.

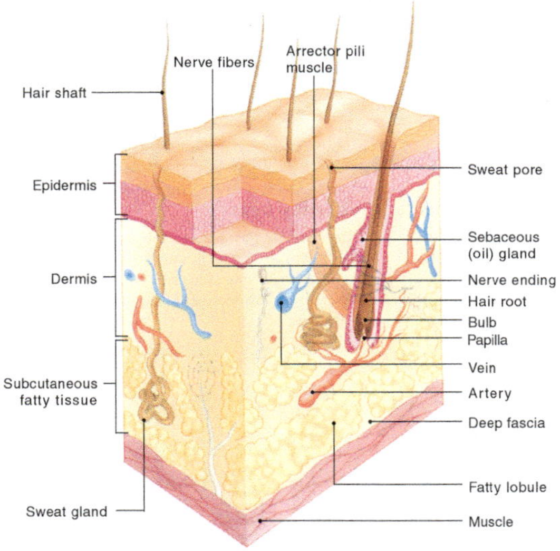

Figure 13.41
Cross section of the integumentary system (skin). What are the glands in the skin?

Apply It

Research a skin disease. You need to know the signs and symptoms for the disease. When you come to class, you must create that disease on a small part of your skin.

Your teacher will assign each of you a patient number. Interview and examine patients (classmates). After writing down the signs and symptoms, come up with the diagnosis and correct treatment. Take a picture of the disease for a medical file.

Structure of the Skin

Skin is made up of three main layers:

- The **epidermis** is the outermost layer and has no blood vessels. These cells are constantly **sloughed** off.
- The *dermis* is just beneath the epidermis and contains many blood vessels. New cells are continually forming to replace those lost from the epidermis. These cells come from the stratum germinativum layer of the epidermis.
- *Subcutaneous* means "under the skin," and this layer connects the skin to muscle.

As noted above, the integumentary system also includes hair, nails, and cutaneous glands. Hair is an outgrowth of protein; it projects from the epidermis, though it grows from hair follicles deep in the dermis. Nails, which are made of a tough protein called keratin, are produced from living skin cells in the fingers and toes. Cutaneous glands include:

- Sweat glands, that excrete sweat to regulate temperature
- Sebaceous glands, oil-producing glands that keep skin and hair moist and soft
- Ceruminous glands, located in the ear canal that produce earwax
- Mammary glands, the milk-producing glands located in the breasts

epidermis
(ep ih DER mus)
Outer layer of skin.

sloughed
(SLUFFED)
Discarded; separated from (e.g., to shed dead cells, as from the outer skin).

Career Connect

Research specialties in which the health care professional limits their expertise to the specific body systems, such as a Physical Therapist who works with the Skeletal and Muscular Systems.

Choose three different specialties and identify the professions that work in those fields. Which appeals to you and why?

ACTIVITY

Have students create a poster or chart that identifies the parts of a cross section of skin. Include the name of the part, its location, and a description of the function it serves in the integumentary system.

Career Connect

- This activity may be done in small groups or individually.
- To facilitate the activity, assign each student or teams of student a different body system.
- Have each student or team identify at least one specialty that limits its practice to the assigned system.

Teaching Tips

- Explain that the skin is the body's largest organ.
- Emphasize that it is the body's first line of defense against infection.
- Point out that the integumentary system includes more than just the skin:
  - Skin
  - Hair
  - Nails
  - Sweat and oil glands
- Explain the main functions of the integumentary system:
  - Protection
  - Regulate body temperature
  - Eliminate waste through sweat
  - Store energy
  - Sense touch, heat, cold, pain, and pressure
  - Produce vitamin D
- Describe the parts of the cross section of skin.

Figure Focus

13.41 Cross section of the integumentary system (skin). What are the glands in the skin?

Answer: Sweat glands and sebaceous glands

Apply It

- Allow enough time to complete this activity. The first part should be completed by the student outside of class, including the research. The rest should be completed in class.
- If you cannot photograph the disease model, have the students draw it.
- Remind students how to use a number to identify a patient and file records.
- Remind students how to record information.
- Emphasize that students must be prepared to diagnose and identify all disorders of the skin, not just the one they are assigned.

What's New?—Artificial Skin

- Discuss the composition of artificial skin.
- Discuss how artificial skin is used, and how it can save lives.

Which part of the skin is permanently replaced by the artificial skin and which part is only temporarily replaced?

Answer: The dermis is permanently replaced by the artificial skin. The epidermis is temporarily replaced until sections of the patient's own epidermis can be grafted to the artificial dermis.

Teaching Tips

- Explain how common disorders of the integumentary system affect the body.
- Review the first part of Table 13.16, and the end of the table on p. 383 together as a class.
- Pronounce the name of each condition out loud:
  - Athlete's foot (tinea pedis)
  - Atopic dermatitis or eczema
  - Boils (furuncle)
  - Skin cancer
- Ask a student to read the description of each disorder.
- Discuss the symptoms of each.
- Review the three types of skin cancer in more detail:
  - Basal cell carcinoma (BCC)
  - Squamous cell carcinoma (SCC)
  - Malignant melanoma

What's New?

Artificial Skin

Third-degree, or full-thickness, burns are the worst kinds of burns. They destroy the deepest layers of skin tissue and make patients vulnerable to infections. Not long ago, if a patient had third-degree burns over more than half of his or her body, that patient had nearly no chance of survival.

Now, a new technology has significantly increased those odds to a 60 percent survival rate. The technology is a permanent, artificial skin. This skin has a dermal replacement layer composed of collagen derived from cow tendons and substances derived from shark cartilage. It also has a temporary epidermal replacement layer made of silicone. About a week after the artificial skin is implanted, blood vessels and proteins start to grow within the dermal layer.

After two or more weeks, the silicone epidermal layer can be removed and replaced with a small graft of the patient's own epidermis. After a month or more, the skin graft looks similar to normal skin.

Which part of the skin is permanently replaced by the artificial skin and which part is only temporarily replaced?

Common Disorders of the Integumentary System

Table 13.16 Common Disorders, Symptoms, and Preventive Measures/Treatment of the Integumentary System

Condition	Disorder	Symptoms	Preventive Measures/ Treatment
Acne	Hair follicles are plugged with dead cells and sebum, becoming infected.	Red, inflamed bumps, may be filled with pus.	Regular cleaning of the skin, topical medications, astringents.
Athlete's foot (tinea pedis)	Caused by a fungus. It usually involves the toes and the soles of the feet but is occasionally found on the hands.	Itching, scaling, and sometimes painful lesions.	For prevention, wearing shoes that do not constrict feet and allow good air circulation. Dry feet well after bathing and lightly apply powder between toes. Treating with (anti-fungal) medication may also be effective.
Atopic dermatitis or Eczema	Reddened areas on the surface of the skin.	Early stage—areas on the skin may be red, swollen, and weeping purulent fluid. Later stage—usually reddened, scaly, itchy areas on the skin.	Avoiding allergens. Topical applications and medication may be helpful as a treatment.
Boils (furuncle)	Skin abscess caused when bacteria enters the hair follicles or sebaceous glands.	Pain, redness, and swelling.	To prevent spreading of infection, it is important to avoid irritating or squeezing the lesion. Treatment may include antibiotics and local moist heat. Incision and drainage may be necessary.

(continued)

382 Chapter 13 | Your Body and How It Functions

ACTIVITY

Have students research and report on a specific condition or illness. Encourage them to review the tables in Chapter 13 that list diseases and conditions for each system. You may wish to assign students a specific condition or disease to report on.

Table 13.16 Common Disorders, Symptoms, and Preventive Measures/Treatment of the Integumentary System (continued)

Condition	Disorder	Symptoms	Preventive Measures/ Treatment
Skin cancer	Rapid growth of cells on the skin that can invade blood vessels, lymph glands, and connecting ducts. The most common types of skin cancer are:	Raised, hard, reddish lesions with a pearly surface. Slightly elevated cells; tumors may become sores that don't heal.	For prevention, applying sunscreen and avoiding excessive exposure to the sun and UV light. Skin cancers can be cured if treated early. Preferred treatment is removal with surgery and radiation. If left untreated, it may cause death.
	Basal cell carcinoma (BCC)	BCC looks like a raised, smooth, pearly bump, usually on the sun-exposed skin of the head, neck, or shoulders. Crusting and bleeding in the center of the tumor frequently develops. It is often mistaken for a sore that does not heal.	Most basal cell carcinomas are removed by surgery.
	Squamous cell carcinoma (SCC)	Commonly a red, scaling, thickened patch on sun-exposed skin. Ulceration and bleeding may occur. When SCC is not treated, it may develop into a large mass.	Most squamous cell carcinomas are removed by surgery, followed by radiaiton.
	Malignant melanoma	Most dangerous type and most likely to metastasize; brown to black looking lesions. Signs include a change in size, shape, color, or elevation of a mole. The appearance of a new mole during adulthood, or new pain, itching, ulceration or bleeding of an existing mole should be checked.	Most malignant melanomas are treated by surgery, followed by up to a year of radiation, and sometimes chemotherapy. Usually must check lymph nodes to make sure condition has not spread.

MEDICAL TERMINOLOGY

acne:	inflammation of the sebaceous gland
alopecia:	baldness
burns:	damage to the skin or other body parts caused by extreme heat, flame, contact with heated objects, or chemicals. Burn depth is generally categorized as first, second, or third degree.
ceraceous:	waxlike in appearance
ceroma:	tumor of waxy appearance
debridement:	removal of dead tissue
decubitus ulcers:	also called bedsores; these are lesions caused by unrelieved pressure to any part of the body
dermatitis:	inflammation of the skin
desquamation:	shedding skin in scales, sheets
erythema:	redness of the skin
keloid:	excessive scarring, resembling a tumor
keratoderma:	scaly skin
keratogenesis:	formation of scaly skin
pustule:	elevation of skin filled with pus
scleroderma:	hardened, thickened skin
sebaceous:	pertaining to oily, fatty matter from the sebaceous gland
sebolith:	stone in a sebaceous gland
seborrhea:	excessive discharge of sebum
squamous:	platelike, scaly
urticaria:	itching wheals on the derma, hives

MEDICAL TERMINOLOGY

Review the terminology:

- Pronounce each word element, and have students repeat.
- Pronounce each term, and have students repeat.
- Allow time for students to write down definitions.
- Select a student to read each definition.
- Assign students to memorize the terms and their definitions.

TEAMWORK

Divide the class into teams of 7 to 10. Describe the symptoms of a disorder of the integumentary system. Award a point to the first team that can identify the disorder. Award a point to the team that can identify the appropriate treatment. The team with the most points at the end of the game wins.

Figure Focus

13.42 What skills and interests do you think might be necessary to become a dermatologist?

Student answers will vary.

Teaching Tips

- Begin a discussion about the jobs and professions that would be suitable for someone interested in the integumentary system.
- Remind students to refer to Chapter 3 for more information on occupations.
- Discuss the skills and requirements for becoming a dermatologist.
- Review the function of the integumentary system and how it protects the body.
- Discuss problems that might arise if the integumentary system cannot function.
- Ask the class to consider what would happen to the parts of the body beneath the skin it the skin was not present.
- Discuss the other body systems that might be affected if the skin was not present, or if it could not function:
    - Endocrine system
    - Skeletal system
    - Muscular system
    - Nervous system
    - Lymphatic system
- Discuss how the intake of water affects the integumentary system.
- Discuss reasons why it is important for all health care workers to have a basic knowledge of the integumentary system and how it functions.
- Discuss the following:
    - What can you tell by looking at the skin of patient?
    - What do you do first when working with a patient with open wounds?
    - What do bluish fingers and toes indicate?
    - Why is the sun harmful to skin?

Related Jobs and Professions

Dermatologist

A dermatologist is a physician trained to treat conditions and diseases of the skin, hair, and nails. (Figure 13.42) This may involve skin allergies, cancer, melanomas, moles, acne, or even some sexually transmitted diseases. Dermatologists must be able to perform various types of dermatologic surgery and be able to analyze and interpret cultures. They must also have a broad base of knowledge that includes things such as allergies and immunology, environmental and industrial medicine, radiology, microbiology, and surgery.

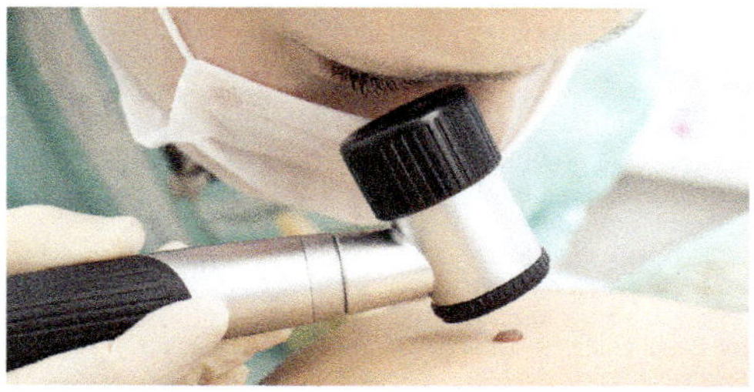

Figure 13.42
What skills and interests do you think might be necessary to become a dermatologist?

To become a dermatologist, you must complete college and medical school. Following medical school, all dermatologists must complete one year of clinical training. Next, they spend three to four years as a resident specializing in dermatology. Those who choose to specialize must train for one more year in that area.

Apply It

One way to check for skin cancer is to apply the "ABCDE" method (research online at skincancer.org). This method is used to look for melanoma, the deadliest form of skin cancer. What does each letter of the mnemonic device represent? Why are each important?

Summary

In this section, you learned the importance of the integumentary system, or skin. The skin helps to protect the body's internal organs from injury or disease. It also helps the body to maintain homeostasis. You have learned that some skin disorders are mild and treatable. However, you have also learned that skin cancer is a life-threatening disorder that can cause death. Skin cancer can be prevented by limiting exposure to the sun and using sunscreen.

Section 13.12 Review Questions

1. What are the six main functions of the skin?
2. What are the three main layers of tissue in skin?
3. Other than skin, what additional structures or tissues are associated with the integumentary system?
4. What is a boil and what causes it?
5. How can skin cancer be prevented?
6. What is acne?
7. A(n) ___________ is a physician trained to treat conditions and diseases of the skin, hair, and nails.

384 Chapter 13 | Your Body and How It Functions

Section 13.12 Review Questions

1. Answer: Protect the underlying body parts from injury and the invasion of pathogens. Regulate body temperature by controlling the loss of body heat. Eliminate wastes through perspiration. Store energy in the form of fat and vitamins. Sense touch, heat, cold, pain, and pressure through receptors. Produce vitamin D.
2. Answer: The epidermis is the outermost layer and has no blood vessels. The dermis is just beneath the epidermis and contains many blood vessels. Subcutaneous means "under the skin," and this layer connects the skin to muscle.

ACTIVITY

Create a resume for a dermatologist looking for a new position. Create a job history, educational credentials, and other relevant information. Refer back to Chapter 4 for information on what to include in a resume.

Genetics

SECTION 13.13

Background

DNA is the genetic material in the cell. It is passed from your father and mother to you through the process of sexual reproduction. DNA and environment influence your hair color, eye color, and other physical traits. DNA can also influence your health. Disorders such as muscular dystrophy and sickle cell anemia are examples of inherited diseases that cause health problems. As a health care worker, you should know how traits are inherited and how these traits may affect health.

Objectives

When you have completed this section, you will be able to do the following:

- Match key terms with their correct meanings.
- Describe the structure of DNA.
- Describe the role of DNA in human heredity.
- Match common genetic disorders with their descriptions.
- Explain why the health care worker's understanding of genetics is important.

deoxyribonucleic acid
(dee AHKS ee rye bow new KLAY ik ASS id)
A molecule found in all living cells that contains information for building proteins and influencing traits.

nucleotides
(NEW klee oh tyde)
Subunits of DNA that each contain a phosphate, sugar, and base.

chromosomes
(KROM uh some)
Structures that contain coiled and condensed portions of the cell's DNA.

Introduction to DNA

DNA, or **deoxyribonucleic acid**, is the genetic material that is present in all living cells. DNA is made of subunits called **nucleotides**. Each nucleotide has a sugar, a phosphate, and a base. The four bases in DNA are *adenine* (A), *thymine* (T), *guanine* (G), and *cytosine* (C). The DNA molecule has the form of a double helix. (**Figure 13.43**)

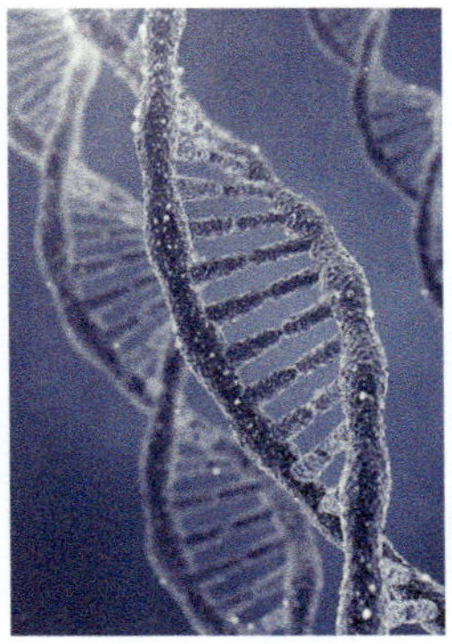

Figure 13.43
The double helix of DNA. What are the two sides of the DNA ladder made of?

Shaped like a twisting ladder, the "rungs" of a double helix are made of bases that pair with each other. In DNA, adenine always pairs with thymine (A-T or T-A) and guanine always pairs with cytosine (G-C or C-G).

DNA is organized into **chromosomes**. Sections of DNA on each chromosome, called **genes**, code for different **traits**. A complete copy of the body's DNA, called the **genome**, is found in each body cell's nucleus. Gene splicing is achieved by using chemicals to "cut" DNA in order to add genetic sequences into the broken chain. The chain is then repaired as a longer chain that now has additional DNA. The purpose of gene splicing is to help with medical conditions such as diabetes, where the gene splicing introduces insulin-producing genes.

genes
(JEENZ)
A portion of DNA that contains instructions for a trait.

traits
(TRAYTS)
Genetically determined characteristics or conditions.

genome
(JEE nohm)
The complete copy of the body's DNA.

Your Body and How It Functions | Chapter 13 385

3. Answer: Hair, nails, and cutaneous glands
4. Answer: A boil is a skin abscess caused when bacteria enters the hair follicles or sebaceous glands.
5. Answer: Apply sunscreen and avoid excessive exposure to the sun
6. Answer: Acne is inflammation of the sebaceous gland.
7. Answer: Dermatologist

TEAMWORK

Divide the class into 13 teams—a team for each of Sections 13.1–13.13 of Chapter 13. Have each team research and report on a new and innovative diagnostic procedure associated with the body system or topic that is described in their section.

FOCUS AND ENGAGE

Introduce the Section

a. Review the content of the Background text, explaining that genetics is the study of how traits are passed from one generation to the next.
b. Emphasize that DNA is the material within genes that carries genetic information.
c. Review the objectives for the section.

Vocabulary Review

a. Direct students to the key terms.
b. Pronounce each word, and have the students repeat the pronunciation out loud.
c. Discuss each definition.

Figure Focus

13.43 The double helix of DNA. What are the two sides of the DNA ladder made of?

Answer: Sugars and phosphates

TEACH

Discuss

- Ask students if they look like their parents, siblings, or cousins.
- If possible, display pictures of relatives that have similar traits.
- Discuss visible traits that are inherited, such as hair color, eye color, and shape of body parts.
- Discuss whether invisible traits, such as tone of voice, physical ability, intelligence are inherited.

Reinforce and Review

- Review the information in Section 13.1: cells, tissues, organs, cavities, and body directions.
- Review the information in Section 13.11, The Reproductive System.

Teaching Tips

- Introduce the topic of DNA.
- Explain that DNA is the molecule in the body that encodes genetic information.

Teaching Tips

- Explain that DNA has subunits called nucleotides.
- Nucleotides are comprised of a sugar, a phosphate, and a base.
- The four bases are:
  - Adenine (A)
  - Thymine (T)
  - Guanine (G)
  - Cytosine (C)
- Describe the structure of DNA:
  - Shaped like a double-helix
  - The "rungs" are made of pairs of bases
  - Adenine always pairs with thymine (A – T or T – A)
  - Guanine always pairs with cytosine (G – C or C – G)
- Explain the role of DNA in human heredity.
- Explain that DNA is organized into chromosomes.
- The sections of DNA on each chromosome are the genes.
- Discuss how gene splicing is achieved and its purpose.
- Describe the human genome:
  - 23 pairs of chromosomes for a total of 46 chromosomes in each cell
  - Explain that one chromosome in each pair comes from the mother, and one from the father.
- Explain the role of alleles.
- Discuss the difference between dominant and recessive alleles.
- Discuss how inherited traits can influence health.
- Explain how common genetic disorders affect the body.

DNA and Heredity

The human genome is organized into 23 pairs of chromosomes for a total of 46 chromosomes in each cell of your body (excluding the sex cells). One chromosome from each pair comes from your mother and from your father. During sexual reproduction, chromosomes from your father's sperm cell combined with chromosomes from your mother's egg cell. Each gene on a chromosome codes for one trait or a set of traits. Because chromosomes come in pairs, you have two forms of the same gene, called **alleles**, coding for each trait. In some cases, both alleles influence a trait. For example, if you have a tall father and a short mother, you may be medium height.

alleles
(uh LEEL)
Forms of a gene that influence a trait or set of traits.

dominant
(DOM uh nuhnt)
Shows influence or control.

recessive
(ri SES iv)
Passive or hidden.

In other cases, one allele has a **dominant** influence over the other, so that you show one trait instead of another. For example, tongue rolling is a dominant trait. Non-tongue rolling is a **recessive** allele. (Figure 13.44)

You inherited genes from both parents, so you are likely to have traits that resemble traits in each parent. For example, you and your father may both be able to roll your tongue. You and your mother may both have a similar nose.

Shared genetic traits can extend to your health. For example, if your mother had breast cancer, you may be more likely to get breast cancer. If your father lived a long life and always had a strong heart, you may be more likely to live long and avoid heart disease. If both parents have an allele for a disorder, such as sickle cell anemia, you might inherit that disorder.

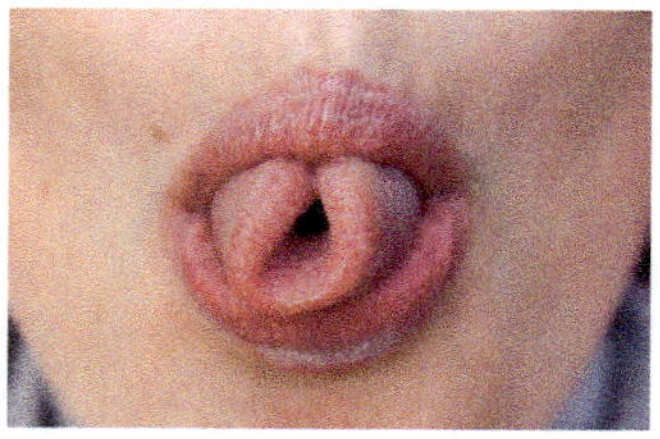

Figure 13.44
Tongue rolling is an inherited trait. Can you roll your tongue?

386 Chapter 13 | Your Body and How It Functions

Figure Focus

13.44 Tongue rolling is an inherited trait. Can you roll your tongue?

Ask students if tongue rolling is a dominant or recessive trait. (Dominant)

Common Inherited Disorders

Table 13.17 Common Inherited Disorders, Symptoms, and Treatment

Condition	Disorder	Symptoms/ Characteristics	Preventive Measures/ Treatment
Cystic Fibrosis	An illness causing serious lung problems that occurs when offspring inherit two recessive alleles for the disease.	Difficulty breathing, frequent respiratory infections, fever, cough, poor appetite.	Medications to reduce airway blockage and infection, bronchial drainage.
Duchene's Muscular Dystrophy	A genetic disorder linked to genes on the X-chromosome that causes muscle weakness and degeneration. Usually affects boys.	Muscle weakness, inability to walk.	Physical therapy, drug therapy. There is no cure for this disease. The patient's muscles may degenerate so that a ventilator or pacemaker is needed.
Down Syndrome	Delayed development and mental retardation caused by an extra copy of chromosome 21.	Low muscle tone and loose joints in infants, slow mental development, distinctive physical features, such as a flat face, enlarged tongue, and small ears.	Some children with Down Syndrome do not have health problems. Others may have heart defects or high blood pressure in the lungs, which can be treated with medication or surgery. Many children with Down syndrome have treatable vision or hearing problems. Other treatable issues include thyroid problems, obesity, seizure disorders, and a higher risk for infection and childhood leukemia.
Sickle Cell Anemia	A blood disorder that creates deformed red blood cells that have trouble carrying oxygen. Caused when offspring inherit two recessive alleles for the disease.	Tiredness; severe pain in chest, stomach, arms, or legs; jaundice.	Folic acid, antibiotics, medications during episodes of pain, blood transfusions. There is no cure for sickle cell anemia.

MEDICAL TERMINOLOGY

genetic amniocentesis: procedure for prenatal diagnosis

carrier: person who does not have a disease, but has one non-functioning gene for a recessive disorder, and so may transmit the disease to offspring

maternal serum screening: blood testing done at 14–20 weeks to assess the risk of a fetus having a disorder

presymptomatic testing: laboratory testing to find out whether a condition will develop in the future, such as breast cancer

risk assessment: using laboratory tests and family history to determine the odds of a certain outcome

X-linked: diseases whose genes are located on the X chromosomes, such as color-blindness, which most often affects males

Your Body and How It Functions | Chapter 13 387

Teaching Tips

- Review Table 13.17 together.
- Pronounce the name of each condition out loud:
  - Cystic Fibrosis
  - Duchene's Muscular Dystrophy
  - Down Syndrome
  - Sickle Cell Anemia
- Ask a student to read the description of each disorder.
- Discuss the symptoms of each.
- Discuss the treatments of each. Note that for the most part, there are no preventive measures for genetic diseases, and often no cures.
- Note that there are other types of inherited diseases, including:
  - Color-blindness
  - Celiac disease
  - Crohn's disease
- Some, such as Tay-Sachs and Sickle Cell Anemia, primarily affect one race or ethnic group.

MEDICAL TERMINOLOGY

Review the terminology:

- Pronounce each word element, and have students repeat.
- Pronounce each term, and have students repeat.
- Allow time for students to write down definitions.
- Select a student to read each definition.
- Assign students to memorize the terms and their definitions.

TEAMWORK

In small groups, prepare a presentation designed to educate people about genetic disorders. Be sure to include the name of the condition and a description, as well as typical symptoms and treatments.

ACTIVITY

Have students discuss their family history of disease and conditions at home. Then ask them to compose a paper on a heritable disease in their own family. Alternatively, assign a heritable disease to each student to research and write a paper about.

Science Link—Human Genome Project

- Review the mission of the Human Genome Project.
- Discuss some of the things scientists learned from the project and some things they hope to learn in the future.
- Refer students to the genome.gov Web site for more information.

Why would it be useful to know whether a disease has a genetic component?

Answer: If you knew that a disease had a genetic component you could examine the genetic code of a patient to look for sequences that are associated with the disease long before the patient has the disease. The patient could then take steps to prevent the disease.

Teaching Tips

- Begin a discussion about the jobs and professions that would be suitable for someone interested in genetics.
- Remind students to refer to Chapter 3 for more information on occupations.
- Discuss the skills and requirements for becoming a geneticist, including the extensive laboratory work that much of the work in genetics involves.
- Review how DNA carries human traits.
- Discuss why it is important for all health care workers to have a basic knowledge of genetics.

Science Link

Human Genome Project

The Human Genome Project is an international scientific research project with the goal of determining the sequence of chemical base pairs that make up human DNA and of identifying and mapping all of the genes of the human genome from both a physical and functional standpoint. It remains the world's largest collaborative biological project. The project was proposed and funded by the U.S. government. Planning started in 1984; the project got underway in 1990; and it was declared complete in 2003.

Researchers determined that humans have approximately 20,500 genes, the same as in mice. Everyone has the same order of nearly all nucleotide bases in their DNA. Genetic tests can show predisposition to a variety of illnesses, including breast cancer, hemostasis disorders, cystic fibrosis, liver diseases, and many others. Also, the etiologies for cancers, Alzheimer's disease, and other areas of clinical interest are considered likely to benefit from genome information and possibly may lead in the long term to significant advances in their management.

The information and technologies produced by the Human Genome Project have helped researchers to study how combinations of genes influence whole body systems. These findings are likely to improve our understanding of the genetic connections to disease.

Working in teams, clarify the relationships about the role of DNA and chromosomes in coding for characteristic traits passed from parents to children. Construct an explanation based on your findings to share with the class.

Why would it be useful to know whether a disease has a genetic component?

Related Jobs and Professions

Geneticist

A geneticist is a scientist who is certified to work in medical and scientific areas related to genes. (Figure 13.45) This work may involve experiments that explore and determine laws and environmental factors that affect the origin, transmission, and development of inherited traits. Geneticists may devise methods to alter traits or produce new traits. A geneticist may specialize in developing resistance methods to disease and disorders, understanding the relationship between heredity and fertility, or evaluating the genetic makeup that has caused a disorder or disability in order to help a patient manage a condition. To become a geneticist a doctoral degree and approximately two years of training in an accredited laboratory for certification are required.

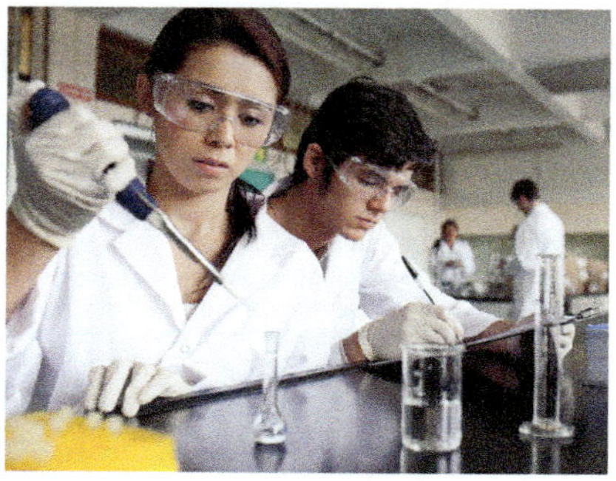

Figure 13.45 What skills and interests do you think might be necessary to become a geneticist?

388 Chapter 13 | Your Body and How It Functions

Figure Focus

13.45 What skills and interests do you think might be necessary to become a geneticist?

Student answers will vary.

Genetic Counselor

Genetic counselors work with families to fully understand risks of certain genetic disorders, such as neuromuscular diseases. A genetic counselor evaluates a family's history and provides information and insight into what that history means from a genetic point of view. The genetic counselor must patiently and thoroughly record details of each patient's medical history and then evaluate that data. This part of the job requires a scientific-based approach, but the job also requires caring support of patients as they go through the evaluation process and learn of risks and difficulties associated with their genetics. A genetic counselor must have a master's degree, preferably in the field of human genetics and/or counseling. Certification is recommended.

Genetic Nurse

Genetic nurses specifically care for the genetic health of patients who have genetic issues, such as Huntington disease, hereditary breast cancer, and cystic fibrosis. Care may includes screening, early detection, risk identification, treatment, and testing. A genetic nurse usually has long-term relationships with patients and their families. The outcomes of patients with genetic problems are often negative, which a genetic nurse must be able to deal with and help families deal with, as well. Genetic nurses need additional training, education, and certification to work in the field.

Summary

In this section, you learned that DNA is the molecule in cells that controls cell function and influences traits. DNA is composed of phosphates, sugars, and a backbone of paired bases. Your DNA was passed down to you by both your mother and your father. Because you inherited their DNA, you also inherited many of the traits that your parents have. Some of these traits may affect your health.

Section 13.13 Review Questions

1. A child inherits a recessive allele for sickle cell anemia and a dominant allele for normal red blood cells. What kind of red blood cells will the child have? Why?
2. What is the cause of Down Syndrome?
3. How are genes, chromosomes, and DNA are related.
4. What is a nucleotide?
5. Why are there generally no cures for genetic disorders?
6. What is cystic fibrosis and how do we treat it?

Teaching Tips

- Discuss the skills and requirements for becoming a genetic counselor.
- Point out that genetic information can affect families in profound ways if there are familial genetic traits for disorders.
- Discuss the skills and requirements for becoming a genetic nurse.
- Review the structure of DNA and the role DNA plays in human heredity.
- Discuss reasons why it is important for all health care workers to have a basic knowledge of genetics.
- Remind students of the importance of collecting medical history information from patients.
- Discuss how information about a parent's medical history might help treat a patient.
- For example, how might knowing that a patient's mother has breast cancer influence treatment?
- How might knowing that a patient's father died of a heart attack influence care?
- You may want to discuss some of the ethical questions involved with genetic medicine.
- Discuss current issues related to genetic research.

ACTIVITY

Using materials such as construction paper, create a model of a strand of DNA. Label the model appropriately by indicating the location of chromosomes, pairs of bases, and other parts of the structure.

Section 13.13 Review Questions

1. Answer: When one allele has a dominant influence, the child will exhibit that specific trait; therefore, the child will have normal red blood cells.
2. Answer: An extra copy of chromosome 21 causes Down Syndrome.
3. Answer: DNA is organized into chromosomes. Sections of DNA on each chromosome, called genes, code for different traits. A complete copy of the body's DNA, called the genome, is found in each body cell's nucleus.
4. Answer: A nucleotide is a subunit of DNA that each contain a phosphate, sugar, and base.
5. Answer: Your DNA was passed down to you by both your mother and your father. Because you inherited their DNA, you also inherited many of the traits that your parents have. Some of these traits may affect your health.
6. Answer: Cystic fibrosis is an illness causing serious lung problems that occur when offspring inherit two recessive alleles for the disease. Medication is used to reduce airway blockage and infection.

CHAPTER 13 REVIEW

Chapter Review Questions

1. Answer: Nerve tissue is located throughout the body and sends impulses to and from the central nervous system and to and from the body systems. Epithelial tissue forms the outer skin and lines body cavities and passages to the outside of the body; this tissue protects, secretes, absorbs, and receives sensations such as hot, cold, and pressure. Connective tissue is bones, tendons, and fat tissue that binds, supports, and connects body tissues. Muscle tissue includes cardiac (heart) that contracts the heart, smooth (internal organs such as the stomach and diaphragm) that contracts the organs, and striated (throughout the body for movement) that contracts and flexes to allow movement.
2. Answer: The appendicular skeleton involves the appendages and includes 126 bones. These bones are in the arms, hands, legs, feet, and pelvis.
3. Answer: Starts in the right atrium; through the tricuspid valve; right ventricle; through the pulmonary valve; pulmonary artery; lungs (oxygen and carbon dioxide exchange); pulmonary veins; left atrium; mitral valve; left ventricle; aortic valve; aorta ("out to the body"); arteries; arterioles; capillaries (oxygen and carbon dioxide exchange); venules; veins; superior or inferior vena cava; right atrium
4. Answer: The spleen filters microorganisms and waste products from the blood. The spleen makes lymphocytes and monocytes to help the body defend itself against microorganisms. The spleen also stores red blood cells and destroys worn-out red blood cells.

CHAPTER 13 REVIEW

Chapter Review Questions

1. Describe the four types of tissue and their functions in the body. (13.1)
2. What is the appendicular skeleton? (13.2)
3. Describe all the structures that blood passes through as it travels between the aorta and the vena cava. (13.4)
4. How does the spleen keep the body healthy? (13.5)
5. The hairlike objects in the bronchial tubes that move mucus out of the lungs are called ________. (13.6)
6. What are the differences between gastritis, enteritis, and gastroenteritis? (13.7)
7. The ____________ contains filtering mechanisms called nephrons. (13.8)
8. How is the function of the thyroid gland different from the function of the parathyroid glands? (13.9)
9. How does the ear help you to hear sound? (13.10)
10. How does muscular dystrophy affect a patient? (13.13)
11. Describe how the lymphatic system helps maintain homeostasis. (13.5)

Activities

1. As a health care worker, your alertness to symptoms and complications associated with the body systems is important for the well-being of your patients. Select and research a chronic disease or an emerging disease or disorder. Write an explanation of potential symptoms and complications. How is the disease diagnosed and treated? Is the disease more prevalent in certain parts of the world? Are there ways to prevent the disease and control health care costs?
2. Work with a partner to test how the skin senses different stimuli. With eyes closed, have your partner report the sensation he or she feels when you apply different stimuli to the skin of the arm. Use objects that are warm and cold. Also apply a light touch, pressure, and a light pinch. Write down your partner's sensations and the objects that caused these sensations. After applying all the stimuli, work together to write down the name of the tactile corpuscle that received each stimulus.
3. You are asked to lift a patient that weighs more than 250 lbs. and has been injured in an automobile accident. Both legs have been broken and the casts have been removed that morning. You will be moving the patient from the bed to a wheelchair and transporting him to physical therapy to begin rehabilitation. Working with a partner, analyze principles of body mechanics—such as forces and the effects of movement, torque, tension, and elasticity of the human body—and demonstrate how you would move the patient.
4. Following rehabilitation, as a physical therapy assistant you are assigned to perform range of motion exercises for both of the patient's legs. Describe how principles of body mechanics such as forces and the effects of movement, torque, tension, and elasticity of the human body will affect the patient's exercises.

390 Chapter 13 | Your Body and How It Functions

5. Answer: Bronchi
6. Answer: Gastritis is the inflammation of the stomach lining and causes pain, indigestion, and burning in the stomach. Enteritis is inflammation of the intestines and causes abdominal cramping and diarrhea. Gastroenteritis is the inflammation of the stomach lining and the intestines and causes vomiting, abdominal cramping, and diarrhea.
7. Answer: Kidney
8. Answer: The thyroid gland controls the rate of metabolism. The parathyroid glands regulate calcium and phosphorus metabolism.
9. Answer: The middle ear is an air space that contains three bones or ossicles. These bones amplify sound waves received by the tympanic membrane. The inner ear contains the semicircular canals, which transmit sound waves received from the middle ear to the nerves that allow us to translate sound. The inner ear is also responsible for equilibrium.

CHAPTER 13 REVIEW

5. Choose a disease of the endocrine system and prepare a presentation on it. In the presentation, summarize how the disease relates to problems with the biological and chemical processes of the system (i.e., homeostasis) and structural or functional problems in the associated glands.
6. With a group, practice these skills related to assisting patients with mobility: positioning, turning, lifting, and transferring patients for treatment or examination.
7. Choose one of the organ systems in this chapter and prepare a presentation on one of the major diseases that affects that system. Explain how the disease relates to problems with homeostasis and structural or functional problems (as a result of trauma or disease) in the associated organs.

Case Studies

1. Ms. Wilson looks confused after her doctor has confirmed and explained her diagnosis of diabetes. You know from talking with her family that they usually call diabetes "sugar." How could you help Ms. Wilson better understand her condition? Brainstorm with classmates to think of other words people use for medical conditions or bodily functions that could cause confusion.
2. A patient complains of painful urination and blood in the urine. He says that he has had these symptoms for a few days. What other information should you get from the patient? What disorders would the symptoms indicate?

Thinking Critically

1. **Communication**—Explain how you think that your understanding of the body systems helps you communicate with patients/clients and co-workers. Your patient/client asks you to explain how the muscles in her upper arm cause the forearm to move. Write how you can communicate this information to a child under 6, an adult over 80, and a teenager.
2. **Patient Education**—Many patients have little knowledge of anatomy and/or the correct terms for body parts. Try to find out if local health care facilities have policies that provide patients with illustrated brochures or diagrams to help explain medical conditions. Working with a partner, create your own brochure or diagram.
3. **Legal and Ethical**—A patient's doctor just told him that he has a serious problem in the gastrointestinal system. The doctor thinks that it is probably a malignant tumor. The patient asks you what you know about his condition. What is your responsibility in this case?

Your Body and How It Functions | Chapter 13 391

10. Answer: Muscular dystrophy causes muscle weakness and degeneration.
11. Answer: Refer students to pages 334 and 335 for further review. The lymphatic system helps to maintain homeostasis (balance in the body) by helping the body to fight disease, build immunity, and prevent the buildup of fluids in the tissues.

Activities

1. Direct students to include information about the system or systems affected by the disease. Encourage students to write a complete report, including a list of sources.
2. You may want students to use scientific methods to complete this activity. Direct students to record the results of their tests in a table and then to create a graph or chart to display the data.
3. Refer the students to pages 526–528 to review the steps of body mechanics, including the importance of teamwork, when bending and lifting a heavy object. They may also want to review the physics of torque and tension and how they relate to the human body.
4. Refer the students to pages 782–786 to review the range of motion procedures particular to the patient's injury described in the activity.
5. (and 7) These presentations can be oral and/or visual using posters. Have the students practice presenting information in different formats.
6. Prior to these activities, have a discussion about body contact, appropriate vs. inappropriate touching, and consent. Have them practice asking for consent before touching another student.

CUSTOMIZED INSTRUCTION

At-Risk Students

For Activity 2, make sure students are partnered with a classmate who is a friend or someone with whom they feel comfortable.

TEAMWORK

Divide the class into teams of five or six students and play "Jeopardy." Each category should correspond to the sections in this chapter. One team will select a category and work together within a time limit to answer a question from that category. If they get it right, they can ask another question. If not, a different team has a turn. Award points for correct answers and subtract points for incorrect answers. The team with the most points when all of the questions have been used wins.

Case Studies

1. Encourage students to be creative with this case study. For example, they may want to perform a skit demonstrating how they would respond, or create a brochure designed to educate people about diabetes.
2. Direct students to Section 13.8 for information on the urinary system.

Thinking Critically

1. Review the importance of clear, concise communication. Direct students to write a general explanation for the first part of the problem, and then refer to the example to write specific information for each of the three patients. Suggest students set up their responses in a table format.
2. Students should telephone, e-mail, or visit the facilities to collect this information. If they locate educational information, allot class time to review and discuss the different examples.
3. Refer students to Chapters 5 and 6 for information about legal and ethical responsibilities. Point out that this problem may not be testing the students' actual knowledge of the diagnosed condition.

CHAPTER 13 REVIEW

Portfolio Connection

Employers look for health care workers who have knowledge of the body and body systems. Assistive personnel work in many different departments and must be able to recognize problems and report them correctly to a supervisor.

Complete the following exercise and put it in your portfolio for review in the future: Identify one body system disorder. Research the objective and subjective symptoms that result from this disorder. Explain your findings in a typed or neatly written paper.

PORTFOLIO TIP

Keep in mind that many cultures find it offensive to directly mention body parts: you may need to prompt your patients/clients as to where they feel discomfort.

392 Chapter 13 | Your Body and How It Functions

Portfolio Connection

- Remind students that this paper will become part of their career portfolio.
- You may want to provide a list of systems and disorders from which each student may select, or approve the topic before the students begin the research.
- Encourage students to write a first draft, use peer review, and then revise the report.
- Check to make sure that students have completed the written assignments and added them to their portfolio.

TEAMWORK

Distribute index cards naming the symptoms of a common disorder covered in this chapter to the students. Label areas of the classroom with the different body systems covered in this chapter. At your signal, instruct students to move to the area labeled with the system that corresponds to the symptoms on his or her index card. Check the groups, and direct students in the incorrect location to try again. When all students are in the correct location, ask each one to read his or her symptoms, and name the condition.

14 Human Growth and Development

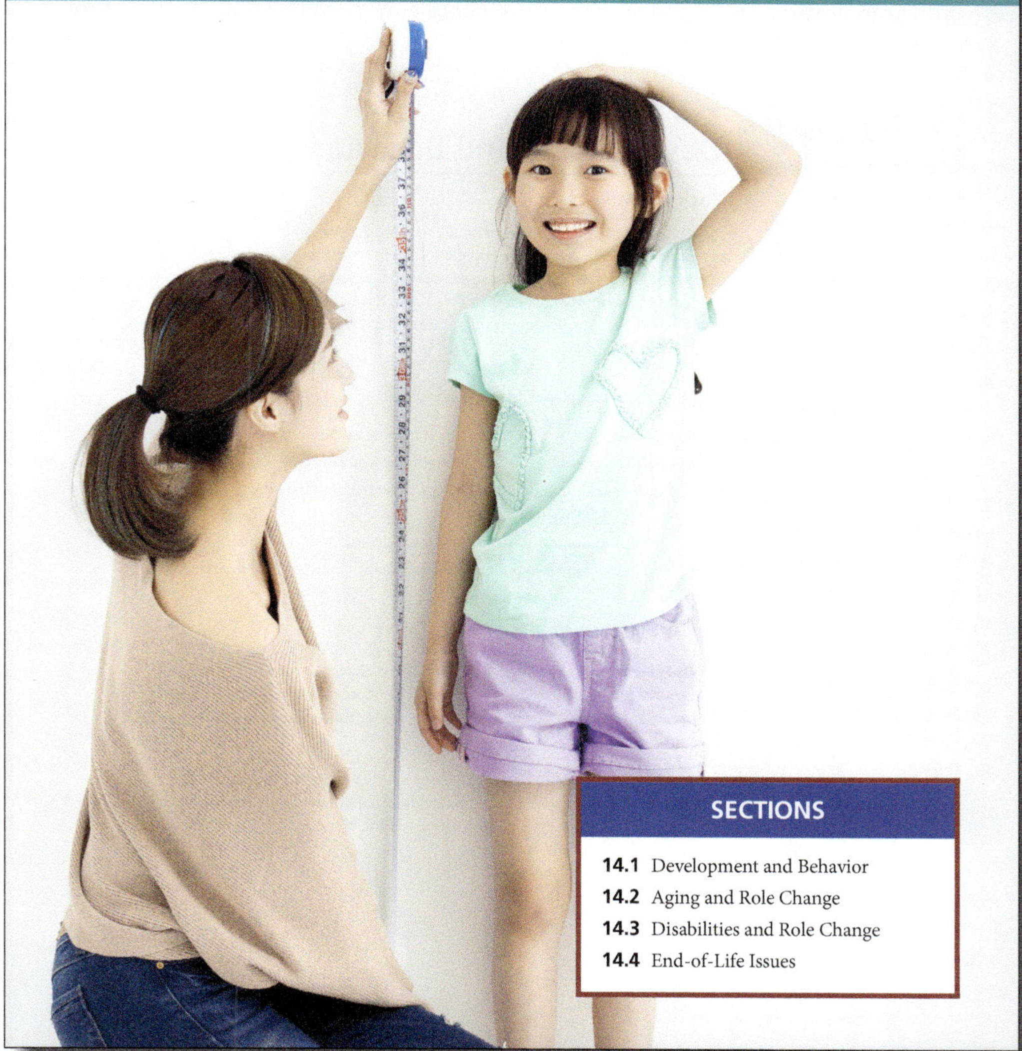

SECTIONS

CHAPTER 14 OVERVIEW

Chapter 14 covers human growth and development. Students learn to recognize normal and abnormal development and behavior. They also learn about the issues confronting people as they age, disabled persons, and persons facing death.

Section 14.1: Section 14.1 covers the physical and emotional stages of life from birth through death.

Section 14.2: In Section 14.2, students are introduced to changes that affect the human body as it ages.

Section 14.3: Section 14.3 covers the physical and emotional changes that occur when people are confronted with life-altering physical and mental disabilities.

Section 14.4: In Section 14.4, students learn how people cope with death and pain, including a lengthy terminal illness, pain management, hospice care, and the ethics of euthanasia.

Advance Preparation	
Review	■ Chapter text for Sections 14.1, 14.2, 14.3, and 14.4.
Contact	■ A local senior center to arrange a tour. ■ A nursery school, preschool, or daycare center to arrange a tour. ■ A support group or political action group for disabled persons to request brochures or educational material. ■ A hospice or organization to request brochures or educational information about end-of-life care and issues. ■ An advocate for senior citizens or disabled persons to speak to the class.
Prepare	■ Examples of music, clothes, and other items from other eras. ■ Photos of people at different stages of life involved in different activities. ■ Cotton balls and gloves to use for activities. ■ Index cards for use as flashcards.

FOCUS AND ENGAGE

Getting Started

- This activity is designed to enable students to experience declining physical ability similar to a senior citizen.
- Help students select a condition that occurs due to aging, such as diminished hearing or eyesight, or weakness in the back or legs.
- Provide materials students can use to simulate the selected condition, or provide a list of materials that they can gather.
- After the exercise, allot class time for discussing the experience.

Introduce the Section

a. Review the content of the Background paragraph, explaining that the life continuum is the cycle of life from birth to death.
b. Emphasize the importance of understanding the stages of growth and development in order to diagnose, treat, and communicate with patients.
c. Review the objectives for the section.

Vocabulary Review

a. Direct students to the key terms.
b. Pronounce each word, and have the students repeat the pronunciation out loud.
c. Discuss each definition.

Getting Started

Spend one school day with a "disabling condition" that may be experienced by an aged person. Select from the following: wheelchair bound, walk with a cane, cotton or other covering to restrict hearing capability, Vaseline covered eyeglasses, one arm bound to your side, or others you might consider. Determine the difficulty of normal daily activities and make suggestions as to how a local public area (shopping mall, restaurant, movie theatre) might improve access and support for those experiencing these conditions.

SECTION 14.1 Development and Behavior

Background

Health care workers provide care for all age groups. It is important to understand the emotional and physical stages of the life continuum. This knowledge assists you in recognizing normal and abnormal development and behavior and to identify the concepts of health and wellness throughout the life span. This awareness of life's stages allows you to be an effective health care worker.

Objectives

When you have completed this section, you will be able to do the following:

- Match key terms with their correct meanings.
- Identify three stages of development between conception and birth.
- List four common developments of growth in the first year of life and the age at which they usually occur.
- Define and describe characteristics of adolescent development.
- Compare your life experiences to each stage described in this chapter.

Development and Behavior

continuum
(kuhn TIN yoo uhm)
Progression from start (birth) to finish (death).

zygote
(ZAHY goht)
Any cell formed by the coming together of two reproductive (sex) cells.

People experience many physical and emotional changes over a lifetime. These changes are part of the normal growth and development process. In this section, we discuss the stages of development and behavior from conception through the life **continuum**.

Conception, or fertilization, occurs when a male sperm and a female ovum combine. This combination causes the single-cell ovum to divide into many cells. This stage of development is called a **zygote**. Within five weeks, the rapidly multiplying cells duplicate into an embryo.

394 Chapter 14 | Human Growth and Development

TEACH

Discuss

- Encourage students to share personal stories of their own growth and development.
- Stories may be positive or negative. For example, acquiring new skills as they grew out of childhood, growth spurts, growth stoppage, etc.
- Discuss that growth, development, and aging are inevitable.

Reinforce and Review

- Review the importance of communication for health care professionals.

CUSTOMIZED INSTRUCTION OVERVIEW	
Less Advanced Students	Pages 398, 415
More Advanced Students	Pages 401, 407
English Language Learners	Pages 395, 405
Special Needs Students	Pages 397, 412
At-Risk Students	Pages 398, 405

- Five weeks after conception, the embryo is about the size of a grain of rice.
- Six weeks after conception, the nervous system, eyes, and ears are visible.
- Twelve weeks, or 3 months after conception, the embryo has grown to about 2½ inches (6 cm) long and is now called a fetus.
- Babies are born 38 to 40 weeks after conception.

Understanding Different Stages of Life

As you work with people, it is helpful to know what to expect in terms of behavior and communication. Everybody is different, but there are stages of development that offer guidelines that you can use to better understand people. Tables 14.1–14.3 on the following pages provide information—by age and developmental stage—that will help you become aware of factors affecting behavior and communication, as well as techniques you can use to enhance communication.

Infancy Through Early Elementary School Age

From infancy through early elementary school, children develop dramatically. They progress from depending completely on others for care to having physical skills that allow them to run and play, along with mental skills that prompt them to look for reasons why things are the way they are in their lives. Use Table 14.1 to better understand infants and children up through the age of eight.

prone
(PROHN)
Lying on the stomach.

supine
(soo PAHYN)
Lying on the back.

Table 14.1 Infant Through Early Elementary School Age Stages

Age	Behavior	Age-Specific Communication Techniques	Effective Communication Techniques During Medical Care
6 Weeks	Baby first begins to smile.	Hold, cuddle, and softly speak frequently to infant.	When possible hold, cuddle, and softly speak frequently to infant.
10 weeks	Infant has the ability to roll from a **prone** to a **supine** position.	Hold, cuddle, and softly speak frequently to infant.	Comfort infants by speaking in a soothing tone and touch them gently to communicate your presence and reassurance.
4 to 6 months	Infant raises head and shoulders while in a supine position.	Talking to infants helps them recognize sounds and make associations. It is helpful to talk slowly and clearly when holding, feeding, or bathing infants at this age. Sudden, strange noise may cause fear.	Comfort infants by speaking in a soothing tone and touch them gently to communicate your presence and reassurance.
6 to 8 months	Infant sits without being supported; when placed on abdomen infant may scoot before mastering a crawl; eye color may change.	Distract or move infants when they are headed for trouble.	When possible perform procedures quickly and efficiently to minimize time the infant is exposed to discomfort. Take time to comfort infants by speaking in a soothing tone and touch them gently to communicate your presence and reassurance. Allow parent or other family members to be present when possible.

(continued)

CUSTOMIZED INSTRUCTION

English Language Learners

Have students write each key term and its pronunciation on one side of an index card and its definition on the other side. Have them read each term and definition aloud to a partner.

TEAMWORK

Read aloud the "All the world's a stage . . ." soliloquy from Shakespeare's play *As You Like It*. (You can find the passage online at many sites, such internetshakespeare.uvic.ca/Library/SLT/life/lifesubj+1.html.) As the students listen, have them write down the seven stages of man. As a class, discuss Shakespeare's interpretation of growth and development.

Teaching Tips

- Introduce the topic of development and behavior.
- Emphasize that there are normal stages of growth and development throughout life.
- Explain the three stages of development between fertilization and birth:
  - Zygote: first five weeks after fertilization
  - Embryo: Five to 12 weeks from fertilization
  - Fetus: 12 weeks from fertilization until birth, usually 38 to 40 weeks from fertilization
- Review the first part of Table 14.1 together as a class.
- Explain that *infant* is used to describe a child from birth to walking, which usually occurs around 12 to 18 months. It is a time of incredible growth and development.
- Discuss average development and behavior during the first year of life.
- Emphasize age-specific communication techniques.
- Encourage students to share personal stories of caring for infants.

Teaching Tips

- Review the second part of Table 14.1 together.
- Explain that *toddler* generally refers to a child who is 18 months to 3 years old, which corresponds roughly to the time between walking and talking.
- Discuss average development and behavior during the toddler years.
- Emphasize age-specific communication techniques.
- Encourage students to share personal stories of interacting with toddlers.
- Review the remainder of Table 14.1 together.
- Explain that the preschool and elementary years encompass ages 4 to 8.
- Discuss average development and behavior during the preschool and elementary years.
- Emphasize age-specific communication techniques.
- Encourage students to share personal stories of interacting with children this age, or things they can remember about their own growth and development.

Table 14.1 Infant Through Early Elementary School Age Stages (continued)

Age	Behavior	Age-Specific Communication Techniques	Effective Communication Techniques During Medical Care
8 to 12 months	Attempts to feed self and begins to crawl, stand, and take steps. As infant becomes toddler, expect frequent falls while learning to walk. Provide a safe environmentfree of sharp edges and, if possible, keep infant on carpeting instead of cement or tile flooring.	Use simple terms to warn them as they head toward trouble: "Hot," "Hurt," or "Tastes bad." Always praise good behavior.	Perform procedures quickly and efficiently to minimize the infant's exposure to discomfort. Comfort infants by speaking in a soothing tone and touch them gently to communicate your presence and reassurance. Allow parent or other family to be present when possible.
1 year	Learning and experimenting absorbs most of infant's waking hours. Understands simple conversation or commands. Most toddlers at this age can say four or five words clearly.	Speak clearly and slowly, using simple words. Children who are spoken to with clear word pronunciation (not baby talk) develop clearer speech. Resist saying "No," constantly and be patient.	Speak in a calming voice tone. Allow parent or family to be available when possible.
18 months	Walks alone, feeds itself, and stacks objects. "Mine" becomes a favorite expression.	Communicate clear limits about acceptable and unacceptable behavior. Reinforce good behavior. Playing easy games and reading simple stories develops vocabulary. Time spent in this way provides positive, nurturing experiences.	*The following is appropriate for children 18 months through 8 years of age:* Refer to the child by his or her favorite name (name or nickname). Use the same words the family uses for toileting. Do not blame or scold if toileting accidents occur. Explain in simple terms what is happening to and around the child. Answer their questions honestly and in terms the child will understand. When possible spend time with the child, talking and playing simple games appropriate to their age. Taking time to communicate and enjoy activities with each child is important in creating a positive sense of well-being during medical care. When possible perform procedures quickly and efficiently to minimize time the child is exposed to discomfort. Following procedures that cause discomfort or emotional tension, take time to comfort child by speaking in a soothing tone and touch them gently to communicate your presence and reassurance.
20 to 24 months	Begins bowel and bladder control. Experiences exploration and a feeling of security. Vocabulary increases rapidly. Pronunciation may take time to develop.	Your patience fosters normal speech development. Resist trying to correct pronunciation too often. Listen carefully and confirm your understanding of the child's words.	
3 to 4 years	Talks in simple, complete sentences. Experiences a span of emotional growth.	Continue following techniques described above.	
4 to 5 years	Dresses and undresses with little assistance. Experiences a span of emotional growth.	*The following is appropriate for children 4 through 8 years of age:* Children require frequent reassurance and truthful, caring conversation. Keep talks short and easy to understand, allowing time for the children to say everything they want. Positive acceptance of what the child says is important, and positive reflection back to them helps the child overcome shyness and withdrawal.	
5 to 6 years	Eye and body **coordination** improves. The child is able to hop, skip, and draw. Awareness of the ability to choose one action over another is present. Child begins to feel guilt and shame.	*(continued from above)*	*(continued from above)*

(continued)

coordination
(koh awr dn EY shuhn)
State of harmonized action, such as eye and hand coordination.

396 Chapter 14 | Human Growth and Development

TEAMWORK

Divide the class into teams of five to seven students. Within a set time limit, such as five minutes, have each team write on a sheet of paper behaviors that develop during the first year of life. When the time is up, see which time has the most correct behaviors. Award extra points for listing a behavior that other teams missed.

ACTIVITY

Make a three-column table comparing the different stages of life between fertilization and birth. One column should describe features of the zygote stage, one of the embryonic stage, and one of the fetus stage. Include the timeframe and key characteristics of development.

Table 14.1 Infant Through Early Elementary School Age Stages (continued)

Age	Behavior	Age-Specific Communication Techniques	Effective Communication Techniques During Medical Care
6 to 8 years	Physical skills continue to improve. Children start school. They begin to look for reasons that explain why they believe certain things. They also compare themselves with others. At about age 7, they may experience emotional withdrawal or shyness.	*(continued from above)*	*(continued from above)*

Adolescence—Preteen Years Through Young Adult

Adolescence occurs from the ages of 11 to 21, or between childhood and adulthood. Development progresses through three stages: early (11–13), middle (14–18), and late (19–21). Each period has its own distinct characteristics of growth and development, but the exact time frame varies from person to person.

Puberty is the process of the body changing into the adult form that is capable of reproduction. Many factors can influence the timing, but the average age for the onset of puberty is 9–14 for girls, and 10–18 for boys.

Reasoning skills improve throughout adolescence. Emotional challenges are also encountered: need for separateness, disagreements with authority figures, changes in long-time friendships, stress from busy schedules, and sexual uncertainty. In later adolescent years, people typically start to become more independent. With maturity, they find that friends' approval is not as important as their own moral sense of right and wrong. Use Table 14.2 to better understand adolescents.

Table 14.2 Preteen Years Through Young Adult Stages

Age	Behavior	Age-Specific Communication Techniques	Effective Communication Techniques During Medical Care
9 to 12 years (preteen or preadolescent years)	Physical growth rate increases, and adult sexual characteristics become noticeable. Girls begin menstruation. Boys develop more hair on their faces and bodies, and voices deepen. Preteens may look to their friends for acceptance and approval rather than to their parents.	Children 9 to 12 years old do best when you listen to them and give them a chance to express themselves. Use positive responses to indicate that you hear what they are saying. It is also important to explain clearly the differences between acceptable and unacceptable behavior. Acknowledge positive actions and discuss why other behaviors are not appropriate.	When appropriate and possible, prior to a medical procedure offer to show them what will be done during procedures. Tell children what to expect concerning how they will physically feel and what they will see and hear. Reassure them by explaining how to get assistance if needed. Explain the importance of asking questions when they are unsure about the way they feel, or what they see or hear.

(continued)

Human Growth and Development | Chapter 14 397

Teaching Tips

- Review the remainder of Table 14.1 together.
- Explain that the preschool and elementary years encompass ages 4 to 8.
- Discuss average development and behavior during the preschool and elementary years.
- Emphasize age-specific communication techniques.
- Encourage students to share personal stories of interacting with children this age, or things they can remember about their own growth and development.
- Review the first part of Table 14.2 together.
- Explain that *preadolescent* generally refers to a child who is between 9 and 11 years old.
- Discuss average development and behavior during the preadolescent years.
- Discuss the onset of puberty.
- Discuss the physical changes that occur at this time.
- Discuss the emotional adjustments that occur at this time.
- Emphasize age-specific communication techniques.
- Encourage students to discuss the changes they experienced in preadolescence, or have witnessed in friends and family members.
- Remind students that when they share stories, they should respect the confidentiality of others.
- Point out some of the overlaps in development between the different stages.
- For example, some children begin puberty at 11, where others do not begin puberty until 13.
- Emphasize that not everyone matures at the same rate.

CUSTOMIZED INSTRUCTION

Special Needs Students

Use consideration when discussing normal growth and development in a classroom that include special needs students. Some may have developmental delays or disabilities that do not fall into the normal range.

Teaching Tips

- Review the remainder of Table 14.2 together.
- Explain that *adolescence* generally refers to the years between childhood and adulthood, roughly 13 to 18.
- Emphasize that it is a time of striving for independence.
- Discuss average development and behavior during the adolescent years.
- Encourage students to discuss the changes they are experiencing or recently experienced in adolescence.
- Again, emphasize age-specific communication techniques.
- Discuss social and health issues that affect teenagers today.
- Review the last item in Table 14.2.
- Explain that young adults are generally between 18 and 20 years of age.
- Emphasize age-specific communication techniques.
- Review the first part of Table 14.3 together.
- Point out that there are many stages of adulthood, roughly broken into 10-year segments:
  - 20 to 30 years of age: new adults trying to find their place in society
  - 30 to 40: established; building families

Table 14.2 Preteen Years Through Young Adult Stages (continued)

Age	Behavior	Age-Specific Communication Techniques	Effective Communication Techniques During Medical Care
13 to 18 years (adolescent or teenage years)	The teenage years are between childhood and adulthood. Teenagers strive for independence. They also experience puberty, a sexual development caused by increased hormone production of certain glands. (Girls may start puberty by age 11; boys usually start at 13.) Puberty is a time of both physical and emotional adjustment.	*The following is appropriate for 13 through 20 years of age:* **Adolescents** need others to listen and reflect their words back to them. This type of communication allows teenagers to hear what they are thinking and gain increased understanding of self. Respect their privacy. Question behavior only when pertinent to their health and well-being.	*The following is appropriate for 13 through 20 years of age:* When appropriate and possible, prior to a medical procedure offer to show them what will be done during procedures. Tell teenagers what to expect concerning how they will physically feel and what they will see and hear. Reassure them by explaining how to get assistance if needed.
18 to 20 years (young adulthood)	People become more independent. As they mature, they begin to seek ways of contributing to society.		

adolescent
(ad l ES uhnt)
The period of life between childhood and maturity.

decade
(DEK eyd)
Period of 10 years.

Adulthood

Adulthood occurs at the age of 21. Although adults' reasoning skills have developed, and they are basically fully grown from a physical standpoint, there are still stages through which adults pass: young adulthood (20s and 30s), middle age (40s and 50s), retirement age (60s and 70s), and old age (80s and beyond). Use **Table 14.3** to better understand adults.

Table 14.3 Adulthood Ages 20 Through 70+ Years Stages

Age	Behavior	Age-Specific Communication Techniques	Effective Communication Techniques During Medical Care
20 to 30 years	This is the beginning of adulthood, when people attempt to build a firm, safe foundation for the future. There is a strong desire to do the right thing. Patterns of living are set during this **decade**, such as: helper patterns (rescuing others), leadership patterns (taking charge, organizing), passive patterns (acting without influence, not taking an active part in things). These are just a few patterns people may fall into; there are many others.	*The following is generally appropriate for ages 20 through the 60s:* Show positive interest in adults' conversation, and interpret and respond to their body language. Use words that are understandable and meaningful to each individual's level. Express your desire to protect privacy; resist questioning personal behaviors and habits unless they are pertinent to the person's health and well-being.	*The following is generally appropriate for ages 20 through the 60s:* Be aware of the impact medical care is having on each person. Be sensitive to fears; honestly explain procedures and expected outcomes. When speaking about a patient, always go to areas away from the patient's view and hearing. Your behavior must communicate respect for others—be aware of your body language and verbal tone; be aware of when words are helpful or silence is preferred.
30 to 40 years	In this decade, people often feel confined by the guidelines that they established for themselves in their 20s. This confined feeling often leads to restructuring of work, family, and social habits. Through this change, people develop more freedom and a new view of self.		

398 Chapter 14 | Human Growth and Development

(continued)

CUSTOMIZED INSTRUCTION

Less Advanced Students

To help less advanced students remember the different stages of human growth and development, have them create a poster or table listing ages from conception through death and the corresponding stage.

At-Risk Students

As you review Table 14.2, ask students to comment on what they consider risky behavior (e.g., giving out personal information online, smoking cigarettes, drinking alcohol, using illegal drugs, or dropping out of school). Discuss some of the unintended consequences of risky behavior, such as getting sick, being punished or arrested, or saying/doing something you regret. Discuss resources available at school and in your community that students can use to help them solve their problems or avoid engaging in risky behaviors.

Table 14.3 Adulthood Ages 20 Through 70+ Years Stages (continued)

Age	Behavior	Age-Specific Communication Techniques	Effective Communication Techniques During Medical Care
40 to 50 years	People often evaluate the first part of their life. They make decisions about future directions. Many find themselves adjusting basic values and their emphasis toward life. This time of adjustment is often referred to as "midlife crisis" or the "deadline decade." Women may develop assertiveness. Men may become more tender and make stronger commitments to ethical issues.	*(continued from above)*	*(continued from above)*
50 to 60 years	These are the years when people may experience a sense of comfort, an acceptance of life, and a new warmth and mellowing. Privacy becomes important, and friends become more cherished. Truth and sincerity become more valued. Renewal of earlier hobbies and interests often sparks new energy and enthusiasm.		
60 to 70 years	These are the years in which people look forward to retirement. For some people there is a gradual change in their work lives. Others prefer full retirement. The additional hours away from work can now be filled with interests or hobbies. This newfound time often allows people to complete lifelong projects or desires. Sharing of oneself with others aids in maintaining a sense of self-worth.	*The following is appropriate for ages 60 and older:* Listening and sharing interest in stories and experiences is a way for younger people to learn and to show gratitude for the mentorship of people of this age. When with a hearing impaired person, use communication techniques that help promote their understanding. For example: go to a quiet area or eliminate unnecessary sounds, always look at the person when talking, and speak clearly. Remember to make sure that the print in documents is large enough for an older person to read.	*The following is appropriate for ages 60 and older:* When appropriate and possible, prior to a medical procedure offer to show them what will be done during procedures. Tell them what to expect concerning how they will physically feel and what they will see and hear. Reassure them by explaining how to get assistance if needed. When possible and if the patient requests, allow a significant other to stay with them.
70 and older	After the 70s, people may continue their daily life in the same adult patterns. The effect of aging on the body is discussed in Section 14.2 of this chapter. If the body loses its resilience and functions become impaired, the individual's lifestyle may change. It is important to note that of the increasing geriatric population, only 5% require in-patient health care. The remaining 95% are **viable**, active seniors.		

viable
(VAHY uh buhl)
Capable of living.

Teaching Tips

- 40 to 50: early midlife
- 50 to 60: midlife
- 60 to 70: approaching or in retirement
- 70 and older: senior years

- Emphasize that the communication techniques for young and middle aged adults are similar, but that changes occur after age 60.
- Explain the meaning of life continuum: A continuous process from birth to death, through many stages.
- Review the stages of life.
- Review communication techniques for different stages of life.
- Emphasize the need for health care workers to adapt their communication techniques to the age of the patient.

ACTIVITY

Write a personal essay about a life cycle experience that influenced your growth and behavior. The essay should include at least four paragraphs: an introduction, two informational paragraphs, and a conclusion. Frame the experience in the context of the human growth and development stages you learned about in Section 14.1.

Teaching Tips

- Point out that there are many different theories about human growth and development.
- Call students' attention to the description of Erik Erikson's theory of human development.

Science Link—Life Cycles in Nature

- Emphasize that life cycle is not limited to humans, but is experienced by all living organisms.
- Review the two types of insect life cycles: Complete metamorphosis and incomplete metamorphosis.
- Categorize different insects according to their life cycles. Incomplete metamorphosis: crickets and grasshoppers; Complete metamorphosis: butterflies and moths.

What is one major way that complete metamorphosis differs from incomplete metamorphosis?

Answer: Complete metamorphosis has four stages and incomplete metamorphosis has three.
The young forms of complete metamorphosis do not resemble the adults but the young forms of incomplete metamorphosis do.

Erik Erikson's Theory of Human Development

Erik Erikson was a psychologist and psychoanalyst who developed a theory of social development in humans that is widely accepted as accurately representing the stages that people go through as they grow and develop and age. Erikson's theory identifies and explains eight stages through which healthy humans pass.

Working with a partner, research Erik Erikson and create a poster or slide show to share with the class.

Summary

In this section, you have learned about development from conception throughout the life continuum. You have also become aware of emotional and behavioral experiences and communication issues related to each decade of life. Communication techniques need to be adapted according to the age and development stage of people with whom you work.

Section 14.1 Review Questions

1. What occurs during the process of fertilization?
2. Relate a zygote to an embryo.
3. How is a prone position different from a supine position
4. What period of life is described as adolescence?
5. Describe the behaviors pertinent to one stage (decade) in adulthood; for example, 30–40 years old or 60–70 years old.
6. What does it mean to say that a person is not a viable senior?

Science Link

Life Cycles in Nature

The life cycle of an organism refers to its sequence of developmental stages between birth and death. Like humans, other mammals, as well as reptiles, amphibians, birds, fish, insects, and other invertebrates have life cycles.

There are two basic types of life cycles for insects. Complete metamorphosis has four stages: egg, larva, pupa, and adult. The female insect lays eggs that hatch into larvae. The larvae usually have a worm-like shape.

Caterpillars, maggots, and grubs are the larval stages of insects. At some point, larvae make a cocoon around themselves. While in the cocoon, larvae do not eat as their bodies develop into an adult shape with wings, legs, and internal organs. This change takes anywhere from several days to many months. When the larvae have changed into adults, they break out of the cocoon. Mealworms, butterflies, and moths go through complete metamorphosis.

Incomplete metamorphosis has three stages: egg, nymph, and adult. In this life cycle, the female insect lays eggs in a protective covering. The eggs hatch into nymphs, which look like the adults but may not have wings.

Nymphs shed, or molt, their outer skeletons several times as they grow. When the nymph reaches its adult size, it stops molting. By this point, it has grown wings. Crickets, grasshoppers, and flower bugs go through incomplete metamorphosis.

What is one major way that complete metamorphosis differs from incomplete metamorphosis?

Describe the four factors that are the basis for the process of evolution.

400 Chapter 14 | Human Growth and Development

Section 14.1 Review Questions

1. Answer: Fertilization occurs when a male sperm and a female ovum combine. This combination causes the single-cell ovum to divide into many cells. This stage of development is called a zygote. Within five weeks, the rapidly multiplying cells duplicate into an embryo.
2. Answer: A zygote is any cell formed by the coming together of two reproductive cells; the cells rapidly multiplying cells duplicate into an embryo, within five weeks after fertilization.
3. Answer: The prone position is lying on your stomach and the supine position is lying on your back.
4. Answer: Adolescence is ages 13–18, or teenage years.
5. Answers will vary.
6. Answer: Viable means capable of living.

ACTIVITY

Have students obtain examples of personality tests to review and discuss.

Aging and Role Change

SECTION 14.2

Background

The population of people over the age of 65 is expanding. Most people over 65 are active, and they adapt well to change. They continue to enjoy physical activities such as tennis, biking, and skiing. Only five percent are in long-term care.

The concept of health and wellness for people over 65 is not the same as for those at other points of the life span. To care adequately for senior citizens with health problems, health care workers must be aware of the emotional and physical changes that occur during the aging process. Understanding these changes allows the health care worker to assist the aging person in adapting more easily to new roles and ability levels.

Objectives

When you have completed this section, you will be able to do the following:

- Match key terms with their correct meanings.
- Identify six body systems and the common physical changes that occur with aging.
- Identify basic human needs that are met through work, environment, socialization, and family relationships.
- Write an "action plan" to assist another person to cope with changes caused by aging.

Physical Changes of Aging

The process of aging begins in every person at the moment of birth. Aging is a very natural process, and the health care worker needs to be aware of the physical changes that take place. Understanding these changes helps you be patient and less frustrated with others.

The older adult (age 70 and older) population is the most **heterogeneous** (different) of all age groups. People vary in how they age depending on their genetics, lifestyle (jobs, choices, habits), and environmental exposures. Health care decisions must be focused on the individual, not the group, because of the wide variability of each person's cognitive and physical status. An easy rule to remember for the aging population is slower and stiffer for all systems.

heterogeneous
(ahet er uh JEE nee uhs)
Different in kind; unlike.

Nervous System

- As the brain ages, a reduction in nerve cells and cerebral blood flow and metabolism are known to occur. These changes cause slower reflexes and delayed response to multiple stimuli. Elderly people may experience memory loss, which can have several causative factors and can affect their problem solving capacity. Also, the older patient learns in a different way and may require repetitive explanations to enable understanding.

Career Connect

Think about some of the special skills a gerontologist or geriatric nurse must have. Create a list of these skills. Compare your list with your classmates. Tally all of the skills listed, and chart the results. Do any skills appear more then others?

Human Growth and Development | Chapter 14 401

FOCUS AND ENGAGE

Introduce the Section

a. Review the content of the Background paragraphs, explaining that people are living longer.

b. Emphasize that in addition to living longer, people are living better and healthier lives.

c. Review the objectives for the section.

Vocabulary Review

a. Direct students to the key terms.

b. Pronounce each word, and have the students repeat the pronunciation out loud.

c. Discuss the definition of each word.

TEACH

Discuss

- Explain that over 65 is the fastest growing segment of the population.
- Discuss how this affects career opportunities in the health care field.

Reinforce and Review

- Review the body systems covered in Chapter 13.
- Review the stages of human growth and development, focusing on later adulthood.

Teaching Tips

- Explain that the process of aging begins at birth.
- Emphasize that people age at different rates, and experience different changes as they age.
- Discuss the fact that people live longer, more active lives.

CUSTOMIZED INSTRUCTION

More Advanced Students

Assign more advanced students to perform statistical research on the life expectancies now and in the past. Have them enter the data in a table and create a graph or chart to display to the class, showing the trends.

Career Connect

- Student answers will vary, but a gerontologist or geriatric nurse must be patient and understanding.

Teaching Tips

- Explain that aging affects body systems.
- Discuss changes to the nervous system:
    - Slower reflexes
    - Memory loss
    - Changes to vision
    - Hearing loss
    - Declining response to taste, smell, and touch
- Discuss changes to the musculoskeletal system:
    - Osteoarthritis, or pain in joints
    - Osteoporosis
    - Loss of muscle
    - Reduced stamina
- Discuss some of the lifestyle changes people can make to reduce the effects of aging on the musculoskeletal system:
    - Proper diet
    - Regular exercise
    - Do not smoke

Community

- Make sure you identify several local physical therapists who might want to volunteer for this activity. Ask the manager of the senior activity center for permission for students to interview their clients.
- Students should check in with the senior citizens and gather a list of the types of songs they would like to hear during their exercise class.
- The physical therapist should come to class to discuss the potential exercise program. Students should provide the list of music and also ask about how the exercises will address specific disabilities.

adaptation
(ad uhp TEY shuhn)
Changing to work better.

Community

Create an exercise program for a class of senior citizens. Some may be in wheelchairs; others may have walkers or canes. Consult with a physical therapist and keep in mind the type of restrictions their clients may have. Research the kind of music their clients would enjoy as part of the class. Then, teach this class at a community senior citizen center.

- *Vision* begins to change with aging:
    - Small print, small items, and things at a distance are more difficult to see
    - Twenty percent more light is needed to see things clearly
    - Night driving may become difficult
    - **Adaptation** to light is more difficult; the eyes take longer to adjust to changes from dark to light and from light to dark
    - All patients over age 65 benefit from annual eye exams
    - Diseases may occur:
        - *Cataract*: clouding of the normally transparent lenses of the eye
        - *Glaucoma*: intraocular pressure causes damage to the optic disks and hardening of the eyeball
- *Hearing* changes become noticeable in the 60s. When speaking to an elderly person with hearing loss remember to sit at eye level and speak clearly and in a lower tone of voice:
    - High-frequency sounds such as a telephone or doorbell may not be heard
    - Loss of understanding of consonants and vowel sounds may result in a person complaining that others mumble or speak too softly
- *Taste*, *smell*, and *touch* senses decline with age:
    - Elderly people may not smell gases, spoiled food, or body odor
    - Taste buds decline 50 percent, and food enjoyment is reduced
    - Elderly people may request extra salt and sugar because they cannot taste well
    - Avoid using excessive heat or cold as the patient may have decreased awareness if an injury should occur
    - Touch and **reflexes** change; the ability to respond to stimuli is decreased; elderly people may burn themselves or hold an ice tray too long and damage tissue or take longer to respond to the directions you give

reflexes
(REE fleks ez)
Result when a nerve is stimulated and an involuntary action occurs (e.g., touch a hot stove, and the muscles react involuntarily to move the fingers away).

Musculoskeletal System

- Osteoarthritis is an inflammation of the joints and causes pain and slowing down of movement.
- Osteoporosis is caused by a loss of calcium in the bone. This is found more in Caucasian women after menopause, when the bones may become very brittle. They may fracture with very little stress.
- Proper diet and exercise throughout the younger years can forestall or minimize osteoporosis symptoms. It is also important to encourage the older patient to remain active. The human body can build muscle up to the ninth decade and weight bearing will diminish bone loss.
- With reduced **stamina**, elderly people are often less active, which results in the muscles becoming smaller. They generally slow down, which may cause the health care worker to feel impatient.

stamina
(STAM uh nuh)
Body's strength or energy.

402 Chapter 14 | Human Growth and Development

TEAMWORK

Divide the class into teams of five to seven students. In turn, give a team a body system and ask them to name one way aging affects that system. Write the response on the board. Continue until all teams have had a chance to address changes for each body system, and the most common physical changes are listed.

Personal Wellness

Hearing Loss

The gradual hearing loss that occurs as you age (presbycusis) is a common condition. However, the number of people experiencing hearing loss at younger ages is gradually increasing.

Each day you are surrounded by a variety of sounds in your environment. Most sounds occur at safe levels that do not affect hearing. However, sounds that are too loud or last for a long time can damage sensitive structures called hair cells in the inner ear. The result is noise-induced hearing loss (NIHL).

Hair cells convert sound energy into electrical signals that travel to the brain. Once damaged, hair cells cannot grow back. Scientists once believed that the force of vibrations from loud sounds caused the damage to hair cells. Recent studies, however, have shown that exposure to harmful noise triggers the formation of molecules that can damage or kill hair cells.

NIHL can be caused by a single exposure to a quick, intense sound such as an explosion, or by long-term exposure to loud sounds over an extended period of time, such as noise generated in a woodworking shop. The loudness of sound is measured in decibels. Sources of noise that can cause NIHL range from 120 to 150 decibels. Examples include motorcycles, firecrackers, and small firearms.

Long or repeated exposure to sounds at or above 85 decibels can also cause hearing loss. The louder the sound, the shorter the time period before NIHL can occur. Sounds of less than 75 decibels, even after long exposure, are unlikely to cause hearing loss.

The good news is that NIHL is 100 percent preventable. In order to protect yourself, you must understand the hazards of noise and how to practice good hearing health in everyday life. To protect your hearing:

- Know which noises can cause damage.
- Wear earplugs or other hearing protective devices when involved in a loud activity.
- Be alert to hazardous noise in the environment.
- Protect the ears of children who are too young to protect their own.
- Make family, friends, and colleagues aware of the hazards of noise.
- If you suspect hearing loss, have a medical examination by an otolaryngologist, a physician who specializes in diseases of the ears, nose, throat, head, and neck. You may also have a hearing test by an audiologist, a health professional trained to measure and help individuals deal with hearing loss.

What are some sources of loud sounds to which you are exposed?

Respiratory and Circulatory System

- The lungs become less elastic, and the **alveolar-capillary** membrane thickens. This makes oxygen exchange more difficult.
- The rib cage does not expand as much.
- The heart becomes less efficient, and the arteries may become narrowed and clogged. The systolic pressure may rise and result in high blood pressure.

alveolar-capillary
(al VEE uh ler) - (KAP uh ler ee)
Pertaining to air sacs in the lungs.

Personal Wellness—Hearing Loss

- Explain the term presbycusis.
- Point out that gradual hearing loss is a normal part of aging.
- Emphasize that noise-induced hearing loss is not a normal part of aging.
- Review the list of steps people can take to protect their hearing.

What are some sources of loud sounds to which you are exposed?

Answer: Loud music, particularly through headphones. Also, machine equipment at a part-time job, or loud street sounds.

ACTIVITY

Make an educational poster about an issue that affects the roles or basic needs of people as they age.

Teaching Tips

- Discuss changes to the respiratory and circulatory systems:
  - Lungs are less elastic, ribs cage expands less: difficulty breathing
  - Heart is less efficient, arteries become clogged: higher blood pressure
  - Heart disease

Teaching Tips

- Discuss changes to the gastrointestinal system:
  - Constipation
  - Loss of teeth
  - Side effects of medication can damage liver
- Discuss changes to the urinary system:
  - Bladder holds less urine
  - Enlarged prostate in men
  - More frequent bladder infections
- Discuss changes to the integumentary system:
  - Less fat to pad bones and keep skin moist
  - Thinning hair
- Discuss importance of health care workers understanding these changes to both better diagnose ailments and to communicate effectively with aging patients.

Apply It

- Divide students into pairs.
- Assist students in compiling their slide presentation.
- Allow class time for presenting students' presentation on age-specific diseases.

Apply It

With a partner, research age-specific diseases. Some diseases are specific to children or young adults, while many are specific to older adults. Decide on one disease to research further, and identify signs and symptoms of the disease.

Prepare two to five presentation slides that describe and explain the disease you researched. Combine slides with those of the rest of the class to create a media presentation on age-specific diseases.

- The heart also becomes a less efficient pump. Heart disease is the number one cause of death in older people. Among these diseases are:
  - Congestive heart failure
  - Ischemic heart disease
  - Cardiac arrhythmias
  - Hypertensive heart disease

Gastrointestinal System

- Many elderly patients/clients experience **constipation**. This can occur because peristalsis of the intestine (the rhythmic contraction of smooth muscles to propel contents through the digestive tract) is often weakened in the elderly, hence they are more prone to constipation. In addition, elderly people may not be taking enough water and fiber in their diet, leading to hard feces.
- Loss of teeth may interfere with chewing and contribute to malnutrition.
- The liver is important in metabolism. With age, the liver loses up to 20 percent of its weight. This is not serious, because the liver can be effective at 50 percent capacity. However, the liver becomes less effective in metabolizing drugs.
- Older people must be monitored carefully and be alert to drug side effects. Encourage the older patient to "brown bag" all of their medications and bring them to their health care appointments at intervals. This would include both prescription and over-the-counter medications. The medications can be evaluated and with the patient's permission any inappropriate or discontinued medication can be discarded. Be alert to any medication which might affect the central nervous system and increase the **propensity** for falls.

constipation
(kon stuh PEY shuhn)
Infrequent or difficult emptying of the bowel.

propensity
(pro PEN sit tee)
A natural inclination or tendency.

retention
(ri TEN shuhn)
Keeping elements within the body that are normally eliminated (e.g., waste products such as urine and feces).

Urinary System

- The bladder holds less urine as a person ages. This may cause an urgent and frequent need to urinate. In addition, an enlarged prostate may also contribute to urinary frequency in males.
- Bladder infections may occur from **retention** of urine in the bladder. This results in urinary urgency and urinary discomfort. Be aware that the first sign of infection, such as a urinary tract infection or respiratory tract infection, may be an increase in confusion.

Integumentary System

- As people age, there is less adipose tissue (also called fat), and therefore, less padding for bones and much drier skin. The hair also thins. It may not be good for elderly patients to bathe every day, as this increases dryness.

Your awareness of these changes helps you be patient and understanding. These physical changes often cause frustration in your patient and in you. Remember that these changes occur because the body is aging. Listen and reflect understanding. Explain procedures in understandable terms.

404 Chapter 14 | Human Growth and Development

TEAMWORK

Ask students to collect pictures of people at different stages of life and bring them to class. The pictures may be photos of family members and friends, or clippings from magazines and newspapers. Organize the pictures into chronological order to illustrate the aging process. Discuss the visual signs of aging throughout the pictures.

Taking the time to understand your patient's baseline function and community support system will enhance your ability to effectively care for these patients. Understanding the process of aging and its complexities will help you to effectively evaluate needs and plan interventions.

Role Changes in People Who Are Aging

Aging persons are experiencing physical and cognitive changes. They want to continue being productive, and they need to feel respected. Understanding these changes will enable the health care worker to provide appropriate interventions to optimize their functional and cognitive status.

All people have basic needs that are met through the roles they have throughout their life span.

- **Work role.** The work a person does provides a sense of independence, security, and self-esteem. Successful aging is enhanced by a life style that provides a sense of accomplishment on a continuous basis.
- **Family relationships.** Being a member of a family meets our needs for emotional warmth, intimacy, and identity. When members of the family begin to leave or die, the person may be left without a means of filling these basic needs. To adapt to these losses, people need help in directing their interests and energies in other areas. Some of these may include social activities, volunteer work, or membership in organizations. When interviewing the older client be sure to inquire about their family situation and their role as a member of the community.
- **Social roles.** Social contacts fill a person's need for interaction with others. Through social contacts, the person feels respected and admired. As the years pass, friends move away or die, and personal relationships change. These losses may cause people to feel that they are no longer socially important. It is very important that the aging person take part in developing new social contacts. Senior centers, churches, and other organizations are available to help meet this need. Becoming involved helps fill the need for interaction with other human beings.
- **Environment.** The home a person lives in is a place where he or she can be in control, where he or she has a feeling of belonging. As aging occurs, it may become necessary to change environments. The home may become a financial burden, or it may be physically impossible to remain there.
- The older person may move into his or her children's home, a nursing home, or a room of his or her own. This change may be very frightening, and the need for control in their environment is threatened. Memory loss or cognitive impairment may worsen when the person's environment changes. Time and patience will be of utmost importance in helping them to make the best adjustment to their new situation.

Community

Interview one adult over the age of 70, perhaps a family member, and ask the following questions:

What is the most significant change you have witnessed during your life?

Do you believe technology has improved life from when you were young? If so, how? If not, why not?

What kind of work did you do when you were young?

Did you participate in sports, dance or other entertaining activities?

What advice would you give to someone my age?

Submit your responses to the teacher for inclusion in a Living History book that can be reproduced and shared with others in the community.

environment
(en VAHY ruhn muhnt)
Surroundings we live in. Environmental disease can occur in any area around us (e.g., hospital, restaurants, public places, home, school).

Human Growth and Development | Chapter 14 405

Teaching Tips

- Review basic needs.
- Explain role changes in people who are aging, discuss how basic needs must still be met:
  - Work role: even in retirement, people want to feel productive.
  - Family relationships: seniors need to feel that they belong to a family or community.
  - Social roles: seniors may need to develop new social contacts as old friends leave or pass away.
  - Environment: seniors need to live in a safe and secure environment, which may require change.

Community

- Allow enough time for students to set up and complete the interview.
- Discuss other questions students might want to ask.
- Encourage students to take a photo of the interviewee to include in the History book.
- Some students may want to videotape or create an audio recording of the interview.
- If so, students may want to compile the results into a multimedia presentation.

CUSTOMIZED INSTRUCTION

English Language Learners

For the Community activity on this page, have students practice asking the questions aloud to a partner before conducting the interview. If they are interviewing a family member who is not a native English speaker, encourage them to do their best to conduct the interview in English.

At-Risk Students

For the Community activity on this page, some students may not know a suitable candidate for the interview. Line up possible candidates ahead of time, such as volunteers at your school and local library, faculty members, or alumni, to be interviewed by the students.

Teaching Tips

- Review the physical and emotional changes confronting the aging.
- Emphasize the effects of frustration on the elderly.
- Ask students to share observations of family members or neighbors who are aging.
- Ask them to discuss how they react to these changes.
- Discuss ways that a health care worker can help people cope with these changes:
  - Listen carefully
  - Observe for changes
  - Provide access to proper nutrition
  - Provide access to social activities
  - Provide access to educational opportunities
  - Provide access to support organizations
- Discuss occupations in the health care field for people interested in helping aging seniors.

Apply It

- Have students identify sources for their research.
- Allow class time to discuss the issues facing senior citizens.
- Guide students in drawing conclusions about why the issues are specific to senior citizens.

Apply It

Find out more about issues that senior citizens currently face. You might use the AARP (American Association of Retired Persons) Web site (www.aarp.org), or one of their publications as a source. You can also do primary research by interviewing an older family member or neighbor. Identify at least three issues and write a brief summary of each.

Participate in a class discussion to share the current issues facing senior citizens that were identified. In your discussion, draw conclusions about why the issues are specific to senior citizens.

As a health care worker, your understanding of these changes helps you develop the necessary skills to work with older clients. Human beings have a great ability to adjust to changes in their life roles. As people age, functional, cognitive, and social role changes occur. These changes affect most body systems. When these changes occur, older patients may experience frustration with their condition.

Summary

As people age, physical changes occur in the body. These changes affect many body systems. When these changes occur, older patients experience frustration with their conditions. The health care worker has an important role in helping the older patient understand and accept changes.

There are many role changes that occur in aging persons. They may no longer have the identity that their work gave them. They may lose a spouse or other important family members, leaving them lonely. Often, their social role changes as they are less involved in activities. They may find it difficult to develop new friendships. They may have to leave the home where they have their roots and move to a strange place. Awareness of these changes helps the health care worker work effectively with older patients.

Section 14.2 Review Questions

1. How does arteriosclerosis affect the thinking abilities of elderly people?
2. What is a cataract?
3. In what ways do a person's reflexes change with age?
4. What organs are directly related to the alveolar-capillary membrane?
5. Why does the need to urinate increase with age?
6. Describe the most common changes in hearing as people age.

406 Chapter 14 | Human Growth and Development

Section 14.2 Review Questions

1. Answer: Arteriosclerosis affects thinking abilities of elderly people because it causes headaches and dizziness and memory changes.
2. Answer: A cataract is the clouding of the normally transparent lenses of the eye.
3. Answer: Reflexes result when a nerve is stimulated and an involuntary action occurs. As a person ages, the ability to respond to stimuli decreases.
4. Answer: Heart and lungs
5. Answer: The need to urinate increases with age because the bladder holds less urine as a person ages. An enlarged prostate can also case the need to urinate more frequently.
6. Answer: Hearing changes become noticeable in the 60s. High-frequency sounds, such as a telephone or doorbell, may not be heard; there is a loss of understanding of consonants and vowel sounds resulting in complaints that others mumble or speak too softly.

Disabilities and Role Change

SECTION 14.3

Background

Physical disabilities can affect any age group. When a disability, injury, or illness changes a person's lifestyle, he or she must adapt to these changes. This is often difficult and causes frustration and depression. As a health care worker, you need to understand these changes. When you understand such changes, you are more effective, and you can be a positive influence as these patients/clients begin to adapt.

Objectives

When you have completed this section, you will be able to do the following:

- Match key terms with their correct meanings.
- Define health.
- List examples of activities of daily living (ADL).
- Define assistive/adaptive devices.
- Identify ways to encourage independence.
- List birth defects and debilitating illnesses.
- Identify common changes that occur following the loss of body functions.
- State the goal of rehabilitation.
- Select a disability and summarize your feelings and expectations concerning:
  - What you think it would be like to live with that disability
  - The type of care you would expect
  - The way others respond to the disability

Definition of Health

The World Health Organization (WHO) defines health as "a state of complete physical, mental, and social well-being and not merely the absence of disease or infirmity." As a health care worker, you strive to help patients/clients reach their highest potential.

Importance of Independence

When a person is ill or injured, they often have limitations. These limitations usually affect their activities of daily living. The activities include:

- Eating
- Hygiene
- Dressing
- Toileting
- Mobility

Human Growth and Development | Chapter 14 407

FOCUS AND ENGAGE

Introduce the Section

a. Review the content of the Background paragraph, explaining that physical disabilities can afflict people of all ages.

b. Emphasize that understanding how to respond to people with disabilities makes a better health care worker.

c. Review the objectives for the section.

Vocabulary Review

a. Direct students to the key terms.

b. Pronounce each word, and have the students repeat the pronunciation out loud.

c. Discuss the definition of each word.

TEACH

Discuss

- Ask students if they have any personal experience interacting with disabled children or adults.
- Ask if they have ever been temporarily disabled—perhaps by a broken bone.
- Discuss the importance of independence in establishing self-worth.

Reinforce and Review

- Review the basic needs, covered in Chapter 7.
- Review the stages of human growth and development.

CUSTOMIZED INSTRUCTION

More Advanced Students

Assign more advanced students to research the World Health Organization and to create a presentation about it to deliver to the class.

Teaching Tips

- Review the definition of health as defined by the World Health Organization.
- Review the role of independence in daily life:
  - Self-esteem
  - Confidence
  - Image

Teaching Tips

- Discuss the daily activities that may be limited due to illness or injury:
  - Eating
  - Hygiene
  - Dressing
  - Toileting
  - Mobility
- Discuss the instrumental activities of daily living (ADL) that may also be affected:
  - Shopping
  - Cooking
  - Laundry
  - Managing finances
  - Transportation
  - Communication (telephone or Internet)
- Emphasize that a goal of all health care workers is to enable everyone—even the disabled—to be as independent as possible.
- Discuss ways health care workers can encourage independence:
  - Encourage patients to try an activity before helping.
  - Let the patient make choices.
  - Be patient and positive.
- Discuss computers as an assistive device:
  - Communication
  - Access to others via the Internet
- Explain assistive or adaptive devices people and explain their value.
- Examine devices for everyday tasks:
  - Hygiene: long handles and holders on everyday objects such as toothbrushes or sponges
  - Dressing: grabbers for pulling up socks, button loops, and zipper aids
  - Eating: grippers for utensils, and feeding cups
  - Daily activities: grippers for doorknobs and faucets

Limitations can also affect what is known as Instrumental Activities of Daily Living. These activities require a higher level of function and cognition. These activities include:

- Shopping
- Cooking
- Laundry
- Managing finances
- Transportation
- Telephone

Some patients/clients can do these activities with little or no help. Others need a lot of help to **adapt**. The goal is to allow each person to be as independent as he or she possibly can be. Always encourage a patient to try an activity. For example, the person may be able to put toothpaste on the brush but needs your help to brush the teeth. You can encourage the client by being patient and positive and by letting him or her make choices. This helps the patient/client feel more independent and increases feelings of well-being and self-respect. There are many assistive/adaptive devices available, such as gripers that extend and reach, gait trainers that facilitate walking mobility, and bath chairs.

adapt
(uh dapt)
To change, to become suitable, to adjust.

Apply It

Divide yourselves into teams of at least four students. Each team will research a different kind of student disability serviced within your school system.

What support organizations exist for these disabilities? Where do they obtain their funding? Consider organizing a class fund-raiser for one organization.

Computers are effective assistive/adaptive devices for children and adults with physical disabilities. People who cannot hold a pencil or speak can use computers with special enhancements to communicate. Individualized computer programs are created to guide learning.

Computers with e-mail and Internet capabilities provide opportunities for people with disabilities to interact with the outside world. The computer enables people with certain disabilities to communicate their needs, thoughts, desires, and intelligence to their parents and caregivers. These devices help the patient be more independent and self-sufficient. They help clients:

- Eat
- Reach objects
- Complete personal care
- Dress and button clothing
- Communicate

Occupational Therapists specialize in assisting with adaptive devices for accomplishing activities of daily living and instrumental activities of daily living.

Physical Disabilities

Physical disabilities may be caused by a congenital condition, a debilitating illness, or an injury. Understanding disabilities helps you give better care to your patients.

Congenital Conditions

Babies who are born with a physical congenital condition, inherited **syndrome**, or other problems have a **congenital condition**. As a health care worker, you need to recognize these conditions in order to give good care and be supportive to family members. Common congenital defects are explained in Table 14.4.

Debilitating illness may occur at any age. Depending on the severity of the disease, physical changes may be minimal or very extensive. Common debilitating illnesses are explained in Table 14.5.

syndrome
(SIN drohm)
A number of symptoms occurring together.

congenital conditions
(kon JEN i tull kon DI shuns)
Existing at or before birth usually through heredity, as a disorder.

debilitating
(di BIL I teyt ing)
Causing weakness or impairment.

408 Chapter 14 | Human Growth and Development

Apply It

- Create teams of five to seven students for this activity.
- You may want to assign the student service each team will research.
- You may want to notify the teacher or administrator in charge of the service about the activity in advance.
- Allot class time for presenting the projects and discussing them.

TEAMWORK

In pairs, use materials such as rolled newspapers and rags to apply splints to elbows so the arms cannot bend. Have students attempt a simple every day activity, such as eating a snack, putting on a coat, or writing a note. After the exercise, have the students write their response and evaluate the experience. Discuss the exercise as a class.

Table 14.4 Congenital Conditions

Condition at Birth	Condition	Identifying Characteristics
Autism	A brain development disorder that impairs social interaction and communication, and causes restricted and repetitive behavior, all starting before a child is three years old.	Makes little or no eye contact; does not speak as well as other children their age; does not use their imagination during play; shows no response when smiled at; can become unusually attached to objects; does not interact with other children; are prone to tantrums for no apparent reason.
Cerebral palsy	A motor function disorder that is caused by a brain defect or lesion present at birth or shortly after.	Spastic hemiplegia; seizures; some degree of mental retardation in some people; impaired vision, speech, and hearing; and stiff, awkward movements.
Cleft lip and/or cleft palate	Fusion of the palate and/or lip takes place during **embryonic** development.	The cleft is often easily seen, but some display an inability to suck or nurse, crying when the child tries to nurse, with fluid coming out of the nose.
Cystic fibrosis	Inherited disorder of the exocrine glands that causes an excessive amount of thick mucus. Most affected are the pancreas, respiratory system, and sweat glands.	Usually diagnosed during infancy or in young children of Caucasian origin. Chronic cough, frequent foul-smelling stools, and persistent upper respiratory infections.
Down syndrome	A chromosomal abnormality known as trisomy 21 and is often associated with advanced maternal age.	Varying degrees of mental retardation and multiple defects; slanted eyes; depressed nasal bridge; low-set ears; large, protruding tongue; short, broad hands with a simian crease and stubby fingers; broad, stubby feet with wide spaces between the first and second toes; prone to respiratory infections, visual problems, and abnormalities in tooth development, and heart problems.
Epilepsy	**Neurological** disorders that may be birth defects but can occur later in life due to cerebral trauma, intracranial infection, brain tumor, **intoxication**, or chemical imbalance.	Recurrent **episodes** of convulsive seizures, sensory disturbances, abnormal behavior, loss of consciousness.
Hydrocephaly	Overproduction or underabsorption of cerebro spinal fluid. May or may not cause increased pressure in the brain.	Globe-shaped head, flat nose bridge, eyes pushed downward and out, becoming widely spread; mild to severe retardation.
Sickle-cell anemia	A **hereditary** disease that is most common among African-American people. The red blood cell is crescent shaped (sickle shaped) and carries an abnormal **hemoglobin**.	Severe joint pain, thrombosis, fever, chronic anemia.
Spinal bifida	A developmental defect. A **hernial** sac containing the meninges, spinal cord, or both protrudes at the end of the vertebral column. This sac is easily ruptured, causing the characteristics at the right.	Leakage of spinal fluid, risk of **meningeal** cystica infection, severe neurological **dysfunction**, paralysis, muscle weakness, retardation.
Tay-Sachs syndrome	An inherited disease caused by an **enzyme deficiency**. It occurs primarily in families of Eastern European Jewish origin.	Difficult breathing and decreased exhange of oxygen and carbon dioxide.

Human Growth and Development | Chapter 14 409

Teaching Tips

- Introduce the topic of physical disabilities.
- May be caused by:
  - Congenital condition
  - Debilitating illness
  - Injury
- Explain congenital conditions (conditions present at birth).
- Review Table 14.4 together as a class.
- Discuss common physical disabilities caused by congenital conditions.
- Discuss the identifying characteristics of each condition.

TEAMWORK

In small groups, prepare a skit demonstrating how a health care worker can encourage independence in a disabled person.

What's New?—Identifying Congenital Conditions

- Review some of the possible causes of congenital conditions:
  - Genetics
  - Organs
  - Body chemistry
- Discuss tests for identifying congenital conditions before birth.
- Discuss pros and cons of such tests.
- Discuss actions that can be taken as a result of identifying a congenital condition prior to birth:
  - Corrective surgery before birth
  - Corrective surgery immediately after birth
  - Education
  - Preparation

How is identifying congenital conditions different today than it was 50 years ago?

Answer: Fifty years ago, technology was not available to detect and treat birth defects before birth.

ACTIVITY

Make a chart categorizing different disabilities as congenital conditions, debilitating illnesses, or debilitating injuries. Give examples of each.

embryonic
(em bree ON ik)
Pertaining to the embryo.

neurological
(noor uh LOG I kuhl)
Pertaining to the nervous system.

episodes
(EP i sod s)
Events in a series.

intoxication
(in tok si KEY shuhn)
State of poisoning or becoming poisoned.

hereditary
(huh RED i ter ee)
Passed from parent to child.

hemoglobin
(HEE muh gloh bin)
An iron-containing protein in red blood cells that combines reversibly with oxygen and transports it from the lungs to body tissues.

hernial
(HUR nee uh)
Pertaining to projection through an abnormal opening in the wall of a body cavity.

meninges
(mi NIN jeez)
Lining of the brain.

dysfunction
(dis FUHNGK shuhn)
Impaired or abnormal functioning.

enzyme
(EN zahym)
Substance that causes a change to occur in other substances.

deficiency
(di FISH uhn see)
Shortage (e.g., a deficient diet causes the body to function poorly because it is missing an important element).

What's New?

Identifying Congenital Conditions

While most babies are born healthy, the risk of having a baby with congenital conditions plagues many women throughout the early stages of pregnancy. Congenital conditions may be related to genetic material, organs, or body chemistry. Some congenital conditions have little impact on the child's life whereas others can be life threatening.

Advancements in technology continue to increase the ability of doctors to identify congenital conditions as early as possible. Just decades ago, doctors who had no forewarning of defects that would be present during delivery can now learn a tremendous amount of information as early as the first trimester of pregnancy (first three months).

Identifying conditions during pregnancy can be important because conditions, such as cleft lip, cleft palate, and some heart problems, can sometimes be surgically corrected shortly after birth or even during pregnancy. In addition, if an abnormality has been identified before birth, health care workers can be prepared to offer any special care needed upon birth.

Some tests performed during pregnancy are screening tests. These tests aim to identify the likelihood of a congenital condition. If the screening test is positive, which means that a problem is identified, a diagnostic test is performed to either confirm or rule out the problem. Keep in mind that no test is 100 percent accurate. In a false negative, test results do not identify congenital conditions when they are actually present. On the contrary, a false positive indicates a condition in a normal baby.

Two common screening tests, maternal serum triple or quad screening, check the pregnant mother's blood for specific substances related to different congenital conditions. These include some brain and spinal cord defects, related neural tube defects, and some chromosome defects. Ultrasound can be used to identify structural defects as well as signs of Down syndrome.

Common diagnostic tests include chorionic villus sampling (CVS) and amniocentesis, in which specific cells are obtained and analyzed for defects. Most recently, combinations of blood tests and ultrasound are being used to identify defects early on in the pregnancy.

How is identifying congenital conditions different today than it was 50 years ago?

Injury

Injuries may occur at any age and cause many different disabilities. Some of the most common are:

- Spinal cord injuries, which may cause paralysis
- Stroke, which may cause paralysis, brain dysfunction, speech impairments, and/or loss of memory
- Head injuries, which may cause coma, loss of memory, and/or paralysis
- Amputation of a limb

Debilitating Illnesses

Elderly patients are more affected by a debilitating illness as they may not have sufficient physical, mental, or financial resources to accommodate recovery. An elderly person experiencing a fall or a hospitalization may experience a spiraling downward effect in their health status.

opportunistic infections
(op er too NIS tik in FEK shen) Infections that occur when the immune system is weakened. Common organisms that the body normally resists cause infection.

disorientation
(dis AWR ee uhn tey shuh n) State of being confused about time, place, and identity of persons and objects.

arteriosclerosis
(ahr teer ee oh skluh ROH sis) Condition of hardening of the arteries.

Table 14.5 Common Debilitating Illnesses

Debilitating Illness	Condition	Identifying Characteristics/Symptoms
Acquired immune deficiency syndrome (AIDS)	Caused by a virus that reduces the immune system's ability to respond to **opportunistic infections**.	Common opportunistic infections that result from AIDS include pneumocystis pneumonia, candidiasis, cryptococcus, and herpes. Cancers that may develop are Kaposi's sarcoma and lymphomas.
Alzheimer's disease	A degenerative disorder that affects the brain generally in later, middle life.	Confusion, memory failure, **disorientation**, restlessness, speech disturbances, inability to carry out purposeful movements, and hallucinations.
Arteriosclerosis	Hardening of the arteries, which reduces the elasticity of the arterial walls.	Elevated blood pressure.
Atherosclerosis	**Lipid**-containing material collects on the inside surfaces of the blood vessels causing thickening of the vessel walls and narrowing of the space that blood flows through, thus inhibiting blood flow. Associated with obesity, hypertension, and diabetes.	Angina pectoris, myocardial infarction (MI), coronary heart disease, strokes.
Cancer	Uncontrolled growth of immature cells that invade normal tissue and travel to other tissues. More than 80 percent of cancers are caused by cigarette smoking, carcinogenic chemicals, radiation, and overexposure to the sun.	Signs of cancer vary, but it is wise to see a physician when the following occurs: change in bowel or bladder habits, a nonhealing sore, unusual bleeding or discharge, a thickening or lump anywhere, indigestion or trouble swallowing, an obvious change in a wart or mole, or a nagging cough or persistent hoarseness.
Cardiovascular disease	Any abnormal heart and/or circulatory condition. Cardiovascular disease remains a leading cause of death in the United States.	Dysfunction of the heart and blood vessels commonly causing angina, shortness of breath, weakness, and general fatigue.

(continued)

Human Growth and Development | Chapter 14 411

Teaching Tips

- Discuss injuries that can cause disability:
  - Spinal cord injuries
  - Stroke
  - Head injuries
  - Amputations
- Explain that such injuries can occur at any age, and can result in different types of disabilities.
- Emphasize that these types of injuries are generally unexpected.
- Some, such as head injuries, may be preventable.
- Discuss prevention, such as helmets or seatbelts.
- Discuss the emotional considerations of an unexpected debilitating injury.
- Explain debilitating illnesses that result in physical and mental disabilities.
- Review Table 14.5 on pp. 411 and 412 together as a class.
- Point out that many debilitating illnesses affect the elderly.
- Discuss the identifying characteristics or symptoms of each condition.
- Emphasize that understanding the cause and characteristics of disabilities helps students become better health care workers.

TEAMWORK

Divide the class into teams of five to seven students. In turn, read the characteristics or symptoms of a debilitating illness or congenital condition to one team. Give the team 30 seconds to name the condition, or offer the question to a different team. Award a point for each correct answer.

Teaching Tips

- Review the basic roles that people require to feel that they are productive members of society:
  - Relationships
  - Work
  - Fitting into the community
- Explain ways that a disability can affect these roles, mentally, emotionally, and physically:
  - Dependence on others
  - Lack of control
  - Loss of body function
- Discuss changes that might occur from the loss of body function:
  - Communication skills may diminish
  - Sensory awareness may diminish
  - Ability to think and comprehend may diminish
  - Ability to move may diminish
  - Elimination of waste products may be affected
  - Ability to eat may be impacted
  - Sexual activity may be impacted

Table 14.5 Common Debilitating Illnesses (continued)

Debilitating Illness	Condition	Identifying Characteristics/Symptoms
Diabetes	Blood glucose, or sugar, levels are too high. With Type 1 diabetes, the body does not make insulin. With Type 2 diabetes, the more common type, the body does not make or use insulin well. Without enough insulin, the glucose stays in your blood. Being obese increases your risk of diabetes.	Excessive thirst and increased urination, flu-like feeling, weight gain or loss, increased fatigue, irritability, blurry vision.
Emphysema	The alveoli in the lungs are overextended and loose their elasticity. The lungs become less and less able to exchange oxygen and carbon dioxide.	Shortness of breath, cough, cyanosis, unequal chest expansion, rapid respiratory rate, elevated temperature. They may also experience, anxiety, restlessness, confusion, and weakness.
Leukemia	Rapid and abnormal growth of immature leukocytes in the blood-forming organs (bone marrow, spleen, and lymph nodes).	Males are affected twice as often as females. Symptoms include fatigue, pallor, weight loss, easy bruising, extreme weakness, bone or joint pain, repeated infections.
Multiple sclerosis	Progressive disease that affects the nerve fibers of the brain and spinal cord. It generally begins in young adulthood and continues throughout life.	Muscle weakness, visual disturbances, and dizziness. It affects the whole body, including emotional stability.
Parkinson's disease	Slowly progressive, degenerative, neurological disorder.	Tremors, shuffling gait, masklike face, forward flexion of the trunk, muscle rigidity, and weakness.

lipid
(LIP id)
Fat.

progressive
(pruh GRES iv)
Moving forward, following steps toward an end product.

Role Changes in People Who Are Physically or Mentally Challenged

When people experience a lengthy disability, they require understanding and patience. Disabled people need to remain a productive part of society and to maintain a sense of well-being. The health care worker can be a positive influence on patients/clients during the period of adjustment and rehabilitation.

People who lose a body part or a part of their body functions experience the same stages of loss as do people with a terminal illness. These are denial, rage and anger, bargaining, depression, and acceptance. Many people who suddenly find themselves disabled are dependent on others for many of their daily needs. Being dependent often leads to feelings of not being in control. Physical losses can cause various body functions to be impaired.

Loss of body function often means that changes may occur in the following:

- Communication skills
- Sensory awareness
- Ability to think and comprehend
- Ability to move
- Elimination of waste products

412 Chapter 14 | Human Growth and Development

CUSTOMIZED INSTRUCTION

Special Needs Students

Encourage special needs students to share personal stories of living with a disability. This may help them feel more comfortable with the class, and will help the other students understand what daily life is like for the disabled. Encourage a discussion.

- Eating
- Sexual activity

Loss of physical functions may cause emotional stability to change. The areas of emotional insecurity usually focus around the following:

- Self-esteem
- Self-confidence
- Self-image

Physical impairments that lead to emotional changes may also create a sense of loss concerning the following:

- Ability to develop relationships with others
- Ability to earn a living
- Ability to be a useful member of society

The health care worker helps patients/clients reach their goals by being understanding and knowledgeable about the process involved in acceptance of a disability and rehabilitation.

Community

Volunteer in a local rehabilitation center. Review a case history (without seeing the existing rehab plan), develop your own rehab plan and design an assistive device for the patient that will meet at least one of their needs. How does your plan match up with the plan created for the patient by licensed professional?

Rehabilitation

When physical changes occur, the goal of rehabilitation is to help the patient/client return to the highest level of functioning possible. Rehabilitation promotes a healthy return to a productive lifestyle. There are many rehabilitation areas involved in this process. The most common are as follows:

- Physical therapy restores the body to normal functioning when possible.
- Occupational therapy restores the ability to be involved in purposeful activity.
- Speech therapy restores the ability to communicate effectively.
- Psychotherapy changes inappropriate behavior patterns, improves interpersonal relationships, and resolves inner conflicts.

There are several groups available to aid the client and family during the recovery and rehabilitation period. These groups, called support groups, are organized to help patients and family members cope with changes during this period. Examples of groups are:

- Breast cancer support group
- Ostomy support group
- Vital Options—a support group for young adults with cancer

You can locate groups in your area by contacting the social services department at hospitals, community centers, and organizations oriented to health care.

Human Growth and Development | Chapter 14 413

Teaching Tips

- Discuss emotional changes that might occur from the loss of body function.
- Patients may feel insecure about:
  - Self-esteem
  - Self-confidence
  - Self-image
- Patients may feel a sense of loss about:
  - Ability to develop relationships with others
  - Ability to earn a living
  - Ability to be a useful member of society
- Discuss ways a health care worker can provide emotional support for the disabled:
  - Educate patient about the process
  - Encourage acceptance
  - Encourage positive action
- Explain the goal of rehabilitation:
  - Help the patient return to the highest level of functioning possible
- Explain that rehabilitation promotes a health return to a productive lifestyle through:
  - Physical therapy
  - Occupational therapy
  - Speech therapy
  - Psychotherapy
- Discuss the role of support groups.

ACTIVITY

Research careers in rehabilitation for the disabled. Write a want ad for one position. Include information about the educational and personal requirements for the position, as well as the location of the job and the salary range.

Community

- Check with a local rehabilitation center to see if they will work with your students on this project.
- Present students with the contact name and appropriate times for them to visit and review the charts. Or, should the center prefer, ask a representative to come to class with case histories (patient names will be deleted) that can be used for this project.

Teaching Tips

- Review the causes of physical disabilities.
- Review the role of a health care worker in helping the disabled.

Section 14.3 Review Questions

1. Answers will vary but may include cerebral palsy, epilepsy, Down syndrome, or spinal bifida
2. Answer: A birth defect exists at or before birth, usually through heredity. A debilitating illness may occur at any age and depending on the severity, physical changes may be minimal or extensive.
3. Answer: Head injury
4. Answer: Nervous system
5. Answer: A hereditary disease is passed from parent to child.
6. Answers will vary. Progressive diseases include Alzheimer's, cancer, Parkinson's diseases, multiple sclerosis, and emphysema.

Language Arts Link—Human Development and Aging

- Note that this activity is designed for pairs.
- You may want to combine this activity with the Community activity on p. 413, or assign students to interview a different subject.
- You may want to have samples of Q&A interviews from newspapers or magazines available for students to look at.
- Encourage students to plan the questions they will ask in advance.
- Direct students to focus on the emotional aspects of aging when planning their interview.

Summary

Physical disabilities, injury, and debilitating illness can occur from birth to old age. There are many different types of disabilities. Some of these are caused by accident, heredity, injury, or illness. When any of these are present, the patient may be frustrated or depressed. As a health care worker, you are responsible for the care and support of these patients. It is important to understand their illness and to be familiar with assistive/adaptive devices and support organizations that are available to help patients and their families.

Section 14.3 Review Questions

1. Give an example of a congenital condition that might limit a person's activities in some way.
2. How is a debilitating illness different from a birth defect?
3. What type of injury is most directly associated with a coma?
4. Which human body system is affected by neurological disorders?
5. What does it mean to say that sickle-cell anemia is a hereditary disease?
6. Give an example of a progressive disease.

Language Arts Link

Human Development and Aging

As people grow, develop and age, they experience a number of changes. For an aging person, some of the changes may be frightening or frustrating. Working with a partner, find a person, such as a friend or family member, who is willing to be interviewed on some of the changes taking place. Initiate the discussion by posing questions that cause your subject to respond with ideas, conclusions, and creative perspectives. Respond thoughtfully to diverse perspectives, recognizing how views differ from generational perspectives.

With your partner, prepare a report on the results of your interview. Develop the topic thoroughly by selecting the most significant and relevant information discussed. Include any thoughts on how you could help your subject manage some of these changes. Revise and edit your document by making it clearer, more concise, or more interesting to read. Try reading your writing aloud so that you and your partner can listen to the flow and clarity of what you've written. Check the spelling and grammar and correct any errors. Working with your partner, prepare a presentation on what you've learned and, if time allows, present your findings to the class.

414 Chapter 14 | Human Growth and Development

- Encourage students to take a photograph of the subject to include in the report and presentation.
- Remind students to write complete sentences and paragraphs and to use proper grammar and spelling.
- Evaluate the reports based on the thoroughness of the interview and the way the students interpret and report the results, as well as on spelling, grammar, and organization.

TEAMWORK

In groups to four to five, research one particular disability and create a presentation about it. Include information such as how the disability might occur, the age of the person who might suffer the disability, and the characteristics and symptoms. Also include the types of physical and emotional challenges people with this disability might encounter in daily life, how health care workers and others might provide care and support, and how people typically respond to someone with this disability.

End-of-Life Issues

SECTION 14.4

Background

As a health care worker, you come in contact with clients who are nearing the end of their life. Your knowledge of the psychological stages experienced by those at the end of life gives you an understanding of their behavior.

Objectives

When you have completed this section, you will be able to do the following:

- Match key terms with their correct meanings.
- Match the psychological stages of a long terminal illness with their names.
- Identify and discuss your feelings about terminal illness.
- Explain the philosophy of hospice care.

Terminal Illness

Patients/clients who have an illness that cannot be cured are terminally ill. They are expected to die. When the patients learn of their illness, they usually pass through five different psychological stages. (Figure 14.1) Elisabeth Kübler-Ross, M.D. (1926–2004), was a Swiss-born psychiatrist who first proposed these Five Stages of Grief as a pattern of phases, most or all of which people tend to go through, in sequence, after being faced with the tragedy of their own impending death. As a health care professional, you will learn techniques to help patients cope with end-of-life issues.

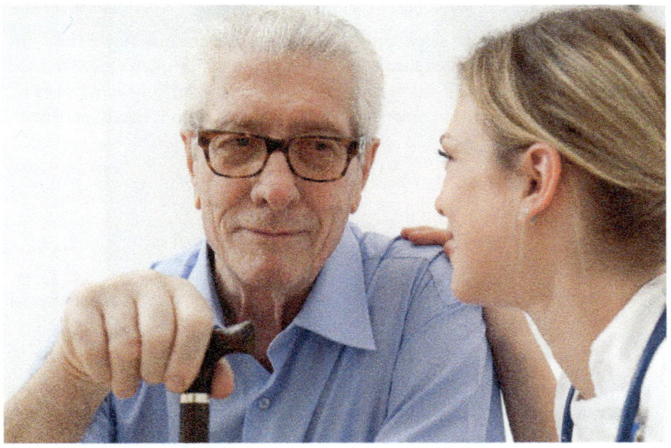

Figure 14.1 Why do most people pass through the five different psychological stages?

Human Growth and Development | Chapter 14 415

FOCUS AND ENGAGE

Introduce the Section

a. Review the content of the Background paragraph, explaining that end-of-life issues concern death and dying.

b. Emphasize that end-of-life issues are most imminent for people who are aging and those with terminal illnesses.

c. Review the objectives for the section.

Vocabulary Review

a. Direct students to the key terms.

b. Pronounce each word, and have the students repeat the pronunciation out loud.

c. Discuss the definition of each word.

TEACH

Discuss

- Ask students if they have experienced the death of a loved one.
- Point out that in some cultures, thinking and talking about death is not encouraged.
- In other cultures, death is considered a natural part of life.
- Discuss different views on death and dying.

Reinforce and Review

- Review the stages of human growth and development.

Teaching Tips

- Explain terminal illness: An illness that cannot be cured.
- Introduce the Kubler-Ross five psychological stages of grief.

CUSTOMIZED INSTRUCTION

Less Advanced Students

To help less advanced students remember the five psychological stages, have them create a flowchart listing them in order to use as a study guide. They might also benefit from flashcards with the stage name on the front and a description of the behaviors associated with the stage on the back.

Figure Focus

14.1 Why do most people pass through the five different psychological stages?

Student answers will vary.

Teaching Tips

- Explain that the Kubler-Ross stages are used to explain the behavior of those facing death.
- Explain that it is the responsibility of the health care worker to recognize the signs of each stage, and respond with the appropriate communication techniques.
- Discuss each stage:
  1. Shock and denial. The health care worker must listen and encourage the patient to express his or her feelings.
  2. Rage and anger. The care worker must not take the anger personally, and must continue to listen and not respond with anger.
  3. Bargaining. The health care worker must express understanding, refrain from judging, and be available to listen.
  4. Depression. The health care worker must be available physically and emotionally, and express concern and understanding.
  5. Acceptance. The health care worker must be able to discuss the facts of the patient's illness and death in a direct and forthcoming manner.
- Point out that some patients skip stages, or regress.
- Note that family and friends may also pass through similar stages.

isolated
(AHY suh leyt ed)
Limited in contact with others.

impending
(im PEN ding)
About to happen.

- **Stage one: Shock and denial.** People find it very difficult to believe that they are really going to die. "No, not me!" During this stage they feel very lonely and **isolated**. *Communication:* If they can discuss these feelings and talk about their **impending** death, they are able to move into the next stage. You may be the only health care worker available to listen to their feelings.
- **Stage two: Rage and anger.** No matter how much kindness you have shown, your client may become very insulting; there might be many complaints about everything you do. You may be tempted to leave them to their anger. *Communication:* If you realize it is not a personal attack, you will be able to listen and to understand that the anger is not directed at you. It is directed at the injustice of the situation. Be a good listener. When patients have exhausted their anger, they will move out of the anger stage.
- **Stage three: Bargaining.** Although they now admit to themselves that they are dying, the clients try to prolong their life with bargaining. For example, they might say, "Just let me live until my children are independent." *Communication:* Listen and reflect what is said, express your understanding, and be aware of your voice tone and body language. Be aware of times when your presence in silence is helpful and when words are not helpful.
- **Stage four: Depression.** Your patients may refuse to talk to you or even look at you. They are experiencing great sadness, for they are losing everyone and everything. *Communication:* Although they may not want to be bothered with friends or visitors, your touch is very important. Your understanding of their feelings of loss enables them to move into the last stage.
- **Stage five: Acceptance.** At last your clients can accept their death. This is a time when your presence lets them know you will not desert them. *Communication:* They may want to discuss their death. Your willingness to be available will help your patients in a very difficult time.

Of course, the patient can skip stages; in addition, he or she may regress back to a stage after they have passed through it. Friends and family often experience the same stages when someone they love and care about is terminally ill. As a health care worker, you need to be understanding. Family and friends may experience the following stages:

- **Shock and denial.** They may continue to make plans for the future that include the dying person.
- **Rage and anger.** They may be irritable and angry and say unkind things occasionally.
- **Bargaining.** They may ask the physician to keep the patient/client alive for a special occasion.
- **Depression.** They feel extreme sadness and even despair.
- **Acceptance.** They finally accept that death is going to occur. They may ask you to recommend someone for them to talk to.

416 Chapter 14 | Human Growth and Development

ACTIVITY

Select one of the five Kubler-Ross stages and create a poster illustrating it. Create a display in the classroom or on a bulletin board using the posters to illustrate all five stages in order.

Decision Making at the End of Life

Decision making related to end-of-life issues must consider all aspects of care. Those decisions must include the patient's culture and spiritual views as well as address issues ranging from living arrangements and dedicated caregivers to preparing a living will, a legal document that defines a patient's wishes should they no longer be able to speak for themselves.

The patient and family's decision making must be supported in an ethical framework of respect for independence and dignity. Without the support of an individual's right to decision making, there is the risk that the patient will be treated as an object rather than as a person.

Health care decision making is built upon a relationship between patient and health care provider that requires mutual respect, trust, honesty, and confidentiality. Manipulation or intimidation must not hinder the resulting free exchange of information. Patients need to know and be informed of the following:

- Their condition
- The proposed treatment
- Expected results
- Alternative treatment options
- Potential risks, complications, and anticipated benefits

Pain Management

When the terminally ill patient decides jointly with health care providers and the family that prolonging life with therapy is no longer possible, then comfort and pain relief becomes the treatment goal.

Many patients with a terminal illness fear physical pain much more than they fear death itself. Pain that is undertreated can have an extreme effect on the patient. It is important to work as a team with your co-workers to address the emotional, physical, spiritual, and psychological effects of pain and relieve discomfort as much as possible.

Relieving pain includes maintaining the patient's personal hygiene and body alignment, and speaking gently and clearly to the patient even if he or she is not able to respond to you. Reporting restlessness, excessive sweating, and rapid respirations to the charge nurse will provide information needed to determine if medication is appropriate.

Scales of 10 are commonly used in health care today for evaluating the level of discomfort. Teaching a patient to use a pain scale gives them a way of evaluating and communicating their pain to a caregiver.

Human Growth and Development | Chapter 14 417

Teaching Tips

- Review the issues involved with decision making.
- Decisions must take into consideration:
  - The patient's perception of death
  - Psychological aspects of culture and spirituality
  - Components of treatment
- Emphasize respect for independence and dignity.
- Review the issues that patients must understand before decisions can be made:
  - Their condition
  - The proposed treatment
  - Expected results
  - Alternative treatment options
  - Potential risks and complications
  - Possible benefits
- Discuss pain management.
- Emphasize that once death is seen as inevitable, the goal of treatment is to provide comfort and pain relief.
- Point out that fear of pain may be greater than fear of death.
- Discuss how to recognize symptoms of pain.
- Discuss the scale of 10 frequently used to assess pain.

TEAMWORK

Divide the class into five groups. Assign each group one of the Kubler-Ross stages. Each group should prepare a skit demonstrating how a patient with a terminal illness might behave in their assigned stage. Present the skits in the order of the stages.

Teaching Tips

- Review the mission of hospice care.
- Explain that the hospice philosophy is to help patients live each day to the fullest.
- Discuss locations for hospice care:
  - In home
  - Hospice facility
- Discuss family involvement in hospice care.
- Introduce the topic of euthanasia.
- Explain that it is the act of ending the life of an individual suffering from a terminal illness or an incurable condition.

Figure Focus

14.2 What are some of the benefits of hospice care?

Student answers will vary.

Hospice Care

philosophy
(fi LOS uh fee)
Theory; a general principle used for a specific purpose.

In many communities, hospice care is available for terminally ill people. The hospice **philosophy** is to help patients/clients nearing the end of life live each day to the fullest. This care is provided in the home or in a hospice facility. Patients are kept comfortable and free from pain. (**Figure 14.2**) When the time for death comes, they are allowed to die peacefully.

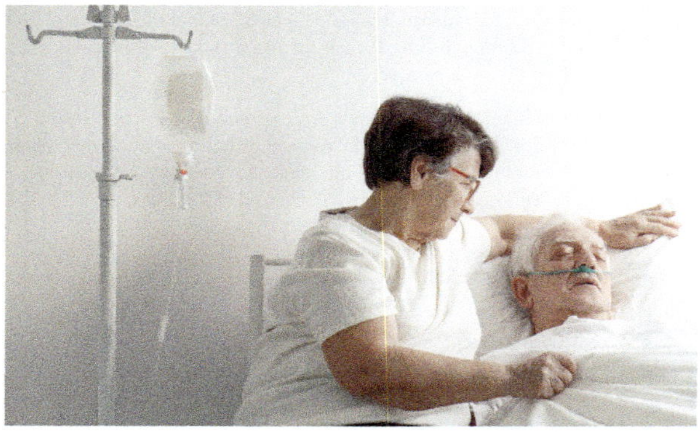

Figure 14.2
What are some of the benefits of hospice care?

An important service of hospice is family involvement. Families are counseled and helped to accept the impending death of a loved one. Following the death, the family has continuing support for at least a year. This support helps make the grieving period more tolerable.

You are an important member of the health care team. Your insight into the patient/client and his or her family and friends provides valuable information to decision makers concerning the care process. This knowledge of what your patients/clients may experience helps you meet their needs.

Euthanasia

Euthanasia, also referred to as a "mercy killing," is the act of ending the life of an individual suffering from a terminal illness or an incurable condition. The word "euthanasia" originated from the Greek language: "eu" means "good" and "thanatos" means "death"; so, it actually means a "good death." If death is not intended, then it is not an act of euthanasia. Euthanasia is carried out by lethal injection or by suspending extraordinary medical treatment. There are different types of euthanasia including:

- **Voluntary euthanasia.** When a person killed requested to be killed.
- **Non-voluntary euthanasia.** When the person killed gave no request or consent to be killed.

- **Involuntary euthanasia.** When the person killed made an expressed wish to the contrary.
- **Assisted suicide.** When someone provides an individual with the information, guidance, and means to take his or her own life with the intention that they will be used for this purpose. When a doctor who helps an individual to kill themselves it is called "physician-assisted suicide."

The issue of euthanasia is very controversial. Some people argue that this is a case of freedom of choice—one that relieves an individual of extreme pain and suffering when their quality of life is low. Others believe that euthanasia devalues human life and can become a means of health care cost containment.

As of November 2021, euthanasia is legal in Belgium, Canada, Colombia, Luxembourg, the Netherlands, New Zealand, Spain, and several states of Australia. In the United States, physician-assisted suicide is legal in California, Colorado, District of Columbia, Hawaii, Montana, Maine, New Jersey, New Mexico, Oregon, Vermont, and Washington.

Organ Procurement and Donation

Organ donation is the removal of tissues of the human body from an individual who has recently died or from a living donor. Organ procurement is the obtaining of organs for transplantation. It includes the transporting of donor organs, after surgical removal, to the hospital for processing and transplant.

The following organs can be procured: heart, intestines, kidneys, lungs, liver, pancreases, bones, and skin. In addition, the following tissues can be procured for donation: tendons, corneas, heart valves, bone marrow, and veins.

Everyone is a potential organ and tissue donor. Age and medical history are not the determining factors; instead, the critical factor is the condition of your organs and tissues at the time of death.

If you are under age 18, a parent or guardian must give permission for you to become a donor. If you are 18 or older, you can agree to be a donor by signing a donor card. It is also important to let your family know your wishes.

Jobs and Professions

- **Geriatrician.** A doctor who specializes in the care for people 65 and older.
- **Hospice worker.** Provides terminally ill patients with services that range from companionship to personal care.
- **Nurse assistant/orderly in long-term care facility.** Works under the supervision of a nurse and provides assistance to patients with daily living tasks.
- **Assistive personnel.** Includes certified nurse's aide, home health aide, and patient care technicians.

Human Growth and Development | Chapter 14 419

Teaching Tips

- Explain that euthanasia is a controversial subject.
- Point out that it is illegal in all states except for Washington, Oregon, Vermont, New Mexico, and Montana. It would result in a criminal charge of murder in all other states.
- Review the types of euthanasia:
  - Voluntary
  - Non-voluntary
  - Involuntary
  - Assisted suicide
- Introduce the topic of organ procurement and donation.
- Explain the organs that may be procured:
  - Heart
  - Intestines
  - Kidneys
  - Lungs
  - Liver
  - Pancreas
  - Bones
  - Skin
- Explain that tissues that may be procured:
  - Tendons
  - Corneas
  - Heart valves
  - Bone marrow
  - Veins
- Discuss who is eligible to donate organs.

ACTIVITY

Contact a hospice facility or hospice care worker in your area. Visit the facility, or invite the worker to speak to your class. If that is not possible, conduct an interview over the phone or via e-mail to learn more about hospice care. Request educational information such as brochures and pamphlets about the facility.

- Emphasize the lifesaving nature of organ donation.
- Discuss the jobs and professions available for health care workers interested in end-of-life issues.
- Encourage the students to discuss death and dying.
- Emphasize that it may be a difficult topic to talk about, but that it is part of the human growth and development life cycle.
- Invite students to share experiences with death and dying.
- Invite them to discuss their fears, and why it is a difficult subject.
- Ask them to consider whether their attitudes are different depending on the circumstances.

Section 14.4 Review Questions

1. Answer: As a health care worker, no matter how much kindness you have shown, your client may become very insulting. You need to realize that it is not a personal attack and that their anger is not directed at you. Be a good listener and offer compassion.
2. Answer: A terminally ill patient tries to bargain to prolong their life.
3. Answer: Touch and your understanding of their feelings and loss can help a patient through the depression stage.
4. Answer: Acceptance
5. Answer: The hospice philosophy is to help patients/clients nearing the end of life live each day to the fullest, to be comfortable and free of pain, and to die peacefully.
6. Answer: Organs that can be procured include: heart, intestines, kidneys, lungs, liver, pancreas, bones, and skin.

ACTIVITY

Euthanasia and organ donation are controversial topics with ethical implications. Select one of the topics and write an essay explaining your view of it. Include a thesis statement, and facts or real-life examples supporting your position. Discuss the essays as a class.

Summary

Most health care workers come in contact with terminally ill patients/clients and are involved in the care of a dying person. The terminally ill patient usually experiences five psychological stages: denial, anger, bargaining, depression, and acceptance. Patients who are terminally ill have an opportunity to choose a hospice for the final days of their illness.

Section 14.4 Review Questions

1. How does knowing that a terminally ill patient will experience anger help a health care worker to perform his or her job?
2. What does a terminally ill patient do during the bargaining stage?
3. In what ways can a health care worker help a patient pass through the depression stage?
4. What is the fifth and final psychological stage experienced by terminally ill patients?
5. Describe the hospice philosophy.
6. Name three organs that can be procured.

420 Chapter 14 | Human Growth and Development

CHAPTER 14 REVIEW

Chapter Review Questions

1. List four common developments of growth that occur in the first year of life. (14.1)
2. What period of adjustment is sometimes described as a midlife crisis? (14.1)
3. What hearing changes often affect people in their 60s? (14.2)
4. Contrast osteoarthritis and osteoporosis and explain how they affect people. (14.2)
5. Why do people often experience a change in environment as they age? How might this affect the person's well being? (14.2)
6. How does a person's work role change throughout life? (14.2)
7. Why does arteriosclerosis result in elevated blood pressure? (14.2)
8. What does it mean for a person with a disability to adapt? (14.3)
9. What is euthanasia? (14.4)
10. How is pain management important to the care of a terminally ill patient? (14.4)

Activities

1. Community resources provide people who are critically or terminally ill with valuable information and assistance. As a health care worker you have the opportunity to share information about available community resources with your patients and their families. Identify community resources with the following basic information about each: services provided, name of the organization, address, telephone number, e-mail address, and all other pertinent information. Summarize your information in a table, like the one shown below, and then create a card file for each resource.
2. A 30-year-old woman suffered a head injury, which left her unable to speak. Her daily care provides a bath, clean clothes, and food. People around her rarely speak to her. She stays in her room and looks out the window most of the time. Compare and differentiate between her day and yours. Make specific recommendations that could assist in moving this person toward health as described by the World Health Organization. Explain how your recommendations would change this client's health status.

Community Resource	Address	E-mail Address	Telephone Number	Services Provided/ Description

Human Growth and Development | Chapter 14 421

CHAPTER 14 REVIEW

Chapter Review Questions

1. Answer: Smile, roll over, sit, feed themselves, crawl, stand, and walk
2. Answer: At 40 to 50 years, people often evaluate the first part of their lives and make decisions about future directions; they adjust basic values and their emphasis toward life; this is sometimes referred to as the deadline decade. Women may develop assertiveness and men may become more tender and make stronger commitments to ethical issues.
3. Answer: High-frequency sounds, such as a telephone or doorbell, may not be heard and the loss of understanding of consonants and vowel sounds may result in a person complaining that others mumble or speak too softly.
4. Answer: Osteoarthritis is an inflammation of the joints and causes pain and slowing down of movement. Osteoporosis is caused by a loss of calcium in the bone. This is found more in Caucasian women after menopause, when the bones may become very brittle. They may fracture with very little stress.
5. Answer: As aging occurs, it may become necessary to change environments. The home may become a financial burden, or it may be physically impossible to remain there. This change may be very frightening, and the need for control in their environment is threatened. Memory loss or cognitive impairment may worsen when the person's environment changes.
6. Answer: The work a person does provides a sense of independence, security, and self-esteem. Successful aging is enhanced by a life style that provides a sense of accomplishment on a continuous basis.
7. Answer: Arteriosclerosis is present when the walls of the arteries become thick and harden, causing vessels to be less elastic. Less blood is able to flow through the arteries because the arteries are narrowed.
8. Answer: They change or make changes to become suitable to their limitations.
9. Answer: Euthanasia, also referred to as a "mercy killing," is the act of ending the life of an individual suffering from a terminal illness or an incurable condition.
10. Answer: Pain management provides comfort. It is important to work as a team with your co-workers to address the emotional, physical, spiritual, and psychological effects of pain and relieve discomfort as much as possible.

Activities

1. Direct students to set up a table or chart similar to the one in the book before beginning the activity. Encourage students to use a telephone book or the Internet to find the information they need.
2. Students may want to use a table to compare their daily activity with the sample woman. Encourage students to write their response to this activity as if they are a social worker or other health care provider assigned to assess the care for the woman and make recommendations.

ACTIVITY

Prepare two sets of cards or pieces of paper. On one set, write ages from birth through 80. On the other set, write a common scenario that might occur in a primary care doctor's office, such as checking heart rate, taking temperature, administering a vaccine. Have a student select one card from each set, and then demonstrate or explain how he or she, as a health care worker, would communicate with a person of the selected age in the selected situation.

CHAPTER 14 REVIEW

Case Studies

1. An elderly husband and wife decide to live in a long-term care facility so that their family won't worry about them. Upon admission, the wife is placed in room 125, and the husband is placed next door in room 126. They ask to share the same room, but the admitting clerk explains that the facility policy doesn't allow men and women to stay in the same room. Working with a partner, role play how you would speak to the couple.
2. Working in the pediatric ward, your team is proud of the progress made with a frightened, withdrawn four-year-old girl. But during visiting hours, her father becomes very angry, telling you that the hospital staff has made his daughter a bad girl because she is having tantrums. How would you handle this situation? With a partner, role play how you would speak to the father.

Thinking Critically

1. **Communication**—Following the medical plan, you are helping Mr. Green learn to use a walker after his stroke. The greatest challenge is that his wife and family tell him that he does not have to bother with learning to get around himself. Now that he is retired due to disability, they tell him that he can just sit in bed and watch television. How would you talk to Mr. Green and his family about the importance of staying mobile?
2. **Patient Education**—A 55-year-old male patient is recovering from a stroke. He is a high school principal and has always been able to take care of himself. His right hand and leg are paralyzed. Each day he is increasingly frustrated because he is unable to bathe or dress himself. Describe devices that could help reduce his frustration. Explain what you would say and do to educate him in the use of assistive/adaptive devices.
3. **Computers**—Patients/clients with disabilities are using computers to communicate and be productive citizens as they live with their disability. Do research on ways computers can be adapted to meet the needs of disabled individuals and write a report explaining what you have learned. Look for assistive technology, alternative input mechanisms, alternative output mechanisms, and computer use with handicapped or disabled children.

422 Chapter 14 | Human Growth and Development

Case Studies

1. Encourage students to contact long-term care facilities to learn about their policies and the reasons behind them. Remind students to use appropriate communications techniques. You may want to allow students to present skits that demonstrate their response to this situation.
2. Direct students to the ages of the patient and her father. Remind students to use appropriate communications techniques. You may want to allow students to present skits that demonstrate their response to this situation.

Thinking Critically

1. Refer students to Section 14.2 for information about aging and role changes. Encourage students to use appropriate communications techniques, and to include specific reasons about why the patient should remain mobile. You may want to let students perform a skit to demonstrate their response to this activity.
2. Refer students to Section 14.3 for information about adaptive devices.
3. Remind students of your school's Internet policies before they go online. Remind them to keep track of their sources to include in a bibliography. Encourage students to include this report in their career portfolio.

CHAPTER 14 REVIEW

Portfolio Connection

Working with people who are ill causes unfamiliar feelings and experiences. Your ability to identify your feelings and understand how you react to those feelings helps you carry on and continue to care for others.

PORTFOLIO TIP

Remember that aging means different things in different cultures.

Select a disability described in this chapter. Imagine that you are diagnosed with this disability. Identify your fears, feelings, and expectations. Explain what each day would be like, what type of care you would need, how others would respond to you, and how you would respond to others.

Your explanation must clearly identify your self-evaluation and new insights about disabilities and behaviors, and must show how you would approach others with disabilities. This assignment helps you investigate your feelings and identify possible behaviors of patients who live with disabilities. Including this assignment in your portfolio gives you easy access to it for review during your training. Comparing assignments throughout your training shows how your experiences have brought about change in your thinking.

Portfolio Connection

- Encourage students to be honest and personal with the first part of this exercise.
- They should work to express their fears, feelings, and expectations clearly in writing.
- For the second part of the exercise, they should provide specific examples and facts about the limitations they would face, the type of care they would need, and their interactions with others.
- Check to make sure that students have completed the written assignment and added it to their portfolio.

ACTIVITY

Contact the Special Olympics or Paralympics in your state or region to learn more about the types of activities and events they sponsor. Find out ways you could become involved.

15 Mental Illness

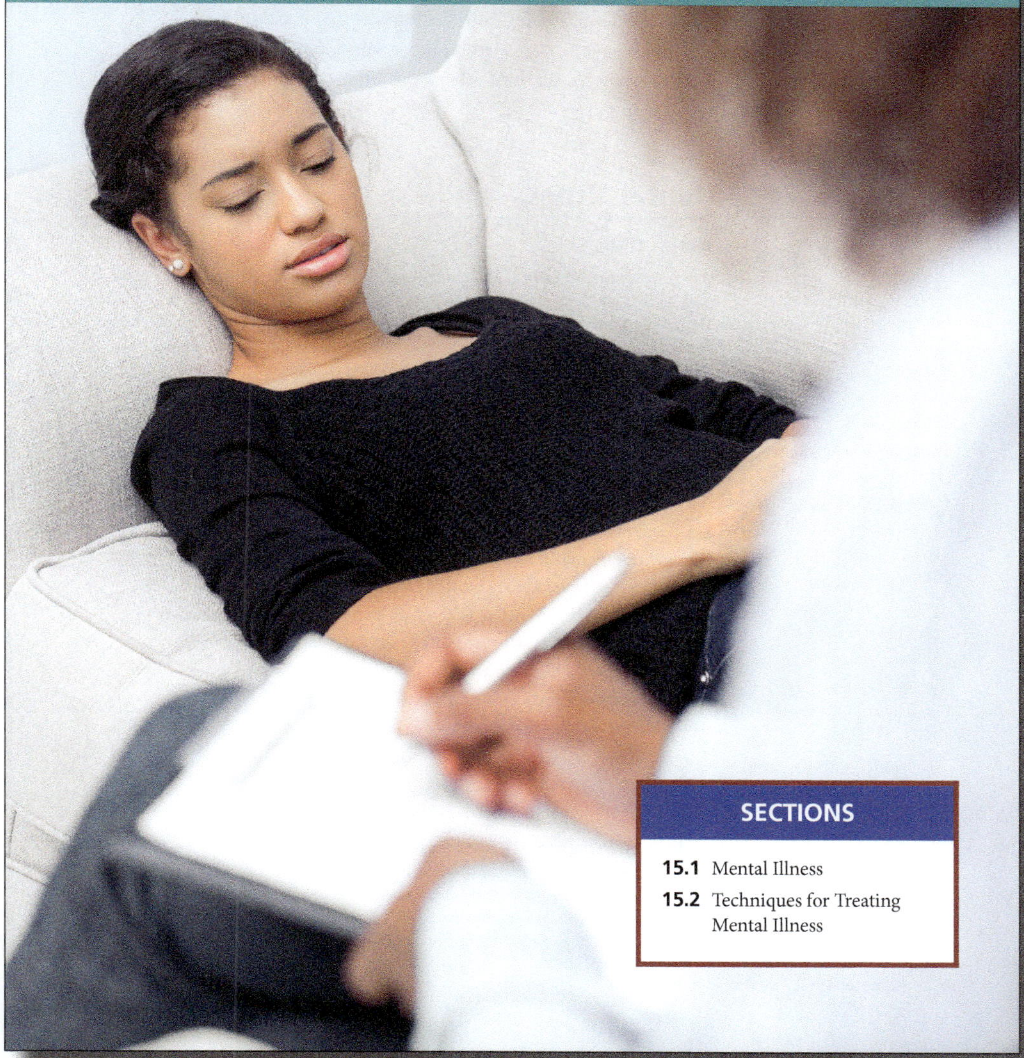

SECTIONS

CHAPTER 15 OVERVIEW

Chapter 15 introduces students to the topic of mental health, including types of common mental illnesses and techniques for treating mental illness.

Section 15.1: Section 15.1 defines and describes mental illness. It introduces different types of mental illness and discusses some of the known causes of mental illness.

Section 15.2: In Section 15.2, students learn about some of the techniques that are used to treat mental illness, such as medication, psychotherapy, and hospitalization. Specific procedures for treating Alzheimer's patients are provided.

Advance Preparation	
Review	■ Chapter text for Sections 15.1 and 15.2, and chapter procedures.
Contact	■ A mental health facility to request educational materials such as pamphlets and brochures. ■ A mental health care worker to set up a class visit.
Prepare	■ Magazine and newspaper articles about mental health diagnoses and treatments. ■ Information about well-known people who suffered from mental illness, such as Abraham Lincoln (depression), Virginia Woolf (bipolar disorder), and John Nash (schizophrenia; if time permits, you may want to show the movie *A Beautiful Mind*). ■ A list of Web sites that provide information about mental illness—such as nimh.nih.gov (National Institutes of Mental Health), nami.org (National Alliance on Mental Illness), alz.org (Alzheimer's Association), and dbsalliance.org (Depression and Bi-Polar Society Alliance).

FOCUS AND ENGAGE

Getting Started

- Ask students to collect and bring in newspaper, Internet, or magazine articles.
- Articles may be as diverse as celebrities checking in to rehab or veterans suffering from posttraumatic stress disorder.
- Provide a bulletin board or large sheets of paper to use as the background for the collage.
- Discuss the displays as a class.

Introduce the Section

a. Review the content of the Background paragraph, explaining that mental illness is a disease.
b. Emphasize the importance of recognizing the signs and symptoms of mental illness in order to provide effective treatment.
c. Review the objectives for the section.

Vocabulary Review

a. Direct students to the key terms.
b. Pronounce each word, and have the students repeat the pronunciation out loud.
c. Discuss each definition.

TEACH

Discuss

- Ask students what they know about mental illness. (They may have preconceived ideas.)
- Discuss pejorative terms used to describe the mentally ill, such as crazy, loony, bonkers, nuts, etc.
- Ask students to consider why these terms are used.

Reinforce and Review

- Review the importance of communication for health care professionals.

Getting Started

People with a mental illness struggle with symptoms ranging from depression and anxiety to powerful delusions and hallucinations. In addition, many have to deal with the stigma associated with mental illness. People with a mental illness often feel isolated, afraid, and alone. As a health care worker, it is essential to recognize the importance of mental health.

Prepare a collage from articles in the newspaper or from the Internet that illustrate poor mental health. Consider entertainment figures, war veterans, those who suffer from obesity or anorexia, or those who have died from suicides or drug-related deaths. Include information on available support resources in your area.

SECTION 15.1 Mental Illness

Background

People react to the world around them in different ways. For most people, daily activities pose few problems. Although these people occasionally feel down or moody, they otherwise feel good about themselves and the people around them. For a small number of people, however, interactions with the world and other people are difficult. Their thoughts and emotions are hard to control, and they may withdraw from daily activities as a result.

Objectives

When you have completed this section, you will be able to do the following:

- Define mental illness.
- Identify the classifications of mental disorders.
- List risk factors for mental disorders.
- State major types of anxiety disorders.
- Define the most prominent features of Obsessive-Compulsive disorder.
- List some disorders associated with traumatic events.
- Identify the features associated with bipolar and depressive disorders.
- State specific types of eating disorders.
- Describe Alzheimer's disease.

mental illness (MEN tuhl IL nuhs) Health condition that changes a person's thoughts, emotions, and behavior and that affects the person's ability to undertake daily functions.

Defining Mental Illness

Emotions and thoughts can be overwhelming. Sometimes, people have a hard time dealing with their emotions and the world around them. When this frequently happens, a person may be diagnosed with a **mental illness**. According to the National Institutes of Mental Health, as many as 26 percent of Americans suffer from a mental illness or know someone who does. A smaller percentage of Americans—about 6 percent—suffer from a serious mental illness.

426 Chapter 15 | Mental Illness

CUSTOMIZED INSTRUCTION
More Advanced Students
Assign more advanced students to research some of the ways patients suffering from mental illness were treated in the past. They should create a presentation to give to the class.

CUSTOMIZED INSTRUCTION OVERVIEW	
Less Advanced Students	Pages 427, 438
More Advanced Students	Pages 426, 437
English Language Learners	Pages 427, 443
Special Needs Students	Pages 431, 444
At-Risk Students	Page 430

Types of Mental Illness

Health care providers diagnose mental health illnesses based on the criteria set forth in the Diagnostic and Statistics Manual of Mental Health Disorders, Fifth Edition (DSM-5). The DSM-5 arranges mental health illnesses into groups known as "classifications" that includes but is not limited to the following:

- **Anxiety Disorders:** Panic attacks and phobias
- **Obsessive Compulsive and Related Disorders:** Obsessive Compulsive Disorder (OCD), Hoarding Disorder, Body Dysmorphic Disorder
- **Trauma and Stressor-Related Disorders:** Post-Traumatic Stress Disorder, Acute Stress Disorder, Adjustment Disorder
- **Bipolar and Related Disorders:** Bipolar I Disorder, Bipolar II Disorder
- **Depressive Disorders:** Major Depressive Disorder
- **Schizophrenia Spectrum and Other Psychotic Disorders:** Schizophrenia, Delusional Disorder
- **Neurodevelopmental Disorders:** Attention-Deficit/Hyperactivity Disorder, Autism Spectrum Disorder
- **Feeding and Eating Disorders:** Anorexia Nervosa, Bulimia Nervosa
- **Substance Related and Addictive Disorders:** Alcohol, Caffeine, Cannabis, Inhalants, Tobacco, Sedatives (and other prescription drugs)
- **Neurocognitive Disorders:** Alzheimer's Disease

Mental illness affects people of all ages, regardless of gender. Some diseases are more common in certain groups. For example, Alzheimer's disease usually affects older adults. Attention disorders are more common in children and young adults.

The Causes of Mental Illness

Scientist do not completely understand the causes of most mental illnesses. However, several risk factors have been found to play a role in the development of mental disorders. These risk factors include:

- **Biological factors:** Mental illnesses occur more often in some families than in others. This may be the result of *genetics*, or the traits passed from parent to child.
- **Environmental factors:** Head injuries, poor nutrition, and exposure to harmful or addictive chemicals can increase the risk of developing a mental illness.
- **Social factors:** Emotional trauma, abuse, exposure to violence, and other stressful events may affect whether someone develops a mental illness.

Anxiety Disorders

Each day, you probably feel some stress. It may be the stress of taking a test, or the stress of playing in an important game. One response to stress is **anxiety**. Because of anxiety, you may feel tense. You may sweat more. Anxiety can help you deal with a stressful situation. However, too much anxiety is unhealthy. People who frequently experience anxiety, often when facing everyday situations, may have an **anxiety disorder**.

anxiety
(ang ZIE i tee)
A feeling of worry and fear that causes physical symptoms, such as sweating, and stress.

anxiety disorder
(ang ZIE i tee DIS ohr duhr)
A mental illness in which a person feels too much anxiety, often in response to everyday situations.

Mental Illness | Chapter 15 427

CUSTOMIZED INSTRUCTION

Less Advanced Students

Take the time to be sure less advanced students understand the difference between the types of anxiety or depression most people experience now and then and actual mental illness.

English Language Learners

Have students write each key term and its pronunciation on one side of an index card and its definition on the other side. Have them read each term and definition aloud to a partner.

Teaching Tips

- Define mental illness: Health condition that changes a person's thoughts, emotions, and behavior.
- Emphasize that mental illness affects a patient's ability to undertake daily functions.
- Emphasize that mental illness can affect people of all ages, genders, races, and economic levels.
- Differentiate between sadness, or periodic problems controlling thoughts and interacting with others, and serious, debilitating mental illness.
- Review the types of mental illness:
  - Anxiety disorders
  - Obsessive-compulsive and related disorders
  - Trauma and stressor-related disorders
  - Bipolar and related disorders
  - Depressive disorders
  - Schizophrenia spectrum and other psychotic disorders
  - Neurodevelopmental disorders
  - Feeding and eating disorders
  - Substance-related and addictive disorders
  - Neurocognitive disorders
- Review the potential risk factors for mental illness:
  - Biological, such as genetic traits
  - Environmental, such as poor nutrition or exposure to chemicals
  - Social, such as exposure to trauma or violence

Figure Focus

15.1 Panic attacks can happen at any time of day. Why do some sufferers of panic attacks refuse to leave their homes?

Answer: Because they live in fear of suffering another attack

Teaching Tips

- Explain that anxiety disorders are characterized by extreme stress and anxiety in everyday situations.
- Describe panic disorder:
  - Sudden attacks of terror
  - Chills, nausea, feeling of being smothered
  - Fear of an attack
- Describe phobias:
  - A fear of something that poses little or no danger
  - Includes social phobias
  - Sometimes accompanied by panic attacks
- Describe obsessive-compulsive disorder:
  - Constant, disturbing thoughts
  - Repetitive behaviors
  - Ranges from mild to severe

Figure Focus

15.2 OCD is a disorder in which people have unwanted and repeated thoughts, feelings, ideas, sensations, or behaviors that make them feel driven to do something. What are the two parts of OCD?

Answer: Constant, disturbing thoughts (obsessions) and repetitive behaviors (compulsions)

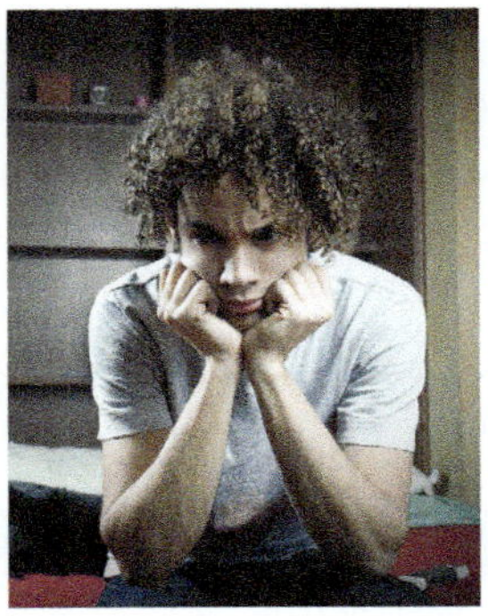

Figure 15.1
Panic attacks can happen at any time of day. Why do some sufferers of panic attacks refuse to leave their homes?

Panic Disorder

Panic disorder is an anxiety disorder that is characterized by sudden attacks of terror. (**Figure 15.1**) People who experience one of these attacks may feel chilled. They may also feel nausea and as though they are being smothered. These panic attacks can occur at any time, even when a person is asleep. Some people have one panic attack and never develop a panic disorder. People who have a panic disorder live in fear of another attack. So, many of these people won't leave their homes or take part in normal activities.

phobia
(FOH bee uh)
An irrational fear of an object or event that poses little or no actual risk.

obsessions
(ahb SESH uhns)
In obsessive-compulsive disorder, undesirable thoughts that occur constantly, causing anxiety.

compulsions
(cuhm PUHL shuhns)
In obsessive-compulsive disorder, behaviors or rituals that develop in response to the anxiety caused by obsessive thoughts.

Phobias

A **phobia** is a fear of something that poses little or no danger. People who suffer from a phobia may be afraid of wild animals (agrizoophobia), high places (acrophobia), open spaces (agoraphobia), or activities such as flying (aviophobia). Some people suffer from a *social phobia*, or a fear of social situations, such as talking to other people, giving speeches, and eating or drinking. Because of their fear, people who have a phobia often suffer from panic attacks. Both men and women are equally affected by phobias. Phobias usually begin during childhood or adolescence.

Obsessive-Compulsive and Related Disorders

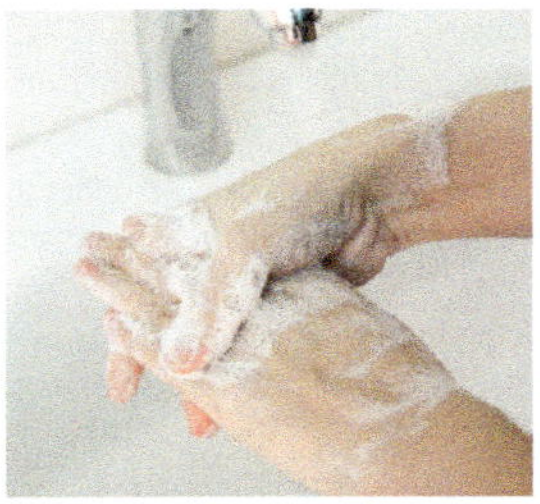

Figure 15.2
OCD is a disorder in which people have unwanted and repeated thoughts, feelings, ideas, sensations, or behaviors that make them feel driven to do something. What are the two parts of OCD?

Obsessive-Compulsive Disorder (OCD) involves constant, disturbing thoughts, or **obsessions**, and repetitive behaviors, or **compulsions**, to control the anxiety caused by the thoughts. For example, someone who obsesses about germs and dirt may respond by compulsively washing his or her hands. A healthy person may also wash his or her hands, but people who have OCD will wash their hands excessively. They may become locked into their compulsion, spending hours washing their hands or cleaning their homes. (**Figure 15.2**) Other obsessive-compulsive related disorders include:

- **Hoarding Disorder:** This is a newly diagnosed mental health disorder characterized by fearful thoughts, a deep-rooted need to keep possessions, and extreme distress when parting with them. The hoarded objects can range from pets and exotic animals to floor-to-ceiling piles of books, papers, and even trash. In some cases, hoarding is sparked by traumatic experiences such as the death of a loved one, a divorce, or the loss of a job.

428 Chapter 15 | Mental Illness

ACTIVITY

Make a chart or table comparing different types of anxiety disorders.

- **Body Dysmorphic Disorder:** Individuals with this disorder spend a great deal of thought and effort in fixing what they perceive to be flaws in their physical appearance. These individuals often subject themselves to costly and expensive reconstructive surgeries (plastic surgery).

The effects of OCD and related disorders may be mild, only partially affecting a person's ability to function. Or, the effects can be extreme, resulting in social isolation and the inability to carry out tasks of daily living. OCD and related disorders affect both men and women and can appear in childhood, adolescence, or early adulthood.

Trauma and Stressor-Related Disorders

People develop **post-traumatic stress disorder (PTSD)** after an incident in which they are harmed or threatened with harm. For example, victims of a violent crime may develop PTSD. Soldiers who have been to war may develop PTSD. People who have PTSD startle easily and are emotionally numb. They lose interest in the things they once enjoyed and may respond aggressively or violently to other people. People suffering from PTSD may relive the incident that caused the PTSD in flashbacks. PTSD affects people of all ages, and affects women more often than it affects men. Other stressor-related disorders include:

post-traumatic stress disorder (PTSD)
(POHST TRAW mat ik STRES DIS ohr duhr)
A mental illness that develops after a terrifying incident that involved physical harm or the threat of harm.

- **Acute Stress Disorder (ASD):** This disorder is characterized by feelings of sadness, confusion, difficulty sleeping, and withdrawal following a traumatic event. ASD symptoms usually last three days to one month following the trauma event. ASD may progress to PTSD if the symptoms persistent for longer than one month.
- **Adjustment Disorder:** The disorder is temporary and subsides following the removal of a stressor. The symptoms include sadness, withdrawal, inability to concentrate, loss of appetite, and trouble sleeping.

Bipolar Disorder

Bipolar Disorder is characterized by severe and prolonged mood swings ranging from heightened joyfulness (mania) to extreme sadness (depression).

bipolar disorder
(BIE puhl uhr DIS ohr duhr)
A mental illness that causes unusual shifts in a person's mood, energy, and ability to function; also known as manic-depressive disorder.

During mania, or a manic episode, a person has increased energy and is more active. He or she will experience racing thoughts and jump from one idea to the next. The person will get easily distracted and won't sleep much. He or she will show poor judgment and deny that anything is wrong.

During depression, a person will experience several negative emotions, including hopelessness, guilt, worthlessness, and helplessness. He or she will lose interest in activities that were once enjoyable. The person will feel tired, but he or she may not get enough sleep. Or, the person will get too much sleep. He or she has difficulty concentrating and making decisions.

Mental Illness | Chapter 15 429

Teaching Tips

- Explain that trauma and stressor-related disorders cause people to have inappropriate emotional reactions.
- Describe bipolar disorder:
  - Severe mood swings
  - Periods of high energy (mania), during which patient shows poor judgment, sleeps little, is easily distracted
  - Periods of low energy (depression), during which patient experiences negative emotions, loses interest in enjoyable activities, sleeps too much, cannot concentrate
  - Sometimes includes psychosis, or hallucinations

Teaching Tips

- Emphasize that everyone feels down or sad at one time or another.
- Explain that depression is a prolonged or permanent state of sadness.
- Describe depression:
  - Frequent sad feelings
  - Hopelessness
  - Irritability and restlessness
  - Loss of interest in activities and hobbies
  - Decreased energy
  - Difficulty sleeping or too much sleep
  - Change in eating habits
  - Thoughts of suicide
  - Body aches, headaches, and other physical problems

Figure Focus

15.3 Depression can decrease a person's appetite. What are three characteristics of depression?

Answer: Depression is characterized by frequent sad feelings, hopelessness, irritability, restlessness, loss of interest in activities, decreased energy, sleep problems, change in eating habits, thoughts of suicide, and physical problems.

ACTIVITY

Write a personal essay about a time when you felt sad or depressed.

Bipolar disorder usually develops in adolescence or early adulthood. It affects both men and women. There are several types of bipolar disorders including:

- **Bipolar I:** This involves periods of mania and depression.
- **Bipolar II:** This is a milder form of mood elevation.
- **Cyclothymic:** This involves mania with brief periods of depression that are not as extensive or long-lasting.

Depressive Disorders

major depressive disorder (MAY juhr DEE pres iv DIS ohr duhr) Mental illness characterized by a combination of symptoms that include prolonged sadness and that interfere with a person's ability to undertake everyday activities.

Depression describes the periods during which people feel sad. (Figure 15.3) Some people experience this for a long period of time or repeatedly as a result of a mental illness called **major depressive disorder**. In his or her lifetime, a person may experience only one episode of major depression, or he or she may experience it several times. Other conditions related to depression include Premenstrual Dysphoric Disorder, a condition where a woman has severe depression symptoms, irritability, and tension before menstruation, and Dysthymia, prolonged and persistent low-level depression lasting for at least two years.

Depression has several characteristics, including the following:

- Frequent sad feelings
- Feelings of hopelessness
- Irritability and restlessness
- Loss of interest in activities and hobbies
- Decreased energy
- Difficulty sleeping or too much sleep
- Change in eating habits
- Thoughts of suicide
- Body aches, headaches, and other physical problems

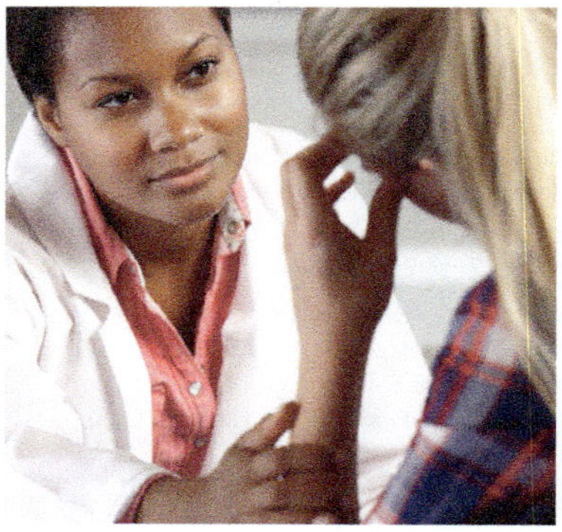

Figure 15.3
Depression can decrease a person's appetite. What are three characteristics of depression?

Depression often occurs with other mental illnesses. It can affect people who suffer from anxiety disorders and who abuse drugs. Depression is also common among people who have serious illnesses, such as cancer, AIDS, and diabetes. Depression is more common among women than it is among men. It can affect people of all ages.

430 Chapter 15 | Mental Illness

CUSTOMIZED INSTRUCTION

At-Risk Students

With a partner, have students research resources in school and in the community that offer help and services to those suffering from depression. In their word processing or desktop publishing program, they should create a list of resources with contact information. Post the lists in the classroom and elsewhere in the school, if appropriate.

Schizophrenia

Schizophrenia is a psychotic disorder in which a person loses touch with reality. He or she may have thoughts that seem unreasonable (delusions) or see and hear things that no one else can (hallucinations). For example, they may hear "voices." These voices may comment on the person's behavior, talk to each other, or warn the person about dangers that do not exist. Other symptoms of schizophrenia include the following:

- **Paranoia**: belief that other people want to harm someone.
- **Thought disorders:** unusual thought processes or difficulty organizing thoughts.
- **Movement disorders:** clumsiness or awkward movement.
- **Flat affect:** little facial expression and a flat voice.
- **Lack of activity:** difficulty starting and engaging in social activities.
- **Poor executive function:** difficulty understanding information and making decisions based on the information.
- **Poor working memory:** inability to remember something just learned.

Schizophrenia usually appears earlier in men than it does in women. Most men show symptoms in their late teens to early 20s. Women show symptoms in their 20s and 30s. Schizophrenia symptoms rarely begin to appear in children before the age of puberty and in adults after age 45.

schizophrenia
(SKIT soh fren ee uh)
Mental illness in which a person loses touch with reality; often characterized by hallucinations, such as voices that other people cannot hear, and delusions.

paranoia
(PAIR ah noy uh)
Unfounded or irrational distrust of other people.

Neurodevelopment Disorders

Children have a tendency to be very active and may be easily distracted. When children are frequently active at inappropriate times or have trouble paying attention, they may be diagnosed with an attention disorder such as **attention deficit hyperactivity disorder (ADHD)**. ADHD affects three to five percent of children in the United States. Even though ADHD is diagnosed mostly in children, it also occurs in adults. (Figure 15.4)

attention deficit hyperactivity disorder
(AH ten shuhn DEF uh sit HIE puhr ak tiv uh tee DIS ohr duhr)
A mental illness characterized by inattention, hyperactivity, and impulsiveness; diagnosed most often in children.

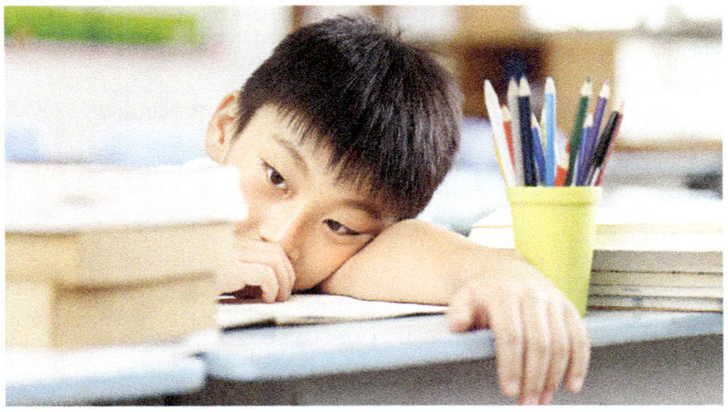

Figure 15.4
One sign of ADHD is excessive daydreaming. What are the three symptoms of ADHD?

Mental Illness | Chapter 15 431

Teaching Tips

- Describe schizophrenia:
  - Lose contact with reality
  - Hear voices
  - Paranoia
  - Difficulty organizing thoughts
  - Clumsiness
  - Lack of facial expression
  - Dull voice
  - Difficulty starting and engaging in social activities
  - Difficulty understanding information
  - Difficulty making decisions
  - Inability to remember something just learned
- Explain that attention disorders usually affect children but can also affect adults.
- Describe attention deficit hyperactivity disorder (ADHD):
  - Easily distracted
  - Inability to concentrate
  - Constant motion
  - Attempts to do multiple tasks at the same time
  - Impulsive behavior and speech

Figure Focus

15.4 One sign of ADHD is excessive daydreaming. What are the three symptoms of ADHD?

Answer: Inattention, hyperactivity, and impulsiveness

CUSTOMIZED INSTRUCTION

Special Needs Students

Some special needs students may suffer from attention disorders. Use care when discussing these disorders to as not to make the students feel uncomfortable or self-conscious.

TEAMWORK

Divide the class into teams of four to six students. Read the symptoms of a disorder to one team. If they correctly identify the disorder within one minute they receive a point, otherwise another team has the opportunity to try. At the end, the team with the most points wins.

Teaching Tips

- Describe the three groups of ADHD:
  - Primarily inattentive
  - Primarily hyperactive and/or impulsive
  - Both inattentive and hyperactive and/or impulsive

Personal Wellness—Diagnosing Mental Illness

- Emphasize that mood swings and emotional outbursts are usually a part of normal life.
- Remind students that adolescents, in particular, experience these type of behaviors.
- Point out that sometimes these behaviors are the result of a physical illness or imbalance.
- Review the symptoms of mental illness and how to recognize them in oneself and others.

How should you deal with the symptoms of mental illness in a friend?

Answer: You should encourage your friend to get professional help. You should be supportive, listen, and help your friend understand that help is available. If your friend won't get help, you should tell a trusted adult about your concerns.

ADHD is characterized by three symptoms:

- **Inattention:** A person cannot concentrate on what is going on around him or her. He or she may become easily bored with a task and not finish it. A person becomes easily distracted and often makes careless mistakes.
- **Hyperactivity:** A person is always in motion. He or she may squirm, fidget, or talk constantly. Older children and adults will feel internally restless and often try to do several things at once.
- **Impulsiveness:** A person lacks the ability to think things through before acting. He or she may say things suddenly and without evaluating the consequences. Adults who experience impulsiveness often do things that have instant results rather than working toward long-term results.

Individuals who have ADHD can be sorted into three general groups. The first group includes people who are primarily inattentive. The second group includes people who are primarily hyperactive and/or impulsive. The third group, or the combined group, is both inattentive and hyperactive and/or impulsive. Even though ADHD is diagnosed mostly in children, the effects of ADHD may continue into adulthood.

Personal Wellness

Diagnosing Mental Illness

The discussion of mental illness may make you worry about your own mental health or the health of the people around you. Keep in mind that mood swings and emotional outbursts can be a normal part of life, especially during adolescence. When these problems occur frequently and interfere with a person's ability to interact with the world around them, then that person should seek care.

While most cases of mental illness are not severe, the symptoms of mental illness should not be ignored. Only a medical professional can diagnose a mental illness. If you are concerned, visit your family doctor or a mental health specialist. The doctor will likely ask you about your family history. He or she may ask you to take a survey or answer a series of questions.

The doctor will examine you and take a blood sample to rule out physical illnesses. Depending on the results of the tests, the doctor will recommend treatment. Don't be afraid to visit the doctor; he or she will work to ensure your privacy.

Sometimes, the people affected by mental illness are your friends or family. You should encourage these people to get professional help, especially if they talk about suicide or other harmful behaviors. Be supportive, listen, and help the person understand that he or she can get help. If you have a friend or family member who won't get help, tell a trusted adult about your concerns.

When you work in health care, you may be exposed to people who have mental illnesses. Because people respond in different ways to an illness and its treatment, you may have to confront very stressful situations. Your facility will likely offer you mental health care to help you deal with these situations.

How should you deal with the symptoms of mental illness in a friend?

432 Chapter 15 | Mental Illness

TEAMWORK

In small groups, prepare a skit demonstrating how friends and family might respond to someone suffering from symptoms of a mental illness. Prepare two versions of the skit: one in which the response will be helpful to the patient, and one in which the response will not be helpful.

Feeding and Eating Disorders

People need to eat to have energy for everyday activities. Sometimes, people eat too little food or too much food. When a person's eating habits have become severely disturbed, a person may be diagnosed with an eating disorder. Eating disorders are considered mental illnesses because they have a psychological, or mental, component. Eating disorders often happen to people who have another mental illness, such as depression, an anxiety disorder, or substance abuse. Eating disorders include the following:

- **Anorexia nervosa:** This eating disorder is characterized by an abnormal fear of gaining weight. People who have anorexia nervosa exercise and diet excessively, or they lose weight by vomiting and by using drugs, such as laxatives and diuretics, that cause their bodies to release more wastes. People who have anorexia have poor body image. They see themselves as overweight even when they are underweight.
- **Bulimia nervosa:** This eating disorder is characterized by cycles of *binging* and *purging*. During a binge, a person eats too much food and feels out of control of his or her eating habits. During a purge, the person gets rid of the food by vomiting or using laxatives and other drugs.

Eating disorders usually appear during adolescence. They affect women more often than they affect men, although there are increased incidences of these conditions in men.

Apply It

Divide yourselves into sets of doctor/patient teams. The patient should describe a variety of specific symptoms and behaviors suggesting a mental disorder, such as OCD, PTSD, etc. The doctor needs to diagnose the disorder, describing why he or she has determined this to be the specific problem.

Substance-Related and Addictive Disorders

A **drug** is any chemical substance that alters the way a person thinks or acts and alters the person's body. Many drugs are helpful. For example, aspirin can be used to treat pain. Other drugs are harmful, and many of these drugs are illegal. These drugs include marijuana (in most states), cocaine, and methamphetamine, to name a few.

drug
(DRUHG)
Any chemical substance that changes a person's physical or psychological state.

Tobacco and alcohol are drugs that are illegal for people under certain ages. Some prescription drugs although legitimately used for treating physical and mental illness can be addictive. The general public often does not recognize the dangers of misuse and overuse of prescription drugs.

Sometimes, people use harmful drugs and lose control of their drug use. At this point, the person is abusing the drug and has a **drug addiction**. Drug abuse is considered a mental illness because of the effect of drugs on the brain. Drug abuse changes the structure and function of the brain. (See the following Science Link.) Because of these changes, a person will have difficulty stopping the use of a drug.

drug addiction
(DRUHG AH dikt shuhn)
The uncontrolled use of a drug.

Drug abuse is often related to other mental illnesses. For example, it can cause anxiety and depression. Or, it may be the result of a person's response to these diseases. For example, a person who feels depressed may decide to use drugs to try to feel better. Both men and women abuse drugs. Drug abuse usually starts in adolescence or early adulthood, but both children and older adults have been found to abuse drugs.

Teaching Tips

- Explain that eating disorders are characterized by severely disturbed eating patterns, such as eating too much or eating too little.
- Describe anorexia nervosa:
  - Abnormal fear of gaining weight
  - Excessive exercise and dieting
  - Poor body image
- Describe bulimia nervosa:
  - Cycles of binging and purging
- Explain that drug abuse is characterized by addiction.
- It occurs when people use harmful drugs and lose control of their drug use.
- Explain that drug abuse changes the structure and function of the brain.

Apply It

- Prepare descriptions or symptoms of an illness for students to use in this exercise.
- Students should work in pairs.
- You should give the "patient" the description, without allowing the "doctor" to see it.
- The doctor should write down the diagnosis.
- Alternatively, the activity could be performed as a skit in front of the class.
- Have the students switch roles for a different illness.

Science Link—The Brain on Drugs

- Explain neurons.
- Explain neurotransmitters.
- Discuss the ways drugs can affect the neurons:
  - Trick the neurons into firing—heroin, marijuana
  - Cause nerve cells to release abnormally large amounts of neurotransmitters—cocaine, methamphetamines
  - Prevent recycling of neurotransmitters—cocaine, methamphetamines
- Discuss dopamine and how a person can become addicted to a drug.

What are three ways in which drugs affect chemical messengers in the brain?

Answer: Trick the neurons into firing, cause nerve cells to release abnormally large amounts of neurotransmitters; and prevent recycling of neurotransmitters

Teaching Tips

- Explain that Alzheimer's disease is a type of dementia that causes the death of brain cells, which results in messages being unable to get from one part of the brain to another.
- Emphasize that some memory loss is a normal part of the aging process, but that Alzheimer's is not.
- The primary risk factors for Alzheimer's are family history (genetics) and aging.

Science Link

The Brain on Drugs

The brain is made up of cells called neurons. Neurons use both electrical signals and chemical messengers to transmit information. An electrical signal is transmitted along the length of a neuron. This signal causes the release of chemical messengers, called neurotransmitters, into the gap between one neuron and the next. Receptors on the next neuron respond to these neurotransmitters by producing an electrical signal and passing it on.

Some drugs, such as heroin and the drug in marijuana, are similar to neurotransmitters. When the drug is used, the neurons are fooled into firing by the drug.

Other drugs, such as cocaine or methamphetamine, cause nerve cells to release abnormally large amounts of neurotransmitters. Or, they prevent the recycling of neurotransmitters, a normal function that shuts off the signal between neurons.

In particular, drugs directly or indirectly affect a neurotransmitter called dopamine. Dopamine causes the euphoric feeling associated with drug use. Excess dopamine is released in response to drug use. As a person abuses a drug, the brain adapts to the excess dopamine. It reduces the amount of dopamine produced or reduces the number of dopamine receptors present. As a result, the drug abuser gets less enjoyment from the drug and uses more of it to get the same sensation.

Create a graphic design to illustrate the organization of interacting systems that provide functions within cellular organisms affected by drug use.

What are three ways in which drugs affect chemical messengers in the brain?

Neurocognitive Disorders (Dementia)

Dementia is a name used to describe a sustained loss of intellectual functions and memory severe enough to cause dysfunction in daily living activities. Although it can occur at any time during the adult years, it most frequently affects the elderly population. Some dementias can be reversed (about 20 percent). For this reason, all patients suffering from memory loss or reduced ability to solve life problems should be medically evaluated and would benefit from an evaluation by a geriatrician (a specialist in elder care).

Alzheimer's disease (AWL sie muhrs DUH seez) Type of dementia that causes the death of brain cells and subsequent impairment of thinking and memory.

Close to 66 percent of all dementias in the geriatric population can be attributed to **Alzheimer's disease**. Family history and increasing age are the primary risk factors for Alzheimer's disease. Research suggests a genetic linkage as a causal factor. Other possible risk factors include previous head injury, female sex, and lower educational level.

Alzheimer's disease is a mental illness that causes the death of cells in the brain. Because of this cell death, parts of the brain become disconnected. As a result, some messages cannot be sent from one part of the brain to another. This interferes with brain functions such as memory and impairs thinking.

434 Chapter 15 | Mental Illness

ACTIVITY

Contact a facility that provides care for Alzheimer's patients and request materials such as brochures or pamphlets. Create a bulletin board or other display to educate your peers about the disease.

Eventually people lose their ability to solve problems. For example, they may become lost while out driving in areas they are familiar with and cannot find their way back home. They may forget how to conduct activities of daily living, such as preparing a meal or even how to eat. Eventually, they may lose their ability to walk or communicate.

Some Alzheimer's patients may become paranoid and express anger and violence towards those around them. This is another expression of their inability to successfully evaluate and solve problems people deal with in their daily lives. The families and caregivers of these patients require an extensive support system. Eventually, many Alzheimer's patients need fulltime professional care.

Unlike many other mental illnesses, the effects of Alzheimer's disease are irreversible. At first, many people don't notice the symptoms of the disease. They think they are forgetful, but the forgetfulness gets worse as the disease progresses.

There are several main stages of Alzheimer's. Patients will progress form one stage to the next; for instance, the memory losses are not random, but reflective of each stage.

- **Early-stage Alzheimer's (Mild):** Memory loss or other cognitive deficits are noticeable, yet the person can compensate for them and continue to function independently. *Example:* Forgets names and words; might make up words; or quit talking to avoid mistakes.
- **Mid-stage Alzheimer's (Moderate):** Mental abilities decline, the personality changes, and physical problems develop so that the person becomes more and more dependent on caregivers. *Example:* Forgets recent events; forgets their own history; increasing difficulty in sorting out names and faces of family and friends.
- **Late-stage Alzheimer's (Severe):** Complete deterioration of the personality and loss of control over bodily functions requires total dependence on others for even the most basic activities of daily living. *Example:* Doesn't recognize familiar people, including their spouse and family members.

Some very rare forms of Alzheimer's disease will affect people as young as their 30s. Otherwise, Alzheimer's disease usually appears in people age 60 or older. Regardless, Alzheimer's disease is not a natural part of aging.

Community

As a member of a team, complete research to determine services and support available to assist those with mental health issues, including the cost to the recipient of services. Put the information in a brochure that you can distribute to homeless shelters, at local mental health facilities, and offices where care may be provided.

Summary

A mental illness is a health condition that changes a person's thoughts, emotions, and behavior. As a result of a mental illness, a person may have difficulty participating in daily activities. Mental illnesses include anxiety disorders, bipolar and depressive disorders, trauma-related disorders, attention disorders, eating disorders, substance abuse, and Alzheimer's disease.

The causes of mental illness are difficult to identify precisely. Biological factors, environmental factors, and social factors all play a role in the development of mental illness.

Mental Illness | Chapter 15 435

Teaching Tips

- Explain that other risk factors include previous head injury, being of the female sex, and lower educational level.
- Symptoms include:
  - Loss of memory
  - Inability to solve problems
  - Forgetting how to do basic tasks
  - Paranoia
  - Aggression
- Emphasize that the symptoms are irreversible.
- Discuss the main stages of Alzheimer's:
  - Early stage (mild): memory loss. Compensation is possible and independence is maintained.
  - Mid-stage (moderate): declining mental abilities. Change in personality, development of physical problems. Depends increasingly on caregivers.
  - Late-stage (severe): Complete loss of memory, personality, and control over bodily functions. Total dependence on caregivers.

Community

- Students should work in teams of three or four.
- Direct students to plan the brochure before conducting the research, so they know what information they need to collect.
- You may want to provide a list of mental health service providers.
- Alternatively, advise students to use the Internet or telephone book to locate the services.
- Direct students on the proper way to identify themselves when they contact the service providers.

Section 15.1 Review Questions

1. Answer: Anxiety disorders; obsessive-compulsive and related disorders; trauma and stressor-related disorders; bipolar and related disorders; depressive disorders; schizophrenia spectrum and other psychotic disorders; neurodevelopmental disorders; feeding and eating disorders; substance-related and addictive disorders; neurocognitive disorders
2. Answer: The risk factors for mental illness include biological factors (genetics), environmental factors (head injuries, poor nutrition), and social factors (trauma, abuse, violence).
3. Answer: Anxiety disorder (panic attacks, phobias, obsessive-compulsive disorder, and post-traumatic stress disorder)
4. Answer: The two phases of bipolar disorder are mania (high energy) and depression (low energy).
5. Answer: ADHD is characterized by inattention, hyperactivity, and impulsiveness.
6. Answer: Anorexia nervosa
7. Answer: Drug abuse is classified as a mental illness because of the effect of drugs on the brain.

Section 15.1 Review Questions

1. List ten types of mental illness.
2. What are three risk factors for mental illness?
3. Which type of disorder might result from a violent event such as a mugging?
4. What are the two phases of bipolar disorder?
5. Describe the three symptoms of ADHD.
6. In which eating disorder does a person exercise or diet excessively?
7. Why is substance abuse classified as a mental illness?

SECTION 15.2 Techniques for Treating Mental Illness

Background

Because the symptoms of mental illness vary from mild to severe, the treatment for mental illness also varies. There are many organizations and health care professionals who are highly trained and committed to helping those with mental health illnesses. Leading the way are the National Institute for Mental Health (NIMH), the American Psychiatric Association (APA), Suicide Prevention Lifeline, and the Substance Abuse and Mental Health Services (SAMHSA) agency. Each has a hotline and Web sites for immediate information and support. Through research and biotechnical advances, the techniques for identifying and treating mental health conditions are continuously evolving.

Objectives

When you have completed this section, you will be able to do the following:

- List ways to treat mental illness.
- List consequences of not treating mental illness.
- Explain why mental illness patients may stop taking medications.
- Define *psychotherapy*.
- List benefits of psychotherapy.
- Explain why treatment for drug abuse involves hospitalization.
- Describe why the treatment for Alzheimer's disease differs from the treatment for most other mental illnesses.

Mental Illnesses Can Be Treatable

Many people have the misconception that people who have mental illnesses are "crazy" or "nuts." This is simply not true. Most cases of mental illness are not severe. These cases can be treated, often with a combination of medication and regular meetings with a medical professional who specializes in treating mental illness.

436 Chapter 15 | Mental Illness

FOCUS AND ENGAGE

Introduce the Section

a. Review the content of the Background paragraph, explaining that flexibility is key in treating mental illness.
b. Emphasize that treatment must be adapted to each individual case because no two cases are exactly the same.
c. Review the objectives for the section.

Vocabulary Review

a. Direct students to the key terms.
b. Pronounce each word, and have the students repeat the pronunciation out loud.
c. Discuss the definition of each word.

TEACH

Discuss

- Ask students if they have read books or seen movies that depict mental illness.
- Discuss their attitudes towards mental illness.
- Explain what stigma means, and discuss why people are often afraid to seek help for mental illness.

Reinforce and Review

- Reinforce the need for patience, understanding, and an open mind when caring for patients with mental illness.

When caught early, the symptoms of most mental illnesses can be reduced or even reversed. In very severe cases, a patient may be dangerous to himself or herself or to other people. So, he or she will need to be hospitalized.

The Consequences of Not Treating Mental Illness

Most people will go to the doctor for an illness such as the flu, asthma, diabetes, or heart disease. But many people hesitate to see a doctor about mental illnesses. Teenagers, especially, do not want to be labeled with a mental illness and have their peers or teachers find out.

Not seeking treatment may result in more advanced symptoms of the mental illness. Untreated mental illness can lead to increased physical illness. A person may think about or attempt suicide. Some mental illnesses cause violent thoughts or actions. In children, untreated mental illness can lead to learning problems and social problems.

Medication

Medicines are often used to treat mental illness. Medicines can be prescribed to treat anxiety disorders, mood disorders, attention disorders, and personality disorders. Medicines can also help some people overcome drug addictions and help treat eating disorders. Many of these medicines need to be taken for several days or weeks. Sometimes, people need the medicines for longer periods.

A doctor must carefully monitor mental illness medications. Some of these medicines have uncomfortable side effects. A doctor can adjust medications or dosages to make a patient more comfortable. Because of the uncomfortable side effects, some patients may decide to stop taking their medicines. As a member of the health care team, you may need to assist with or monitor a patient's medicines.

Psychotherapy

During **psychotherapy**, a patient will meet with a medical professional such as a counselor, **psychiatrist**, or **psychologist** to discuss their feelings. Discussion helps patients understand their mental illness and work through their problems. Psychotherapy helps patients in the following ways:

- It can change thought patterns and behaviors.
- It can help patients recognize how past experiences affect their current behaviors.
- It can help the patient learn skills to deal with their mental illness.
- It can help medical professionals monitor a patient's response to treatment and medication.

psychotherapy
(SIE koh ther uh pee)
Treatment method in which a mental health professional and a patient discuss problems and feelings related to a mental illness.

psychiatrist
(SIE kie uh trist)
A medical professional who specializes in the prevention, diagnosis, and treatment of mental illness; has a medical degree (M.D.) and can prescribe medication as part of treatment.

psychologist
(SIE kahl uh jist)
A medical professional who specializes in the prevention, diagnosis, and treatment of mental illness; can only use talk therapy for treatment.

Mental Illness | Chapter 15 437

ACTIVITY

Create a poster to educate your peers about mental illness. Select one disorder or disease, and include symptoms they should be aware of. Display the posters in an appropriate place, such as the nurse's office.

Teaching Tips

- Emphasize that most mental illnesses can be treated.
- List the most common and effective forms of treatment:
  - Medication
  - Psychotherapy
  - Hospitalization
- Explain the consequences of not treating mental illness:
  - More advanced symptoms
  - Increased physical illness
  - Suicidal thoughts or attempts
  - Violent thoughts or actions
  - Learning problems
  - Social problems
- Discuss medication as a treatment for mental illness.
- Explain that it can be successfully used to treat many types of mental illness:
  - Anxiety disorders
  - Mood disorders
  - Attention disorders
  - Personality disorders
  - Eating disorders
  - Addictions
- Emphasize the need for monitoring patients on medication.
- Discuss the effects of unpleasant side effects:
  - Patient may stop taking medication
  - Changes in symptom
  - Physical illness
- Explain psychotherapy: Treatment method in which a mental health professional and a patient discuss problems and feelings related to a mental illness.
- Review the four ways talking can help patients suffering from mental illness.
- Emphasize that psychotherapy is often used in combination with medication.

CUSTOMIZED INSTRUCTION

More Advanced Students

More advanced students might enjoy learning about the types of medications used to treat mental illness. They could create a chart of medications, what they treat, and what the side effects are.

Figure Focus

15.5 Psychotherapy gives patients a chance to discuss their problems and helps the therapist evaluate the patients' progress. What are four benefits of psychotherapy?

Answer: Psychotherapy can help patients change thought patterns and behaviors, recognize how past behaviors affect current behaviors, learn skills to deal with mental illness, and help medical professionals monitor the patient's response to treatment and medication.

Language Arts Link—Mental Health and Social Services Career Paths

- You may want to provide a list of resources such as Web sites or local facilities that students can use to research this project.
- Remind students about your school's Internet policy, how to recognize a reputable source, and to keep a list of sources for a bibliography.
- For evaluation, you should verify that the information is correct, and you should mark spelling and grammatical errors.

Psychotherapy can occur individually or in a group setting. (**Figure 15.5**) Usually, it involves talking, but it may involve activities such as art or music. Talking, art therapy, and music therapy help patients express themselves in healthy ways. Group therapy can help patients learn how to interact with other people.

Like medications, psychotherapy must occur over a period of time. Some people only need a few visits. Other people, who have more severe mental illnesses, will spend years in psychotherapy. When used with medication, psychotherapy has been shown to help patients more than medicines alone.

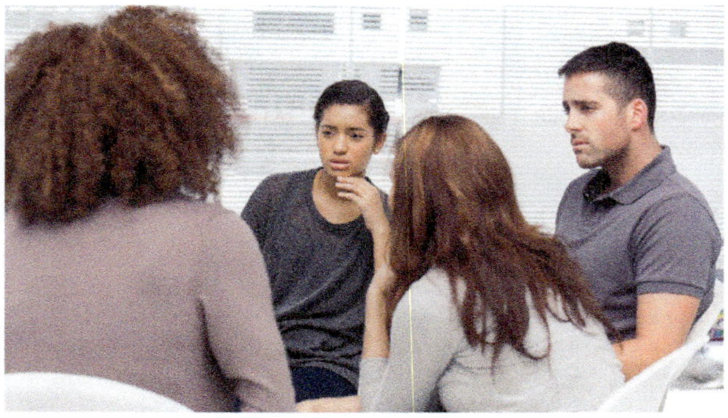

Figure 15.5
Psychotherapy gives patients a chance to discuss their problems and helps the therapist evaluate the patients' progress. What are four benefits of psychotherapy?

Language Arts Link

Mental Health and Social Services Career Paths

Mental health is all about how we think, feel, and interact with others as we manage the pressures of daily life. Everyone experiences some stress, sadness, or anxiety from time to time, but for a person with mental illness, these feelings do not go away.

There are health care professionals that specialize in working with people with mental illness. They require specialized training to work in these professions, including psychiatrists, psychologists, therapists, social workers, and counselors.

Working with a partner, research various mental health careers. Using multiple sources of information, presented in diverse formats and media, determine the education and skills needed to practice in one of these careers. The research could include an interview with someone working in mental health. The interview should include: how he or she became interested in working in mental health, his or her particular job requirements and working environment, and the benefits and challenges of working in mental health.

After you've completed your research, create a document with several paragraphs on each career that you learned about. Be sure to proofread your work to see if you can improve it by making it clearer, more concise, or more interesting to read. Check the spelling and grammar and correct any errors.

438 Chapter 15 | Mental Illness

CUSTOMIZED INSTRUCTION

Less Advanced Students

Many of the vocabulary terms in this chapter are similar—psychotherapy, psychologist, psychotherapist, etc. Allow enough time for less advanced students to learn the vocabulary and provide assistance so they can differentiate between the similar terms.

Hospitalization

For very severe mental illnesses, patients may require constant care. As a result, they will be placed in a facility that specializes in the treatment of mental illnesses. In some cases, people only need a short hospitalization period and may never need to go back. In the most severe cases, some people cannot recover enough from their mental illness to leave a hospital.

Hospitalization for Drug Abuse

Hospitalization is often a treatment for drug abuse. Drug addiction creates a physical and psychological dependence on a drug. When a person stops taking the drug, he or she will experience **withdrawal**. The symptoms of withdrawal are often painful and uncomfortable and may even cause death. As a result, a drug addict should be monitored by medical professionals as he or she goes through withdrawal.

withdrawal
(with DRAW uhl)
Uncomfortable physical and psychological symptoms that arise when a drug addict stops using a drug.

Treating Alzheimer's Disease

Unlike most other mental illnesses, the effects of Alzheimer's disease cannot be reversed. If caught early, the disease can be treated with medications that slow the progress of the disease. However, the symptoms will continue to worsen. In addition to memory problems, the patient may experience depression and anger. A patient may eventually forget basic skills, such as hygiene and the ability to read.

Eventually, an Alzheimer's patient will need fulltime care. He or she will need home care or will need to be placed in a care facility. As a health care worker, you may need to take care of the patient's basic needs, such as dressing, bathing, brushing teeth, or shaving.

Many of the treatments for Alzheimer's disease are designed to stimulate the memory and to keep a patient engaged with the people around him or her. Activities, art therapy, and music therapy have been used to reinforce memories.

Care for Alzheimer's patients requires a great deal of patience. On some days, a patient may seem completely normal. On other days, the patient will have difficulty remembering even simple things. As a member of the health care team, you will need to use listening skills and communication skills to help the patient deal with his or her day-to-day needs.

Career Connect

Research mental health professionals who have been in the news lately for evaluating or treating famous personalities. What is their training and background? Do they have a specialty?

Mental Illness | Chapter 15 439

Teaching Tips

- Explain hospitalization as a treatment for those suffering from severe mental illness.
- Emphasize that there are facilities that specialize in customized care for the mentally ill.
- Discuss hospitalization for patients suffering from addiction to drugs or alcohol.
- Explain that the symptoms of withdrawal may be physically harmful, so the patient should be monitored 24/7.
- Review the description of Alzheimer's disease in Section 15.1.
- Discuss reasons why Alzheimer's may require different treatment than other mental illnesses:
  - Effects cannot be reversed
  - Currently incurable
- Emphasize that the goal of Alzheimer's treatment is to slow the progression of the disease in order to slow the advance of the symptoms.
- Explain that many treatments attempt to stimulate memory and keep the patient interacting with other people.
- Discuss the difference between treatment and care for Alzheimer's patients.
- Explain that care of patients with advanced Alzheimer's usually requires providing basic needs, such as hygiene.
- Discuss the personal characteristics required for health care workers responsible for treating Alzheimer's patients:
  - Patience
  - Compassion
  - Strong listening and communication

Career Connect

- Direct students to Chapter 3 for information on careers in mental health.
- You may want to combine this activity with the Language Arts Link on p. 438.
- You might ask students to create a table or chart comparing three or four of the occupations in the mental health care field.

Procedure Tips

15.1 Activities with Alzheimer's Patients

- Review the background information, discussing how activities can benefit the patients:
  - Structure time
  - Improve self-esteem
  - Provide social interaction
- Review Standard Precautions.
- Remind students of the importance of patience.
- Explain the preprocedure steps.
- Explain the procedure steps.
- Explain the postprocedure steps.

PROCEDURE PRACTICE

- Demonstrate the steps for Procedure 15.1, Activities with Alzheimer's Patients, as many times as necessary, or ask students to demonstrate the steps. Have students practice and perform the procedure until they are competent.

Procedure Tips

15.2 Music Therapy

- Review the background information, discussing the benefits of music therapy:
  - Activate memories
  - Ward off depression
  - Stimulate brainwaves
- Review Standard Precautions.
- Remind students of the importance of patience.
- Explain the preprocedure steps.
- Explain the procedure steps.
- Explain the postprocedure steps.
- Direct students to Web sites, such as musictherapy.org, for more information.

Procedure 15.1 Activities with Alzheimer's Patients

BACKGROUND: For people who have Alzheimer's disease, activities help structure the time. Activities also improve a patient's self-esteem.
ALERT: Follow Standard Precautions (see Section 17.2).

Preprocedure

1. Wash hands.
2. Identify the patient and the activity in which he or she will be participating. Pay attention to:
   a. the patient's skills and abilities
   b. what the patient enjoys
   c. physical problems
   d. the physician's recommendations
3. Gather equipment for the activity (if needed).
4. Break the activity into small, measurable steps.

Procedure

5. Greet the patient, and tell him or her what you are going to do today.
6. Help the patient get started with the activity.
7. Explain each step of the activity using simple terms. It may be necessary to repeat the explanation or to clarify in terms the patient understands.
8. Help the patient through difficult steps or if he or she appears frustrated. As much as possible, let the patient do most of the activity on his or her own.
9. Do not criticize or correct the patient.

Postprocedure

10. Put away equipment.
11. Wash hands.
12. Record the patient's response to the activity.

Procedure 15.2 Music Therapy

BACKGROUND: Music helps Alzheimer's patients recall memories and emotions.
ALERT: Follow Standard Precautions (see Section 17.2).

Preprocedure

1. Identify the patient.
2. Identify the type of music that the patient enjoys.
3. Provide a comfortable space in which the patient can listen to the music.
4. Gather and set up equipment. Choose music, something to play it on, and pictures that mean something to the patient to help them recall memories.
5. Block other sources of sound. Close windows and doors, turn off televisions and other radios, and reduce background noise as much as possible.

Procedure

6. Start the music.
7. Encourage the patient to clap or sing along with the music. When appropriate, encourage the patient to dance or move with the music.
8. While playing the music, show the patient pictures to help with memories.

Postprocedure

9. Put away equipment.
10. Wash hands.
11. Record the patient's response to the activity.

440 Chapter 15 | Mental Illness

PROCEDURE PRACTICE

- Demonstrate the steps for Procedure 15.2, Music Therapy, as many times as necessary, or ask students to demonstrate the steps. Have students practice and perform the procedure until they are competent.

TEAMWORK

In pairs or small groups, practice the steps in the procedures. Have one student act as the caregiver while the other(s) act as the patient(s).

Procedure 15.3 **Art Therapy**

BACKGROUND: Like music, art can help an Alzheimer's patient reconnect with the world around him or her. Art provides a way for the patient to express himself or herself.
ALERT: Follow Standard Precautions (see Section 17.2).

Preprocedure

1. Identify the patient.
2. Assemble materials. Avoid potentially harmful materials, such as sharp blades and tools. Materials may include the following:
   a. nontoxic acrylic paints or watercolor paints
   b. brushes and canvases or watercolor paper
   c. clay
3. Prepare a work area for the patient. Neatly arrange materials and cover surfaces to protect them from spillage.

Procedure

4. Help the patient start the project.
5. Encourage the patient to talk about what he or she is doing. Ask the patient to remember events related to the project or to tell a story about the project.
6. Help the patient through difficult steps or if he or she appears frustrated. As much as possible, let the patient do most of the project on his or her own.
7. Do not criticize or correct the patient.
8. When the patient is finished with the project, help him or her clean up.

Postprocedure

9. Put away equipment.
10. Clean work space, and wash hands.
11. Record the patient's response to the activity.

Summary

Mental illness is treated with a combination of medication and psychotherapy. Medication will treat symptoms of mental illness, but uncomfortable side effects may cause some patients to stop taking their medicine. Psychotherapy gives patients a chance to talk about and understand their illness. In extreme cases, mental illness patients will be hospitalized. Unlike other mental illnesses, at this time, Alzheimer's disease cannot be cured. Eventually, an Alzheimer's patient may need home care or hospitalization.

Section 15.2 Review Questions

1. What are three ways in which mental illness is treated?
2. What might happen if mental illness is not treated?
3. Define psychotherapy.
4. What are four benefits of psychotherapy?
5. Why do drug abuse patients need to be hospitalized during treatment?
6. How is Alzheimer's disease different from most other mental illnesses?

Mental Illness | Chapter 15 441

Section 15.2 Review Questions

1. Answer: Mental illness is treated with medication, psychotherapy, or hospitalization.
2. Answer: Untreated mental illness can lead to physical illness, suicide, learning problems, or social problems.
3. Answer: Psychotherapy is the treatment method in which a mental health professional and a patient discuss problems and feelings related to a mental illness.
4. Answer: Psychotherapy can change a patient's thought patterns and behaviors, help patients recognize how past experiences affect their current behavior, help the patient learn to deal with their mental illness, and help medical professionals monitor a patient's response to treatment and medication.

Procedure Tips

15.3 Art Therapy

- Review the background information, discussing the benefits of art therapy:
  - Connect with others
  - Creative outlet
  - Exercise cognitive abilities
- Review Standard Precautions.
- Remind students of the importance of patience.
- Explain the preprocedure steps.
- Explain the procedure steps.
- Explain the postprocedure steps.
- Direct students to Web sites, such as arttherapy.org, for more information.

PROCEDURE PRACTICE

- Demonstrate the steps for Procedure 15.3, Art Therapy, as many times as necessary, or ask students to demonstrate the steps. Have students practice and perform the procedure until they are competent.

Teaching Tips

- Review the treatments for mental illness:
  - Medication
  - Psychotherapy
  - Hospitalization
- Discuss the risks and benefits of treating mental illness.

ACTIVITY

Write a short story or draw a picture demonstrating the consequences of allowing mental illness to go untreated.

5. Answer: Drug abuse patients are hospitalized during treatment because drug addiction creates a physical and psychological dependence on a drug. When a drug addict stops taking the drug, he or she will experience withdrawal. Withdrawal symptoms are often painful and uncomfortable and for this reason they should be monitored by medical professionals.
6. Answer: Alzheimer's disease is different from most other mental illnesses because the effects of Alzheimer's cannot be reversed.

What's New?—New Alzheimer's Disease Therapies

- Review the risk factors for Alzheimer's.
- Direct students to Section 13.13 for more information on genetics.
- Emphasize that Alzheimer's is currently incurable.
- Explain that treatments focus on slowing the course of the disease.
- Discuss advances that bring hope for treatments that will be able to prevent the disease.
- Review the preventive treatments researchers are working on.
- You may want to discuss scientific research in general.

For which of the above potential therapies might it be possible to use a treatment that does not involve drugs?

Answer: Cardiovascular therapies

What's New?

New Alzheimer's Disease Therapies

Once people develop Alzheimer's disease, the disease cannot be cured. Most of the drugs currently used to treat Alzheimer's slow the course of the disease, but they do not stop it.

According to the Mayo Clinic, the focus of future Alzheimer's treatments will be on preventing it in people who have a risk for the disease, but do not yet have it. Risk factors include age and genetics. Approximately 5 percent of Americans between the ages of 65 to 74, and almost half of those 85 years and older suffer from Alzheimer's disease. And, early-onset Alzheimer's has been clearly shown to be genetic in origin.

While mutations on chromosomes 9 and 19 have been linked with late-onset Alzheimer's (the most common form), not everyone with the mutations develops the disease. The relationship between genetics and late-onset Alzheimer's is not fully known.

Other possible factors *may* include prior traumatic head injury, lower education level, and female gender. Scientists are working on the following preventive measures:

- **Alzheimer's vaccine:** A vaccine was developed and tested, but it caused dangerous side effects. Scientists continue to look for a vaccine that won't cause these side effects.
- **Secretase inhibitors:** Secretase is an enzyme, or protein, that causes the formation of plaques in the brain. These plaques have been thought to be the cause of Alzheimer's disease. Secretase inhibitors will prevent the formation of secretase and, thus, plaques. Unfortunately, the inhibitors are large molecules that do not easily pass from the blood to the brain. Scientists are working to fix this problem. In addition, new research is indicating that the role of plaques is more complex than originally thought, which is prompting other ideas in the hunt for a drug treatment for Alzheimer's disease.
- **Cardiovascular therapies:** The term *cardiovascular* refers to the heart and blood vessels. Cardiovascular diseases include high blood pressure and high cholesterol. These diseases often result from poor eating habits and lack of exercise. In some people, genetics plays a role in high blood pressure and high cholesterol. Some evidence indicates that controlling these diseases may also reduce the risk of Alzheimer's disease.
- **Anti-inflammatory drugs:** Some drugs, such as ibuprofen, may reduce the risk of Alzheimer's disease. However, these drugs have caused stomach and intestinal problems.

For which of the above potential therapies might it be possible to use a treatment that does not involve drugs?

CHAPTER 15 REVIEW

Chapter Review Questions

1. Which type of mental illness includes panic attacks and phobias? (15.1)
2. What is a focus of treatment for Alzheimer's disease? (15.1)
3. How does Alzheimer's disease cause memory problems? (15.1)
4. Compare anorexia nervosa and bulimia nervosa. (15.1)
5. ________ is a mental illness in which sufferers may hear voices that other people cannot hear. (15.1)
6. What are the three groups into which people who have ADHD may be classified? (15.1)
7. Obsessive-compulsive disorder is a mental illness characterized by _______ and _______
8. Why might some people stop taking medications for mental illness? (15.2)
9. Why might people who have a mental illness be hospitalized? (15.2)
10. A(n) _______ can prescribe medications when providing psychotherapy. (15.2)

Activities

1. Write a public service announcement about mental illness. Your public service announcement should inform people about the frequency of mental illness and how it is treated. It should also make people aware of the risks of avoiding treatment. Perform your public service announcement for the class.
2. With a group of your classmates, discuss the positive and negative effects of relationships on physical and emotional health. Come up with strategies for how to enhance the positive effects and mitigate the negative effects for patients suffering from mental health disorders.
3. Create a table that compiles mental health statistics for people in the United States. Your table should provide information about the illnesses discussed in the chapter. Use the table below as a sample upon which you can base your table.

Mental Illness	Percentage of Americans Affected	Suggested Treatments

Case Studies

1. Mr. Gomez seems to be forgetting things lately. He couldn't find his car keys and had trouble remembering his neighbor's name. His family thinks Mr. Gomez forgets things because of his age. Why should they be concerned? Should Mr. Gomez seek medical help? Why or why not? What might eventually happen to Mr. Gomez?
2. Sheila noticed lately that her friend Nan has stopped coming to social events. When she goes to Nan's house, Nan doesn't want to leave her bedroom and she seems sad. Additionally, Sheila noticed that Nan isn't eating much during lunch, and Nan told her that she hasn't been sleeping well. Based on this information, which mental illness might Nan have? What are some other symptoms of this illness? What kind of help does Nan need?

Mental Illness | Chapter 15 443

CHAPTER 15 REVIEW

Chapter Review Questions

1. Answer: Anxiety disorders
2. Answer: The focus of treatment for Alzheimer's disease is to slow the progress of the disease. Many treatments simply try to stimulate the patient's memory and keep the patient engaged with other people. There is currently no cure and eventually the patient will need full-time care.
3. Answer: Alzheimer's causes the death of brain cells, which leads to parts of the brain being disconnected so messages are not sent from one part of the brain to another.
4. Answer: Anorexia nervosa is characterized by an abnormal fear of gaining weight. People who have anorexia nervosa exercise and diet excessively, or they lose weight by vomiting and by using drugs. Bulimia nervosa is an eating disorder characterized by cycles of binging and purging.
5. Answer: Schizophrenia
6. Answer: Inattentive, hyperactive, and impulsive
7. Answer: Obsessions and compulsions
8. Answer: Some patients stop taking medications for mental illness because of the uncomfortable side effects.
9. Answer: Some patients with mental illness require constant care, and patients going through drug abuse withdrawal need to be monitored by health care professionals because of the painful side effects of withdrawal.
10. Answer: Psychiatrist

Activities

1. Direct students to write the announcement as a script, so they can perform it for the class. Encourage creativity by allowing students to videotape the announcements. They may be able to upload them to a school Web site, or air them on local access cable.
2. Have students brainstorm a list of positive and negative effects of relationships on physical and emotional health.
3. You might want to provide a list of resources where the students will find the statistics, such as nimh.nih.gov. Advise students to set up the table in a spreadsheet or on paper before beginning the research, so they can enter the data directly into the table.

CUSTOMIZED INSTRUCTION

English Language Learners

Some English Language Learners may be uncomfortable presenting their announcement to the entire class in Activity 1. Allow them the option to share it with a small group or a partner.

Case Studies

1. Direct students to the parts of Section 15.1 on Alzheimer's disease for more information. You may want to allow students to present skits demonstrating their response to this situation.
2. Direct students to the parts of Section 15.1 on depression for more information. Remind them to consult Section 15.2 for information about appropriate treatments. You may want to allow students to present skits to demonstrate their response to this situation.

ACTIVITY

Investigate a celebrity who has recently undergone rehabilitation or hospitalization for drug or alcohol addiction. What were the symptoms that indicated treatment was necessary? Was this the first time he or she tried hospitalization? Write a report or create a poster about the situation.

Thinking Critically

1. Refer students to Chapters 5 and 6 for more information about legal and ethical responsibilities. Direct students to write the response in proper essay form, including a thesis statement and supporting facts and examples.
2. Direct students to consider what they have learned about the way families and friends respond to a patient's illness. They should also consider genetics, and other risk factors of mental illness.

CHAPTER 15 REVIEW

Thinking Critically

1. **Legal and Ethical**—As a health care provider, you will be asked to protect the privacy of your patients. Why is this especially important for people who suffer from mental illnesses?
2. **Cause and Effect**—Emanuel's mother has been treated for depression in the past. She received medication and psychotherapy. She responded well to the treatment and currently doesn't have any symptoms of depression. How might his mother's depression affect Emanuel's mental health?
3. **Identifying Relationships**—Art and music therapy are used to treat Alzheimer's patients. These activities often involve creativity and interaction. Describe how these activities likely benefit patients.
4. **Research**—Biomedical therapies are physiological interventions that are used to reduce the symptoms associated with psychological disorders. Three procedures used are drug therapies, such as anti-anxiety drugs and antidepressants, electroconvulsive (shock) therapy, and psychosurgery, which is rarely used. Select a disorder and research the types of biomedical therapy that could be used to treat or prevent the disorder and how it relates to the pathology of the disorder.

Portfolio Connection

Volunteer with an organization that helps people who have mental illnesses. For example, some organizations will visit nursing homes to work with people who have Alzheimer's disease. Other organizations work with children who have ADHD or other behavioral disorders.

Keep a journal as you work with the organization. Describe the activities that you participate in. Ask the medical professionals with whom you work to identify how the activity helps the patient. Record your observations about the patient's response to the activity. (Note: Protect the patient's privacy by not using the patient's name in your journal.) Once you have finished your journal, write a short essay discussing how your thoughts about the care process and how the care benefits the patient.

PORTFOLIO TIP

Record keeping is one of the most important steps of patient care. Records must be accurate and private. When recording your observations, avoid adding personal comments that won't help a medical professional treat the patient. Be precise and informative, and avoid including judgmental statements or opinions.

3. Direct students to the part of Section 15.2, "Treating Alzheimer's Disease," and to Procedures 15.1, 15.2, and 15.3. Students may also want to consult Web sites, such as musictherapy.org and arttherapy.org, for information.
4. Student research and results will vary.

Portfolio Connection

- Point out that volunteering is an excellent way to find out whether a particular job or environment is appealing.
- Also, emphasize that there are many different ways to volunteer.
- Students might want to be involved in hands-on interaction with patients.
- Others might prefer fundraising, administration, or education.
- The types of volunteer activities they select might indicate the types of careers they should pursue.
- Check to make sure that students have completed both the journal and the essay and added them to their portfolio.

CUSTOMIZED INSTRUCTION

Special Needs Students

If any students in your class are being treated for an attention disorder, ask if they are willing to discuss it with the class. They may take medication, or make use of behavior modification, nutritional, or other type of treatment to control the symptoms. Alternatively, ask the students to write a personal essay about it.

16 Nutrition

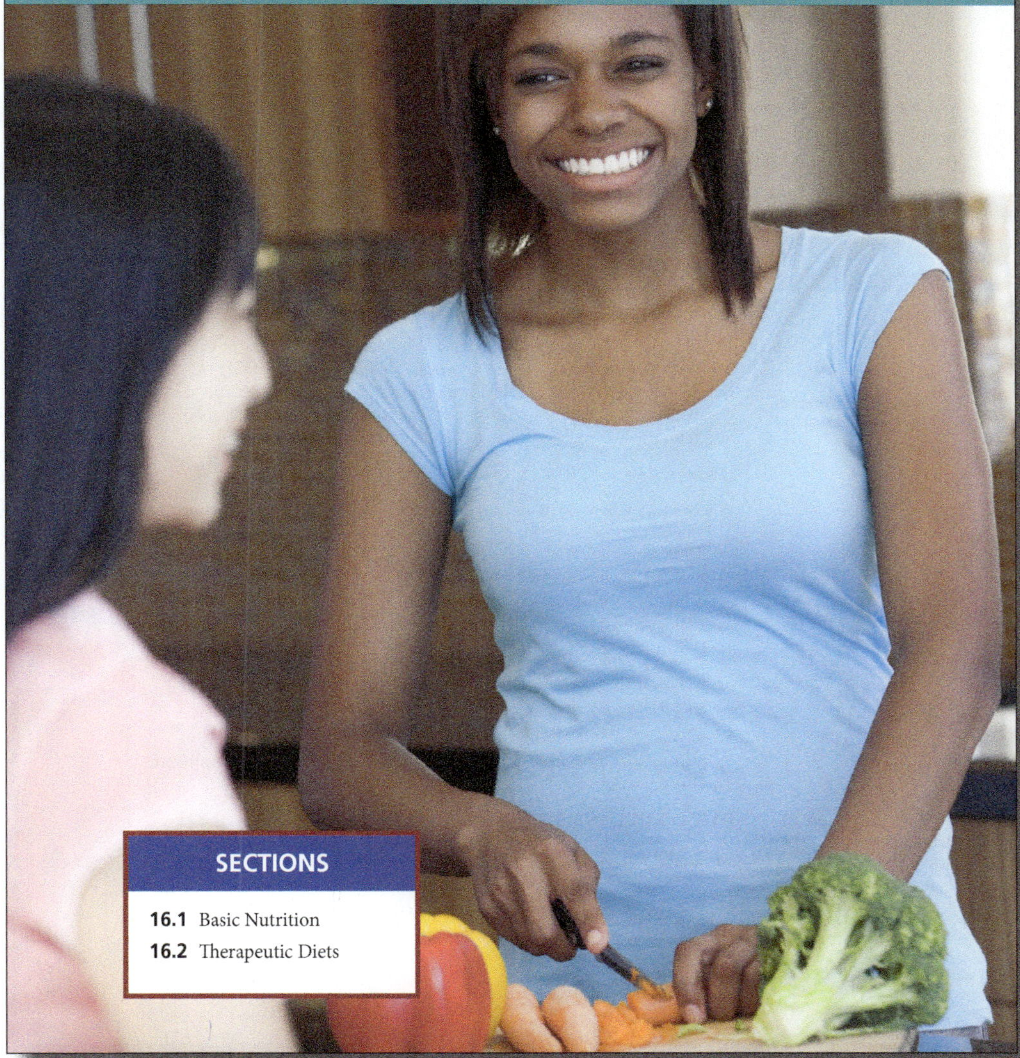

SECTIONS

CHAPTER 16 OVERVIEW

Chapter 16 provides an introduction to nutrition. Students learn about how the body uses food, how nutrients affect the body, and the types of diets that might be recommend for patients in a health care setting.

Section 16.1: Section 16.1 covers basic nutrition, such as the function of food, basic nutrients, and issues and conditions that might arise from poor nutrition.

Section 16.2: Section 16.2 introduces students to therapeutic diets. It covers factors that influence food habits, characteristics and treatment of common eating disorders, and the circumstances under which therapeutic diets that might be prescribed.

Advance Preparation	
Review	■ Chapter text for Sections 16.1 and 16.2.
Contact	■ General Food Consumer Center, 250 North St., White Plains, NY 10625, to request brochures and other educational material. ■ A nutritionist at a hospital, senior center, school, or other facility to schedule a class visit to a kitchen, or to invite the professional to the class.
Prepare	■ Magazine and newspaper articles about nutrition. ■ Food labels listing nutritional content. ■ A list of Web sites that provide information about nutrition—such as American Dietetic Association at eatingright.org and School Nutrition Organization at schoolnutrition.org.

FOCUS AND ENGAGE

Getting Started

- Emphasize that it is important for health care workers to model a healthy lifestyle and to emphasize proper nutrition.
- Encourage students to be honest when keeping the food journal.
- Explain that the goal is to provide insight into eating habits that might not be healthy and inspire change, as well as to educate students to recognize proper nutrition in others.

Introduce the Section

a. Review the content of the Background paragraph, explaining that proper nutrition provides the fuel bodies need to function.
b. Emphasize the importance of recognizing symptoms of poor nutrition and being able to communicate the benefits of proper nutrition are important for providing effective care.
c. Review section objectives.

Vocabulary Review

a. Direct students to the key terms.
b. Pronounce each word, and have the students repeat the pronunciation out loud.
c. Discuss each definition.

TEACH

Discuss

- Ask students what they have eaten so far today.
- Discuss the food groups and what is meant by a well-balanced diet.

Reinforce and Review

- Review Section 7.1, Wellness and Preventive Health Care, focusing on nutrition.

Getting Started

Health care workers must be healthy workers. It is well documented that those with good health habits miss fewer work days, are able to meet the required schedule more efficiently, and maintain a more rigorous work ethic. Eating right is a major factor in reaching and maintaining good health.

Keep a journal for one week of everything you eat. Analyze the strengths and weaknesses of your dietary habits, including potential diseases/disorders that might result from eating habits.

Keep a journal for the second week, eating a well-balanced diet; add a little exercise, and then calculate your body mass index (BMI) chart to see if you are in the normal range (see What's New on p. 456). If you are not in the normal range, continue your well-balanced nutrition and exercise to obtain a healthy BMI, making these things part of your health habits.

SECTION 16.1 Basic Nutrition

Background

vitality
(vahy TAL i tee)
The ability of an organism to go on living.

Health care workers must maintain good health in order to be efficient in their work. When you eat the proper foods, you have the energy and **vitality** to function effectively. Patients need a healthy diet to maintain or restore good health. Knowledge of nutrition helps you understand how to maintain good health for yourself and your patients/clients.

Objectives

When you have completed this section, you will be able to do the following:

- Match key terms with their correct meanings.
- Name the four functions of food.
- Name the five basic nutrients and explain how they maintain body function.
- Perform basic volume conversions.
- List five problems associated with obesity.
- Explain the U.S. Dietary guidelines and the role of MyPlate.
- Understand therapeutic diets.
- Describe common disorders associated with nutrition and other substances.

Introduction to Basic Nutrition

resistance
(ri ZIS tuhns)
The ability of the body to protect itself from disease.

Good nutrition promotes a healthier body and mind. It also aids in **resistance** to illness. When we eat a healthy diet, our energy and vitality are increased. The right foods speed the healing process and help a person feel better and sleep better.

446 Chapter 16 | Nutrition

CUSTOMIZED INSTRUCTION
Special Needs Students
Some special needs students may need help keeping track of everything they eat for a week. Assign a study partner to help.

CUSTOMIZED INSTRUCTION OVERVIEW	
Less Advanced Students	Pages 449, 458
More Advanced Students	Pages 450, 465
English Language Learners	Pages 447, 464
Special Needs Students	Pages 446, 463
At-Risk Students	Page 454

Your patients/clients are all from different cultural and religious backgrounds. Each culture and religion has dietary differences. Appetites, food budgets, cultural food preferences, and religious restrictions influence some of these differences. You and your patients need the same basic nutrients provided by a balanced, healthy diet. The health care worker must understand about foods and their effect on the body in order to assess his or her own diet and the patient's diet.

The Function of Food

When food is taken into the body, it is used in many different ways. The right combination of nutrients work together in the body to:

- Provide heat
- Promote growth
- Repair tissue
- **Regulate** body processes

regulate
(REG yuh leyt)
To control or adjust.

Basic Nutrients

Nutrients are chemical compounds found in food. When the food we eat enters the digestive tract, it is changed into a simple form and absorbed into the blood. The blood carries these nutrients to body cells, where they are used to maintain body functions. Table 16.1 lists the essential nutrients.

Water is **essential** to the body. Found in all body tissues, water makes up most of blood plasma. It carries nutrients to the body cells and carries waste products away from the body cells. It also lubricates the joints and helps regulate body temperature and body processes. The average person should drink 6–8 glasses of water daily.

essential
(uh SEN shuhl)
Necessary (e.g., certain food elements are necessary for the body's functions).

Fiber

Fiber adds bulk to the diet and helps prevent bowel and colon diseases. **Cellulose** is often referred to as dietary fiber or roughage. It is not digestible by humans and acts as a bulking agent by absorbing water; this helps to prevent constipation.

The diet many people eat is high in protein, fats, and carbohydrates but very low in fiber. To keep the bowel healthy, a person should eat several servings of fiber each day. Fiber is found in greens, kale, cabbage, celery, vegetable salads, raw and cooked fruits, whole-grain food, and cereals.

Good nutrition enhances your appearance and increases your stamina. It is important to plan meals and snacks that include all of the basic nutrients each day. Poor nutrition can lead to **malnutrition**.

cellulose
(SEL yo loz)
The primary component of plant cell walls which provides the fiber and bulk necessary for optimal functioning of the digestive tract.

malnutrition
(mal noo TRISH un)
Poor nutrition caused by an insufficient or poorly balanced diet or by a medical condition.

Calories

Food is the source of energy for our bodies. The body **metabolizes** food nutrients to create energy. As the body creates energy, it produces heat. Energy ensures that all of the body systems function. The amount of energy created by the food we eat is measured in **calories**. Calorie needs vary from person to person. A large, active person needs more calories than a smaller, inactive person does.

Basal metabolic rate (BMR) is the amount of energy, or calories, your body uses when it is at rest in a neutral environment. BMR is usually calculated after 12 hours of fasting so that the body is not even using energy to digest food. The temperature is set so that the environment is not hot or cold enough for the body to have to try and stay cool or warm.

metabolize
(mi TAB e liz)
To break down substances in cells to obtain energy.

calorie
(KAL uh ree)
Unit of measurement of the fuel value of food.

Nutrition | Chapter 16 447

Teaching Tips

- Discuss the reasons proper nutrition is so important.
- Explain the functions of food:
  - Provide heat
  - Promote growth
  - Repair tissue
  - Regulate body processes
- Explain that nutrients are chemical compounds found in food.
- Review the way the body extracts nutrients from food and delivers it to the body.
- Emphasize the role of water.
- Discuss the need for fiber to maintain digestive health.
- Explain that fiber adds bulk to the diet but is not digested.
- Discuss the foods that are high in fiber:
  - Greens
  - Kale
  - Cabbage
  - Celery
  - Raw and cooked fruits
  - Whole-grain foods
  - Cereals
- Explain that calories are a unit of measure for calculating the fuel value of food.
- Discuss basal metabolic rate (BMR) in relation to how the body burns calories during all types of activities.
- Discuss how gender, weight, height, and age affect BMR.
- Explain the relationship between calories and diet.
- Explain that we take calories into our bodies in the form of food and that we expend calories when we exercise.
- Emphasize that the balance of intake and expenditure affects body mass or weight.

TEAMWORK

Have students work in small groups to research BMR in depth, including ways to calculate it. Then have them calculate their personal BMR.

CUSTOMIZED INSTRUCTION

English Language Learners

Have students write each key term and its pronunciation on one side of an index card and its definition on the other side. Have them read each term and definition aloud to a partner.

ACTIVITY

Select one type of food and make a poster that identifies its nutritional value. Include the basic nutrients such as vitamins and elements derived from the food. On the poster, illustrate or explain why this food should or should not be part of a healthy, well-balanced diet.

Apply It

- Assign students to pairs.
- Point out to students that there is more than one way to arrive at calorie needs. For example, they may want to calculate BMR as part of the process.
- You may wish to bring in samples of food packaging to discuss nutrition labels.
- Allow time for students to discuss their comparisons of actual calorie intake and the daily calorie needs they calculated.
- You may wish to follow up the activity by having students analyze the nutritional value of their personal daily food intake for inadequate or excessive intake of nutrients.

Teaching Tips

- Point out that the balance of calories and exercise is a simply formula:
  - Intake more than we burn—gain body mass or weight
  - Expend more than we intake—lose body mass or weight
- Review Table 16.1 together as a class.
- Describe the basic nutrients listed in the left column of the chart and explain how they maintain body function (right column).
- Proteins:
  - Build and renew body tissue
  - Provide heat
- Carbohydrates:
  - Provide the basic source of energy for body heat and body activities
  - May be simple or complex
- Fats:
  - Provide fatty acids for normal growth and development
  - Provide energy

Apply It

With a partner, research factors that affect calorie needs. Based on your findings, calculate your own daily calorie needs. Using nutrition labels and other resources for calorie amounts, add up your calorie intake for three days. Compare those amounts to the average daily total that you calculated that you needed.

The number of calories we eat and the amount of exercise we do balance weight. If we eat more calories than we burn, we gain weight. If we burn more calories than we eat, we lose weight. The FDA food labeling standard adopts the Recommended Dietary Allowances (RDAs) from the average USDA 2,000 calorie dietary guidelines.

When a patient is inactive and feels ill, he or she may not want to eat. It is your responsibility to encourage the patient to take in enough calories to produce the energy needed to heal the body.

protein
(PROH teen)
Complex compound found in plant and animal tissues, essential for heat, energy, and growth.

amino acids
(ah MEE no a sid)
Any of a large number of compounds found in living cells that contain carbon, oxygen, hydrogen, and nitrogen, and join together to form proteins.

Complementary Proteins

Complete proteins are found in animal and soy products; other plant-based sources of protein are incomplete. Many vegetarians combine foods containing complementary with incomplete proteins. For example, combining rice (which is limited in lysine) with red beans (which are high in lysine but deficient in tryptophan) results in a complete protein.

Table 16.1 Essential Nutrients

Nutrient	What It Does
Proteins	■ Build and renew body tissues. ■ Provide heat energy. ■ Help produce antibodies. ■ Formed by organic compounds called **amino acids**. ■ Made up of 22 amino acids: 9 are essential, which means the body cannot produce these amino acids and they must be supplemented through the diet. They are found in almost all animal sources. ■ Main sources/complete proteins: meat, fish, milk, cheese, and eggs. ■ Incomplete proteins: cereal/soybeans, dry beans, peas, and peanuts. ■ Complementary incomplete proteins can be combined to form complete proteins. ■ 1 gram of protein = 4 calories
Carbohydrates	■ Provide the basic source of energy for body heat and body activities. ■ Starches or sugars. ■ Main sources: bread, cereal, pasta, crackers, potatoes, corn, peas, fruits, sugars, and syrups. ■ Simple carbohydrates are molecules made when one or two smaller sugar molecules (called saccharides) combine: found in raw and cooked fruits, some cooked vegetables, and refined sugar and its products (soda or candy). ■ Complex carbohydrates are long chains of glucose molecules bonded together. The chains may be straight, but usually branch and connect more than one chain together: found in grains, grain products (like bread or pasta), legumes, and some cooked vegetables and fruits. ■ Complex carbohydrates absorb slowly and provide a steady supply of energy; simple carbohydrates absorb so quickly, they are usually converted to fat. ■ 1 gram of carbohydrates = 4 calories
Fats	■ Provide fatty acids for normal growth and development. ■ Provide energy. ■ Carry vitamins A and D to the cells. ■ Help maintain body temperature by providing insulation; helps cushion organs and bones; provides flavor to foods. ■ Essential component of every cell membrane. ■ Main sources: butter, margarine, oils, creams, fatty meats, cheeses, and egg yolk. ■ Classified as saturated (solid at room temperature) or polyunsaturated (liquid at room temperature). ■ Sometimes called **lipids**. ■ 1 gram of lipid = 9 calories

(continued)

448 Chapter 16 | Nutrition

  - Carry vitamins A and D to cells
  - Help maintain body temperature
- Discuss sources of simple and complex carbohydrates.
- Make a differentiation between the functions of simple and complex carbohydrates.
- List sources of each type of carbohydrate.
- Discuss complete and complementary proteins. Identify complete and incomplete proteins.

TEAMWORK

Have students work in pairs to produce combinations of complementary proteins. Discuss their combinations as a class.

ACTIVITY

Using food labels, compare the nutritional value of two or more similar types of food products, such as Special K cereal and Fruit Loops. Include the serving size, number of calories, and breakdown of nutritional components. Make a chart, table, or graph depicting the results.

Table 16.1 Essential Nutrients (continued)

Nutrient	What It Does
Elements	■ Regulate the activity of the heart, nerves, and muscles. ■ Build and renew teeth, bones, and other tissues. ■ Inorganic (nonliving) elements found in all body tissue. ■ More than $\frac{1}{3}$ of the dietary nutrients needed each day are elements. ■ Major dietary elements: calcium, chloride, magnesium, phosphorus, potassium, sodium, sulfur. ■ Trace dietary elements: chromium, copper, fluoride, iodine, iron, manganese, molybdenum, selenium, zinc. ■ See Figure 16.1.
Vitamins	■ Essential for normal metabolism, growth, and body development. ■ Inorganic (non-living) elements found in all body tissues. ■ Regulate body functions: • Metabolism; help release energy from other nutrients • Vital role in almost every chemical reaction within the body • Co-enzyme for normal health/growth (some behave like hormones) ■ Only a small amount required—a well balanced diet provides required vitamins. ■ Excess or deficiency can cause poor health. ■ Water soluble or fat soluble (A, D, E, K). ■ See Figure16.2.
Water	■ All cells in the body must be bathed in water. ■ Water is active in most chemical reactions and is needed to carry other nutrients, to regulate body temperature, and to help eliminate wastes. Water makes up about 60 percent of an adult's body weight. ■ Lost through evaporation, urination, and respiration so it must be replaced every day. ■ Remove toxins and wastes from your body. ■ Dehydration, or under-hydration, is when the body loses more water than it takes in; may occur during hot weather when there is profuse sweating or as a result of prolonged exertion; older people may not recognize that they are becoming dehydrated because of their bodies not registering thirst, though thirst isn't the only sign. ■ Over-hydration is when the body takes in more water than it loses; may occur in people whose kidneys do not excrete urine normally or in athletes who drink more water than they need when trying to avoid dehydration.

lipids
(LIP id z)
Any of a group of organic compounds, including the fats, oils, triglycerides, etc. that—together with carbohydrates and proteins—constitute the principal structural material of living cells.

elements
(EL e ment s)
Regulate the activity of the heart, nerves, and muscles. Build and renew teeth, bones, and other tissues.

vitamins
(VAHY tuh min s)
Group of substances necessary for normal functioning and maintenance of health.

Too Much or Too Little?

A *deficiency* is a disease caused by lack of a nutrient; toxicity is a disease caused by too much of a nutrient. There is a range between the two that is optimal for most humans. Vitamin intake, for instance, should fall within a range that assists the body in achieving optimal good health. There are Recommended Dietary Allowances (RDAs) for each nutrient to help you prevent diseases associated with getting too much or too little of a specific vitamin or nutrient.

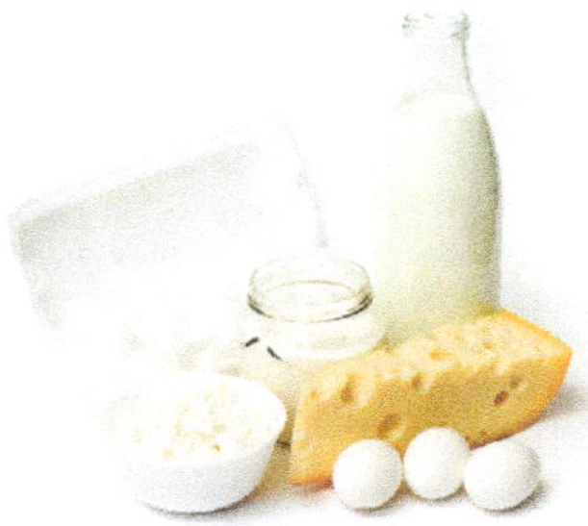

Figure 16.1
Calcium is an important element. Besides for dairy foods, what are other good dietary sources of calcium?

Teaching Tips

- Have students give examples of sources that contain complete proteins.
- Discuss health risks associated with inadequate or excessive intake of protein.
- Elements:
  - Regulate activity of heart, nerves, and muscles
  - Build and renew teeth, bones, and other tissues
- Discuss and describe the classifications of minerals: trace and major.
- Discuss and predict possible health risks of inadequate or excessive intake of each mineral.
- Vitamins:
  - Essential for normal metabolism, growth, and body development
- Discuss and predict possible health risks of inadequate or excessive intake of each vitamin.
- Water:
  - Carries other nutrients
  - Regulates body temperature
  - Helps eliminate wastes
- Distinguish between underhydration and overhydration. Have students predict the health risks associated with under- or overhydration.
- Discuss deficiency and toxicity. Have students predict the health risks associated with inadequate and excessive intake of each essential nutrient.
- Discuss the types of foods that provide vitamins and elements:
  - Calcium: Milk and most dairy products
  - Iron: Meat, fish, some vegetables
  - Iodine: Fish

ACTIVITY

Have students analyze their personal daily food intake for any vitamin deficiencies. Have them determine food sources to address any deficiencies they identify.

CUSTOMIZED INSTRUCTION

Less Advanced Students

You may want to provide less advanced students with handouts explaining the difference between vitamins and elements.

Figure Focus

16.1 Calcium is an important element. Besides for dairy foods, what are other good dietary sources of calcium?

Answer: Many vegetables, such as collard greens, kale, and broccoli, and some seafood, such as canned sardines with bones, are high in calcium.

Figure Focus

16.2 Vitamins include A, B complex, B_1, B_2, B_{12}, C, D, and niacin. Why are vitamins an important part of our diet?

Answer: Vitamins are essential for normal metabolism, growth, and body development.

Teaching Tips

- Vitamin A: Apricots, cantaloupe, milk, cheese, eggs, meat organs, butter, fish-liver oils, and dark green and deep yellow vegetables
- Vitamin B_1: Whole-grain and enriched grain products; meats, dry beans, and peas; milk, cheese, and eggs
- Vitamin B_2: Whole-grain and enriched grain products, dark green vegetables
- Vitamin B_{12}: Liver, cheese, eggs, and milk
- Vitamin C: Fresh, raw citrus fruits, and vegetables
- Vitamin D: Fish-liver oils, eggs, and sunshine
- Niacin: Liver, meat, fish, poultry, eggs; peanuts; dark green vegetables; whole-grain and enriched cereal products
- Explain digestion and absorption:
  - Saliva breaks down food
  - Tongue pushes food into esophagus
  - Food enters stomach
  - Small particles and proteins enter small intestine
  - Body absorbs basic nutrients
  - Waste travels through colon and is excreted from body

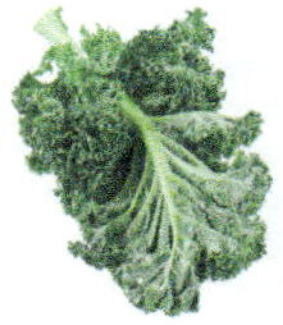

Vitamin A
One form of vitamin A is yellow and one form is colorless. Foods rich in vitamin A include apricots, cantaloupe, milk, cheese, eggs, meat organs (especially liver and kidney), fortified margarine, butter, fish-liver oils, and dark green and deep yellow vegetables.

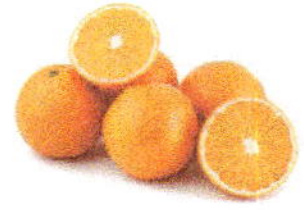

Vitamin C (Ascorbic Acid)
Foods rich in vitamin C are fresh, raw citrus fruits and vegetables—oranges, grapefruits, cantaloupe, strawberries, tomatoes, raw onions, cabbage, green and sweet red peppers, and dark green vegetables.

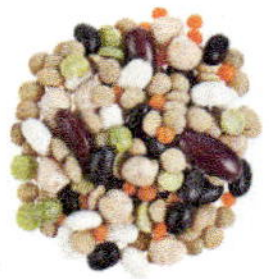

Vitamin B Complex & Vitamin B_1 (Thiamine)
Foods rich in vitamins B and B_1 include whole-grain and enriched-grain products, meats (especially pork, liver, and kidney), dry beans, and peas.

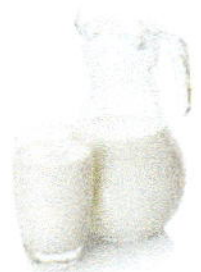

Vitamin D
Foods rich in vitamin D include milk, margarine, fish-liver oils, and eggs. Certain foods are now fortified with vitamin D to add the nutrient. Sunshine is also a source.

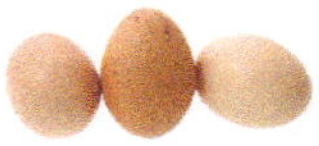

Vitamin B_2 (Riboflavin)
Foods rich in vitamin B_2 include milk, cheese, eggs, meat (especially liver and kidney), whole-grain and enriched-grain products, and dark green vegetables.

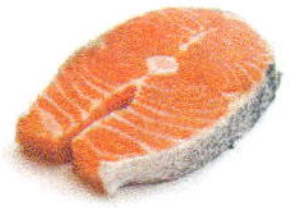

Niacin
Foods rich in niacin include meat, fish, poultry, eggs, peanuts, dark green vegetables, whole-grain, and enriched cereal products.

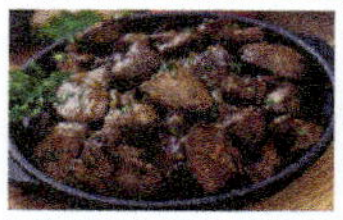

Vitamin B_{12}
Foods rich in vitamin B_{12} include liver, other organ meats, cheese, eggs, and milk.

Figure 16.2
Vitamins include A, B complex, B_1, B_2, B_{12}, C, D, and niacin. Why are vitamins an important part of our diet?

digestion
(di JES chuh n)
The process of making food absorbable by dissolving it and breaking it down into simpler chemical compounds that occur in the living body chiefly through the action of enzymes secreted into the alimentary canal.

cholesterol
(kuh LES tuh rawl)
A type of lipid, or fat, found in the body; produced by the liver or eaten in food.

absorption
(ab SAWRP shuh)
To take up liquid or other matter.

Digestion and Absorption

Digestion is a complex process of turning the food we eat into the energy that we need to survive. Digestion begins before you even put food your mouth. Saliva forms in your mouth when you smell, see, or think of food. Saliva helps to break down the chemicals, specifically carbohydrates, in food.

The tongue pushes food to the esophagus, which then carries the food to the stomach. The stomach acts as a mixer by grinding the food into smaller pieces and breaking down proteins which then go into the small intestine.

Cholesterol is often thought of only as a factor in heart disease. However, cholesterol is a component in digestion. It is a lipid made by the liver and, in addition to being involved in digestion, cholesterol is part of the transport process for nutrients. The job of the small intestine is to break the food down even more, so that our body can absorb all the vitamins, minerals, proteins, carbohydrates, and fats. This is the process of **absorption**. Although most nutrients are absorbed by the body, there is waste left. The waste travels through the colon, where any excess water is absorbed, and the waste becomes solid. The solid waste, stool, then is **excreted** from the body.

450 Chapter 16 | Nutrition

- Explain what cholesterol is.
- Discuss the body's role in producing cholesterol, and explain the functions of cholesterol in the body.
- Discuss the effects of cholesterol on the body, including effects of excessive intake of cholesterol.
- Have students predict and describe the health risks associated with excessive intake of cholesterol.

CUSTOMIZED INSTRUCTION

More Advanced Students

Assign more advanced students to learn more about the ways vitamins and minerals affect the body. For example, recent students credit vitamin D with numerous health benefits. Have students report their findings to the class.

Our body gets the energy it needs from food through a process called **metabolism**. Metabolism is a constant process that occurs from the beginning of life to the end of life.

Estimated Energy Requirement (EER)

The EER is the average dietary energy intake that is predicted to maintain energy balance in a healthy adult. In other words, if the individual is currently a healthy weight, this amount of intake will cause him or her to maintain that healthy weight. EER deals with overall calorie intake; it does not specify which nutrients should comprise that total. The overall number of calories a person needs depends on their age, gender, weight, height, and physical activity level and health status. For many generic dietary calculations, such as the percentages of RDA met by a particular food as noted on the nutrition label, 2,000 calories is the usual "assumed" amount. However, in actual practice, this varies greatly from person to person.

U.S. Dietary Guidelines and MyPlate

A healthy diet along with physical activity help to ensure and maintain good health. The U.S. Department of Agriculture (USDA) has provided MyPlate as a reminder of healthy eating practices regarding the types and amounts of food on our plates. (**Figure 16.3**) Although this new symbol has replaced the food pyramid, the food groups have remained the same. They include vegetables, fruits, grains, proteins, and diary.

MyPlate illustrates the five food groups using a place setting. When building healthy meals, half of your "plate" should contain fruits and vegetables; half of your grains should be whole grains; twice a week seafood should be the protein on your plate; beans, a natural source of fiber, is a good protein option; meat and poultry portions should be small and lean, and milk products should be fat-free or low-fat (1%). It is advised that foods high in solid fats—such as ice cream, cookies, cakes, pizza, and hot dogs—are not every day foods, but something you enjoy once in a while. The guidelines also suggest that sodium levels, especially in packaged foods and frozen meals, should be checked and lower-sodium or reduced-sodium items selected, and water is recommended instead of sugary drinks. Follow these guidelines for yourself and your patients/clients. The food choices of all cultures fit into these guidelines when you plan carefully.

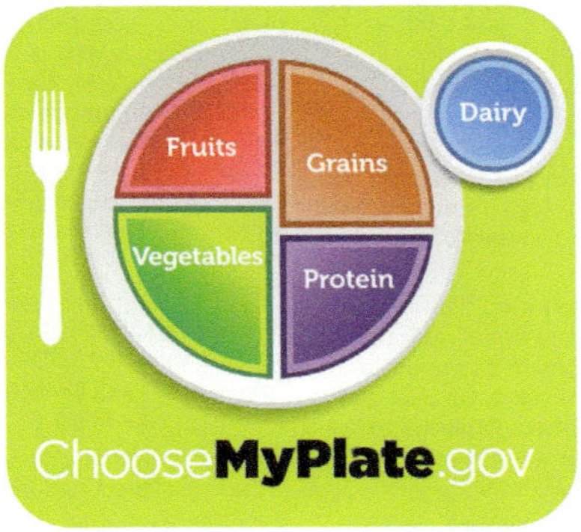

Figure 16.3
The MyPlate graphic. Why do you think MyPlate uses a familiar mealtime image to represent the food groups?

excreted
(ik SKREE ted)
When waste matter is discharged from the blood, tissues, or organs.

metabolism
(mi TAH buh lih zum)
Collection of chemical reactions that takes place in the body's cells to convert the fuel in the food we eat into the energy needed to power everything we do.

Apply It

Factors that take into account a person's energy intake, energy expenditure, age, gender, weight, height, and physical activity level (PAL) are used to calculate EER. Research online for the information and equations appropriate for your personal factors, and compute your EER. In groups of 3–5, discuss your EER findings and whether you need to adjust your activity levels.

Nutrition | Chapter 16 451

ACTIVITY

Divide the class into four groups. Assign each group one of these four minerals: calcium, magnesium, potassium, and sodium. Each group should plan a day's menu that incorporates foods high in their assigned mineral. As a class, compare the differences and overlap in foods that have each of the minerals.

TEAMWORK

Have students use old magazines to clip pictures of food or alternatively, they can find pictures of food on the Internet and print them. Then, working in pairs, have students identify which of their pictures show foods that contain cholesterol.

Teaching Tips

- Explain metabolism.
- Discuss estimated energy requirement (EER) and how it is calculated and computed.
- Discuss how sex, weight, age, and height affect EER so that everyone's personal EER is different.
- Explain that the MyPlate was created by the United States Department of Agriculture.
- Emphasize that the size of portions—servings—depends on the individual.
- Discuss the importance of eating more whole grains, fruits, and vegetables and lesser amounts of protein and dairy.
- Emphasize the importance of minimizing the intake of fats and sweets.

Figure Focus

16.3 The MyPlate graphic. Why do you think MyPlate uses a familiar mealtime image to represent the food groups?

Answer: The plate image is a symbol that everyone recognizes, and it shows proportionality how much of each food group people should eat.

Apply It

- Direct students to appropriate sources for information and equations for calculating and computing EER.
- Verify that students have the information they need to accurately calculate EER.
- Arrange for students to discuss their findings and computed EERs in small groups.

Teaching Tips

- Explain types of fats:
  - Saturated fats: Fats from animals; fully hydrogenated
  - Trans fats: Fat created by adding hydrogen atoms to liquid fat to transform it into a solid; fully hydrogenated
- Discuss the effects of saturated fats and trans fats on the body, including effects of excessive intake.
- Have students predict and describe the health risks associated with excessive intake of saturated fats and trans fats.
- Discuss why it is important to educate children on proper nutrition.

What's New?—Food Pyramids and MyPlate

- Review the history of nutritional guidelines, and the introduction of the 1992 food pyramid.
- If possible, show a picture of the 1992 food pyramid (everydiet.org/food_pyramid_old.htm).
- Compare some of the old recommendations with new recommendations.
- Discuss why MyPlate was introduced.

Why do you think the meat, dairy, and sugar industry would care about the USDA food guidelines?

Answer: The meat, dairy, and sugar industry care about the USDA recommendations because millions of people read them and use them. If the government advises U.S. citizens to cut down on dairy, meat, or sugar, this would affect the profits of their industry. Also, government institutions (such as the military and public schools) generally follow the recommendations of the USDA. So, food industry representatives lobby the government to make sure that their particular food group is not slighted in the government recommendations.

The Department of Health and Humans Services (HHS) and the Department of Agriculture (USDA) jointly publish the Dietary Guidelines for Americans every five years and is intended for people above the age of two years old. According to The Dietary Guidelines for Americans, 2015, a healthy diet emphasizes fruits, vegetables, whole grains, and fat-free or low-fat milk and milk products. It also includes lean meats, poultry, fish, beans, eggs, and nuts, and is low in saturated fats, and trans fats.

NOTE: Saturated fats are fats from animal products—a fat in which the carbon atoms are fully hydrogenated. A diet heavy in saturated fat is thought to raise cholesterol in the bloodstream. Trans fats are a specific type of fat formed when liquid fats are made into solid fats by the addition of hydrogen atoms, a process known as hydrogenation. They increase bad cholesterol and decrease good cholesterol.

What's New?

Food Pyramids and MyPlate

The U.S. government has been issuing dietary recommendations for more than 100 years. In 1992, the U.S. Department of Agriculture (USDA) released a nutrition guide known as the American food pyramid. This illustration suggested how much of each food category a person should eat each day.

Many nutritional experts, however, complained that the 1992 pyramid was not accurate based on the latest nutrition research. They believed it was heavy on beef and dairy and did not put enough emphasis on fruit and vegetables. In addition, the pyramid lumped all members of the protein-rich group ("Meat, Poultry, Fish, Dry Beans, Eggs, and Nuts") together and made no distinction between whole grains and refined products.

As a result, in 2005, the USDA released a new nutritional guide known as MyPyramid. There were no foods pictured on the new MyPyramid image and no text. Instead, the new logo emphasized the importance of physical activity by showing a sort of stick figure climbing the stairs of the pyramid.

In 2011 after reviewing and updating the dietary guidelines of 2010, the MyPlate symbol replaced the food pyramid. This was done in a joint initiative involving The First Lady, Michelle Obama, and the USDA. The goal of the MyPlate symbol is to serve as a reminder of portions and types of foods to include on our plates at meal time.

Like the food pyramid, MyPlate does not suggest serving sizes but it does emphasize proportions recommended for the five basic food groups. It is color-coded, red for Fruits, green for vegetables, orange for grains, purple for proteins, and blue for diary. The size of the food group symbols on the plates represent the proportions. The reason MyPlate does not not suggest specific serving sizes is because people have different nutritional needs based on age, gender, height, weight, physical activity level, and health status. The MyPlate Web site (ChooseMyPlate.gov) provides information to personalize your food intake and exercise plans.

The Harvard School of Public Health has issued their own "Healthy Eating Plate" as an alternative to the one provided by the USDA. The Harvard plate can be accessed at www.hsph.harvard.edu/nutritionsource. Harvard's plate includes healthy oils, and, where MyPlate has a glass of dairy, Harvard recommends water or coffee or tea with little or no sugar. At the bottom of Harvard's Healthy Eating Plate is a running figure with the text "Stay Active," suggesting—as do the USDA guidelines—that in order to maintain a healthy weight, you need to consider what you eat and also exercise.

Harvard's Healthy Eating Plate is far from the only alternative to the USDA recommendations. The "plate wars" will likely continue in the nutrition community for years to come.

Why do you think the meat, dairy, and sugar industries would care about the USDA food guidelines?

452 Chapter 16 | Nutrition

ACTIVITY

Have students identify sources of fat in their personal diets. Remind them to check the nutrition labels of the foods they eat to determine how much and what kind of fat is in the foods.

TEAMWORK

Working in pairs, use the Web site choosemyplate.gov to develop a personalized nutrition plan for yourself and your partner. Explore the tools available on the Web site, and then use them accordingly. Print out the results, and discuss them with the class.

Math Link

Liquid Conversions

Even after the United States became independent, the people continued to use the English system of measurement. This system had grown naturally for hundreds of years. People used familiar objects and parts of the body, such as "feet," as measuring devices. They measured liquid volume with common household items such as teaspoons, cups, and pails (the word "gallon" comes from an old name for a pail). Although this system could be quite confusing, it is still used in the United States today.

The metric system was developed in France during the French Revolution in the 1790s. The metric system has several advantages over the English system. The metric system was based on a decimal system, which made it much easier to do calculations. The scientific community adopted the metric system almost from its inception. It came to be used by most other nations of the world.

The dual systems create problems for Americans. Liquid measurement seems to be an incomprehensible whirl of drams, milliliters, cups, and tablespoons. The situation is not helped by the fact that one cubic centimeter (cc) equals one milliliter (ml); they are the same. Here's a conversion chart to help you out on the trickier volume conversions:

- one teaspoon = 5 cc = 5 ml
- one tablespoon (tbl) = three teaspoons
- one tablespoon = 15 cc = 15 ml
- one fluid ounce (U.S. liquid) = 30 cc = 30 ml = 2 tablespoons = 6 teaspoons
- one cup = eight fluid ounces = 16 tablespoons
- one pint = 2 cups = 16 fluid ounces

Actually, one teaspoon equals 4.928921594 milliliters, but the chart has rounded it off to make things easier. Similarly, one fluid ounce (U.S.) equals 29.573529562 milliliters. Believe it or not, it actually makes a difference. At some point, "rounding off" errors would become serious. However, for the problems below, you can use the easier equivalents.

Example 1

Billy must drink 2,250 cc of water each day. How many pints of water will he drink? Round to the nearest tenth of a pint.

1 pint = 16 oz.
1 oz = 30 cc
16 oz × 30 cc = 480 cc
2,250 cc divided by 480 cc = 4.688 pints
4.7 pints

Example 2

Convert 55 tbsp into an equal volume of cups.

Round to the nearest tenth of a cup.

1 cup = 6 tbs
55 divided by 6 = 9.167 cups
9.2 cups

1. A dose of a specific medicine is 1 tbs. How many doses does an 8 oz bottle contain?
2. A bottle of juice contains 2 liters. If 1 liter equals 33.8 fl. oz, how many cc of juice are there in the 2-liter bottle?
3. The humidifier for the nursing station holds 14 pints of water.
   a. How many ounces will completely fill the reservoir?
   b. How many 8-oz bottles will be needed to fill the reservoir?
4. U.S. fluid ounces and British fluid ounces are not the same volume. One British fluid ounce equals only 28.41 milliliters. Why is this evidence that the metric system is easier to use than the English system of measurement?

Choose a level of accuracy appropriate to solve the problem when reporting quantities.

Nutrition | Chapter 16 453

Math Link—Liquid Conversions

- Review types of measurement in Section 12.2, and review the metric system in Section 11.2.
- Emphasize the importance of accurate measurements in the health care field.
- What might happen if a measurement is inaccurate?
- Emphasize the importance of liquid measurements in health care.
- When are liquid measurements used?
- Review the equivalents of metric and standard volume measures.
- Discuss how rounding up might cause problems.
- Review the examples together.
- Read each question out loud.

Answers:

1. 1 oz = 2 tbs 8 oz = 16 tbs
   16 doses
2. 1 oz = 30 cc 33.8 oz [1 liter] = 1014 cc
   1014 × 2 (liters) = 2028 cc

3a. 1 pint = 16 fl. oz
14 pints × 16 fl. oz = 224 oz

3b. 224 oz divided by 8 oz bottles = 28 eight-ounce bottles

4. It is obviously a difficult system when one measurement term means two different things! Some believe the metric system is easier to use because it is based on the number 10, which makes it easier to calculate measurements.

TEAMWORK

Imagine you work for a company or organization responsible for increasing the consumption of vegetables. In a small group, select one vegetable and create a marketing brochure designed to encourage people to eat more of that vegetable. You might include facts about the vegetable, recipes for cooking with the vegetable, personal endorsements for the vegetable, etc. Include pictures to make the brochure more appealing. Display the brochures in the classroom.

Teaching Tips

- Describe conditions that might arise from poor nutrition:
  - Anemia
  - Anorexia nervosa
  - Bulimia
  - Constipation
  - Dull hair and eyes
  - Mental slowdown
  - Obesity
  - Osteoporosis
  - Rickets
  - Poor skin conditions
- Explain why poor nutrition often strikes the elderly:
  - Lack of appetite
  - Dental problems
  - Difficulty obtaining food
  - Difficulty preparing food
  - Low income
  - Illness
- Discuss ways to insure that the elderly achieve proper nutrition:
  - Assistance from family and friends
  - Quality health care

Apply It

Form nutrition teams of five or six students. Create a profile of a person, including how tall he or she is, weight, activity level, and so forth. Use MyPlate to plan a day's menus, including meals, snacks, and beverages, for the person you profiled. Before planning, you may find it helpful to calculate the person's BMI, their daily calorie needs and/or their EER. Be sure to consult nutrition labels for information about the nutrients found in the foods you are including in the menus. When the day's menus are complete, present them to the class.

A nutrition label provides information about how much, and what type of, fats you are eating in a food. Nutrition labels also alert you to how much cholesterol is in foods.

Good food habits are learned and should be taught to children. To ensure children have good food habits:

- Give children enough time at the table, don't rush the meal.
- Be a good role model and practice what you preach.
- Don't reward, punish, or appease children with food so you can avoid food problems later on in life.

How Poor Nutrition Affects the Body

When we do not supply our bodies with the proper nutrients, many things can go wrong. We lose stamina and vitality. An unhealthy diet often results in illness and disease. Not having the proper nutrients for good health may come from either excessive or inadequate intake of essential nutrients. The following are a few of the problems that poor nutrition can cause:

- Anemia, a decreased number of red blood cells or a decreased amount of **hemoglobin**, results in:
  - Fatigue
  - Paleness
  - Rapid heartbeat
  - Dyspnea (shortness of breath) on exertion
  - Headache
  - Indigestion
  - Insomnia (inability to sleep)
- Constipation is infrequent, difficult defecation. It is commonly caused by lack of activity and by not eating enough vegetables, fruit, or water.
- Dull hair and eyes are symptoms of poor diet.
- Mental slowdown can occur when nutrition is poor.
- **Obesity** occurs when a person takes in more calories than the body uses. This results in increasing amounts of fatty tissue.
- Osteoporosis occurs when bones become porous, causing them to break easily. This is caused by inadequate calcium intake or absorption.
- Rickets is a softening of the bones in children, potentially leading to fractures and deformity. This occurs from a lack of vitamin D.
- Dehydration occurs when more water is lost than taken in. This can be caused by not drinking enough liquids, diarrhea, vomiting, excessive sweating, and some diseases such as diabetes.
- Poor skin condition results from poor nutrition.

hemoglobin
(HEE muh gloh bin)
Complex chemical in the blood; carries oxygen and carbon dioxide.

obesity
(oh BEE sih tee)
Extreme fatness; abnormal amount of fat on the body.

Community

Help a food distribution agency such as Meals on Wheels or the Salvation Army or another group plan and serve a well-balanced nutritious menu for one day.

454 Chapter 16 | Nutrition

Apply It

- Divide students into teams.
- Make sure students take as many factors into account as possible, as they plan the day's menus.
- Remind students to analyze the nutritional value of the daily food intake they are planning for inadequate or excessive intake of nutrients.
- Allow class time for discussion of the challenges the students encountered as they planned the days menu for their fictional person.

Community

- You might want to provide a list of agencies in your area where your students can volunteer.
- Some students may already participate in programs like these—ask them to invite classmates to join them.
- Allot class time to discuss the experience.

CUSTOMIZED INSTRUCTION

At-Risk Students

Students learn how poor nutrition can affect a person's physical well-being. Have them research how it can also affects one's emotional and intellectual well-being. For example, going without food or proper nutrition can cause depression, aggression, anxiety, and poor social skills. Have students create a poster or slideshow presentation that describes or illustrates the effects poor nutrition can have on a person's ability to perform well in school or on the job. Have them share their posters or presentations with the class.

Malnutrition in the Elderly Population

Due to a variety of factors, malnutrition is prominent among the elderly population. As people age they experience sensory loss, especially in taste and smell leading to decreased appetite. Poor dentition also may put the patient at risk because the patient will select foods high in carbohydrates and sugars which are easier to chew. The presence of disease in the elderly can also affect their dietary intake.

Another factor can be an alteration in functional status which prevents the patient from obtaining food (grocery shopping) or preparing food (cooking). These patients will require assistance in obtaining and preparing food. They may benefit from the home delivery of prepared meals or the purchase of pre-packaged meals which can be easily prepared in a microwave.

Personal Wellness

Obesity in the U.S.

Americans, especially young people, are getting fatter. In past years, there has been a dramatic increase in obesity in the United States. In 1980, 25 percent of adults in the United States were overweight. By 2011–2012, this figure had risen to 35.1 percent percent of adults age 20 years and over.

In a way, the numbers are even bleaker for children. The number of overweight children between the ages of 6 and 19 tripled between 1980 and 2004. An estimated 9 million children over the age of six (about 15 percent) are currently obese. About four out of every five of these obese children will remain overweight into adulthood.

So what is so bad about being overweight? The answer is quite simple. Overweight and obese people have an increased risk for many diseases and health conditions such as the following:

- Hypertension (high blood pressure)
- Diabetes
- Coronary heart disease
- Stroke
- Gallbladder disease
- Sleep apnea and respiratory problems
- Some cancers (endometrial, breast, and colon)
- Osteoarthritis (a degeneration of cartilage and its underlying bone within a joint)

The U.S. government estimates that the cost of obesity in the United States was more than $190 billion. That's the amount of added medical costs every year that are estimated to stem from obesity-related problems. It's nearly 21 percent of total U.S. health care costs. Obesity is now considered one of the major health crises affecting the United States.

The solution to the problem is simple, but instituting it is not. People have to eat less, eat smarter, and exercise more. Fatty, sugary diets have contributed to growing waistlines. Fast food and junk food are not nutritionally sound.

More than half of all Americans do not get the recommended amount of physical activity—thirty minutes daily for adults; sixty minutes daily for children. Kids spend more time staring at television and computer screens than they do in physical play; nearly one quarter of American children eight or older spend more than five hours a day watching television or playing computer/video games.

Both children and adults have to limit their time in front of the television or computer and follow the recommendations of the MyPlate program.

Personal Wellness—Obesity in the U.S.

- Define obesity.
- Emphasize that there is a difference between being overweight and being obese.
- Review the statistics that show the trend toward more obese people.
- Point out that obesity is particularly problematic for children.
- Review the health problems associated with obesity.
- Explain why the costs associated with obesity should concern everyone.
- Discuss reasons for the increase in obesity:
  - Fast food
  - Sedentary lifestyle—more television and less exercise
  - Processed food
  - Cutting back on physical education programs in schools

What are some ways to stop the increase in the number of obese people of all ages in the U.S., and ways for people who are currently obese to lose weight?

Answer: Both children and adults have to limit their time in front of the television or computer and follow the recommendations of the MyPlate guidelines.

ACTIVITY

Have students analyze the nutritional value of their personal daily intake for any inadequate or excessive intake of a nutrient.

TEAMWORK

Divide the class into groups corresponding to the food groups on the MyPlate. Ask each member of the class to bring in a healthy recipe that includes the food in his or her assigned food group. Compile the recipes into a cookbook.

Teaching Tips

- Review the importance of proper nutrition in maintaining a healthy body.
- Review ways to use the MyPlate food guidelines.

What's New?—Body Mass Index

- Explain that weight is not the only way to measure whether a body is a healthy size.
- Describe Body Mass Index (BMI).
- Explain that it is a formula that helps estimate how much of the body is made of fat.
- Emphasize that, although it is not accurate for everyone, it is a good tool for most people.
- Review the formula, but explain that there are charts already set up so people do not have to actually do the math. (Students may have used a BMI chart in Chapter 12.)
- Review the Weight Status classifications:
  - Underweight
  - Normal
  - Overweight
  - Obese

How can BMI be used to help people understand when they need to change their lifestyle?

Answer: Many people are sensitive about their weight, and do not like to discuss it. They become defensive when told they are overweight or obese, or even underweight. Using BMI can help point out body size problems without focusing on actual weight. Once people are aware of their BMI they can make lifestyle changes as necessary. For example, they can eat a more balanced diet to gain or lose body mass, and learn to incorporate proper exercise into their daily routine.

What's New?

Body Mass Index

Looking at height and bone structure is one way of assessing appropriate body weight. Another method that is gaining wide acceptance with many health practitioners is the body mass index (BMI).

BMI is a number based on a person's weight and height that provides an indication of the percent of the body that is made up of fat. Because the percentage of body fat is a truer indication of health than weight alone, BMI is a useful diagnostic tool that can be used to determine if a person is overweight and by how much. BMI is an estimate of body fat. It may not be accurate for older people or for athletes that have a great amount of muscle. However, it closely tracks the amount of fat the normal person has.

BMI can be calculated with this formula:

$\text{weight} \div \text{height}^2 \times 703 = \text{BMI}$

For example, you would calculate the BMI for a person who weighs 150 pounds and is 5 feet 5 inches (65 inches total) tall like this:

$150 \div 65^2 \times 703 = 24.96$

Next, you find the BMI on this chart:

BMI	Weight Status
Below 18.5	Underweight
18.5–24.9	Normal
25.0–29.9	Overweight
30.0 and above	Obese

How can BMI be used to help people understand when they need to change their lifestyle?

Summary

A balanced, healthy diet is essential for maintaining health and stamina. Everyone needs certain basic nutrients in his or her diet. When you plan your daily meals using the guidelines in the MyPlate program, you meet your body's nutritional needs and help maintain good health. All individuals must eat a healthy diet that provides balanced nutrients and meets cultural and religious needs.

Section 16.1 Review Questions

1. What are nutrients?
2. What foods are good to eat in order to get a large supply of fiber?
3. What is anemia?
4. What are the problems associated with obesity?
5. How many teaspoons are there in two fluid ounces?
6. What is the goal of MyPlate?

456 Chapter 16 | Nutrition

TEAMWORK

In small groups, prepare a skit that demonstrates how poor nutrition can affect the body, and what a caregiver should do to help a patient suffering from poor nutrition. Present the skit to the class.

Section 16.1 Review Questions

1. Answer: Nutrients are chemical compounds found in food.
2. Answer: Fiber is found in greens, kale, cabbage, celery, cereals, whole grains, raw and cooked fruit, and vegetable salads.
3. Answer: Anemia is a decreased number of red blood cells or a decreased amount of hemoglobin. It can result in fatigue, headache, paleness, indigestion, rapid heartbeat, dyspnea (shortness of breath) on exertion, and insomnia (inability to sleep).

Therapeutic Diets

SECTION 16.2

Background

Some patients/clients have illnesses that require special diets. Therapeutic diets are diets that modify a patient's normal diet in order to treat an illness. Understanding why the diet has been changed helps you to encourage clients to eat the food prepared for them. When you are knowledgeable about their diet, you are able to explain how important it is to their recovery.

Objectives

When you have completed this section, you will be able to do the following:

- Match key terms with their correct meaning.
- List three factors that influence food habits.
- Select a correct therapeutic diet for physical disorders.
- Discuss characteristics and treatment of common eating disorders
- List four commonly abused substances and their negative impacts on the human body.

Introduction to Therapeutic Diets

It is especially important to remember the factors that influence food habits for patients who are on a therapeutic diet. Always respect the patient's personal attitudes and preferences, nationality, race, and religious needs.

A therapeutic diet is often very different from the foods the patient normally eats. Your understanding of the reason for the diet and your patients' special needs helps ease their concerns. The dietitian will talk with the patient and try to adapt a therapeutic diet to meet a patient's nutritional and personal needs. An example of a special or personal need is religious restrictions.

Many religions of the world follow specific dietary laws. These guidelines are very important to clients. The stress caused by breaking the law when clients are on a therapeutic diet may cause added worry. Always be respectful of the dietary requests that your clients make, and report their requests to your supervisor. Ask your clients what diet they normally follow. If there is a problem with the diet, report it to your supervisor, who will talk with the dietitian. Table 16.2 lists a few of the restrictions that you may observe.

Purposes of Therapeutic Diets

Therapeutic diets are given to:

- Regulate the amount of food in metabolic disorders.
- Prevent or restrict edema by restricting sodium intake.
- Assist body organs to regain and/or maintain normal function.
- Aid in digestion by avoiding foods that irritate the digestive tract.
- Increase or decrease body weight by adding or eliminating calories.

metabolic
(met uh BOL ik)
Pertaining to the total of all the physical and chemical changes that take place in living organisms and cells.

deficient
(di FISH uhnt)
Lacking something (e.g., a deficient diet causes the body to function poorly because it is missing an important element).

gastrointestinal
(gas troh in TES tuh nuhl)
Pertaining to the stomach and intestine.

colitis
(kuh lahy tis)
Inflammation of the colon.

ileitis
(il ee AHY tis)
Inflammation of the ileum (the lower three-fifths of the small intestine).

diabetes mellitus
(dahy uh BEE teez mel uh thus)
Condition that develops when the body cannot change sugar into energy; there is an insufficient amount of insulin, leading to an increased amount of sugar in the blood.

4. Answer: Diabetes, coronary heart disease, stroke, gallbladder disease, sleep apnea and respiratory problems, some cancers (endometrial, breast, and colon), and osteoarthritis
5. Answer: 12 teaspoons (one fluid once = 6 teaspoons)
6. Answer: MyPlate illustrates the recommended proportions of each food group.

FOCUS AND ENGAGE

Introduce the Section

a. Review the content of the Background paragraph, explaining that a therapeutic diet is designed to treat an illness or disorder.
b. Emphasize the importance of understanding therapeutic diets in order to provide quality patient care.
c. Review the objectives for the section.

Vocabulary Review

a. Direct students to the key terms.
b. Pronounce each word, and have the students repeat the pronunciation out loud.
c. Discuss each definition.

TEACH

Discuss

- Discuss attitudes toward eating that might affect the amount and type of food people eat.
- Discuss cultural differences toward food. Students may be willing to share stories of the role food plays in their own families.
- Ask students if they have ever been "on a diet," or if they have helped someone "stick to a diet."
- Discuss the relationship between food, social interactions, and pleasure.
- Discuss why it can be hard to change eating habits.

Reinforce and Review

- Review Section 16.1.
- Review Section 15.1, Eating Disorders.

ACTIVITY

Prepare a menu for your family for one week. Use MyPlate as a guide to insure proper nutrition. Take into consideration the age, size, and health of all family members. At the end of the week, record whether the menu was successful. Total the food group services for each day, and explain whether the daily intake was balanced.

Teaching Tips

- Explain factors that influence food habits:
  - Personal attitudes
  - Ethnic background
  - Religion
- Explain that therapeutic diets are used to modify a patient's normal diet to treat an illness.
- Emphasize that many patients may resist a therapeutic diet, for the reasons mentioned above.
- Also, changing a diet is difficult. It often requires the support of all family members and friends with whom the patient usually eats.
- Explain the purpose of a therapeutic diet:
  - Regulate the amount of food
  - Prevent or restrict edema
  - Assist the body in regaining and maintaining normal function
  - Aid in digestion
  - Increase or decrease body weight
- Explain religious dietary restrictions and how they might impact a therapeutic diet.
- Review Table 16.2 together as a class.
- Review the name of the religion and the type of restriction usually enforced.
- Explain that not all people who observe the listed religions also observe the dietary restrictions.
- Emphasize the importance of communicating with patients to ascertain their beliefs and observances.

soluble
(SOL yuh buhl)
Able to break down or dissolve in liquid.

atherosclerosis
(ath uh roh skluh ROH sis)
Condition of hardening of the arteries due to fat deposits that narrow the space blood flows through.

anorexia nervosa
(an uh REK see uh nur VOH suh)
Loss of appetite with serious weight loss. It is considered a mental disorder.

hypertension
(hahy per TEN shuhn)
High blood pressure.

lactation
(lak TEY shuhn)
Body's process of producing milk to feed newborns.

Table 16.2 Religious Dietary Restrictions

Religion	Restriction
Christian Science	Avoid alcohol, coffee, tea.
Church of Latter-Day Saints (Mormons)	Avoid alcohol, coffee, tea.
Conservative Protestants	Avoid alcohol, coffee, tea.
Greek Orthodox	No meat or dairy products on fast days.
Muslim (Moslem)	No alcohol, pork, or pork products.
Orthodox Jewish	No shellfish, pork, or non-kosher meats. No serving milk and milk products with meat. No eating leavened bread during Passover. Abstain from eating on specific fast days.
Roman Catholic	No food one hour before communion and no meat on Ash Wednesday, Good Friday, and all the Fridays during Lent.
Buddhist	Generally vegetarian.
Hindu	Generally vegetarian.

Types of Therapeutic Diets

Table 16.3 describes the various types of therapeutic diets and their purposes.

The physician may order other diets. Always check the diet that has been ordered for the patient/client. If you have any question about it, ask the person in charge. Correct diets are essential in maintaining good health, and only those foods allowed should be served.

Table 16.3 Some Therapeutic Diets and Their Purposes

Type of Diet	Purpose of Diet	Description
Clear liquid Nutritionally inadequate	Replaces fluids lost from vomiting, diarrhea, surgery	Plain gelatin, ginger ale, tea, coffee (no cream), fruit or apple juice (no pulp), fat-free broth
Full liquid May be **deficient** in iron	Trouble chewing or swallowing, **gastrointestinal** disturbances	All clear liquids, fruit or vegetable juices, strained soup, custard, ice cream, sherbet, milk, cream, eggs, buttermilk, carbonated beverages, eggs, cocoa, eggnog
Soft Nutritionally inadequate	For patients who have trouble chewing, postsurgically	Foods that are soft in consistency, such as fish, ground beef, broth, pureed vegetables, strained cream soup, tender cooked vegetables, fruit juices, cooked fruit, refined cereals, pasta, sherbet, ices, ice cream, custard, plain cookies, angel food cake, tea, coffee, cocoa, carbonated beverages, cheese, cottage cheese
Bland Nutritionally adequate	Soothes gastrointestinal tract, avoids irritation in ulcers, **colitis**	Foods low in fiber and connective tissue that are mild flavored and easy to digest, such as bananas, prune juice, applesauce, custard, pudding, ice cream, plain cookies, sponge cake, decaffeinated coffee, milk, cheese, yogurt

(continued)

458 Chapter 16 | Nutrition

CUSTOMIZED INSTRUCTION

Less Advanced Students

If less advanced students have not heard of the religions listed in Table 16.2, take the time to describe the religion and explain some of its customs, or provide a handout with more information.

Table 16.3 Some Therapeutic Diets and Their Purposes (continued)

Type of Diet	Purpose of Diet	Description
Restricted residue Nutritionally adequate	Reduces normal work of the intestine, in cases of rectal diseases, colitis, **ileitis**	Foods low in fiber and low in bulk, such as milk, buttermilk, cottage cheese, butter, margarine, eggs (not fried), tender poultry, fish, lamb, ground beef (broiled, boiled, baked), broth, refined bread, cereals, pasta, gelatin, angel food or sponge cake, mild-flavored cooked vegetables, lettuce, vegetable and fruit juice, applesauce, canned fruit, citrus fruit without membranes
Low carbohydrate (diabetic) Nutritionally adequate	Matches food intake with insulin uptake and nutritional requirements, used for patients with hyperinsulism and **diabetes mellitus**	Foods that supply enough protein, fat, and carbohydrate to maintain health and activities; requires a balance of carbohydrates, protein, and fat to meet the individual need of the patient; restricts sugar, cookies, pies, candies, etc.
Low fat Deficient in fat **soluble** vitamins	For patients with gallbladder and liver disease, obesity, and heart conditions	Foods high in carbohydrates and proteins; all fats are limited; skim milk, buttermilk, cottage cheese, lean fish, poultry, meats, fat-free soup broths, cooked vegetables, lettuce, fruit juice, bananas, citrus fruits, gelatin, angel food cake, coffee, tea, carbonated beverages, jelly, honey as desired
Low cholesterol Nutritionally adequate	Regulates amount of cholesterol in the blood for patients with coronary disease and **atherosclerosis**	Foods low in fat, such as lean muscle meat, fish, poultry without skin or fat, skim milk, vegetables, fruits
Low calorie Nutritionally adequate (800–2,000 cal)	Reduces number of calories for overweight patients and for clients with arthritis or cardiac conditions	Foods low in fats and calories: skim milk, buttermilk, lean meats, clear soup, vegetables, fresh fruit, coffee, tea, herbs, onions, garlic
High calorie Nutritionally adequate (2,000+ cal)	For persons 10 percent or more below desired weight; for patients with **anorexia nervosa** and hyperthyroidism	All foods with nutritionally balanced proteins, carbohydrates, fats, vitamins, minerals
Low sodium Nutritionally adequate	Reduces salt intake for patients with kidney disease, cardiovascular disorders, edema, and **hypertension**	Natural foods prepared without salt, such as fresh fruits, fresh vegetables, foods without salt added
High protein Nutritionally adequate	For children and adolescents needing additional protein for growth; during pregnancy and **lactation**; postsurgically; during illnesses resulting in protein loss	Foods high in protein, such as milk, cheese, eggs, lean meats, fish, and poultry; fruit, cereals, vegetables

Eating Disorders

Eating disorders are not due to a failure of will. They are real and treatable medical illnesses. The three main types of eating disorders are anorexia nervosa, bulimia, and binge-eating. All three can affect a person's health including causing serious heart conditions, kidney failure, and electrolyte imbalance. The cause of eating disorders is not entirely clear. They seem to have a basis in biology but they are also affected by emotions, genes, and culture.

Eating is controlled by many factors including a person's appetite; the availability of food; family, peer, and cultural practices; advertisements; and attempts at voluntary control. An eating disorder involves a serious disturbance in eating behavior, such as extreme reduction of food intake, severe overeating, or

Apply It

Working in pairs, choose a therapeutic diet and pretend it has been prescribed to you. Create a menu for one week, based on this diet.

Go to several different grocery stores and collect the store circulars. Keep track of grocery costs and compare your menu to the MyPlate recommendations to see if it is well-balanced.

Nutrition | Chapter 16 459

Teaching Tips

- Review the types of therapeutic diets.
- Discuss ways physicians communicate the need for a therapeutic diet with other members of the caregiving team.
- Discuss the role members of the team play in planning and administering the diet.
- For example, who is responsible for communicating the reason for the diet to the patient and the family? Who is responsible for planning meals? Who is responsible for delivering the meals?
- Review Table 16.3 together as a class.
- Pronounce the type of diet out loud.
- Read the purpose of the diet.
- Ask a student to read the description of the diet.
- Point out that problems or deficiencies that might be part of the diet are listed along with the diet type.
  - Example: Full liquid may be deficient in iron.
- Explain what is meant by inadequate and adequate.

ACTIVITY

Have students obtain copies of therapeutic diets from local health care facilities.

Apply It

- You may want to bring in the grocery store flyers so students can plan their menus in class.
- You may want to set a budget ahead of time and direct students to stay within it.
- You may want to assign specific diets to each pair.
- Direct students to create a varied, interesting menu.
- Allot class time to discuss and compare the diets.

TEAMWORK

In small groups, use pictures from magazines, brochures, or the Internet to create a poster illustrating a specific therapeutic diet. Be sure the poster includes the foods that should be consumed as part of the diet. Display the name of the diet, and why it might be necessary. Share the posters with the class, and then display them in the room or another area of the school.

Teaching Tips

- Explain the symptoms of anorexia nervosa.
- Discuss the personality types most at risk:
  - Perfectionists
  - Controllers
  - Individuals with low self esteem

Language Arts Link—Dietary Careers

- You may want to provide a list of resources, such as Web sites or local facilities, that students can use to research this project.
- Remind students about your school's Internet policy, how to recognize a reputable source, and to keep a list of sources for a bibliography.
- For evaluation, you should verify that the information is correct, and you should mark spelling and grammatical errors.

intentional vomiting. Eating disorders frequently develop during adolescence or early adulthood and can often be found with other problems such as depression, substance abuse, and anxiety disorders.

Women are much more likely than men to develop an eating disorder. Magazines, fashion trends, and some activities and professions promote dieting to achieve the "perfect" lean body. This can lead to pressure on women to be thin. Eating disorders are sometimes triggered by the stress of being unable to reach an unattainable goal. Males make up only about 10 percent of people with anorexia or bulimia.

Anorexia Nervosa

Anorexia nervosa is a mental condition in which the person develops intense fear of gaining weight, causing them to use unhealthy practices to achieve a body weight of less than 85 percent of what it should be. Most people with this disease are young females. (**Figure 16.4**) Anorexia nervosa is a very serious illness, with a high mortality rate. According to the APA, it develops in 0.5 to 1 percent of U.S. females, and between 5 and 20 percent of these will die from it.

Career Connect

Participate in a job shadow of a Dietician in either an acute care or long-term care facility and learn about the therapeutic diets required for specific conditions such as diabetes, high blood pressure, or hypoglycemia.

People who have anorexia nervosa are so fearful of being fat that they develop an unrealistic perspective of their weight; they think they are fat when they are—in fact—very thin. They may fast completely, eat only minimal calories per day, or eliminate certain food groups. As a result of the too-low body weight, females may stop having menstrual periods, or, if they have not begun menstruation yet, they may not begin at all.

Anorexia nervosa is so deadly because the body shuts itself down due to starvation. When there is no fat left to burn for energy, the body turns on itself, burning muscle mass and even organ tissue. In addition, people with anorexia nervosa are at great

Language Arts Link

Dietary Careers

Proper nutrition is vital for both health care workers—so that they maintain the stamina and health required for the job—and patients—so that they grow stronger or stay healthy. Eating a balanced diet is important for both the brain and the body. As many Americans do not follow a healthy diet, the role of those working in dietary professions is becoming more and more important to the health of the population. There are different types of dietary careers, including Registered Dietitians, Dietetic Technicians, and Food Service Workers.

All of those working in health care must be informed of the special dietary requirements of patients during treatment and follow-up care.

Working with a partner, research the education, certification, licensure or degree, continuing education requirements, and salary potential for a dietary career. If possible, include in your analysis an interview with a dietary professional to identify how they became interested in this field, their current job responsibilities and benefits of working in a dietary career.

After you've completed the research, create several paragraphs that describe your findings. Use precise language and dietary career-specific vocabulary for each career investigated. Present your findings to your class.

risk for heart problems, including irregular heartbeats, rapid heart rate, low blood pressure, and even heart failure and death. There can also be gastrointestinal problems, such as irritable bowel syndrome, constipation, and stomach pain.

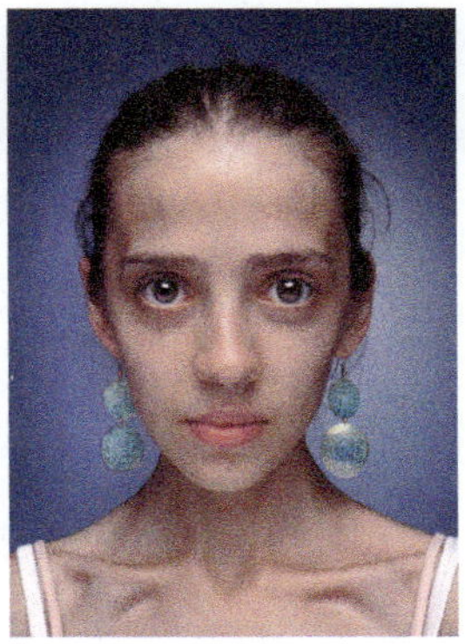

Figure 16.4
Anorexia nervosa most often affects young women. Why do you think young women are more susceptible to this disease than men or older women?

Bulimia Nervosa

Bulimia nervosa is an eating disorder in which the person eats an abnormal amount (binge eating), and then vomits, uses laxatives to expel it from their system before it is digested, or indulges in excessive exercise to burn off the calories. During the binge portion of the cycle, the person feels unable to control their eating; then, during the purge portion, they feel great remorse that leads them to the purge behaviors.

Bulimia nervosa is even more common than anorexia nervosa; it affects between 1 and 4 percent of women. Many people who have bulimia nervosa also have anorexia nervosa. People who have only bulimia, however, are less likely to die from it; only 1 percent of those with bulimia die within 10 years of diagnosis.

Bulimia is characterized by recurrent episodes of binge eating, followed by compensating behavior such as vomiting, on a regular and ongoing basis. The health risks include electrolyte imbalance (leading to heart problems); stomach and esophagus inflammation and ulceration; tooth erosion, staining, and decay; mouth sores; and swelling of the cheeks or jaw area.

Binge Eating Disorder/Food Addiction

Binge eating disorder occurs when someone has the first part of bulimia nervosa—the binge eating—but not the purging part. Individuals who have it tend to be obese, and may describe their relationship with food as an addiction. Between 1 and 2 percent of the population suffers from this disease. However, it's hard to estimate because not everyone who has it seeks medical or psychological assistance.

Treatment

Treatment for eating disorders is multi-faceted. A variety of behavioral and psychological treatments can be used. Treatment is considered a "success" when harmful behaviors cease, and the patient learns new ways to deal with the emotions or psychological events that trigger the behavior in the first place. Some facets of treatment may include:

- Individual counseling or psychotherapy
- Group counseling sessions
- Behavior modification
- Cognitive/behavioral therapy
- Nutrition study
- Relaxation activities, such as yoga, meditation, or exercise
- Medications (especially in patients who also suffer from depression or anxiety)
- Inpatient care and monitoring (especially in extreme cases of anorexia nervosa, where the patient's weight is dangerously low)

Nutrition | Chapter 16 461

Teaching Tips

- Explain the symptoms of bulimia.
- Review binging and purging.
- Emphasize that bulimics often have "normal" body weight, so they may be better able to hide their eating disorder than anorexics.
- Point out that both those suffering from anorexia and bulimia frequently attempt to keep their behavior secret.
- Explain the symptoms of binge-eating disorder.
- Differentiate it from bulimia:
  - No purging
  - Overweight
- Explain the difficulties in treating eating disorders:
  - Denial on the part of the sufferer
  - Denial on the part of the family
  - Resistant to change
  - Misunderstandings
- Emphasize that treatment can be successful.
- Emphasize that treatment usually requires multiple types of care:
  - Medical care
  - Psychological care
  - Nutritional counseling
  - Medication

TEAMWORK

In small groups, research the food requirements and traditions of an ethnic or religious group that is represented in your area. Find a recipe that meets the requirements. If possible, prepare the recipe and bring it in to share with the class. Alternatively, bring a picture of the dish to class. Explain to the class whether the dish is nutritionally balanced.

Personal Wellness—Substance Abuse

- Explain substance abuse. Refer to Section 15.1 for more information.
- Emphasize that both legal and illegal substances can be abused.
- Point out that cigarettes are included in this category.
- Explain addiction: a compulsion to continue a behavior even though it has negative consequences.
- Review the symptoms of withdrawal.
- Discuss alcohol abuse.
- Explain the effects of alcohol.
- Explain the health risks associated with alcohol abuse.
- Discuss tobacco abuse.
- Emphasize the number of deaths that can be attributed to tobacco.
- Describe nicotine.
- Emphasize the addictive nature of nicotine.
- Review the associated diseases:
  - Heart disease
  - Lung cancer
  - Emphysema
  - Stroke
- Emphasize other drawbacks:
  - Cost
  - Smell
  - Effects on hair and skin
- Discuss products other than cigarettes:
  - Chewing tobacco
  - Cigars
  - Pipes

Personal Wellness

Substance Abuse

Substance abuse refers to the use of legal or illegal substances that cause harm to a person's health or life. Abused substances usually produce some form of intoxication that alters judgment, perception, or physical control.

Substance abuse in the United States is widespread. In 2012, an estimated 23.9 million Americans aged 12 or older—or 9.2 percent of the population—had used an illicit drug, and 17 million adults were heavy alcohol users. About one out of five Americans smokes cigarettes.

People use alcohol and other drugs because they like the way these substances make them feel. However, substance abuse may lead to addiction. Addiction is a compulsion to continue using a substance even though it has negative consequences. People can become addicted to illegal drugs, drugs that doctors prescribe, or to things they may not think of as drugs, such as alcohol and the nicotine in cigarettes.

Many abused substances can produce a phenomenon known as tolerance. This means a person would have to use a larger amount of the drug to produce the same level of intoxication. Once a person is addicted to a drug, it becomes harder and harder to stop using it. Sometimes, when people stop using a drug, they experience withdrawal. Withdrawal can range from mild anxiety to seizures and hallucinations.

Alcohol

Despite the focus on illegal drugs, alcohol remains the main drug problem in the United States. Alcohol lessens a person's inhibitions, slurs speech, and decreases coordination. Many people use alcohol without any negative consequences. However, there are approximately 17 million people in the country addicted to alcohol; more than 5.7 million of them are women.

Alcohol is the most common cause of liver failure in the U.S. The drug can also cause heart enlargement and cancer of the pancreas, esophagus, and stomach. Alcohol abuse is associated with nearly half of all fatal motor vehicle accidents. Every year in the United States, alcohol abuse also causes 500,000 injuries, 600,000 assaults, and 70,000 sexual assaults.

Tobacco

Cigarettes kill more Americans than alcohol, car accidents, suicide, AIDS, homicide, and illegal drugs combined. Yet, amazingly, people continue to smoke. Cigarettes and other forms of tobacco contain nicotine, one of the most addictive of all drugs. Despite the rising cost of cigarettes, more than 42 million U.S. adults are smokers. This is almost 20 percent of all American adults.

About half of all Americans who continue to smoke will die because of the habit. Each year about 443,000 people die in the United States from illnesses related to cigarette smoking such as heart disease, lung cancer, emphysema, and stroke.

Although 70 percent of smokers want to quit and 35 percent attempt to quit each year, fewer than 5 percent succeed. This is because smokers not only become physically addicted to nicotine but they also become psychologically addicted. Nicotine withdrawal symptoms of smoking include anxiety, hunger, sleep disturbances, and depression. All these factors make it very difficult for a person to stop smoking once he or she starts.

Illegal Drugs

Marijuana comes from the plant Cannabis sativa and is the most commonly used drug in the United States. Marijuana is a popular drug because it produces a feeling of pleasure and relaxation without a high risk of addiction. More than 83 million Americans have tried marijuana. However, there are dangers associated with it. Like anything that is smoked, it can irritate a person's lungs.

Smoking marijuana also impairs coordination and memory. Perhaps most importantly, possession of even small amounts of marijuana in the United States remains a crime in most states. However, as of January 2015, 23 states and the District of Columbia currently have laws legalizing marijuana in some form. In 2010, 52 percent of all drug arrests were for marijuana.

Americans in large numbers use many other types of illegal drugs. Cocaine, derived from the coca plant of South America, is the most abused major stimulant in America. Almost 1 million Americans use heroin despite the very real danger of death through overdose.

(continued)

462 Chapter 16 | Nutrition

- Discuss symptoms of physical and psychological nicotine withdrawal.
- Discuss illegal drug abuse.
- Review the types of illegal drugs.

Personal Wellness (continued)

Methamphetamines are a powerful stimulant that increases alertness and decreases appetite. An assortment of so-called "club drugs" have also become popular in the last two decades, including Ecstasy, PCP, GHB, Rohypnol, Ketamine, and LSD.

Most of these drugs deliver a feeling of happiness, excitement, and energy. However, most of them are physically and/or psychologically addictive. Withdrawal symptoms can be particularly harrowing for some drugs such as heroin. In addition, prolonged use of any of them can lead to serious health problems including coronary problems, dangerously high blood pressure, and stroke.

Steroids

Anabolic steroids are artificial versions of the hormone testosterone. Testosterone brings out male sexual traits. Steroids are often used to treat delayed puberty and the wasting of the body caused by diseases. However, anabolic steroids also help the growth of skeletal muscle. For this reason, these compounds have been abused by bodybuilders, weightlifters, and athletes in many other sports.

By the 2000s, the use of steroids was becoming epidemic among college and high school athletes. A study done in 2012, found that about one in twenty teenagers had used steroids to increase their muscle mass.

Anabolic steroids can be injected, taken by mouth, or rubbed on the skin when in gels or creams. Anabolic steroid abuse has been associated with a wide range of adverse side effects such as irritability, aggression, acne, breast development in men, liver cancer, and heart attacks. Most of the effects are reversible if the abuser stops taking the drug, but some can be permanent.

Summary

There are many factors that influence food habits. Some of these factors are personal attitudes, nationality, race, and religious restrictions. A health care worker must be aware of these factors in order to help the patient/client adapt to therapeutic diets.

The therapeutic diet is prescribed for various ailments. It is important to understand why the diet was prescribed and how it helps in regaining a healthier state. The health care worker should be aware of the foods allowed and not allowed in therapeutic diets and serve only proper foods to his or her patients.

Section 16.2 Review Questions

1. What is a therapeutic diet?
2. What is a common dietary restriction for Muslims?
3. What is the purpose of a clear liquid diet?
4. If a patient has ulcer problems, what kind of therapeutic diet would be most helpful?
5. What foods are high in protein?
6. What types of care might be included in a treatment program for eating disorders?

Nutrition | Chapter 16 463

CUSTOMIZED INSTRUCTION

Special Needs Students

Encourage special needs students to spend time on the choosemyplate.gov Web site investigating whether their special needs affect their nutritional requirements.

Personal Wellness (cont.)

- Discuss health problems from using illegal drugs.
- Discuss the abuse of legal drugs.
- Discuss abuse of steroids.
- Explain that anabolic steroids are artificial versions of testosterone.
- Discuss health problems from using steroids. Review the factors that influence eating habits.

Teaching Tips

- Review the types of therapeutic diets.
- Discuss eating disorders.
- Discuss substance abuse and how it can impact the body.

Section 16.2 Review Questions

1. Answer: A therapeutic diet is prescribed for a patient to treat a medical condition such as heart disease or diabetes and may contain foods that the patient usually does not eat.
2. Answer: No alcohol, pork, or pork products
3. Answer: A clear liquid diet replaces fluids lost during vomiting, diarrhea, or surgery.
4. Answer: A person with ulcer problems would benefit from a bland (nutritionally adequate) diet.
5. Answer: Foods high in protein include milk, cheese, eggs, beans, lean meats, fish, poultry, fruits, cereals, and vegetables.
6. Answer: Patients with eating disorders might be given medical care, psychological treatment, nutritional counseling, and medication.

CHAPTER 16 REVIEW

Chapter Review Questions

1. Answer: Water is found in all body tissues and makes up most of blood plasma. It carries nutrients to the body cells and carries waste products away from the body cells. It also lubricates the joints and helps regulate body temperature and body processes.
2. Answer: It depends on the person's level of activity. The number of calories we eat and the amount of exercise we do balance weight. If we eat more calories than we burn, we gain weight. If we burn more calories than we eat, we lose weight.
3. Answer: Vitamins are essential for normal metabolism, growth, and body development.
4. Answer: The new MyPlate icon uses a familiar object to represent a balanced diet.
5. Answer: The metric system was invented in France during the French Revolution in the 1790s.
6. Answer: Purposes of therapeutic diets include: regulating the amount of food in metabolic disorders; preventing or restricting edema by restricting sodium intake; assisting body organs to regain and/or maintain normal function; aiding in digestion by avoiding foods that irritate the digestive tract; and increasing or decreasing body weight by adding or eliminating calories.
7. Answer: A low-carbohydrate diet matches food intake with insulin uptake and nutritional requirements.
8. Answer: Foods low in cholesterol include fish, poultry without skin or fat, lean muscle meat, beans, skim milk, vegetables, and fruits.
9. Answer: Bulimics have bouts of binge-eating but purging follows so they maintain a normal weight. Binge-eaters eat an excessive amount of food in a short period of time without purging.
10. Answer: Anabolic steroid use can cause irritability, aggression, acne, breast development in men, liver cancer, and heart attacks.

CHAPTER 16 REVIEW

Chapter Review Questions

1. Why is water important to the human body? (16.1)
2. If a person consumes 2,000 calories a day, will he or she gain weight or lose weight? What factors play a role beside calorie intake? (16.1)
3. How do vitamins affect the human body? (16.1)
4. What does the new MyPlate icon attempt to do? (16.1)
5. Where and when was the metric system invented? (16.1)
6. What are three purposes of a therapeutic diet? (16.2)
7. Why would a low carbohydrate (diabetic) diet work best for a patient with diabetes? (16.2)
8. What kinds of food can be found in a low cholesterol diet? (16.2)
9. What is the difference between bulimia and binge-eating disorder? (16.2)
10. What are some problems associated with the use of anabolic steroids? (16.2)

Activities

1. Research a religious group listed on Table 16.2: Religious Dietary Restrictions. You can use an encyclopedia or the Internet. Discuss the religion's dietary laws in more detail than the chart provides. Make sure you quote directly from the religion's scriptures or holy book that regulates diet.
2. Make a list of five questions you would ask a psychologist about eating disorders. Then, look up "psychologist" in the phone book or the Internet. Find someone who specializes in eating disorders and ask or e-mail your questions. When you get your responses, create a newspaper article on eating disorders. Work the quotations directly into the article. Don't forget to include citations.

Case Studies

1. Mrs. Cohen, an Orthodox Jew, has been in St. Andrews Nursing Home for several years. This evening the staff in the kitchen sent her a dinner with mashed potatoes, pork roast, green beans, and custard. She is very upset and is crying: She is hungry, but does not want to eat because of her dietary restrictions. You know that the staff in the kitchen is new. What steps can you take to remedy this problem?
2. Richard is your patient. He is on a low-fat diet because of coronary difficulties. Richard is feeling disgruntled and is complaining about everything on his tray. He says the "food here stinks," and keeps asking family members to sneak him donuts. How can you help Richard understand the reason for the diet?

464 Chapter 16 | Nutrition

CUSTOMIZED INSTRUCTION

English Language Learners

For Activity 2, have students practice asking their questions to a partner before speaking with a psychologist. If they are e-mailing the questions, they should ask a partner to edit the questions before sending them.

CHAPTER 16 REVIEW

Thinking Critically

1. **Communication**—As you are distributing meal trays, you notice that one of your patients is trying to exchange food with the patient next to him. This patient is supposed to be on a bland diet because he has ulcers. Instead of raising your voice and asking, "What do you think you are doing?," how would you explain to the patient about the importance of following the diet prescribed for him?
2. **Cultural Competency**—An Orthodox Jewish patient is upset because the hospital keeps bringing her kosher chicken and milk for her dinner. She is supposed to be on a bland diet, but refuses to eat. Why is the patient upset? How would you calm her down? What steps would you take?
3. **Cause and Effect**—Each year about 443,000 people die in the United States from illnesses related to cigarette smoking. Cigarettes kill more Americans than alcohol, car accidents, suicide, AIDS, homicide, and illegal drugs combined. Yet smoking cigarettes is legal in the United States while smoking marijuana is illegal in most states. Why do you think this is?

Portfolio Connection

When you care for patients, it is important to know if they are eating a healthy diet. Therapeutic diets do not always meet the standards of a healthy diet.

Choose an illness that requires a therapeutic diet. Write a paragraph about the illness. Explain the symptoms, how the body is affected, and the treatment. Use the MyPlate recommendations as a guide to evaluating the therapeutic diet required. Describe in what ways the diet is nutritionally healthy or deficient.

Place this exercise in your portfolio to help you review MyPlate, healthy diets, and therapeutic diets.

PORTFOLIO TIP

Food preferences and diet can be more of a source of distress and conflict for patients than the actual illness. Make a large photocopy of the MyPlate icon and keep it in your portfolio.

Write notes for yourself demonstrating how you would explain to patients the importance of a varied diet.

Nutrition | Chapter 16 465

CUSTOMIZED INSTRUCTION

More Advanced Students

Ask more advanced students to create a chart or table comparing the guidelines at MyPlate (choosemyplate.gov) and Harvard's Healthy Eating Plate (hsph.harvard.edu/nutritionsource). They should include a picture of each "plate," as well as information about the food groups, the recommended daily servings, and the goal of the food recommendations.

Activities

1. Remind students of the school's Internet policy before they go online, and direct them to use reputable Web sites. Remind them to keep a list of sources so they can create a bibliography.
2. You might want to provide a list of providers who are willing to speak with the students. Advise the students on how to approach the professional. It is important that the professional understand this is a class assignment, and not a student reaching out for help. If students cannot contact a professional, advise them to write the article using source material they find in magazines, books, or the Internet. You might have the students publish a newsletter with their articles and distribute it to the class and to other classes.

Case Studies

1. Direct students to Section 16.2 for more information on religious dietary restrictions. You may want to allow students to present skits demonstrating their responses to this situation.
2. Remind students of proper communications techniques. You may want to allow students to present skits to demonstrate their responses to this situation.

Thinking Critically

1. Remind students of the importance of using appropriate communication skills. Discuss the importance of patient education.
2. Direct students to start by identifying why the patient is upset about the food.
3. Direct students to write the response in proper essay form, including a thesis statement and supporting facts and examples.

Portfolio Connection

- Remind students to select an illness or condition that benefits from a therapeutic diet.
- Direct students to include specific references to MyPlate.
- Remind students to proofread and revise their work.
- Encourage students to use a peer review to find ways to improve the document.
- Check to make sure that students have completed the assignment and added it to their portfolio.

TEAMWORK

Divide the class into teams of five to seven students. Name a therapeutic diet, and allow two or three minutes for each team to write down as many food items they can think of that could be consumed as part of the diet. Compare responses, and award points for any unique foods (items that only one team wrote down). Allow one to two minutes for teams to write the purpose of the diet. Award one point to each team that writes the correct purpose.

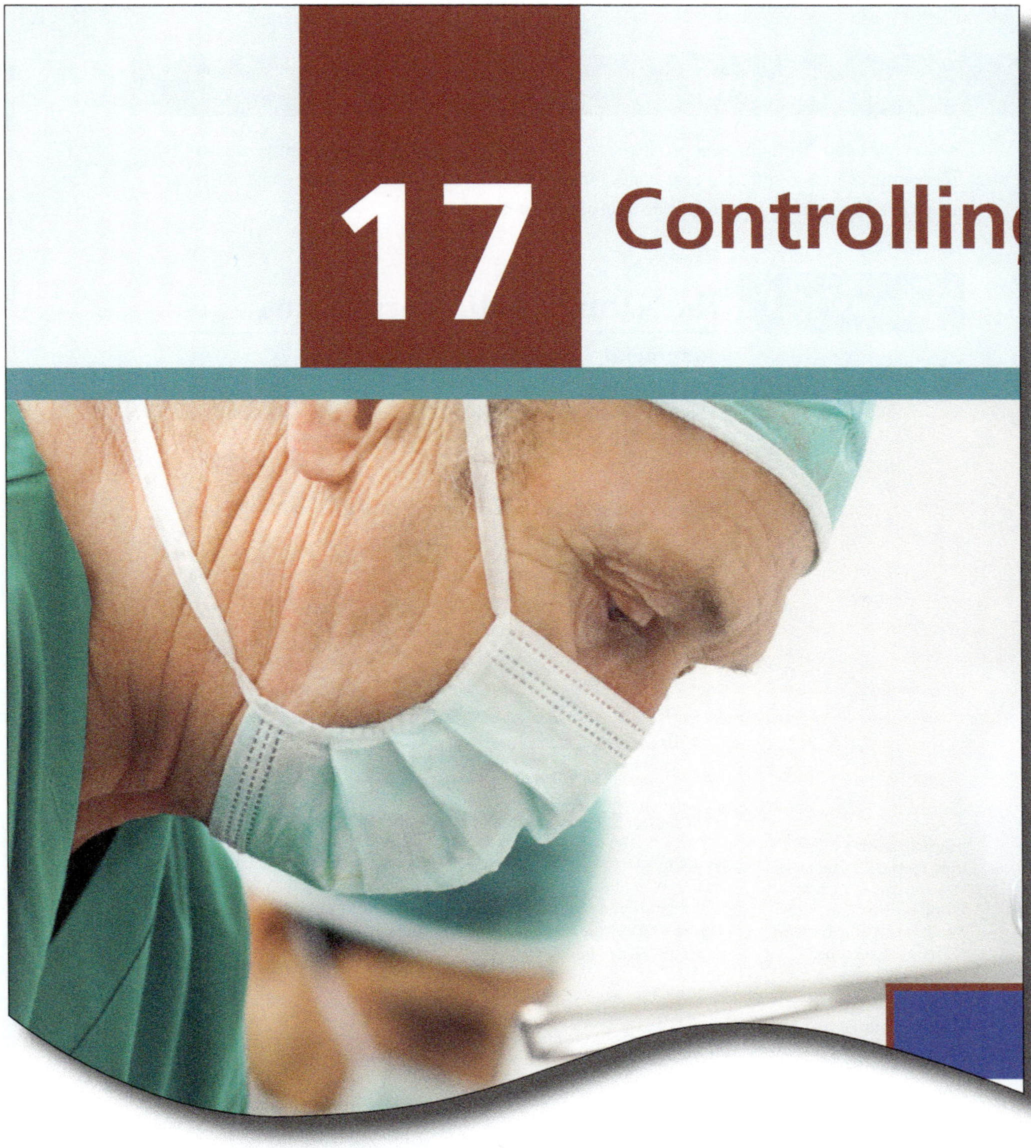

Advance Preparation

- Review: Chapter text for Sections 17.1, 17.2, 17.3, and 17.4; and chapter procedures.

Contact:
- An infection control nurse or other infection specialist to speak to the class.
- Local health care facilities to request brochures or other documents about handwashing and other infection control techniques.

Prepare:
- Agar plates, microscopes, and slides for looking at microorganisms.
- Samples of personal protective wear and equipment.
- Samples of both bactericidal and bacteriostatic disinfectant containers.
- Magazine and newspaper articles about the spread of infection.
- Handwashing facilities with soap and running water.
- A list of Web sites that provide information about infection control—such as the Centers for Disease Control and Prevention at cdc.govnutrition, and the National Institute of Health at nlm.nih.gov/medlineplus/infectioncontrol.html.

CHAPTER 17 OVERVIEW

Chapter 17 addresses the very important topic of how to control infection. It includes information about microorganisms and viruses, asepsis and standard precautions, transmission-based precautions, and precautions for bloodborne diseases.

Section 17.1: Section 17.1 introduces students to the nature of organisms. It defines different types of organisms, and examines the way they cause illness and how they spread. Students learn how they can prevent them from spreading, and how to recognize infections.

Section 17.2: Section 17.2 covers the skills health care workers will need to restrict the spread of pathogenic microorganisms. It includes aseptic techniques and the Standard Precaution guidelines. Procedures cover handwashing, using personal protective equipment, caring for soiled linens, disposing of sharps, and wrapping instruments for the autoclave.

Section 17.3: In Section 17.3, students learn techniques to protect themselves and others from the spread of transmission-based infections. Procedures include how to put on and remove sterile gloves, applying personal protective equipment, and changing a sterile dressing.

Section 17.4: Section 17.4 provides information about how students can protect themselves and others from the spread of bloodborne diseases. They learn how bloodborne diseases spread, Universal Precautions, and ethical and legal issues related to bloodborne diseases.

FOCUS AND ENGAGE

Getting Started

- Consult the science department at your school for information about obtaining and using agar plates, and interpreting the results.
- Divide the class and have each group use different products to wash. Also have one control group not wash at all.
- Determine the identity of the microorganisms that are present.
- As a class, discuss the results of the cultures that the students prepared.

Introduce the Section

a. Review the content of the Background paragraph, explaining that microorganisms spread infection and disease through contact.

b. Emphasize that not all microorganisms are "bad."

c. Review the objectives for the section.

Vocabulary Review

a. Direct students to the key terms.

b. Pronounce each word, and have the students repeat the pronunciation out loud.

c. Discuss the definition of each word.

TEACH

Discuss

- Ask students whether they wash after using the restroom. Then, ask if they touch the doorknobs on the way out.
- Discuss how casual contact such as touching a light switch, doorknob, or telephone can transfer microorganisms.

Getting Started

Wash your hands with different products: soap, betadine, alcohol, and hand sanitizer. Then, make finger impressions in different agar plates for each product used. After 24 hours, check to see which product worked best to kill the microorganisms.

SECTION 17.1 The Nature of Microorganisms

Background

Microorganisms are all around us, but we cannot see them. There are both good and bad microorganisms. To help prevent the spread of infection and disease, you must be aware of microorganisms and how they are spread.

Objectives

When you have completed this section, you will be able to do the following:

- Match key terms with their correct meanings.
- Define *pathogenic* and *nonpathogenic*.
- List conditions affecting the growth of bacteria.
- List ways that microorganisms and viruses cause illness.
- List ways that microorganisms and viruses spread.
- List five ways to prevent the spread of microorganisms and viruses.
- Describe generalized and localized infections.
- Explain the difference in signs and symptoms of generalized and localized infections.

Introduction to Microorganisms

microorganisms
(mie kroh ORG uhn izms)
Tiny organism, such as a fungi, protists, or bacteria, that can only be seen under a microscope.

viruses
(VAHY ruhs es)
Genetic material that is surrounded by a protective coat and that can only reproduce inside a host cell; can only be seen under a microscope.

We are surrounded by tiny **microorganisms** and **viruses**. They are in the air we breathe, on our skin, in our food, and on everything we touch. You cannot see these organisms and viruses without a microscope because they are so small. (**Figure 17.1**) Viruses are much smaller than microorganisms. So, stronger microscopes are used to look at viruses.

Some microorganisms and viruses cause illness, infection, or disease and are called *pathogenic*. Some microorganisms help keep a balance in the environment and in the body. These microorganisms are called *nonpathogenic*.

Viruses do not have all of the characteristics of living organisms. For example, viruses do not eat. They also cannot reproduce on their own. So, viruses are not considered living as microorganisms are. For microorganisms to live, they must have certain elements in their environment. Some organisms require oxygen in

468 Chapter 17 | Controlling Infection

Reinforce and Review

- Review Chapter 13, Your Body and How It Functions.

ACTIVITY

Make a chart or table listing examples of nonpathogenic microorganisms and how they are useful to humans. Use a reference book or the Internet to locate the information.

CUSTOMIZED INSTRUCTION OVERVIEW	
Less Advanced Students	Pages 486, 491
More Advanced Students	Pages 481, 501
English Language Learners	Page 470
Special Needs Students	Pages 469, 483
At-Risk Students	Page 477

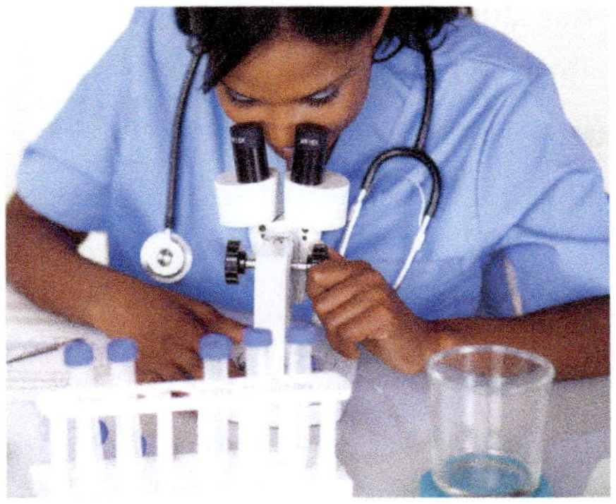

Figure 17.1
A microscope is needed to see microorganisms. Stronger microscopes are needed to see viruses, which are much smaller than microorganisms. List a step you might need to take to ensure that a microscope works properly.

order to survive. These are called **aerobic**. Other microorganisms live in an environment without oxygen. These are called **anaerobic**.

Most microorganisms that cause illness thrive in warm temperatures—about the temperature of the body. All organisms need moisture, and most microorganisms prefer a dark area to grow in. (**Figure 17.2**) Microorganisms also need food to survive. Some of these organisms live on dead matter or tissues and are called **saprophytes**. Other organisms that live on living matter or tissues are called **parasites**. (**Figure 17.2**)

aerobic
(uh ROH bik)
Require oxygen in order to survive.

anaerobic
(an uh ROH bik)
Able to grow and function without oxygen.

saprophytes
(SAP ruh fahyts)
Organisms that live on dead organic matter.

parasites
(PARE uh sahyts)
Organisms obtaining nourishment from other organisms they are living in or on.

Figure 17.2
Conditions affecting the growth of bacteria. What are three things that you can do to help prevent the growth of bacteria in patient's room?

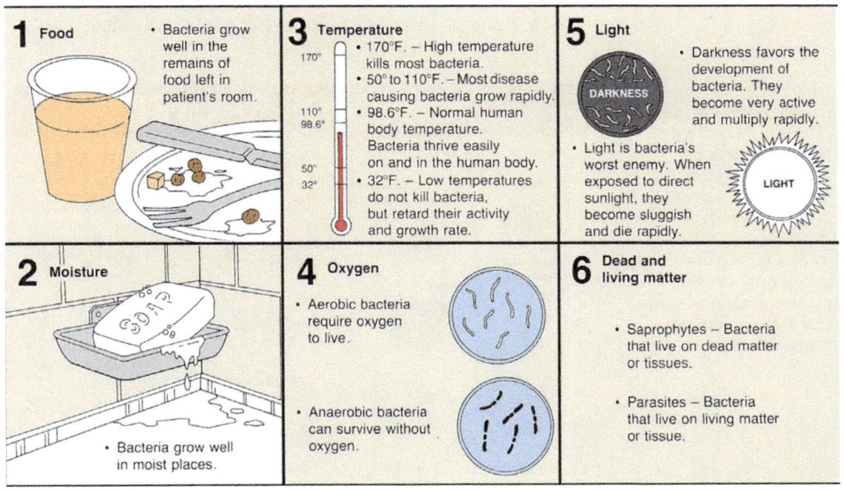

Controlling Infection | Chapter 17 469

Teaching Tips

- Explain microorganisms. Emphasize:
  - Microorganisms are all around us
  - Good microorganisms are called nonpathogenic
  - Bad microorganisms are called pathogenic
- Explain the difference between microorganisms and viruses:
  - Viruses are not living organisms
  - Viruses are much smaller
  - Viruses do not eat
  - Viruses cannot reproduce on their own
- Explain that aerobic organisms require oxygen but anaerobic organisms do not.
- Define nonpathogenic.
- Emphasize that nonpathogenic microorganisms are vital to maintaining balance in the human body and the environment.

Figure Focus

17.1 A microscope is needed to see microorganisms. Stronger microscopes are needed to see viruses, which are much smaller than microorganisms. List a step you might need to take to ensure that a microscope works properly.

Answer: Make sure that the lenses of the microscope stay clean.

CUSTOMIZED INSTRUCTION

Special Needs Students

You may be able to obtain microscopes customized for use by special needs students.

Figure Focus

17.2 Conditions affecting the growth of bacteria. What are three things that you can do to help prevent the growth of bacteria in patient's room?

Answer: Dispose of food right away after the patient has eaten; replace bar soap with a dispenser; help the patient wash his or her hands.

Teaching Tips

- Define pathogenic.
- Differentiate between different types of pathogenic microorganisms.
- Bacteria cause many diseases, including strep throat and staph infections.

Figure Focus

17.3 Common shapes and groupings of bacteria. The cocci and bacilli can be single, pairs, and higher-order assemblies. The streptococci is a string of bacteria, whereas the staphylococci is a cluster of bacteria. A unique shape among bacteria is the spirochete. What precautions should health care workers take to avoid coming in contact with bacteria?

Answer: Use appropriate protective equipment (see Section 17.2); wash hands

ACTIVITY

Have students research and identify common microorgnisms such as fungus, bacteria, and protozoa.

Nonpathogenic Microorganisms

There are many microorganisms that are not disease causing, or **pathogenic**. These microorganisms, called **nonpathogenic**, are "good" microorganisms that are used in different ways. For example, these microorganisms can be used in the following ways: to make buttermilk, to ferment grain for alcoholic beverages, to make bread rise, and so on. Many nonpathogenic organisms also **decompose** organic materials in nature.

pathogenic
(path oh JEN ik)
Disease causing.

nonpathogenic
(nahn path oh JEN ik)
Not disease causing.

decompose
(dee kuhm POES)
To decay, to break down.

In the body, nonpathogenic microorganisms work in the digestive system to break down food elements that the body cannot use. This broken down food is eventually eliminated as a part of feces. Nonpathogenic microorganisms also help control the growth of pathogenic organisms.

Pathogenic Microorganisms and Viruses

Health care workers must be aware of the different kinds of pathogens that cause disease. There are several kinds of disease-causing microorganisms: bacteria, protozoa, fungi, and **rickettsiae**. Viruses are also pathogens.

rickettsiae
(rih KET see ee)
Parasitic microorganisms that live on another living organism and cause disease.

spirochetes
(SPAHY ruh keets)
Slender, coil-shaped organisms.

- **Bacteria.** Bacteria are responsible for many diseases. (Figure 17.3) For example, strep throat is caused by streptococci, staph infection is caused by staphylococci, and syphilis is caused by **spirochetes**. These are only a few of the diseases that bacteria cause.

  Staphylococcus and streptococcus are organisms that are always present in health care environments. Staphylococcus (staph) infections can have a serious impact on patients, caregivers, and families. An uncontrolled or untreated staph infection in a newborn nursery, for example, can cause infants to die. People who have a stressed immune system have trouble fighting a staph infection and may die.

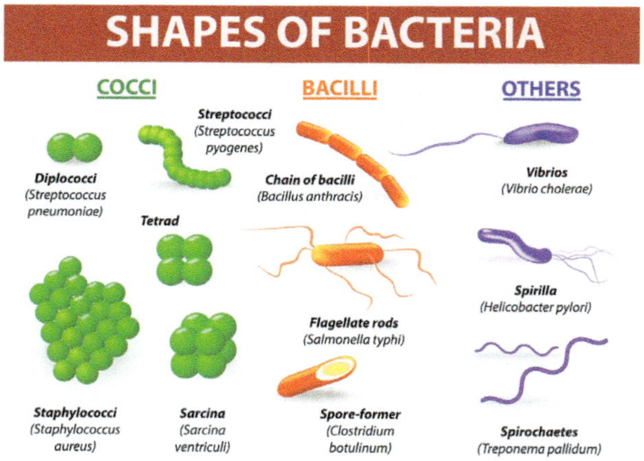

Figure 17.3
Common shapes and groupings of bacteria. The cocci and bacilli can be single, pairs, and higher-order assemblies. The streptococci is a string of bacteria, whereas the staphylococci is a cluster of bacteria. A unique shape among bacteria is the spirochete. What precautions should health care workers take to avoid coming in contact with bacteria?

CUSTOMIZED INSTRUCTION

English Language Learners

Have students write each key term and its pronunciation on one side of an index card and its definition on the other side. Have them read each term and definition aloud to a partner.

Hospital stays are prolonged because of staph infections. Staph is usually the cause of pimples or boils found on the skin. All drainage from a pimple or boil should be handled according to Standard Precautions to prevent the spread of infection. Patients who have staph infections are always treated with Standard Precautions.

- **Protozoa.** Protozoa are larger than viruses but also grow within a **host** cell. They cause trichomoniasis, amebic dysentery, and malaria. Most protozoa are too small to be seen with the naked eye, but can easily be found under a microscope. Protozoa are found in water and soil environments and play an important role in their ecology.
- **Fungi.** Microscopic fungi include molds and yeasts. Some fungi can cause disease, such as athlete's foot, thrush, vaginitis, and serious lung diseases.
- **Rickettsiae.** Rickettsiae are parasites that live in lice, fleas, ticks, and mites. When one of these organisms is infected with rickettsiae, the disease is transferred to a person after he or she is bitten. Rickettsiae are responsible for many of the world's worst epidemics, including various types of typhus and spotted fever. Rodent and insect control helps prevent rickettsiae infection.
- **Viruses.** Viruses are much smaller than bacteria. They cannot reproduce until they have taken over a living cell. Viruses cause the common cold and many upper respiratory infections. They also cause smallpox, chickenpox, measles, mumps, influenza, and fever blisters. One of the most serious viruses is human immunodeficiency virus (HIV), which causes acquired immunodeficiency syndrome (AIDS). These are only a few of the illnesses caused by viruses.

host
(ho st)
The organism from which a microorganism takes nourishment. The microorganism gives nothing in return and causes disease or illness.

When nonpathogenic microorganisms leave their normal environment in the body and move into other areas, they become pathogens. Some common examples are:

- **Escherichia coli** or *E. coli*. *E. coli* is a normally nonpathogenic bacterium found in the intestine of many animals and humans. *E. coli* from the colon can come in contact with other parts of the beef, thus contaminating the meat. *E. coli* infections may cause food poisoning and even death. *E. coli* infections can be prevented by cooking meat until it reaches a temperature of about 160°F (71.1°C).

  Poor personal hygiene can allow *E. coli* to spread from the human colon to the urethra causing urinary tract infections known as **urethritis** and **cystitis**. Health care workers who have dirty hands—especially hands that are not washed after using the toilet—can spread *E. coli* to patients' food or onto equipment used to provide care.
- **Salmonella**. Salmonella infections are caused by bacteria. Salmonella infections may cause food poisoning or death. Salmonella infections can be caused by eating chicken that is undercooked or from eating foods that contain raw eggs. Salmonella can be spread to food when food service workers do not wash their hands. Salmonella is also spread when cooking utensils or surfaces are not cleaned properly after preparing raw meat, chicken, or egg dishes in particular.

urethritis
(yoor uh THRAHY tihs)
Inflammation of the urethra.

cystitis
(sis TAHY tihs)
Inflammation of the urinary bladder.

salmonella
(sal muh NEL uh)
A rod-shaped bacterium found in the intestine that can cause food poisoning, gastroenteritis, and typhoid fever.

Controlling Infection | Chapter 17 471

Teaching Tips

- Protozoa are tiny organisms found usually in water and soil.
- Fungi include mold and yeast.
- Rickettsiae are parasites that live in small insects, such as lice and fleas.
- Emphasize that viruses are also pathogens and they cause common colds, and upper respiratory illnesses.
- Explain that some types of nonpathogenic organisms become pathogenic when they leave their normal environments:
  - *E. coli*
  - Salmonella
- Discuss the difference between acute and chronic infections.

TEAMWORK

In pairs or small groups, look at prepared slides under a microscope to observe microorganisms such as fungus, bacteria, and protozoa. Have students illustrate the microorganisms they observe.

Teaching Tips

- Explain that an endogenous infection grows or develops from within an organism, tissue, or cell when an individual is in an already weakened state.
- Explain that an exogenous infection originates from outside the body.
- Explain that an opportunistic infection occurs when there is weakness or compromise in the immune defenses of an individual.

Science Link—Prions

- Explain prion: An infectious protein molecule.
- Explain how they differ from microorganisms and viruses: They do not replicate themselves.
- Discuss how they infect people.
- Discuss the types of diseases they cause.

Proteins are denatured, or inactivated, by heat. How does this reaction to heat apply to the prevention of prion infection?

Answer: Heat can be used to denature prions. So, equipment should be sterilized with heat.

ACTIVITY

Create a public service poster about one way members of your school community can help stop the spread of infection. Display the posters in an appropriate place, such as a main hallway, the nurse's office, the cafeteria, or the restrooms.

Chronic vs. Acute

Acute infections occur suddenly or last a short time. Chronic infections happen slowly over a long period of time and may last months, or even years.

We know that infections are caused by pathogens. Infections fall into two groups: *endogenous* and *exogenous.* An endogenous infection grows or develops from within an organism, tissue, or cell when an individual is in an already weakened state. An endogenous infection is caused by an infectious agent already present in the body, with the previous infection having been dormant or non-apparent.

An exogenous infection originates from outside the body. Examples of exogenous infections include salmonella poisoning after eating an uncooked egg or poultry, catching a cold after eating off of someone else's fork, or contracting rabies after getting bit by a dog.

An opportunistic infection occurs when there is weakness or compromise in the immune defenses of an individual. Opportunistic infections may be caused by bacteria, fungi, viruses, or parasites. These infections can be fought off by people with strong immune systems; however, they can be fatal for AIDS patients.

toxins
(TAHKS ihns)
Poisonous substances.

enterotoxin
(ehn tuhr oh TAHKS uhn)
Poisonous substance that is produced in, or originates in, the contents of the intestine.

How Microorganisms Affect the Body

Pathogens cause disease in several different ways. Some microorganisms produce **toxins** that affect the body. For instance, staphylococcus produces an **enterotoxin** that is the cause of food poisoning. The toxin causes fatigue, diarrhea, and vomiting. The tetanus bacilli produce a toxin that enters the bloodstream and attacks the central nervous system, causing severe damage and frequently death.

Science Link

Prions

Unlike bacteria, protists, and fungi, viruses are not living organisms. Another type of nonliving pathogen is called a *prion.* Prions are infectious protein molecules. Prions are a defective version of a protein found in normal brain cells. They cause several brain diseases, including Creutzfeld-Jakob disease and mad cow disease.

Unlike viruses and microorganisms, prions do not replicate themselves. So, how do they infect people and animals? According to one theory, the prion is taken into the body. In the case of mad cow disease, humans eat infected beef. The prions enter brain cells, and the cells begin producing the prion instead of the normal protein. This happens because the prion comes in contact with normal proteins. The normal proteins become prions, which in turn spread to other cells.

Prions cause the death of the brain cells that send signals to and from the body. Over time, the cell death keeps the body from sending signals to and from the brain. So, the body stops functioning properly, eventually leading to death.

Prion infections are rare. In the case of mad cow disease, they can be prevented by avoiding raw meat, especially meat that has been or may have been contaminated with the prion. Steps can be taken by groups or individuals to ensure the survival of affected species. These steps can include ensuring disease is not transmitted through the use of contaminated equipment during medical procedures. Proper cleaning and sterilization of equipment prevents the spread of prions. Some prion diseases are inherited, so little action can be taken to prevent the disease.

Proteins are denatured, or inactivated, by heat. How does this reaction to heat apply to the prevention of prion infection?

Describe how specific changes in the environment such as use of fertilizer, drought, or flood affect distribution or disappearance of traits in species.

472 Chapter 17 | Controlling Infection

Some microorganisms and all viruses invade living cells and destroy them; this is called *cell invasion*. For example, there is a **protist** that invades the red blood cells of the host. As the protists grow, the cells rupture and cause chills and fever.

The presence of some microorganisms causes a violent *allergic reaction* in the body. A runny nose, watery eyes, and sneezing can be caused by the presence of a microorganism to which the host is allergic.

How Microorganisms and Viruses Spread

Now that you know something about microorganisms and viruses, you need to know how they are spread and how they enter the body. This helps you protect yourself and your patients/clients from infection.

For microorganisms or viruses to cause disease or infection, they must have a **susceptible** host. This host is unable to fight off infection because its resistance to the pathogen is low. Low resistance may be caused by poor diet, fatigue, inadequate rest, stress, or poor health. Table 17.1 shows five primary ways by which microorganisms and viruses are spread.

A model used to understand the infection process is the **chain of infection**. (Figure 17.4) This model represents each component in the cycle. Each component must be present and in sequential order: infectious agent, reservoir, portal of exit from the reservoir, mode of transmission, and portal of entry into the susceptible host.

Understanding the characteristics of each link provides the health care professional with methods to support vulnerable patients, prevent the spread of infection, and protect themselves.

protist
(PRO tis t)
An organism belonging to the kingdom that includes protozoans, bacteria, and single-celled algae and fungi.

susceptible
(suh SEHP tuh buhl)
Capable of being affected or infected (e.g., body can be attacked by microorganisms and become ill).

chain of infection
(CHAY in ove in FEC shun)
A chain of events all interconnected is required for an infection to spread.

Career Connect

If possible, contact an Infection Control Nurse and ask him or her to discuss the Chain of Infection as related to appropriate hand washing and other preventive techniques. Working with a classmate, create a poster to share with the class.

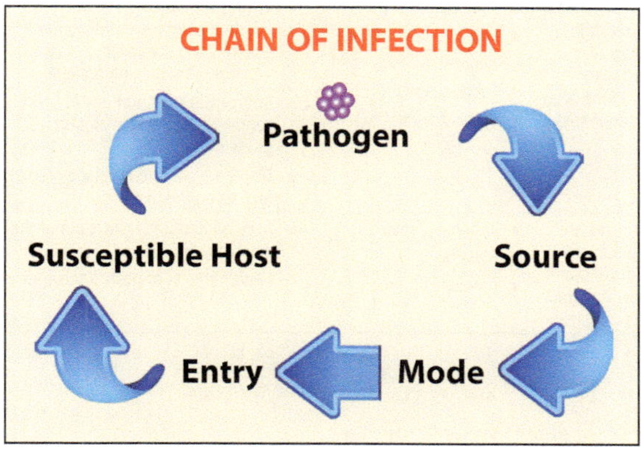

Figure 17.4
The chain of infection must include all of these events. How can health care workers interrupt one or more links in the chain?

Controlling Infection | Chapter 17 473

Teaching Tips

- Explain how microorganisms cause illness.
- Discuss shapes and growth patterns:
  - Coccis
  - Clusters
  - Chains
  - Rods
  - Spirochetes
- Discuss how microorganisms affect the cells and tissues of the body:
  - Toxins
  - Cell invasions
  - Allergic reactions
- Review how microorganisms and viruses spread.
- Discuss the conditions required for the growth of microorganisms.
- Explain that transmission requires three elements:
  1. A source of pathogen.
  2. A susceptible host with a source of entry receptive to the pathogen.
  3. A mode of transmission for the pathogen.
- Discuss the chain of infection:
  - Infectious agent
  - Reservoir
  - Portal of exit from the reservoir
  - Mode of transmission
  - Portal of entry into the susceptible host
  - Susceptible host

Career Connect

- Direct students to Chapter 3 for information on career paths.
- If you are unable to arrange a class visit, provide information about the requirements and responsibilities of an Infection Control Nurse.
- Alternatively, assign students to research the position, including educational requirements, career ladder, and salary range.

Figure Focus

17.4 The chain of infection must include all of these events. How can health care workers interrupt one or more links in the chain?

Answer: Kill or remove agent; eliminate or reduce reservoir; do not allow germs to escape and travel; wash hands

Teaching Tips

- Explain how microorganisms are spread.
- Review Table 17.1 together.
- Explain each of the five methods:
    - Direct contact
    - Indirect contact
    - Airborne
    - Oral route
    - Insects and pests
- Emphasize the difference between indirect and direct contact.
- Ask students to read the information and examples for each method.
- Emphasize the prevention guidelines for each method.
- Discuss examples of how people spread micro-organisms.
- Discuss some of the reasons why infections are prevalent in hospitals and other health care facilities:
    - Staph in the nursery
    - Pseudomonas in wounds

ACTIVITY

Draw a flowchart illustrating the chain of infection.

Table 17.1 Five Ways Microorganisms and Viruses Are Spread

Method	Information	Examples	Prevention Guidelines
Direct contact	Occurs when organisms or viruses are transmitted directly from one person to another.	■ Physical contact by touch on open or closed skin or a body opening ■ Sexual contact ■ Breathing in pathogens directly from an infected person	■ Abstain from sex. ■ Do not drink or eat from dishes or utensils used by another person. ■ Stay an appropriate distance away from individuals who are coughing or sneezing. ■ Do not, without proper protection, touch objects used by someone who has an infection. ■ Wash your hands.
Indirect contact	Occurs when organisms or viruses are transferred from one object to another.	■ Contaminated substances and objects, such as food, air, soil, feces, clothing, and equipment	■ Do not, without proper protection, touch objects used by someone who has an infection. ■ Hold contaminated linen, belongings, or other items away from your uniform.
Airborne	Some microorganisms and viruses are carried in the air. Coughing and sneezing project droplets into the air, and these droplets are carried on air currents until they find a place to land. The droplets cling to hair, uniforms, and medical equipment, or they fall on the floor. As you move from place to place, you may spread these pathogens.	■ Influenza ■ Chickenpox ■ Wound infections	■ Keep your hair short or tied back so that it does not swing around, spreading microorganisms. ■ Cover your mouth and nose with your sleeve when you sneeze or cough, then wash your hands. ■ Change out of your uniform after working and before going anywhere other than home. ■ Consider anything dropped on the floor as contaminated. DO NOT USE IT. ■ Stay home when you are sick with an acute respiratory infection.
Oral route	Microorganisms or viruses enter the body through the mouth by way of **contaminated** water and food, dirty hands, and from other contaminated objects.	■ Food poisoning ■ Polio ■ Hepatitis ■ Salmonellosis ■ Typhoid fever	■ Wash your hands: – before eating or handling food – after using the toilet – before/after helping patients ■ Refrigerate food properly to prevent contamination and microorganism growth. ■ Dispose of wound drainage promptly and according to policy.
Insects and pests (**vectors**)	Organisms or viruses are picked up by insects and other pests from contaminated areas and carried to water, food, and people.	■ Bubonic plague ■ Malaria ■ Amoebic dysentery	■ Keep all flies and insects out of the environment. ■ Report insects or pests immediately.

contaminated
(kuhn TAM uh nayt uhd)
Soiled, unclean, not suitable for use.

vector
(VEK ter)
An entity that can transmit a pathogen to another location.

474 Chapter 17 | Controlling Infection

Fallacies of Disease Transmission

In the nineteenth and twentieth centuries, developments such as the culture plate method of identifying disease-causing organisms, pasteurization, vaccines, antiseptics, and asepsis dramatically lowered the incidence of disease. A common fallacy, however, is to think that an infectious disease is completely controlled. In January 2015, a resurgence of measles in the Unites States was a reminder that effective immunization requires diligence. Another example of a fallacy related to disease transmission is the assumption that bats carry rabies—bats are mammals and can contract rabies, but that does not make them specific carriers of the disease. There are also many fallacies and misunderstandings concerning the transmission of bloodborne diseases, but standard precautions have been developed to effectively address realistic risks.

Protection from Microorganisms

Standard Precautions and Transmission-Based Precautions were created to provide guidelines that prevent the spread of microorganisms. These guidelines are described in Sections 17.2 and 17.3 of this chapter. Section 17.4 provides guidelines regarding bloodborne diseases. Read the guidelines carefully and follow them whenever infectious microorganisms are present.

Signs and Symptoms of Infection

An infection may be **generalized**, or it may be **localized**. If the infection is generalized, there is usually headache, fatigue, fever, and increased pulse and respiration. There may also be vomiting and/or diarrhea. If the infection is localized, you can see and feel one or more of the following: redness, swelling, heat, and/or drainage. There is usually pain at the site of the infection.

Summary

We are surrounded by microorganisms and viruses. They are in the air we breathe, on our skin, in our food, and on everything we touch. Some microorganisms and viruses are pathogens; other microorganisms are nonpathogens. Pathogens include some bacteria, some protists, some fungi, rickettsiae, and viruses. Since pathogens cause illness, it is important to understand how they are spread and how they can be controlled. Learning the signs and symptoms of infection will help you provide better patient care.

It is the responsibility of every health care worker to help prevent the spread of infection. Every year thousands of patients have extended stays in the hospital because they have acquired an infection while hospitalized. It is vital that all health care workers practice good techniques to prevent the spread of infection.

Career Connect

Epidemiologist

Epidemiologists are health care professionals who study diseases and how they spread. Their goal is to reduce the risk of diseases and how often they occur. Epidemiologists collect vast amounts of data and then share their observations and recommendations with public health officials and the community.

As infectious diseases become more prevalent and as many antibiotics are no longer effective against many microorganisms, the job of an epidemiologist becomes more important. As infectious diseases, such as ebola, Zika virus, and drug-resistant bacteria increase, the demand for the skills of the epidemiologist are emerging.

Using the Occupational Outlook Handbook (www.bls.gov/OOH/), investigate what it takes to become an epidemiologist, what skills are required of an epidemiologist, and the work environment of the epidemiologist. Share your findings with your class.

generalized
(JEN uhr uhl ahyzd)
Affecting all of the body.

localized
(LOH kuhl ahyzd)
Affecting one area of the body.

Apply It

Play medical charades in class. Take turns acting out a specific pathogen or a different way in which viruses are spread.

Teaching Tips

- Discuss fallacies of disease transmission.
- Explain that precautions have been established as guidelines that health care workers can follow to minimize the spread of infection.
- Emphasize handwashing.
- Explain that a generalized infection affects the whole body, while a localized infection affects just one area.
- Symptoms of generalized infection:
  - Headache
  - Fatigue
  - Fever
  - Increased pulse and respiration
  - Possibly vomiting and/or diarrhea
- Symptoms of localized infection:
  - Redness
  - Swelling
  - Heat and/or drainage
  - Pain at the site

Apply It

- You may want to divide the class into teams for this activity.
- You could have each students write a pathogen, method of transmission, or preventive measure on a slip of paper, then put all the slips into a bucket.
- Students can select a slip from the bucket without the rest of the team seeing.
- Put a time limit on each person.
- Award points to teams that guess the answer within the time limit.

Section 17.1 Review Questions

1. Define the terms *pathogenic* and *nonpathogenic*.
2. A microorganism that doesn't need oxygen is called what?
3. List five disease-causing pathogens.
4. What are five ways by which microorganisms and viruses spread?
5. Compare generalized and localized infections.
6. What conditions affect the growth of bacteria?

SECTION 17.2 Asepsis and Standard Precautions

Background

The environment of the health care worker contains larger numbers of microorganisms than do most other environments. The health care worker must acquire the knowledge and skills required to restrict the spread of pathogenic microorganisms. The health care worker who practices good aseptic technique and follows Standard Precautions protects patients, co-workers, and the community from infection.

Objectives

When you have completed this section, you will be able to do the following:

- Match key terms with their meanings.
- Define *medical asepsis.*
- Match terms related to medical asepsis with their correct meanings.
- List five aseptic techniques.
- List some of the Standard Precaution guidelines concerning the use of protective equipment.
- Demonstrate appropriate handwashing techniques.
- Explain the difference between *bactericidal* and *bacteriostatic.*
- List reasons why asepsis is important.

Introduction to Asepsis

Health care facilities are filled with people who are ill. Some of their illnesses are caused by body dysfunctions; other illnesses are caused by infections or injury. Thus, health care environments are constantly contaminated with the pathogens carried by patients, visitors, and staff.

This constant presence of pathogens requires the staff to wage an all-out battle against these microorganisms and viruses. This battle is waged by the continual use of medical asepsis, or the destruction of the environment that allows pathogens to live, breed, and spread. Medical asepsis is accomplished by using

476 Chapter 17 | Controlling Infection

Section 17.1 Review Questions

1. Answer: *Pathogenic* means disease-causing and *nonpathogenic* means not disease-causing.
2. Answer: Anaerobic
3. Answer: Bacteria, protozoa, fungi, rickettsiae, and viruses
4. Answer: Direct contact, indirect contact, airborne, oral route, insects and pests
5. Answer: Generalized infections affect all of the body. A patient may experience headache, fatigue, fever, vomiting, and diarrhea. A localized infection affects one area of the body. A patient will see or feel redness, swelling, heat, or drainage.
6. Answer: Food, moisture, temperature, oxygen, light, dead and living matter

FOCUS AND ENGAGE

Introduce the Section

a. Review the content of the Background paragraph, explaining that asepsis is the state of being free of pathogenic microorganisms.
b. Emphasize the importance of understanding how to maintain asepsis in order to provide quality patient care.
c. Review the objectives for the section.

Vocabulary Review

a. Direct students to the key terms.
b. Pronounce each word, and have the students repeat the pronunciation out loud.
c. Discuss each definition.

TEACH

Discuss

- Ask students what they think is the first and best defense against the spread of infection in the health care environment.
- Discuss their reactions when you say it is handwashing.

Reinforce and Review

- Review Chapter 13, Your Body and How It Functions.
- Reinforce the nature of microorganisms and how infection spreads, from Section 17.1.

Teaching Tips

- Define medical asepsis: The destruction of the environment that allows pathogens to live, breed, and spread.

ACTIVITY

Make flashcards to use as a study aid in learning the medical terminology associated with asepsis, as covered in Section 17.2.

aseptic technique. Aseptic technique is very important when you are working with patients/clients. The practice of aseptic technique helps to prevent:

- Cross infection, which is caused by infecting the patient with a new microorganism or virus from another patient or health care worker (**nosocomial infection**)
- Reinfection with the same microorganism or virus that caused the original illness
- Self-inoculation by the patient's own organisms, such as *E. coli* from the intestines entering the urethra
- An illness passing from the patient to the health care worker or from the health care worker to the patient

Aseptic technique includes:

- Proper handwashing
- Employees being clean and neat
- Proper handling of all equipment
- Using sterile procedure when necessary
- Using proper cleaning solutions: *bacteriostatic* solutions, which slow or stop the growth of bacteria, or *bactericidal* solutions, which kill bacteria
- Following **Standard Precautions**

The health care team must strive toward achieving an aseptic environment to reduce the infection rate in the health care setting.

aseptic technique
(ay SEP tihk tek NEEK)
Method used to make the environment, the worker, and the patient as germ-free as possible.

nosocomial infection
(nohs uh KOH mee uhl ihn FEHKT shuhn)
An infection acquired while in a health care setting, such as a hospital.

Standard Precautions
(STAN derd prih KAW shuhn)
Guidelines designed to reduce the risk of transmission of microorganisms from recognized and unrecognized sources of infection in the hospital.

transmitting
(trahnz MIHT ihng)
Causing to go from one person to another person.

Standard Precautions

Transmission of infectious agents requires three elements: 1) a source of infectious agents; 2) a susceptible host with a source of entry receptive to the agent; and 3) a mode of transmission for the agent. All blood, body fluids, secretions, excretions—except sweat—nonintact skin, and mucous membranes may contain contagious infectious agents.

Because of the risk of **transmitting** these infections agents, a set of standard precautions were developed. In 1985, health care isolation practices in the United States changed to defend against the increased risk of exposure to hepatitis B virus (HBV) and human immunodeficiency virus (HIV). For the first time, all blood and body fluids were treated as infected substances.

The Occupational Safety and Health Administration (OSHA) of the U.S. Department of Labor established mandatory guidelines published in the *Occupational Exposure to Bloodborne Pathogens; Needlestick and Other Sharps Injuries; Final Rule*. These guidelines ensure that all employers provide personal protective equipment to employees at risk of exposure to body fluids. In 1992, OSHA increased its mandate to employers, insisting that training and immunization be provided to all employees within 10 days of hire. This means that employees at risk for exposure to body fluids must:

- Be offered hepatitis B vaccine (HBV) at no charge
- Be trained to use the appropriate protective equipment to prevent exposure to body fluids
- Receive an annual update and review

State Board of Health

In addition to national agencies that deal with safety guidelines in regard to transmission of infectious agents, each state has a board of health. A state board of health licenses health care facilities and requires compliance with OSHA and CDC guidelines.

Locate your state board of health online and learn what the expectations are for preventing the transmission of infectious agents.

Controlling Infection | Chapter 17 477

Teaching Tips

- Explain why aseptic techniques are necessary.
- Discuss what aseptic techniques accomplish:
  - Prevent cross-infection
  - Prevent reinfection
  - Prevent self-inoculation
  - Prevent illness exchange between patient and health care worker
- Describe aseptic techniques:
  - Proper handwashing
  - Clean and neat employees
  - Proper handling of all equipment
  - Use of sterile equipment
  - Use of proper cleaning solutions
  - Following Standard Precautions
- Explain that Standard Precautions help lower the risk of transmitting pathogens.
- Discuss OSHA guidelines requiring the use of personal protective wear when contact with body fluids is possible, and access to vaccines at no charge.
- Discuss a state board of health's role, along with the federal government's role, in standard precautions.
- Emphasize that noncompliance with Standard Precautions can results in loss of job, but if the worker becomes infected, it may result in serious illness or even death.

CUSTOMIZED INSTRUCTION

At-Risk Students

Have students create a poster that illustrates things they can do in their normal day-to-day activities to minimize or eliminate the spread of infection. Have students share with the class.

ACTIVITY

Make a poster demonstrating one or more of the Standard Precaution guidelines concerning the use of protective equipment.

Teaching Tips

- Explain that Standard Precautions protect health care providers, patients, family, and visitors from exposure to pathogens which may be in body fluids.
- Review the types of body fluids:
  - Blood
  - Vaginal secretions
  - Pericardial fluid
  - Body fluids containing visible blood
  - Amniotic fluid
  - Peritoneal fluid
  - Tissue specimens
  - Cerebrospinal fluid
  - Interstitial fluid
  - Semen
  - Pleural fluid
- Review the methods of transmission of HBV and HIV:
  - Through a needle
  - Contact of infected body fluids with mucous membranes
  - Sexual contact
  - From pregnant woman to fetus
- Emphasize the high risk of infection in a hospital or other health care environment.
- Emphasize that all health care workers should assume every patient is infected, and act accordingly in terms of Standard Precautions.
- Discuss what is the same and what is different between medical asepsis and surgical asepsis.

amniotic fluid
(am nee AH tihk FLOO ihd)
Liquid that surrounds the fetus during pregnancy.

peritoneal fluid
(per ih toh NEE uhl FLOO ihd)
Liquid in the peritoneal cavity.

cerebrospinal fluid
(suh ree broh SPAHYN uhl FLOO ihd)
Liquid that flows through and around brain tissue.

interstitial fluid
(ihnt uhr STIHSH uhl FLOO ihd)
Liquid that fills the space between most of the cells of the body.

semen
(SEE muhn)
Fluid from the testes, seminal vesicles, prostate gland, and bulbourethral glands.

pleural fluid
(PLOOR uhl FLOO ihd)
Liquid that surrounds the lungs.

In 1996, the Centers for Disease Control and Prevention (CDC) expanded the bloodborne pathogen guidelines to assist in the prevention of nosocomial infections. These expanded guidelines are known as Standard Precautions. The CDC updated these Standard Precautions in 2007 to include a new section on Respiratory Hygiene/Cough Etiquette, primarily in response to the SARS virus outbreak in 2003.

Standard Precautions are appropriate for all patients receiving care or service in a health care environment regardless of their diagnosis. Standard Precautions provide protection from contact with blood, mucous membranes, nonintact skin, and all body fluids. Body fluids include the following:

- Blood
- Vaginal secretions
- Pericardial fluid
- Body fluids containing visible blood
- **Amniotic fluid**
- **Peritoneal fluid**
- Tissue specimens
- **Cerebrospinal fluid**
- **Interstitial fluid**
- **Semen**
- **Pleural fluid**

Infection with HBV and HIV occur through:

- Direct injection of infected blood or a contaminated needle that punctures the skin
- Contact of infected body fluids with mucous membranes such as the eye or inside of the mouth
- Sexual contact
- Pregnancy—when the mother is infected, the infection is transferred to the newborn infant

The risk of being infected in the health care setting is high. It is important for you to treat all patients as though they were infected. If you provide hands-on care to patients, you must follow all Standard Precaution guidelines (**Table 17.2**) to protect yourself and others. Make it a habit to follow each step in the Standard Precaution guidelines.

These include practices that apply to all health care providers, patients, visitors, and family members. Hand hygiene is the single-most effective way to prevent the spread of infections. Other safe practices may involve the use of gloves, goggles, face shield, and/or a gown when there is a risk of splashing or spray of blood or body fluids. Safe handling of soiled linens also reduces the risks of spreading infectious agents. Listed below are procedures to follow to minimize the risk of spreading infectious agents.

ACTIVITY

Divide the class into two groups. Have one group prepare a presentation that demonstrates medical asepsis and one group prepare a presentation that demonstrates surgical asepsis.

TEAMWORK

In small groups, prepare skits demonstrating the consequences of not following Standard Precautions in a health care environment.

Table 17.2 Standard Precaution Guidelines

Protective Equipment	When to Use Personal Protective Equipment (PPE)
Gloves	■ Wear when in contact with: – Any body fluid – Nonintact skin and mucous membrane, or potentially contaminated intact skin (e.g., of a patient incontient of stool or urine) ■ Wear when your hands are chapped, when a rash is present, or when you have open sores.
Nonpermeable gowns or aprons	■ Wear during procedures that are likely to expose you to: – Any body fluid – Nonintact skin and mucous membrane
Mask and protective eyewear or face shield	■ Wear when: – Body fluid droplets or splashes are likely – Patients are coughing continuously
Special masks and eyewear that seal against face	■ Wear when assisting with procedures that cause body tissues to be aerosolized (e.g., laser treatments).
Handwashing	■ Wash hands before putting on and after removing gloves and before and after working with each patient, with his or her equipment, or both.
Shared equipment/multiple-use patient care equipment (e.g., blood pressure cuff, stethoscope, aural thermometer)	■ Remove all shared equipment for cleaning after use on each patient. ■ Need to clean shared equipment between every patient—not just when exposed to body fluids or non-intact skin.

Surgical Asepsis

Medical asepsis includes all practices used to limit the number of microorganisms, their growth, and their transmission and to confine them to a specific area. Surgical asepsis, or sterile technique, includes all practices that keep an area completely free of microorganisms.

Controlling the Spread of Infection

Skin and hair cannot be **sterilized** because any solutions or procedures that kill microorganisms are harmful to skin. You use a bacteriostatic solution for cleaning skin. Bacteriocidal solutions are used on equipment. This method of controlling the spread of infection is called **disinfection**.

There are a variety of methods of disinfection. You can use boiling water to kill germs. You can add a 10% solution of household bleach to disinfect items that tolerate exposure to mild bleach solution. You can use stronger disinfection for cleaning inanimate items, such as floors, walls, tables, and patient care equipment.

There are also ultrasonic cleaners, which offer a fast, consistent, and inexpensive way to remove contaminants from all kinds of surfaces. Ultrasonic cleaners are especially useful for precision cleaning of small parts that contain contamination in small hard-to-reach crevices. These machines mean you use less cleaning solution.

Caution: Never use bleach on any item that will be put into the body or with any other product (e.g., cleansers, sprays).

sterilized
(STEHR uhl ahyzd)
Made free from all living microorganisms.

disinfection
(dis ihn FEHKT shuhn)
Process of freeing from microorganisms by physical or chemical means.

Community

In a team of three or four students, prepare a presentation for elementary or middle school students on proper hand washing. Design a poster on how germs are transmitted and how proper hand washing techniques limit transmission of germs.

Teaching Tips

- Review Table 17.2 together as a class.
- Ask a student to read out loud the type of protective equipment listed in the left column.
- Then discuss when to use the specific type of equipment, as described in the right column.
- If possible, display examples of protective equipment, such as gloves, aprons, masks, and eye protection.
- Explain disinfection.
- Differentiate between bacteriostatic (to slow the growth of bacteria) and bactericidal (to kill bacteria).
- Explain the uses of each:
  - Bacteriostatic is used on skin and hair
  - Bactericidal is used on equipment
- Discuss different methods of disinfection:
  - Boiling water
  - Bleach
  - Disinfecting solutions
  - Ultrasonic cleaners
- Discuss reasons for using bleach: kills AIDS and other viruses.

Community

- You may want to allow class time for students to practice delivering their presentations.
- Remind students to create their presentations for the appropriate age group.
- Students may use a presentation graphics program to create a slideshow or to create posters.
- You might want to contact the teachers at the elementary school to set up the visit.
- Students could also present at a day care center, after school program, or senior center.

TEAMWORK

Divide the class into small groups. Give each team an empty disinfectant container (have containers of different types of disinfectants available). In a set amount of time, such as three minutes, have each group identify the active ingredient, the recommended usage, and whether the disinfectant is bactericidal or bacteriostatic. When time is up, pass the containers to a different group. Repeat until each group has had a chance to identify each container. Discuss the activity as a class.

Teaching Tips

- Explain sterilization.
- Discuss bacteria that are spore formers, such as tuberculosis.
- Emphasize the difficulty of destroying spores—must use steam.
- Describe use of an autoclave.
- Discuss different types of autoclaves, and when they are used:
  - Steam
  - Gas
  - Chemical baths
  - Dry heat
- Reiterate the importance of proper handwashing techniques.
- Review Table 17.3 together as a class.
- Ask students to take turns reading out loud the directions (left column) and the information (right column).
- Discuss each item in the chart, insuring that students understand it before moving on.
- Point out some of the items that are different from normal handwashing:
  - Hold hands lower than elbows
  - Use a dry paper towel to turn faucets off and on
  - Rewash if you touch the sink or faucet
  - Dry hands completely
- Discuss hand cleansing and when it is an appropriate procedure to use instead of hand washing.

exposed
(eks POEZD)
Left unprotected.

autoclaves
(AH toh klayvz)
Sterilizers that use steam under pressure to kill all forms of bacteria on fomites (objects that pathogens live on and can transfer infection).

Sterilization is the process of killing all microorganisms, even spores (bacteria that have a protective shell around them). Sanitization is the process of removing most microorganisms, whether pathogenic or non-pathogenic. Antisepsis is the destruction of disease-producing microorganisms to prevent infection. Spores are killed when they are **exposed** to steam under pressure at high temperatures. **Autoclaves** are used to produce steam. Gas autoclaves and chemical baths are used to sterilize equipment that would be damaged by steam, such as plastic and rubber devices and fiber optics. Items needing sterilization are those that are put into the body or around an open wound.

Handwashing

Handwashing is the process of removing microorganisms from contaminated hands. Proper handwashing is the most effective way to prevent infecting yourself or others. See Table 17.3 for proper handwashing guidelines.

Table 17.3 Handwashing Guidelines

Directions	Information
Always wash your hands: – Before and after contact with a patient and/or patient's belongings – Before and after eating – After using the bathroom – After handling any contaminated fluid or object – After touching body fluids, even if wearing gloves	Handwashing is the most effective way to reduce the spread of microorganisms.
Use enough soap from dispenser to make a good lather.	A bar of soap is considered contaminated after it is opened.
Interlace your fingers together and rub all sides of fingers and hands to produce friction for **10 seconds**. Be sure to clean beneath fingernails and around knuckles. If no nail brush is available, rub fingernails on palms of hands.	Lather and friction help remove microorganisms.
Hold hands lower than elbows and rinse thoroughly to remove pathogens.	This prevents lather and water from running over arms and causing contamination.
Turn on and off faucets with dry paper towel.	Faucets and sink are considered contaminated.
Rewash your hands if you touch the sink or faucet.	Touching a contaminated area recontaminates your hands.
Dry hands completely from tips of fingers to wrist.	Reddened and chapped hands easily leave open areas that can become infected.

Hand Cleansing

If hands are not visibly soiled, a facility's procedures may allow the use of an alcohol-based hand rub for cleansing hands instead of washing them. According to CDC guidelines, situations where hand cleansing, instead of washing, may be appropriate include:

- Before having direct contact with patients
- After contact with a patient's intact skin, for example after taking a pulse or blood pressure, or after lifting a patient

480 Chapter 17 | Controlling Infection

TEAMWORK

Have students put on a "protective equipment" fashion show. They should work together or in small groups to write a brief description of each item, including why and when it should be used. Students can take turns modeling and reading the descriptions during the show. Use a digital camera or video camera to record the event.

- After removing gloves
- After contact with inanimate objects, including medical equipment, when near a patient.

A facility-approved hand lotion should be used to prevent irritation and chapping from frequent hand washing or cleansing because repeatedly using an alcohol-based hand-rub can irritate the skin; irritated skin poses a risk of an individual becoming infected or infecting others.

What's New?

Antibiotic Resistant Bacteria

Bacterial diseases are treated with drugs called antibiotics. Antibiotics can be highly effective in treating bacterial infections, but many bacteria have developed a resistance to antibiotics. As a result, these infections are more difficult to treat.

Why does antibiotic resistance occur? Some bacteria are naturally resistant to antibiotics or mutate to develop a resistance. Sometimes, these bacteria survive to produce more antibiotic resistant bacteria. Resistant bacteria arise when antibiotics are used incorrectly:

- A prescription for antibiotics is not completed. Some people stop taking their antibiotics after they feel better. Doing so increases the chance that resistant bacteria will survive. Often, these patients become ill again.
- Antibiotics are taken when a patient does not need them; for example, a patient who has the flu. The antibiotics will not help the patient get over the flu because the flu is caused by a virus, which is not affected by antibiotics. As a result, resistant bacteria may arise. Doctors often avoid prescribing antibiotics in such a case.
- The widespread use of antibiotics in cleaning products has been linked to antibiotic resistance. Repeated exposure to an antibiotic can result in strains of bacteria that are resistant to the drug.

Several bacteria that were once easily controlled by antibiotics are now major health threats. Examples of these bacteria include:

- Tuberculosis: Tuberculosis is a contagious disease that affects the lungs. About one percent of tuberculosis cases involve a strain of bacteria that is resistant to multiple antibiotics. These cases need almost four times more recovery time than nonresistant strains of tuberculosis. Treatment of resistant strains is also more expensive and has more uncomfortable and dangerous side effects.
- Methicillin-resistant staphylococcus aureus (MRSA): Resistant forms of S. aureus were first noted in the 1960s. Since, it has become one of the most common antibiotic resistant bacteria found in hospitals. Infection by S. aureus has been linked to longer hospital stays and increased risk of death from secondary infections. In addition to the ongoing incidence of MRSA in hospitals, there also have been school-based outbreaks of the infection. Although not considered a superbug by public health officials, MRSA is a threat that should be respected.
- Streptococcus: Various species of streptococci are resistant to antibiotics. These bacteria cause diseases such as pneumonia, meningitis, and arthritis.

While some antibiotics have little effect on bacteria, some substances, such as alcohol and bleach are effective. Additionally, some equipment can be autoclaved to destroy bacteria. Regardless, careful monitoring of antibiotic use and proper equipment care are needed to prevent the development of resistance and the spread of resistant bacteria.

One of your patients is refusing to finish his antibiotic prescription. What would you tell him to make sure that he finishes his medicine?

Controlling Infection | Chapter 17 481

What's New?—Antibiotic Resistant Bacteria

- Explain antibiotics.
- Discuss some infections for which antibiotics are usually prescribed:
  - Strep throat
  - Pneumonia
  - Urinary tract infections
  - Bladder infections
- Review reasons for the growth of antibiotic resistant bacteria.
- Review the bacteria that are becoming increasingly resistant to antibiotics.
- Discuss why antibiotic resistant bacteria, such as MRSA, is a serious problem.
- Discuss steps that can help stop the increase of antibiotic-resistant bacteria.

One of your patients is refusing to finish his antibiotic prescription. What would you tell him to make sure that he finishes his medicine?

Answer: Explain to the patient that he may become sick again if he doesn't finish his medicine. Tell him that not taking all of his antibiotics may also result in antibiotic-resistant pathogens.

CUSTOMIZED INSTRUCTION

More Advanced Students

Assign more advanced students to research antibiotics. They can prepare a table or chart listing types of antibiotics and the pathogens they are used to fight, and share the information with the class.

Procedure 17.1 Hand Hygiene (Washing)

BACKGROUND: Contaminated hands are the most common cause of infection. Proper handwashing technique is the most effective way to prevent the spread of infection.

Preprocedure

1. Wash your hands between patient contacts.
2. Wash your hands after removing protective gloves.
3. Wash your hands after contact with body fluids, even if gloves have been worn.

Procedure

4. Stand at sink. Avoid contact of your uniform with the sink. Roll a paper towel out to have ready to use after washing your hands.
5. Turn on water and adjust water temperature.
6. Wet the hands and wrist area. Keep hands lower than elbows.
7. Using soap from dispenser, lather thoroughly.

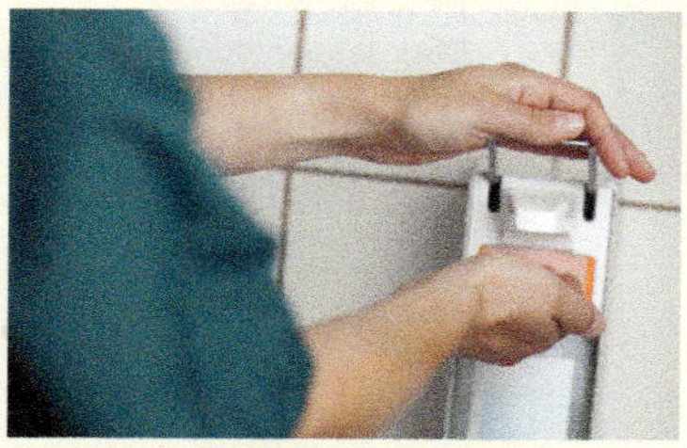

8. Using soap and friction, wash the palms, backs of the hands, fingers, between the fingers, knuckles, wrists and forearms. Clean nails. If no nail brush is available, rub nails across palms of hands.
9. Continue washing for at least 15 seconds.
10. Rinse thoroughly with fingertips downward.

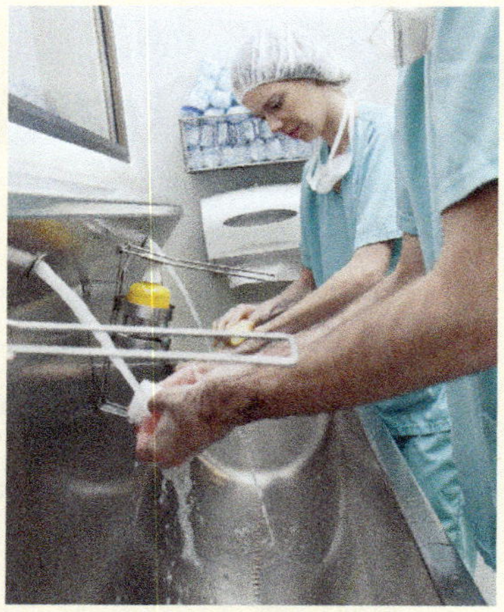

11. Dry hands.
12. Use a paper towel to turn off faucets and open door if necessary.

482 Chapter 17 | Controlling Infection

Procedure Tip

17.1 Hand Hygiene (Washing)

- Review the background information, emphasizing the ease with which pathogens can be transmitted by hand.
- Point out that the first three steps are directives for when hands should be washed.
- Review the procedure steps.
- Step 6: Emphasize that hands should be lower than elbows. Explain that this keeps the water from running down the arms and spreading contaminants.
- Step 8: Explain the need for friction.
- Step 9: Demonstrate how to count to identify 15 seconds.
- Demonstrate the steps.
- Have students practice and perform the procedure.

PROCEDURE PRACTICE

- Demonstrate the steps for Procedure 17.1, Hand Hygiene (Washing), as many times as necessary, or ask students to demonstrate the steps. Have students practice and perform the procedure until they are competent.

ACTIVITY

Teach a younger student or family member proper handwashing procedures. Use the steps in Procedure 17.1 as a guide, and refer to Table 17.3 for additional information and explanations.

Procedure 17.2 **Personal Protective Equipment**

BACKGROUND: Personal protective equipment (PPE) are a variety of barriers and respirators used alone or in combination to protect mucous membranes, airways, skin, and clothing from contact with infectious agents.

Preprocedure

1. Determine the expected level of exposure.
2. Refer to the CDC guidelines for the use of Personal Protective Equipment to determine the appropriate PPE equipment to use.
3. Always practice safe work practices, which includes:
   a. Keep hands away from face.
   b. Work from clean to dirty.
   c. Limit surfaces touched.
   d. Change when torn or heavily contaminated.
   e. Perform hand hygiene.

Procedure

NOTE: When using Personal Protective Equipment, don in the order the procedures are given. Prior to donning protective equipment:

1. Remove your watch or push it well up your arm.
2. Wash your hands.

Gown

1. Untie the gown's waist strings; then put the gown on and wrap it around the back of your uniform.
2. Tie or snap the gown at the neck and at the waist making sure your uniform is completely covered.

Mask

Surgical-type masks are used to cover the nose and mouth and provide protection from contact with large infectious droplets (over 5 mm in size). For protection from inhalation of small particles or droplet nuclei, particulate respirators are recommended. The health care worker must be fitted for these masks prior to use in order to maintain appropriate seal and protection. The infection control department staff will do fit testing for the employee during the employees orientation period.

1. Determine the appropriate type of face mask to be used.
2. Place the mask snugly over your nose and mouth. Secure the mask by tying the strings behind your head or placing the loops around your ears.
3. If the mask has a metal strip, squeeze it to fit your nose firmly.
4. If you wear eyeglasses, tuck the mask under their lower edge.

Goggles/Face Shield

Goggles or face shield should be worn when there is a risk of contaminating the mucous membranes of the eyes.

Mouthpieces, Resuscitation Bags, and Other Ventilation Devices

Use a ventilation device, which provides protection for the caregiver from oral contact and secretions, as alternative to mouth to mouth resuscitation.

Gloves

Gloves should be worn when there is risk of touching blood or body fluids. Gloves are worn only once and are discarded according to agency policy. Some care activities for an individual patient may require changing gloves more than once. Hands should be thoroughly washed after gloves are removed.

1. Use clean, disposable gloves.
2. Select a glove that provides appropriate fit.
3. Place the gloves on the hands so that they extend to cover the wrist of the isolation gown.

(continued)

Controlling Infection | Chapter 17 483

Procedure Tip

17.2 Personal Protective Equipment

- Review the background information, emphasizing the importance of protecting the body from contact with infectious agents.
- Explain that a barrier is equipment such as a gown, goggles, or face shield.
- Explain that a respirator is equipment such as a mouthpiece, resuscitation bag, or other ventilation device.
- Review the preprocedure steps.
- Step 2: Discuss CDC guidelines.
- Step 3: Review safe work practices.
- Review the procedure steps.
- Emphasize that equipment should be put on in the proper order.
- Point out that watches and other wrist adornments may transmit pathogens and should be removed.
- Emphasize the need for proper handwashing.
- Review the procedures for each piece of equipment, including removal.
- Demonstrate the procedures using proper equipment.
- Emphasize that gloves are worn only once.
- Emphasize that proper care must be taken when removing protective equipment, so as to avoid contamination.
- Have students practice and perform the procedure.

CUSTOMIZED INSTRUCTION

Special Needs Students

If necessary, provide customized equipment for special needs students to use for the procedures, such as a handicap-accessible sink for handwashing.

PROCEDURE PRACTICE

- Demonstrate the steps for Procedure 17.2, Personal Protective Equipment, as many times as necessary, or ask students to demonstrate the steps. Have students practice and perform the procedure until they are competent.

Procedure Tip

17.3 Caring for Soiled Linens

- Review the background information, emphasizing that the hospital laundry is responsible for disinfecting linens.
- Emphasize the importance of following precautions when handling soiled linens.
- Point out that many bodily fluids come in contact with linens, including:
  - Mucous
  - Blood
  - Urine
- Review the preprocedure steps.
- Note that the prepocedure steps include the procedures for washing hands and donning protective equipment.
- Review the procedure steps.
- Step 3: Explain that folding the linens helps trap contaminants within the sheets.
- Step 4: Emphasize the importance of preventing contact with the linens.
- Demonstrate the procedure using clean linens.
- Have students practice and demonstrate the procedure.

PROCEDURE PRACTICE

- Demonstrate the steps for Procedure 17.3, Caring for Soiled Linens, as many times as necessary, or ask students to demonstrate the steps. Have students practice and perform the procedure until they are competent.

Procedure 17.2 Personal Protective Equipment (continued)

Removing Personal Protective Equipment

Remember that the outside surfaces of your Personal Protective Equipment are contaminated.

1. While wearing gloves, untie the gowns waist strings.
2. With your gloved left hand, remove the right glove by pulling on the cuff, turning the glove inside out as you pull.
3. Remove the left glove by placing two fingers in the glove and pulling it off, turning it inside out as you remove it. Discard. Wash your hands.
4. Untie the neck strings of your gown. Grasp the outside of the gown at the back of the shoulders and pull the gown down over your arms, turning it inside out as you remove it.
5. Holding the gown well away from your uniform, fold it inside out. Discard it in the laundry hamper.
6. Wash your hands. Turn off the faucet using a paper towel and discard the towel in trash container.
7. Remove the mask/goggles to avoid contaminating your face or hair in the process. Untie your mask and/or remove your goggles by holding only the strings/strap. Discard.
8. Wash your hands and forearms with soap or antiseptic after leaving the room.

Procedure 17.3 Caring for Soiled Linens

BACKGROUND: The hospital laundry uses water temperature and cleaning products capable of destroying any pathogens that might be present in patient's bed linens.
ALERT: Follow Standard Precautions

Preprocedure

1. Wash hands.
2. Don disposable gloves.

Procedure

3. Fold the soiled bed linens inward upon themselves when removing them from the bed.
4. Hold the linens away from your uniform when removing from room.
5. Place in the nearest hamper.
6. Should the outside surface of the linen hamper bag become soiled it should be placed in a clean outer bag prior to pickup by the laundry staff.

484 Chapter 17 | Controlling Infection

ACTIVITY

Make a list of all the people in a health care facility who might come in contact with soiled linens in the course of a day. Write a paragraph explaining why all these people should be educated in the use of aseptic techniques.

Procedure 17.4	Disposing of Sharps

BACKGROUND: Because of the danger inherent in handling sharp objects or contaminated needles, the health care industry has moved towards needleless systems whenever possible. When a needleless system cannot be provided, needles with have a protective sheath used to cover before and after use. There is no longer any need to recap used needles.
ALERT: Follow Standard Precautions

Preprocedure

1. Select the safest method of using sharps, using a needleless system whenever possible.
2. Wash hands.
3. Don disposable gloves.
4. Locate the closest sharps container to the area you will be working in.

NOTE: Gloves are not meant to protect the caregiver from needle stick or sharps injuries.

Postprocedure

5. After the use of any needle, place the protective sheath before leaving the patient area.
6. If sharps are used during a procedure, carefully separate them from other items on the tray and cover them with the procedure tray cover.
7. Place any disposable sharps items in the closest sharps container.
8. For non-disposable sharps items, place them in the designated area of the closest dirty utility room.
9. Remove and discard disposable gloves.
10. Wash hands.

Procedure 17.5	Wrapping Instruments for Autoclave

BACKGROUND: Reusable items used for providing patient care must be cleaned and sterilized before re-use. This requires that the item be cleaned and appropriately wrapped prior to being sterilized. This will include instruments, basins, glassware, patient care equipment, and any other items deemed necessary. The facility will provide an area, known as the Decontamination Room, for this activity.
ALERT: Follow Standard Precautions

Preprocedure

1. Retrieve/receive instruments and equipment to be decontaminated.
2. Don appropriate attire:
   a. scrub uniform
   b. head cover
   c. cover gown
   d. gloves
   e. goggles and/or face mask

Procedure

3. Sort grossly soiled instruments from those less soiled.
4. Soak instruments that have gross soil in approved enzymatic hospital cleaner. If manual scrubbing is necessary, a soft bristled brush will be used below the water line to decrease the possibility of aerosol contamination.

(continued)

Controlling Infection | Chapter 17 485

TEAMWORK

Hold up items, or pictures of items, that are commonly found in a health care facility. Have students respond as to what type of disinfection or sterilization method is appropriate for cleaning that particular item.

PROCEDURE PRACTICE

- Demonstrate the steps for Procedure 17.5, Wrapping Instruments for Autoclave, as many times as necessary, or ask students to demonstrate the steps. Have students practice and perform the procedure until they are competent.

Procedure Tip

17.4 Disposing of Sharps

- Review the background information.
- Explain that sharps refers to any sharp object that could puncture the skin, but usually refers to needles.
- Explain a needleless system.
- Review the preprocedure steps.
- Emphasize that gloves will not protect the wearer from a puncture.
- Review the procedure steps.
- Demonstrate the procedure.
- Have students practice and demonstrate the procedure.

PROCEDURE PRACTICE

- Demonstrate the steps for Procedure 17.4, Disposing of Sharps, as many times as necessary, or ask students to demonstrate the steps. Have students practice and perform the procedure until they are competent.

Procedure Tip

17.5 Wrapping Instruments for Autoclave

- Review the background information, emphasizing that any equipment that is used more than once must be sterilized between uses.
- Explain that the location of the sterilization equipment depends on the facility.
- Review the purpose of an autoclave.
- Review the preprocedure steps.
- Review the procedure steps.
- Step 3: Explain the difference between grossly soiled and less soiled.

Procedure Tip

17.5 Wrapping Instruments for Autoclave, continued

- Discuss why items must be cleaned before being sterilized.
- Point out responsibilities include more than cleaning:
  - Sorting
  - Assembling
  - Inventory
- Review postprocedure steps.
- If possible, demonstrate the procedure.
- Have students practice and demonstrate the procedure.

Teaching Tips

- Reinforce major factors in aseptic techniques used to control microorganisms:
  - Sterilization
  - Bactericidal solutions
  - Bacteriostatic solutions
  - Handwashing
- Review reasons for sterilizing.
- Review items that need sterilizing.
- Discuss protective isolation.

Section 17.2 Review Questions

1. Answer: Asepsis is a sterile condition, free from all germs.
2. Answer: Proper handwashing; employees being clean and neat; proper handling of all equipment; using sterile procedure when necessary; using proper cleaning solutions; and following Standard Precautions.
3. Answer: Any five of the following: Blood, vaginal secretions, pericardial fluid, body fluids containing visible blood, amniotic fluid, peritoneal fluid, tissue specimens, cerebrospinal fluid, interstitial fluid, semen, or pleural fluid
4. Answer: Bacteriostatic solutions slow or stop the growth of bacteria. Bactericidal solutions kill bacteria.
5. Answer: It is important to maintain asepsis to control the spread of infection.

Procedure 17.5 Wrapping Instruments for Autoclave (continued)

5. Place instruments with moving parts or hard to reach areas in Sonic Cleaner in open position for cycle. All large surface instruments, retractors and elevators will be cleaned manually.
6. Rinse all instruments, washed mechanically or manually, in standing tap water, and running tap water.
7. Immerse instruments with moving parts in instrument lubricant for 45 seconds.
8. Wash instrument trays, washbasins, and rubber items in warm water.
9. Rinse items in standing tap water and running tap water, and dry before wrapping.
10. Wash glassware, such as syringes, in warm water and appropriate cleaner. Rinse in standing, running tap water, and distilled water.
11. Air-dry syringes before preparing for sterilization.
12. After the cleaning process, move all instruments to the assembly table in the clean processing room.
13. Assemble, using the appropriate item list for each tray. Note any shortages and try to locate any missing instruments.
14. Make note of any sets with missing instruments.
15. Place tray with items onto designated wrapper. Fold each side of the wrapper in towards the middle. Secure the wrapper with autoclave tape.
16. Notify autoclave personnel of trays, items when readied for sterilizing.

Postprocedure

17. Personnel are responsible for maintaining a clean area.
18. Hand washing is mandatory prior to leaving the area.

Summary

Infection control is critical in health care environments. Asepsis is the method used to destroy the environment that allows pathogens to live, breed, and spread. Major factors in the control of microorganisms are handwashing, disinfection, sterilization, and following Standard Precautions. The effective health care worker always strives to provide an aseptic environment by following aseptic technique procedures and Standard Precautions.

Section 17.2 Review Questions

1. Define the term *asepsis*.
2. What are five aseptic techniques?
3. List five body fluids that should be handled using Standard Precautions.
4. What is the difference between bactericidal and bacteriostatic substances?
5. Why is it important to maintain asepsis?
6. What are the guidelines for handwashing?

486 Chapter 17 | Controlling Infection

6. Answer: Always wash your hands before and after contact with a patient and/or patient belongings; before and after eating; after using the bathroom; after handling any contaminated fluid or object; and after touching body fluids. Use enough soap to make a good lather. Interlace your fingers together and rub all sides of fingers and hands to produce friction for 15 seconds. Be sure to clean beneath fingernails and around knuckles. If no nail brush is available, rub fingernails on palms of hands. Hold hands lower than elbows and rinse thoroughly to remove pathogens. Turn on and off faucets with dry paper towel. Rewash hands if you touch the faucet or sink. Dry hands completely from tips of fingers to wrist.

CUSTOMIZED INSTRUCTION

Less Advanced Students

Provide adequate time for less advanced students to learn the procedures. They may require more time to review the steps and to practice them.

Transmission-Based Precautions

SECTION 17.3

Background

As a health care worker, you are exposed to patients, equipment, and supplies that are contaminated with pathogens. An estimated 1.7 million hospital-acquired infections occur in the United States each year. These infections may cause as many as 90,000 deaths annually. Use the techniques taught in this chapter to protect yourself and other people and to help prevent the spread of infection to patients, co-workers, and the community.

Objectives

When you have completed this section, you will be able to do the following:

- Match key terms with their meanings.
- Name primary levels of precautions identified in the guidelines developed by the Centers for Disease Control and Prevention (CDC).
- Identify three types of Transmission-Based Precautions.
- Demonstrate the correct procedure for entering and leaving an area where Transmission-Based Precautions are followed.
- Differentiate between Standard Precautions and Transmission-Based Precautions.

Introduction to Standard and Transmission-Based Precautions

The 2007 guidelines from the CDC established the need for two levels of protection: Standard Precautions and Transmission-Based Precautions. Standard Precautions are the primary strategy for successful hospital-acquired (nosocomial) infection control. Standard Precautions are appropriate for all patients receiving care or service in a health care environment, regardless of their diagnosis. These precautions provide protection from contact with blood, mucous membranes, nonintact skin, and all body fluids. Transmission-Based Precautions are designed for patients suspected to be infected with pathogens spread by **airborne** or **droplet** transmission, contact with dry skin, or contact with contaminated surfaces.

Sterile technique is first and foremost about minimizing possible sources of infection. *Sterile* means free of bugs that can infect people. Sterility will apply to surfaces of objects or to substances that will be introduced into a patient's body. Some objects, like hands or surgical masks, can be clean, but not sterile. Only specific prepared surfaces or substances, like surgical tools, are considered sterile.

airborne
(EHR born)
Articles that float in the air.

droplet
(DRAWP leht)
A small drop of fluid.

Controlling Infection | Chapter 17 487

TEAMWORK

Divide the class into teams of five to seven students. Play Hangman using the vocabulary words for Section 17.3.

FOCUS AND ENGAGE

Introduce the Section

a. Review the content of the Background paragraph, explaining that Transmission-Based Precautions are specifically for preventing pathogens from airborne or droplet transmission.

b. Emphasize that Transmission-Based Precautions are used in addition to Standard Precautions.

c. Review the objectives for the section.

Vocabulary Review

a. Direct students to the key terms.

b. Pronounce each word, and have the students repeat the pronunciation out loud.

c. Discuss the definition of each word.

TEACH

Discuss

- Ask students if they or a family member ever had a communicable disease, such as strep throat.
- Discuss how these types of illnesses spread.
- Discuss precautions they might have taken to avoid catching the illness.

Reinforce and Review

- Review Chapter 13, Your Body and How It Functions.
- Reinforce the importance of asepsis, aseptic techniques, and steps to prevent the transmission of pathogens, as covered in Section 17.2.

Teaching Tips

- Explain the two primary levels of precautions: Standard Precautions (Section 17.2) and Transmission-Based Precautions.
- Explain that Transmission-Based Precautions are designed for patients suspected to be infected with pathogens spread by:
  - Airborne or droplet transmission
  - Contact with dry skin
  - Contact with contaminated surfaces
- Emphasize that Transmission-Based Precautions are used in addition to—not in place of—Standard Precautions.
- Explain that there are three types of Transmission-Based Precautions:
  - Airborne, which reduces the spread of airborne droplet nuclei or dust particles containing the pathogen
  - Droplet, which reduces the risk of transmission by contact between mucous membranes and large particle droplets
  - Contact, which reduces the risk of transmission through direct or indirect contact

ACTIVITY

Make a chart or table comparing the three types of Transmission-Based Precautions.

Transmission-Based Precautions are used in addition to Standard Precautions when some contagious diseases are present. There are three types of Transmission-Based Precautions:

- Airborne Precautions
- Droplet Precautions
- Contact Precautions

Follow the guidelines in **Table 17.4** when working with patients in Transmission-Based Precaution environments.

Communicable Diseases

The AIDS Patient

AIDS (Autoimmune deficiency syndrome) is a chronic, life threatening condition caused by the human immunodeficiency virus (HIV). HIV destroys the cells of the immune system, which affects the body's ability to fight bacteria, fungi, and viruses. This makes the body more susceptible to certain types of cancers and opportunistic infections that the body would normally resist, such as pneumonias, Kaposi's sarcoma, and tuberculosis.

The first cases of this disease were reported in the 1980s. When first discovered, there was rampant fear of anyone with HIV or AIDS. People avoided contact with infected people. Even some health care workers devoted to the care of the ill refused to care for them. The homosexual population was particularly affected by this isolation, and even those that were not infected were sometimes treated as outcasts.

AIDS has become a global epidemic—35 million people are living with HIV. In 2013, an estimated 2.1 million people were newly infected with HIV and 1.5 million people died from AIDS; 39 million have died of AIDS since the epidemic began. Progress has been made in the treatment of and improved access to care. However, our best hope for stemming the spread of the virus lies in prevention, treatment and education.

On a positive note, the recognition of this disease was instrumental in the creation of Standard Precautions and the continuing revision of precautions for Occupational Health and Bloodborne Pathogens. Education about the causes and treatment of the disease has progressed to the point that health care workers and the general public are more accepting and much less fearful of those infected. Famous people who have become infected with this virus have done much to quell the fear and isolation of this population.

488 Chapter 17 | Controlling Infection

Table 17.4 Transmission-Based Precautions

Common Communicable Diseases Requiring Special Precautions	Type of Precautions	Precaution Guidelines
Chickenpox (Varicella zoster) Tuberculosis Herpes zoster (Shingles, Varicella zoster)	**Airborne:** Reduces the spread of airborne droplet nuclei (5 **microns** or smaller in size) or dust particles containing the pathogen	■ Standard Precautions ■ Private room with specific ventilation criteria ■ Keep the room door closed ■ Wear respiratory protection ■ Wash hands: – before entering the room – before leaving the room – after leaving the room
Haemophilus influenzae Some forms of meningitis Diphtheria Pertussis Adenovirus Mumps Some forms of pneumonia Severe viral infections	**Droplet:** Reduces the risk of transmission by contact of the mucous membranes of the eye, nose, or mouth with large particle droplets	■ Standard Precautions ■ Private room or room with another patient with same pathogen ■ Wear a mask when working within three feet of the patient ■ Wash hands: – before entering the room – before leaving the room – after leaving the room
Multidrug-resistant infections of: ■ Gastrointestinal system ■ Respiratory system ■ Integumentary system (skin)	**Contact:** Reduces the risk of transmission through direct or indirect contact	■ Standard Precautions ■ Private room or room with another patient with same pathogen ■ Use personal protective equipment (PPE) such as gloves and gowns ■ Wash hands – before entering the room – before leaving the room – after leaving the room

Use the following precautions against HIV and AIDS:

- Use clean needles. Dispose of used needles appropriately in designated sharps boxes. Never re-cap needles.
- Report and receive follow-up care for any needle sticks or exposures to bloodborne pathogens.
- Remember the importance of following the procedure for Standard Precautions.

When treating HIV positive or AIDS patients, be sure to:

- Educate yourself and the patient.
- Help the patient understand options for treatment.
- Be supportive.
- Promote the patient's role as an individual and a member of the community.

microns
(MAHY krohns)
Units equaling one millionth of a meter.

Controlling Infection | Chapter 17 489

Teaching Tips

- Review Table 17.4 together as a class.
- Focus on the common communicable diseases that require special, Transmission-Based Precautions (left column).
- Identify the type of Transmission-Based Precautions that should be used for each (middle column).
- Note the explanation of how each type of Transmission-Based Precaution reduces risk (middle column).
- Review the Precaution Guidelines (right column).
- Note that Standard Precautions are always used in addition to the specific Transmission-Based Precautions.
- Explain the additional risk posed by patients with communicable diseases.
- Explain AIDS, and how research into the treatment of AIDS helped lead to the development of precautions.
- Review precautions that should be taken when working with patients infected with HIV or AIDS.

TEAMWORK

Divide the class into teams of four to six students. Have each team write the types of Transmission-Based Precautions on three separate pieces of paper. You name a disease. Each team holds up the paper with the corresponding type of Transmission-Based Precaution that should be used when treating patients with the disease. Award a point to each team that answers correctly.

Teaching Tips

- Review the information about patients with communicable diseases.
- Emphasize that it may be necessary to isolate patients with known communicable diseases.
- Review the need for Standard Precautions.
- Explain that you can prioritize Standard Precautions based on the level of risk of transmission, and take the appropriate steps:
  - Category I: High Risk
  - Category II: Low Risk
  - Category III: No Risk
- Point out that priorities should be set based on:
  - Potential for contact with blood
  - Potential for contact with any body fluids
  - Tasks (procedures) that will be performed
- Review Table 17.5 together as a class.
- Note the category of risk and the contact required for each task.
- Review the necessary precautions.
- Review the necessary equipment.

TEAMWORK

In small groups, create a three-dimensional model of one type of Transmission-Based Precaution room.

When treating HIV positive or AIDS patients, do NOT:

- Avoid personal contact.
- Isolate patient from human contact.
- Exhibit personal prejudices.

Note: There is no need to wear protective gloves when directly interacting with these patients. Only use gloves when there is a danger of contact with blood or body fluids, mucous membrane, or non-intact skin. As with any other patient, practicing good hand washing techniques is always appropriate and in the caregiver and patient's best interest.

Patients with Communicable Diseases

Patients who can contaminate the area with known communicable diseases should be in a private room or isolated from other patients. There will be a list of diseases which are communicable and the cautions which should be taken available on the patient unit. The infection control department will monitor all admissions and advise staff of any additional precautions that need to be taken.

Before you start to measure vital signs or work with patients, you must remember to follow the basic Standard Precautions necessary to protect yourself when contact with blood or body fluids is possible. Make sure you review Tables 17.5 and 17.6.

Table 17.5 Standard Precautions with Risk Categorization

Infection-control guidelines exist to protect employees and patients against infectious viruses and bacteria. The Standard Precautions you take depend on the (1) potential for contact with blood, (2) potential for contact with any body fluids, and (3) tasks (procedures) that you perform. This table tells you what to wear when you are doing various tasks. Follow these guidelines to protect yourself and others from infection.

Category	Task Requires	Protect Yourself By	Have Available
I: High risk	Direct contact with blood or other bodily fluids	■ Washing hands: – If you touch blood/body fluids – After removing gloves ■ Wearing: – Apron or gown – Eye protection – Face mask ■ Never recapping needles or bending/breaking them ■ Placing used needles in a sharps container ■ Cleaning off blood/body fluids immediately ■ Disposing of waste materials in biohazard container ■ Being vaccinated for hepatitis B	Gloves Apron Eye protection Face mask
II: Low risk	When you have close contact with patients but are not likely to come in contact with blood/body fluids	Washing hands	Mask Eye protection Gloves
III: No risk	Your routine work requires no contact with blood/body fluid	Washing hands, as a general rule	

Table 17.6 Standard Precautions: Examples of Tasks and Use of Protective Equipment

Task	Gloves	Gown	Mask	Protective Eyewear
Controlling spurting blood	Yes	Yes	Yes	Yes
Controlling minimal bleeding	Yes	No	No	No
Blood drawing	Yes	Yes	Yes	Yes
Oral or nasal suction	Yes	No	Yes	Yes
Handling/cleaning contaminated instruments	Yes	Yes	Yes	Yes
Measuring blood pressure	No	No	No	No

Transmission-Based Precaution Rooms

Figures 17.5 and 17.6 illustrate precautions that should be taken within the room when contagious diseases are present. When entering or leaving a Transmission-Based Precaution room, follow the specific directions on the precaution card at the door.

Reverse or Protective Isolation

There is also another type of isolation: reverse or protective isolation. This is the type of isolation used for patients who are not contagious, but whose immune system is so weak that they must be protected from other people that might be carrying disease. Some examples of these are patients on chemotherapy, leukemia, burn patients, etc.

Psychosocial Issues During Special Precautions

Transmission-Based Precautions may be difficult for patients. The patients are alone most of the time. Visitors must wear personal protective wear. Hugs or touching may not be allowed. The health care worker cannot stay and visit because there is other work to do. This may cause the patient to feel angry, depressed, and frustrated.

Take as much time as you can to listen to the patient's feelings and concerns. Encourage communication, and be supportive. If the patient seems unusually upset, report it to your supervisor.

Taking steps to educate patients and their families on procedures during special precaution situations can help reduce anxiety for everyone involved. You can make a difference by staying attuned and responding to patients' feelings and moods, always treating each person with dignity, and by providing the very best care. Some age-specific considerations for patients/clients requiring Transmission-Based Precautions are listed in Table 17.7.

Controlling Infection | Chapter 17 491

CUSTOMIZED INSTRUCTION

Less Advanced Students

Less advanced students may find the many tables in this chapter confusing, and have trouble differentiating the information they provide. Provide adequate time for them to read and understand each table before moving on to a new table.

Teaching Tips

- Review Table 17.6 together as a class.
- Note that it provides information about the protective equipment required for specific tasks.
- Explain that rooms housing patients with known contagious diseases are known as Transmission-Based Precaution rooms.
- Health care providers must follow Transmission-Based Precautions on entering and leaving Transmission-Based Precaution rooms.
- Emphasize that Infection Control personnel should post specific directions on a precaution card at the entrance to each room.
- Discuss types of isolation:
  - Strict isolation
  - Protective isolation
- Discuss psychosocial issues that might affect patients who are treated with Transmission-Based Precautions.
- Explain that patients may feel:
  - Isolated
  - Lonely
  - Angry
  - Depressed
  - Frustrated
- Review a care giver's responsibility to communicate effectively with patients to help them understand and cope with anxiety resulting from the precautions.
- Washing hands is one of the best ways health workers can prevent the spread of infection and protect themselves and others.

Figure Focus

17.5 Transmission-Based Precautions. How do precautions for airborne and droplet transmission differ?

Answer: Unlike airborne precautions, a mask is not always needed and a gown is not needed for droplet precautions.

Teaching Tips

- Advise students to turn the page on its side so they can view the figure correctly.
- Point out that the left half of the figure displays droplet precautions, and that the right half of the figure displays airborne precautions.

TEAMWORK

Divide the class into teams of four to six students. You name a task that a medical professional might perform when working with a patient in a Transmission-Based Precaution room. Each team writes down whether the task is High Risk, Low Risk, or No Risk. Compare results and award point for correct answers.

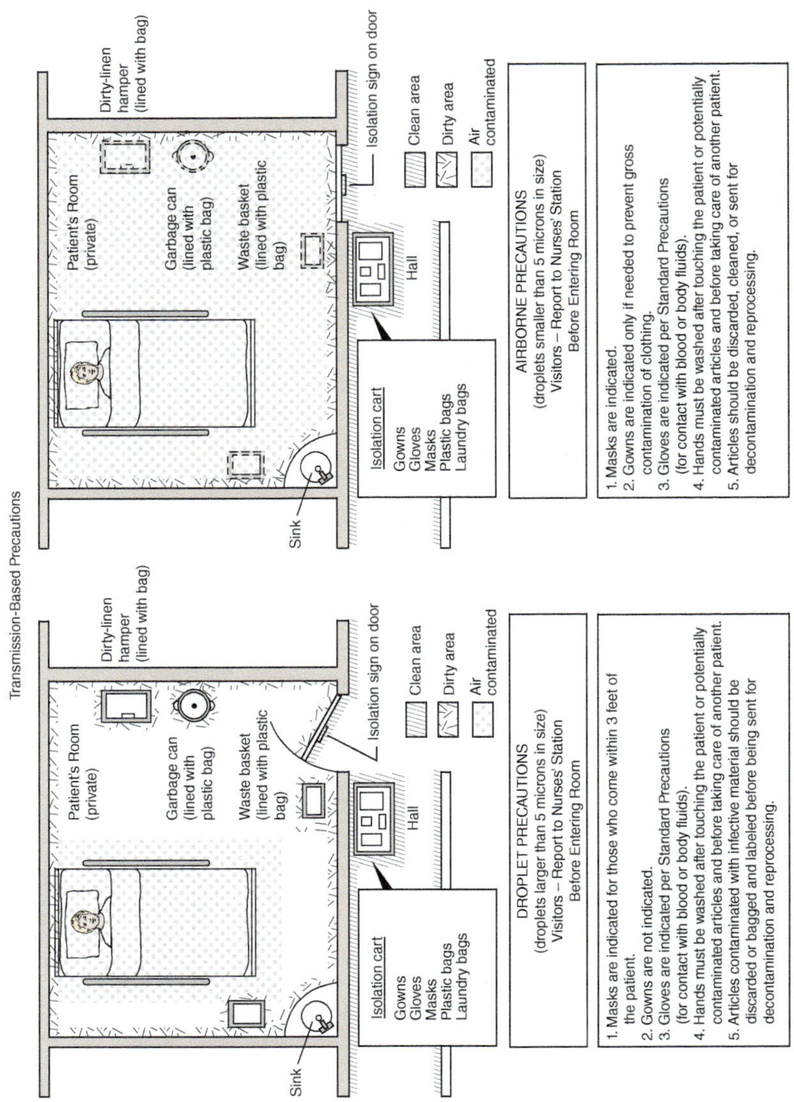

Figure 17.5
Transmission-Based Precautions. How do precautions for airborne and droplet transmission differ?

492 Chapter 17 | Controlling Infection

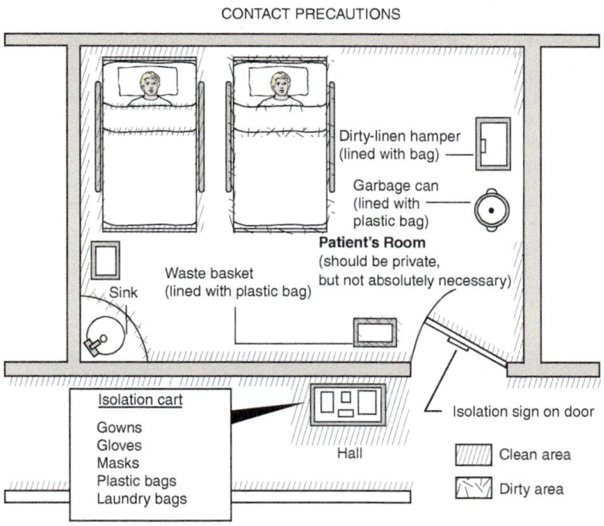

Figure 17.6
Contact precautions. When do you need to use gloves, gowns, and masks for a patient undergoing contact precautions?

CONTACT PRECAUTIONS
Visitors – Report to Nurses' Station
Before Entering Room

1. **Masks** are not indicated.
2. **Gowns** are indicated if soiling is likely.
3. **Gloves** are indicated for touching infective material.
4. **Hands must be washed after touching the patient or potentially contaminated articles and before taking care of another patient.**
5. **Articles** contaminated with infective material should be discarded or bagged and labeled before being sent for decontamination and reprocessing.

A private room is indicated for Contact Precautions if patient hygiene is poor. A patient with poor hygiene does not wash hands after touching infective material, contaminates the environment with infective material, or shares contaminated articles with other patients. In general, patients infected with the same organism may share a room.

Controlling Infection | Chapter 17 493

Figure Focus

17.6 Contact precautions. When do you need to use gloves, gowns, and masks for a patient undergoing contact precautions?

Answer: Gowns should be used if soiling is likely. Gloves should be used if touching infective material. Masks are not indicated.

TEAMWORK

In small groups or as a class, conduct an experiment using an adjustable spray bottle to determine the difference between mist and droplets. Fill the bottle with water and adjust the nozzle to the finest mist setting. Place paper towels on the counter or table and spray water into the air over the towels. Record observations about the spray and the condition of the towels. Adjust the nozzle to provide droplet-sized spray. Place new, dry paper towels in a different location and spray water into the air over the towels. Record observations about the spray and the condition of the towels. The experiment should indicate that droplets fall quickly, while mist stays in the air longer. Discuss the results as a class, including how this might impact the spread of pathogens.

Teaching Tips

- Review Table 17.7 together as a class.
- Discuss the importance of effective communication for the patient's emotional well-being.
- Review the communication techniques for each age group.
- Note the importance of educating the patient and family members on proper precaution procedures.

Procedure Tip

17.6 Putting on Sterile Gloves and Removing Gloves

- Review the background information, emphasizing that sterile gloves prevent transmission of pathogens from one area of the patient to another.
- Explain that the goal is to keep the gloves free from contamination so that treatment may proceed without risk of transmission.
- Review the preprocedure steps.
- Emphasize proper handwashing.
- Review the procedure steps.
- Step 7: Explain how to maintain the sterility by avoiding contact with non-sterile surfaces.
- Step 9: Emphasize the need to touch only the inside of the glove.
- Step 14: Emphasize that touching one glove with the other glove does not impact the sterility.
- Step 17: Emphasize that touching the outside of either glove to skin or any non-sterile surface contaminates the glove.
- Step 21: Emphasize that new gloves must also be used if the gloves become contaminated.
- Review the postprocedure.
- Step 22: Emphasize that the gloves should be turned inside out in order to keep any contaminants within the gloves when they are removed.

Table 17.7 Age-Specific Considerations

Isolation is difficult for patients of any age. Understanding the special needs of each group gives the patient a sense of security and improves the healing process.

Age	Communication	Comfort	Safety
Birth–5 years	Explain the reason for isolation to the parents and family members.	Keep child with parent or family member to increase feeling of security.	Teach family the procedures that must be followed in an isolation area.
5–12 years	Explain the reason for isolation and the importance of staying in the isolation unit.	Keep child with parent or family member to increase feeling of security.	Teach patient, parent, or family member the procedures.
12+ years	Explain the reason for isolation and the importance of staying in the isolation unit.	Encourage peer, parent, or family member to stay as much as possible.	Teach patient, peer, and family members the procedures for isolation.

Procedure 17.6 Putting on Sterile Gloves and Removing Gloves

BACKGROUND: Sterile gloves cover the hands and allow treatment of open skin areas. Following the procedure is essential to prevent contamination of the gloves. Contamination allows bacteria to enter the treatment area and may cause infection.

Preprocedure

1. Assemble equipment.
2. Wash hands.

Procedure

3. Pick up wrapped gloves.
4. Check to be certain that they are sterile:
   a. Package intact
   b. Seal of sterility
5. Place on clean, flat surface.
6. Open wrapper by handling only the outside.
7. Maintain sterility of wrap and gloves.
8. Position with cuff end toward self.
9. Use your left hand to pick up the right-handed glove at folded cuff edge, touching only the inside of glove.
10. Grasp inside of glove with thumb and forefinger.
11. Lift glove out and insert other hand.
12. Put on glove while maintaining sterility.
13. Put glove on right hand.
14. Use gloved right hand to pick up left-handed glove.
15. Place finger of gloved right hand under cuff of left-handed glove.
16. Lift glove up and away from wrapper to pull onto left hand.
17. Continue pulling left glove under wrist. (Be certain that gloved right thumb does not touch skin or clothing.)
18. Place fingers under cuff of right glove and pull cuff up over right wrist with gloved left hand.
19. Adjust fingers of gloves as necessary.
20. Keep hands in view and above waist while sterile gloves are on.
21. If either glove tears, remove and discard. Begin with new gloves.

Postprocedure

22. Turn gloves inside out as you remove them.

494 Chapter 17 | Controlling Infection

- Demonstrate the procedure.
- Have students practice and perform the procedure.

PROCEDURE PRACTICE

- Demonstrate the steps for Procedure 17.6, Putting on Sterile Gloves and Removing Gloves, as many times as necessary, or ask students to demonstrate the steps. Have students practice and perform the procedure until they are competent.

ACTIVITY

Create an educational poster illustrating the importance of using sterile gloves in a Transmission-Based Precaution room.

ACTIVITY

Teach a younger student or family member the way to properly put on and remove sterile gloves.

Procedure 17.7 Transmission-Based Precautions: Applying Personal Protective Equipment

BACKGROUND: A primary responsibility of all health care workers is to prevent the spread of pathogenic microorganisms. Wearing appropriate protective equipment is one way health care workers can protect themselves and others from being infected by pathogenic microorganisms.
ALERT: Follow Standard Precautions

Preprocedure

1. Assemble equipment.
2. Wash hands.

Procedure

3. Cover all hair on head with a paper cap.
4. Put on a mask by:
   a. Unfolding mask if appropriate.
   b. Cover mouth and nose with mask.
   c. Secure mask by:
      - Pulling elastic on each side of mask over ear, or
      - Tying top string at sides of mask at back of head and tie lower string at back of neck.

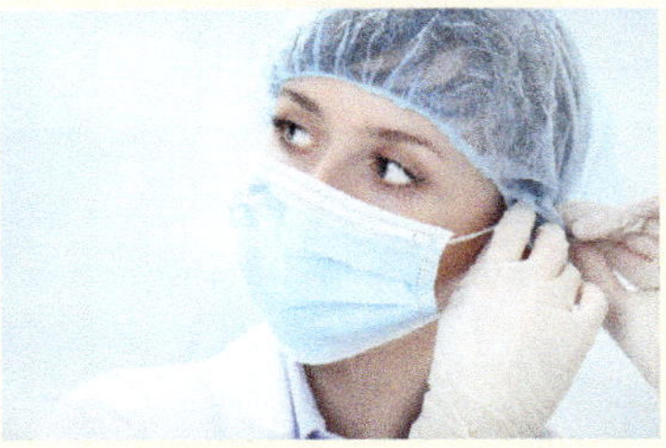

5. Put on gown with opening at back. Slip arms into sleeves of gown:
   a. Tie bow at back of neck.
   b. Overlap gown edges.
   c. Tie at waist with bow or fasten with Velcro strip.
   d. Make sure that uniform is completely covered.

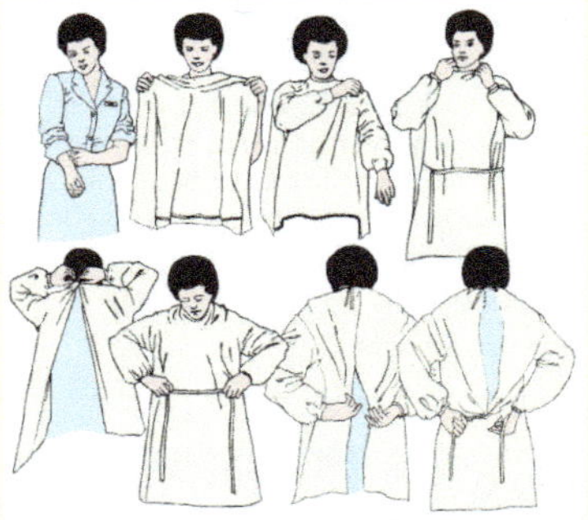

Controlling Infection | Chapter 17 495

Procedure Tip

17.7 Transmission-Based Precautions: Applying Personal Protective Equipment

- Review the background information, emphasizing that protective equipment should be used correctly to prevent the spread of infection.
- Point out that the type of equipment required may vary, depending on the type of Transmission-Based Precautions.
- Emphasize that Standard Precautions must be followed in all instances.
- Review the preprocedure steps.
- Emphasize proper handwashing.
- Review the procedure steps.
- Emphasize the importance of the order in which equipment is donned.
- Demonstrate the procedure.
- Have students practice and perform the procedure.

PROCEDURE PRACTICE

- Demonstrate the steps for Procedure 17.7, Transmission-Based Precautions: Applying Personal Protective Equipment, as many times as necessary, or ask students to demonstrate the steps. Have students practice and perform the procedure until they are competent.

TEAMWORK

You may have to adjust this activity depending on the number of students in your class. Select one of the Transmission-Based Precautions procedures. Have each student write one step of the procedure on a piece of paper, or illustrate the step in a drawing. They should not write the step number on the paper. Shuffle the papers and hand out them randomly. Have the students arrange themselves in the proper procedure order.

Procedure Tip

17.8 Transmission-Based Precautions: Removing Personal Protective Equipment

- Review the background information, emphasizing the importance of proper disposal of equipment after use.
- Emphasize that Standard Precautions must be followed in all instances.
- Review the preprocedure steps.
- Emphasize proper handwashing.
- Review the procedure steps.
- Emphasize the importance of the order in which equipment is removed.
- Step 2c: Point out the importance of not touching the outside of the contaminated glove with an unprotected hand.
- Step 3: Emphasize the need to wash hands.
- Step 5b: Point out that the gown is folded inside out to keep contaminants contained.
- Step 5c: Emphasize proper disposal of the gown.
- Step 6: Emphasize the need to wash hands.
- Review the postprocedure steps.
- Step 10: Emphasize the need to wash hands.
- Demonstrate the procedure.
- Have students practice and perform the procedure.

PROCEDURE PRACTICE

- Demonstrate the steps for Procedure 17.8, Transmission-Based Precautions: Removing Personal Protective Equipment, as many times as necessary, or ask students to demonstrate the steps. Have students practice and perform the procedure until they are competent.

Procedure 17.8 Transmission-Based Precautions: Removing Personal Protective Equipment

BACKGROUND: A primary responsibility of all health care workers is to prevent the spread of pathogenic microorganisms. Removing and disposing of protective equipment appropriately is one way health care workers prevent the spread of pathogenic microorganisms.

ALERT: Follow Standard Precautions

Preprocedure

1. Untie waist tie of gown.

Procedure

2. Remove gloves by:
   a. With dominant hand, remove other glove by grasping it just below wrist.
   b. Pulling the first glove inside out as you remove it from hand.
   c. With first two fingers of ungloved hand, reach inside glove without touching outside of glove—pull glove off hand covering the first glove. (The second glove removed surrounds the first and both are inside out.) Discard.
3. Wash hands.
4. Untie gown at neck.
5. Remove gown by:
   a. Crossing arms and grasping shoulder of gown with each hand.
   b. Pull gown forward causing it to fold inside out.
   c. Roll gown so that all contaminated portions are inside of roll, and place in dirty hamper marked *Toxic Waste* or *Hazardous Waste* inside room.
6. Wash hands.
7. Remove cap and mask, and discard.

Postprocedure

8. Use paper towel to open door.
9. Discard towel inside room.
10. Wash hands immediately after leaving the room.

Procedure 17.9 Changing a Sterile Dressing

BACKGROUND: Proper technique in changing a sterile dressing prevents wound infection and contamination to the health care worker.

ALERT: Follow Standard Precautions

Preprocedure

1. Wash hands.
2. Assemble supplies:
   a. Pair of nonsterile examination gloves
   b. Pair of sterile examination gloves
   c. Sterile dressing material
   d. Tape
   e. Biohazardous waste container
3. Explain procedure to patient.
4. Position patient/client.

Procedure

5. Put on nonsterile gloves.
6. Remove soiled dressing and examination gloves. Note appearance of wound (size, color, drainage).
7. Discard in biohazardous waste container.
8. Wash hands.
9. Designate a site to be used as a sterile field:
   a. Place sterile drape on site.
   b. Open and place all sterile dressing supplies on sterile field.

(continued)

Procedure Tip

17.9 Changing a Sterile Dressing

- Review the background information, emphasizing the importance of making sure both the worker and the wound are protected from infection.
- Emphasize that Standard Precautions must be followed in all instances.
- Review the preprocedure steps.
- Review the list of supplies, and emphasize the need to assemble them before beginning the procedure.
- Steps 2 and 3: Emphasize the use of effective communication techniques.
- Review the procedure steps.
- Step 5: Note the use of nonsterile gloves.
- Step 8: Emphasize the need to wash hands.
- Step 9: Define sterile field and explain the importance of creating a sterile field.

Procedure 17.9 | **Changing a Sterile Dressing (continued)**

c. Pour wound-cleaning solution or antiseptic into sterile container.

10. Put on sterile gloves.
11. Medicate wound as directed by physician.
12. Apply a double layer of gauze to wound or incision.

NOTE: If moderate to heavy drainage is expected, reinforce dressing. If drainage seeps through to outer layer, wound will be contaminated.

Postprocedure

13. Remove gloves and place in biohazardous waste container.
14. Wash hands.
15. Secure dressing with tape.
16. Document the following:
    a. Date
    b. Time
    c. Type of dressing applied
    d. Appearance of wound
    e. Your name and certification

Summary

In this section you learned about Transmission-Based Precautions, which are designed for patients suspected to be infected with pathogens. In the preceding section you learned about Standard Precautions, which are required for the care of all patients. Your careful use of these precautions prevents transmission of infectious agents that cause disease and illness in yourself and other people.

Section 17.3 Review Questions

1. List three types of Transmission-Based Precautions.
2. Describe the procedure for entering and leaving an area where Transmission-Based Precautions are followed.
3. Compare Standard Precautions and Transmission-Based Precautions.
4. How might a patient respond to Transmission-Based Precautions?
5. Describe an age-related concern for Transmission-Based Precautions.
6. What is the meaning of *sterile*?

Controlling Infection | Chapter 17 497

17.9 Changing a Sterile Dressing, continued

- Review the postprocedure steps.
- Step 14: Emphasize the need to wash hands.
- Step 16: Review proper documentation techniques.
- Demonstrate the procedure.
- Have students practice and perform the procedure.

PROCEDURE PRACTICE

- Demonstrate the steps for Procedure 17.9, Changing a Sterile Dressing, as many times as necessary, or ask students to demonstrate the steps. Have students practice and perform the procedure until they are competent.

TEAMWORK

In small groups, prepare skits demonstrating problems that might arise from failing to follow Transmission-Based Precautions.

Teaching Tips

- Review the difference between Standard Precautions and Transmission-Based Precautions.
- Review the three types of Transmission-Based Precautions.
- Review precautions for entering and leaving an area where Transmission-Based Precautions are followed.

Section 17.3 Review Questions

1. Answer: Airborne precautions, droplet precautions, and contact precautions
2. Answer: Masks are not indicated. Gowns are indicated if soiling is likely. Gloves are indicated for touching infective material. Hands must be washed after touching the patient or potentially contaminated articles and before taking care of another patient. Articles contaminated with infective material should be discarded or bagged and labeled before being sent for decontamination and reprocessing.
3. Answer: Standard Precautions are the primary strategy for successful hospital acquired infection control. Standard Precautions are appropriate for all patients receiving care or service in a health care environment, regardless of their diagnosis. Transmission-Based Precautions are for patients suspected to be infected with pathogens spread by airborne or droplet transmission, contact with dry skin, or contact with contaminated surfaces.
4. Answer: A patient isolated because of Transmission-Based Precautions will be alone most of the time. Visitors will need to wear gloves and gown and are not allowed to hug or touch the patient. A patient may feel sad, angry, depressed, and frustrated.
5. Answers will vary, but should address the issue of children understanding the reason for isolation and importance of staying in the isolation unit.
6. Answer: Sterile means free of the bugs that can infect people.

FOCUS AND ENGAGE

Introduce the Section

a. Review the content of the Background paragraph, explaining that bloodborne diseases require their own set of precautions.

b. Emphasize the importance of understanding how to prevent the transmission of bloodborne diseases to protect oneself and the patient from infection.

c. Review the objectives for the section.

Vocabulary Review

a. Direct students to the key terms.

b. Pronounce each word, and have the students repeat the pronunciation out loud.

c. Discuss the definition of each word.

TEACH

Discuss

- Ask students if they have received vaccinations for any diseases, and to name the diseases.
- Discuss the types of vaccinations that are recommended or required for health care providers.

Reinforce and Review

- Review Section 17.1, The Nature of Microorganisms.
- Reinforce the importance of preventing the spread of pathogens.

SECTION 17.4 Bloodborne Diseases and Precautions

Background

Bloodborne diseases are a potential risk in the health care setting. A caregiver must understand how to protect him- or herself from blood and body fluids that are contaminated with blood. Additional precautions are required to prevent the spread of bloodborne pathogens.

Objectives

When you have completed this section, you will be able to do the following:

- Describe three bloodborne diseases.
- Define the term *vaccine*.
- List three ways by which bloodborne diseases are accidentally passed.
- List two behaviors that increase the risk of contracting bloodborne diseases.
- Describe Universal Precautions.
- List six pieces of equipment used in Universal Precautions.
- Discuss ethical and legal issues related to bloodborne diseases.

bloodborne
(BLUHD born)
Carried in the blood.

hepatitis B (HBV)
(hep uh TAHY tuhs BEE)
Bloodborne viral disease that affects the liver; transmitted by blood exposure, sexual contact, sharing needles, or from infected mother to infant.

vaccine
(vak SEEN)
Harmless form of a pathogen that helps the body develop immunity to a disease.

hepatitis C (HVC)
(hep uh TAHY tuhs SEE)
Bloodborne viral disease that affects the liver; transmitted by blood exposure, sharing needles, or from infected mother to infant; rarely transmitted by sexual contact.

human immunodeficiency virus (HIV)
(HYOO man i MYOO noe dih FIHSH uhn see VAHY ruhs)
Virus that infects cells of the immune system, reducing the immune system's ability to fight disease; transmitted by blood exposure, sexual contact, sharing needles, or from infected mother to infant.

Types of Bloodborne Illnesses

Sometimes, pathogens are transmitted through contact with blood, body fluids contaminated with blood, semen, or vaginal secretions. These pathogens are called **bloodborne** pathogens. In the health care setting, you may be exposed to the following three bloodborne pathogens:

- **Hepatitis B (HBV)**: Hepatitis B is a viral disease that attacks the liver. It causes scarring of the liver and liver cancer and can eventually lead to death. There is no cure for HBV, but health care personnel should receive a **vaccine** against the disease. (Figure 17.7)
- **Hepatitis C (HCV)**: Like HBV, HCV is a virus that attacks the liver, causing many of the same problems as HBV does. The HBV vaccine may help prevent HCV infection, but there is no vaccine for HCV.
- **Human immunodeficiency virus (HIV)**: HIV is a viral disease that attacks the immune system. It breaks down the body's immune defenses, making it easier for other infections to occur. HIV does not kill a patient, but it weakens the immune system so much that the patient may die from an opportunistic infection. HIV causes **acquired immunodeficiency syndrome (AIDS)**.

498 Chapter 17 | Controlling Infection

Teaching Tips

- Explain bloodborne pathogens.
- Differentiate between bloodborne pathogens and other types of pathogens.

ACTIVITY

Make flashcards to use as study aids for the vocabulary terms in Section 17.4.

Transmission of Bloodborne Diseases

In the health care setting, bloodborne diseases are rarely passed between caregiver and patient. However, the risk is still present, so precautions should be taken. Direct contact with infected blood and blood-contaminated body fluids can introduce a bloodborne disease. The following accidents may result in bloodborne disease infection:

- Accidental needlesticks: Puncture wounds from needles contaminated with diseased blood.
- Cuts from sharp instruments: Cuts from sharp instruments that have been in contact with infected blood.
- Direct contact with infected blood: Infected blood comes in contact with the eyes, nose, mouth, or skin.

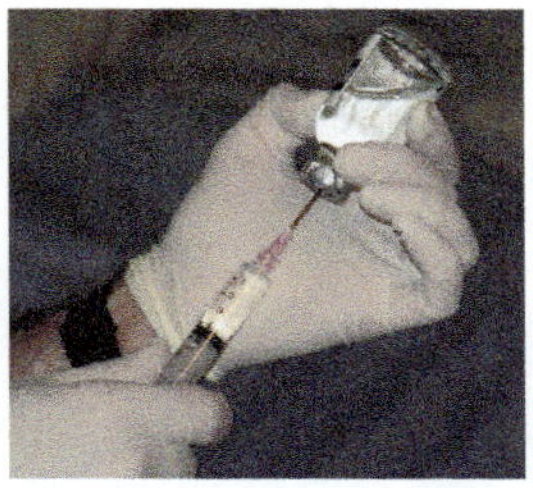

Figure 17.7 Vaccines prevent diseases such as HBV. Who should be vaccinated against HBV?

acquired immunodeficiency syndrome (AIDS) (uh KWAHY uhrd i myoo noh dih FIHSH uhn see SIHN droem) Late stages of HIV infection; characterized by secondary infections.

Bloodborne diseases are sometimes passed from an infected mother to her infant. In the past, these diseases were transmitted to people through blood transfusions and organ donations from infected donors. New testing methods have made this mode of infection rare.

Bloodborne diseases are **not** spread through casual contact, hugging, or kissing. Additionally, they cannot be spread by food or water, sharing utensils and dishes, coughing, or sneezing.

At-Risk Behaviors

Some behaviors put people at greater risk of contracting a bloodborne disease. Those behaviors include the following:

- Unprotected sex, including oral sex
- Sharing needles to inject illegal drugs

Each of these behaviors puts people in contact with blood, semen, or vaginal fluids, all of which can carry bloodborne pathogens. (A notable exception is HCV, which is rarely spread through sexual contact. Instead, HCV is spread by transmitted by blood-to-blood contact, such as unsterilized injection equipment or infusion of inadequately screened blood and blood products.)

Universal Precautions

As a health care worker, you should follow Standard Precautions in dealing with patients. Additionally, you should use **Universal Precautions** to prevent the transmission of bloodborne diseases. Universal Precautions are similar to Standard Precautions. You should avoid direct contact with blood, vaginal secretions, semen, pericardial fluid, amniotic fluid, peritoneal fluid, interstitial fluid, and pleural fluid. You do not need to take Universal Precautions for feces, nasal secretions, sputum, sweat, tears, urine, vomit, or saliva unless it is contaminated with blood.

Universal Precautions (yoo nuh VER suhl pree KAHW shuhns) A set of precautions that prevents the transmission of HIV, HBV, HCV, and other bloodborne pathogens when providing health care.

Controlling Infection | Chapter 17 499

Teaching Tips

- Emphasize the three types of bloodborne pathogens that are common in hospitals and other healthcare facilities:
  - Hepatitis B (HBV)
  - Hepatitis C (HCV)
  - Human Immunodeficiency Virus (HIV)
- Emphasize that there is a vaccine that protects against HBV.
- Describe the transmission methods of bloodborne diseases:
  - Accidental needlesticks
  - Cuts from sharp instruments
  - Direct contact with infected blood
- Emphasize that bloodborne diseases are rarely passed from patient to caregiver.
- Emphasize how bloodborne diseases are NOT transmitted:
  - Casual contact, hugging, kissing
  - In food or water
  - Sharing utensils or dishes
  - Coughing or sneezing
- Discuss at-risk behavior.

Figure Focus

17.7 Vaccines prevent diseases such as HBV. Who should be vaccinated against HBV?

Answer: All health care workers should be vaccinated against HBV.

TEAMWORK

In small groups, plan and create an educational handout about the ways bloodborne diseases are and are not transmitted. The handout could be a brochure, flyer, or poster. Make the handout available to students at your school in the nurse's office, or at an event such as back-to-school night.

Teaching Tips

- Explain Universal Precautions: A set of precautions that prevents the transmission of HIV, HBV, HCV, and other bloodborne pathogens.
- Describe the protective equipment required by Universal Precautions:
  - Gloves
  - Gowns
  - Aprons
  - Masks
  - Protective eyewear
  - Resuscitation equipment that prevents the spread of pathogens
- Emphasize the need to avoid injuries caused by contaminated sharps, and contact with contaminated surfaces.
- Discuss testing for bloodborne diseases.
- Discuss legal and ethical issues surrounding bloodborne diseases.
- Emphasize confidentiality.

Figure Focus

17.8 Personal protective clothing and gear includes gloves, masks, earplugs, and goggles.

Emphasize the importance of using protective clothing and gear.

CAUTION: You should always wear gloves when handling body fluids to prevent the spread of diseases, both bloodborne and not.

Universal Precautions require the use of the following protective equipment (**Figure 17.8**):

- Gloves
- Gowns
- Aprons
- Masks
- Protective eyewear
- Resuscitation equipment that prevents the spread of pathogens

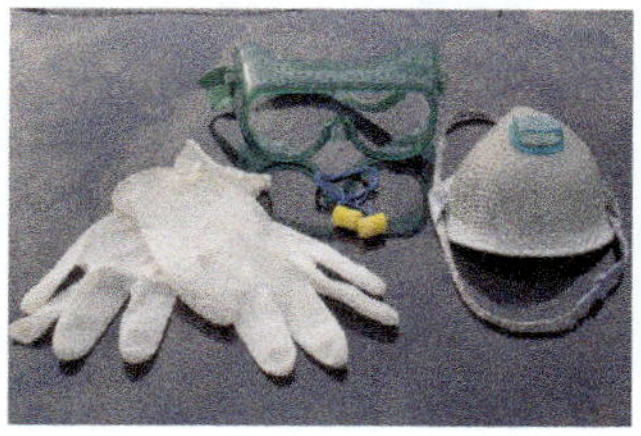

Figure 17.8
Personal protective gear includes gloves, masks, earplugs, and goggles.

Under Universal Precautions, you should also take steps to avoid injuries caused by contaminated scalpels, needles, and other sharp instruments. Surfaces and equipment that come in contact with infected blood should be sterilized using a bleach solution or as dictated by facility guidelines.

Testing for Bloodborne Diseases

There are some external symptoms of HBV and HCV infections, such as jaundiced (yellowed) skin. However, HIV infection may not have external symptoms. A blood test can confirm the presence of any of these three diseases. A false positive is possible, so multiple tests are required to verify infection.

As a health care worker, your facility likely has a routine blood testing procedure in place. You will need to undergo regular blood testing. If you are exposed to infected blood, you likely will need to be tested more often.

Ethical and Legal Issues

As a health care worker, your employer has certain obligations to keep you safe. The employer should provide protective equipment at all times. Your employer should also have practices in place that reduce your risk of exposure. You should also be vaccinated with the HBV vaccine.

If you are exposed to a bloodborne disease, your employer should offer management and treatment for the disease. Exposure, whether you contract the disease or not, will be recorded in your confidential medical records. It may be reported to government agencies for disease tracking and research purposes. Regardless, your personal information will remain private.

500 Chapter 17 | Controlling Infection

ACTIVITY

Make a chart or table listing the protective equipment required by Universal Precautions. Include information about how the equipment protects the caregiver.

People who have a bloodborne disease, including health care workers, have certain legal rights. A health care facility must maintain a patient's confidentiality. Participation in any treatment and testing must be voluntary. A facility should also offer adequate information, support, and referrals to help an infected individual and his or her family understand the disease and its treatment. Depending on state and federal laws, a health care facility must report bloodborne diseases and make an effort to warn other people who are at risk in a confidential manner.

Personal Wellness

What to Do After Exposure to Bloodborne Pathogens

Imagine that you are exposed to blood during work. Do you know what to do? You should first take theses steps:

- Wash accidental needlesticks and cuts with soap and water.
- If your nose, mouth, or skin is exposed, flush the affected area with water.
- If your eyes are exposed, flush with water, saline, or other sterile solutions as mandated by your facility.
- Always report the exposure to your manager. You will need to discuss the exposure with your facility's exposure management department to evaluate your risks and post-exposure treatment.

Post-exposure treatment depends on the type of exposure. Because health care workers are given the HBV vaccine, the risk of infection is low. Workers should be tested within a couple months of vaccination to make sure immunity is complete. Hepatitis B immune globulin and/or the HBV vaccine can be given after exposure to prevent infection. Treatment should start within 24 hours of exposure. Because postexposure treatment is usually effective, routine follow-up is not recommended unless there are symptoms.

For HCV, there is no vaccine. Also, there is no postexposure medical treatment. So, preventative measures are important in the case of HCV. However, the incidence of HCV infection after exposure is relatively low when compared to HBV. A person who is exposed to HCV should be tested immediately after exposure and 4 to 6 months after exposure to see if he or she is infected.

As with HCV, although under investigation and research, there is currently no vaccine for HIV. The use of antiretroviral drugs after exposure has been shown to reduce the transmission of HIV. However, these drugs have serious side effects, so they are not used unless exposure is significant. Treatment should start as soon as possible. A person exposed to HIV should be tested for the virus as soon as possible after exposure. Testing should be repeated at 6 months and then again at one year.

Compare the postexposure treatments for HBV, HCV, and HIV.

Personal Wellness—What to Do After Exposure to Bloodborne Pathogens

- Emphasize that there is no need for panic.
- Review the steps for cleaning accidental needlesticks or other cuts caused by sharp instruments.
- Review the steps for flushing nose, mouth, or skin with water.
- Review the steps for flushing eyes, as directed by the facility.
- If possible, demonstrate these procedures.
- Discuss testing procedures and timetables.

Compare the postexposure treatments for HBV, HCV, and HIV.

Answer: HBV is treated with immunoglobulin and the HBV vaccine. HCV cannot be treated. HIV may be treated with antiretroviral drugs, depending on the type of exposure.

CUSTOMIZED INSTRUCTION

More Advanced Students

Assign more advanced students to research the history of HIV and AIDS, including information about how attitudes and care have changed over the years.

Language Arts Link—Employers and Safety Standards

- Review the correct formatting of a business letter.
- Show examples.
- Allow students to handwrite the letters, or to use a word processing program.
- Students may be creative in terms of the names of people and facilities, but remind them to use facts and examples of situations that really could occur.
- Remind them to include suggestions for improvements.
- Encourage peer review by having students exchange letters for critique and editing.
- Evaluate the letters based on proper formatting, spelling, grammar, and content.

Teaching Tips

- Review the types of diseases that are transmitted by bloodborne pathogens.
- Review the ways bloodborne pathogens may be transmitted.
- Review the types of behavior that increases risk.
- Review the equipment and behavior required by Universal Precautions.

Language Arts Link

Employers and Safety Standards

Imagine that you work for a company that disposes of medical waste. You are well aware that much of medical waste is highly toxic. You are concerned that your employer is not taking proper precautions for the safety of the employees and for those living in the surrounding community.

Write a letter to the manager in charge of safety standards. Develop the topic thoroughly by citing the most significant specific examples and relevant facts. Gather relevant information from authoritative print and digital sources. Offer several suggestions to correct the problem using precise examples and citing sources for the information you gathered to create your suggestions.

Check the spelling and grammar and correct any errors. When you've completed your letter, exchange it with a classmate. Provide feedback on your classmate's letter, and then exchange back. Read your classmate's comments and revise your letter as necessary.

Summary

Bloodborne diseases include HBV, HCV, and HIV. These diseases are rarely passed between a patient and caregiver, but they still pose a significant risk. A caregiver must follow not only Standard Precautions, but also Universal Precautions. Universal Precautions reduce exposure to blood and blood-contaminated fluids, thus reducing exposure to bloodborne diseases. Additionally, a health care facility is obligated to provide protection and confidentiality to both its patients and its employees.

Section 17.4 Review Questions

1. List three bloodborne diseases.
2. What is a vaccine?
3. In the health care setting, how are bloodborne diseases passed from one person to another?
4. What two risky behaviors increase the risk of contracting a bloodborne disease?
5. What are six pieces of equipment used in Universal Precautions?
6. What legal rights are afforded to health care workers who have a bloodborne disease?

502 Chapter 17 | Controlling Infection

Section 17.4 Review Questions

1. Answer: Hepatitis B, Hepatitis C, and HIV
2. Answer: A vaccine is a harmless form of a pathogen that helps the body develop immunity to a disease.
3. Answer: Accidental needle sticks, cuts from sharp instruments that have been in contact with infected blood, and direct contact with infected blood
4. Answer: Unprotected sex, including oral sex, and sharing needles to inject illegal drugs
5. Answer: Gloves, gowns, aprons, masks, protective eyewear, resuscitation equipment that prevents the spread of pathogens
6. Answer: If you are exposed to a bloodborne disease, your employer should also offer management and treatment for the disease. Exposure, whether you contract the disease or not, will be recorded in your confidential medical records. Your personal information will remain private.

TEAMWORK

In small groups, prepare a skit demonstrating how a caregiver might be exposed to a bloodborne pathogen, and what steps should be taken in case of exposure.

CHAPTER 17 REVIEW

Chapter Review Questions

1. What is the difference between generalized and localized infections? (17.1)
2. As a health care worker, what preventative measures can you take to avoid contracting microorganisms that are airborne? (17.1)
3. What does the practice of aseptic techniques prevent? (17.2)
4. List some examples of items that require sterilization. (17.2)
5. Why is it important to dry your hands completely after washing them? (17.2)
6. What transmission-based guidelines should a health care worker take when working with a patient that has tuberculosis? (17.3)
7. Why is it important for health care workers to provide time and frequent communication to patients that are placed in special precaution rooms or separated from other patients and staff? (17.3)
8. List three types of accidents that could result in bloodborne disease infection. (17.4)
9. Explain Universal Precautions. (17.4)
10. What are an employer's obligations to keep employees safe? (17.4)

Activities

1. Create a table similar to the one below in order to interpret technical material. In the table, describe three bloodborne diseases, their effects, how they are treated, what personal protective equipment the health care worker should use, and how a health care worker should respond to exposure. Use this table to create a pamphlet to educate health care workers about bloodborne diseases.
2. Imagine that you are writing questions for a quiz show. Write ten questions that relate to Standard Precautions, Transmission-Based Precautions, and Universal Precautions. After writing your questions, test them out on your classmates to see how well they work.

Pathogen	Description of Infection	Treatment	Appropriate PPE	Postexposure response
1.				
2.				
3.				

Case Studies

1. Patients in restricted Transmission-Based Precautions feel isolated and locked away from everyday life. Mrs. Grey was just admitted for a tuberculosis infection. Her condition requires her to be in Transmission-Based Airborne Precautions. Write a plan describing how you will explain these protocols to your patient. Include details about how you will identify and satisfy her special needs.
2. One of your coworkers accidentally cuts her hand with a scalpel after treating a patient who has HCV. How should your coworker respond to the cut?

Controlling Infection | Chapter 17 503

CHAPTER 17 REVIEW

Chapter Review Questions

1. Answer: Generalized infections affect all of the body. A patient may experience headache, fatigue, fever, vomiting, and diarrhea. A localized infection affects one area of the body. A patient will see or feel redness, swelling, heat, or drainage.
2. Answer: Wash hands before entering the room; wash hands before leaving the room; wash hands after leaving the room; and wear a gown, mask, and gloves when with the patient.
3. Answer: Aseptic techniques are used to make the environment, the worker, and the patient as germ-free as possible.
4. Answers will vary but might include: floors, walls, tables, patient care equipment, toilets.
5. Answer: Reddened and chapped hands easily leave open areas that can become infected.
6. Answer: Wash hands before entering the room; wash hands before leaving the room; wash hands after leaving the room; and wear respiratory protection.
7. Answer: Patients in isolation or precaution rooms feel separated and may experience anger, frustration, and depression.
8. Answer: Accidental needlesticks, cuts from sharp instruments that have been in contact with infected blood, and direct contact with infected blood.
9. Answer: Universal Precautions prevent the transmission of bloodborne diseases. Universal Precautions are similar to Standard Precautions. You should avoid direct contact with blood, vaginal secretions, semen, pericardial fluid, amniotic fluid, peritoneal fluid, interstitial fluid, and pleural fluid. You do not need to take Universal Precautions for feces, nasal secretions, sputum, sweat, tears, urine, vomit, or saliva unless it is contaminated with blood.
10. Answer: Employers should provide protective equipment at all times, have practices in place that reduce your risk of exposure, and offer HBV vaccine.

Activities

1. Direct students to first set up the table on paper or using a computer program. You may want to allow students to work in small groups to create the brochure.
2. Encourage students to include questions related to all types of precautions. You might want to allow class time to play a quiz-show game using the students' questions.

Case Studies

1. Direct students to Section 17.3 for more information on Transmission-Based Precautions. In addition to writing a specific and detailed plan, you may want to allow students to present skits demonstrating their responses to this situation.
2. Direct students to Section 17.4 for information on postexposure procedures. In addition to writing a specific and detailed plan, you may want to allow students to present skits demonstrating their responses to this situation.

TEAMWORK

Divide the class into teams of five to seven students. You name a disease. Each team confers and writes down the correct type of precautions that should be used when treating patients with the disease. Award a point to each team that answers correctly.

Thinking Critically

1. Encourage students to describe the specific patient they are addressing, including age, culture, etc. Remind students of the importance of using appropriate communication techniques.
2. Review the importance of patient education. Remind students of the importance of using appropriate communication techniques.
3. Encourage students to write a complete essay, including a thesis statement supported by facts and real-life examples.

CHAPTER 17 REVIEW

Thinking Critically

1. **Communication**—Write a half-page scenario describing how you would explain to a patient the precautionary measures taken daily to control infection in the health care environment. Think in simple terms, such as replacing handkerchiefs with disposable tissues.
2. **Patient Education**—A patient in a Transmission-Based Precaution room requests fresh water immediately after you have cleaned her wound. After you wash your hands and return to get the water jug it becomes clear from her distressed silence that she is offended. Think of ways to talk to her about asepsis and passing on infection so that she understands that this is not a personal matter.
3. **Computers**—Advances in medicine are continually changing the way health care workers protect themselves and treat infections. Explain how computers help keep the medical community informed about the latest medical progress. Describe ways you can access this information if you do not own a computer.

Portfolio Connection

The medical community is constantly finding new information about how microorganisms affect our lives. This constant flow of new information makes it necessary to research how new findings affect us. Conduct your own research and write a paper about a microorganism. Select a microorganism from those mentioned in this chapter or from another source. Explain how the microorganism affects society and describe its shape, size, color, and pattern of growth. Describe its nature (aerobic or anaerobic), its effect on the body, and the physical symptoms it causes.

Contact a local hospital or the County Health Department infection control manager. Develop questions to ask during the interview that will provide insight into the greatest infectious health risks in the hospital or community and find out why the risk is so high. Write a report and place it in the section of your portfolio labeled "Written Reports and Assignments."

PORTFOLIO TIP

Health care levels of cleanliness may be more demanding than some households. Patients are not necessarily dirty when noncompliant and must not be shamed. It is important to show patients and their families respect in all situations.

Role-play with a classmate and record for your portfolio the rationales you would give two patients. One patient wants to bathe morning and night while the other patient prefers bathing only once a week. Without quoting facility policy, how would you explain to each patient what the acceptable levels of hygiene are and the reasons for them?

504 Chapter 17 | Controlling Infection

Portfolio Connection

- For the first activity, direct students to write a complete research paper, including source information.
- You may want to provide a list of microorganisms, as well as a list of Web sites and printed resources.
- Encourage students to include pictures to illustrate the report.
- For the second activity, if it is not possible for a professional to visit, encourage students to make contact and conduct an interview by phone or e-mail.
- Remind students to proofread and revise their work.
- Encourage students to use peer review to find ways to improve the documents.
- Check to make sure that students have completed the assignments and added them to their portfolio.

18 Patient and Employee Safety

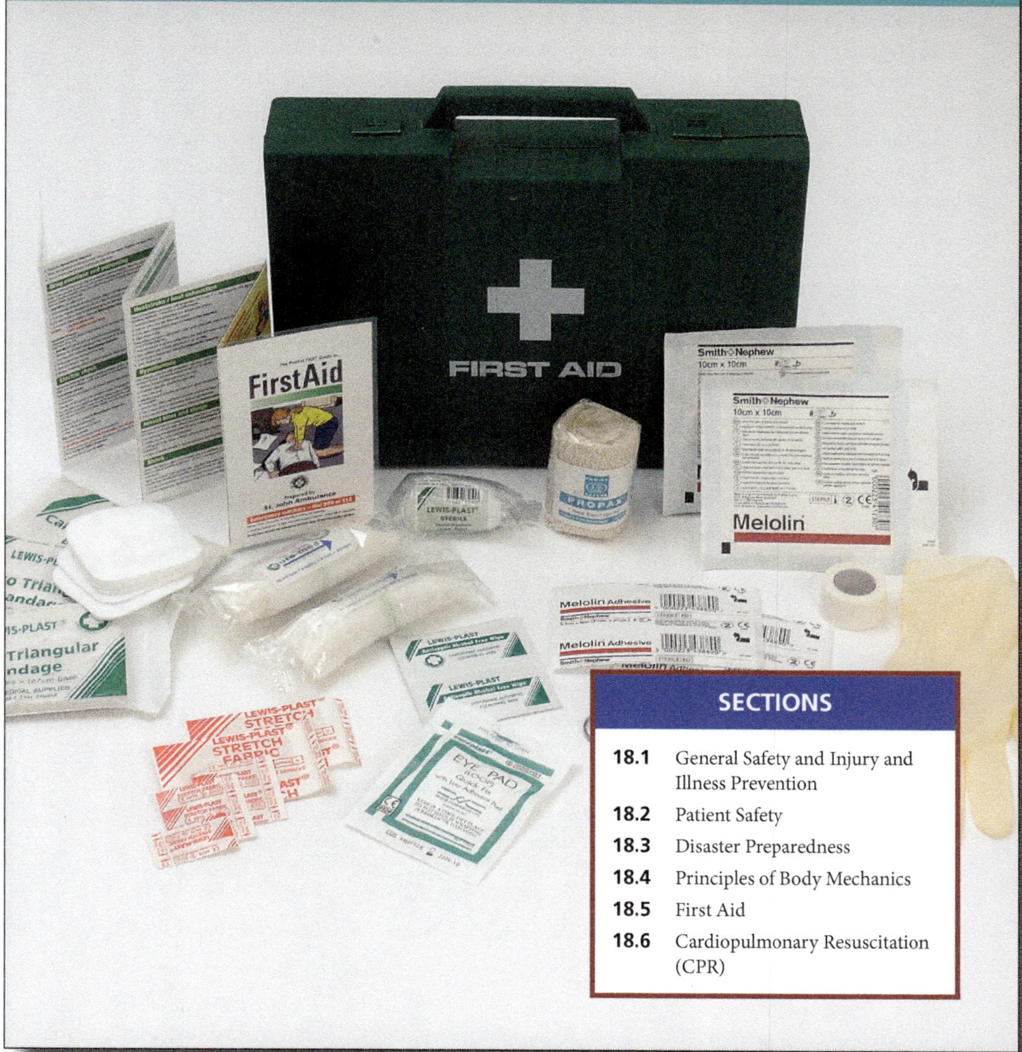

SECTIONS

18.1	General Safety and Injury and Illness Prevention
18.2	Patient Safety
18.3	Disaster Preparedness
18.4	Principles of Body Mechanics
18.5	First Aid
18.6	Cardiopulmonary Resuscitation (CPR)

CHAPTER 18 OVERVIEW

Chapter 18 reviews methods of preparing for and reacting to emergency situations.

Section 18.1: The first section discusses OSHA standards and reviews the responsibilities of both employers and employees in creating a safe work environment.

Section 18.2: This section covers procedures for ensuring the safety of patients. It reviews proper procedures for using ambulation devices, transporting devices, postural supports, and side rails, and reinforces the importance of safety measures.

Section 18.3: This section addresses plans for disaster response and fire prevention. It also summarizes safety requirements and equipment.

Section 18.4: This section presents principles of body mechanics and relates these principles to methods of avoiding injury.

Section 18.5: This section introduces several life-saving first aid skills and discusses situations in which each would be required.

Section 18.6: The final section summarizes the steps of cardiopulmonary resuscitation (CPR).

Advance Preparation	
Review	■ Chapter text for Sections 18.1, 18.2, 18.3, 18.4, 18.5, and 18.6; and chapter procedures.
Contact	■ Local hospital, clinic, and elementary schools to arrange visits. ■ Guest speakers to discuss specific topics and perform demonstrations.
Prepare	■ A list of volunteer, government, and other health agency Web sites—such as redcross.org (American Red Cross) and npsf.org (National Patient Safety Foundation).

FOCUS AND ENGAGE

Getting Started

- Divide students into teams of eight and instruct them to create the index cards as described.
- Show the students how the game is played by using an example condition such as diabetes or a heart attack.
- Play the game with the students.

Introduce the Section

a. Have students prepare the index cards described in the Getting Started feature. Set the cards aside until you complete the chapter.

b. Review the content of the Background paragraphs, explaining the importance of OSHA and its role in maintaining safety.

c. Point out that both employers and employees are responsible for establishing a safe work environment.

d. Discuss the objectives for the section.

Vocabulary Review

a. Direct students to the key terms.

b. Pronounce each word, and have the students repeat the pronunciation out loud.

c. Discuss the definition of each word.

Getting Started

Your teacher will present information on several conditions that requires immediate and temporary care. At the end of the lesson, your teacher will divide the class into teams of eight students. Each team will prepare a set of 3 × 5 cards of the alphabet; five cards for each vowel (five of letter A, five of letter E, etc.) and three cards for each consonant (three of letter B, three of letter C, three of letter D, etc.).

The teacher will begin reading signs and symptoms that may require immediate and temporary care. As each team identifies the condition being described, they use the cards to correctly spell the condition. So, if a student thinks they know the answer, they would pick the first letter. Once the team agrees that they've guessed the correct answer, they complete the word and raise their hands. The teacher keeps score for the first team to identify and correctly spell the condition being described.

SECTION 18.1 General Safety and Injury and Illness Prevention

Background

A health care worker is responsible for maintaining a safe environment for him- or herself, for co-workers, and, most importantly, for patients. You must know your employer's policies and procedures and be able to respond quickly to workplace incidents. Your employer is also obligated to maintain safety policies, ongoing training, and to supply protective equipment.

The Occupational Safety and Health Administration (OSHA) of the U.S. Department of Labor determines, develops, and monitors safe practices for each industry. If you or your employer fails to provide appropriate safety for all, OSHA will penalize your employer with a large fine or lock the doors of the facility until the safety violation is corrected. If you are at fault for not providing safe conditions, you could lose your job.

Objectives

When you have completed this section, you will be able to do the following:

- Match key terms to their correct meanings.
- Define *OSHA* and explain the agency's role in safety.
- Differentiate between IIPP, hazard communication, and exposure control.
- Name places to find information about hazards in a facility.

506 Chapter 18 | Patient and Employee Safety

CUSTOMIZED INSTRUCTION
Less Advanced Students
Provide additional time for less advanced students to learn the vocabulary.

CUSTOMIZED INSTRUCTION OVERVIEW	
Less Advanced Students	Pages 506, 508, 516, 519, 521, 523, 540, 541, 552, 556, 559, 565
More Advanced Students	Pages 509, 517, 523, 531, 534, 538, 547, 550, 555, 558, 559, 567
English Language Learners	Pages 507, 532
Special Needs Students	Pages 507, 511, 519, 522, 527, 538, 542, 551, 557, 566
At-Risk Students	Page 513

- Explain the health care worker's role in maintaining a safe workplace.
- Discuss the employer's role in maintaining a safe workplace.
- Identify general safety rules.
- Summarize the importance of safety in a health care environment.

OSHA Standards

The Occupational Safety and Health Administration (OSHA) is part of the U.S. Department of Labor. OSHA establishes the guidelines for a safe work environment for all employers and their employees. The OSHA standards say that employees have the "right to know" what hazards are present in their environment.

OSHA regulations require employers to train and offer immunizations to high-risk employees in the first 10 days of a new job. A committed partnership between the employer and employee is necessary to provide a safe environment for everyone. This section explains the areas with which health care agencies and facilities must **comply**. They are the:

- Ergonomic Program
- Injury and Illness Prevention Program
- Hazard Communication Program
- Exposure Control Plan

comply
(kum PLAHY)
To follow directions, do what you are asked to do.

Ergonomic Program

Employers are changing the work environment to meet the expected OSHA **ergonomic** standards. You spend a large portion of your day in the work environment. You should be comfortable, use good posture, and learn exercises to prevent getting stiff and sore.

ergonomic
(erg uh NOM ik)
An object or practice designed to reduce injury.

The safety officer where you work will help you adjust your environment to accomplish this. If you sit in a workstation during the day, your chair, desk, and computer must be adjusted to fit your needs. If patients need to be lifted and moved in your workplace, there should be procedures and equipment in place to facilitate lifts and movements.

You should get into the routine of stretching frequently during the day if you sit at a work station. Stretching and other simple exercises can reduce the risk of injury due to repetitive activities. The following exercises can reduce eyestrain, headaches, and tension in your back, neck, shoulders, and wrists:

1. **Deep Breathing.** Close your eyes. Inhale deeply and slowly through your nose. Exhale slowly through your mouth. Repeat at least four times.
2. **Changing Focus.** Look up from your computer screen and focus your eyes on a distant object. Look back at an object that is close and allow your eyes to focus on it. Repeat this exercise four times.

Patient and Employee Safety | Chapter 18 507

TEACH

Teaching Tips

- Ask students to define OSHA as the Occupational Safety and Health Administration.
- Explain that OSHA establishes and monitors safety in the work environment.
- Tell students that OSHA standards define employer and employee responsibilities.
- Let students know that OSHA has the power to levy large fines or to close a facility in which OSHA standards are not being met.
- Explain OSHA's Ergonomic Program.

Reinforce and Review

- Remind students that they have been learning safety rules with all of the procedures they have encountered.
- Ask volunteers to recall some examples of safe practices when working with patients.

CUSTOMIZED INSTRUCTION

Special Needs Students

Have students demonstrate each of the seven exercises presented in the text. Ask a volunteer to lead the demonstration of each exercise. Tell students to follow along for only those exercises that they can do comfortably.

After they have completed the exercises, ask students to discuss how these brief activities made them feel. Encourage them to consider how stretching can increase their health and well-being in a work environment.

You may wish to play relaxing or soothing music. Extend the discussion to consider the role of music in relaxation and workplace safety.

CUSTOMIZED INSTRUCTION

English Language Learners

Have students write each key term and its pronunciation on one side of an index card and its definition on the other side. Have them read each term and definition aloud to a partner.

Teaching Tips

- Explain that the IIPP mandates that employers implement a safety program.
- Stress the fact that safety is everyone's responsibility. Employees should not rely upon or blame employers, but employers should provide a safe work environment.

Discuss

- Ask students to discuss why an IIPP is important.
- Ask students to give examples of good or poor safety in the health care environment.

ACTIVITY

Find out how to report an injury or illness during work hours at a specific facility and what documentation to complete.

3. **Arm and Hand Shake.** Drop your arms and hands to your side and let them relax. Shake your relaxed hands for a few seconds. Then shake your hands and arms.
4. **Finger Stretch.** Grab the edge of your desk with your palms down and your thumb below the edge. Press down for a few seconds. Then press up for a few seconds. Turn your hands upside-down, so palms are facing up and your four fingers are below the edge. Repeat the exercise.
5. **Ankle Stretch.** Sit upright in your chair. Rotate both feet to the right, so that your ankles are stretched. Then rotate both feet to the left.
6. **Body Stretch.** Lock your hands behind your head. Lean back in your chair and arch your back.
7. **Shoulder Shrug.** Bring your shoulders up to your ears and try to press your shoulders and ears together. Hold for a few seconds. Let go of your shoulders and allow them to drop. Repeat four times.

Injury and Illness Prevention Program

mandates
(MAN dayts)
Orders or commands.

implement
(IM pluh ment)
To carry out a rule or procedure.

The Injury and Illness Prevention Program (IIPP) **mandates** that every employer establish, **implement**, and maintain an effective IIPP.

As a student or employee, you are responsible for:

- Knowing who is responsible in the facility for the IIPP.
- Practicing policies and procedures that ensure safe and healthy work practices.
- Understanding the communication system used to keep you informed of hazards.
- Knowing what hazards are present and how to prevent injury from them.
- Knowing to whom to report an injury or illness during work hours and what documentation to complete.
- Knowing where the safety bulletin board (or communication book) is in your facility. You are responsible for reading all items posted each month.

Your school or employer will test you for signs of tuberculosis (TB). Exposure to tuberculosis is determined by a TB skin test. If your TB test indicates exposure, additional tests will be necessary. You will also be offered hepatitis B vaccine, which protects you from getting hepatitis B while working in the health care environment.

Hazard Communication Program

The Hazard Communication Program mandates that employers inform employees of:

- Chemicals or hazards in the environment
- Where chemicals or hazards are stored and used
- How to interpret chemical labels and hazard signs
- Methods and equipment for cleaning chemical spills
- Personal protection equipment and its storage location
- The hazard communication system

508 Chapter 18 | Patient and Employee Safety

CUSTOMIZED INSTRUCTION

Less Advanced Students

Have students research tuberculosis and hepatitis B. Ask them to report to the class on these diseases, why they pose a hazard in health care environments, and how they can be prevented or treated.

As a student or employee, you are responsible for knowing:

- What chemicals or hazards are in your work area
- Where the chemicals or hazards are stored or used
- Waste management and recycling protocols
- How to read and interpret container signs and labels
- What to do when a chemical or **biohazard** spills
- What personal protective equipment (PPE) to wear when working with or around chemicals and biohazards
- Your facility's system for informing you of hazards in the work area

Apply It

Being able to read and understand safety signs, symbols, and labels is an essential skill at school, on the job, and at home. Working with a partner, research laboratory safety symbols or other types of safety signs and symbols. Create a poster that illustrates these. Display the posters in the classroom.

biohazard
(BAYH o haz uhrd)
Biological materials or infectious agents that may cause harm to human, animal, or environmental health.

Hazard Categories

The way that harm is caused determines the hazard category:

- *Chemical hazards* cause harm when a chemical is mixed with another chemical, causing a reaction. When a chemical reacts with another substance or because of temperature change, it creates a new chemical. For example: Chlorine bleach mixed with ammonia creates a harmful (even deadly) gas called chloramines.
- *Health hazards* have the potential to harm a healthy body. For example, acid burns and destroys skin.

Science Link

Biohazardous Material

Biohazardous materials are defined as biological materials or infectious agents that may cause harm to human, animal, or environmental health. Viruses that cause disease (such as the human immunodeficiency virus, or HIV) are biohazards. So are disease-causing bacteria (such as *E. coli*).

Plant toxins, allergens (such as pollen), and snake venom are biological agents that may cause disease, so they may be classified as biohazards. Certain types of recombinant DNA may also be classified as biohazards. This is DNA that has the potential to harm plants or animals if it escapes into the environment.

Viruses, bacteria, and other biohazardous material can be spread by blood or other body fluids. Therefore, care must be taken to minimize patient and health care worker exposure to body fluids. Any equipment that is used on a patient must be sterilized before it is used on any other patient. Health care professionals must wear gloves, protective clothing, and (in some cases) masks when working with patients. Needles must be used carefully and discarded in a designated container after use.

Any clothes or linens exposed to blood or other body fluids must be stored in properly labeled biohazard containers until they can be washed. Drawn blood must be transported carefully and stored in labeled safety cabinets or containers.

OSHA has developed procedures for the proper handling and disposal of biohazardous materials. These procedures must be followed in every health care facility, for the safety of patients, visitors, and staff.

What is the difference between a biohazard and a chemical hazard?

Design a poster display of the various methods for reducing the impacts of the use of biohazardous materials in the health care environment.

Patient and Employee Safety | Chapter 18 509

Teaching Tips

- Review the Hazard Communication Program.

Science Link—Biohazardous Material

- Write the word biohazard on the board. Point out that the word contains the prefix bio-. Tell students that this prefix means "life." Ask students to relate the prefix to the word. Lead them to conclude that it means dangers related to living things or materials from living things.
- The United States Centers for Disease Control and Prevention (CDC) categorizes biohazards into four levels. Ask students to conduct research on the Internet or using other sources to identify these levels. Have them share their findings with the class. Verify that the information is correct.
- Allow students to discuss locations in which they may have seen the biohazardous material symbol.

CUSTOMIZED INSTRUCTION

More Advanced Students

Ask students to investigate the transport of biohazardous materials. The shipment of hazardous materials is regulated by the U.S. Department of Transportation (DOT) and the International Air Transport Association (IATA). Tell students to find out information such as whether biohazardous materials can be shipped, how they must be transported, who can ship them, and why such laws are in effect.

Teaching Tips

- Differentiate between chemical and health hazards.
- Explain material safety data sheet (MSDS) communication.
- Review the information that must be presented by the Hazard Communication Program.

Apply It

- You may want to contact the environmental services technician or a custodian to facilitate this project.
- Students may also make posters or a slide presentation illustrating what they have learned.

TEAMWORK

Have the class work together to create a safety bulletin board. Students should list the information discussed in class in a clear and accessible manner.

Material Safety Data Sheets (MSDSs)/ Safety Data Sheets (SDS)

Product manufacturers prepare material safety data sheet (MSDS) forms to provide the information needed to handle chemicals safely. Employers must make the MSDSs available to employees. **Figure 18.1** identifies the type of information discussed on the MSDS.

The Hazard Communication Program explains how the employer plans to keep people safe when chemicals are present. The communication system must explain:

- What hazards are present and where they are stored and used
- What precautions to take when hazardous products are present. These precautions include:
  - Wearing appropriate personal protective equipment (PPE)
  - Proper room ventilation
  - Keeping flammable products away from flames or other heat sources
- How to use potentially hazardous products safely
- Proper cleanup and disposal of hazardous products
- First aid if exposure occurs
- How to label containers with a chemical, by always including:
  - Product name
  - Chemicals in the product
  - Precautions for use of the product

As a student or employee you are responsible for knowing where hazard communications are kept and how to access them. You find hazard information on manufacturer's literature. You may receive memorandums from your employer alerting you to new hazards in the environment. Most facilities keep hazard communications:

- In safety policy and procedure manuals
- In material safety data sheet (MSDS) books
- On the safety bulletin board
- On product labels
- On signs

Apply It

While at school, ask to meet with the environmental services technician or a custodian, and interview him or her regarding the types of hazardous chemicals that are on site. Ask if you can see the material data safety sheets, also known as safety data sheets. Ask what the most common hazards are at your school and what safety policies and procedures does the school use to keep you and everyone else safe. Report your findings back to the class.

510 Chapter 18 | Patient and Employee Safety

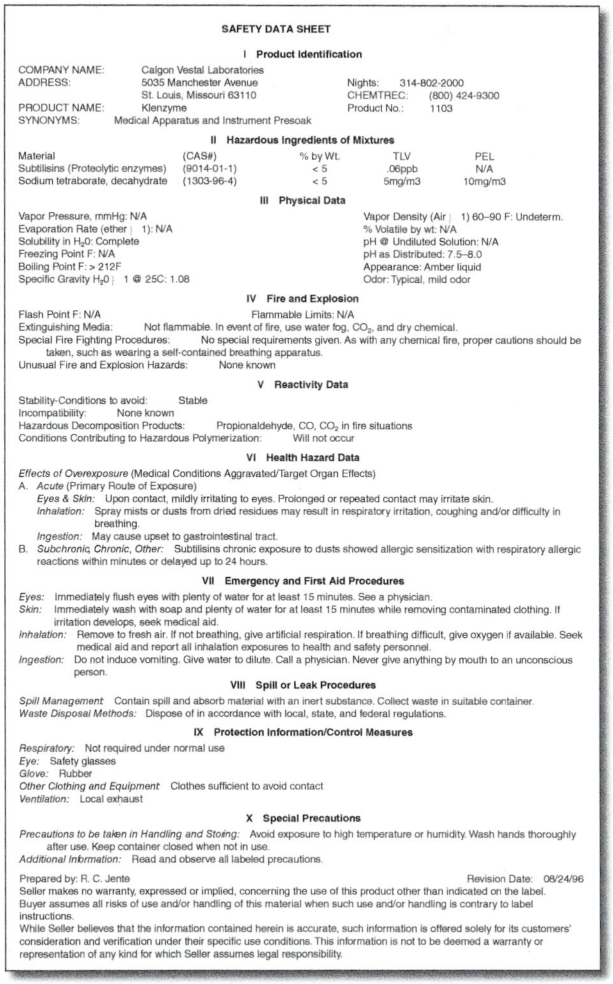

SAFETY DATA SHEET

I Product Identification

COMPANY NAME: Calgon Vestal Laboratories
ADDRESS: 5035 Manchester Avenue, St. Louis, Missouri 63110
Nights: 314-802-2000
CHEMTREC: (800) 424-9300
PRODUCT NAME: Klenzyme
Product No.: 1103
SYNONYMS: Medical Apparatus and Instrument Presoak

II Hazardous Ingredients of Mixtures

Material	(CAS#)	% by Wt.	TLV	PEL
Subtilisins (Proteolytic enzymes)	(9014-01-1)	< 5	.06ppb	N/A
Sodium tetraborate, decahydrate	(1303-96-4)	< 5	5mg/m3	10mg/m3

III Physical Data

Vapor Pressure, mmHg: N/A
Evaporation Rate (ether 1): N/A
Solubility in H_2O: Complete
Freezing Point F: N/A
Boiling Point F: > 212F
Specific Gravity H_2O 1 @ 25C: 1.08
Vapor Density (Air 1) 60–90 F: Undeterm.
% Volatile by wt: N/A
pH @ Undiluted Solution: N/A
pH as Distributed: 7.5–8.0
Appearance: Amber liquid
Odor: Typical, mild odor

IV Fire and Explosion

Flash Point F: N/A
Flammable Limits: N/A
Extinguishing Media: Not flammable. In event of fire, use water fog, CO_2, and dry chemical.
Special Fire Fighting Procedures: No special requirements given. As with any chemical fire, proper cautions should be taken, such as wearing a self-contained breathing apparatus.
Unusual Fire and Explosion Hazards: None known

V Reactivity Data

Stability-Conditions to avoid: Stable
Incompatibility: None known
Hazardous Decomposition Products: Propionaldehyde, CO, CO_2 in fire situations
Conditions Contributing to Hazardous Polymerization: Will not occur

VI Health Hazard Data

Effects of Overexposure (Medical Conditions Aggravated/Target Organ Effects)
A. *Acute* (Primary Route of Exposure)
Eyes & Skin: Upon contact, mildly irritating to eyes. Prolonged or repeated contact may irritate skin.
Inhalation: Spray mists or dusts from dried residues may result in respiratory irritation, coughing and/or difficulty in breathing.
Ingestion: May cause upset to gastrointestinal tract.
B. *Subchronic, Chronic, Other:* Subtilisins chronic exposure to dusts showed allergic sensitization with respiratory allergic reactions within minutes or delayed up to 24 hours.

VII Emergency and First Aid Procedures

Eyes: Immediately flush eyes with plenty of water for at least 15 minutes. See a physician.
Skin: Immediately wash with soap and plenty of water for at least 15 minutes while removing contaminated clothing. If irritation develops, seek medical aid.
Inhalation: Remove to fresh air. If not breathing, give artificial respiration. If breathing difficult, give oxygen if available. Seek medical aid and report all inhalation exposures to health and safety personnel.
Ingestion: Do not induce vomiting. Give water to dilute. Call a physician. Never give anything by mouth to an unconscious person.

VIII Spill or Leak Procedures

Spill Management Contain spill and absorb material with an inert substance. Collect waste in suitable container.
Waste Disposal Methods: Dispose of in accordance with local, state, and federal regulations.

IX Protection Information/Control Measures

Respiratory: Not required under normal use
Eye: Safety glasses
Glove: Rubber
Other Clothing and Equipment Clothes sufficient to avoid contact
Ventilation: Local exhaust

X Special Precautions

Precautions to be taken in Handling and Storing: Avoid exposure to high temperature or humidity. Wash hands thoroughly after use. Keep container closed when not in use.
Additional Information: Read and observe all labeled precautions.

Prepared by: R. C. Jente
Revision Date: 08/24/96
Seller makes no warranty, expressed or implied, concerning the use of this product other than indicated on the label. Buyer assumes all risks of use and/or handling of this material when such use and/or handling is contrary to label instructions.
While Seller believes that the information contained herein is accurate, such information is offered solely for its customers' consideration and verification under their specific use conditions. This information is not to be deemed a warranty or representation of any kind for which Seller assumes legal responsibility.

Figure 18.1
Example of a Safety Data Sheet form. Which portions of the Safety Data Sheet form may be most useful for health professionals?

Figure Focus

18.1 Example of a Safety Data Sheet form. Which portions of the MSDS form may be most useful for health professionals?

Answer: Health hazard data and the emergency and first aid procedures

Teaching Tips

- Direct students to the figure. Point out that not all MSDSs look the same, but the information required is mandated.

CUSTOMIZED INSTRUCTION

Special Needs Students

If students are intimidated by the MSDS, walk them through the information presented. Explain that they can still learn from the sheet, even if they are unfamiliar with some terms on it. Encourage them to summarize the information they can pick out of the sheet.

What's New?—Green Cleaning

- Have students interview two or three people about their opinions of eco-friendly products at home. As a class, discuss whether people are concerned about the cleaning ability of the products or are eager to switch to a safer product. Select volunteers to relate opinions (right or wrong) to the widespread use of the product.
- Ask students to compare the labels of an ecofriendly product and a traditional product. They may have the products at home or they can compare them in the aisle of a grocery or hardware store. Have them report on the different types of ingredients and warnings between the two products.

What additional benefits can you see in the use of eco-friendly products?

Student answers will vary, but may include that green products may be better for people with allergies to strong chemicals.

Discuss

- Begin a class discussion by asking: Why are all these controls necessary?
- Ask: Do you think they protect everyone?

TEAMWORK

Have the class, or groups within the class, work together to create an advertisement for eco-friendly cleaners. Tell them to be creative as they highlight the benefits of such products.

What's New?

Green Cleaning

Most traditional cleaning supplies, even the mildest of them, come with warnings. They may cause blindness, vomiting, or even death if swallowed. Although they are effective cleaners, they seem to be an odd choice to use around extremely sick people. At least that's the thinking that has inspired some institutions to search for green cleaning supplies and other eco-friendly products. These products, which are made from natural resources, are often far safer for use around people and have a lower impact on the environment.

Green cleaning goes beyond just using natural products. It sometimes also means using less of the chemicals that have always been used. Frequently, we simply use more cleaners than we need for a particular job. For instance, new ways of cleaning using microfibers can reduce the need for chemicals. Microfiber mops require less water, and less chemical cleaners, than do traditional cotton mops.

In the past, many facilities have stayed away from green products because they thought they would be more costly. Green products do not have to be more expensive, particularly when all costs are taken into account. Government agencies closely regulate many toxic chemicals. With green products, there are fewer toxic chemicals to track, which cuts regulatory costs and results in fewer injuries due to chemical accidents.

While green cleaning is not yet widespread, more and more institutions are beginning to see its advantages. Look for even more hospitals and environmental services departments to begin considering green cleaning in the future.

What additional benefits can you see in the use of eco-friendly products?

Exposure Control Plan

An exposure control plan provides steps to reduce employee or student exposure to bloodborne pathogens. The plan includes the following:

- Determining the possibility of exposure under each position description
- Developing a schedule and method for ensuring that the plan is enforced
- Postexposure evaluation

General Safety

Hospitals and other healthcare settings can present numerous safety risks to patients, visitors, and healthcare staff. To be a safe worker and to protect everyone, learn the rules listed here:

- **Take a moment to assess each space you enter for safety risks.** Check for spills and leaks that could present a slipping hazard. Make sure any essential equipment is working correctly. Check for objects such as furniture that may be blocking travel paths. Ensure that all medications and controlled substances are secured.
- **Walk! Never run in hallways.** If you run, you may fall and injure yourself. You can collide with another person or object. You can injure someone else, or you might create panic.

What's New?

Safety Equipment

Some health care institutions are providing new safety equipment designed to keep health professionals safe. Respirators filter air to keep health care workers safe from SARS, influenza, and other contagious diseases that are spread when infected patients cough or sneeze.

Needle safety devices and personal protective gear help to reduce the risk of being stuck by a needle. A needle stick doesn't just hurt. It can spread bloodborne pathogens, such as HIV, from infected patients.

Needle safety devices either provide built-in needle shields or containers that separate the needle from the syringe right after blood is drawn. Puncture-resistant finger or arm guards also help to eliminate needle sticks.

Most facilities are now using needleless systems. Although it may be impossible to remove all use of needles from health care facilities, the use of needleless systems for intravenous fluid systems and covered needle systems for any necessary needle use has decreased the incidence of needle stick injuries. There is no longer any need to recap needles.

Why is it important to handle needles safely?

- **Walk on the right-hand side of the hall not more than two abreast.** It is important to leave hallways open so that there are no traffic jams. In an emergency, a traffic jam can cause a delay and mean the difference between life and death.
- **Use handrails when using the stairs.** This prevents falling and injuring yourself.
- **Watch out for swinging doors.** Be certain that someone is not on the other side of a swinging door. You might injure yourself or someone else.
- **Horseplay is not tolerated.** It is disturbing to others, may lead to accidents, causes confusion, and shows a lack of respect for patients and personnel.

abreast
(a BREST)
Side by side.

horseplay
(HAWS play)
Rowdy behavior; acting inappropriately in a work environment.

Community

Create a poster that provides safety information pertinent to a local afterschool center or program. Review the safety tips with the program participants. Ask if they have any other suggestions and add them to the poster with credit to person who suggested the idea.

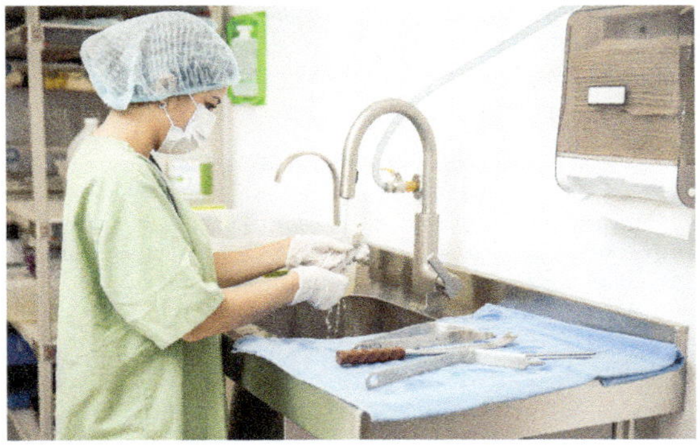

Figure 18.2
Safety is everyone's responsibility. Why is this so important?

Patient and Employee Safety | Chapter 18 513

CUSTOMIZED INSTRUCTION

At-Risk Students

Ask students to consider the general safety of their neighborhoods. Do they include sidewalks and green space? Are lawns well-kept and litter-free? Are streets and walkways well-lit? Are traffic and pedestrian signs clearly visible? They should prepare a list of guidelines they think would contribute to the general safety and security of a neighborhood and make suggestions on how to improve the safety and security of their own neighborhoods.

What's New?—Safety Equipment

- Explain that a respirator is a device that is worn over the mouth and nose. It consists of filters that trap incoming dust, debris, and other particles in the air. It may also use a mechanical or chemical cartridge that purifies the air before it reaches the nose and mouth.
- Ask students to research needleless systems. Challenge them to find out how they are used and for what types of situations they can be used. Students may use research materials, such as on the Internet, or they might speak with employees at a local health care facility.

Why is it important to handle needles safely?

Discuss answers to the question. Make sure students recognize that being pricked by a needle can pose life-threatening dangers.

Teaching Tips

- Discuss each of the general safety rules and explain why each one is important.

Figure Focus

18.2 Safety is everyone's responsibility. Why is this so important?

Student answers will vary.

Community

- In advance, tell students to bring in materials to make a poster, such as poster board, markers, and stickers.
- Allow students to draw pictures or cut them out from magazines.
- Encourage students to be both accurate and creative with their posters.

Teaching Tips

- Ask volunteers to discuss any bad experiences they may have had with a swinging door. They are sources of more injuries than may be expected.
- A swinging door should be approached slowly in case it is being opened from the other side. It should also be pushed slowly so as to avoid someone on the other side.
- If a swinging door is readily available, have pairs of students demonstrate the proper technique for approaching a swinging door.

Emergency Codes

- Discuss emergency terms and codes and their purposes.
- Have students explain emergency codes with which they are familiar.
- Compare and contrast the codes that students explain.
- Emphasize that codes and terms vary in different settings.

Apply It

- You may want to contact local elementary schools in advance to gain permission.
- Students may need to visit the school in small groups at different times or different days so as not to provide a distraction.
- Encourage students to note how the behavior of the students changes with their ages and how adults must supervise younger children more carefully than older ones.

Apply It

Pretend you are a school "hall monitor." Make a list of all of the dangerous actions/activities/situations you see during a day at school. Then, go to the local elementary school and conduct the same activity with an elementary school partner. Can the younger students identify potentially dangerous situations?

frayed
(frayd)
Worn or tattered (e.g., electrical cords may be worn, causing wires to be exposed).

shock
(SHAHK)
Convulsion of muscles and extreme stimulation of nerves when an electric current passes through the body.

malfunctioning
(mal fungk shen ing)
Not working as it is supposed to.

Emergency Codes

There are emergency terms that are common to all health care facilities, such as "no code" or "DNR." However, each facility has its own emergency terminology with which employees must be familiar. Many health care facilities combine the word code with other words or numbers to communicate particular kinds of emergencies when calling emergency medical teams to an area of the hospital (e.g., *code zero, code blue*, or *code 99*). It is important that you become familiar with the codes used in your place of work.

- **Always check labels.** Never use anything from containers that are not labeled. Using the wrong contents can cause injury or death to a patient. Using the wrong contents may also damage or ruin equipment.
- **Wipe up spills and place litter in containers.** A wet floor can cause someone to slip and fall. If there is litter on the floor, someone may trip and be seriously injured.
- **Dispose of sharps in designated containers.** Used needles, broken glass, and other sharp objects should be deposited in specially marked safety containers, to minimize injury.
- **Follow instructions carefully.** If you do not understand instructions or do not know how to do a task, always ask for instructions. If you do something incorrectly, you may cause a serious problem.
- **Report any injury to yourself or others to your supervisor immediately.** Reporting an injury ensures treatment for the injured without delay and correction of the potential hazard.
- **Do not use electrical cords that are frayed or damaged.** Frayed or damaged cords can cause shocks, burns, or fire.
- **Report a shock you receive from electrical equipment to your supervisor.** This prevents fire or a shock to someone else.
- **Do not use malfunctioning equipment.** It is dangerous and may cause serious injury to you or someone else.
- **Make sure all medical supplies and equipment are secure.** Sharp instruments, drugs, and chemicals may cause harm if taken by patients or other visitors to the health care facility. Keep these and other supplies in locked drawers or closets, if possible.
- **Follow Standard Precaution guidelines.**
- **Use proper body mechanics.** It is important to use proper body mechanics when lifting, position, or moving patients, such as lifting with your knees, keeping the center of gravity of anything carry close to your own, and keeping your legs spread to maintain a wide base of support.
- **Report unsafe conditions to your supervisor immediately.** Safety is everyone's business. Be aware of your environment. Assess whether there are any unsafe conditions.

Summary

Safety is the responsibility of all health care workers. Employers must inform employees of workplace risks and take steps to minimize those risks. Employees must follow rules and practice safe behavior to minimize risks of injury to themselves, co-workers, and patients. OSHA is very strict about enforcement of regulations that keep the work environment safe.

514 Chapter 18 | Patient and Employee Safety

ACTIVITY

Divide students into teams of two. Have them look for hazardous conditions in the classroom, on campus, or at a healthcare facility. Tell students to list the conditions they find and suggest ways to correct the problems. Bring any hazardous conditions to the attention of someone in charge to make sure they are corrected.

Personal Wellness

Slips, Trips, and Falls

Slipping on wet surfaces, falling, and tripping over obstacles are among the most common injuries suffered by workers. The Occupational Safety and Health Administration (OSHA), a U.S. Department of Labor agency, provides guidelines to help workers avoid some of these accidents. The following are some OSHA recommendations:

- Clean only one half of a hallway or staircase at a time so that staff, visitors, and patients have a dry surface to walk on.
- Clean all spills immediately and thoroughly.
- Keep floors dry and clean. This can be especially important in entry ways when people walk in out of the rain. Put down mats to help reduce slipping. Use warning signs to alert people to slippery floors.
- Do not leave buckets, mops, or other supplies sitting in hallways when they are not in use.
- Use appropriate ladders or step stools to reach hard-to-reach places or to perform maintenance, such as when cleaning light fixtures.
- Use non-skid waxes in toilets and shower areas to reduce slipping.
- Immediately report damaged surfaces, poor or ineffective lighting in halls, stairways, or other areas, and other conditions that can lead to injury.
- Areas that are frequently wet or moist—such as an outside walkway with poor drainage—can become especially slippery due to the growth of mold and fungi. Report such areas to your supervisor. Additionally, keep these areas clean. Use appropriate cleaners to reduce the growth of molds and fungi.
- Wear functional shoes with good grip.

Why are EVS (Environmental Services Technician)/housekeeping workers especially at risk for slipping, tripping, and falling?

Section 18.1 Review Questions

1. What does OSHA do?
2. How does the Hazard Communication Program help employees to stay safe at work?
3. What is an exposure control plan?
4. Name six behaviors that might increase the risk of a workplace injury.
5. Why is it important to use ergonomic equipment?
6. Where can you usually find hazard communications in a health facility?

Patient and Employee Safety | Chapter 18 515

Personal Wellness—Slips, Trips, and Falls

- Ask students if anyone has ever slipped on a wet floor. Discuss the fact that friction is reduced when a floor is wet. This can make the surface very slippery.
- Discuss the types of shoes worn by health care professionals. If possible, inspect the bottoms of a few examples of shoes. Note that they are often made of rubber to provide a grip on the floor. They also often have grooves in them through which water can pass while allowing part of the shoe to retain a good grip.

Why are EVS (Environmental Services Technician)/housekeeping workers especially at risk for slipping,tripping, and falling?

Discuss answers to the question. Help students recognize that these workers spend more time in situations with wet floors, spills, and cleaning supplies and therefore are in greater danger of related accidents.

Section 18.1 Review Questions

1. Answer: OSHA establishes the guidelines for a safe work environment for all employers and their employees.
2. Answer: The Hazard Communication Program mandates that employers inform employees of: Chemicals or hazards in the environment; where chemicals or hazards are stored and used; how to interpret chemical labels and hazard signs; methods and equipment for cleaning chemical spills; personal protection equipment and its storage location; and the hazard communication system.
3. Answer: An exposure control plan provides steps to reduce employee or student exposure to bloodborne pathogens. The plan includes the following: determining the possibility of exposure under each position description, developing a schedule and method for ensuring that the plan is enforced, and postexposure evaluation.
4. Answer: Running in hallways; walking on the left-hand side of the hall and more than two abreast; not using handrails when using the stairs; not watching out for swinging doors; horseplaying; not checking labels; not wiping up spills and not placing litter in containers; not disposing of sharps in designated containers; not following instructions carefully; not immediately reporting injury to yourself or others to your supervisors; using electrical cords that are frayed or damaged; not reporting a shock you receive from electrical equipment to your supervisor; using malfunctioning equipment; not making sure all medical supplies and equipment are secure; not reporting unsafe conditions to your supervisor immediately; and not following Standard Precaution guidelines.

5. Answer: Ergonomic equipment is designed to reduce injury, and while working you should be comfortable, use good posture, and learn exercises to prevent getting stiff and sore.
6. Answer: In safety policy and procedure manuals; in material safety data sheet (MSDS) books; on the safety bulletin board; on product label; and on signs

FOCUS AND ENGAGE

Introduce the Section

a. Review the content of the Background paragraph, highlighting each topic that will be covered.

b. Point out that many accidents involving patients can be avoided by following procedures properly.

c. Discuss the objectives for the section.

Vocabulary Review

a. Direct students to the key terms.

b. Pronounce each word, and have the students repeat the pronunciation out loud.

c. Discuss the definition of each word.

ACTIVITY

Have students research patient safety at the Joint Commission's Web site (jointcommission.com) and download the latest National Patient Safety Goals (NPSGs). Allow time for students to have a round-table discussion about how they will meet those goals as health care workers. Encourage students to consider patient safety as they move through Chapter 18.

SECTION 18.2 Patient Safety

Background

Health care workers are responsible for the safety of patients. If you do not follow Standard Precautions and basic safety precautions, patients can be seriously injured. Accidents involving patients are reduced if simple safety measures are followed. In this section, we explain rules to follow when using ambulation devices, transporting devices, postural supports, and side rails.

Objectives

When you have completed this section, you will be able to do the following:

- Match key terms with their correct meaning.
- Explain how to use ambulation devices, transporting devices, postural supports, and side rails safely.
- Match descriptions and principles associated with ambulation devices, transporting devices, postural supports, and side rails.
- Explain the importance of safety measures.
- Follow safe practice guidelines when caring for patients.

Identifying the Patient

When you work directly with a patient, you must identify him or her to avoid a mistake. Errors are avoided if you follow these *important* steps:

- Check with the nurse's station for the right room number.
- Check the requisition or physician's order, which has the patient's name on it, against the patient's identification band.
- In ambulatory care, confirm chart name and information with each patient.

Ambulation Devices

ambulation devices (am byoo LAY shun duh VYS iz) Canes, crutches, walkers, or other equipment that help a patient to walk.

Ambulation devices are devices used to assist in walking. The most common devices in the health care setting are canes, crutches, and walkers. These devices give the patient additional support and aid in balancing while walking or standing.

516 Chapter 18 | Patient and Employee Safety

CUSTOMIZED INSTRUCTION

Less Advanced Students

Provide additional time for less advanced students to learn the vocabulary.

Safe Practice Guidelines When Using Ambulation Devices

It is essential that all devices be in good condition, because patients depend on these items:

- Devices must always be structurally safe, without dents or cracks. For example, wooden crutches are unsafe if the wood is split or cracked. A loose joint in a walker allows it to wobble or break, and the patient can fall.
- Areas touching the ground must be covered with rubber tips to prevent slipping.
- The devices must always be clean and free of blood or body fluids.

Transporting Devices

Transporting devices include equipment used to move patients from one place to another. The most common transporting devices are wheelchairs and **gurneys**. Gurneys and wheelchairs make it easy to move patients who are unable to walk. Follow these basic principles to ensure the patient's safety. (Figure 18.3)

gurney
(GUR nee)
A stretcher on wheels.

Safe Practice Guidelines When Using Gurneys and Wheelchairs

- Always lock the brakes except when you are moving.
- Back a wheelchair over indented or raised doorways, such as an elevator or any ridges on the floor.
- Always back a patient in a wheelchair or a gurney down a hill.
- Always secure straps or put side rails up on a gurney.
- Lock brakes when moving the patient on or off a gurney.
- Always back the patient on a gurney headfirst into an elevator.
- Never leave a patient on a gurney unattended.
- Always keep the gurney free of blood and body fluids.

Postural Supports

Postural supports are devices that **restrict** a patient's movement. This type of restriction is necessary only when the patient's safety is in jeopardy. Occasionally, patients become disoriented due to a change of environment or as a response to medication. When this occurs, postural supports are used to keep patients safe.

Postural supports are more common in long-term care facilities. *Example:* A confused patient may not realize that he is too weak to walk to the bathroom without falling. Use a postural support to remind patients to call for assistance when they need to get out of bed. There are many types of supports. The most common are vest supports, wrist supports, and ankle supports. When you use postural supports, certain **principles** must be observed.

postural supports
(POS chuh ruhl suh PORTS)
Soft restraints used to protect residents.

restrict
(ree STRIKT)
To keep within limits; to confine.

principles
(PRIN suh puhl)
Codes of behavior.

Patient and Employee Safety | Chapter 18 517

TEACH

Discuss

- As a class, discuss the importance of identifying the patient.
- Have students consider dangers of making a mistake. For example, a patient who should not be moved might be moved, or treatment might be given to the wrong patient.

Teaching Tips

- Define different types of ambulation devices and their use.
- Define different types of transporting devices and their use.
- Discuss precautions when using ambulation and transporting devices.

ACTIVITY

Arrange for a physical therapist to be a guest speaker. Ask the speaker to demonstrate the use of ambulation devices and transporting devices. Have students practice what the speaker has demonstrated.

CUSTOMIZED INSTRUCTION

More Advanced Students

Have students research the prefix of the word *ambulatory*. Challenge students to identify and define other words with this prefix.

Figure Focus

18.3 How should you move a patient in a gurney or wheelchair down a hill?

Review each part of the figure. Discuss the question. Make sure students realize that a patient should be backed down a hill when using a wheelchair or gurney.

TEAMWORK

Arrange to have a wheelchair in the classroom. Have students work together to identify all of the parts of the device. Ask volunteers to demonstrate such activities as how to lock and unlock the breaks or how to fold and unfold the chair. Then, have pairs of students work together to demonstrate how to transport a patient using the wheelchair.

Figure 18.3
Principles in the use of gurneys and wheelchairs. How should you move a patient in a gurney or wheelchair down a hill?

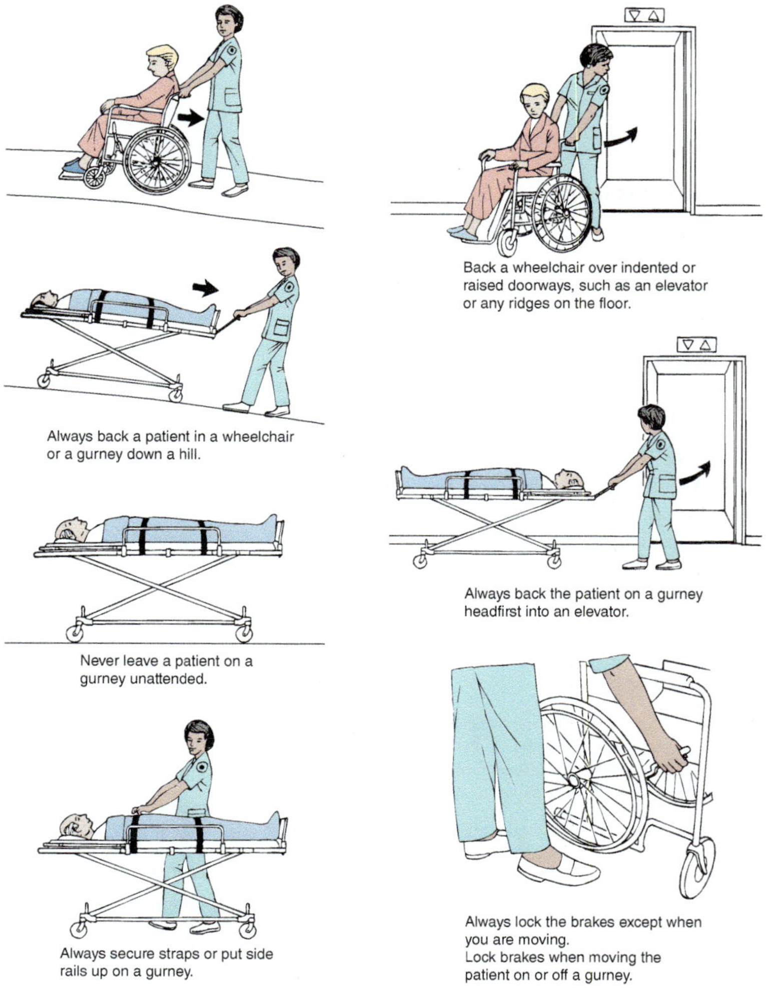

518 Chapter 18 | Patient and Employee Safety

Safe Practice Guidelines When Using Postural Supports

- A physician's order is required by law.
- Never use a postural support on a patient in a chair or bed without wheels.
- Patients requiring postural supports must be checked frequently. The support must be released or loosened every two hours.
- Use a half-bow knot to secure the support.
- Leave at least two fingers' ease between the patient's skin and the support so his or her circulation is not restricted.
- Never secure supports to side rails; always attach to the framework of a bed or gurney.
- Secure the half-bow knot out of the patient's reach.
- Discard supports that have touched blood or body fluids, following Standard Precautions.
- Always try alternative methods of supporting patients before applying physical restraints.
- Postural supports are of valid use when a patient is at high risk of injuring self or others, such as in the procedure or operating room, while undergoing conscious or unconscious sedation, when moving could cause significant injury.
- Follow the guidelines under your facilities restraint policy and procedure.

Side Rails

Side rails are not to be used as a restraint. Research has shown that the use of side rails as a restraining device can actually increase the risk of falls and injuries from falls. Placing a side rail up with the intent of securing a confused patient will only increase the probability of a patient becoming caught in a side rail or falling from an even greater height.

There have been incidents where a patient has become caught and severely injured from the use of side rails with the intent to restrain. Half side rails may be used to facilitate the use of bed controls or turning by the patient.

Safe Practice Guidelines When Using Side Rails

- A form releasing the facility of responsibility must be completed if a patient and/or family requests the use of full side rails.
- Side rails must be locked securely if used. Patients may lean on the rail for support and fall, if not secured.
- Precautions must be taken when side rails are put up or down. Tubing and the patient's legs and arms must be away from the rail.
- Side rails should always be clean and free of body fluids.

Patient and Employee Safety | Chapter 18 519

ACTIVITY

Demonstrate tying a half-bow knot. Then, have students practice tying half-bow knots. You may wish to refer students to the procedures in Chapter 19.

Teaching Tips

- Discuss the use of postural supports.
- Emphasize that there must be a physician's order to use them.
- Explain that they must be absolutely the only alternative to keep the patient safe.
- Stress that the supports must be loosened and released at least every two hours.
- Explain the importance of side rails.
- Review safe practice guidelines when using side rails.

CUSTOMIZED INSTRUCTION

Less Advanced Students

Have students make a diagram comparing examples of ambulation devices, transporting devices, postural supports, and side rails to make sure they know the differences among them.

Special Needs Students

Some students may benefit from a demonstration of these devices. Gather materials to demonstrate the use of postural supports. Allow student volunteers to be involved in the demonstrations.

Section 18.2 Review Questions

1. Answer: Transporting devices are equipment used to move patients from one place to another including wheelchairs and gurneys.
2. Answer: Ambulation means walking.
3. Answer: Postural supports are used to restrict a patient's movement and are used when the patient is danger of hurting themselves.
4. Answer: If a patient is in a wheelchair, back the wheelchair in; if the patient is on a gurney, back the patient headfirst into the elevator.
5. Answer: A form releasing the facility of responsibility must be completed if a patient and/or family requests the use of full side rails; side rails must be locked securely if used; precautions must be taken when side rails are put up or down; tubing and the patient's legs and arms must be away from the rail; side rails should always be clean and free of body fluids; half side rails may be used to facilitate the use of bed controls or turning by the patient; side rails should not be used a method of restraint.
6. Answer: Always lock the brakes except when you are moving; back a wheelchair over indented or raised doorways; always back a patient in a wheelchair or a gurney down a hill; always secure straps or put side rails up on a gurney; lock brakes when moving the patient on or off a gurney; always back the patient on a gurney headfirst into an elevator; never leave a patient on a gurney unattended; always keep the gurney free of blood and body fluids.

Summary

By following each of the simple principles discussed in this section, you provide safe conditions for your patients. You have learned to identify the patient to prevent errors and to keep your patients safe when using ambulation devices, transporting devices, postural supports, and side rails.

Section 18.2 Review Questions

1. What are transporting devices?
2. What does *ambulation* mean?
3. Under what circumstances might postural supports be used?
4. How would you move a patient in a transporting device onto an elevator?
5. What are the safe practice guidelines for using side rails?
6. What are the safe practice guidelines when using gurneys and wheelchairs?

SECTION 18.3 Disaster Preparedness

Background

Disasters can occur anywhere and at any moment. As a health care worker, you are expected to respond quickly according to your agency disaster plan. You must be familiar with the practices that are detailed in that plan and be able to follow them if a disaster occurs.

A disaster is anything that causes damage and injury to a group of people. Examples are flood, earthquake, tornado, explosion, fire, and bioterrorism. Be alert to emergency equipment, exits, and the disaster plan. They provide the essentials necessary to respond effectively to a disaster.

Be particularly aware of instructions in the disaster plan telling you how to cooperate with first responders, police and fire personnel, and disaster-specific instructions from local, state, and federal officials.

Objectives

When you have completed this section, you will be able to do the following:

- Match key terms with their correct meaning.
- Identify what you are responsible for knowing and doing when a disaster occurs.
- List the three elements required to start a fire.
- Explain four ways to prevent fires.
- Summarize all safety requirements that protect the employee/student, patient, and employer.

520 Chapter 18 | Patient and Employee Safety

FOCUS AND ENGAGE

Introduce the Section

a. Review the content of the Background paragraphs, defining a disaster and relating it to the role of a health care worker.
b. Tell students that health care workers need to know how to interact with local, state, and federal officials as well as first responders.
c. Discuss the objectives for the section.

Vocabulary

a. Direct students to the key terms.
b. Pronounce each word, and have the students repeat the pronunciation aloud.
c. Discuss the definition of each word.

ACTIVITY

To help students recognize safety procedures and policies, have them research accident prevention methods and disaster plans of the local school district. Allow time for students to discuss and describe methods and plans.

Disaster Plan

Your facility is required to have a disaster plan. You are responsible for knowing the plan and responding when a disaster occurs. To be prepared for any type of disaster you need to know the following:

- The floor plan of your facility
- The nearest exit route
- The location of alarms and fire extinguishers
- How to use alarms and fire extinguishers
- Your role as a health care worker when a disaster occurs

The following are some basic rules to remember when a disaster strikes:

- Assess the situation; count to 10 to calm yourself.
- Be sure that you are not in danger. (Placing yourself in danger only makes the situation worse.)
- Remove those who are in immediate danger, if it is safe to do so.
- Notify others of the emergency according to facility policy.
- Use stairs, *not* the elevator.

Fire Causes and Prevention

Fire is often the result of a disaster. It is your responsibility to be alert to causes of fire and act to prevent fire when possible. There are three elements that must be present before a fire can start:

- Oxygen
- Heat
- Fuel

Most fires can be prevented if everyone is **observant** and careful. The following are some ways you can help prevent fires:

- Smoking is restricted to **designated** outdoor areas.
- Monitor garbage containers.
- Check electrical equipment for proper functioning and frayed electrical cord. If there is any problem, report it immediately. (Figure 18.4)
- When using **flammable** liquids, take only the amount needed to complete the task. You would spill only the amount you poured, not the whole container.
- Keep flammable liquids in a container approved by the Underwriters' Laboratories.

observant
(ob ZUR vent)
Quick to see and understand.

designated
(DEZ ig nay ted)
Chosen for a specific purpose.

flammable
(FLAM uh buhl)
Catches fire easily or burns quickly.

Patient and Employee Safety | Chapter 18 521

TEACH

Teaching Tips

- Tell students that every facility must have a disaster plan and must have disaster drills.
- Review the basic rules to remember during a disaster.
- Make sure students understand that heat and oxygen can cause a flammable material to burn.
- If possible, show students a frayed electrical cord. Discuss the dangers of using such cords.
- Then, discuss ways that fires can be prevented.

ACTIVITY

Have students draw a floor plan of the classroom and nearby section of the facility. Tell them to mark exits, alarms, and fire extinguisher locations.

TEAMWORK

Divide students into small groups. Identify places in the room for each group where there is an imaginary fire. Have students work together to explain in writing how they would react to the fire. Have each group report to the class.

CUSTOMIZED INSTRUCTION

Less Advanced Students

Provide additional time for less advanced students to learn the vocabulary.

Figure Focus

18.4 Why is an overloaded power strip a potential hazard?

Answer: An overloaded power strip can result in failure or fire.

Teaching Tips

- Describe a fire extinguisher
- Assign Procedure 18.1.

Procedure Tip

18.1 How to Operate a Fire Extinguisher

- Review the background information, discussing the importance of safety inspections and fire drills.
- Discuss the preprocedure.
- Explain the acronym RACE.
- Explain the difference between the different classes of fire extinguishers.
- Review the procedure steps.

PROCEDURE PRACTICE

- Demonstrate the steps for Procedure 18.1, How to Operate a Fire Extinguisher, as many times as necessary, or ask students to demonstrate the steps. Have students practice and perform the procedure until they are competent.

Figure 18.4
Why is an overloaded power strip a potential hazard?

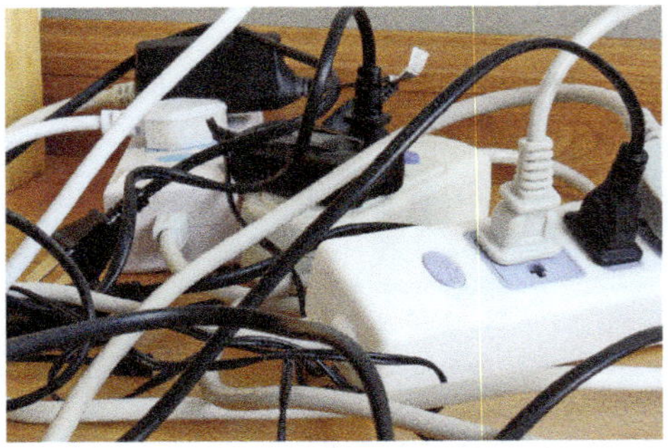

Procedure 18.1 How to Operate a Fire Extinguisher

BACKGROUND: Health care facilities are required by law to establish safety boards and to inspect the facility regularly for any type of potential fire hazard. Equipment must be checked regularly and escape routes must be kept open. Fire drills are performed at specific intervals to assure that the facility and its staff are equipped to handle any fire emergency. Health professionals are educated and tested annually on their knowledge of the procedures for response to a fire and how to remove patients from danger. Fire extinguishers can be used for types A, B, or C fires.

A Trash, wood, or paper
B Liquids
C Electrical equipment
ABC Use on all fires

Preprocedure

1. First Response: RACE
   Rescue
   Alert appropriate facility officials
   Contain Fire
   Extinguish Fire

Procedure

PASS
P Pull the pin.
A Aim the fire extinguisher at the base of the fire.
S Squeeze the handle of the fire extinguisher.
S Sweep from side to side at the base of the fire.

2. Locate fire extinguisher and check type.

NOTE: All personnel should know the location of the closest fire extinguisher to his or her workstation and be trained and ready to use it when necessary.

3. Hold fire extinguisher upright. Pull ring pin.
4. Stand back six to ten feet and direct flow toward base of the fire.
5. Squeeze lever, sweeping side to side.

Postprocedure

6. Replace or have extinguisher recharged after use.

522 Chapter 18 | Patient and Employee Safety

CUSTOMIZED INSTRUCTION

Special Needs Students

Allow students to handle a fire extinguisher. Make sure they know the parts and how it operates.

Classes of Fire Extinguishers

There are four classes of fire extinguishers. Each type extinguishes a different type of fire:

- **Class A** extinguishers are the most common and put out fires in ordinary combustibles, such as wood, paper, cloth, and many plastics. These extinguishers contain pressurized water. Class A extinguishers have a green triangle marking of an "A" and depict a garbage can and wood pile burning.
- **Class B** extinguishers should be used on fires involving flammable liquids, such as grease, gasoline, and oil. These extinguishers contain carbon dioxide. Class B extinguishers have a red square marking of a "B" and depict a gasoline can with a burning puddle.
- **Class C** extinguishers should be used on energized electrical equipment or wiring where the electric non-conductivity of the extinguishing agent is important. These extinguishers contain potassium bicarbonate or potassium chloride. Class C extinguishers have a blue circle marking a "C" and depict an electric plug with burning outlet.
- **Class D** extinguishers are designed for use on combustible metals such as sodium, titanium, and magnesium. These extinguishers contains either sodium chloride or copper powder and are pressurized with nitrogen. Class D extinguishers have a yellow star marking of a "D." There is no picture designator for Class D extinguishers and they are not given a multi-purpose rating for use on other types of fires.

In addition, there is a **Class ABC** extinguisher that can be used on wood, cloth, paper, flammable liquids, gasoline, grease and electrical equipment. A Class ABC fire extinguisher is designed to extinguish Class A, B, and C fires. It contains a graphite type chemical that is irritating to the skin.

Apply It

Partner with a classmate and review the disaster relief plans in local buildings—schools, government offices, libraries, museums, etc.

Compare your results. What are the best features of each plan? Has your school's plan been updated recently? Is there anything you think should change?

Bioterrorism

Everyone must be aware of the dangers of chemical or biological disasters. Facilities have plans to provide for the safety of patients, physicians, staff, and visitors. These plans include shelter-in during a possible exposure.

Shelter-in is a nationally accepted term indicating the need to remain inside of the facility during a potential exposure to chemical and biological hazards. These plans include securing entrances and exits to the building and securing outside air sources. Your responsibility is to learn what your facility plan is and to follow the procedures that are in place.

Patient and Employee Safety | Chapter 18 523

Teaching Tips

- Explain that bioterrorism is another threat for which health care workers need to be prepared.
- Define the term *shelter-in*. Your school may have practice drills for sheltering-in, so students may be familiar with this procedure.

Apply It

- Point out that disaster plans need to be re-evaluated and updated frequently.
- As a class, make a list of the best features of all the plans proposed.
- If possible, review your school's plan to consider situations that the class may have overlooked.

ACTIVITY

Have students research information about Community Emergency Response Team (CERT) at HOSA. The Web site is hosa.org. Allow students to share their finding orally with the class.

CUSTOMIZED INSTRUCTION

Less Advanced Students

Have students make a chart comparing the types of fire extinguishers.

More Advanced Students

While any type of disaster is always possible, have students identify at least one type of disaster that is more specific to where you live. For example, hurricanes are more likely in Florida, earthquakes in California, tornadoes in the Mid-west, and snowstorms in the northern states. Ask students to report any information they find interesting related to this type of threat and preparedness for it.

Language Arts Link—Job Safety

- You may want to provide some resources to the class. Consider suggesting OSHA's Web site: osha.gov.
- You may want to have students draft an outline, story web, or list questions they need to answer to organize their ideas.
- Remind students about your school's Internet policy before having them go online to find information. Emphasize that they should use reputable Web resources, such as sites sponsored by the government or educational institutions.
- Remind them to keep a list of sources to use for a bibliography.
- If students do not have access to the Internet, be sure to direct them to other resources, such as books, periodicals, or videos.
- For evaluation, verify that the information is correct and in the correct order, and you should mark spelling and grammatical errors.

Language Arts Link

Job Safety

Whether you work in a hospital, clinic, paramedic unit, or office, safety is a highly important workplace consideration. The Occupational Safety & Health Administration (OSHA) is a branch of the U.S. Department of Labor, responsible for assuring the safety and health of America's workers.

OSHA sets the standards for on the job safety that every business in the United States is required to follow. In addition, many health care facilities have their own safety standards, and provide education for employees on proper behavior and precautions. They also institute plans and procedures to follow in case of an emergency, including fires and natural disasters.

Evaluate multiple sources of information, presented in diverse formats and media, to determine the primary causes of work-related accidents and injuries in hospitals or other health care facilities. Locate statistics that list the types of injuries such as falls, repetitive stress, or back strains. Include the costs of such accidents in terms of lost productivity, worker's compensation, or insurance claims.

After you've completed the research, create a chart that includes the different statistical data collected. When the chart is completed, create a brochure that the human resource department can distribute to employees. Include suggestions on ways to prevent accidents and notes on the facility's emergency response plans. Use precise language and specific vocabulary for safety practices and facility type.

Summary

potential
(puh TEN chul)
Possible.

Disaster preparedness is everyone's responsibility. Each person is responsible for responding to a disaster and being alert to **potential** hazards.

There are three elements required to start a fire: oxygen, heat, and fuel. There are at least three ways to help prevent fires. These include checking for frayed electrical cords and malfunctioning equipment, careful handling of flammable liquids, and following proper oxygen procedures.

Know the disaster plan of your agency or facility. Move patients to safety if they are in danger. Know where to find the fire extinguishers and which exits to use. Do not use an elevator. Be calm. Do not panic!

Section 18.3 Review Questions

1. Why would you want to be observant during a disaster?
2. What are three ways that you can prevent fires in a health care facility?
3. What should the staff of a health care facility do to ensure their safety and the safety of patients during a possible bioterrorism attack?
4. What are the basic rules to follow during a disaster?
5. When you are working in a health care facility, what do you need to know in order to be prepared for a disaster?
6. What is the generally accepted term indicating the need to remain inside of the facility during a potential exposure to chemical and biological hazards?

524 Chapter 18 | Patient and Employee Safety

Section 18.3 Review Questions

1. Answer: If a disaster occurs, everyone is responsible for responding and to be alert to the potential hazards. As a health care worker, you should know the floor plan of your facility, the nearest exit route, the location of alarms and fire extinguishers, how to use alarms and fire extinguishers, and your role as a health care worker when a disaster occurs.
2. Answer: Restrict smoking to designated outdoor areas; monitor garbage containers; check electrical equipment for proper functioning and frayed electrical cord; when using flammable liquids, take only the amount needed to complete the task; keep flammable liquids in a container approved by the Underwriters' Laboratories.
3. Answer: Staff is responsible for knowing their facility's plan for a bioterrorism attack.
4. Answer: Be alert; assess the situation; count to 10 to calm yourself; be sure that you are not in danger; remove those who are in immediate danger, if it is safe to do so; notify others of the emergency according to facility policy; use stairs, not the elevator.
5. Answer: The floor plan of your facility; the nearest exit route; the location of alarms and fire extinguishers; how to use alarms and fire extinguishers; your role as a health care worker when a disaster occurs
6. Answer: Shelter-in

Principles of Body Mechanics

SECTION 18.4

Background

As a health care worker, you lift, move, and carry many different objects and patients. It is important to use ergonomic practices and proper body mechanics when you are lifting or moving anything. Ergonomic practices prevent both fatigue and injury. If you injure yourself, you then become ineffective in your job. Worker injuries can cost a large facility thousands of dollars each year.

Objectives

When you have completed this section, you will be able to do the following:

- Match key terms with their correct meanings.
- Define *body mechanics.*
- List the rules of correct body mechanics.
- List the principles of body mechanics.
- Demonstrate correct lifting and moving of objects.

Body Mechanics

Health care workers move, lift, and carry all types of equipment and supplies. They also help position or move patients. Moving patients can be particularly hazardous to your back, as the patient may struggle or twist during movement.

Ergonomic practices suggest the use of specialized equipment for moving patients. Special equipment could include wheelchairs, walkers, canes, hydraulic lifts, or gait belts.

Every facility should have gait belts available for use in all patient areas. (Figure 18.5) Gait belts combined with good body mechanics allow the health care worker to safely lift, transfer, and ambulate the heavier and disabled patients with less personal strain or danger of injury.

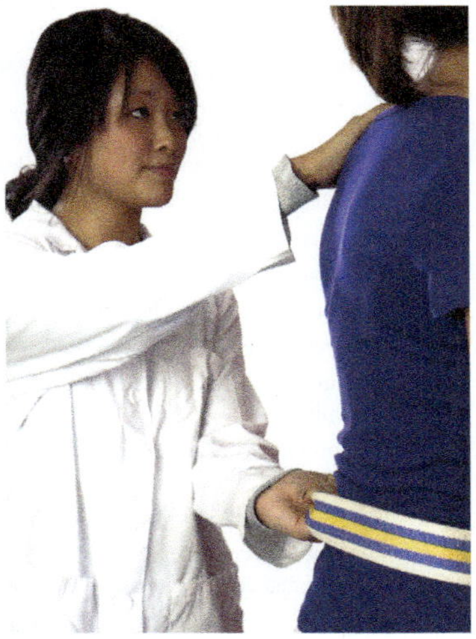

Figure 18.5
The simplest and possibly most effective item for decreasing injuries to both the patient and the health care worker is the gait belt. How can using a gait belt help prevent injuries?

FOCUS AND ENGAGE

Introduce the Section

a. Review the content of the Background paragraph, explaining that one way to avoid injury is to move your body correctly.

b. Discuss the objectives for the section.

Vocabulary Review

a. Direct students to the key terms.

b. Pronounce each word, and have the students repeat the pronunciation out loud.

c. Discuss the definition of each word.

Figure Focus

18.5 The simplest and possibly most effective item for decreasing injuries to both the patient and the health care worker is the gait belt. How can using a gait belt help prevent injuries?

Discuss student answers to the question.

TEACH

Teaching Tips

- Define body mechanics: coordination of body alignment, balance, and movement to prevent injury.
- Review the principles of body mechanics.

Discuss

- Discuss the importance of using correct body mechanics.
- Ask students about experiences they have had lifting heavy objects.
- Help students realize that they can damage their backs if they try to lift a heavy load using back muscles instead of leg muscles.

ACTIVITY

Have students stand with their feet together and try to pick up something from the floor. Then have them move their feet 12 inches apart and bend to pick up the object again. Ask them to explain which felt more balanced.

TEAMWORK

Divide the class into groups of two. Have each student demonstrate the correct procedure for lifting and moving objects. Allow time for both students to demonstrate while the other student critiques the demonstration and makes suggestions for improvement.

When equipment is unavailable, ergonomic practices emphasize proper body mechanics during movement. When you use proper body mechanics, you save energy, prevent muscle strain, and increase your **efficiency**. Body mechanics is the coordination of body alignment, balance, and movement. When you use your body and your muscles properly, you are practicing good body mechanics.

efficiency
(ee FISH uhn see)
Ability to accomplish a job with the least possible difficulty.

Using Proper Body Mechanics

Good body mechanics require you to keep your body in a neutral, upright position. You should keep your back straight at all times. You should let your leg muscles do most of the work. You should never twist your body. You should never strain as you perform work.

It is essential to practice good body mechanics when you are lifting or moving patients, in order to prevent strain and injury. You should also practice good body mechanics when you are performing simple tasks, such as checking blood pressure or entering data into a computer. Injuries from these simple tasks can develop over time if you use poor body mechanics. The following principles will help you to maintain good body mechanics.

1. Stoop. Do not bend.
   - Stand close to the object. Create a base of support by placing your feet wide apart.
   - Place one foot slightly forward.
   - Bend at your hips and knees with your back straight, lower your body, and bring your hands down to the object.
   - Use the large muscles in your legs to return to a standing position.
2. Lift firmly and smoothly after you size up the **load**.
   - If you cannot easily pull the object to you (i.e., the load is too heavy), *get help!*
   - Grasp the load firmly.
   - Lift by using the large muscles of your legs.
   - Keep the load close to your body.
   - Do not twist your body.
   - To change direction, shift your feet in the direction you want to go.
3. Always use the center of **gravity** when carrying a load.
   - Keep your back as straight as possible.
   - Keep the weight of the load close to the body and centered over your hips.
   - Put down the load by bending at the hips and knees. Keep your back straight and the load close to your body.
   - If the load is too heavy, *get help!*
   - When two or more people carry the load, assign one person as the leader so that he or she can give commands.

load
(LOHD)
Weight of an object or person that is to be moved.

gravity
(GRAV i tee)
Natural force or pull toward the earth. In the body, the center of gravity is usually the center of the body.

4. Pulling: Push or pull rather than lift the load.
   - Place your feet apart with one foot slightly forward. Keep close to the object you are moving.
   - Grasp the object firmly, close to its center of gravity.
   - **Crouch**; lean away from the object.
   - Pull by straightening your legs. Keep your back straight.
   - Walk backwards. Your leg muscles should do all the work.
5. Pushing: Push or pull rather than lift the load.
   - Stand close to the object to be moved.
   - Crouch down with your feet apart.
   - Bend your elbows and put your hands on the load at chest level.
   - Lean forward with your chest and shoulders near the object. (Figure 18.6)
   - Keep your back straight.
   - Push with your legs.
6. Reaching: Carefully evaluate the distance.
   - Always use a stool or a ladder to reach objects that are too high.
   - Stand close to the object.
   - If you are standing on the floor, place your feet wide apart, one foot slightly forward.
   - Maintain good body **alignment**. Move close to the object. Do not reach to the point of straining.
   - When reaching for an object that is above your head, grip it with your palms up, and lower it. Keep it close to your body on the way down.

crouch
(KROWCH)
To stoop, using the large muscles of the legs to help maintain balance.

alignment
(uh LAHYN ment)
Keeping the body in proper position—in a straight line without twisting.

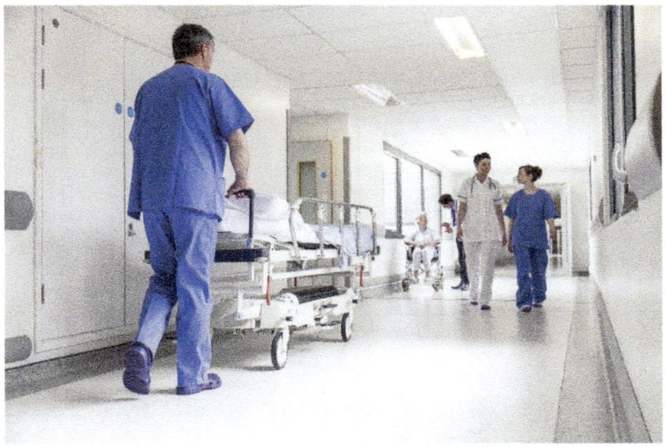

Figure 18.6
To push an object, such as a moveable hospital bed, lean forward with your chest and shoulders near the bed as you push forward.

Patient and Employee Safety | Chapter 18 527

Teaching Tips

- Help students conclude that if they do not use safe lifting techniques, they can injure themselves and/or their patients.
- Tell students that even if they do not feel discomfort immediately from lifting an object, an injury may develop over time. The best way to avoid a problem is to use the proper technique every time.

Figure Focus

18.6 To push an object, such as a moveable hospital bed, lean forward with your chest and shoulders near the bed as you push forward.

Discuss with students why it is important to always use good body mechanics.

CUSTOMIZED INSTRUCTION

Special Needs Students

Have students demonstrate what it means to crouch. Let them show how this helps them to move an object by pushing or pulling rather than lifting.

Discuss

- Talk about the importance of evaluating the actions of co-workers.
- Explain that evaluation can help students and their co-workers correct bad habits and avoid injury.
- Invite students to share their feelings about this issue.

Apply It

- Assign students in pairs.
- Allow time for students' research.
- As a class, discuss the safety issues students determined are associated with various health care career areas.

Personal Wellness—Staying Fit

- Discuss student answers to the question. Help students relate the importance of physical fitness to working in the health care profession.
- Invite students to discuss their favorite ways of keeping fit.
- Ask students to talk about how they manage to fit regular exercise into their busy schedules. Encourage students to suggest ways of maintaining a regular schedule.

Apply It

Nearly all areas of health care are physically demanding. There are also risks associated with many types of health care occupations. With a partner, select a health care career and research the safety issues within that career area. Use the Internet for your research, and, if possible, interview one or more person who works in the area you are researching. Share your findings with the class, and compare and contrast the safety issues found for different career areas.

Evaluating Ergonomics to Avoid Injury

Using the principles of body mechanics can help you to avoid injury. As you are working, however, it is sometimes hard to determine whether your body is in the proper position. One aspect of ergonomics is self-evaluation or evaluation by supervisors or co-workers.

Evaluation can help you and your co-workers to correct bad habits and avoid injury. Evaluation can also help to identify problems in the workplace that may lead to poor body mechanics. You can do the following to evaluate ergonomic practices:

1. **Watch each other.** Tell your co-workers if they are twisting their bodies or bending their backs when working with patients. Ask co-workers to watch your body mechanics as well.
2. **Check equipment.** Equipment that is faulty or hard to operate can cause you to strain muscles. Make sure brakes on wheelchairs are working, so that you do not hurt your back while moving a patient. Make sure other equipment is at the correct height (between the waist and the shoulders), so you do not have to bend to use it.
3. **Discuss procedures.** In some situations, good body mechanics alone may not be enough to prevent injury. Discuss whether you need to create lifting teams instead of having staff move patients by themselves. Also discuss how you can use equipment to help move patients.

Personal Wellness

Staying Fit

Maintaining fitness is important when you are a health care professional. A fit body is strong and flexible and can help you to move patients and equipment without fatigue or injury. A fit mind can help you to handle the stresses of caring for people. Exercise can help you to maintain both a fit body and a fit mind.

Lifting weights can help you to build strength in your arm, leg, and back muscles. Pilates, yoga, or dance can help you to strengthen core muscles, improve balance, and focus your mind. Running or biking can help to increase your endurance. Any exercise can help you to work off stress.

Choose an exercise that appeals to you. Make sure you exercise at least three times per week. Incorporate a variety of exercises into your weekly routine for different physical and mental benefits.

How can an exercise program help a health care worker to avoid injury on the job?

528 Chapter 18 | Patient and Employee Safety

Summary

In this section, you learned that by following basic principles, you prevent fatigue and injury. There are six important rules to remember when following the basic principles of body mechanics.

Six Rules to Remember:

1. Keep your back straight.
2. Bend at the hips and knees.
3. Keep your feet approximately 6 to 8 inches apart to provide a wide base of support.
4. Use the strongest muscles of your legs.
5. Do not twist your body.
6. Use the weight of your body to help push or pull.

When you learn to lift and move correctly, you protect yourself and others from injury.

Section 18.4 Review Questions

1. What does the term *body mechanics* mean?
2. What are the six principles of body mechanics?
3. Where is your center of gravity?
4. Describe how you would safely pull a load.
5. How can using proper body mechanics help you to stay healthy and perform well in a health care position?
6. How can you evaluate ergonomic practices?

Patient and Employee Safety | Chapter 18 529

Section 18.4 Review Questions

1. Answer: Body mechanics is the coordination of body alignment, balance, and movement.
2. Answer: Keep your back straight; bend at the hips and knees; keep your feet approximately 6 to 8 inches apart to provide a wide base of support; use the strongest muscles of your legs; do not twist your body; use the weight of your body to help push or pull.
3. Answer: In the body, gravity is located in the center of the body.
4. Answer: Place your feet apart with one foot slightly forward; keep close to the object you are moving; grasp the object firmly, close to its center of gravity; crouch; lean away from the object; pull by straightening your legs; keep your back straight; walk backwards; your leg muscles should do all the work.
5. Answer: Using proper body mechanics helps to avoid injury.
6. Answer: To evaluate ergonomic practice, watch each other, evaluate equipment, and discuss procedures.

FOCUS AND ENGAGE

Introduce the Section

a. Review the content of the Background paragraph, discussing the need to be able to deal with sudden illness or injury.

b. Discuss the objectives for the section.

Vocabulary

a. Direct students to the key terms.

b. Pronounce each word, and have the students repeat the pronunciation out loud.

c. Discuss the definition of each word.

TEACH

Teaching Tips

- Discuss the importance of being well trained before an emergency arises.
- Define first aid as quick emergency care until advanced care arrives.

SECTION 18.5 First Aid

Background

In or out of the clinical setting, the health care worker is expected to respond quickly and effectively when there is a sudden illness or injury. As a health care worker you are responsible for seeking information and becoming competent in first-aid skills. This knowledge enables you to be a well-prepared and effective health care worker.

Objectives

When you have completed this section, you will be able to do the following:

- Match key terms with their correct meanings.
- Demonstrate the procedures for:
  - Mouth-to-mouth breathing
  - Obstructed airway
  - Serious wounds
  - Preventing shock
  - Splints
  - Slings
  - Bandaging

Introduction to First Aid

This section is an overview of commonly used first-aid techniques. It is recommended that everyone attend a basic first-aid class and a heart saver or **cardiopulmonary** resuscitation (CPR) class in order to become proficient. These classes are given by the American Red Cross and the American Heart Association.

Appropriate first aid can save a life and prevent a permanent disability. Most situations requiring first aid need prompt, **definitive** action. To gain understanding and a high skill level, you need supervised practice for each of the procedures listed.

First aid is the emergency care given to a victim of an accident or a sudden illness. This treatment is required immediately and continues as needed until advanced medical care is available.

cardiopulmonary
(kahr dee oh PUHL muh ner ee)
Having to do with the heart and lungs.

definitive
(di FIN i tiv)
Clear, without question, exacting (e.g., when giving emergency care, each treatment should be done in a definitive manner).

General Principles of First Aid

1. Never panic; always remain calm. Unfortunately, often this is easier said than done. Here are some basic rules that help you remain calm:
   - Take a few slow, deep breaths.
   - Survey the surrounding area and ensure that it is safe before approaching.
   - Determine what resources are available and what is needed.
2. Evaluate the situation by:
   - Checking the victim's level of consciousness.
   - Opening the victim's airway.
   - Checking for breathing.
   - Checking circulation, including pulse and bleeding.
3. Determine if the victim is in a safe environment, free from danger.
4. Determine **priorities** of treatment (i.e., decide which condition requires the most immediate care).
   - Urgent care is required in life-threatening situations, such as stopped breathing, heart attack, shock, serious wounds, poisoning, and burns.
   - A victim may need first aid, but the situation may not be life threatening. Nonlife-threatening conditions include **fracture** of an arm or leg and a minor **contusion** or **laceration**.
5. Decide how to provide the care that is needed and begin providing any care you are trained or permitted to give. Never provide emergency care for which you have not been trained.
6. Call or send for help as soon as possible. If an adult patient is conscious, you must get their permission to help them. If the patient is a child and a parent is available, you must get a parent's permission to help the child.
7. Stay with the injured victim until emergency medical services or more qualified caregiver arrives.

priorities
(prah AWR i tee)
Those things that are most important.

fracture
(FRAK cher)
Broken bone.

contusion
(cuhn TOO shuhn)
Condition in which the skin is bruised, swollen, and painful, but is not broken.

laceration
(las uh RAY shuhn)
Wound or tear of the skin.

CAUTION: Carry disposable gloves. Also carry a pocket mask for delivering rescue breaths. Use these items to prevent exposure to body fluids. Always follow Standard Precautions.

Life-Threatening Situations

Most cities have an emergency medical system (EMS) that responds immediately with emergency care providers. The most common number used to alert the EMS system is 911. If this is not in place, dial 0 and ask local operator to connect you to the Emergency Medical System. The following situations are considered life threatening and require emergency medical care.

Oxygen is necessary for brain cells to live. Permanent brain damage can occur if oxygen is not present for four to six minutes. You have only a few minutes to save the life of a person who has stopped breathing.

Patient and Employee Safety | Chapter 18 531

Teaching Tips

- Discuss the general principles of first aid.
- Discuss the value of being trained in first aid by the American Red Cross.

Discuss

- Begin a class discussion by asking the following questions:
  - Why are these principles important?
  - Do they protect the rescuer?
  - What emergency care is available in your community?
  - How do you access it?

CUSTOMIZED INSTRUCTION

More Advanced Students

Have students research CPR information from the American Red Cross and the American Heart Association. Suggest the following Web sites: redcross.org and americanheart.org. Ask volunteers to present their findings to the class.

Teaching Tips

- Explain the importance of oxygen to the brain cells. Emphasize that four to six minutes without oxygen causes brain damage or death.
- Review life-threatening situations that require emergency medical care:
  - Stopped breathing
  - Heart attack
  - Shock
  - Serious wounds
  - Poisoning
  - Burns
- Explain what an obstructed airway is.
- Compare a partial obstruction with a complete obstruction.

ACTIVITY

Have students prepare a visual way to compare the signs of partial and complete obstructed airways.

Obstructed Airway (Closed Airway, Stopped or Not Breathing)

An obstructed airway occurs when an object blocks the airway leading to the lungs. This occurs when a piece of food or other object lodges in the back of the throat or in the windpipe. Early detection of an airway obstruction is important in determining your plan of action. There are two types of obstructions:

- *Partial obstruction* or *mild obstruction* occurs when some air can be exchanged. There may be *good air exchange* when the victim coughs forcefully or wheezes between coughs. Do not interfere with the victim's attempt to cough the object out. A mild or partial obstruction can progress to a severe obstruction. With severe partial obstruction, the victim:
  - Becomes weak
  - Has an ineffective cough
  - Has a crowing or high-pitched noise during inhalation
  - Has increased difficulty breathing
  - Turns bluish around the mouth and fingernails
- *Complete obstruction* occurs when there is no air exchange or there is poor air exchange. The signs of complete obstruction are present when the victim:
  - Is suddenly unable to breathe, cough, or speak
  - Clutches neck or throat—this is the universal choking sign and a way of telling people around you that you are choking (see photograph in Procedure 18.3)
  - Is struggling to breathe

When you observe these signs, follow the procedure for obstructed airway.

532 Chapter 18 | Patient and Employee Safety

CUSTOMIZED INSTRUCTION

English Language Learners

Have students role-play a situation in which they must call 911 to report that a family member is choking. The goal is to have them speak clearly in English to provide the necessary information, such as the reason for the call and their address.

Procedure 18.2 Rescue Breathing—Adult

BACKGROUND: Rescue breathing is used when a victim is no longer breathing on his or her own. Rescue breathing delivers essential oxygen to the brain cells of the victim. This procedure explains how to administer rescue breathing to an adult.
ALERT: Follow Standard Precautions

Preprocedure

1. Put on disposable gloves and obtain disposable CPR mask if available.
2. Check for consciousness by shaking victim's shoulder gently and asking if he or she is OK. If there is no response, activate EMS system.

Procedure

3. Open airway by placing one hand at victim's chin and the other hand on victim's forehead; gently lift chin by supporting jawbone with fingertips and lifting upward to open mouth. (Do not put pressure on throat; this may block airway.) This is called the *head tilt/chin lift.*
4. Check for pulse by palpating the carotid artery for at least 5 but no more than 10 seconds. If you find a pulse, proceed to step 5.
5. Check for effective breathing. If the patient is gasping or not breathing, place a pocket mask over mouth and nose. Put apex (point) over bridge of nose and base between lip and chin. Give two breaths (1½ to 2 seconds per breath) through the one-way valve. Allow lungs to empty between each breath. (If dentures obstruct the airway, remove them.) If air does not inflate lungs: retilt head to ensure an open airway and repeat the two breaths. Watch for chest to rise. Allow for exhalation between breaths. (If lungs still do not inflate, treat victim for an obstructed airway; see the Obstructed Airway procedures.)
6. Check carotid pulse.
7. If breathing is absent and pulse is present, keep the airway open and give one breath to victim every 5 seconds. If there is no pulse, cardiopulmonary resuscitation (CPR) is needed to circulate oxygenated blood through body. Continue to check the pulse frequently.

   See Section 18.6 for CPR procedures.

Postprocedure

8. Ensure that victim has follow-up treatment or assessment by Emergency Medical Technicians or hospital personnel.
9. Discard gloves and wash hands (follow hand-washing guidelines).

Patient and Employee Safety | Chapter 18 533

Teaching Tips

- Discuss situations when rescue breathing is necessary.
- Review how students find the carotid pulse.
- Assign Procedure 18.2.

Procedure Tip

18.2 Rescue Breathing—Adult

- Review the background information.
- Explain the reasons why rescue breathing is important.
- Guide students through the preprocedure.
- Demonstrate the procedure.
- Point out the postprocedure.

PROCEDURE PRACTICE

- Demonstrate the steps for Procedure 18.2, Rescue Breathing—Adult, as many times as necessary, or ask students to demonstrate the steps. Have students practice and perform the procedure until they are competent.

ACTIVITY

Have students investigate equipment that can be used to protect themselves when administering rescue breathing (e.g., gloves and a pocket mask). Allow volunteers to bring in examples and explain the reasons for their use.

Discuss

- Begin a discussion about the Heimlich maneuver.
- Find out how many students are familiar with this procedure.
- Ask if anyone has ever used it or seen it used.
- Discuss why the procedure must be adjusted for pregnant or obese victims.
- Assign Procedure 18.3.

Procedure Tip

18.3 Obstructed Airway in a Conscious Victim—Adult

- Review the background information.
- Guide students through the preprocedure.
- Demonstrate the procedure.
- Point out the postprocedure.
- Discuss why it is important for a choking victim to receive follow-up treatment.

PROCEDURE PRACTICE

- Demonstrate the steps for Procedure 18.3, Obstructed Airway in a Conscious Victim—Adult, as many times as necessary, or ask students to demonstrate the steps. Have students practice and perform the procedure until they are competent.

Procedure 18.3 **Obstructed Airway in a Conscious Victim—Adult**

BACKGROUND: An obstructed airway may occur if a victim inhales food or drink. This procedure explains how to apply pressure from an abdominal thrust (also called the Heimlich maneuver) to force an obstruction out of an adult victim's airway.

ALERT: Follow Standard Precautions

Preprocedure

When signs of choking are present:

1. Ask "Are you choking?" Observe victim for coughing or wheezing. Do *not interfere* if good air exchange is present.

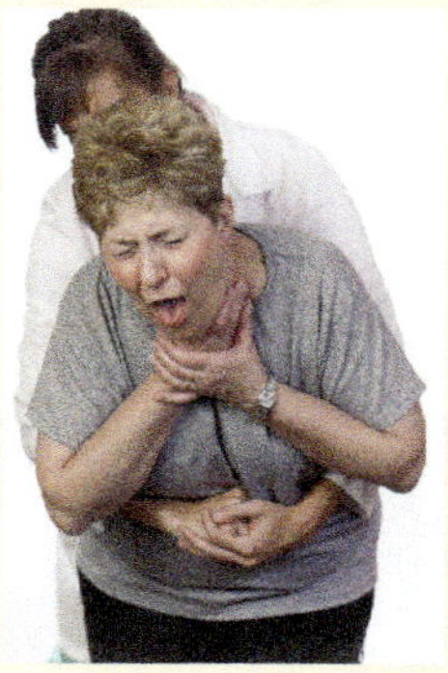

Procedure

2. Give **abdominal thrust**, sometimes called the **Heimlich maneuver**. Stand in back of victim; put your arms around victim's waist. Make a fist with one hand and put the thumb side of the fist slightly above the navel and well below the breast bone.

   Take your other hand and grasp fist; pull into victim's abdomen with quick upward thrust. Repeat separate, rapid inward and upward thrusts until airway is cleared or patient becomes unconscious. (Use chest thrusts for a pregnant or obese victim.)

Postprocedure

3. Ensure that victim has follow-up treatment or assessment by Emergency Medical Technicians or hospital personnel, if needed.
4. Wash hands (follow hand-washing guidelines).

abdominal thrust or **Heimlich maneuver** (HYM lik muh noo ver) Forceful thrust on the abdomen, between the sternum and the navel, in an upward motion toward the head.

534 Chapter 18 | Patient and Employee Safety

CUSTOMIZED INSTRUCTION

More Advanced Students

Tell students that if a person is alone and is choking, that person may have to perform the Heimlich maneuver on him- or herself. Have students find and present the procedure for performing the Heimlich maneuver on oneself.

Procedure 18.4 Obstructed Airway in a Victim Who Becomes Unconscious—Adult

BACKGROUND: An airway obstruction can cause the victim to become unconscious due to lack of oxygen. This procedure explains how to clear an obstructed airway in an unconscious adult.
ALERT: Follow Standard Precautions

Preprocedure

If the victim becomes unconscious:

1. Activate the EMS system.
2. Put on disposable gloves.

Procedure

3. Assist the victim to the floor and begin CPR using the C-A-B sequence. Begin by checking pulse and giving compressions. If pulse is present, go to step 4.
4. Attempt to ventilate. Open the airway and ventilate through a pocket face mask with a one-way valve. If no air enters, retilt head and try to ventilate again. Every time you give a breath, open mouth wide and look for object. If you see an object, remove it with fingers. If you do not see an object, proceed with CPR. See Procedures 18.24 and 18.25 for CPR procedures.

Postprocedure

5. Ensure that victim has follow-up treatment or assessment by Emergency Medical Technicians or hospital personnel.
6. Discard gloves and wash hands (follow hand-washing guidelines).

Procedure 18.5 Rescue Breathing—Infant

BACKGROUND: It is important to quickly deliver oxygen to an infant who has stopped breathing. An infant's brain is actively developing and may become damaged if it lacks oxygen. This procedure explains how to deliver rescue breaths to an infant who has stopped breathing.
ALERT: Follow Standard Precautions

Preprocedure

1. Put on disposable gloves.
2. Check for consciousness. Shake baby's shoulders gently and speak baby's name. If no response, shout for help.

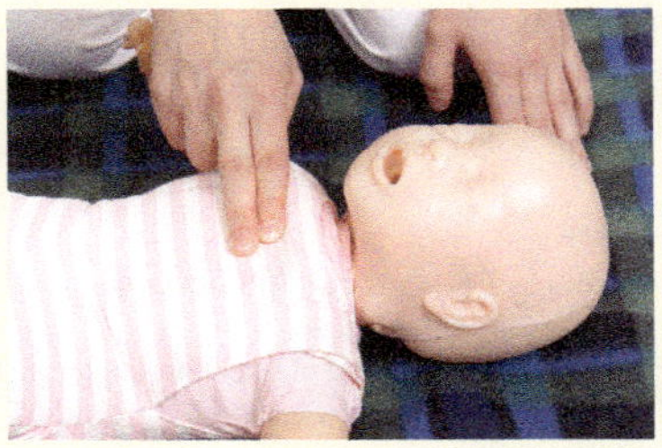

Procedure

3. Check for brachial pulse for at least 5 but no more than 10 seconds. If the pulse is present and is faster than 60 beats per minute proceed to step 4.
4. Check for effective breathing. Look, listen, and feel.

(continued)

Teaching Tips

- Explain that the Heimlich maneuver cannot be performed on an unconscious victim.
- Point out that different attempts must be made to clear the obstructed airway in this case.
- Assign Procedure 18.4.

Procedure Tip

18.4 Obstructed Airway in a Victim Who Becomes Unconscious—Adult

- Review the background information.
- Guide students through the preprocedure.
- Demonstrate the procedure.
- Point out the postprocedure.

PROCEDURE PRACTICE

- Demonstrate the steps for Procedure 18.4, Obstructed Airway in a Victim Who Becomes Unconscious—Adult, as many times as necessary, or ask students to demonstrate the steps. Have students practice and perform the procedure until they are competent.

Teaching Tips

- Explain the importance of restoring oxygen flow to an infant.
- Emphasize the importance of protecting the delicate organs of an infant.
- Assign Procedure 18.5.

Procedure Tip

18.5 Rescue Breathing—Infant

- Review the background information.
- Discuss the differences between administering CPR to an adult versus an infant.
- Guide students through the preprocedure.
- Demonstrate the procedure.
- Point out the postprocedure.

TEAMWORK

Have students review the relationship between the circulatory and respiratory systems. Oversee students as they create a diagram outlining these systems. Volunteers should present information about the two systems and how they work together to bring oxygen to cells and remove wastes.

PROCEDURE PRACTICE

- Demonstrate the steps for Procedure 18.5, Rescue Breathing—Infant, as many times as necessary, or ask students to demonstrate the steps. Have students practice and perform the procedure until they are competent.

Teaching Tips

- Discuss objects that could obstruct an infant's airway.
- Assign Procedure 18.6.

Procedure Tip

18.6 Obstructed Airway in a Conscious Infant

- Review the background information.
- Discuss the differences between administering CPR to an unconscious infant versus a conscious infant.
- Guide students through the preprocedure.
- Demonstrate the procedure.
- Point out the postprocedure.

TEAMWORK

Small tubes are available for parents and caregivers to test whether or not an object can fit into an infant or toddler's throat. Have students obtain such a tube and design a safety poster around it for a school or daycare facility.

Procedure 18.5 Rescue Breathing—Infant (continued)

Procedure (cont)

If not breathing:

5. Place an infant-sized barrier device on the infant's face.* Ventilate through the one-way valve and give rescue breathing. Give two slow breaths using only air in your cheeks. (Too much air may overinflate an infant's lungs.)

   Watch for chest to rise and allow chest to fall or deflate between each breath. If air does not inflate lungs.

   Retilt head to ensure open airway. Repeat the two breaths. If lungs still do not inflate, treat infant for an obstructed airway.

If lungs do inflate:

5. Keep airway open, and give one breath to infant every 3 seconds. After 1 minute activate EMS.
6. Check pulse. Place three fingers over brachial artery/pulse. The baby's heart may have stopped. In this event, only cardiopulmonary resuscitation (CPR) will help to circulate oxygenated blood throughout the body. See Procedure 18.23 for CPR procedures.

Postprocedure

7. Ensure that victim has follow-up treatment or assessment by Emergency Medical Technicians or hospital personnel.
8. Discard gloves and wash hands (follow hand-washing guidelines).

* Adult-sized pocket face masks can be adapted by inverting (reversing) them. See manufacturer's guidelines.

Procedure 18.6 Obstructed Airway in a Conscious Infant

BACKGROUND: The procedures for clearing an obstructed airway in an infant are different from the procedures for an adult. Care must be taken to protect the smaller, more delicate organs and bones of the infant. This procedure explains how to clear an obstructed airway in a conscious infant.
ALERT: Follow Standard Precautions

Preprocedure

1. Put on disposable gloves
2. Observe to determine infant's ability to cry, cough, or breathe. If there is no evidence of air exchange, shout for help.

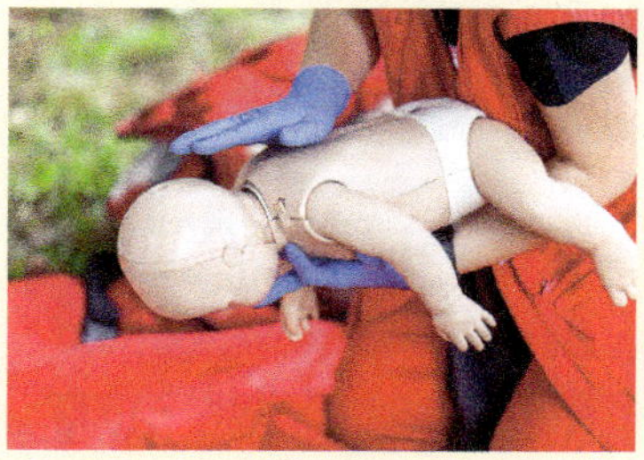

Procedure

3. Give five back blows. Place infant face down, supporting head and neck and tilting infant so that the head is lower than rest of body. Give five firm hits with heel of your hand over backbone and between shoulder blades.

(continued)

536 Chapter 18 | Patient and Employee Safety

Procedure 18.6	Obstructed Airway in a Conscious Infant (continued)

Procedure (cont)

4. Give five chest thrusts by turning infant on its back with head lower than rest of body. Using two to three fingers, push five times on midsternum, which is about one finger's width below nipple line at midchest at a rate of about one per second.
5. Continue procedure until obstruction is clear or infant becomes unconscious. If infant becomes unconscious, stop giving black blows and start CPR.

Postprocedure

6. Ensure that victim has follow-up treatment or assessment by Emergency Medical Technicians or hospital personnel.
7. Discard gloves and wash hands (follow hand-washing guidelines).

Procedure 18.7	Obstructed Airway in an Infant Who Becomes Unconscious

BACKGROUND: It is important to deliver oxygen to an infant who is not breathing as soon as possible to prevent brain damage. This procedure explains how to clear an obstructed airway in an unconscious infant.
ALERT: Follow Standard Precautions

Preprocedure

1. Put on disposable gloves
2. Check for responsiveness. If no response, send bystanders to activate EMS.

Procedure

3. Begin chest compressions at a rate of 100 per minute. After every set of 30 compressions, open the airway and look for object. Remove the object if you see it, otherwise attempt to ventilate and continue compressions.
4. Once the airway is clear, ventilate once every 3 seconds.

Postprocedure

5. Ensure that victim has follow-up treatment or assessment by Emergency Medical Technicians or hospital personnel.
6. Discard gloves and wash hands (follow hand-washing guidelines).

Patient and Employee Safety | Chapter 18 537

PROCEDURE PRACTICE

- Demonstrate the steps for Procedure 18.6, Obstructed Airway in a Conscious Infant, as many times as necessary, or ask students to demonstrate the steps. Have students practice and perform the procedure until they are competent.

Teaching Tips

- Compare the situation of a conscious infant with that of an unconscious infant when it comes to an obstructed airway.
- Assign Procedure 18.7.

Procedure Tip

18.7 Obstructed Airway in an Infant Who Becomes Unconscious

- Review the background information.
- Guide students through the preprocedure.
- Demonstrate the procedure.
- Compare the steps for administering CPR to a conscious versus unconscious infant. What are the differences and why?
- Point out the postprocedure.

PROCEDURE PRACTICE

- Demonstrate the steps for Procedure 18.7, Obstructed Airway in an Infant Who Becomes Unconscious, as many times as necessary, or ask students to demonstrate the steps. Have students practice and perform the procedure until they are competent.

Teaching Tips

- Describe a heart attack and its symptoms.
- Point out that the first two hours after a heart attack are critical.
- Discuss how denial of a heart attack is common.
- Stress that quick action can save lives.
- Review Table 18.1 with students.
- Make sure students understand the information provided in each column of the table.
- Divide the class into seven groups. Assign one condition to each group.
- Tell students to make a brief presentation to the class about the condition, its possible treatments, and patient education.
- Encourage students to supplement the information in the table with additional research.

Review and Reinforce

- Review the meaning of blood pressure.
- Discuss what the numbers in a blood pressure measurement mean.
- Review the procedure for measuring blood pressure.
- Relate high blood pressure to cardiovascular conditions.

Heart Attack

The first two hours after the onset of a heart attack are the highest-risk period. Recognition of early warning signs alerts you to an impending heart attack. Early warning signs are:

- Squeezing feeling in the chest ("feels like a band is around my chest"), pressure, or tightness ("feels like an elephant is sitting on my chest").
- Persistent discomfort that spreads to shoulders, arms, neck, jaw, or across the chest.
- Sweating, nausea, vomiting, shortness of breath, or feeling faint.

When one or all of these signs are present, call for advanced life support systems (doctor or paramedics depending upon the health care setting). If signs continue, the heart and breathing may stop, and it will be necessary to start CPR.

Table 18.1 Common Cardiovascular Conditions, Possible Treatments, and Patient Education

Condition	Possible Treatments	Patient Education
Coronary artery disease; also called arteriosclerosis (narrowing of arteries of the heart).	Medication Surgery Diet	1. Explain importance of low-salt, low-fat diet; weight control; prescribed exercise program. 2. Reduce stress factors. 3. Stress importance of taking prescribed medication. 4. Provide written information on condition.
Myocardial infarction (MI, heart attack)	Medication Rehabilitation	1. Encourage patient to follow prescribed diet, medication program, and exercise program. 2. Provide written instructions and information about condition.
Congestive heart failure (CHF, tissues of heart and lungs are edematous)	Medication Rest Diet Antiembolism stocking	1. Encourage patient to follow prescribed diet and medication program. 2. Provide written instructions and information about condition.
Hypertension (blood pressure above 140/90)	Medication Diet therapy Exercise program	1. Warn patient not to stop medication without seeing physician. 2. Stress importance of diet and exercise. 3. Explain why blood pressure increases with weight gain and poor dietary habits.
Varicose veins (veins that allow blood to pool and not return to the heart)	TED (thromboembolic devices) Warm soaks Surgery	1. Explain importance of changing position frequently (sitting, standing). 2. Explain application of elastic stockings and their purpose. 3. Stress importance of elevating legs. 4. Stress importance of loose clothing so that circulation is not impaired.
Thrombophlebitis	Medication Surgery Warm compresses	1. Instruct in application of warm compresses. 2. Instruct in elevation of legs. 3. Teach to watch for danger signs.
Cerebral vascular accident (CVA, stroke)	Hospitalization Physical therapy Occupational therapy Speech therapy Medication	1. Encourage patient to reach highest potential. 2. Teach awareness of adaptive devices and assist in selection.

538 Chapter 18 | Patient and Employee Safety

CUSTOMIZED INSTRUCTION

More Advanced Students

Have students research and present statistics related to heart attacks and heart disease.

Special Needs Students

Be sure to give students who have difficulty reading enough time to understand the table.

Wound Care and Observation

Patients who have suffered a trauma or surgery have very specific needs. Their wounds may be life threatening and must be cared for properly. As a nurse assistant, your primary responsibility in caring for wounds includes careful, specific observations and reporting.

You must understand wounds in order to make good observations and reports. Always observe and report the location, size, appearance, and odor of the wound; the condition of the surrounding skin; and the type and amount of drainage.

Wounds often have drainage, and there are other complications to watch for.

Wounds may be described by color:

- **Red wounds.** Red is the color of healthy tissue and indicates normal healing.
- **Yellow wounds.** Yellow is the color of exudates produced by microorganisms. Too many organisms in accumulated exudates causes the wound to have drainage and appear yellow.
- **Black wounds.** Black wounds signify necrosis or dead tissue.
- **Multicolored wounds.** There may be more than one color present in a wound. In this case describe it by the least healthy color. An example of this would be a wound that is both yellow and black should be described as a black wound.

Types of Wounds

Wounds are described as being either *open* or *closed* (**Figure 18.7**):

- **Closed wounds.** Tissue is injured, but the skin is not broken. These wounds can be caused by bruising, sprains, and twists.
- **Open wounds.** The skin or mucous membrane is broken. These wounds can be caused by bites, cuts, and incisions. Whenever there is an open wound there is a chance of infection. Open wounds can be either partial thickness or full thickness wounds:
  - **Partial thickness wounds.** The dermis and epidermis are broken.
  - **Full thickness wounds.** The dermis, epidermis, and subcutaneous tissue are penetrated. Muscle and bone may be involved.

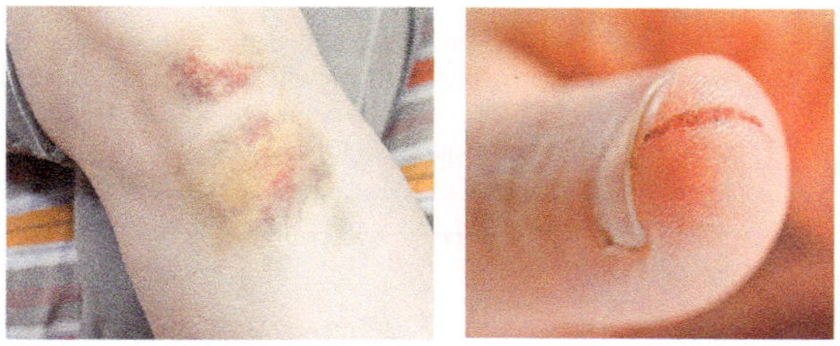

Figure 18.7
Closed wound on the knee and open wound on the finger. Which type of wound carries the most risk for infection?

Teaching Tips

- Review how to describe a wound by color.
- Discuss what each color might indicate about the wound.
- Compare closed wounds and open wounds.

Review and Reinforce

- Direct students back to Section 9.4 to review what they learned about observation and charting.
- Tell students that they would use these skills when attending to a patient's wounds.

Figure Focus

18.7 Closed wound on the knee and open wound on the finger. Which type of wound carries the most risk for infection?

Answer: Open wounds carry the most risk of infection because the skin is broken, allowing bacteria to enter the body.

Teaching Tips

- Help students recognize that an open wound carries the most risk for infection.
- Compare the sources of each type of wound.

Teaching Tips

- Explain that wounds heal in different ways.
- Discuss primary intention, secondary intention, and third intention.
- Review major complications in wound healing:
  - Dehiscence
  - Evisceration
  - Hemorrhage

ACTIVITY

Have students write each of the seven common types of wounds on individual index cards. Tell them to describe the wound on the back of the index card. Students can use these as study cards to make sure they are familiar with the differences among them.

The following are some common types of wounds:

- **Abrasion.** Partial thickness wound caused by scraping the skin away.
- **Amputation.** Removal of all or part of a limb or digit of the body, as by surgery.
- **Contusion.** Closed wound caused by a blow to the body.
- **Incision.** Intentional wound made with a scalpel.
- **Laceration.** Open wound with jagged edges and torn tissue.
- **Penetrating wound.** Open wound caused by piercing the underlying tissues of the skin.
- **Puncture wound.** Open wound caused by a sharp object entering the skin and underlying tissues.

How Wounds Heal

Types of Healing

Wounds are allowed to heal in different ways:

- **Primary (first) intention.** The wound is pulled together by suturing, stapling, taping, clipping, or gluing. This is a clean wound that usually heals quickly.
- **Secondary (second) intention.** The wound edges are not brought together. The wound is cleaned, and dead tissue is removed. This method is often used in infected and contaminated wounds. The closure of the wound with granulations means that there is formation in wounds of small, rounded masses of tissue during healing.
- **Third intention.** The wound is left open and may be closed at a later time. Poor circulation and infection are common reasons for using this method. In this case, you would choose to treat the grossly contaminated wound by delaying closure until after contamination has been markedly reduced and inflammation has subsided.

Medical Emergencies in Wound Healing

Wound healing is dependent on many factors, including the type of wound and the patient's age, nutrition, and lifestyle. The patient's medical history is also very important. Poor circulation, diabetes, some medications, and a weakened immune system can cause complications. The following are major complications:

- **Dehiscence.** The skin layer and/or the underlying tissues separate, reopening the wound. Stress to the wound from coughing, vomiting, and abdominal distension is usually the cause of dehiscence. This is a surgical emergency. Notify your supervisor immediately.
- **Evisceration.** The skin layer is separated by the protrusion of an internal organ through the wound. The causes are the same as in dehiscence. This is also a surgical emergency. Notify your supervisor immediately.

protrusion
(proh TROO shuhn)
Pushing through.

540 Chapter 18 | Patient and Employee Safety

CUSTOMIZED INSTRUCTION

Less Advanced Students

Have students look up the words primary and secondary in a dictionary. Ask them to relate the definitions they found to primary, secondary, and third intention wounds.

- **Hemorrhage.** Excessive bleeding that is life threatening. Hemorrhage is a medical emergency and must be reported to your supervisor immediately. The patient is in immediate danger:
  - *External hemorrhage* is easily seen. Dressings soak with blood and blood may flow under the body. Always check under the patient for pooling blood when you see saturated dressings.
  - *Internal hemorrhage* cannot be seen. The bleeding is in the tissue of the body and in the body cavities. Signs of internal bleeding include the patient's vomiting blood or coughing up blood, shock, and loss of consciousness. A hematoma may form (i.e., blood collects under the skin, causing swelling and discoloration).

Types of Drainage

Wound drainage occurs during the inflammatory stage of healing when healing fluid and cells escape from the surrounding tissues. The overlying skin heals, but the underlying tissue does not. Drainage that is trapped in the wound and underlying tissue causes swelling and pain and may cause infection. The doctor puts in a drainage tube when large amounts of drainage are expected.

There are several different types of drainage, including the following:

- **Purulent drainage.** Thick green, yellow, or brown drainage
- **Sanguineous drainage.** Bloody drainage; large amounts may indicate hemorrhage
- **Serous drainage.** Watery, clear drainage
- **Serosanguineous drainage.** Thin, watery, blood-tinged drainage

Remember to always follow Standard Precautions when in contact with any type of drainage.

Severe Wounds

Serious wounds, or severe wounds, are life threatening because heavy bleeding is frequently present. Bleeding that pulsates or **spurts** with each heartbeat is from an artery. The victim will bleed to death if the bleeding is not controlled. Venous bleeding is also serious and must be controlled. An open wound allowing a constant flow of blood from a vein can also cause death. The open area is also susceptible to infection and needs to be covered.

spurts
(SPURTZ)
Forces out in a burst; squirts.

Wound Infection

Wounds often get infected because they become contaminated with dirt and bacteria. Deep scrapes and puncture wounds are the most likely wounds to become infected. The following are signs that a wound has become infected:

- Pus or cloudy fluid draining from the wound
- Pimple or yellow crust appears
- Increased scab size
- Red streak spreading beyond the wound

Patient and Employee Safety | Chapter 18 541

Teaching Tips

- Explain different types of drainage.
- Discuss the dangers of serious wounds.

Discuss

- Ask students to discuss common reasons why wounds become infected.
- Have volunteers list signs that a wound has become infected.

ACTIVITY

Wound centers often deal exclusively with wounds that won't heal or take long periods of time to heal. Have students find local wound centers. Have class representatives contact individual centers to learn about what they do and what types of wounds they care for.

CUSTOMIZED INSTRUCTION

Less Advanced Students

Have students set up a demonstration to show what it means if something spurts. They might consider such supplies as balloons and water for their demonstrations.

Procedure Tip

18.8 How to Treat Serious Wounds

- Review the background information.
- Guide students through the preprocedure.
- Demonstrate the procedure.
- Explain that the wound should be elevated and direct pressure applied to it.
- Point out the postprocedure.

PROCEDURE PRACTICE

- Demonstrate the steps for Procedure 18.8, How to Treat Serious Wounds, as many times as necessary, or ask students to demonstrate the steps. Have students practice and perform the procedure until they are competent.

dressings
(DRES ing)
Gauze pads that are used to cover a wound.

saturated
(SACH uh reyt id)
Soaked; filled to capacity.

- Increased tenderness
- Increased pain or swelling
- Wound becomes blistered
- Appearance of black dead tissue around the wound
- Fever

Procedure 18.8 How to Treat Serious Wounds

BACKGROUND: To stop bleeding and minimize infection, apply direct pressure with your gloved hand and some type of **dressing** or pad. Sterile gauze pads/gauze dressings are very effective. If gauze dressings are not available, use a piece of clean cloth, a handkerchief, or toweling. Even though the cloth is not sterile, it aids in controlling the bleeding.
ALERT: Follow Standard Precautions

Preprocedure

1. Follow the Procedure 18.9 in order to prevent shock.

Procedure

2. Apply direct pressure over the wound with gauze or clean material and your gloved hand. Apply a pressure dressing and secure with a roll bandage. Hold for 5–10 minutes. If blood soaks through, apply second dressing on top of original dressing.
3. Elevate the wounded area if you do not think there are broken bones and continue to apply pressure.

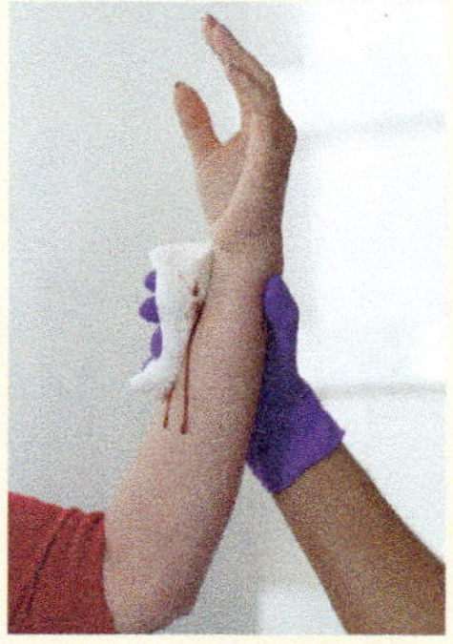

4. Check pulse below pressure bandage to check for circulation.
5. If direct pressure and elevation do not control bleeding:
   a. Apply pressure to the appropriate pressure point above the wound. (Figure 18.8) The pressure point must be on the same limb or the same side of the body.
   b. Continue to apply direct pressure and maintain elevation to the wound. Do not remove the dressings and bandages when they are **saturated**. Apply dry dressings over the saturated bandage.
   c. When bleeding is under control, gradually release pressure at the pressure point. Keep applying direct pressure over the pressure dressing.
6. Remove gloves and wash hands thoroughly.
7. Call or send for help as soon as possible.

Postprocedure

8. Ensure that victim has follow-up treatment or assessment by Emergency Medical Technicians or hospital personnel.
9. Discard gloves and wash hands (follow hand-washing guidelines).

542 Chapter 18 | Patient and Employee Safety

CUSTOMIZED INSTRUCTION

Special Needs Students

Show an example of what it means to elevate a body part. Let students practice feeling a pulse in different locations so they can easily find the pulse below an elevated wound.

Shock

Shock is life threatening. Shock is usually caused by major loss of body fluids or blood; it can be caused by vomiting and diarrhea. If it is due to major blood loss, body cells and organs are deprived of oxygen, which is carried by the blood. Shock slows body functions and keeps the major organs from functioning normally.

Anyone with a serious injury should seek advanced medical care immediately. A victim can be treated appropriately for an injury, yet die from shock because of the fluid or blood and oxygen loss. Treat every victim for a life-threatening injury until the victim is stabilized and emergency care providers or doctors arrive. Follow the procedure to prevent shock.

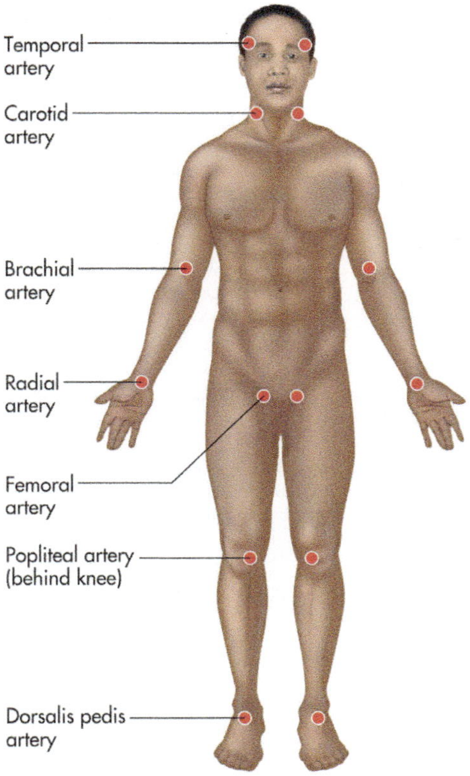

Figure 18.8
Use of pressure points to control profuse bleeding from the upper extremity, lower extremity, and neck. Where is the pressure point to stop bleeding in the leg?

Patient and Employee Safety | Chapter 18 543

Teaching Tips

- Discuss shock as the shutdown of body functions, preventing major organs from functioning normally.
- Make sure students appreciate the seriousness of shock.
- Assign Procedure 18.9 on the next page.

Figure Focus

18.8 Use of pressure points to control profuse bleeding from the upper extremity, lower extremity, and neck. Where is the pressure point to stop bleeding in the leg?

Answer: Direct students to see that the pressure point is on the femoral artery.

Review and Reinforce

- Review the difference between arteries and veins.
- Discuss the role of each in the circulatory system.

TEAMWORK

Have pairs of students bring in dolls or similar items. Ask them to use tape to label each of the pressure points identified in Figure 18.8.

Procedure Tip

18.9 Preventing Shock

- Review the background information.
- Describe the symptoms of shock.
- Discuss why it is so important to prevent and treat shock immediately.
- Guide students through the preprocedure.
- Demonstrate the procedure.
- Reinforce to students that a victim with a potential head or neck injury should not be moved.
- Point out the postprocedure.

PROCEDURE PRACTICE

- Demonstrate the steps for Procedure 18.9, Preventing Shock, as many times as necessary, or ask students to demonstrate the steps. Have students practice and perform the procedure until they are competent.

Teaching Tips

- Explain that poisoning often involves sudden collapse, vomiting, and difficulty breathing.
- Talk about the ways that poisoning can occur.
- Assign Procedure 18.10 on the next page.

Discuss

- Lead a class discussion with the following questions:
  - Why should you try to find the poison container?
  - Do you know how to reach the local poison center?

Procedure 18.9 Preventing Shock

BACKGROUND: Shock is a life-threatening condition that must be treated immediately. A victim who remains in shock could die. The most common symptoms of shock include an extremely low blood pressure; fast but weak pulse; dizziness, faintness, or light-headedness; feeling weak or nauseous; moist, clammy skin; profuse sweating; unconsciousness; rapid, shallow breathing; feeling anxious, agitated, or confused; chest pain; and/or blue lips and fingernails. This procedure explains how to stabilize a victim and prevent shock.

ALERT: Follow Standard Precautions

Preprocedure

1. If patient is located in the field (not in a health care facility), contact EMS.

Procedure

2. Provide comfort, quiet, and warmth.
3. Maintain normal body temperature by covering with blanket.
4. Keep victim calm.
5. Keep victim lying down on back if possible. Elevate feet and arms. Do not elevate an unsplinted arm or leg that is fractured.
6. If victim is vomiting, bleeding from mouth, or feels like vomiting, position victim on side. Do not move the victim if there is any possibility of a spinal injury or if the victim complains of numbness, tingling, lack of sensation, or inability to move limbs.
7. If person has a head injury, neck injury, or breathing problem, feet should not be elevated and the victim should not be turned on his or her side.
8. Do not give the victim anything to eat or drink.
9. Provide oxygen as soon as possible if you have the training and equipment to do so; otherwise, call immediately for someone who does.

Postprocedure

10. Discard gloves and wash hands (follow handwashing guidelines).

Poisoning

ingestion (in JES chuhn) Take in by mouth.

Poisoning often causes sudden collapse, vomiting, and difficult breathing. Poisoning can occur in various ways—for example, **ingestion**, inhalation (which is breathing in a poisonous substance), absorption through the skin, or injection, insect stings or animal bites, or from needles that puncture the skin. Look for items near the victim that may be the source of poisoning, such as an empty container or a needle. To care for a poisoning victim follow the procedure for a conscious victim.

An *unconscious victim* who is suffering from poisoning may be convulsing and vomiting. Follow the procedure for an unconscious poison victim.

544 Chapter 18 | Patient and Employee Safety

TEAMWORK

Victims suspected of going into shock should be placed in specific positions. Have students investigate these positions. Then, have pairs or small groups demonstrate the position according to the cause of the shock. Begin with the standard position.

Procedure 18.10 | **Treating a Conscious Poison Victim**

BACKGROUND: A poison victim should get emergency treatment as soon as possible. A person who has ingested poison may experience organ damage, shock, or death. This procedure explains how to treat a conscious poison victim.
ALERT: Follow Standard Precautions

Preprocedure

1. Put on disposable gloves.
2. Try to locate poison container (try to identify source of poisoning); do not waste time. Check victim's body and clothes for signs of poisoning.
3. Position victim on his side to let mouth drain.

Procedure

4. Call 911 to get an ambulance as soon as possible; then call the nearest poison center, hospital, or physician.* (Directions on poison containers and for ingested substances are not always correct.) When you call, state that you have a poisoning emergency. If you have the container, be prepared to read ingredients. Follow the directions from the poison center.
5. If poison is on skin, wash with water.
6. If poison is from a snakebite: Cover and wrap the affected snakebite area. Continue wrapping the entire affected limb and apply a splint. This is called the pressure immobilization technique. Remember to make sure the wound does not swell enough to make the splint a tourniquet, cutting off the blood flow. Get person to an emergency care center as soon as possible.
7. If poison is from an insect bite: Apply cold compresses. A doctor may prescribe calcium gluconate for muscle pain and an anti-anxiety drug for spasms. For any poisonous insect bite, be sure your tetanus immunization is current.
8. Be alert for breathing problems. If breathing stops, you will perform mouth-to-mask (rescue breathing) resuscitation as discussed earlier.
9. Follow procedure for preventing shock.

Postprocedure

10. Ensure that victim has follow-up treatment or assessment by Emergency Medical Technicians or hospital personnel.
11. Discard gloves and wash hands (follow hand-washing guidelines).

* Ambulance personnel can communicate directly with the hospital and the poison control center. They can start lifesaving procedures with special equipment and poison treatment medications.

Patient and Employee Safety | Chapter 18 545

Procedure Tip

18.10 Treating a Conscious Poison Victim

- Review the background information.
- Discuss why a poison victim should get emergency treatment immediately.
- Guide students through the preprocedure.
- Explain why it is important to know what poisoned a victim.
- Demonstrate the procedure.
- Point out the postprocedure.
- Discuss why a poison victim should receive follow-up treatment.

PROCEDURE PRACTICE

- Demonstrate the steps for Procedure 18.10, Treating a Conscious Poison Victim, as many times as necessary, or ask students to demonstrate the steps. Have students practice and perform the procedure until they are competent.

Procedure Tip

18.11 Treating an Unconscious Poison Victim

- Review the background information.
- Discuss the differences between treating a conscious versus an unconscious poison victim.
- Guide students through the preprocedure.
- Demonstrate the procedure.
- Point out the postprocedure.

PROCEDURE PRACTICE

- Demonstrate the steps for Procedure 18.11, Treating an Unconscious Poison Victim, as many times as necessary, or ask students to demonstrate the steps. Have students practice and perform the procedure until they are competent.

Teaching Tips

- Explain that some burns result from inhalation.
- Review signs that may indicate this type of burn.
- Emphasize that an absence of pain does not indicate a mild burn.

Figure Focus

18.9 Severity of burns. What is a third-degree burn?

Answer: Full thickness burns are deep and destroy tissue. Make sure students recognize that a third-degree burn is a full-thickness burn, destroying both surface and underlying tissue.

Procedure 18.11 Treating an Unconscious Poison Victim

BACKGROUND: An unconscious poison victim must receive emergency medical treatment as quickly as possible to prevent damage to organs, shock, or death. This procedure explains how to treat an unconscious poison victim.
ALERT: Follow Standard Precautions

Preprocedure

1. Put on disposable gloves.
2. Do *not* give any fluids.

Procedure

3. Position victim on his or her side in a safe place.
4. Try to identify the poison source; do not waste time.
5. Call 911 to get an ambulance as soon as possible; then call the nearest poison center, hospital, or physician. Follow their directions.*
6. If chemicals have gotten on skin, wash with water. Remove clothes and jewelry that are contaminated.
7. Be alert for breathing problems.
8. Follow procedure for preventing shock.

Postprocedure

9. Ensure that victim has follow-up treatment or assessment by Emergency Medical Technicians or hospital personnel.
10. Discard gloves and wash hands (follow hand-washing guidelines).

* Ambulance personnel can communicate directly with the hospital and the poison control center. They can start lifesaving procedures with special equipment and poison treatment medications.

Burns

The seriousness of a burn is determined by the degree or depth of the burn. (Figure 18.9)

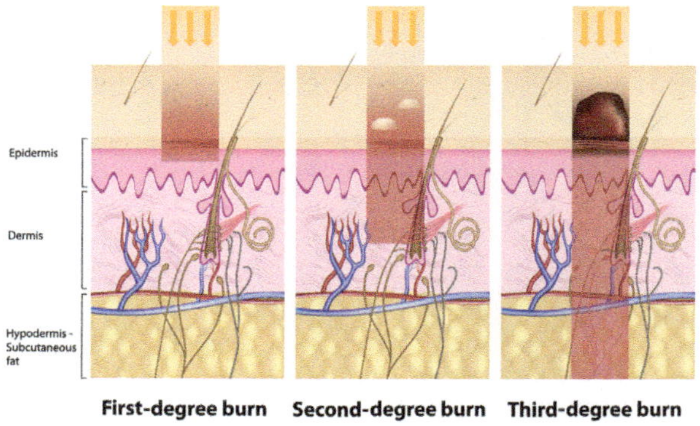

Figure 18.9 Severity of burns. What is a third-degree burn?

546 Chapter 18 | Patient and Employee Safety

ACTIVITY

Have students make a model to represent the layers of the skin.

TEAMWORK

Have students brainstorm a "Do-Not" list, which is a list of things that should not be done to a burn. For example, "Do not pierce blisters," "Do not peel off dead skin," or "Do not peel off clothing stuck to the burn."

Severity of Burns

- Superficial or *first-degree burns* are surface burns.
- Partial thickness or *second-degree burns* are deeper or just below the surface of the skin, and blistering occurs.
- Full thickness or *third-degree burns* are even deeper, destroying both surface and underlying tissue.

Burns around the mouth or nose may indicate that the airway is burned. This can cause swelling that may obstruct the airway. If breathing stops, follow the procedure for rescue breathing as discussed at the beginning of this section. However, if the airway is swollen causing breathing to stop, rescue breathing may be ineffective. Call emergency care providers immediately. Blistering and swelling may not appear until later.

A full thickness burn destroys nerve endings, so a burn victim may not feel pain in that area, but surrounding areas may be painful. The absence of pain does not indicate a mild burn. Do the following for a burn victim as described in the following procedure:

- Relieve pain.
- Minimize the chance of infection.
- Prevent shock (Procedure 18.9).

Procedure 18.12 Treating Burns

BACKGROUND: A burn destroys tissue and may send a victim into shock. This procedure explains how to treat victims of first-degree, second-degree, or third-degree burns. You must identify the degree of the burn:

- *First-Degree Burn* (superficial partial-thickness burn): Appears pink or red; sensitive to touch
- *Second-Degree Burn* (deep partial-thickness burn): Appears pink or red with a mottled appearance; blisters and edema; touching causes severe pain
- *Third-Degree Burn* (full-thickness burn): Appears red, waxy white, brown or black; insensitive to touch; loss of hair in area

ALERT: Follow Standard Precautions

Preprocedure

1. Put on disposable gloves.

Procedure

First-Degree Burn

2. Apply cool water to burn area, submerge burn site in cool water, or cover the area with cool damp cloths; this will reduce pain.
3. Large surface burns should never be wet as this causes shock. Large burns may be dried with sterile dressing. Apply a cold pack over dressing to reduce discomfort. Partial thickness or deeper burns (full thickness) require the following procedure.

Second- and Third-Degree Burns

2. Stop the burning process by smothering or dousing with water and removing smoldering or hot clothing. Remove any sources of heat such as metal jewelry, belts, etc.

(continued)

CUSTOMIZED INSTRUCTION

More Advanced Students

Many people believe myths related to burn treatments, such as putting butter on a burn. Have students investigate such myths and discuss why they are not true.

Teaching Tips

- Discuss why burns require immediate attention.
- Assign Procedure 18.12.

Procedure Tip

18.12 Treating Burns

- Review the background information.
- Review the different degree of burns.
- Guide students through the preprocedure.
- Demonstrate the procedure.
- Reinforce the different steps for each type of burn.
- Point out the postprocedure.
- Discuss why it is important to receive follow-up treatment after being burned.

PROCEDURE PRACTICE

- Demonstrate the steps for Procedure 18.12, Treating Burns, as many times as necessary, or ask students to demonstrate the steps. Have students practice and perform the procedure until they are competent.

Teaching Tips

- Discuss non-life-threatening situations.
- Compare closed fractures and open fractures.
- Point out that a fracture should be splinted to prevent further injury.

Procedure 18.12 **Treating Burns (continued)**

Procedure (cont)

3. Cover burned area with dry, sterile, nonstick dressing to help prevent infection. Do not pull away clothing that is stuck to burn site.
4. Check the patient's airway and breathing. Perform CPR if necessary.
5. Contact emergency medical service.
6. Cover with a dry sterile dressing if available. A non-fuzzy clean sheet or tablecloth could be substituted if sterile dressing is not available.
7. If you can elevate the burned area to decrease swelling, especially if head is involved and victim is having trouble breathing.
8. Follow procedure to prevent shock.

Postprocedure

9. Ensure that victim has follow-up treatment or assessment by Emergency Medical Technicians or hospital personnel.
10. Discard gloves and wash hands (follow hand-washing guidelines).

Non-Life-Threatening Situations

The bone fractures described below are examples of non-life-threatening conditions. Such conditions require first aid or medical care but not urgent care.

Bone Fractures

A *closed fracture* means the skin is closed even though the bone is broken. *Open fractures* involve both opened skin and the broken bone is exposed. Types of fractures include:

- **Comminuted Fracture (crush).** These fractures result from objects falling on bones and splintering or crushing them, such as seen when buildings collapse on victims of disasters (i.e. earthquakes, tornadoes).
- **Greenstick Fracture.** A partial bone fracture, usually occurring in children, in which the bone is bent but only broken on one side.
- **Compound Fractures.** Also known as open fractures, in these fractures broken bone pierces the skin.
- **Impacted Fracture.** One part of the bone is driven into another part, often occurs in motor vehicle accidents.
- **Colles' Fractures.** Fracture of the radial bone near the wrist, which often results when a person falls backwards and tries to catch themselves using an out-reached hand to brace their fall.
- **Compression Fractures.** Caused by pressure on bones, most seen in the vertebrae among elderly and post-menopausal women.

Fractures are injuries and as such they will have the following signs:

- Swelling
- Pain
- Change in the color of the skin (redness and heat)
- Deformity

Call or send for advanced medical help if you believe a fracture is present.

A fracture of the arm usually requires a sling. Apply a triangle sling so that the victim's hand and forearm are slightly higher than the elbow. This helps to minimize the swelling. A sling is a triangular bandage used to support the arm. Once the patient's arm is placed in a sling, a **swathe** can be used to hold the patient's arm against the side of the chest. (**Figure 18.10**)

swathe (SWOTH) Bandage.

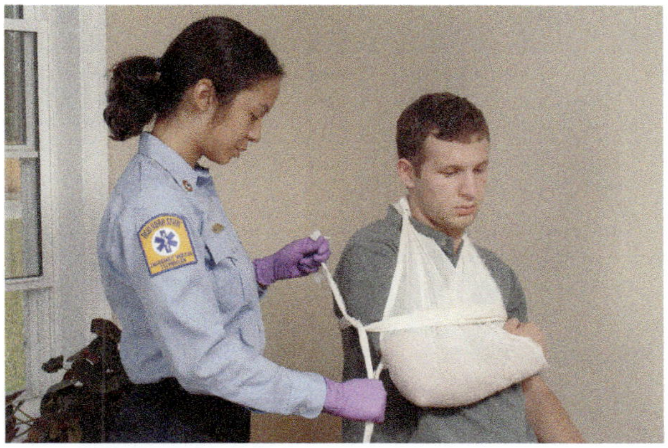

Figure 18.10 An EMT ties a swathe around a patient with his arm in a sling. Why would you use a swathe on a patient?

Commercial slings are available. Roller bandage can be used to form a sling and swathe. Velcro straps can be used to form a swathe. Use whatever materials you have on hand, provided that they will not cut into the patient as will narrow cords or wire. Remember: Shirts, ties, and wide belts can be used to make both sling and swathe.

Dislocations

A dislocation is when there is the separation of two bones where they meet a joint. Dislocations temporarily deform and immobilize joints and may cause ligament or nerve damage. They may occur from a fall, sports injury, or other trauma such as a motor vehicle accident. The hip, shoulder, knee, fingers, and toes are the most common places to have a dislocation. You have to immobilize the joint and seek immediate medical attention. DO NOT try to pop the bones back in place.

Patient and Employee Safety | Chapter 18 549

Figure Focus

18.10 An EMT ties a swathe around a patient with his arm in a sling. Why would you use a swathe on a patient?

Answer: Holds the extremity in place. Explain that a swathe can be used to hold a patient's arm against the side of the chest. This helps to prevent swelling and further injury.

Teaching Tips

- Explain what a dislocation is.
- Review the symptoms of dislocation.
- Warn against trying to pop a dislocated bone back into place.

ACTIVITY

Have students use the Internet to research different kinds of splints.

TEAMWORK

Challenge small groups of students to work together to use articles of clothing to make a sling and a swathe.

Teaching Tips

- Compare strains and sprains.

The following are symptoms of a dislocation:

- Visibly out of place
- Limited movement
- Swollen or discolored
- Intense pain
- Tingling or numbness

To diagnose a dislocation, an x-ray or MRI might be necessary.

Strains and Sprains

A strain is when a muscle or tendon is stretched or torn. This is also known as a pulled muscle. Strains are caused by overuse or misuse of a muscle. The most common strains occur in the hamstring or back. The symptoms of a strain include pain, stiffness, swelling, and bruising.

A sprain is when a ligament is stretched or torn. Sprains are caused when a joint is forced into an unnatural position. The most common sprains occur in the ankles and knees. The symptoms of a sprain include rapid swelling, joint and muscle pain, and bruising.

Dressings and Bandages

Dressings cover wounds and help prevent infectious bacteria from entering a wound. Also use dressing to apply direct pressure over a wound to control bleeding. There are many types of dressings used for various body locations. Bandages hold dressings in place.

Principles of Bandaging

- Always wear disposable gloves and follow Standard Precautions.
- Never encircle a wound with a non-elastic bandage. If swelling occurs a restrictive bandage may cause undue pressure and circulatory impairment.
- The bandage needs to be snug enough to hold the dressing in place but not tight enough to stop the circulation.
- When applying dressings and bandages to wounds on arms or legs, leave fingers and toes exposed so that you can watch for discoloration of the skin or swelling.
- Check pulse below bandage.
- Check the skin temperature. Cold skin may indicate poor circulation caused by a bandage that is too tight. Check the bandage to be certain it is not too tight. You should be able to insert a finger under the bandage.
- Loosen bandages if the patient complains of numbness or a tingling feeling.
- Do not remove a dressing once it has been applied. If blood soaks through, add another layer of dressings and secure with a bandage.

550 Chapter 18 | Patient and Employee Safety

CUSTOMIZED INSTRUCTION

More Advanced Students

Have students investigate Web sites for medical supplies companies to learn about different types of bandages.

Procedure 18.13 **Applying a Splint**

BACKGROUND: A splint helps to stabilize a broken bone and prevent further injury to tissues. This procedure explains how to make a splint out of a variety of materials.
ALERT: Follow Standard Precautions

Preprocedure

1. Put on disposable gloves.
2. Move fractured area as little as possible.

Procedure

3. Splint area with a firm object, such as newspapers, magazines folded flat, wood, or a commercially made splint. The **splint** should extend from the fingertips to the elbow. Need to immobilize joints above and below injury. Pad splint with clothing or towels if possible. Place padding or roller gauze in the hand for support and comfort.
4. Secure splint in place using roller gauze, wrapping it snugly and overlapping about two-thirds each wrap, or secure splint to extremity with strips of cloth at distal and proximal ends of the arm. You can wrap roller gauze over the fracture site. Do not exert any pressure over the injury.
5. If it is an open fracture, apply dressing over wound and secure in place with tape or with roller gauze that holds splint in place.

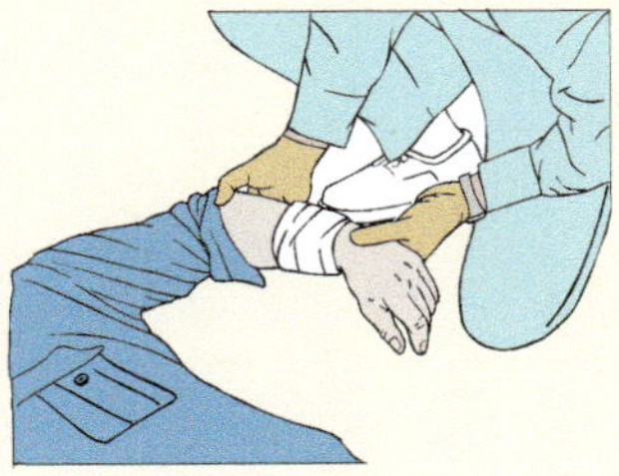

Postprocedure

6. Ensure that victim has follow-up treatment or assessment by Emergency Medical Technicians or hospital personnel.
7. Discard gloves and wash hands (follow handwashing guidelines).

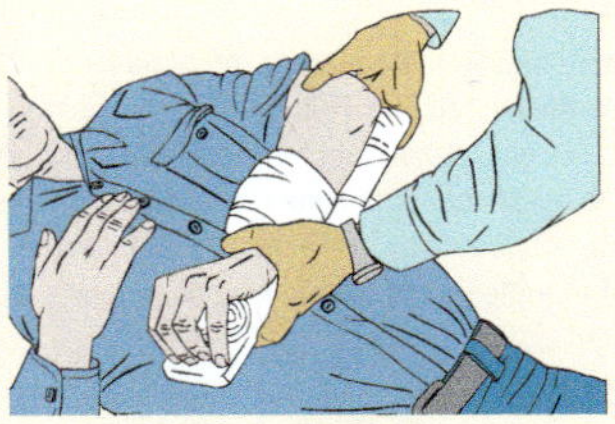

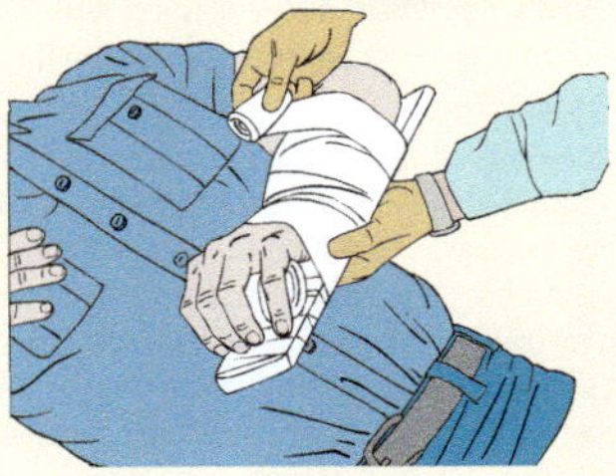

splint
(SPLINT)
Firm object used to support an unstable body part.

Patient and Employee Safety | Chapter 18 551

Teaching Tips

- Explain that splints can be applied to different parts of the body.
- Assign Procedure 18.13.

Procedure Tip

18.13 Applying a Splint

- Review the background information.
- Guide students through the preprocedure.
- Demonstrate the procedure.
- Explain to students the purpose of applying a splint.
- Point out the postprocedure.

PROCEDURE PRACTICE

- Demonstrate the steps for Procedure 18.13, Applying a Splint, as many times as necessary, or ask students to demonstrate the steps. Have students practice and perform the procedure until they are competent.

ACTIVITY

Have students practice applying a splint to a finger.

CUSTOMIZED INSTRUCTION

Special Needs Students

Emphasize that splints can be made from household objects. Help students make splints from common objects, such as magazines or wooden sticks.

Teaching Tips

- Describe reasons for using a sling.
- Assign Procedures 18.14 and 18.15.

Discuss

- Begin a class discussion by asking the following questions:
  - Why is it important to know how to make a sling out of common materials?
  - Why is the size of the material important?
  - What kinds of materials can you use to make a triangular sling?

Procedure Tip

18.14 Applying a Triangular Sling

- Review the background information.
- Guide students through the preprocedure.
- Demonstrate the procedure.
- Point out the postprocedure,

PROCEDURE PRACTICE

- Demonstrate the steps for Procedure 18.14, Applying a Triangular Sling, as many times as necessary, or ask students to demonstrate the steps. Have students practice and perform the procedure until they are competent.

Procedure 18.14 Applying a Triangular Sling

BACKGROUND: A sling is a bandage that holds up and stabilizes an injured arm. This procedure explains how to make a sling out of any long piece of cloth.
ALERT: Follow Standard Precautions

Preprocedure

1. Put on disposable gloves.
2. Make a sling from a piece of cloth, clothing, towel, or sheet; fold or cut this material into shape of a triangle. The ideal sling is about 50 to 60 inches long at its base and 36 to 40 inches long on each side.

Procedure

3. Position triangular material over top of patient's chest opposite the injured arm. Fold patient's arm across chest. If patient cannot hold his or her own arm, have someone assist you, or provide support for patient's arm until you are ready to tie sling. Note that one point of triangle should extend beyond patient's elbow on injured side.
4. Take bottom point of triangle and bring this end up over patient's arm. When you are finished, take this bottom point over top of patient's shoulder on the side of injured arm.
5. Draw up on ends of sling so that patient's hand is about 4 inches above elbow. Tie the two ends of the sling together, making sure that the knot does not press against back of patient's neck. Place a flat pad of dressing or a handkerchief under the knot. Leave patient's fingertips exposed so that you can see any color changes that indicate lack of circulation. Check for radial pulse. If pulse is absent, take off sling and attempt to reposition arm to regain pulse, then repeat procedure.
6. Take point of material at patient's elbow and fold it forward. Pin it to front of sling. This forms a pocket for the elbow. If you do not have pin, twist excess material and tie knot in point. This will provide a shallow pocket for patient's elbow.
7. Create a swathe by folding a triangular bandage in half and then folding it to a 4-inch width. This swathe is tied around chest and injured arm, over sling. Do not place this swathe over patient's arm on uninjured side.

Postprocedure

8. Ensure that victim has follow-up treatment or assessment by Emergency Medical Technicians or hospital personnel.
9. Discard gloves and wash hands (follow hand-washing guidelines).

552 Chapter 18 | Patient and Employee Safety

CUSTOMIZED INSTRUCTION

Less Advanced Students

Have students describe the procedure for making a triangular sling in their own words. Allow students to describe the procedure to another student to see if the second student can make the sling from the directions.

Procedure 18.15 Triangular Bandaging of an Open Head Wound

BACKGROUND: A triangular bandage can be used to hold a dressing on a wound. This procedure explains how to fold a triangular bandage to bandage an open head wound.
ALERT: Follow Standard Precautions

Preprocedure

1. Put on disposable gloves.
2. Fold triangular bandage to make 2-inch hem along base.

Procedure

3. Apply gauze pad over wound. With folded edge facing out, position bandage on patient's forehead, just above eyes. Make certain that point of bandage hangs down behind patient's head.
4. Draw ends of bandage behind patient's head and tie them.
5. Next, pull ends to front of patient's head and tie them together.
6. Tuck in the tail at back.

Postprocedure

7. Ensure that victim has follow-up treatment or assessment by Emergency Medical Technicians or hospital personnel.
8. Discard gloves and wash hands (follow hand-washing guidelines).

Procedure 18.16 Circular Bandaging of a Small Leg or Arm Wound

BACKGROUND: Circular bandaging holds a dressing in place over a wound and applies pressure to the wound. This procedure explains how to apply a circular bandage to a small leg or arm wound.
ALERT: Follow Standard Precautions

Preprocedure

1. Put on disposable gloves.

Procedure

2. Apply dressing to wound and elevate extremity.
3. Place end of gauze roll (1 to 2 inches wide) on dressing. Anchor end of gauze roll over dressing with two initial wraps. (Place end of gauze over the dressing. Wrap gauze around the area once. Fold angled corner of gauze back over wrapped gauze.) Continue to wrap from distal (far) end of extremity to proximal (near the torso) end until entire dressing is covered. Bandage will overlap dressing on both sides. Pull bandage snug as you wrap. Overlap each wrap by about two-thirds. Cut gauze and tape end or tie gauze to secure in place.

Postprocedure

4. Ensure that victim has follow-up treatment or assessment by Emergency Medical Technicians or hospital personnel.
5. Discard gloves and wash hands (follow hand-washing guidelines).

Patient and Employee Safety | Chapter 18 553

Teaching Tips

- Explain that head wounds can be bandaged using a triangular bandage.

Procedure Tip

18.15 Triangular Bandaging of an Open Head Wound

- Review the background information.
- Discuss the types of head wounds that would benefit from a triangular bandage.
- Guide students through the preprocedure.
- Demonstrate the procedure.
- Point out the postprocedure.

PROCEDURE PRACTICE

- Demonstrate the steps for Procedure 18.15, Triangular Bandaging of an Open Head Wound, as many times as necessary, or ask students to demonstrate the steps. Have students practice and perform the procedure until they are competent.

Teaching Tips

- Describe that it is important to cover a wound and to apply pressure.
- Assign Procedure 18.16.

Procedure Tip

18.16 Circular Bandaging of a Small Leg or Arm Wound

- Review the background information.
- Guide students through the preprocedure.
- Demonstrate the procedure.
- Point out the postprocedure.

PROCEDURE PRACTICE

- Demonstrate the steps for Procedure 18.16, Circular Bandaging of a Small Leg or Arm Wound, as many times as necessary, or ask students to demonstrate the steps. Have students practice and perform the procedure until they are competent.

Teaching Tips

- Explain that large wounds and wounds near the feet require special bandaging.
- Assign Procedures 18.17 and 18.18.

Procedure Tip

18.17 Spiral Bandaging of a Large Wound

- Review the background information.
- Discuss why spiral bandaging is better for large wounds.
- Guide students through the preprocedure.
- Demonstrate the procedure.
- Explain that gauze rolls come in different sizes.
- Point out the postprocedure.

PROCEDURE PRACTICE

- Demonstrate the steps for Procedure 18.17, Spiral Bandaging of a Large Wound, as many times as necessary, or ask students to demonstrate the steps. Have students practice and perform the procedure until they are competent.

Procedure Tip

18.18 Bandaging of an Ankle or Foot Wound

- Review the background information.
- Guide students through the preprocedure.
- Demonstrate the procedure.
- Point out the postprocedure.

Procedure 18.17 Spiral Bandaging of a Large Wound

BACKGROUND: Spiral bandaging can be used to hold on a dressing and apply pressure to a large wound of the arm or leg. This procedure explains how to use spiral bandaging on a large wound.
ALERT: Follow Standard Precautions

Preprocedure

1. Put on disposable gloves.

Procedure

2. Apply dressing to wound.
3. Place end of gauze roll (3 to 6 inches wide) on lower edge of dressing.
4. Anchor end.
5. Wrap gauze around arm or leg at an angle and overlap the edges.
6. If you use up the gauze, continue the wrap with another roll.
7. Secure end by taping or tying off.

Postprocedure

8. Ensure that victim has follow-up treatment or assessment by Emergency Medical Technicians or hospital personnel.
9. Discard gloves and wash hands (follow hand-washing guidelines).

Procedure 18.18 Bandaging of an Ankle or Foot Wound

BACKGROUND: A bandage can be wrapped around the ankle or foot, to secure a dressing and apply pressure to a wound. This procedure explains how to bandage an ankle or foot wound.
ALERT: Follow Standard Precautions

Preprocedure

1. Put on disposable gloves.

Procedure

2. Apply dressing to wound.
3. Place end of gauze roll (1 to 2 inches wide) on top of foot just above toes, and anchor ends.
4. On second wrap around foot, bring gauze around back of ankle and over top of foot. Bring gauze under foot and over top of foot again. Wrap around ankle and over top of foot, then under foot. Continue these steps until dressing is covered, and secure gauze by tying off or taping.

Postprocedure

5. Ensure that victim has follow-up treatment or assessment by Emergency Medical Technicians or hospital personnel.
6. Discard gloves and wash hands (follow hand-washing guidelines).

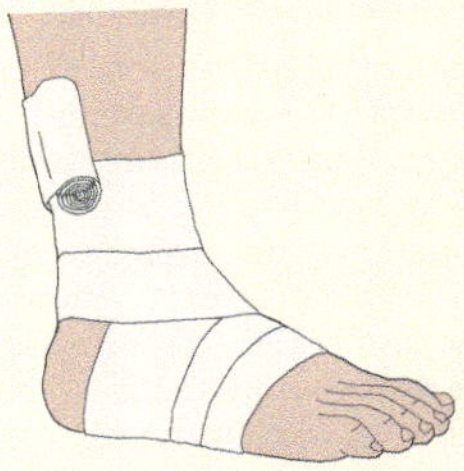

554 Chapter 18 | Patient and Employee Safety

PROCEDURE PRACTICE

- Demonstrate the steps for Procedure 18.18, Bandaging of an Ankle or Foot Wound, as many times as necessary, or ask students to demonstrate the steps. Have students practice and perform the procedure until they are competent.

Procedure 18.19 How to Care for a Dislocation

BACKGROUND: A dislocation occurs when excessive stress in an abnormal direction on one or more bones near a joint disrupts the continuity of joint configuration and articulation. When this occurs, the bones' articulating surfaces no longer contact each other. Most dislocations result from trauma. Damage to ligaments and soft tissue may complicate these injuries.

ALERT: Follow Standard Precautions

Preprocedure

Expect the patient to complain of pain and decreased range of motion around the affected joint. Dislocations generally occur during a traumatic event so expect that the patient may have other injuries, which could include a fracture of the joint. Depending on the nature of the injury, the patient may require closed reduction of the injured joint or a surgical intervention to properly realign the affected joint. Expect that an x-ray of the affected joint will be necessary.

1. Determine the traumatic event leading to the injury.
2. Inspect the patient's affected joint for swelling, bruising, odd configuration of joint anatomy, and altered mobility.
3. Gently palpate the joint noting any tenderness. Palpate nearby pulses to assess the circulatory status. Obtain medical assistance right away.

Procedure

Closed Reduction

NOTE: Closed Reduction and Surgical Correction will occur in a hospital or other care facility and will be done by physicians.

4. Provide support for the patient during the examination and any procedure that may be indicated.
5. Assist with the application of an external immobilization device.
6. Apply ice for at least the first 24 hours.
7. Monitor the patient's neurovascular status by checking for pulses, warmth, color, and sensory function of the region around the injury site. Also note any increased swelling.

NOTE: The patient will be medicated with prescribed pain medication only by licensed individuals.

8. Use a pain rating scale, such as a scale of 1 to 10, to evaluate the effectiveness of the pain medication.
9. Provide education to the patient/family regarding any ongoing care necessary and any rehabilitative exercise program prescribed for after the immobilizing device is removed.

Surgical Correction

10. Monitor the patient closely in the immediate post-operative period for:
    - neurovascular status
    - pain
    - alteration in vital signs
11. Expect the patient to have either a cast or an external immobilizer.
12. Provide pain medication as directed by the physician.
13. Apply ice as directed by the physician.
14. Use a pain rating scale, such as a scale of 1 to 10, to evaluate the effectiveness of the pain medication and other interventions provided to relieve discomfort.
15. Prepare the patient for the rehabilitation period.

Note: Possible complications of a joint dislocation and its treatment include:

- Vascular impairment
- Nerve injury
- Residual joint laxity with chronic joint instability.
- Degenerative arthritis
- Thromboembolic complications
- Neurovascular compromise
- Skin breakdown from extended wearing of an immobilization device

Patient and Employee Safety | Chapter 18 555

Procedure Tip

18.19 How to Care for a Dislocation

- Review the background information.
- Guide students through the preprocedure.
- Discuss why patients may complain.
- Demonstrate the procedure.
- Discuss the different types of dislocations.
- Review the procedure steps.

PROCEDURE PRACTICE

- Demonstrate the steps for Procedure 18.19, How to Care for a Dislocation, as many times as necessary, or ask students to demonstrate the steps. Have students practice and perform the procedure until they are competent.

ACTIVITY

Have students use a drawing of a skeleton to label common places for dislocations.

CUSTOMIZED INSTRUCTION

More Advanced Students

Challenge students to find out why dislocations are uncommon in younger children. Instead younger children are more prone to fractures than dislocations.

Teaching Tips

- Review the three grades of strains.
- Explain the meaning of the acronym RICE when it comes to treating strains and sprains.
- Assign Procedure 18.20.

Procedure Tip

18.20 How to Care for a Strain

- Review the background information.
- Describe how strains occur and how they differ from sprains.
- Compare the three levels of strains.
- Explain the meaning of the acronym RICE.
- Guide students through the preprocedure.
- Demonstrate the procedure.

PROCEDURE PRACTICE

- Demonstrate the steps for Procedure 18.20, How to Care for a Strain, as many times as necessary, or ask students to demonstrate the steps. Have students practice and perform the procedure until they are competent.

Procedure 18.20 How to Care for a Strain

BACKGROUND: A strain occurs when partial, microscopic muscle tears result from overuse or overstretching of a single muscle, muscle group, or tendon. A strain can be acute or chronic. An acute strain arises from a sudden forced movement that overstretches a muscle; a chronic strain results from the cumulative effects of repeated muscle overuse. Strains commonly result from injury suffered while playing active sports or from poor body mechanics, such as improper lifting and carrying techniques. Strains are classified into three grades of injury:

- *Grade I* (mild): microscopic muscle and/or tendon tear with no strength loss
- *Grade II* (moderate): incomplete muscle and/or tendon tear with bleeding into muscle tissue and some strength loss
- *Grade III* (severe): complete muscle and/or tendon tear usually resulting from separation of muscle from muscle, muscle from tendon, or tendon from bone

It is worth remembering RICE when it comes to the treatment of uncomplicated soft tissue, such as strains and sprains. This stand for:

R (rest)
I (ice)
C (compression)
E (elevate)

ALERT: Follow Standard Precautions

Preprocedure

Expect the patient to complain of pain, decreased mobility, and strength loss at the site of injury. Important points to remember when assessing the patient are:

1. Ask how the injury occurred.
2. Ask about prior joint injuries.
3. Inspect the injured joint for swelling or bruising.
4. Palpate the joint, noting any tenderness. Palpate nearby pulses to assess the circulatory status.
5. To rule out a fracture, the physician will order x-rays.

Procedure

6. Consult with the physician for any specific instructions related to the injury.
7. Apply a compression bandage as ordered by the physician.
8. Elevate the affected joint.
9. Check with the physician. Apply ice or heat as directed. If injury is several days old, the physician may order heat rather than ice to reduce pain.
10. Elevate the affected extremity.
11. Monitor the patient's neurovascular status by checking for pulses, warmth, color, and sensory function of the region around the injury site. Also note any increased swelling.
12. Medicate as directed by the physician. In most cases, analgesics, anti-inflammatory drugs, or a muscle relaxant will be prescribed. These should be dispensed by licensed heath care professionals.
13. Use a pain rating scale, such as a scale of 1 to 10, to evaluate the effectiveness of the Pain medication and other interventions.
14. Advise the patient to rest and avoid using the strained muscle.
15. Educate the patient on prescribed exercises to follow after healing has begun.
16. Advise the patient to resume activities gradually.

556 Chapter 18 | Patient and Employee Safety

CUSTOMIZED INSTRUCTION

Less Advanced Students

Help students differentiate between strains and sprains. Encourage students to make a visual demonstration to show the difference.

Procedure 18.21 **How to Care for a Sprain**

BACKGROUND: A sprain occurs when a ligament or the capsule surrounding a joint becomes stretched or torn. A moderate or severe sprain can cause joint instability and loss of function. Sprains are classified into three grades of injury:

- *Grade I* (mild): minor or partial ligament tear with normal joint stability and function
- *Grade II* (moderate): partial ligament tear with mild joint laxity and function loss
- *Grade III* (severe): complete ligament tear or complete separation of ligament from bone, causing total joint laxity and function loss

ALERT: Follow Standard Precautions

Preprocedure

Expect the patient to complain of pain around the affected joint. The patient may also complain of diminished function of the joint. Important points when assessing this patient are:

1. Ask how the injury occurred.
2. Ask about prior joint injuries.
3. Observe the patient as he or she stands, walks, and sits, noting abnormalities such as change in gait or inability to bear weight on joint.
4. Inspect the injured joint for swelling and bruising.
5. Palpate the joint, noting any tenderness. Palpate nearby pulses to assess the circulatory status.

NOTE: Be sure to compare extremities on both sides of the body when assessing musculoskeletal injuries. The patient needs to be seen by a physician and have x-rays to rule out fracture.

Procedure

6. Consult with the physician for any specific instructions related to the injury.
7. Immobilize the joint, using a splint or aircast.
8. Monitor the patient's neurovascular status by checking for pulses, warmth, color, mobility, and sensory function of the region around the injury site. Also note any increased swelling.
9. Elevate the injured extremity to reduce swelling and pain.
10. Apply ice to the injury.
11. Medicate the patient with prescribed pain medication. Remember: Only licensed people can give medication.
12. Use a pain rating scale, such as a scale of 1 to 10, to evaluate the effectiveness of the pain medication and other interventions.
13. Provide education to the patient/family regarding any ongoing care necessary.

Patient and Employee Safety | Chapter 18 557

Teaching Tips

- Review the three grades of sprains.
- Explain the difference between a sprain and a fracture.
- Assign Procedure 18.21.

Procedure Tip

18.21 How to Care for a Sprain

- Review the background information.
- Discuss the three levels of sprains.
- Explain why it is important to know when and how a sprain occurred.
- Guide students through the preprocedure.
- Demonstrate the procedure.

PROCEDURE PRACTICE

- Demonstrate the steps for Procedure 18.21, How to Care for a Sprain, as many times as necessary, or ask students to demonstrate the steps. Have students practice and perform the procedure until they are competent.

CUSTOMIZED INSTRUCTION

Special Needs Students

Allow students with special needs extra time to complete the procedure properly.

Teaching Tips

- Describe a cast and its use.
- Discuss some of the materials from which casts are made.
- Assign Procedure 18.22.

Procedure Tip

18.22 Cast Care

- Review background information.
- Describe the different types of casts.
- Explain why a fracture has to be set.
- Guide students through the preprocedure.
- Demonstrate the procedure.

PROCEDURE PRACTICE

- Demonstrate the steps for Procedure 18.22, Cast Care, as many times as necessary, or ask students to demonstrate the steps. Have students practice and perform the procedure until they are competent.

Procedure 18.22 Cast Care

BACKGROUND: A cast is a hard mold that encases a body part, usually an extremity, to provide immobilization without discomfort. It can be used to treat injuries such as fractures, correct orthopedic conditions such as deformities, or promote healing after general or plastic surgery, amputation, or nerve and vascular repair.

Casts may be constructed of plaster, fiberglass, or other synthetic materials. Typically, a physician applies a cast and a nurse prepares the patient and the equipment and assists during the procedure. The orthopedic technician, after special training, may apply or change a standard cast but the orthopedist must reduce and set the fracture.

ALERT: Follow Standard Precautions

Preprocedure

Prior to the application of the cast the nurse should establish a baseline assessment of the area to be casted. This would include:

- Palpation of the distal pulses
- Assessment of the color, temperature, and capillary refill of the skin
- Neurologic function, including sensation and motion in the affected area

Special Considerations: A fiberglass cast dries immediately after application. A plaster cast dries in approximately 24 to 48 hours. During this drying period, the cast must be properly positioned to prevent a surface depression that could cause pressure areas or dependent anemia.

Procedure

1. Assess your patient frequently.
2. Check the casted area for drainage stains.
3. Elevate the extremity above patient's heart level.
4. Place absorptive pads between the moist cast and any bedding to absorb moisture.
5. Periodically check the cast for flat spots or dents. These may cause pressure areas, resulting in skin breakdown.
6. Reposition the patient every 2 hours to ensure even cast drying. Use the palm of the hand, not the fingers for repositioning in order to avoid denting the cast. Make sure bony prominences, such as heels, ankles, and elbows are pressure free.
7. Routinely assess your patient's neurovascular status. Check for swelling, pallor, numbness, tingling, loss of pulses, and cool skin areas around the cast. Notify the doctor immediately for any of these signs.
8. Notify the doctor for:
   - Drainage from the wound on the cast
   - Malodor from the cast
9. Protect the cast from getting wet.
10. Provide skin care.

558 Chapter 18 | Patient and Employee Safety

CUSTOMIZED INSTRUCTION

More Advanced Students

Have students contact a representative from the office of an orthopedic surgeon. Ask them to find out about the kinds of casts that are used, the treatment they require, and the reasons for selecting one over the other. Ask volunteers to present their findings.

Diabetes Mellitus

Diabetes Mellitus is an endocrine disorder that manifests as a carbohydrate intolerance. This disease is caused when the islets (islands) of Langerhans in the pancreas do not produce enough insulin. When there is an insulin imbalance, you must watch the resident carefully for signs of diabetic shock or **insulin shock**. Diabetic shock occurs when the diabetic resident does not have enough insulin, when there is an infection, or if there is increased stress. The following are symptoms of diabetic shock:

insulin shock
(IN suh lin shok)
Condition caused by too much insulin.

- Loss of appetite
- Abdominal discomfort or pain
- Dry skin
- Flushed skin
- Sweet or fruity odor of the breath
- Soft eyeballs (also known as sunken eyeballs, caused by excessive dehydration)
- Generalized aches
- Increased urination
- Air hunger (the feeling of not being able to get a satisfying breath), increased respiration, labored breathing
- Nausea and/or vomiting
- Dulled senses
- Weakness
- Excessive thirst

Diabetes is classified as:

1. Diabetes Mellitus.
   a. Insulin-Dependent Type I (DM): Usually genetically determined abnormality
   b. Non-Insulin Dependent (NIDDM) Type II: Adult onset—altered production and use of insulin
2. Impaired Glucose Tolerance (IGT).
3. Gestational Diabetes (GDM): Onset during pregnancy due to altered secretion of hormones.

When there is an endocrine disorder such as diabetes, the patient must monitor their blood glucose levels. A blood glucose level over 115 is called *hyperglycemia*. A glucose level under 80 is called *hypoglycemia*. Hyperglycemia is caused by lack of adequate insulin, infection, and increased stress. The symptoms of hyperglycemia include:

- Altered mental state
- Excessive thirst
- Flushed skin
- Sweet or fruity breath

Teaching Tips

- Define diabetes mellitus.
- Review the symptoms of diabetic coma.
- Differentiate among the types of diabetes.
- Contrast hyperglycemia with hypoglycemia.

ACTIVITY

Write each of the four types of diabetes on separate pieces of paper. Divide the class into four groups. Have a member from each group select a piece of paper at random. The group should prepare and present a report on the type they selected.

CUSTOMIZED INSTRUCTION

More Advanced Students

Have students compare the prefixes *hyper-* and *hypo-*. Ask them to relate the prefixes to their study of diabetes.

Teaching Tips

- Explain the dangers of too much glucose in the blood.
- Describe tests to provide indications of glucose control.
- Review the guidelines for testing blood for glucose.

TEAMWORK

Diabetes has been related to obesity. Have students find information about recent trends in diabetes as it relates to obesity. Tell students to prepare a presentation of their information.

- Increased urination
- Blurred vision
- Weakness
- Abdominal discomfort
- Loss of appetite
- Labored breathing

Hypoglycemia is caused by excessive insulin, decreased nutritional intake, and excessive exercise. The symptoms of hypoglycemia include:

- Hunger
- Blurred vision
- Irritability
- Weakness
- Headache
- Tremors

One of your responsibilities in caring for the diabetic patient is monitoring blood sugars with a glucose monitor at designated intervals, usually before meals and at bedtime. Documenting these results accurately and notifying the nurse about too high or too low blood sugars is very important.

These patients should also be monitored for physical and cognitive signs of hypo- or hyperglycemia. If these symptoms are present, the patient should be immediately tested with the blood glucose monitor.

Patients with higher than normal blood sugar levels may need additional insulin. Patients with lower than normal blood sugar levels may need additional oral nutrition or glucose.

A blood glucose of 40 or less is a medical emergency. The patient with severe hypoglycemia must receive instant glucose either by mouth or through their intravenous site if present. You may find this patient unconscious. If so, seek immediate medical assistance.

ALERT: Blood sugars that are either too high or too low can cause irreversible loss of system functions. These injuries are cumulative over time and may cause such problems as diabetic retinopathy, renal failure, or failure to heal with loss of limbs.

Blood Glucose Testing

Diabetic Patient

The diabetic patient does not produce enough insulin. This causes glucose to remain in the blood. Too much glucose in the blood can cause:

- Circulatory problems
- Poor healing of lesions on legs and feet
- Changes in the retina (which can lead to blindness)
- Nerve disorders

Some patients with diabetes can successfully control sugar levels in the blood with diet and exercise. Others need medication to control their sugar levels.

The diabetic patient controls the disease with diet, exercise, and medication. A clinical study conducted between 1983 and 1993 called the Diabetes Control and Complications Trial (DCCT) showed that controlling glucose levels reduces the risk of eye, kidney, nerve, and cardiovascular disease. New studies confirm the DCCT findings.

A laboratory test called Glycosolated Hemoglobin (HbA_1C) provides indications of glucose control. Each number above 7 grams HbA_1C means an increase in the risk of disease for patients with diabetes. Patients who need insulin must check the level of glucose in their blood. The level of glucose tells them how much insulin they need. Patients use a glucose meter to measure the sugar level in their blood before taking insulin.

General Guidelines for Testing Blood for Glucose

1. Complete quality control checks at prescribed times.
2. Store reagent strips according to instructions.
3. Keep the lid on the reagent bottle tightly closed.
4. *Do not touch* the pad on the reagent strip.
5. Use careful technique in obtaining blood specimen.

There are many different glucose meters. Each one is a little different from the others. Learn the steps for the meter that is used in your facility.

Understanding and Handling Fainting

The term *syncope* is another term for fainting. It is caused when the brain does not have an adequate supply of blood. Symptoms of syncope include: feeling of uneasiness; lightheadedness; pale, cool, clammy skin; or dilated pupils. Several things can cause this: fear of pain; sight of blood or needles; emotional disturbance; pain; long periods without movement causing poor blood circulation; dehydration; or standing up too fast.

Take proper precautions to prevent an accident or injury to a resident or to yourself. Have the resident put his or her head between the knees, with arms hanging loose at the side. Place your hands on the back of the resident's head. Instruct resident to apply upward pressure with the head.

Break open a spirits of ammonia ampule and place under the resident's nose. Have the resident lie down, with head lower than legs, if possible. Place a cold towel on the forehead and loosen any tight clothing.

Convulsions

Convulsions are when a person's body shakes rapidly and uncontrollably. This is caused by the muscles contracting and relaxing repeatedly. Most convulsions are harmless and last anywhere from 30 seconds to two minutes.

The symptoms of convulsions include blacking out, confusion, loss of bladder or bowel control, clenching teeth, uncontrollable muscle spasms, drooling, and grunting.

When a person experiences a convulsion, it is important to protect the person from injury. To do this, clear the area around the person, lay the person on the ground, cushion the person's head, loosen any tight clothing, turn the person on their side, and call for medical help. A person experiencing low blood glucose is susceptible to have convulsions, If this occurs, seek medical treatment immediately.

Adverse Drug-Related Emergencies

As a result of increasing over-dosages of opioids and other drugs in many communities, emergency medical services and specially trained providers carry drugs that reverse the actions of the opioid. Drugs, such as naloxone, can rapidly restore breathing of a victim who has overdosed on an opioid or heroin. Each state establishes laws that determines who can give the drug and if a prescription is needed to obtain the naloxone.

Patient and Employee Safety | Chapter 18 561

Teaching Tips

- Discuss what happens to a person experiencing convulsions.
- Explain how to care for a person experiencing convulsions.
- Explain why the margin note on syncope, or fainting, is shown here. Explain to students that low blood sugar can lead to fainting.

ACTIVITY

Investigate types of testing processes for people with diabetes. Find out what the test involves and how often the blood must be tested.

Section 18.5 Review Questions

1. Answer: Closed wound
2. Answer: Assess the person to see if the airway is obstructed, call 911, and perform the procedure for obstructed airway (Heimlich maneuver).
3. Answer: Squeezing feeling in the chest; persistent discomfort that spreads to shoulders, arms, neck, jaw, or across the chest; sweating, nausea, vomiting, shortness of breath, or feeling faint
4. Answer: Give five back blows. Place infant face down, supporting head and neck and tilting infant so that the head is lower than rest of body. Give five firm hits with heel of your hand over backbone and between shoulder blades. Give five chest thrusts by turning infant on its back with head lower than rest of body. Using two to three fingers, push five times on midsternum, which is about one finger's width below nipple line at midchest at a rate of about one per second. Continue procedure until obstruction is clear or infant becomes unconscious. If infant becomes unconscious, stop giving black blows and start CPR.
5. Answer: Mandibular artery, brachial artery, femoral artery
6. Answer: Shock is usually caused by major loss of body fluids or blood; it can be caused by vomiting and diarrhea.

Summary

In this section, you learned very basic first-aid skills. You were introduced to the general principles of handling both life-threatening and non-life-threatening situations. You learned about rescue breathing, obstructed airway, and heart attack.

We discussed the treatment for shock, poisoning, serious wounds, and burns. It is very important for you to become proficient in first aid. To do this, you should attend a class given by a qualified American Red Cross instructor.

Section 18.5 Review Questions

1. What word describes the condition in which the skin is bruised, swollen, and painful, but is not broken?
2. A person in a restaurant starts coughing and wheezing after eating some chicken. What should you do?
3. What are the early warning signs of a heart attack?
4. How would you clear an obstruction from the airway of a conscious infant?
5. What are three pressure points that can be used to stop bleeding?
6. What causes shock?
7. How is a second-degree burn different from a first-degree burn?
8. What kind of bandaging would you use to cover a small wound on the leg?

562 Chapter 18 | Patient and Employee Safety

7. Answer: First-degree burn (superficial partial-thickness burn) appears pink or red; sensitive to touch; second-degree burn (deep partial-thickness burn) appears pink or red with a mottled appearance; blisters and edema; touching causes severe pain
8. Answer: Circular bandaging

Cardiopulmonary Resuscitation (CPR) — SECTION 18.6

Background

Cardiopulmonary resuscitation (CPR) is a rapid life-saving technique that pumps blood through the body and provides oxygen until advanced life-support (ALS) becomes available. CPR originated in Paris during the 1700s as mouth-to-mouth breathing for drowning victims. During the late 1800s, chest compressions were added to address the absence of heartbeats in unconscious victims.

Although initially limited to physicians, over the years, the American Heart Association (AHA) has expanded CPR guidelines to include basic life support (BLS) training for all health care professionals and simple techniques such as "hands-only" CPR for the general public at large. CPR is performed until the heart can be shocked back into a normal rhythm, using a defibrillator. As a health care professional, you should know how to perform CPR.

Community

Prepare a poster board with the questions below. Make a presentation to elementary students about making an emergency call.

One of the team members acts as the 911 dispatcher, asking the following questions: Who is the injured person? Did you see the accident happen? Can the person move? Is the person bleeding? Can the person speak to you? Does the person have a bump on the head? Where is it located? What other injuries can you see? Students participate in a team-led discussion about their responses.

Objectives

When you have completed this section, you will be able to do the following:

- Match key terms with their correct meanings.
- Demonstrate the procedures for cardiopulmonary resuscitation (CPR).
- Explain the role of the automated external defibrillator in delivering CPR.

Cardiac Arrest and CPR

Cardiac arrest, or heart attack, can cause the heart to change rhythm and ultimately stop beating. During sudden cardiac arrest, a normal beat changes to ventricular fibrillation (VF). The rhythm of a heart in VF is fluttery and irregular. The heart needs a shock to bring it back into a normal rhythm.

Cardiopulmonary **resuscitation** (CPR) provides body cells with **oxygenated** blood, in order to keep the cells alive. (Figure 18.11) The technique combines chest compressions, which attempts to restore circulation, with artificial breathing (mouth-to-mouth, which forces air into the lungs). In 2010, the American Heart Association updated CPR guidelines to recommend that if there are not CPR-trained individuals present, untrained bystanders should attempt chest compressions until a trained respondent arrives. This is called Hands-Only CPR. CPR does not cause the heart to start beating again with a normal beat. It helps keep oxygenated blood circulating to the heart and brain until the heart can be shocked back into a normal rhythm, by a device called a **defibrillator**. In 2015, the AHA updated the guidelines again to confirm and enhance the 2010 recommendations.

The American Heart Association Guidelines for CPR and ECC (Emergency Cardiovascular Care) recommend calling for emergency assistance immediately, and then commencing C-A-B (Chest compressions, Airway, Breathing) for adults, children, and infants. (Figure 18.12)

cardiac
(KAR dee ack)
Relating to the heart.

resuscitation
(ri suhs i TAY shuhn)
Bringing back to life, reviving.

oxygenated
(OK si juh nayt ed)
Containing oxygen.

defibrillator
(dee FIB ruh lay ter)
A device that administers an electric shock to restore normal heartbeat.

Patient and Employee Safety | Chapter 18 563

FOCUS AND ENGAGE

Introduce the Section

a. Review the content of the Background paragraphs, introducing the content of the section.

b. Discuss the objectives for the section.

Vocabulary Review

a. Direct students to the key terms.

b. Pronounce each word, and have the students repeat the pronunciation out loud.

c. Discuss the definition of each word.

TEACH

Teaching Tips

- Explain what happens during a cardiac arrest.
- Discuss the importance of CPR.
- Assign Procedures 18.23 through 18.25.

Community

- Provide students with necessary materials.
- Arrange a visit to a local elementary school.
- Review presentation beforehand. Although the topic is serious, be sure that the presentation will be helpful, but not frightening, to younger students.
- You may want to bring a doll or stuffed animal for elementary students to use as a victim.
- Discuss responses upon returning to your classroom.

Figure Focus

18.11 CPR pumps the heart to keep oxygenated blood flowing to organs after cardiac arrest. Why is it important to keep oxygen flowing to organs?

Answer: Oxygen keeps cells alive. Make sure students recognize that cells need a constant supply of oxygen. Oxygen is required for most cellular processes. Without oxygen, cells will begin to die.

Figure 18.11
CPR pumps the heart to keep oxygenated blood flowing to organs after cardiac arrest. Why is it important to keep oxygen flowing to organs?

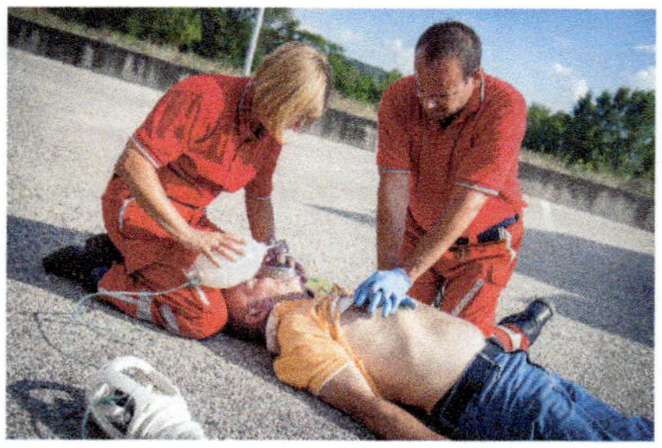

Table 18.2 Summary of Key BLS Components for Adults, Children, and Infants

Component	Adults and Adolescents (Puberty to Adulthood)	Children (Age 1 Year to Puberty)	Infants (Age Less Than 1 Year, Excluding Newborns)
Scene Safety	■ Make sure the environment is safe for rescuers and victim		
Recognition of Cardiac Arrest	■ Check for responsiveness ■ No breathing or only gasping (i.e., no normal breathing) ■ No definite pulse felt within 10 seconds ■ Breathing and pulse check can be performed simultaneously in less than 10 seconds		
Activation of Emergency Response System	■ If you are alone with no mobile phone, leave the victim to activate the emergency response system and get the AED before beginning CPR ■ Otherwise, send someone and begin CPR immediately; use the AED as soon as it is available	**Witnessed Collapse:** ■ Follow steps for adults and adolescents on the left **Unwitnessed Collapse:** ■ Give 2 minutes of CPR ■ Leave the victim to activate the emergency response system and get the AED ■ Return to the child or infant and resume CPR; use the AED as soon as it is available	
Compression-Ventilation Ratio *without* Advanced Airway	■ **1 or 2 Rescuers:** 30:2	■ **1 Rescuer:** 30:2 ■ **2 or More Rescuers:** 15:2	
Compression-Ventilation Ratio *with* Advanced Airway	■ Continuous compressions at a rate of 100–120/min ■ Give 1 breath every 6 seconds (10 breaths/min)		
Compression Rate	■ 100–120/min		
Compression Depth	■ At least 2 inches (5 cm)	■ At least one-third AP diameter of chest ■ About 2 inches (5 cm)	■ At least one-third AP diameter of chest ■ About 1½ inches (4 cm)
Hand Placement	■ 2 hands on the lower half of the breastbone (sternum)	■ 2 hands or 1 hand (optimal for very small child) on the lower half of the breastbone (sternum)	**1 Rescuer:** ■ 2 fingers in the center of the chest, just below the nipple line **2 or More Rescuers:** ■ 2 thumb-encircling hands in the center of the chest just below the nipple line
Chest Recoil	Allow full recoil of chest after each compression; do not lean on the chest after each compression		
Minimizing Interruptions	Limit interruption in chest compressions to less than 10 seconds		

Abbreviations: AED = Automated External Defibrillator; AP = Anterior-Posterior; CPR = CardioPulmonary Resuscitation

564 Chapter 18 | Patient and Employee Safety

Procedure 18.23 Cardiopulmonary Resuscitation—Child and Infant

BACKGROUND: The most common cause of unresponsiveness in infants and children is due to respiratory arrest. CPR can keep oxygen flowing to organs until help arrives. The American Heart Association defines an infant as birth to 1 year of age and a child as 1 year of age until puberty.

ALERT: Follow Standard Precautions

Preprocedure

1. Put on disposable gloves and get disposable CPR mask if available.
2. Assess the victim for unresponsiveness. If there is no response, activate EMS system by shouting for someone to call 9-1-1 and get an AED (automated external defibrillator). If multiple people are present then give orders to specific individuals.

Procedure

3. Give two rescue breaths:
   - For infant: Make complete seal over infant's mouth and nose and blow in air over 1 second until you see chest rise.
   - For child: Pinch the nose shut and then make a complete seal over the child's mouth and blow in air over one second until you see chest rise.
   - Give a total of 2 rescue breaths, one after the other.
4. Deliver high quality CPR chest compressions (this should be done within 10 seconds of identifying cardiac arrest).

   For infant:
   - Place two fingers in the center of the infant's chest, just below the nipple line.
   - Deliver 30 compressions at 1½ inches depth to 2 breaths (one rescuer).

   For child:
   - Place the heel of one hand on the center of the chest, then place the heel of the other hand on top of the first hand, and lace your fingers together.
   - Deliver 30 compressions at 2 inches depth.

   NOTE: Child or infant must be on firm, flat surface.
5. Continue to deliver high quality CPR at a ratio of 30 compressions to 2 breaths until help arrives. Compressions should be at a rate of at least 100 per minute. Be sure infant or child is on a firm, flat surface. CPR should not be interrupted for more than 10 seconds.

Postprocedure

6. Ensure that victim has follow-up treatment or assessment by Emergency Medical Technicians or hospital personnel.
7. Discard gloves and wash hands (follow handwashing guidelines).

Community

Prepare a poster showing the importance of prompt bystander CPR and AED use. Your poster should include survival statistics and how these statistics improve with early CPR. Consider displaying the posters around your school or presenting them to other classes.

Patient and Employee Safety | Chapter 18 565

CUSTOMIZED INSTRUCTION

Less Advanced Students

Point out that many terms associated with health care are known by their abbreviations, such as CPR. Ask students to create a small poster that creatively relates the term cardiopulmonary resuscitation to its abbreviation.

Procedure Tip

18.23 Cardiopulmonary Resuscitation—Child and Infant

- Review the background information.
- Explain CPR.
- Guide students through the preprocedure.
- Demonstrate the procedure.
- Point out the postprocedure.

PROCEDURE PRACTICE

- Demonstrate the steps for Procedure 18.23, Cardiopulmonary Resuscitation—Child and Infant, as many times as necessary, or ask students to demonstrate the steps. Have students practice and perform the procedure until they are competent.

Community

- Encourage students to research the topic using the Internet or library.

Teaching Tips

- Make sure students know that adult CPR is different from infant CPR.
- Explain that guidelines for CPR are updated from time to time. It is important to keep up on CPR guidelines and be aware of changes.
- Emphasize the importance to students of taking a CPR course taught by the AHA or another certified instructor.

ACTIVITY

Have students write a letter to parents stressing the importance of learning infant CPR.

Procedure Tip

18.24 Cardiopulmonary Resuscitation—Adult

- Review the background information.
- Explain CPR.
- Guide students through the preprocedure.
- Demonstrate the procedure.
- Point out the postprocedure.

PROCEDURE PRACTICE

- Demonstrate the steps for Procedure 18.24, Cardiopulmonary Resuscitation—Adult, as many times as necessary, or ask students to demonstrate the steps. Have students practice and perform the procedure until they are competent.

ACTIVITY

Invite a speaker to demonstrate proper methods of CPR. Invite students to ask questions. Have students write a brief summary of what they learn.

Procedure 18.24 Cardiopulmonary Resuscitation—Adult

BACKGROUND: CPR allows you to circulate blood and oxygen to the organs when a patient's heart has stopped. This procedure explains how to perform CPR on an adult victim using the C-A-B sequence. NOTE: Your teacher can provide information on the most current American Heart Association CPR guidelines. The American Heart Association defines an adult as after the age of puberty.

ALERT: Follow Standard Precautions

Preprocedure

1. Put on disposable gloves and disposable CPR mask or barrier device if available.
2. Check for consciousness by shaking victim's shoulder gently and asking if he or she is OK. If there is no response, activate EMS system.

Procedure

3. Check for pulse by palpating the carotid pulse for at least 5 but no more than 10 seconds.
4. If pulse is absent, begin high quality chest compressions. Kneel on one side of the victim. Place the **heel** of one hand in the center of the victim's chest on the lower half of the breastbone. Place the other hand on top. Push straight down on the chest for 30 **compressions.** The chest should be pushed down at least 2 inches during each compression. Compressions should be faster than one per second, so that blood is pumped through the body at a rate of 100 pumps per minute. Be sure to allow complete chest recoil between compressions.

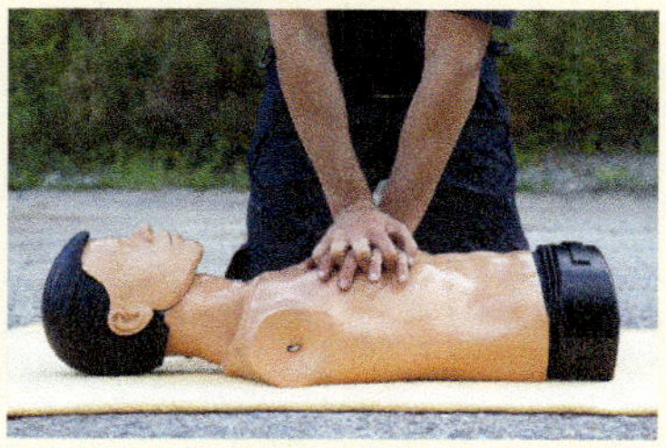

5. Open airway by placing one hand at victim's chin and the other hand on victim's forehead; gently lift chin by supporting jawbone with fingertips and lifting upward to open mouth. (Do not put pressure on throat; this may block airway.) This is called the head tilt/chin lift.
6. Ventilate. Place a pocket mask over mouth and nose. Put apex (point) over bridge of nose and base between lip and chin. Give two breaths for each set of 30 compressions (1½ to 2 seconds per breath) through the one-way valve. Allow lungs to empty between each breath. (If dentures obstruct the airway, remove them.) If air does not inflate lungs: retilt head to ensure an open airway and repeat the two breaths. Watch for chest to rise, allow for exhalation between breaths. If no CPR mask available, you may do "hands-only" CPR by giving compressions but no breaths.
7. Continue to deliver high quality CPR until help arrives.

Postprocedure

8. Ensure that victim has follow-up treatment or assessment by Emergency Medical Technicians or hospital personnel.
9. Discard gloves and wash hands (follow handwashing guidelines).

heel
(HEEL)
Part of the hand between the palm and the wrist.

compressions
(kuhm PRESH uhns)
The act of pressing on the chest to pump blood through the body of a cardiac arrest.

566 Chapter 18 | Patient and Employee Safety

CUSTOMIZED INSTRUCTION

Special Needs Students

Many CPR instructors will customize training to those who need it. Training mannequins, for example, can be placed on tabletops for those who have difficulty bending down to the ground. Allow students with special needs to customize their procedure as necessary.

Procedure 18.25 **Performing CPR, Two Person**

BACKGROUND: Sudden cardiac arrest is a leading cause of death in the United States. The provision of cardiopulmonary resuscitation can improve a victim's chance of survival.

ALERT: Follow Standard Precautions

Preprocedure

The provider should understand that the critical concepts of quality CPR include:

- Push hard, push fast: compress at a rate of 100 compressions per minute.
- Allow full chest recoil after each compression.
- Minimize interruptions in chest compressions.
- Avoid hyperventilation

Procedure

When a second rescuer is available to help, that second rescuer should activate the emergency response system and get the AED if available. The first rescuer should remain with the victim to begin CPR immediately.

After the second rescuer returns, the rescuers should take turns doing chest compressions, switching after every 5 cycles of CPR. Follow the procedure for one person cardiopulmonary resuscitation assigning tasks as follows:

Rescuer 1:

- Location should be at victim's side.
- Performs chest compressions.
- Switches duties with rescuer 2 every 5 cycles, taking less than 5 seconds to switch.
- Maintains an open airway.

Rescuer 2:

- Location should be at the victim's head.
- Gives breaths, watching for chest rise.
- Encourages rescuer 1 to perform compressions that are fast and deep enough to allow full chest recoil between compressions.
- Switches duties with rescuer 1 every 5 cycles taking less than 5 seconds to switch.

Automated External Defibrillator

Automated external defibrillators (AEDs) are designed to be used by lay rescuers and function to assess the heart for a shockable rhythm. They are a vital part of the chain of survival for victims of sudden cardiac arrest due to ventricular fibrillation (V-fib/VF) or pulseless ventricular tachycardia (VT).

Although AED training classes are offered by qualified American Heart Association or American Red Cross instructors, the goal of this device is to be simple enough for non-trained lay rescuers. Always remember to request an AED when activating the Emergency Response System for unresponsive victims. High quality chest compressions and AED early defibrillation saves lives.

Career Connect

Participate in either a ride-along with a first responder, paramedic, police officer, or fire service professional, or job shadow an emergency dispatcher to determine the response for different emergency situations.

As an alternative opportunity, consider joining an EMT Explorer Post, or invite one of these professionals to speak to your class.

Patient and Employee Safety | Chapter 18 567

CUSTOMIZED INSTRUCTION

More Advanced Students

Have student find local facilities that teach CPR. Ask them to find out when and where the classes are held and to whom they are offered.

Teaching Tips

- Discuss the use of a defibrillator.
- Assign Procedure 18.26.
- Emphasize the importance of knowing the differences between performing CPR on children and adults. This can be a matter of life and death for a child. Discuss the advantage of two-person CPR in that it gives each rescuer a small break.
- Point out that this procedure functions basically the same way as CPR by one person.

Procedure Tips

18.25 Performing CPR, Two Person

- Review the background information.
- Discuss the concepts of CPR.
- Explain when two-person CPR is appropriate.
- Guide students through the preprocedure.
- Demonstrate the procedure.
- Discuss the actions of CPR.

PROCEDURE PRACTICE

- Demonstrate the steps for Procedure 18.25, Performing CPR, Two Person, as many times as necessary, or ask students to demonstrate the steps. Have students practice and perform the procedure until they are competent.

ACTIVITY

Invite a speaker to show the class a defibrillator. Ask the speaker to discuss how and why it is used.

Teaching Tips

- Review the conditions that warrant the use of an AED.

Procedure Tip

18.26 Demonstrating the Use of AED (Automated External Defibrillator)

- Review the background information.
- Explain AED.
- Discuss when it is appropriate to use an AED.
- Demonstrate the procedure.

PROCEDURE PRACTICE

- Demonstrate the steps for Procedure 18.26, Demonstrating the Use of AED, as many times as necessary, or ask students to demonstrate the steps. Have students practice and perform the procedure until they are competent.

TEAMWORK

Have students prepare a presentation on AED programs. Assign pairs or small groups of students to find out different information, such as who can purchase an AED, how much does an AED cost, what steps can an organization take to purchase an AED, can it be used on children, why should local EMS be notified about the purchase of an AED, as well as any other pertinent information.

Procedure 18.26 Demonstrating the Use of AED (Automated External Defibrillator)

BACKGROUND: The interval from collapse to defibrillation is one of the most important determinants of survival from cardiac arrest.

AEDS are computerized devices that are attached to a pulseless victim with adhesive pads. They will recommend shock delivery only if the victim's heart rhythm is one that a shock can treat. AEDS give rescuers visual and voice prompts to guide rescuer actions.

AEDs are reliable and simple to operate, allowing laypersons and health care providers to attempt defibrillation safely.

Use AEDs only when victims have the following three clinical findings:

- No response
- No breathing
- No pulse

ALERT: Follow Standard Precautions

Procedure

Once the AED arrives, put it at the victim's side, next to the rescuer who will operate it. This will allow a second rescuer to perform CPR from the opposite side of the victim without interfering with AED operation. The following are four universal steps for operating an AED:

1. Power on the AED:
   - Open the carrying case.
   - Turn the power on.
2. **ATTACH** electrode pads to the victim's bare chest:
   - Choose correct pads for size/age of victim. Child pads will be used for children less than 8 years of age. Adult pads are used for the victim who is over 8 years of age.
   - Peel the backing away from the electrode pads.
   - Quickly wipe the victim's chest dry if covered with sweat or water. If the chest is covered with hair and electrode pads will not stick, pull the pad away from chest. This should take the hair with it. If still will not stick, shave area with razor included in the AED Kit.
   - Attach the adhesive electrode pads to the victim's bare chest.
     - — Place one electrode pad on the upper-right side of the bare chest to the right of the breastbone, directly below the collarbone.
     - — Place the other pad to the left of the nipple, a few inches below the left arm pit.
   - Attach the AED connecting cables to the AED box (some are preconnected).
3. "Clear" the victim and **ANALYZE** the rhythm:
   - Always clear the victim during the analysis. Be sure that no one is touching the victim, not even the person in charge of giving breaths.
   - Some AEDS will tell you to push a button to allow the AED to begin analyzing the heart rhythm; others will do that automatically. The AED may take about 5 to 15 seconds to analyze.
   - The AED then tells you if a shock is needed. Remember, if the victim is not in ventricular fibrillation, there will be no advice to shock.
4. If the AED advises a shock, it will tell you to be sure to clear the victim:
   - Clear the victim before delivering the shock; be sure no one is touching the victim to avoid injury to rescuers.
     - — Loudly state a "clear the patient" message, such as "I'm clear, you're clear, everybody's clear."
     - — Perform a visual check to ensure that no one is in contact with the victim.
   - Press the SHOCK button.
   - The shock will produce a sudden contraction of the victim's muscles.
5. As soon as the AED gives the shock, begin CPR starting with chest compressions.
6. After 2 minutes of CPR, the AED will prompt you to repeat steps 3 and 4.
7. DO NOT remove the pads once they are placed on the victim. This will allow the AED to continue to monitor patient.

568 Chapter 18 | Patient and Employee Safety

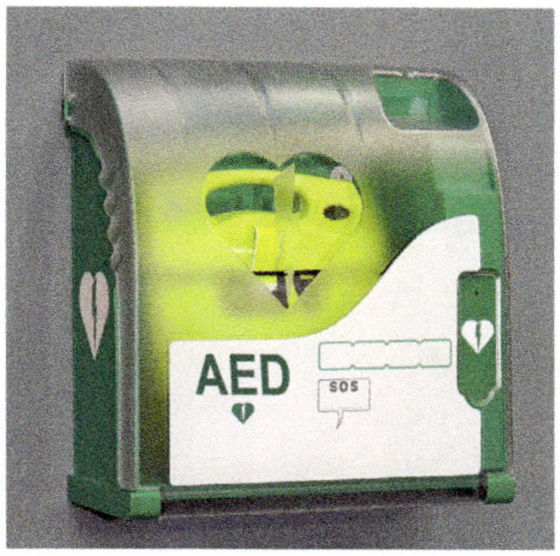

Figure 18.12 More and more often AEDs have become available in the community setting. How has this improved the overall outcomes of cardiopulmonary resuscitation?

Career Connect

Both the American Red Cross and the American Heart Association offer multiple CPR courses. If you are taking CPR certification as a requirement for a job or as a part of a medical course, be sure that you are taking the correct level course from the proper organization.

Summary

CPR is an important technique that can keep organs alive until the heart can be shocked with a defibrillator. All health professionals must become proficient in CPR. To do this, you should attend a class given by a qualified American Heart Association or American Red Cross teacher.

Section 18.6 Review Questions

1. What does a defibrillator do?
2. How many compressions should be given per minute during CPR?
3. Describe the position of your hands when performing CPR on an adult.
4. What are the basic steps for performing CPR on an adult?
5. How do you deliver a chest compression to an infant who has no heartbeat?

Figure Focus

18.12 More and more often AEDs have become available in the community setting. How has this improved the overall outcomes of cardiopulmonary resuscitation?

Discuss the topic with students.

Career Connect

- Contact local organizations to find out about certification courses.

Section 18.6 Review Questions

1. Answer: A defibrillator administers an electric shock to restore normal heartbeat.
2. Answer: Compressions should be faster than one per second, so that blood is pumped through the body at a rate of 100 pumps per minute.
3. Answer: Place the heel of one hand in the center of the victim's chest on the lower half of the breastbone. Place the other hand on top.
4. Answer: Check for consciousness and for pulse. If pulse is absent, begin high quality chest compressions. Open airway and ventilate. Continue until help arrives.
5. Answer: Place an infant-sized barrier device on the infant's face. Ventilate through the one-way valve and give rescue breathing. Give two slow breaths using only air in your cheeks. (Too much air may overinflate an infant's lungs.) Watch for chest to rise and allow chest to fall or deflate between each breath. If air does not inflate lungs, retilt head to ensure open airway. Repeat the two breaths. If lungs still do not inflate, treat infant for an obstructed airway.

CHAPTER 18 REVIEW

Chapter Review Questions

1. Answer: A wet floor can cause someone to slip and fall. If there is litter on the floor, someone may trip and be seriously injured.
2. Answer: MSDS forms provide the information needed to handle chemicals safely.
3. Answer: Side rails should be used on a bed to keep a patient safe from falling out of bed. Side rails should not be used to restrain a patient.
4. Answer: Postural supports
5. Answer: Using a lightweight electrical cord with heavily powered equipment, defective outlets, frayed wires, and overloading circuits with too many electrical cords.
6. Answer: Restrict smoking to designated outdoor areas. Monitor garbage containers. Check electrical equipment for proper functioning and frayed electrical cords. When using flammable liquids, take only the amount needed to complete the task.
7. Answer: Lift firmly and smoothly after you size up the load. If you cannot easily pull the object to you (i.e., the load is too heavy), get help! Grasp the load firmly. Lift by using the large muscles of your legs. Keep the load close to your body. Do not twist your body. To change direction, shift your feet in the direction you want to go.
8. Answer: Spiral bandaging
9. Answer: Shock is life-threatening because of fluid or blood and oxygen loss.
10. Answer: 30 compressions to 2 breaths

CHAPTER 18 REVIEW

Chapter Review Questions

1. Why is it important to clean up litter and wipe up spills on the floor? (18.1)
2. What is the purpose of MSDS forms? (18.1)
3. Under what circumstances should side rails be used on a bed? (18.2)
4. Devices that restrict a patient's movement are called ____________. (18.2)
5. What are four ways that electricity can be used incorrectly? (18.3)
6. What are four ways to prevent a fire? (18.3)
7. Describe the correct way to pick up a load, using the principles of body mechanics. (18.4)
8. What kind of bandaging procedure would you perform for a large leg wound? (18.5)
9. Why is it important to treat seriously injured patients for shock? (18.5)
10. When performing CPR on an infant, the ratio of chest compressions to rescue breaths is ____________. (18.6)

Activities

1. Have a classmate pretend to have three different types of wounds. Perform the correct bandaging procedure for each type of wound.
2. Disposing of waste properly and recycling is not only important for maintaining a safe and clean facility, but it is good for the environment and it can help lower some operating costs. Working with a classmate, create a poster or presentation on waste management.
3. Find an object in your classroom that is moderately heavy (20–30 lbs) but that you can lift safely. Demonstrate proper body mechanics as you lift and move the object to another location in the class. Have your classmates critique your form. Discuss with your classmates how you would apply these techniques to lift even heavier objects, such as an unconscious patient.

Case Studies

1. Your facility is being evacuated due to a small fire. You are in charge of moving a patient who is unable to sit up or walk. What kinds of precautions should you take to make sure the patient is safe as she is being moved? How will you determine what type of equipment your patient will need?
2. Mr. Benton is a patient who is in the hospital after suffering a heart attack. He is hooked up to a heart monitor and has an IV in his arm that delivers fluids and medications. He has also been prescribed a medication in pill form. You are assigned to give Mr. Benton his pill and check his vital signs. You enter his room and see that he is in bed with the side rails up. How do you make sure that Mr. Benton safely receives his medicine and remains safe after you leave the room?
3. Search the Internet for a video demonstrating how to perform CPR and use an automated external defibrillator. Take notes and study them. Try to explain to a friend what you have learned without looking at your notes.

570 Chapter 18 | Patient and Employee Safety

Activities

1. Have the necessary materials available in advance. Divide students into pairs. Have each member of the pair take a turn bandaging. Review each bandage before students take them off. Allow other students to observe correct procedures as well as common mistakes.
2. Encourage students to be creative in their presentations. Also discuss ways that students can recycle and manage waste at home.
3. The students may not have a good sense for how heavy is too heavy. Keep an eye out for students that might hurt themselves trying to choose an unreasonably large object.

CHAPTER 18 REVIEW

Thinking Critically

1. **Medical Terminology**—Use the following medical terms in two or three sentences related to first aid: cardiopulmonary, priorities, laceration, and dressings.
2. **Customer Service**—In a home care environment you notice that your patient is very careless with the kitchen stove. Describe how you could demonstrate safer stove use while assisting the patient with meal preparation.
3. **Patient Education**—Mrs. Green is not happy about her lengthy stay at the hospital and is not listening to the hospital staff. Her behavior, such as getting out of bed on her own, has put her at risk. How will you get her to cooperate with specific industry safety standards? Describe how you would talk to her about safety requirements and what is necessary for patients to understand and to do.

Portfolio Connection

Reading and understanding product labels and being able to understand safety signs and symbols is a necessary skill. We need to know if products will do what we want them to do. We need to know if there is a risk in using a product.

In this chapter, we discussed MSDS (material safety data sheet) forms. You learned that MSDSs provide all the primary information needed for any product in the work environment. If you become a home health aide, you work in patients' homes. There will not be an MSDS book to refer to. You will have to read the labels on products for the information you need.

Choose three household products from home—for example, toothpaste, a cleaning product, a synthetic food product—and create your own MSDS form for each of these three products. Use the following headings in your forms:

1. Product Identification
2. Hazardous Ingredients of Mixture
3. Physical Data
4. Fire and Explosion
5. Reactivity Data
6. Health Hazard Data
7. Emergency and First-Aid Procedures
8. Spill or Leak Procedures
9. Protection Information/Control Measures
10. Special Precautions
11. Symbols or Safety Signs Included on the Label

Completion of this assignment for your portfolio shows your ability to assimilate information and transfer your knowledge into a usable format for your daily use. When you appropriately apply each step of your learning, you show others that you are capable of taking responsibility in a work environment. Place these three forms in the section of your portfolio labeled "Written Reports and Assignments."

PORTFOLIO TIP

You can use your word processing, spreadsheet, or database programs to create basic forms that are easy to read and evaluate. Most computer applications provide professionally designed templates for all types of documents, including lists and inventories. Explore options for creating your own MSDS forms in electronic format. Remember, employers look for employees who have experience using computer applications. These are transferable skills that will serve you well in any career you choose.

Patient and Employee Safety | Chapter 18 571

Case Studies

1. Remind students not to panic in an emergency situation. Encourage students to consider the appropriate transporting devices as well as any necessary postural supports.
2. Ask the students why it is everyone's responsibility to maintain a safe environment. You may wish for students to work with a partner on this project.
3. You may ask students to present their findings to the class.

Thinking Critically

1. Verify that students use the terms correctly.
2. Remind students to take a patient's feelings and concerns into account when trying to instruct them about safety at home or in a health care facility.
3. Answers should be presented clearly, with a topic sentence and examples when appropriate.

Portfolio Connection

- Students should include as much information as possible for each product.
- Students can look back to Figure 18.1 as an example of an MSDS form.

19 Measuring Vital Signs and Other Clinical Skills

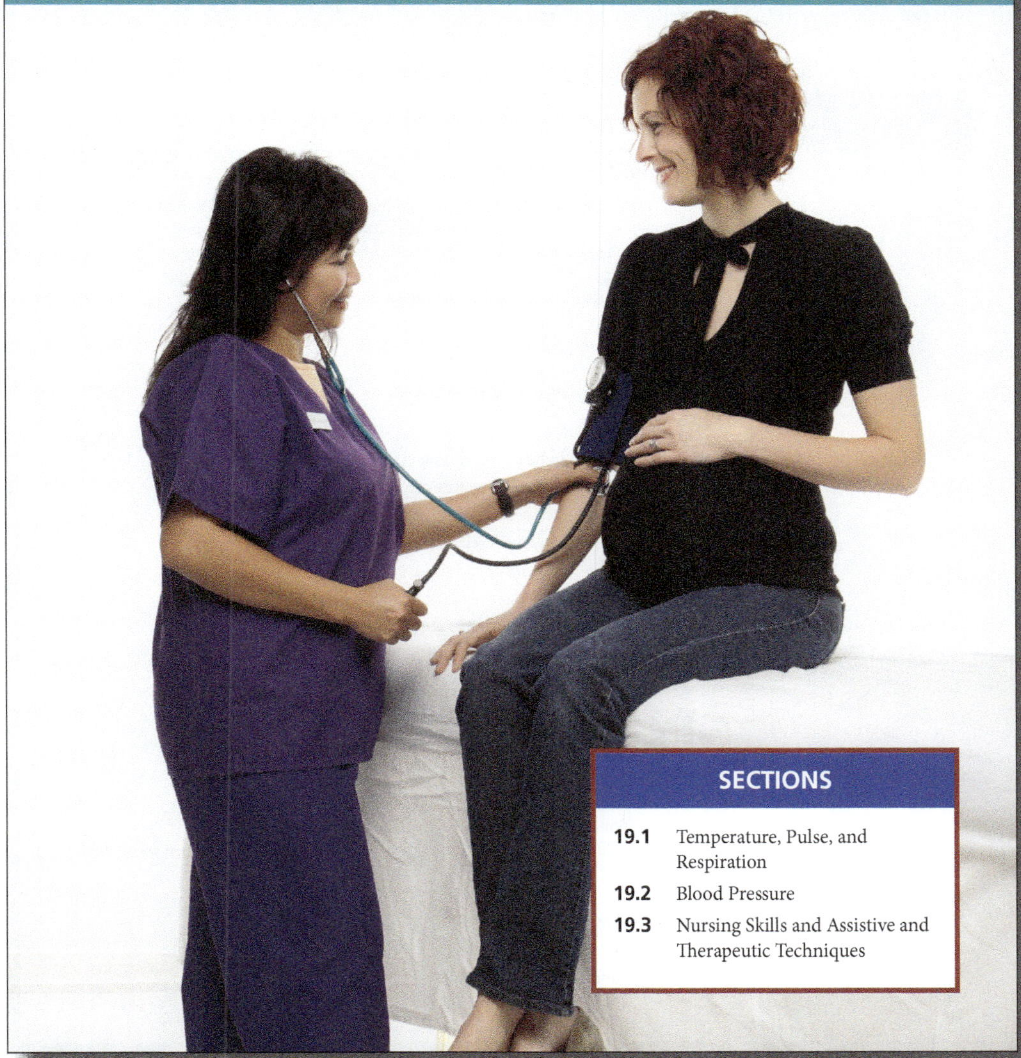

SECTIONS

CHAPTER 19 OVERVIEW

Chapter 19 provides general information and specific skill procedures for measuring vital signs as well as other medical skills.

Section 19.1: Section 19.1 explains temperature, pulse, and respiration and the devices used for measuring them. Procedures include different methods of measuring temperature, counting a pulse, and counting respiration.

Section 19.2: Section 19.2 covers blood pressure and how to measure it.

Section 19.3: In Section 19.3, students are introduced to nursing skills and assistive and therapeutic techniques. Procedures cover morning and evening care routines, skin care, oral hygiene, elimination care, movement and ambulation skills, positioning and body alignment, application of restraints, bathing, bedmaking, feeding, measuring intake and outtake, special procedures, and postmortem care.

Advance Preparation	
Review	■ Chapter text for Sections 19.1, 19.2, and 19.3; and chapter procedures.
Contact	■ Medical professionals willing to address the class or demonstrate procedures relating to vital signs and clinical skills. ■ Medical facilities or associations, such as the American Heart Association, to request brochures and other educational material about the risks of high blood pressure. ■ Long-term care facilities and mortuaries to request a tour or possibility of job shadows.
Prepare	■ Materials for procedures, including (but not limited to): urine cups and Clinistix, graduates and other measuring devices, thermometers, toothbrushes, toothpaste, combs, and brushes.

FOCUS AND ENGAGE

Getting Started

- This activity allows students to practice measuring pulse rate.
- It also demonstrates how pulse rate can vary depending on the current activity level and condition of the patient.
- You may want to delay this activity until after Section 19.1, in which students learn more about pulse rate and how to measure it.

Introduce the Section

a. Review the content of the Background paragraph, explaining that vital signs provide information about how the body is functioning.

b. Emphasize the importance of understanding vital signs and how to measure them.

c. Review the objectives for the section.

Vocabulary Review

a. Direct students to the key terms.

b. Pronounce each word, and have the students repeat the pronunciation out loud.

c. Discuss the definition of each word.

Getting Started

With a partner, take and record each others' pulse at the beginning of class. Next, as a class, lie still for 5 minutes and obtain a resting pulse. Then, take and record each others' pulse rate again to determine any change. Next, complete 20 jumping jacks or a similar exercise, and then take and record each other's pulse. At the end of the class, take and record the final pulse to compare how the different activities impacted your pulse rate.

SECTION 19.1 Temperature, Pulse, and Respiration

Background

Vital signs are important indicators of your patient's health status. Vital signs give you information about breathing, body temperature, and the heart. They indicate how well the body systems are functioning. As a health care worker, you need to observe patients whenever you are near them. Your knowledge of vital signs and how to measure them helps you know when to report that a patient is having problems.

Objectives

When you have completed this section, you will be able to do the following:

- List the vital signs.
- List factors that influence body temperature.
- Name the sites where temperature can be measured.
- Tell how normal temperature differs depending on the site.
- Describe how to measure oral, rectal, and axillary temperature.
- Describe a common method for measuring a pulse.
- List the factors that influence the pulse rate.
- Demonstrate counting and recording a radial pulse.
- Recognize the parts of a respiration.
- List the factors that affect respiration.

Vital Signs

Vital signs are monitored at prescribed times for the hospitalized patient. The frequency of these measurements is increased with any change in the patient's physical condition or whenever an invasive procedure is performed. It is the nurse's responsibility to be able to interpret these vital signs and to know when an

574 Chapter 19 | Measuring Vital Signs and Other Clinical Skills

TEACH

Discuss

- Ask students to think about when they have had their own vital signs measured.
- Discuss the type of information that a medical provider can learn from measuring vital signs.

Reinforce and Review

- Review Chapter 13, Your Body and How It Functions.

ACTIVITY

Make a table or chart listing the vital signs and their abbreviations, along with descriptions of each, and what information can be learned from taking each vital sign.

CUSTOMIZED INSTRUCTION OVERVIEW	
Less Advanced Students	Pages 593, 618
More Advanced Students	Pages 575, 696
English Language Learners	Pages 575, 700
Special Needs Students	Pages 580, 625
At-Risk Students	Page 588

intervention is necessary—such as notifying the physician, medicating the patient, or altering any physical activity prescribed for the patient.

Another important indicator of body functioning is the oxygen concentration in the hemoglobin of the arterial blood. This can be measured through a noninvasive technique called **pulse oximetry**.

Pain is considered the fifth cardinal sign. Because it is sometimes difficult to relate to the patient's report of pain, it is best to teach the patient how to use a valid and reliable scale for objectively measuring and reporting pain. This is most frequently a scale of 1–10 with 10 being the patient's highest level of discomfort.

For children or others unable to relate to a numerical scale, the use of differing degrees of the happy face from very happy to very sad is used. For the cognitively impaired patient, it is important that we use our observation skills to determine level of comfort. Look for crying, moaning, grimacing, or restlessness. Most importantly, we must allow the patient to rate and report their own pain and not use our subjective views to determine their need for pain relief.

pulse oximetry
(puhls ok SIM I tree)
Procedure used to determine the oxygen concentration in the hemoglobin of the arterial blood.

It is extremely important that vital signs be measured and recorded accurately, either in a paper or electronic file. Be sure to verbally report to the nurse in charge of the patient's care any alteration from norms in vital signs, reports or displays of discomfort, or perceived alterations in the patient's physical or mental status. The nurse will rely on the assistant's ability to communicate this information.

Remember that other health care workers depend on this information when making decisions about the patient's treatment. In this section, you will learn how to measure body temperature and count the pulse rate and respiratory rate. Together, these measurements are referred to as **TPR**. Section 19.2 teaches you to measure blood pressure.

Height and Weight

Often the first thing you will measure from your patient is their height and weight. The average height in the U.S. is 69 inches for adult males and 64 inches for adult females. Heights far from these averages could indicate pituitary problems such as gigantism or dwarfism. What is considered a "normal" weight depends on age and height, so body mass index (BMI) is more often used to assess issues with weight. Generally a BMI below 18.5 would be considered underweight, while a BMI above 25 would be overweight or obese.

TPR
(TEE PEE R)
An abbreviation that stands for "temperature, pulse, respiration."

oxidation
(ok si DAY-shun)
The mixing of oxygen and another element.

excretion
(ex SKREE-shun)
The process of eliminating waste material.

Temperature

Temperature is the measure of body heat. Heat is produced in the body by the muscles and glands and by the **oxidation** of food. Heat is lost from the body by respiration, perspiration, and **excretion**. The balance between the heat produced and the heat lost is the body temperature.

Measuring Vital Signs and Other Clinical Skills | Chapter 19 575

Teaching Tips

- Describe vital signs:
  - T = body temperature
  - P = pulse rate
  - R = respiratory rate
  - BP = blood pressure
- Emphasize the abbreviations: TPR and BP.
- Explain why monitoring vital signs is important: They indicate normal or abnormal function.
- Explain that when signs are normal, the body is in homeostasis—balanced.
- Explain that obtaining accurate measurements of vital signs can mean the difference between life and death.
- Explain that pulse oximetry and degree of pain may also be considered vital indications of a patient's state.
- Explain that pain is usually measured on a scale from 0 to 10.

CUSTOMIZED INSTRUCTION

More Advanced Students

Ask more advanced students to research hypothermia, including what it is, how it is caused, who is at risk, and treatments. Have them prepare a presentation for the class on the information they have learned.

English Language Learners

Have students write each key term and its pronunciation on one side of an index card and its definition on the other side. Have them read each term and definition aloud to a partner.

Teaching Tips

- Explain that temperature is the measure of body heat:
  - Heat is produced by muscle activity, food oxidation, and glands.
  - Heat is lost through respiration, perspiration, and excretion.
- Review terminology used in describing body temperature:
  - Afibrile is a temperature within the normal range.
  - Febrile is a temperature elevated above the normal range.
  - Hypothermia is a temperature below the normal range.
  - Pyrexia is a temperature above the normal range.
- A substance that produces a fever is called a pyrogenic.
- Emphasize that a fever is not an illness. It is a sign of abnormal conditions within the body.
- Review the most common abnormal conditions: viral and bacterial infections, colds or flu-like illnesses, sore throats and strep throats, ear infections, viral gastroenteritis or bacterial gastroenteritis, acute bronchitis, infectious mononucleosis, urinary tract infections (UTIs), upper respiratory infections such as tonsillitis or laryngitis.
- Review more serious abnormal conditions: pneumonia, appendicitis, tuberculosis, meningitis, rheumatoid diseases, autoimmune disorders, AIDS, ulcerative colitis, and cancer.
- Review Table 19.1 together as a class.
- Explain that elevated body temperature is caused by friction between cells rubbing together.

afebrile
(ey FEE bruhl)
Referring to temperature within a normal range.

febrile
(FEE bruhl)
Referring to elevated temperature.

hypothermia
(hahy puh THUR mee uh)
Below-normal temperature.

pyrexia
(pahy REK see uh)
Above-normal temperature.

pyrogenic
(pahy ruh JEN ik)
Producing fever.

If body temperature is within a normal range, it is **afebrile**. Normal body temperature will vary among individuals from .5 to 1 degree Fahrenheit. Using a chart for recording temperatures will allow you to reference the current temperature against past readings to determine the status of the patient. If temperature is elevated, usually considered one degree over the patient's norm, it is **febrile**. Temperature below normal, usually below 95°F, is called **hypothermia**. Temperature above normal is called **pyrexia** (this is another word for fever). Any substance that produces fever is called **pyrogenic**. **Table 19.1** shows the factors that influence temperature.

Table 19.1 Factors That Influence Temperature

Increase Temperature	Decrease Temperature
Exercise	Sleep
Digestion of food	Fasting
Increased environmental temperature	Exposure to cold
Illness	Certain illnesses
Infection	Decreased muscle activity
Excitement	Mouth breathing
Anxiety	Depression

Abnormal Conditions

Fever is not an illness. Actually, it is an important part of the body's defense against infection. Many infants and children develop high fevers with minor viral illnesses. The older adult loses some thermoregulatory control and an elevated temperature will not be the first presenting symptom of infection. While a fever signals that a battle might be going on in the body, the fever is fighting for the person, not against.

Most bacteria and viruses that cause infections in people thrive best at 98.6°F. Raising the temperature a few degrees can give your body the winning edge. In addition, a fever activates the body's immune system to make more white blood cells, antibodies, and other infection-fighting agents.

Although infections are the most common causes of elevated body temperature, fevers have a long list of other causes, including toxins, cancers, and autoimmune diseases. Unexplained fevers that continue for days or weeks are called fevers of undetermined origin (FUO).

The most common causes of fevers are "abnormal" conditions, such as:

- Viral and bacterial infections
- Colds or flu-like illnesses
- Sore throats and strep throats
- Ear infections

576 Chapter 19 | Measuring Vital Signs and Other Clinical Skills

- Discuss the factors that cause body cells to be more active, thereby increasing body temperature: exercise, digestion of food, increased environmental temperature, illness, infection, excitement, and anxiety.
- Explain that lowered body temperature is caused by reduced friction between cells rubbing together.

ACTIVITY

Discuss the factors that cause body cells to be less active, thereby decreasing body temperature: sleep, fasting, exposure to cold, depression, decreased muscle activity, certain illnesses, and mouth breathing.

- Viral gastroenteritis or bacterial gastroenteritis
- Acute bronchitis
- Infectious mononucleosis (“mono”)
- Urinary tract infections (UTIs)
- Upper respiratory infections, such as tonsillitis or laryngitis

Occasionally, fevers indicate more serious problems, such as pneumonia, appendicitis, tuberculosis, meningitis, rheumatoid diseases and autoimmune disorders, AIDS, ulcerative colitis, and cancer.

Thermometers

A thermometer is an instrument used to measure temperature. There are several types of thermometers: glass thermometers, aural thermometers, temporal artery thermometers, chemically treated paper or plastic thermometers, and electronic/digital thermometers.

Glass Thermometers

A glass thermometer is used mainly for home care. It is a hollow glass tube with **calibration** lines on it. The liquid in the glass thermometer is heat sensitive and rises up the hollow tube when exposed to heat. This enables you to read the patient’s temperature. The two most common types of glass thermometers are the **oral** thermometer and the **rectal** thermometer. (Figure 19.1) The oral thermometer has a long, slender tip, and the rectal thermometer has a shorter, stubby, and rounded tip.

calibration
(KAL i bray-shun)
Standard measure (e.g., each line on a thermometer or a ruler is a calibration).

oral
(AWR uhl)
Referring to the mouth.

rectal
(REK tl)
Referring to the far end of the large intestine just above the anus.

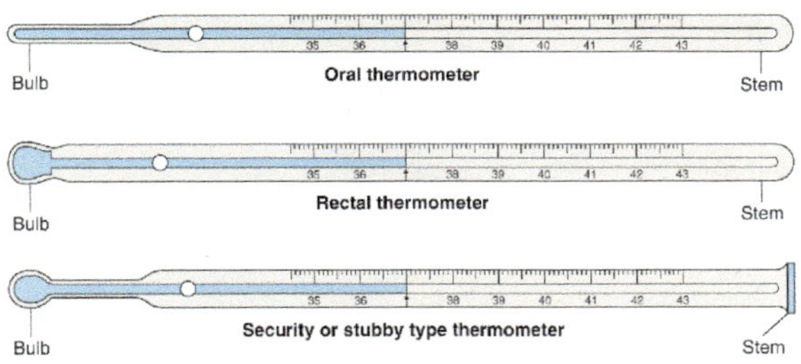

Figure 19.1
Types of glass thermometers. The rectal thermometer has a rounded bulb that helps prevent perforation of tissue. Security or stubby thermometers are used for infants. How do these thermometers work?

ACTIVITY

Make a public service poster identifying factors that influence body temperature, explaining when people should seek medical treatment and when an increase in body temperature is normal.

Teaching Tips

- Explain that body temperature is measured using a thermometer, and that there are different types of thermometers:
  - Glass
  - Electronic/digital
  - Aural
  - Temporal artery
  - Chemically treated strips

Figure Focus

19.1 Types of glass thermometers. The rectal thermometer has a rounded bulb that helps prevent perforation of tissue. Security or stubby thermometers are used for infants. How do these thermometers work?

Answer: The liquid in the glass thermometer is heat sensitive and rises up the hollow tube when exposed to heat.

TEAMWORK

In pairs, have students sit back to back. Have one student rub his or her hands together for at least 30 seconds, and describe the feeling to their partner, who will document it. Reverse roles. As a class, discuss the generation of heat from friction.

Teaching Tips

- Explain how a glass thermometer works.
- Discuss the difference between Celsius and Fahrenheit measurements.
- Assign Procedure 19.1.

Procedure Tip

19.1 Reading a Glass Thermometer

- Review the background information, discussing the importance of reading a thermometer correctly.
- Explain the preprocedure steps.
- Explain the procedure steps.
- Explain the postprocedure steps.

PROCEDURE PRACTICE

- Demonstrate the steps for Procedure 19.1, Reading a Glass Thermometer, as many times as necessary, or ask students to demonstrate the steps. Have students practice and perform the procedure until they are competent.

Figure Focus

19.2 Are Fahrenheit and Celsius thermometers read in the same way?

Answer: Fahrenheit and Celsius thermometers are read according to the same principles. However, Celsius calibration is usually measured at $^{1}/_{10}$ of a degree while Fahrenheit calibration is $^{2}/_{10}$ of a degree.

Procedure 19.1 | Reading a Glass Thermometer

BACKGROUND: Although still available, mercury thermometers are rarely used because of the risks of mercury poisoning if they should break. Mercury-free glass thermometers and digital thermometers are replacing glass mercury thermometers. Exposure to high levels of mercury can cause respiratory and digestive problems and renal (kidney) damage. Even exposure to low levels of mercury can cause chest pains, chills, nausea, and diarrhea.
ALERT: Follow Standard Precautions

Procedure

1. Hold the thermometer by the stem at eye level. Rotate the thermometer until you can see the line indicating the temperature reading.
2. Look at the lines on the scale at the upper side of the liquid. Each line represents a whole degree. There are four short lines between each of the long lines. The short lines represent $^{2}/_{10}$ (0.2) of a degree. Only even numbers are shown on a **Fahrenheit** clinical thermometer, for example 96°, 98°, 100°. (Figure 19.2)
3. If the liquid ends at one of the short lines, look to see which long line is just before it. This tells you the degree of temperature. Then, add $^{2}/_{10}$ of a degree for each short line.
4. Read a **Celsius** thermometer the same way. Each long line represents a degree. Each short line represents $^{1}/_{10}$ (0.1) of a degree. (Figure 19.2)

Figure 19.2
Are Fahrenheit and Celsius thermometers read in the same way?

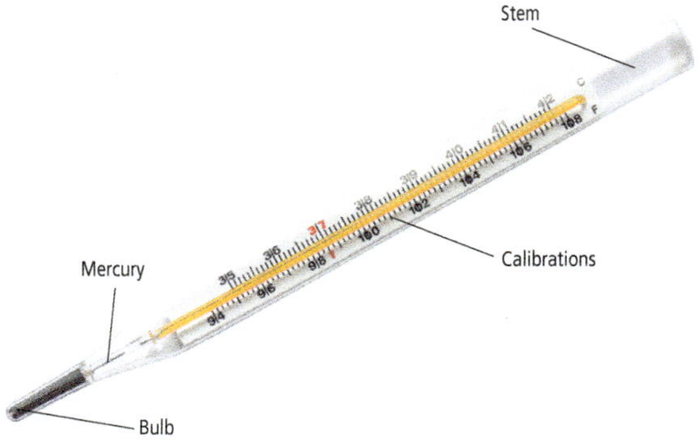

Fahrenheit
(FEHR uhn hite)
Measure of heat; in medicine a Fahrenheit thermometer is often used to measure body heat.

Celsius
(SEHL see uhs)
Measure of heat; in medicine a Celsius thermometer is sometimes used to measure body heat. Also called centigrade.

Many thermometers, like the one shown above, contain both Celsius and Fahrenheit. You may be asked to change a temperature from Celsius to Fahrenheit or from Fahrenheit to Celsius. If you need to make these changes, use the information in **Table 19.2**.

578 Chapter 19 | Measuring Vital Signs and Other Clinical Skills

Table 19.2 Fahrenheit and Celsius Comparison

Fahrenheit	Celsius/Centigrade	Fahrenheit	Celsius/Centigrade
32	0	100.4	38
95	35	101.2	38.4
96	35.5	102.2	39
96.8	36	103	39.4
97.8	36.5	104	40
98.6	37	105	40.5
99.6	37.5	105.8	41
		106.8	41.5

Aural Thermometers (Ear)

The aural thermometer is commonly used because it is accurate, fast, easy to use, and safe. It is especially effective for babies and children. The probe from the aural thermometer is positioned in the aural canal of the ear. Some aural thermometers can take a temperature in just one second. (**Figure 19.3**) Although aural temperatures are commonly used in children, there is some question about the accuracy of the reading, especially in children younger than 6 years of age.

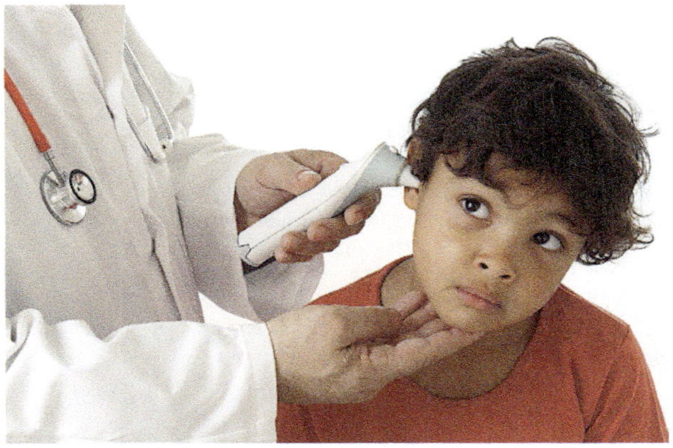

Figure 19.3
Aural, or ear, thermometer. What are the advantages of an aural thermometer?

Liquid Crystal Thermometer (Forehead)

This type of thermometer uses heat-sensitive liquid crystals in a plastic strip that is applied to the forehead. Temperature changes affect the color of the crystals. The color change indicates the patient's temperature based on the heat emitted from the surface of the skin. A liquid crystal thermometer can be used on children and babies. The strip can be left on the forehead for a continuous update on temperature changes.

Measuring Vital Signs and Other Clinical Skills | Chapter 19 579

Teaching Tips

- Review Table 19.2 together.
- Explain how an aural thermometer works.
- Explain how a temporal artery thermometer works.
- Explain how chemically treated strips and plastic thermometers are used.
- Explain how electronic/digital thermometers are used.

Figure Focus

19.3 Aural, or ear, thermometer. What are the advantages of an aural thermometer?

Answer: It is accurate, fast, easy to use, and safe. It is especially effective for babies and children.

ACTIVITY

Distribute glass thermometers to each student, or small groups of students. Have them identify the parts of the thermometer.

Figure Focus

19.4 Electronic/digital thermometer. What is the main advantage of this type of thermometer?

Answer: Electronic/digital thermometers are quick and easy to use.

Math Link—Converting Between Celsius and Fahrenheit

- Remind students that they may have learned the formula for converting Celsius to Fahrenheit in Chapter 12.
- Emphasize that most measurements will be in Fahrenheit.
- Explain that Centigrade is the same as Celsius.
- Review the examples together as a class.
- Answers:
  a. $F = (37.2 \times 1.8) + 32$ $F = (66.96) + 32$ $F = 98.96°$
  b. $C = (101.6 - 32) / 1.8$ $C = (69.6) / 1.8$ $C = 38.67°$
  c. $C = (96 - 32) / 1.8$ $C = 64 / 1.8$ $C = 35.56°$
  d. $F = (41 \times 1.8) + 32$ $F = (73.8) + 32$ $F = 105.8°$

Why is it very important for you to double-check your results when you make temperature conversions?

Answer: Because a small error can make a big difference. You want to make sure a careless math error does not radically affect a patient's care or outcome.

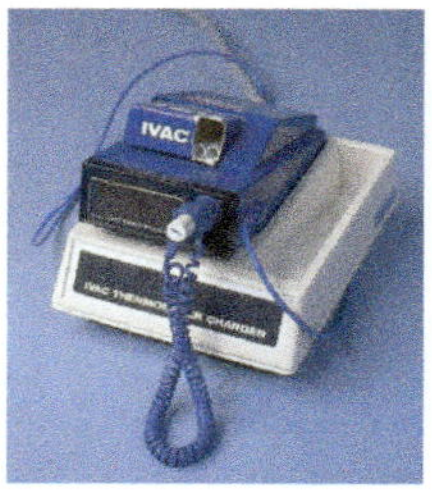

Figure 19.4
Electronic/digital thermometer. What is the main advantage of this type of thermometer?

Chemically Treated Paper or Plastic Thermometers

This type of thermometer is read by noting its change in color. It is discarded after one use.

Electronic/Digital Thermometers

This thermometer has a probe that is covered with a protective, disposable shield. (**Figure 19.4**) The temperature is measured and displayed digitally on a screen. Electronic thermometers are quick and easy to use. There are various types of electronic equipment available and different probes for oral and rectal temperatures. Always follow the manufacturer's instructions.

Math Link

Converting Between Celsius and Fahrenheit

In science, the Celsius scale is used more often than the Fahrenheit scale. Since many health care processes and practices are based in the sciences, it is expected that the Celsius scale would have wide use as well. However, there are a number of health care processes and practices that are measured and reported using the Fahrenheit scale. With that in mind it is important to have the ability to convert from Celsius to Fahrenheit and vice versa.

If you do not have a reference like Table 19.2, you will need to know how to convert a Celsius (C) reading to a Fahrenheit (F) and a Fahrenheit reading to a Celsius. You may sometimes hear the word "centigrade." It is just another word for "Celsius."

Fahrenheit is based on 32 degrees at the freezing point of water and 212 degrees at the boiling point of water. Celsius, on the other hand, is based on 0 degrees at the freezing point of water and 100 degrees at the boiling point. Here are the formulas for converting from one to another.

To convert Celsius to Fahrenheit:

$F = (C \times 1.8) + 32$

To convert Fahrenheit to Celsius:

$C = (F - 32) / 1.8$

Example 1

Convert 35° C to degrees Fahrenheit:

$F = (35 \times 1.8) + 32$

$F = (63) + 32$

$F = 95°$

Example 2

Convert 104°F to degrees Celsius:

$C = (104 - 32) \times 1.8$

$C = 72 / 1.8$

$C = 40°$

What are the conversions for the following temperatures?

a. 37.2°C
b. 101.6°F
c. 96°F
d. 41°C

Why is it very important to double-check your results when you make temperature conversions?

Identify a multi-step medical process that is commonly measured and recorded using the Celsius scale. Convert the Celsius scale measurement to the Fahrenheit scale to guide the solution of the multi-step process.

TEAMWORK

Display drawings of different thermometers displaying different readings. Have students record the readings accurately. Have students practice reading different thermometers by running the thermometers under warm water and/or shaking down the thermometers to change the temperature. Verify that they are accurately recording the readings.

CUSTOMIZED INSTRUCTION

Special Needs Students

You may be able to obtain thermometers customized for use by special needs students.

Sites to Take Body Temperature

Oral

The simplest and most common, convenient, and comfortable site to take a temperature is the oral (referring to the mouth) cavity. The average normal oral temperature is 98.6°F or 37°C. The normal range is 97.6°F to 99.6°F, or 36°C to 37.5°C. Use the oral cavity whenever possible and when the patient has:

- Diarrhea
- Rectal surgery
- Fecal impaction

Rectal

Rectal temperature is the most accurate way to measure body temperature. When measuring a rectal temperature of an infant or small child, always have a second person assist you by holding the child in an appropriate position to prevent the child from being injured. A normal rectal temperature is 98.6°F or 37.5°C.

Rectal temperature is taken when patients:

- Are less than six years of age
- Have difficulty breathing
- Are extremely weak
- Are confused, unconscious, or senile
- Are being given oxygen
- Are mouth breathers
- Are experiencing partial paralysis of the face caused by a stroke or accident

Aural

The aural (referring to the ear) site, like the oral cavity, is also accurate and easy to use. The aural site can be used in place of the oral cavity and for the same types of patients. To measure an aural temperature, an aural probe is positioned in the ear canal. A normal aural temperature is 98.6°F or 37°C.

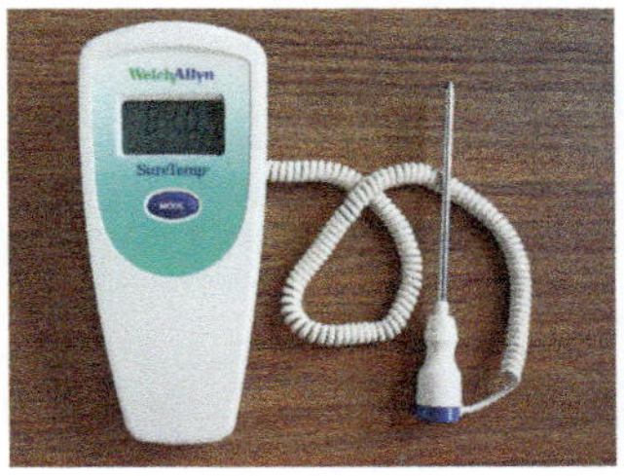

Figure 19.5
Axillary or oral thermometer. When is an axillary thermometer used to take a patient's temperature?

Axillary

The least accurate temperature is taken in the armpit. The normal temperature for this site is 97.6°F or 36.4°C. The normal range is 96.6°F to 98.6°F or 35.9°C to 37°C. Use the **axillary** technique only when the temperature cannot be taken orally, aurally, or rectally. **Figure 19.5** shows a thermometer that can be used for measuring axillary or oral temperature. Always report a temperature that is above normal to your supervisor.

axillary
(AK suh lair ee)
Referring to the armpit.

Teaching Tips

- Review the sites for taking a body temperature:
  - Oral
  - Rectal
  - Aural
  - Axillary
- Give the normal temperature readings for each site:
  - Oral = 98.6°F (37°C)
  - Aural = 98.6°F (37°C)
  - Axillary = 97.6°F (36.4°C)
  - Rectal = 99.6°F (38°F)

Figure Focus

19.5 Axillary or oral thermometer. When is an axillary thermometer used to take a patient's temperature?

Answer: The least accurate temperature is taken in the armpit. For this reason, the axillary technique is used only when the temperature cannot be taken orally, aurally, or rectally.

TEAMWORK

Play a game similar to pin-the-tail-on-the-donkey to identify the normal temperatures at different body sites. Using a poster or diagram of the body, hand a student a sticky note with a normal temperature written on it. Have the student stick the note to the correct body site.

Procedure Tip

19.2 Using an Electronic Thermometer

- Review the background information, emphasizing that this procedure is used for electronic thermometers only.
- Explain how to check the batteries.
- Point out that Standard Precautions must be followed.
- Review the preprocedure steps.
- Step 1: Emphasize proper handwashing.
- Step 2: Emphasize the use of gloves.
- Steps 3–5: Emphasize effective communication techniques.
- Review the procedure steps.
- Step 8: Explain how thermometer will indicate reading is complete.
- Review the postprocedure steps.
- Step 10: Review steps for properly documenting temperature.
- Step 12: Emphasize importance of handwashing.
- Step 14: Emphasize importance of observation and reporting.

PROCEDURE PRACTICE

- Demonstrate the steps for Procedure 19.2, Using an Electronic Thermometer, as many times as necessary, or ask students to demonstrate the steps. Have students practice and perform the procedure until they are competent.

Procedure 19.2 **Using an Electronic Thermometer**

BACKGROUND: There are many different kinds of thermometers. The electronic thermometer is the most commonly used in the hospital setting. If another kind of thermometer is used, refer to the procedure manual provided by the facility. This procedure explains how to use an electronic thermometer to measure body temperature. When you use an electronic thermometer, it is very important to check to see that the batteries are charged. A low battery can cause an inaccurate temperature reading.

ALERT: Follow Standard Precautions. Also, for this and all procedures involving patient movement, see Section 18.4 for information on proper body mechanics.

Preprocedure

1. Wash hand (follow hand-washing guidelines).
2. Assemble equipment:*
   a. Plastic thermometer cover/sheath
   b. Electronic thermometer with appropriate probe (blue for oral and axillary; red for rectal)
3. Identify patient. Pull privacy curtain or close the door to provide for the patient's privacy.
4. Explain procedure to patient.
5. Ask the patient if they have had anything to eat, drink, or smoke in the last 15 minutes. If they have, you need to wait 15 minutes to take an oral temperature.

Procedure

6. Place plastic thermometer cover over probe to prevent contamination.
7. Insert probe in proper position to measure body temperature (blue-tipped probe under tongue or in axilla; red-tipped probe in rectum). If taking axillary temperature, need to hold arm down.
8. Hold probe in place until thermometer indicates reading is complete.
9. Remove plastic sheath and discard it into a biohazardous waste container.

Postprocedure

10. Record temperature. Health care professionals will record a patient's temperature on their chart. Report elevated temperature to a supervisor.
11. Position patient for comfort. Open curtain or door.
12. Wash hands (follow hand-washing guidelines).
13. Return electronic thermometer to its storage place.
14. Report any unusual observation immediately.

Charting Example:

12/15/24 1900
T– 97.4°F oral
S. Jones CNA

* Wear gloves when measuring rectal temperatures. Follow facility policy for measuring oral temperature.

582 Chapter 19 | Measuring Vital Signs and Other Clinical Skills

TEAMWORK

After each procedure encourage discussion of the importance of identifying baseline vital signs and any changes from that baseline that might indicate a change in the patient's status. Discuss what could cause the changes. Build teamwork skills by emphasizing the role of reporting findings to the appropriate persons on the team. Emphasize the importance of integrating information such as the patient's age, diagnosis, previously recorded vital signs, and any other factors that might be influencing vital sign readings. This will discourage "routine vital signs" and encourage the integration of patient care delivered in a holistic manner.

Procedure 19.3 | **Measuring an Oral Temperature Using a Mercury or Nonmercury Thermometer**

BACKGROUND: This procedure explains how to measure temperature with an oral probe.
ALERT: Follow Standard Precautions

Preprocedure

1. Wash hands (follow hand-washing guidelines).
2. Assemble equipment:*
   a. Clean oral (reusable or disposable) thermometer
   b. Alcohol wipes
   c. Watch with second hand
   d. Disposable thermometer cover
3. Identify patient and preferred route to be used. Pull privacy curtain or close door.
4. Explain procedure to patient.

Procedure

5. Apply disposable probe cover.
6. Ask the patient if they have had anything to eat, drink, or smoke in the last 15 minutes. If the answer is yes, wait 15 minutes before taking temperature.
7. Place thermometer under tongue and to the side of the mouth.
8. Instruct patient to hold thermometer with closed lips. You might need to help the patient hold the thermometer.
9. Leave in mouth until thermometer indicates reading is complete.
10. Remove from mouth.
11. Remove and discard disposable cover in a biohazardus waste container.
12. Note thermometer reading correctly.
13. Open curtain or door.

* Follow facility policy for wearing gloves.

Postprocedure

14. Wash thermometer in cool water and dry. Discard thermometer if it is disposable.
15. Wash hands (follow hand-washing guidelines).
16. Record temperature correctly on pad.
17. Report any unusual observation immediately.

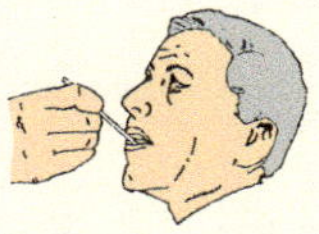

A Insert the thermometer gently into the client's mouth under the tongue.

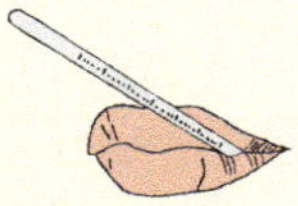

B Position the thermometer to the side of the mouth.

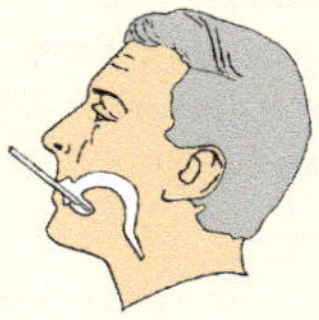

C Instruct the client to keep the thermometer under the tongue by gently closing the lips around the thermometer.

Charting Example:

12/03/24 1600
T– 99.6°F oral
S. Jones CNA

Measuring Vital Signs and Other Clinical Skills | Chapter 19 583

Procedure Tip

19.3 Measuring an Oral Temperature Using a Mercury or Nonmercury Thermometer

- Review the background information.
- Refer students to the information on pages 577–578 for information on reading a glass thermometer.
- Point out that Standard Precautions must be followed.
- Review the preprocedure steps.
- Step 1: Emphasize proper handwashing.
- Step 2: Emphasize the use of gloves.
- Steps 3 and 4: Emphasize effective communication techniques.
- Review the procedure steps.
- Step 6: Explain why waiting is necessary.
- Step 12: Point out the need to note the reading immediately.
- Review the postprocedure steps.
- Step 15: Emphasize importance of handwashing.
- Step 16: Review steps for properly documenting temperature.
- Step 17: Emphasize importance of observation and reporting.

PROCEDURE PRACTICE

- Demonstrate the steps for Procedure 19.3, Measuring an Oral Temperature Using a Mercury or Nonmercury Thermometer, as many times as necessary, or ask students to demonstrate the steps. Have students practice and perform the procedure until they are competent.

Procedure Tip

19.4 Measuring a Rectal Temperature

- Review the background information, emphasizing the information in the CAUTION paragraph.
- Point out that Standard Precautions must be followed.
- Review the preprocedure steps.
- Step 1: Emphasize proper handwashing.
- Steps 3 and 4: Emphasize effective communication techniques.
- Step 5: Emphasize the required use of gloves.
- Review the procedure steps.
- Step 7: Explain need for proper positioning.
- Step 14: Point out the need to note the reading immediately.
- Review the postprocedure steps.
- Step 17: Emphasize importance of handwashing.
- Step 18: Review steps for properly documenting temperature.
- Step 19: Emphasize importance of observation and reporting.

PROCEDURE PRACTICE

- Using a mannequin, demonstrate the steps for Procedure 19.4, Measuring a Rectal Temperature, as many times as necessary, or ask students to demonstrate the steps. Have students practice and perform the procedure using a mannequin until they are competent.

Procedure 19.4 Measuring a Rectal Temperature

BACKGROUND: This procedure explains how to measure a temperature using a rectal thermometer probe.

CAUTION: Do not take a rectal temperature if a patient has had recent rectal surgery, rectal injury, or has had recent treatment that causes body tissues to become thin and fragile. For example, do not take a rectal temperature on a patient who has been undergoing chemotherapy or radiation or has been taking steroids. Rectal temperatures can also be dangerous for people with heart disease because the thermometer can stimulate the vagus nerve in the rectum, which can slow down the heart rate.

ALERT: Follow Standard Precautions

Preprocedure

1. Wash hands (follow hand-washing guidelines).
2. Assemble equipment:
   a. Clean rectal (reusable or disposable) thermometer
   b. Alcohol wipes
   c. Watch with second hand
   d. Lubricant
   e. Disposable nonsterile gloves
   f. Disposable thermometer cover
3. Identify patient and preferred route to be used.
4. Explain procedure to patient. Pull privacy curtain or close the door.
5. Put on disposable gloves.

Procedure

6. Remove thermometer from container and apply disposable cover.
7. Lower backrest on bed. Have patient lie on their left side with right leg bent at the knees.
8. Apply lubricant to probe end.
9. Separate buttocks by pulling up on upper buttock.
10. Insert thermometer 1.5 inches into rectum, or 1 to 1.2 inch for an infant. Do not force thermometer.
11. Hold in place until thermometer indicates reading is complete.
12. Remove thermometer. Wipe anal area to remove excess lubricant and any feces. Cover the patient.
13. Remove and discard disposable cover in a biohazardous waste container.
14. Read thermometer correctly. Open curtain or door.

Postprocedure

15. Clean equipment and return to appropriate storage place.
16. Remove and discard disposable gloves.
17. Wash hands.
18. Record temperature correctly. Remember to indicate that it is a rectal temperature with an Ⓡ.
19. Report any unusual observation immediately.

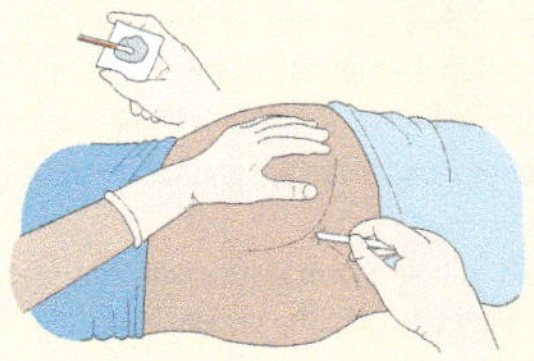

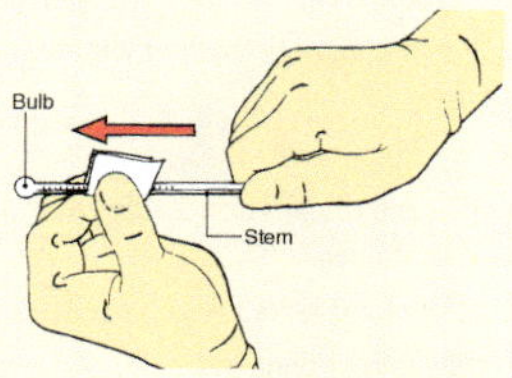

Charting Example:

12/14/24 1500
T– 99.2°F Ⓡ
J. Gonzalez CNA

584 Chapter 19 | Measuring Vital Signs and Other Clinical Skills

Procedure 19.5 Measuring an Axillary Temperature

BACKGROUND: This procedure explains how to measure a temperature using an axillary probe.
ALERT: Follow Standard Precautions

Preprocedure

1. Wash hands (follow hand-washing procedure).
2. Assemble equipment:
   a. Clean reusable or disposable thermometer
   b. Alcohol wipes
   c. Watch with second hand
   d. Disposable thermometer cover
3. Identify patient and preferred route to be used. Pull privacy curtain or close the door.
4. Explain procedure to patient.

Procedure

5. Remove thermometer from container and apply disposable cover.
6. Dry the axilla with a towel.
7. Place the thermometer in axilla. Hold the arm close to the body. Leave in place until thermometer indicates reading is complete.
8. Remove thermometer.
9. Remove and discard disposable cover in biohazardous waste container.
10. Read thermometer correctly. Open curtain or door.

Postprocedure

11. Clean equipment and return to appropriate storage space.
12. Wash hands (follow hand-washing guidelines).
13. Record temperature correctly. You must indicate it was an axillary temperature.
14. Report any unusual observation immediately.

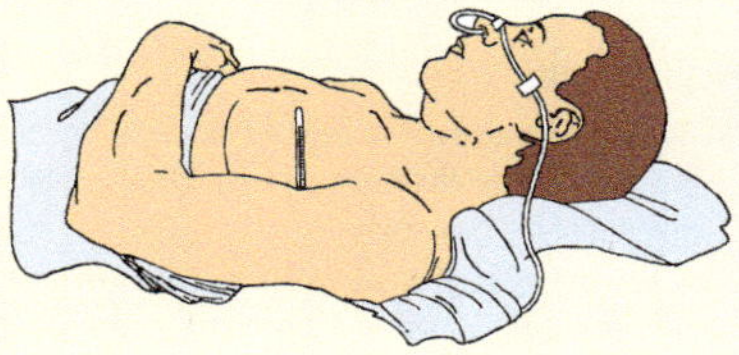

Charting Example:

6/14/24 0400
T– 97°F AX
H. Ferguson RMA

Procedure Tip

19.5 Measuring an Axillary Temperature

- Review the background information, reminding students that an axillary probe is used in the armpit.
- Point out that Standard Precautions must be followed.
- Review the preprocedure steps.
- Step 1: Emphasize proper handwashing.
- Steps 3 and 4: Emphasize effective communication techniques.
- Review the procedure steps.
- Step 10: Point out the need to note the reading immediately.
- Review the postprocedure steps.
- Step 12: Emphasize importance of handwashing.
- Step 13: Review steps for properly documenting temperature.
- Step 14: Emphasize importance of observation and reporting.

PROCEDURE PRACTICE

- Demonstrate the steps for Procedure 19.5, Measuring an Axillary Temperature, as many times as necessary, or ask students to demonstrate the steps. Have students practice and perform the procedure until they are competent.

Procedure Tip

19.6 Measuring an Aural (or Tympanic) Temperature

- Review the background information.
- Remind students that they should always follow Standard Precautions.
- Review the preprocedure steps.
- Step 2: Explain reasons for reviewing chart.
- Review the procedure steps.
- Step 3: Emphasize proper handwashing.
- Step 4: Emphasize effective communication techniques.
- Step 7: Point out the need to note the reading immediately.
- Review the postprocedure steps.
- Emphasize importance of handwashing.
- Step 10: Review steps for properly documenting temperature.
- Steps 11 and 12: Emphasize importance of observation and reporting.

PROCEDURE PRACTICE

- Demonstrate the steps for Procedure 19.6, Measuring an Aural (or Tympanic) Temperature, as many times as necessary, or ask students to demonstrate the steps. Have students practice and perform the procedure until they are competent.

Procedure 19.6 Measuring an Aural (or Tympanic) Temperature

BACKGROUND: The human body has a homeostatic mechanism that regulates all systems and maintains normal function. One of the body's homeostatic mechanisms is the control of body temperature. Body temperature is the balance between heat production and heat loss.

The hypothalamus is the main regulator of body temperature. Factors such as loss of skin integrity with an extensive burn, exposure to extreme weather conditions, disease states such as tumors, or strokes involving the hypothalamus can affect our ability to maintain normal body temperature. An elevated temperature, pyrexia, is a protective mechanism for the body, believed to aid the body in fighting disease.

The elderly patient may have difficulty maintaining **homeostasis**. For that reason an elevated temperature may not be their first sign of infection. The pediatric patient has greater variation in temperature control and may respond to a disease state with a more elevated degree of pyrexia.

ALERT: Follow Standard Precautions

Preprocedure

1. Determine the device to be used for measuring the patient's temperature. Special devices are available for use in the outer ear canal.

NOTE: While the use of an aural (tympanic) thermometer has proven easiest for use in the pediatric patient, research is still in progress to determine its reliability.

2. Review the patient's graphic record to determine baseline temperature and any recent alterations from baseline.

Procedure

3. Wash hands.
4. Explain procedure to patient.
5. Gently pull the ear straight back for children under age 1, or up and back for age 1 or older. Insert the covered probe gently but firmly into the external ear.
6. Activate the device.
7. Note the temperature reading.
8. Remove the device and discard the probe cover in a biohazardous waste container.

Postprocedure

9. Assure that the patient is comfortable and has no further needs before leaving the area.
10. Record the reading on the designated form. Remember to indicate that this was an aural route.
11. Note if the temperature is elevated. Compare the reading with previous temperature readings.
12. If temperature is elevated, communicate that information to the nurse in charge of the patient's care.

Charting Example:

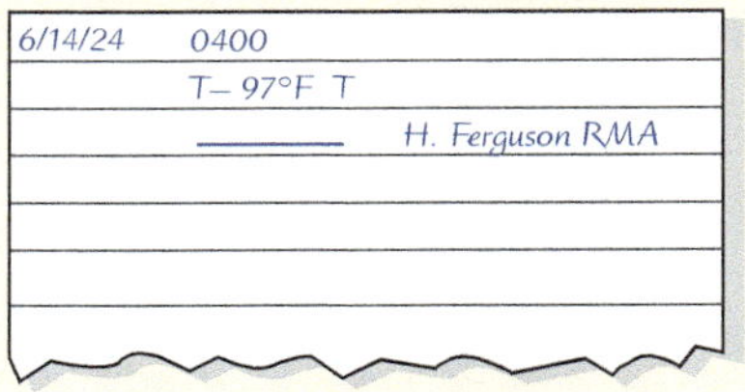

homeostasis
(hoh mee uh STEY sis)
A state of balance, when vital signs are within normal limits.

586 Chapter 19 | Measuring Vital Signs and Other Clinical Skills

Pulse

The pulse is caused by the pressure of the blood pushing against the wall of an artery as the heart contracts and relaxes. (Figure 19.6) It is the throbbing of an artery as the human heart beats. The pulse rate is an important vital sign because it indicates how well the blood is circulating through the body. When you check the pulse rate, you count the number of beats (heartbeats) in 1 minute. This is called beats per minute (bpm).

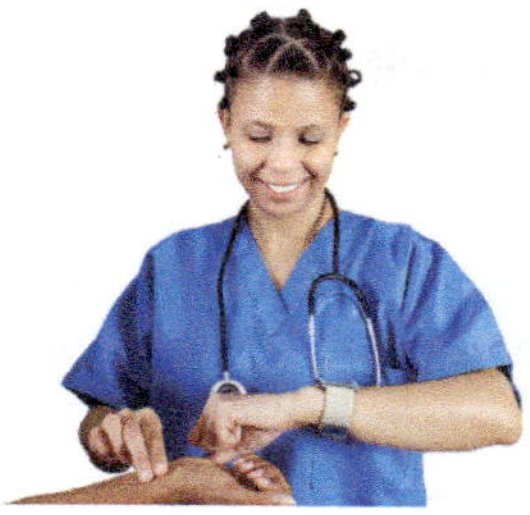

Figure 19.6
The pulse rate is a measure of the heartbeat. A pulse is usually taken for how long a period of time?

Location of Pulse Points

When you count the pulse, place your fingers over an artery and squeeze gently against the bone. Figure 19.7 shows the locations on the body where the pulse may be taken. The pulse rate should be the same at all pulse sites. Table 19.3 shows the factors that affect pulse rate.

Pulse Characteristics

Just counting the beats is not enough. It is important to observe the characteristics of the pulse. This means that you must also note the:

- **Rate.** Number of pulse beats per minute. Table 19.4 lists normal pulse rates for different ages.
- **Rhythm.** Regularity of the beats. Is the rhythm steady or irregular, slow or fast? Sometimes there are uneven intervals between the beats. It is also important to identify if the uneven intervals are regular or irregular. If the uneven interval is irregular, it is called an irregular rhythm. This condition is called **arrhythmia**. Always report a heartbeat below 60 or over 100 beats per minute (bpm).
- **Volume.** Strength or pressure felt with each beat. Note a gentle normal pulse, or a **bounding** forceful pulse. You might also feel a weak pulse that may feel like a thin thread. This is called a **thready** pulse.

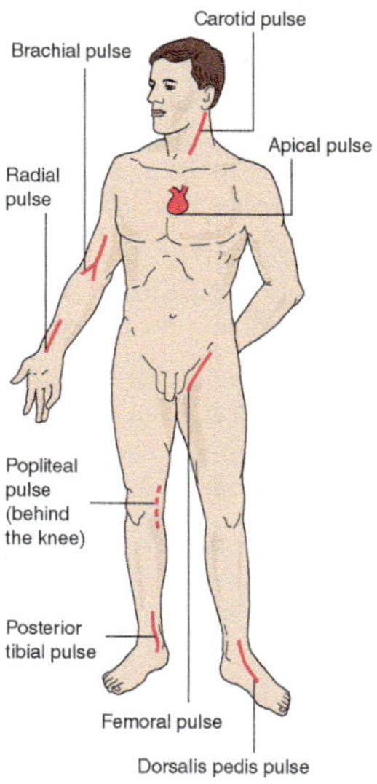

Figure 19.7
Pulse points of the body. Which site is used most often?

arrhythmia
(uh RITH mee uh)
An irregular pulse rate.

bounding
(BAUND ing)
Leaping, strong, or forceful pulse.

thready
(THRED ee)
Weak, barely felt pulse; thin, like a thread.

Measuring Vital Signs and Other Clinical Skills | Chapter 19 587

Teaching Tips

- Explain that pulse:
  - Is the number of times the heart beats in a minute
  - Indicates that blood is circulating through the body
- Explain that when counting a pulse, you feel the pressure of blood against the artery as the heart contracts.
- Describe the location of pulse points on the body.
- Explain that a pulse should be the same rate at every pulse site.
- Emphasize that a missing pulse could indicate a circulatory problem.
- Explain how to determine the characteristics of a pulse:
  - Rate
  - Rhythm
  - Volume

Figure Focus

19.6 The pulse rate is a measure of the heartbeat. A pulse is usually taken for how long a period of time?

Answer: One minute

Figure Focus

19.7 Pulse points of the body. Which site is used most often?

Answer: The radial pulse site

ACTIVITY

Ask students to locate their own carotid pulse. On your signal, have them count the pulse, and then record the count. Have them use their right hand for the right carotid and then the left hand for the left carotid.

Teaching Tips

- Review Table 19.3, discussing the factors that increase and decrease pulse rate.
- Review Table 19.4, explaining that the table lists a normal range for each age group.
- Discuss the factors that increase pulse rate:
  - Exercise
  - Illness
  - Anxiety
  - Medication
  - Shock
- Discuss the factors that decrease pulse rate:
  - High level of aerobic or cardiovascular fitness
  - Depression
  - Medication
  - Cardiac dysfunction
  - Sleep
- Explain that pulse rate varies for different ages.
- Emphasize that a pulse below 60 (bradycardia) or over 100 (tachycardia) should always be reported, as it might indicate a serious problem.
- Review the formulas for calculating a pulse rate.
- Explain how to count a pulse.
- Review the difference between radial and apical.
- Emphasize that a thumb should never be used to count a pulse rate.

ACTIVITY

Have students note the characteristics of their own radial pulse. First, have them count their resting pulse and note the characteristics. Then, have them exercise for one minute, count their pulse, and note the characteristics. Discuss the results as a class.

Table 19.3 Factors That Affect Pulse Rate

Increase Pulse Rate	Decrease Pulse Rate
Exercise	High level of aerobic fitness
Illness	Depression
Anxiety	Medication
Medication	Cardiac dysfunction
Shock	Sleep

Table 19.4 Normal Pulse Rates

Age	Rate
Before birth	140–150
At birth	90–160
First year of life	115–130
Childhood years	80–115
Adult	60–80

Pulse Rate

hemorrhage (HEM er rij or HEM-rij) Large amount of bleeding.

tachycardia (tak i KAHR dee uh) Pulse rate over 100 beats per minute (for adults).

bradycardia (brad i KAHR dee uH) Pulse rate below 60 beats per minute.

Pulse rate generally increases with exercise, emotional excitement, **hemorrhage**, or elevated temperature. Drugs can increase or decrease the heart rate. When the rate is over 100 beats per minute, it is called **tachycardia**. When the rate is below 60 beats per minute, it is called **bradycardia**. When the rate is irregular, it is called arrhythmia.

The pulse rate is determined by counting the number of times you feel a pulse in 1 minute. You can determine the rate by counting the pulse for:

- 15 seconds and multiply by 4 (there are four 15-second periods in 1 minute). For example, 22 beats (in 15 seconds) × 4 = 88 beats per minute.
- 30 seconds and multiply by 2 (there are two 30-second periods in 1 minute). For example, 44 beats (in 30 seconds) × 2 = 88 beats per minute.

If you count the pulse for 60 seconds, this will give you the beats per minute (bpm). When the pulse rate is irregular, it is important to count the pulse for a full 60 seconds to be sure that the count is accurate. Be sure to follow your facility's policy on how long to count the pulse.

ALERT: When you record the pulse rate, always report to your supervisor anything that is abnormal. This includes rate (Table 19.4), rhythm, and force.

588 Chapter 19 | Measuring Vital Signs and Other Clinical Skills

CUSTOMIZED INSTRUCTION

At-Risk Students

Ask students to count their own pulse and that of two to three other family members, friends, or teachers. Refer them to Procedure 19.7 on p. 589. They should take the pulse for each person at least twice in a 24-hour period. Have them create a short journal in which they note the age of the person and what he or she was doing before each count was taken. Have them compare the results to the rates listed in Table 19.4. Do any of the rates appear to be abnormal? If so, encourage students to discuss with the individual.

Radial Pulse

The radial pulse is the most common site for counting the pulse rate. This pulse is counted on the thumb side of the wrist. Do not use your thumb to count a pulse because you have a pulse in your thumb.

Apical Pulse

You may be asked to count an apical pulse. This is the pulse counted at the **apex** (pointed end) of the heart. Count the apical heartbeat by placing the **stethoscope** 2 to 3 inches to the left of the sternum, just below the nipple on the chest.

apex
(AY peks)
Pointed end of something (for example, the pointed end of the heart is called the apex of the heart).

stethoscope
(STETH uh skohp)
Instrument used to amplify sound.

Procedure 19.7 Counting a Radial Pulse

BACKGROUND: It is important for health care workers to monitor the patient's physical status. One way to determine this status is by counting the patient's pulse rate. This procedure explains how to count a radial pulse.
ALERT: Follow Standard Precautions

Preprocedure

1. Wash hands (follow hand-washing guidelines).
2. Assemble equipment:
   a. Watch with second hand
   b. Pad and pencil
3. Identify patient. Pull privacy curtain or close the door.
4. Explain procedure to patient.

Procedure

5. Place three fingers on the radial artery—do not use thumb.
6. Count pulse (number of beats or pulsations) for 1 minute.
7. Record pulse rate on pad immediately. Open curtain or door.

Postprocedure

8. Wash hands (follow hand-washing guidelines).
9. Record pulse rate on chart.
10. Immediately report any unusual observation. Examples include an irregular pulse, a bounding or weak pulse, or a pulse rate less than 60 bpm or more than 100 bpm.

NOTE: If the pulse is difficult to assess, irregular, weak, or rapid, the apical rate should be assessed.

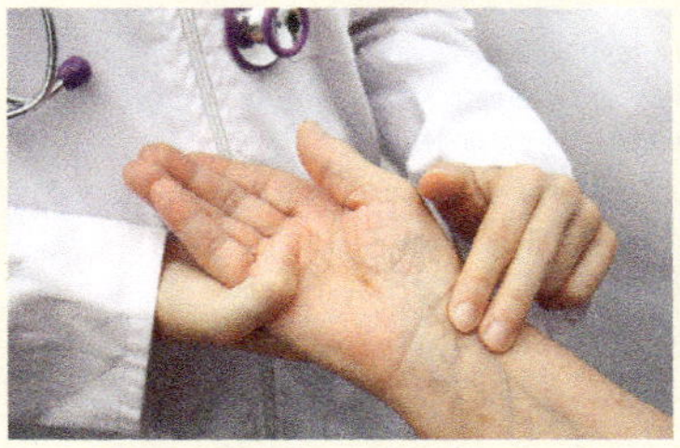

Charting Example:

2/14/24	1300
	Pulse = 72
	Regular and strong
	________ T. Morales CNA

Measuring Vital Signs and Other Clinical Skills | Chapter 19 589

Procedure Tip

19.7 Counting a Radial Pulse

- Review the background information, emphasizing that pulse rate is one indication of the patient's physical status.
- Emphasize the importance of following Standard Precautions.
- Review the preprocedure steps.
- Step 1: Emphasize the importance of proper handwashing.
- Step 2: Emphasize the need for a second hand.
- Steps 3 and 4: Emphasize effective communication techniques.
- Review the procedure steps.
- Step 5: Emphasize that the thumb should not be used.
- Step 7: Point out the need to note the count immediately.
- Review the postprocedure steps.
- Step 8: Emphasize importance of handwashing.
- Step 9: Review steps for properly documenting pulse rate.
- Step 10: Emphasize importance of observation and reporting.

PROCEDURE PRACTICE

- Demonstrate the steps for Procedure 19.7, Counting a Radial Pulse, as many times as necessary, or ask students to demonstrate the steps. Have students practice and perform the procedure until they are competent.

Procedure Tip

19.8 Counting an Apical Pulse

- Review the background information, emphasizing the situations in which an apical pulse count is used.
- Emphasize the importance of following Standard Precautions.
- Review the preprocedure steps.
- Step 2: Emphasize the importance of proper handwashing.
- Steps 3 and 4: Emphasize effective communication techniques.
- Review the procedure steps.
- Step 7: Point out that a stethoscope is not necessary for infants.
- Step 8: Emphasize that in addition to count, it is important to note strength, rate, and rhythm of beat.
- Step 10: Point out the need to note the count immediately.
- Review the postprocedure steps.
- Step 11: Emphasize importance of handwashing.
- Step 12: Review steps for properly documenting apical pulse rate.
- Step13: emphasize importance of observation and reporting.

PROCEDURE PRACTICE

- Demonstrate the steps for Procedure 19.8, Counting an Apical Pulse, as many times as necessary, or ask students to demonstrate the steps. Have students practice and perform the procedure until they are competent.

Procedure 19.8 Counting an Apical Pulse

BACKGROUND: The apical pulse is assessed upon admission, when the peripheral pulse is difficult to assess, and also when giving medications that alter heart rate and rhythm, such as digoxin.
ALERT: Follow Standard Precautions

Preprocedure

1. Assemble equipment:
   a. Stethoscope
   b. Alcohol swabs
2. Wash hands (follow hand-washing guidelines).
3. Identify patient. Pull privacy curtain or close door.
4. Explain procedure to patient.

Procedure

5. Uncover left side of patient's chest.
6. Locate the apex of the heart between the fifth and the sixth rib, about 3 inches to the left of the median line and slightly below the nipple.
7. Place stethoscope over apical region and listen for heart sounds. The apical rate of an infant is easily palpated with the fingertips.
8. Count the beats for 1 minute; note rate, rhythm, and strength of beat.
9. Cover patient. Open the curtain or door.
10. Record pulse rate on pad.

Postprocedure

11. Wash hands (follow hand-washing guidelines).
12. Record apical pulse rate on chart. Remember to indicate that it was an apical pulse.
13. Report any unusual observation immediately.

Charting Example:

12/14/24	1000
	82 / 78 AP
	Pulse deficit = 4
	Quality of beat strong regular rhythm
	———— S. Padlewski RMA

Respiration

respiration (res puh REY shuhn) Taking oxygen into the body and expelling carbon dioxide (CO_2) from the body.

Respiration is the process of taking oxygen (O_2) into the body and expelling carbon dioxide (CO_2) from the body. One inspiration (breathing in) and one expiration (breathing out) are considered as one respiration. (**Figure 19.8**)

When you count a patient's respiration, you do not want the patient to be aware of what you are doing. If the patient realizes that you are counting respirations, he or she may not breathe normally. Count the respiration rate after you finish counting the pulse. **Table 19.5** shows the factors that affect respiration.

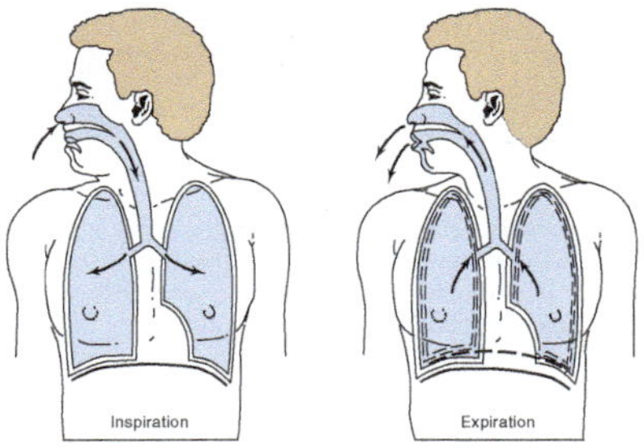

Figure 19.8
One respiration. Breathing in once (inspiration) and breathing out once (expiration) make up one respiration. What is expelled from the body by expiration?

Table 19.5 Factors That Affect Respiration

Increase Respiration	Decrease Respiration
Exercise	Relaxation
Anxiety	Depression
Respiratory disease	Head injury
Medication	Medication
Pain	
Heart disease (e.g., congestive heart failure)	

Pulse Oximetry

Pulse oximetry is a procedure used to determine the oxygen (O_2) saturation of arterial blood. Pulse oximetry is useful for monitoring patients at risk for hypoxia (a condition in which the body or a region of the body is deprived of adequate oxygen supply) and postoperative patients. The device that measures the oxygen in the blood is called a pulse oximeter. (Figure 19.9)

Figure 19.9
Digital pulse oximeter. When would you use a digital pulse oximeter?

Blood O_2 content is an important indicator of a patient's respiratory and cardiac condition. The oximeter sends red and infrared light through a pulsating arterial vascular bed through a sensor attached to the fingertip, earlobe, bridge of the nose, or toe. This measures the O_2 content of the blood and the pulse rate and displays the reading on a monitor.

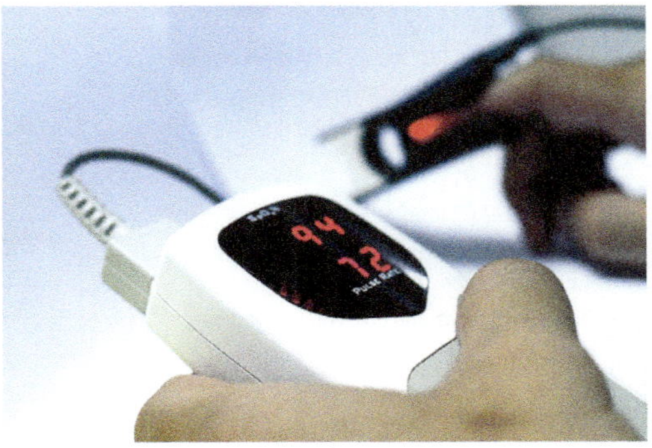

Low readings cause an alarm to sound. The normal range is considered to be between 95 and 100 percent. Any reading below 90 percent may indicate that oxygenation to the tissues is inadequate. Interventions such as increasing oxygen therapy, providing nebulizer treatments or changing the mode of oxygen delivery may be necessary.

Measuring Vital Signs and Other Clinical Skills | Chapter 19 591

Figure Focus

19.8 One respiration. Breathing in once (inspiration) and breathing out once (expiration) make up one respiration. What is expelled from the body by expiration?

Answer: Carbon dioxide

Teaching Tips

- Explain that respiration is the process of:
  - Taking in oxygen
  - Expelling carbon dioxide
- Emphasize that one respiration is made of two parts:
  - One inspiration (breathing in)
  - One expiration (breathing out)
- Explain that respirations help regulate body temperature and eliminate waste products.
- Review Table 19.5.
- Discuss factors that increase respiration:
  - Exercise
  - Anxiety
  - Respiratory disease
  - Medication
  - Pain
  - Heart disease
- Discuss factors that decrease respiration:
  - Relaxation
  - Depression
  - Head injury
  - Medication
- Point out that rate may also be affected by age and the presence of fever.

Figure Focus

19.9 Digital pulse oximeter. When would you not use a digital pulse oximeter?

Answer: Do not use a digital pulse oximeter over a break in the skin, a swollen area, or an area where the circulation is poor.

TEAMWORK

In pairs, have students practice counting each other's respirations. Have each student list five words that describe how it felt knowing the other person was counting his or her respirations. Discuss how knowing affects the way you breathe, and why it is important that the patient not know when his or her respirations are being counted.

Personal Wellness—Asthma

- Explain asthma.
- Ask if any students have asthma, and if they are willing to discuss it.
- Review the symptoms.
- Review the treatments.

What can you do to help a friend or relative who has asthma?

Answer: If a friend or relative has asthma, it is important to encourage him or her to see a doctor and get medical help. Help your friend or relative follow the doctor's treatment plan and remind them to take their medicine at the proper times. Encourage people who suffer from asthma to take their inhaler with them at all times, but only to use it when they have asthma symptoms.

Procedure Tip

19.9 Counting Respirations

- Review the background information, emphasizing why it is important to know the respiration rate of a patient.
- Emphasize the importance of following Standard Precautions.
- Review the preprocedure steps.
- Step 1: Emphasize the importance of proper handwashing.
- Step 2: Emphasize the need for a second hand.
- Step 4: Explain why it is important to tell patient pulse rate is being counted. Point out that patients may change their respiration rate unconsciously if they know it is being counted.
- Review the procedure steps.
- Step 5: Explain that placing your finger on the pulse rate is to distract the patient.

Personal Wellness

Asthma

Asthma is a chronic condition that occurs when the main air passages of the lungs, known as the bronchial tubes, become inflamed. The muscles of the bronchial walls tighten and extra mucus is produced. This causes the airways to narrow.

In the United States, asthma sufferers number about 25 million. According to the Mayo Clinic, about 4,000 Americans die each year from asthma, and another 500,000 people are hospitalized.

Symptoms of asthma include:

- Shortness of breath or wheezing
- Disturbed sleep caused by shortness of breath, coughing, or wheezing
- Chest tightness or pain

Asthma is a very treatable disease. However, if left untreated, asthma can result in reduced lung function and possibly permanent lung damage. Therefore, if you have symptoms of asthma, the first step is a visit to your doctor.

The doctor will develop a treatment plan. If you have persistent asthma, the doctor may prescribe an inhaled anti-inflammatory medication. A doctor may also prescribe a quick-relief inhaler to be used only when you have asthma symptoms. Remember to always keep your inhaler with you.

What can you do to help a friend or relative who has asthma?

Procedure 19.9 Counting Respirations

BACKGROUND: It is important for health care workers to monitor the patient's physical status. One way to determine this status is by counting the patient's respiratory rate. This procedure explains how to count the number of times a patient breathes in a minute.
ALERT: Follow Standard Precautions

Preprocedure

1. Wash hands (follow hand-washing guidelines).
2. Assemble equipment:
   a. Watch with second hand
   b. Pad and pencil
3. Identify patient. Pull privacy curtain or close door.
4. Explain to the patient that you are going to take their pulse.

Procedure

5. Relax fingers on pulse point.
6. Observe rise and fall of chest.
7. Count respirations and calculate rate.
8. Note rate, rhythm, and quality of respirations.

Postprocedure

9. Open curtain or close door.
10. Wash hands (follow hand-washing guidelines).
11. Record the respiratory rate accurately. Make sure you take it for 30 seconds and multiply times two. If respirations are irregular, take for one full minute.
12. Report any unusual observation immediately. This could include irregular respiration, noisy breathing, and pain with or difficulty breathing.

Charting Example:

5/22/24 0930
Resp. 20 and regular
M. Taylor CNA

592 Chapter 19 | Measuring Vital Signs and Other Clinical Skills

- Step 8: Emphasize that in addition to count, it is important to note rate, rhythm, and quality of respirations.
- Review the postprocedure steps.
- Step 10: Emphasize importance of handwashing.
- Step 11: Review steps for properly documenting respiration rate.
- Step12: Emphasize importance of observation and reporting.

PROCEDURE PRACTICE

- Demonstrate the steps for Procedure 19.9, Counting Respirations, as many times as necessary, or ask students to demonstrate the steps. Have students practice and perform the procedure until they are competent.

TEAMWORK

In small groups, create a presentation to educate younger students about asthma. Include information such as causes, factors that make it worse, and treatments.

Respiratory Characteristics

Age influences respiration. The rate of newborns may be 40 respirations per minute. The suggested normal adult rate is 12 to 20 respirations per minute. When you measure respiration, always note the following:

- **Rate**. The number of respirations per minute.
- **Rhythm**. The regularity, or irregularity, of breathing.
- **Quality**. The amount of air exchanged and the effort it takes to breathe.
- **Dyspnea**. Shortness of breath. Is breathing difficult?
- **Tachypnea**. Abnormally fast respirations.
- **Apnea**. Has breathing stopped?
- **Cheyne-Stokes**. Are there periods of labored respirations followed by apnea?
- **Rales**. Can you hear bubbling or rattling sounds caused by mucus in the air passages?

ALERT: Always report any unusual or abnormal respirations to your supervisor.

rate of respirations
(reyt of resp puh REY shuhn)
The number of respirations per minute.

rhythm of respirations
(RITH uh m of res puh REY shuhn)
The regularity, or irregularity, of breathing.

quality of respirations
(KWOL i tee of res puh REY shuhn)
The amount of air taken into the body and expelled from the body and the effort it takes to do this.

Recording Vital Signs

Always write the temperature, pulse, and respiration (TPR) in the same order:

T	P	R
98.6	72	16

Since all health care workers write vital signs in the same way, you do not need to put T P R above the figures. Write 98.6/72/16 for an oral temperature, or write 98.6°. Put an Ⓡ next to a rectal temperature (for example, 99.6Ⓡ) and an AX next to an axillary temperature (for example 97.6AX).

Some facilities may have a policy requiring that a T be placed next to the aural temperature (for example, 98.6T). These symbols tell other health care workers where you measured the temperature, and this helps ensure accuracy. Some health care workers include BP (blood pressure) after TPR. *Always report abnormal or unusual vital signs to your supervisor.*

Taking vital signs may seem routine, but the information is important to the well-being of the patient. Careful recording of vital signs is essential for the protection of the patient.

Always compare most recent reading to those in the recent past. Look for patterns in the readings, such as temperature always elevated at a particular time of day, or blood pressure elevated during an episode of acute discomfort. Reporting the patterns, as well as the current reading, will help the nurse determine the significance of the current data.

Teaching Tips

- Describe normal respiration rates:
  - Adult: 12 to 20 respirations per minute
  - Infant: approximately 40 per minute
- Emphasize the need to note:
  - Rate
  - Rhythm
  - Quality
- Describe some abnormal respirations:
  - Dyspnea
  - Apnea
  - Cheynes-Stokes
  - Rales
- Describe some abnormal lung sounds:
  - Rales
  - Crackling
  - Diminished sounds
  - No sounds at all
- Explain how to record vital signs.
- Emphasize that there is a standard method for recording vital signs.

CUSTOMIZED INSTRUCTION

Less Advanced Students

If less advanced students have difficulty identifying the characteristics of respirations and pulses, they might benefit from specific examples. Play recordings of abnormal sounds and rhythms as well as normal ones. Provide descriptive words such thready, weak, and uneven, to help students understand how to communicate the characteristics.

What's New?—Obtaining and Recording Temperatures with Accuracy

- Explain why an elevated temperature signals a change in health status. Our blood and lymphatic systems produce white blood cells which fight off infection. As our white blood cells increase in number, they go faster and faster attacking the germs. This causes our bodies to heat up, giving us a fever or rise in body temperature.
- There are been concerns about the accuracy of tympanic thermometers. Some of these concerns reflect the "offsets" (or internal calculations) set by the manufacturer to convert the ear temperature to an equivalent oral or rectal temperature. Other concerns address the variables that impact ear-based temperature measurement, such as the ear canal structure or the positioning of the probe itself.

Teaching Tips

- Review the types of vital signs.
- Review the purpose of vital signs.
- Explain that vital signs provide clues that indicate signs of wellness or disease.
- Emphasize that abnormal vital signs may point to specific disease processes and that routine measurement of vital signs allows treatment for conditions before a crisis.
- For example:
  - Reducing a high body temperature prevents brain damage.
  - Increasing a slow pulse or reducing a fast pulse provides an even flow of blood to deliver oxygen to organs.
  - Maintaining a respiratory rate provides the body with adequate oxygen and eliminates carbon dioxide.

What's New?

Obtaining and Recording Temperatures with Accuracy

Caregivers monitor a patient's temperature at intervals and use the readings to determine health status of their patients. An elevated temperature may be the first indication of a change in health status. An elevated temperature is one of the body's protective mechanisms used to fight infection or to indicate that an inflammatory process is present.

There have been some recent concerns regarding the accuracy of tympanic thermometers. In some instances, facilities are replacing tympanic thermometers with newer versions of the electronic oral and rectal thermometers. Because of the importance of accurately determining the temperature of your patients, it is very important to use appropriate technique and the most accurate instruments available for measurement.

Summary

Vital signs are important indicators of the body's condition. Three of these vital signs are temperature, pulse, and respiration (TPR). Many factors influence TPR in the human body, and it is important to be aware of them. You have learned the steps for taking temperature, pulse, and respiration, and you know how to recognize a normal TPR and an abnormal TPR.

You may also be responsible for accurately measuring oxygen (O_2) in the blood. You also know that pain is an important sign in how the body is functioning. All this information is essential in giving good patient care and in recognizing problems with your own personal health.

Section 19.1 Review Questions

1. Name four different types of thermometers.
2. Identify four sites on the body where temperature may be taken.
3. When would you not take an oral temperature?
4. What vital sign indicates how well the blood is circulating through the body?
5. Where is the most common site on the body for counting the pulse rate?
6. What are the two components, or parts, of one respiration?
7. What does TPR stand for?

594 Chapter 19 | Measuring Vital Signs and Other Clinical Skills

- Review factors that influence temperature.
- Review factors that influence pulse rate.
- Review factors that influence respiration rate.
- Review how to recognize abnormal vital signs.

Section 19.1 Review Questions

1. Answer: Glass (clinical), aural (ear), temporal artery (forehead), chemically treated paper or plastic, electronic/digital
2. Answer: Oral (mouth), rectal, aural (ear), axillary (armpit)
3. Answer: Do not take an oral temperature if the patient has had anything to eat, drink, or smoke in the last 15 minutes.
4. Answer: Pulse
5. Answer: Radial pulse is the most common and is counted on the thumb side of the wrist.
6. Answer: Inspiration (breathing in) and expiration (breathing out)
7. Answer: Temperature (T), Pulse (P), Respiration (R)

Blood Pressure

SECTION 19.2

Background

You have learned that temperature, pulse, and respiration are signs that indicate whether the body is functioning within normal limits. Blood pressure is the fourth vital sign. Measuring the patient's blood pressure gives you a complete picture of his or her vital signs. A complete record of all vital signs helps in the diagnosis and treatment of the patient.

Objectives

When you have completed this section, you will be able to do the following:

- Match key terms with their correct meanings.
- Define *blood pressure*.
- Match descriptions of systolic and diastolic blood pressure.
- List factors that increase blood pressure.
- List factors that can reduce blood pressure.
- State the normal range of blood pressure.
- Demonstrate how to measure and record a blood pressure accurately.
- Explain how vital signs provide information about the patient's health.

Blood Pressure

Blood pressure is the force of the blood pushing against the walls of the blood vessels. The **systolic pressure** is the greatest force exerted on the walls of the arteries by the heart. This pressure is exerted when the heart is contracting. You hear the first beat when contraction occurs. The **diastolic pressure** is the least force exerted on the walls of the arteries by the heart. This pressure occurs as the heart relaxes between contractions. When the heart relaxes, there is no sound (beat). The normal systolic blood pressure is below 135. For the diastolic pressure, it is below 85.

Blood pressure depends on the volume of blood in the circulating system, the force of the heartbeat, and the condition of the arteries. When arteries lose their elasticity, they give more resistance, and the blood pressure increases.

When the blood pressure is below the normal range, it is called hypotension. A very low blood pressure can indicate decreased perfusion, which can cause a decrease in organ function such as to the brain. When this occurs the patient may lose consciousness. **Table 19.6** shows the factors that affect blood pressure.

blood pressure (BP)
(bluhd PRESH er)
Highest and lowest pressure of the blood pushing against the walls of the arteries.

systolic pressure
(sis TAHL ic)
Highest pressure against blood vessels. It is represented by first heart sound or beat heard when taking a blood pressure.

diastolic pressure
(DIE es tahl ic)
Lowest pressure against the blood vessels of the body. It is measured between contractions.

Measuring Vital Signs and Other Clinical Skills | Chapter 19 595

ACTIVITY

Make flashcards to use as a study aid in learning the medical terminology associated with blood pressure, as covered in Section 19.2.

FOCUS AND ENGAGE

Introduce the Section

a. Review the content of the Background paragraph, explaining that blood pressure is one of the vital signs.

b. Emphasize the importance of monitoring blood pressure to identify normal or abnormal conditions in the body.

c. Review the objectives for the section.

Vocabulary Review

a. Direct students to the key terms.

b. Pronounce each word, and have the students repeat the pronunciation out loud.

c. Discuss the definition of each word.

TEACH

Discuss

- Ask students to share personal stories of having blood pressure checked.
- Discuss the problems that are indicated by blood pressure that is too high (e.g., clogged arteries), or too low (e.g., internal bleeding).

Reinforce and Review

- Review Chapter 13, Your Body and How It Functions.
- Reinforce the importance of monitoring vital signs (Section 19.1).

Teaching Tips

- Explain that blood pressure is the force of the heart's action and the elasticity of the arteries when blood is pushed through the blood vessels.

Teaching Tips

- Differentiate between systolic pressure and diastolic pressure.
- Explain that systolic pressure is the greatest pressure exerted on the walls of the arteries during the contraction of the heart.
- Explain that diastolic pressure is the lowest pressure against the arteries during the heart's rest between contractions.
- Review Table 19.6.
- Discuss factors that increase blood pressure: loss of elasticity in the arteries, exercise, eating, stimulants, or anxiety.
- Discuss factors that reduce blood pressure: depressants, fasting, shock, hemorrhage, inactivity, or suppressants.
- Define normal blood pressure:
  - Systolic: 90–140 mm
  - Diastolic: 60–90 mm
- Explain how to communicate blood pressure rates: systolic over diastolic. For example, 120 over 80, which is written 120/80.
- Always report hypotension (blood pressure below the normal range) and hypertension (blood pressure above the normal range).

Table 19.6 Factors That Affect Blood Pressure

Increase Blood Pressure	Decrease Blood Pressure
Loss of elasticity in the arteries (arteriosclerosis)	Hemorrhage
Exercise	Inactivity
Eating	Fasting
Stimulants (e.g., medication, coffee)	Suppressants (e.g., medications that cause blood pressure to lower)
Anxiety	Depression
	Shock

Normal Blood Pressure

millimeters
(MILL ih mee tehr)
Measure of length.

The normal blood pressure range is between 90 and 140 **millimeters** (mm) mercury for the *systolic pressure*. For the *diastolic pressure*, it is between 60 and 90 millimeters (mm) of mercury. When you record a blood pressure, it is written:

$$120/80 = \frac{120\text{ systolic}}{80\text{ diastolic}}$$

In addition, the normal pulse pressure range is 30–40 mm of Mg. You find this by subtracting diastolic from systolic.

hypertension
(hahy per TEN shuh n)
High blood pressure.

asymptomatic
(ey simp tuh MAT ik)
Without visible symptoms.

hypotension
(hahy puh TEN shuhn)
Low blood pressure.

When the blood pressure is above the normal range, it is called **hypertension**, or high blood pressure. Hypertension is called the silent killer. It is a disease that is **asymptomatic** in most cases. This condition is discovered only when a patient's blood pressure is measured.

Heredity plays a major role in patients who develop hypertension. Some of the effects are stroke, kidney problems, changes in the retina, and heart disease. When the blood pressure is below the normal range, it is called **hypotension**.

Blood Pressure Apparatus

sphygmomanometer
(sfig moh muh NOM i ter)
A device used to measure the pressure against the arteries of the body.

apparatus
(ap uh RAT uhs)
Equipment needed to perform a task. For example, blood pressure apparatus includes a blood pressure cuff and a stethoscope.

Blood pressure is measured with an instrument called a **sphygmomanometer**. In the word *sphygmomanometer*:

- **Sphygmo** refers to pulse.
- **Mano** refers to pressure.
- **Meter** refers to measure.

Most health care workers refer to the sphygmomanometer as a BP cuff or blood pressure cuff. There are different kinds of blood pressure **apparatus**:

- Aneroid
- Electronic/digital

596 Chapter 19 | Measuring Vital Signs and Other Clinical Skills

ACTIVITY

Read examples of systolic and diastolic blood pressure readings out loud to the class, and have each student correctly write the blood pressure for each example. Check to be sure they wrote them correctly.

The aneroid apparatuses have a **gauge**, which is marked with a series of long and short lines. The long lines are at 10-mm (millimeter) intervals. The short lines are between the long lines and indicate 2 mm (millimeters) each. When you measure a blood pressure, you must do two things at one time. You listen to the heartbeat as it pulses through the artery. You also watch the gauge in order to take a reading.

gauge
(GAYJ)
Standard scale for measurement.

The blood pressure cuff is a cloth-covered rubber bladder that fills with air as the bulb is squeezed. When the cuff is **inflated** around the arm, it stops the flow of blood. As the pressure is relieved, the flow returns and you hear a beat. This is the systolic pressure. As the cuff continues to deflate, you hear a last beat and then silence. The last beat you hear is the diastolic pressure.

inflated
(in FLEY tid)
To swell or fill up with air.

Stethoscope

When you listen to pulse sounds, you use a stethoscope. A stethoscope picks up sound when it is placed against the body. The stethoscope has earpieces, a spring to help keep the earpieces in the ears, flexible rubber tubing that carries sound, a bell, and a diaphragm that magnifies sound.

Palpating Blood Pressure

You may be asked to take a blood pressure by first palpating (feeling) the radial pulse. This allows you to determine the correct inflation pressure when inflating the cuff.

What's New?

Holter Monitors

A Holter monitor is a machine that continuously records the heart's rhythms. The monitor is usually worn for 24 hours during normal activity. It may also be called an ambulatory electrocardiography.

One of the problems with Holter monitors is the refusal of many patients to wear them. Traditional Holter monitors were bulky and had to be worn and attached for 24 to 48 hours at a time. These requirements reduced the willingness to wear this important device.

New technology has now been developed to increase patient compliance by making the Holter monitor more user-friendly. Some newer monitors weigh only 1 ounce (28g) and are no bigger than a single AAA battery. This monitor is so small and lightweight that it may be worn comfortably underneath clothing and patients hardly notice they are wearing the device. Another company has experimented with a wireless monitor that eliminates the need for electrodes.

Modern monitors record onto digital flash memory devices. The data is then uploaded into a computer through a secure USB connection. The computer analyzes the input and calculates summary statistics such as average heart rate, and minimum and maximum heart rate.

The new technology in Holter monitors makes sure doctors get the quick results they need. The report can be returned to the referring physician within 24 hours to help them diagnose the nature of their patient's potential heart problem.

Teaching Tips

- Display a sphygmomanometer.
- Explain that most people call it a blood pressure cuff.
- Remove the bladder to show how it fits into the sleeve.
- Point out the fastener.
- Show students how the manometer attaches to the cuff.
- Demonstrate how to hold the bulb and turn the thumbscrew valve.
- Describe the aneroid cuff as a dial with numbers and an indicator that shows blood pressure readings.
- Display a stethoscope and explain its use to hear the beats when checking blood pressure.
- Explain palpating blood pressure.

What's New?—Holter Monitors

- Explain that using a Holter Monitor to track the heart's function during normal activity over a long period of time can help medical providers determine the effectiveness of treatment and diagnose problems.
- Emphasize the use of technology for medical applications, such as flash drives to store and upload the data.

TEAMWORK

Distribute blood pressure equipment and alcohol wipes to the students (the wipes are for cleaning the stethoscope ear pieces). Instruct students to work in pairs to practice applying the cuff to their partner's arm. Have them use communication skills to let each other know if they are pumping too high and leaving pressure in the cuff.

Procedure Tip

19.10 Palpating a Blood Pressure

- Review the background information, emphasizing that palpating the blood pressure lets you know how high to inflate the blood pressure cuff.
- Emphasize the importance of following Standard Precautions.
- Emphasize the need to listen carefully and not be distracted by anything.
- Review the preprocedure steps.
- Step 1: Emphasize the importance of proper handwashing.
- Step 2: Emphasize the need to use effective communication techniques.
- Review the procedure steps.
- Step 3: Explain proper sizing.
- Step 6: Explain proper positioning.
- Step 8: Explain that this is when student palpates the radial pulse.
- Step 12: Emphasize that a thumb should not be used to hold the stethoscope in place.
- Review the postprocedure steps.
- Step 20: Review steps for properly documenting blood pressure.
- Step 22: Emphasize importance of handwashing.
- Step 23: Emphasize importance of observation and reporting.

PROCEDURE PRACTICE

- Demonstrate the steps for Procedure 19.10, Palpating a Blood Pressure, as many times as necessary, or ask students to demonstrate the steps. Have students practice and perform the procedure until they are competent.

Procedure 19.10 Palpating a Blood Pressure

BACKGROUND: As a health care worker, it is important to monitor the patient's physical status. One way to determine this status is by measuring the patient's blood pressure. This procedure explains how to palpate a blood pressure so you will know how high to inflate the blood pressure cuff.
ALERT: Follow Standard Precautions

Preprocedure

1. Wash hands (follow hand-washing guidelines).
2. Explain procedure to patient. Pull privacy curtain or close door.

Procedure

3. Select the appropriate cuff for your patient. A cuff that is too small may cause a false-high reading and a cuff that is too large may cause a false-low reading.
4. Support patient's arm, palm side up, on a firm surface.
5. Roll up patient's sleeve above elbow, being careful that it is not too tight.
6. Wrap wide part of cuff around patient's arm directly over brachial artery. Most cuffs have an arrow to position over the brachial artery. The lower edge of cuff should be 1 or 2 inches above bend of elbow.
7. Find radial pulse with your fingertips.
8. Inflate cuff until you can no longer feel radial pulse. Continue to inflate another 30 mm of mercury.
9. Open valve and slowly deflate cuff until you feel the first beat of radial pulse again.
10. Observe mercury or dial reading. This is the placatory systolic pressure. It is recorded, for example, as B/P 130 (P).
11. Deflate cuff rapidly and squeeze out all the air.
12. Using your first and second fingers, locate brachial artery. You will feel it pulsating. Place bell or diaphragm of stethoscope directly over artery. You will not hear the pulsation. Do not hold the stethoscope in place with your thumb.
13. Tighten thumbscrew of valve to close it. Turn to the left.
14. Hold stethoscope in place and inflate cuff until the dial points to about 30 mm above the palpated B/P.

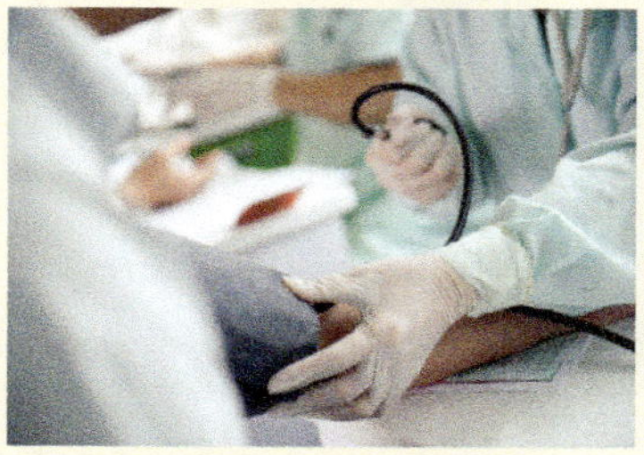

15. Open valve counterclockwise. Let air out slowly until you hear first beat.
16. At this first sound, note reading on sphygmomanometer. This is the systolic pressure.
17. Continue to release air slowly. Note number on the indicator at which you hear last beat or the sound changes to a dull beat. This is the diastolic pressure.
18. Open valve and release all the air.
19. Remove cuff. Open curtain or door.

Postprocedure

20. Record time and blood pressure.
21. Clean stethoscope—earpieces and diaphragm.
22. Wash hands.
23. Report any unusual observation immediately.

598 Chapter 19 | Measuring Vital Signs and Other Clinical Skills

Procedure 19.11 **Measuring Blood Pressure**

BACKGROUND: As a health care worker, it is important to monitor the patient's physical status. One way to determine this status is by measuring the patient's blood pressure. This procedure explains how to determine the patient's systolic (highest pressure) and diastolic (lowest pressure) blood pressure.
ALERT: Follow Standard Precautions

Preprocedure

1. Wash hands (follow hand-washing guidelines).
2. Assemble equipment:
   a. Alcohol wipes
   b. Sphygmomanometer
   c. Stethoscope
   d. Pad and pencil
3. Identify patient. Pull privacy curtain or close the door.
4. Explain procedure to patient.

Procedure

5. Delay obtaining the blood pressure if the patient is in acute pain, has just exercised, or is emotionally upset, unless there is an urgent reason to obtain a blood pressure reading.
6. Select the appropriate arm for application of the cuff. Limbs that have an intravenous infusion, breast or axillary surgery on that side, arteriovenous shunt, or are injured or diseased should not be used.
7. Apply cuff correctly. This should be about one inch above the anticubital space. (Refer to steps 4 and 5 in Procedure 19.10, "Palpating a Blood Pressure.")
8. Clean earpieces on stethoscope.
9. Place earpieces in ears.
10. Locate brachial artery. Place stethoscope over it.
11. Tighten thumbscrew on valve. (Remember the two clues: righty tighty and lefty loosey.)
12. Hold stethoscope in place. Do not use your thumb.
13. Inflate cuff to 170 mm.
14. Open valve. If systolic sound is heard immediately, reinflate cuff to 30 mm mercury above systolic sound.
15. Note systolic at first beat.
16. Note diastolic.
17. Open valve and release air.
18. Record time and blood pressure reading correctly on pad. Open curtain or door.

Postprocedure

19. Wash hands.
20. Wash earpieces on stethoscope.
21. Put away equipment.
22. Record blood pressure in chart.
23. Report any unusual observation immediately.

Charting Example:

7/29/24 0900
B/P 134/88
left arm, sitting
R. Martin CNA

Measuring Vital Signs and Other Clinical Skills | Chapter 19 599

Procedure Tip

19.11 Measuring Blood Pressure

- Review the background information, emphasizing that systolic is the highest pressure and that diastolic is the lowest pressure.
- Emphasize the importance of following Standard Precautions.
- Emphasize the need to listen carefully and not be distracted by anything.
- Review the preprocedure steps.
- Step 1: Emphasize the importance of proper handwashing.
- Steps 3 and 4: Emphasize the need to use effective communication techniques.
- Review the procedure steps.
- Step 5: Discuss why BP should not be checked under these conditions.
- Step 7: Explain proper positioning.
- Step 18: Emphasize importance of recording the data immediately.
- Review the postprocedure steps.
- Step 19: Emphasize importance of handwashing.
- Step 22: Review steps for properly documenting blood pressure.
- Step 23: Emphasize importance of observation and reporting.

PROCEDURE PRACTICE

- Demonstrate the steps for Procedure 19.11, Measuring Blood Pressure, as many times as necessary, or ask students to demonstrate the steps. Have students practice and perform the procedure until they are competent.

Math Link—EKG Graph Paper Speed

- Describe an EKG machine.
- Explain how it is used to monitor the heart's rhythms over time.
- Explain how the speed of the paper equates to the length of time the heart is monitored.
- Explain that the paper speed is important to the technician who is responsible for reading the EKG.
- Answers:
  a. 5 large blocks × 50 = 250 large blocks × 5 (small blocks) = 1,250 small blocks
  b. 1.5 minutes = 90 seconds × 5 × 5 = 2,250 small blocks
  c. 998 × 0.20 seconds = 199.6 seconds; or 3 minutes and 19.6 seconds
  d. 50,000 × 0.04 = 2,000 seconds; or 331/3 minutes; or 33 minutes and 20 seconds

Why would it matter if the EKG paper speed were 25 mm per second or 50 mm per second?

Answer: As the speed of the EKG paper increases, the reading on the graph paper becomes more compressed. A reading at 50 mm/second would take up only half the space of a reading at 25 mm/second.

Math Link

EKG Graph Paper Speed

ECG/EKG graph paper can be run through the EKG machine at different speeds. The standard speed is 25 mm per second. However, faster speeds are sometimes used.

Each small block of EKG paper equals 1 square mm. At a standard paper speed of 25 mm per second, one small block of EKG paper equals 1/25th of a second or 0.04.

If five small blocks equal one large block, how many seconds are represented by one large block?

5 blocks × 0.04 seconds = 0.20 seconds

If one large block equals 0.20 seconds, how many large blocks equal one second?

1 large block = 0.20 seconds

1 second divided by 0.20 seconds = 5

5 × 1 large block = 5 large blocks

Example 1

A sample EKG reading takes 5½ minutes. How many large blocks of graph paper would that take up 25 mm per second? How many small blocks?

5.5 minutes = 330 seconds

330 seconds × 5 blocks/second = 1,650 large blocks

1 large block = 5 small blocks

1,650 large blocks = 8,250 small blocks

Example 2

A sample EKG reading at 25 mm per second takes up 427 large blocks. How long did the EKG procedure take?

1 large block = 0.20 seconds

427 × 0.20 = 85.4 seconds

85.4 seconds = 1 minute and 25.4 seconds

How many small blocks would be used in an EKG procedure at 25 mm per second for the following times?

a. 50 seconds

b. 1.5 minutes

If an EKG reads at 25 mm per second, how long were the following procedures?

a. 998 large blocks

b. 50,000 small blocks

Why would it matter if the EKG paper speed were 25mm per second or 50 mm per second?

Fluently add, subtract, multiply, and divide multi-digit decimals to determine the solution to a problem similar to the examples given.

Community

Have a blood pressure clinic at lunch for students and faculty. Make and display posters that list the blood pressure risk factors and the dangers of hypertension.

600 Chapter 19 | Measuring Vital Signs and Other Clinical Skills

Community

- You may want to allow class time for students to make posters and handouts.
- Students may be able to obtain educational materials, such as brochures, from a local health care facility.
- They may be able to invite a medical professional, who is certified to check blood pressure, to attend the session and check the blood pressure of attendees.
- Encourage students to plan the event in advance, and to distribute flyers announcing the event.

Personal Wellness

Warning Signs of a Heart Attack

An EKG (electrocardiogram) is a graphic produced by an electrocardiograph, which records the electrical activity of the heart over time. An EKG can determine if there is narrowing in an artery leading to the heart muscle. This narrowing is a warning sign of a possible heart attack.

Cardiovascular disease affects more than 50 million Americans and coronary heart disease is the main cause of death in the United States. Stroke is the third leading cause of death and a major cause of serious disability.

Unfortunately, all the EKGs in the world won't help you if you ignore the warning signs of heart attacks. Some heart attacks are very sudden and there is no doubt about what is happening. However, most heart attacks begin slowly with only mild discomfort.

People who experience these symptoms often are not sure what's wrong and wait too long before getting help. Sometimes they don't want to "bother" the doctor, or they don't want to appear "weak," or they have too many "important things" to do. These can be fatal mistakes.

Here are some of the indications that a heart attack is occurring:

- **Chest discomfort.** Most heart attacks involve pain in the center of the chest that lasts more than a few minutes. Sometimes the discomfort goes away and comes back again. It can feel like uncomfortable pressure, squeezing, fullness, or pain.
- **Discomfort in other areas of the upper body.** Symptoms can include pain or discomfort in one or both arms, the back, neck, jaw, or stomach.
- **Shortness of breath.** Sudden difficulty breathing may occur with or without chest discomfort.
- **Breaking out in a cold sweat.**
- **Nausea.**
- **Lightheadedness.**
- **Extreme fatigue.** This is particularly important for women who may not have other symptoms.

Even if you are not sure if it is a heart attack, have it checked out. In the event of any these symptoms the appropriate action is to keep the patient still and call 911. Every minute, and even every second, matters during a heart attack. Fast action can save lives—maybe even your own.

Summary

Blood pressure is the fourth vital sign. Many factors influence blood pressure, and an abnormal blood pressure may indicate a serious condition. It is important to be accurate in following the step-by-step instructions for taking a blood pressure, recording the blood pressure of your patient, and reporting any abnormalities immediately.

Section 19.2 Review Questions

1. What is blood pressure?
2. What is the difference between systolic and diastolic pressure?
3. What factors lead to increased blood pressure?
4. What is the normal range of blood pressure?
5. How is blood pressure written?
6. Why is hypertension called "the silent killer"?

Measuring Vital Signs and Other Clinical Skills | Chapter 19 601

Section 19.2 Review Questions

1. Answer: Blood pressure is the force of the blood pushing against the walls of the blood vessels.
2. Answer: The systolic pressure is the greatest force exerted on the walls of the arteries by the heart. This pressure is exerted when the heart is contracting. You hear the first beat when contraction occurs. The diastolic pressure is the least force exerted on the walls of the arteries by the heart. This pressure occurs as the heart relaxes between contractions.
3. Answer: Factors that lead to increased blood pressure include loss of elasticity in arteries, exercise, eating, stimulants, and anxiety.
4. Answer: The normal blood pressure range is between 90 and 140 millimeters (mm) mercury for the systolic pressure. For the diastolic pressure, it is between 60 and 90 millimeters (mm) of mercury.
5. Answer: 120/80
6. Answer: Hypertension is "the silent killer" because symptoms are asymptomatic, meaning without visible symptoms. Hypertension is discovered only when blood pressure is taken.

Personal Wellness—Warning Signs of a Heart Attack

- Review the purpose of an EKG: To monitor the heart's rhythms over time.
- Explain that an EKG can help identify narrowing of the arteries, which is a warning sign of a heart attack.
- Explain that other signs do not require a diagnostic test, but are frequently ignored, or attributed to something else.
- Explain that women and men often experience different warning signs.
- Review the signs:
  - Chest discomfort
  - Discomfort in the upper body
  - Shortness of breath
  - Cold sweat
  - Nausea
  - Lightheadedness
  - Extreme fatigue
- Emphasize the importance of seeking medical attention if one or more of these symptom is present.

ACTIVITY

Create a resume for an EKG technician looking for a new position. Create a job history, educational credentials, and other relevant information. Refer back to Chapter 4 for information on what to include in a resume.

FOCUS AND ENGAGE

Introduce the Section

a. Review the content of the Background paragraph, explaining that the skills and techniques in this section are usually performed by a nurse assistant.

b. Emphasize the importance of performing these procedures accurately in order to insure effective patient care.

c. Review the objectives for the section.

Vocabulary Review

a. Direct students to the key terms.

b. Pronounce each word, and have the students repeat the pronunciation out loud.

c. Discuss the definition of each word.

TEACH

Discuss

- Discuss daily routines.
- Discuss reasons why patients might need assistance with daily routines.

Reinforce and Review

- Review Standard Precautions (Section 17.2).
- Reinforce the importance of effective communication techniques.

TEAMWORK

Divide the class into teams. Play Hangman using the vocabulary words from Section 19.3.

SECTION 19.3 Nursing Skills and Assistive and Therapeutic Techniques

Background

Each morning you do many things to get ready for the day, such as taking a shower and brushing your teeth. You likely also have nighttime habits. Patients in the hospital also have daily habits and other needs. As a nurse assistant, you will need to know how to help patients undertake these activities. Also, you will be responsible for their safety and comfort.

Objectives

When you have completed this section, you will be able to do the following:

- Match key terms with their correct meanings.
- Identify the following:
  - Responsibilities of the nurse or nurse assistant
  - Skin conditions requiring special attention
  - Areas on the body where pressure sores usually develop
  - Antipressure aids
  - Occupied bed, closed bed, and open bed
  - Causes and symptoms of dehydration
  - Common types of specimens collected for analysis
  - Common prosthetic devices
- List the following:
  - Types of bathing
  - Body areas requiring special attention during the bathing process
  - Changes in the skin that may indicate the beginning of a pressure sore
  - Techniques for positioning patients
  - Reasons why ambulation is important
  - Steps to preparing a patient for a meal
  - Ways to prevent pressure sores
  - Causes and symptoms of edema
  - Conditions that may develop when using postural supports
  - Things you must do when using postural supports
- Explain the following:
  - Reasons to give mouth care
  - Reasons for routine bathing
  - Why patients who have diabetes must have their toenails cut by a podiatrist

602 Chapter 19 | Measuring Vital Signs and Other Clinical Skills

- Why a urinary drainage bag is not raised above the level of insertion
- Causes of incontinence
- Procedures for bowel and/or bladder training
- Important observations about urine
- Important observations about stool

- Define the following terms:
  - AM and PM care
  - Good body alignment
  - Postural supports
- Calculate in cc's and record fluid intake properly.
- Demonstrate each procedure in this chapter.

Nursing Responsibilities

Nurses and nurse assistants are important members of the health care team. They are responsible for giving personal care to the patient. They spend more time with the patient than the other members of the team. This gives them an opportunity to give extra support and understanding to the patient. They may work in an acute care hospital or in long-term care.

As a nurse or nurse assistant you will be responsible for assisting patients with activities of daily living:

- Provide AM and PM care
- Provide oral hygiene
- Offer the bedpan and urinal
- Monitor the patient's elimination functions
- Assist with dressing and undressing
- Bathe patients
- Provide effective skin care
- Follow the patient care plan (**Figure 19.10**)
- Perform range of motion
- Provide body alignment and positioning
- Care for hair and nails
- Shave the patient
- Apply hot and cold applications
- Make the bed
- Assist patients to move and ambulate
- Apply prosthetic devices and supports
- Assist with feeding the patient
- Record intake and output

Measuring Vital Signs and Other Clinical Skills | Chapter 19 603

Teaching Tips

- Review the nurse assistant's responsibilities:
  - AM and PM care
  - Oral hygiene
  - Offer bedpan and urinal
  - Monitor patient's elimination
  - Dressing and undressing
  - Bathing
  - Skin care
  - Follow patient care plan
  - Perform range of motion
  - Provide body alignment and positioning
  - Hair and nails
  - Shaving
  - Apply hot and cold
  - Make the bed
  - Assist patients to move and ambulate
  - Apply prosthetic devices and supports
  - Feeding
  - Record intake and output
  - Care for incontinent patient
  - Understand tubes and catheters
  - Collect specimens
  - Height and weight
  - Seizure precautions
  - Stoma care
  - Postmortem care

TEAMWORK

In pairs, have students discuss how they like to be awakened in the morning. Have each pair select one example to share with the class.

Teaching Tips

- Emphasize that the nurse assistant provides personal care.
- Emphasize that the nurse assistant spends a lot of time with each patient.
- Explain that procedures will be practiced in the classroom.

Figure Focus

19.10 Components of the patient care plan. Why is a patient care plan important?

Answer: A patient care plan provides a comprehensive guide to the treatment and care that the patient will receive during his or her stay.

incontinent
(in KAHNT uh nuhnt)
Unable to control the bowel or bladder.

catheters
(KAHTH uh tuhrs)
Tubes inserted into body opening or cavity.

stoma
(STOH muh)
Opening, e.g., opening in abdomen in an ostomy.

postmortem
(POHST mor tuhm)
After death.

- Care for the **incontinent** patient
- Understand tubes and **catheters**
- Collect specimens
- Measure height and weight
- Take seizure precautions
- Give **stoma** care
- Do **postmortem** care

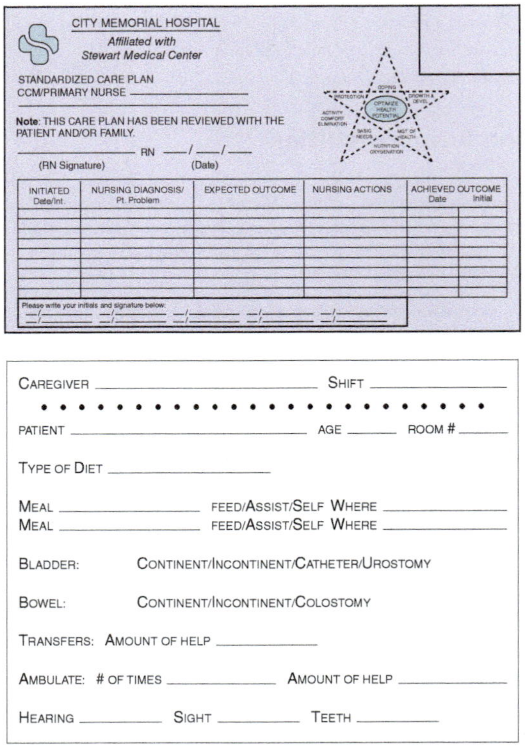

Figure 19.10
Components of the patient care plan. Why is a patient care plan important?

Standard Precautions

Always follow Standard Precautions when caring for a patient. You must evaluate the situation before you start a procedure to determine when you must wear protective gear. The following procedures indicate when to put on gloves and when to discard them. However, you are responsible for determining when to wear gloves. There are times when you need gloves to protect yourself from body fluids that may not be addressed in a procedure. Carefully think through the care you are giving and protect yourself and others.

Morning and Evening Care (AM and PM Care)

The beginning of the day is very important. How you care for the patient when he or she first awakens sets the tone for the entire day. This care is called AM care and is given before breakfast.

Awaken the patient quietly; never be loud or abrupt. Do not shake the person by the shoulder. Touch him or her on the arm and say the person's name. After the person is awake, there are several steps in the care you give. Follow the AM care procedures.

The PM care given to patients just before sleep is also important. Use this time to make patients comfortable for the night. Unhurried care allows the patients to feel relaxed, and they sleep better. If you take care of all their needs before you leave the room, it gives you time to finish your other duties. If you do not make them comfortable (e.g., see if they need to go to the bathroom), you have to return frequently to their rooms. Follow the PM care procedures.

Measuring Vital Signs and Other Clinical Skills | Chapter 19 605

Teaching Tips

- Reinforce Standard Precautions.
- Emphasize the use of protective equipment when necessary.
- Explain morning (AM) and evening (PM) care.
- Emphasize the importance of a calm, relaxed manner.
- Explain the importance of starting the day in a pleasant manner.
- Describe how to awaken residents gently in the morning.
- Explain key things to do when preparing a resident for sleep.

ACTIVITY

Have students write a personal essay about how they like to relax before going to bed at night. Have them include rituals they might perform and other details about what they do to make sure they get a good night's sleep.

Procedure Tip

19.12 AM Care

- Review the background information, emphasizing the importance of starting the day in a pleasant manner.
- Discuss the importance of hygiene for the patient.
- Emphasize the importance of following Standard Precautions.
- Review the preprocedure steps.
- Step 1: Emphasize the importance of proper handwashing.
- Step 4: Emphasize the need to use effective communication techniques.
- Step 5: Emphasize the importance of privacy.
- Review the procedure steps.
- Step 11: Emphasize the importance of independence for the patient.
- Review the postprocedure steps.
- Step 21: Emphasize importance of handwashing.
- Review responsibilities for observation and reporting.

PROCEDURE PRACTICE

- Demonstrate the steps for Procedure 19.12, AM Care, as many times as necessary, or ask students to demonstrate the steps. Have students practice and perform the procedure until they are competent.

Procedure 19.12 AM Care

BACKGROUND: AM care refreshes the patient. Clean teeth, clean hands, morning elimination, and other comfort measures help improve appetite and enjoyment of breakfast.
ALERT: Follow Standard Precautions

Preprocedure

1. Wash hands.
2. Gently awaken patient.
3. Assemble equipment:
   a. Washcloth and towel
   b. Toothbrush and toothpaste
   c. Emesis basin
   d. Glass of water
   e. Denture cup, if needed
   f. Clean gown, if necessary
   g. Clean linen, if necessary
   h. Comb and brush
   i. Disposable gloves (two pair)
4. Explain what you plan to do.
5. Provide privacy by pulling privacy curtain.
6. Elevate head of the bed if allowed.
7. Put on disposable gloves.

Procedure

8. Provide a bedpan or urinal if needed, or escort patient to bathroom.
9. Empty bedpan or urinal, rinse it, and dispose of gloves.
10 Put bedpan or urinal out of sight.
11. Allow patient to wash hands and face.
12. Put on disposable gloves.
13. Assist with oral hygiene.
14. Provide a clean gown, if necessary.
15. Smooth sheets if patient remains in bed.
16. Transfer to a chair if patient is allowed out of bed.
17. Allow patient to comb hair; assist, if necessary.
18. Prepare the overbed table:
   a. Clear tabletop
   b. Wipe off
19. Position overbed table and make sure call bell is within reach if patient is to remain in the room, or transport patient to dining room.

Postprocedure

20. Remove and discard gloves.
21. Wash hands.

Charting Example:

10/06/24	0630
	AM care given
	Patient looking forward to breakfast
	No complaints
	S. Gomez CNA

606 Chapter 19 | Measuring Vital Signs and Other Clinical Skills

Procedure 19.13 PM Care

BACKGROUND: PM care refreshes, relaxes, and comforts a patient, providing a quiet time before sleep.
ALERT: Follow Standard Precautions

Preprocedure

1. Wash hands.
2. Tell patient what you are going to do.
3. Provide privacy.
4. Assemble equipment:
   a. Washcloth and towel
   b. Toothpaste and toothbrush
   c. Glass of water
   d. Emesis basin
   e. Denture cup, if necessary
   f. Night clothes
   g. Lotion
   h. Linen as needed
   i. Disposable gloves

Procedure

5. Encourage patient to do his or her own care if capable.
6. Assist if unable to do his or her own care.
7. Put on disposable gloves.
8. Provide bedpan or urinal, if necessary, or escort to bathroom.
9. Empty bedpan or urinal.
10. Rinse and place in a convenient place for nighttime use.
11. Remove and dispose of gloves.
12. Wash patient's hands and face.
13. Put on gloves.
14. Provide for oral hygiene.
15. Change gown, if soiled.
16. Transfer patient from chair or wheelchair into bed, if out of bed.
17. Give back rub with lotion.
18. Observe skin for irritations or breakdown.
19. Smooth the sheets.
20. Change draw sheets, if necessary.
21. Provide extra blankets, if necessary.
22. Position side rails as ordered after patient is in bed.

Postprocedure

23. Remove and discard gloves.
24. Wash hands.
25. Provide fresh drinking water.
26. Place bedside table within patient's reach.
27. Secure call light within patient's reach.

Charting Example:

8/30/24	*2045*
	PM care given
	No complaints
	________ *S. Gomez CNA*

Measuring Vital Signs and Other Clinical Skills | Chapter 19 **607**

Procedure Tip

19.13 PM Care

- Review the background information, emphasizing the importance of relaxation before sleep.
- Discuss the importance of hygiene for the patient.
- Emphasize the importance of following Standard Precautions.
- Review the preprocedure steps.
- Step 1: Emphasize the importance of proper handwashing.
- Step 2: Emphasize the need to use effective communication techniques.
- Step 3: Emphasize the importance of privacy.
- Review the procedure steps.
- Step 5: Emphasize the importance of independence for the patient.
- Review the postprocedure steps.
- Step 24: Emphasize importance of handwashing.
- Review responsibilities for observation and reporting.

PROCEDURE PRACTICE

- Demonstrate the steps for Procedure 19.13, PM Care, as many times as necessary, or ask students to demonstrate the steps. Have students practice and perform the procedure until they are competent.

Teaching Tips

- Explain the importance of observing the skin during a bath.
- Describe changes that should be noted: dryness, bruising, broken skin areas, redness, heat, tenderness, or any unusual condition.
- Explain that broken skin areas may indicate pressure sores (decubitis).
- Emphasize the seriousness of pressure sores.
- Review the primary areas on the body where pressure sores usually appear: shoulders, elbows, hips, sacrum, heels, ankles, ears, or toes.
- Describe ways to prevent pressure sores:
  - Change patient's position at least every two hours.
  - If patient is up in chair, ask the patient to shift their weight at least every two hours.
  - Keep skin clean.
  - Massage reddened areas over sharp, bony areas to increase circulation.
  - Provide back rubs to increase circulation and relax the patient.
  - Keep linen dry and free of wrinkles.
  - Consider the use of specialized equipment.

Skin Management

Skin is the first defense against infection. When you bathe your patients, you have an opportunity to observe their skin. You should look for:

- Dryness
- Bruising
- Any unusual condition
- Broken area (pressure sore/decubitus)

Pressure sores/decubiti are very serious. Patients must be moved to help remove pressure on the skin, or pressure sores develop. This pressure can occur when patients are in bed or when they are sitting. They must be moved at least every 2 hours. The following areas are very sensitive to pressure:

- Shoulders
- Elbows
- Hips
- Sacrum
- Heels
- Ankles
- Ears
- Toes

Watch these areas carefully. (**Figure 19.11**) The bones press against the skin and stop circulation of blood. This causes the skin and tissue to break down. Pressure sores/decubiti are very painful and are difficult to heal. They can become quite deep and require a surgical procedure to help them heal. They can be prevented! Report any changes, such as redness, heat, tenderness, or broken skin, to the charge nurse.

To help prevent pressure sores/decubiti:

- Change the patient's position or turn them at least every 2 hours.
- If patient is up in a chair, ask the patient to shift their weight at least every two hours.
- Keep skin clean.
- Massage reddened areas over sharp, bony areas to increase circulation.
- Provide back rubs to increase circulation and relax the patient.
- Keep linen dry and free of wrinkles.
- Consider the use of specialized beds or gel-filled pads for the patient at high risk of a break in skin integrity.

If a patient should develop a break in skin integrity, the area should be documented as to: 1) stage of breakdown; 2) size of breakdown in centimeters; and 3) steps taken to care for breakdown.

608 Chapter 19 | Measuring Vital Signs and Other Clinical Skills

ACTIVITY

Create a career ladder for a nurse assistant. Refer to Chapter 3 for more information, and consult reference books, the Internet, or people who are currently employed as a nurse assistant. Include job descriptions, educational requirements, and salary ranges.

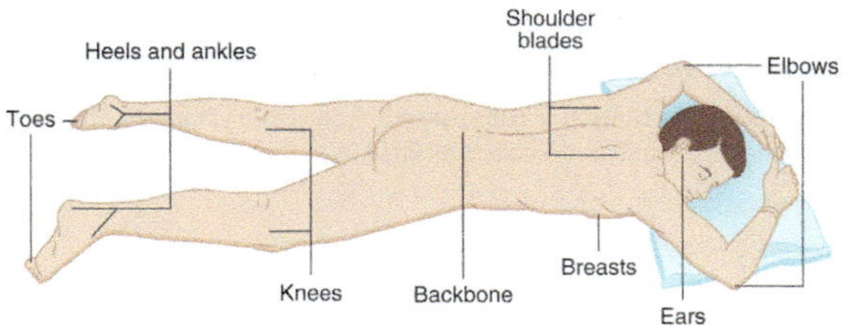

Figure 19.11
Places to check for signs of pressure sores. Why are these areas prone to pressure sores?

Patients who are stationary for long periods of time can easily develop pressure sores. In the past, egg crate mattresses were thought to provide protection. We now know that the at-risk patient will need other therapeutic measures to help in avoiding skin integrity problems. These include:

- **Low-Air-Loss Beds.** Composed of segmented cushions covered by a low friction fabric. The cushions inflate reducing pressure on skin surfaces and diminish sheering forces when patients are turned. Low-air-loss beds circulate cool air which helps to evaporate moisture and reduce temperature, thereby excess skin moisture and preventing additional breakdown. These beds are indicated for patients with skin grafts, pressure ulcers, edema, and advanced arthritis.
- **Rotation Beds.** These beds rotate from side to side in a cradle like motion. They are especially useful for patients with spinal cord injury, multiple trauma, or severe burns.
- **Air-Fluidized Beds.** This bed allows for minimal contact between the bed and the patient. They sometimes have a low-air-loss component as well. The fluid-like surface reduces pressure on the skin helping to prevent pressure ulcers and to promote wound healing.
- **Gel Pad.** These specialized pads are useful for patients who sit in chairs for prolonged periods of time and have difficulty shifting their body positions. They reduce the pressure placed on the sacral area.

Measuring Vital Signs and Other Clinical Skills | Chapter 19 609

Teaching Tips

- Explain how to report a break in skin integrity.
- Describe anti-pressure aids, and display them, if possible:
  - Low-air-loss beds
  - Rotation beds
  - Air-fluidized beds
  - Gel pads

Figure Focus

19.11 Places to check for signs of pressure sores. Why are these areas prone to pressure sores?

Answer: These are areas where, if the patient is stationary for a long period of time, bones press against the skin and stop circulation of blood, causing the skin and tissue to break down.

ACTIVITY

Label a diagram or draw a poster identifying the areas on the body that are most prone to pressure sores.

Procedure Tip

19.14 Skin Care—Giving a Back Rub

- Review the background information, emphasizing the importance of checking the skin.
- Discuss the importance of listening to the patient's comments and concerns.
- Emphasize the importance of obtaining permission for the procedure.
- Emphasize the importance of following Standard Precautions.
- Review the preprocedure steps.
- Step 1: Emphasize the importance of proper handwashing.
- Step 3: Emphasize the need to use effective communication techniques.
- Step 4: emphasize the importance of privacy.
- Review the procedure steps.
- Review the postprocedure steps.
- Step 27: Emphasize importance of handwashing.
- Step 28: Emphasize the importance of proper observation and reporting.

PROCEDURE PRACTICE

- Using a mannequin, or a volunteer if permission has been obtained, demonstrate the steps for Procedure 19.14, Skin Care—Giving a Back Rub, as many times as necessary, or ask students to demonstrate the steps. Have students practice and perform the procedure until they are competent.

Procedure 19.14 **Skin Care—Giving a Back Rub**

BACKGROUND: Giving a back rub provides an opportunity to help the patient relax and to check for any skin changes. It is also a good time to listen to any complaints or concerns the patient might have.

CAUTION: Check with team leader for permission to give a back rub.

ALERT: Follow Standard Precautions

Preprocedure

1. Wash hands.
2. Assemble equipment:
   a. Lotion
   b. Powder
   c. Towel
   d. Washcloth
   e. Soap
   f. Water (105°F)
   g. Disposable gloves
3. Tell patient what you are going to do.
4. Provide privacy by pulling privacy curtains.

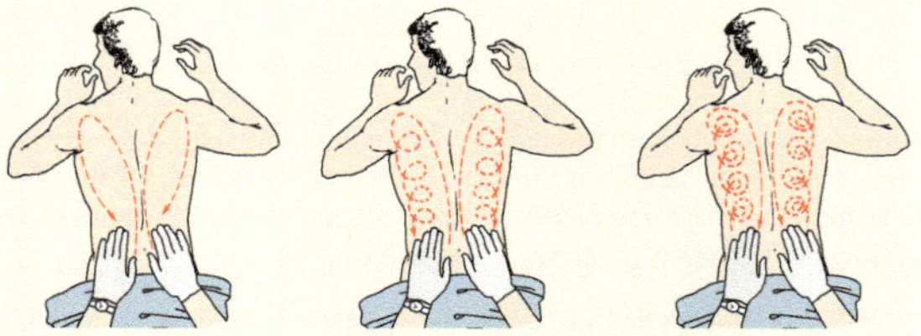

Procedure

5. Place lotion container in warm water to help warm it.
6. Raise bed to a comfortable working height.
7. Lower side rail on the side you are working on.
8. Put on disposable gloves.
9. Position patient on side or in prone position.
10. Place a towel along back to protect linen if patient is in a side-lying position.
11. Wash back thoroughly.
12. Rub a small amount of lotion into your hands.
13. Begin at base of spine and apply lotion over entire back.
14. Use firm, long strokes, beginning at buttocks and moving upward to neck and shoulders.
15. Use firm pressure as you stroke upward, and light circular strokes returning to buttocks.

NOTE: Pay special attention to bony prominences.

16. Use a circular motion over each area (shoulder blades, backbone).
17. Observe skin for irritation or breakdown.

NOTE: Do not rub or apply lotion to any open area on the skin.

18. Repeat several times (3 to 5 minutes).
19. Dry back.
20. Adjust gown for comfort.
21. Remove towel.
22. Position patient comfortably.
23. Return bed to lowest height.
24. Put up side rail if required.
25. Secure call light in reach of patient.

Postprocedure

26. Remove and discard gloves.
27. Wash hands.
28. Record procedure and any observations (e.g., redness, broken areas, dry skin).

Charting Example:

7/15/24	1350
	Back rub given
	No skin change noted
	Rails up
	R. Johnson CNA

610 Chapter 19 | Measuring Vital Signs and Other Clinical Skills

Oral Hygiene

Good mouth care should be provided at least three times a day: before breakfast when you give AM care, after lunch, and after dinner. It is important because it:

- Reduces odor
- Helps prevent tooth decay
- Is refreshing
- Relieves dry lips and mouth, especially if the patient has an elevated temperature or breathes through the mouth

Procedure 19.15 Giving Special Mouth Care to the Unconscious Patient

BACKGROUND: The mouth must be cared for during illness. If the patient is helpless, the nurse needs to make certain the patient receives the care necessary to keep the mouth clean and moist, every 1 to 2 hours as necessary.
ALERT: Follow Standard Precautions

Preprocedure

1. Wash hands prior to and after administering care.
2. Put on disposable gloves.

Procedure

3. Assemble equipment within reach—toothbrush, toothpaste, emesis basin, normal saline solution, cup with cool water, towel, mouthwash, sponge toothette, padded tongue blade, irrigating syringe with rubber tip, petroleum jelly, suction catheter with suction apparatus.
4. Provide privacy for the patient. Adjust the height of the bed to a comfortable position for the nurse. Lower the side rail next to the nurse and position the patient on their side with the head of the bed lowered. Place the towel across the patient's chest and emesis basin in position under the chin.
5. Open the patient's mouth and gently insert a padded tongue blade between the back molars if necessary.
6. If teeth are present, brush carefully with toothbrush and paste. If dentures are present, remove gently and cleanse before replacing. Use a toothette moistened with normal saline to gently cleanse gums, mucous membranes, and tongue.
7. If necessary, use the irrigating syringe with rubber tip and rinse mouth gently with a small amount of water. Position the patient's head to allow for the return of water or use suction apparatus to remove the water from the oral cavity.
8. Apply petroleum jelly to the patient's lips.
9. Remove equipment and return the patient to a comfortable position. Raise the siderail and lower the bed.

Postprocedure

10. Document the nursing assistant's oral assessment and any unusual findings.

Charting Example:

6/14/24	0640
	Brushed teeth;
	provided oral hygiene.
	_______ S. Gomez CNA

Measuring Vital Signs and Other Clinical Skills | Chapter 19 611

Teaching Tips

- Explain reasons for routine oral hygiene:
  - Reduces odor
  - Helps prevent tooth decay
  - Is refreshing
  - Relieves dryness

Procedure Tip

19.15 Giving Special Mouth Care to the Unconscious Patient

- Review the background information, emphasizing that this procedure is for the helpless patient.
- Emphasize the importance of following Standard Precautions.
- Review the preprocedure steps.
- Step 1: Emphasize the importance of proper handwashing.
- Review the procedure steps.
- Review the postprocedure steps.
- Step 10: Emphasize the importance of proper observation and reporting.

PROCEDURE PRACTICE

- Demonstrate the steps for Procedure 19.15, Giving Special Mouth Care to the Unconscious Patient, as many times as necessary, or ask students to demonstrate the steps. Have students practice and perform the procedure until they are competent.

Procedure Tip

19.16 Oral Hygiene—Self-Care

- Review the background information, emphasizing that this procedure is for the patient who has the capacity to care for him or herself, but must remain in bed.
- Emphasize the importance of following Standard Precautions.
- Review the preprocedure steps.
- Step 1: Emphasize the importance of proper handwashing.
- Step 3: Emphasize the importance of effective communication techniques.
- Step 4: Emphasize the importance of privacy.
- Review the procedure steps.
- Review the postprocedure steps.
- Step 13: Emphasize the importance of proper handwashing.
- Step 14: Emphasize the importance of proper observation and reporting.

PROCEDURE PRACTICE

- Demonstrate the steps for Procedure 19.16, Oral Hygiene—Self-Care, as many times as necessary, or ask students to demonstrate the steps. Have students practice and perform the procedure until they are competent.

Procedure 19.16 Oral Hygiene—Self-Care

BACKGROUND: A clean mouth and clean teeth help prevent oral problems, freshen the breath, and give an overall feeling of well-being.

ALERT: Follow Standard Precautions

Preprocedure

1. Wash hands.
2. Assemble equipment:
   a. Toothbrush
   b. Toothpaste
   c. Mouthwash
   d. Cup of water with straw, if needed
   e. Emesis basin
   f. Bath towel
   g. Tissues
3. Identify patient and explain what you are going to do.
4. Screen patient by pulling privacy curtain around bed.

Procedure

5. Raise head of the bed if patient is allowed to sit up.
6. Place towel over blanket and patient's gown.
7. Place toothbrush, toothpaste, mouthwash, emesis basin, and glass of water on overbed table.
8. Remove overbed table when patient has completed brushing.
9. Put away towel and make patient comfortable.
10. Put up side rails if required.
11. Secure call bell within patient's reach.
12. Put away all equipment and tidy unit.

Postprocedure

13. Wash hands.
14. Chart procedure.

Charting Example:

6/14/24	*0640*
	Set up equipment on overbed table
	Brushed teeth without assistance
	________ S. Gomez CNA

612 Chapter 19 | Measuring Vital Signs and Other Clinical Skills

Procedure 19.17 **Oral Hygiene—Brushing the Patient's Teeth**

BACKGROUND: A clean mouth and clean teeth help prevent oral problems, freshen the breath, and give an overall feeling of well-being.
ALERT: Follow Standard Precautions

Preprocedure

1. Wash hands.
2. Assemble equipment:
   a. Toothbrush
   b. Toothpaste
   c. Mouthwash
   d. Cup of water with straw, if needed
   e. Emesis basin
   f. Bath towel
   g. Tissues
   h. Disposable nonsterile gloves
3. Identify patient and explain what you are going to do.
4. Screen patient by pulling privacy curtain around bed.

Procedure

5. Raise head of bed if patient is allowed to sit up.
6. Place a towel over blanket and patient's gown.
7. Put on gloves.
8. Pour water over toothbrush; put toothpaste on brush.
9. Insert brush into the mouth carefully.
10. Place brush at an angle on upper teeth and brush in an up-and-down motion starting at rear of mouth.
11. Repeat on lower teeth.
12. Give patient water to rinse mouth. If necessary, use a straw.
13. Hold emesis basin under chin. Have patient expectorate (spit) water into the basin.
14. Offer tissues to patient to wipe mouth and chin. Discard tissues.
15. Provide mouthwash if available. Use emesis basin and tissues as above.
16. Put up side rails before turning away from patient.
17. Return all equipment.
18. Remove gloves and put in hazardous waste.

Postprocedure

19. Wash hands.
20. Tidy up unit.
21. Secure call bell within patient's reach.
22. Make patient comfortable before leaving the room.
23. Chart procedure and how patient tolerated it.

Charting Example:

5/14/24	0825
	Brushed teeth, provided oral hygiene
	Tolerated well
	No oral problems noted
	______ *R. Johnson CNA*

Measuring Vital Signs and Other Clinical Skills | Chapter 19 613

Procedure Tip

19.17 Oral Hygiene—Brushing the Patient's Teeth

- Review the background information, emphasizing that this procedure is for the patient who requires assistance with personal hygiene, and must remain in bed.
- Emphasize the importance of following Standard Precautions.
- Review the preprocedure steps.
- Step 1: Emphasize the importance of proper handwashing.
- Step 3: Emphasize the importance of effective communication techniques.
- Step 4: Emphasize the importance of privacy.
- Review the procedure steps.
- Review the postprocedure steps.
- Step 19: Emphasize the importance of proper handwashing.
- Step 23: Emphasize the importance of proper observation and reporting.

PROCEDURE PRACTICE

- Demonstrate the steps for Procedure 19.17, Oral Hygiene—Brushing the Patient's Teeth, as many times as necessary, or ask students to demonstrate the steps. Have students practice and perform the procedure until they are competent.

Procedure Tip

19.18 Oral Hygiene—Ambulatory Patient

- Review the background information, emphasizing that this procedure is for the patient who is able to walk to the sink and perform his or her own personal hygiene.
- Emphasize the importance of following Standard Precautions.
- Review the preprocedure steps.
- Step 1: Emphasize the importance of proper handwashing.
- Step 2: Emphasize the importance of effective communication techniques.
- Review the procedure steps.
- Review the postprocedure steps.
- Step 5: Emphasize the importance of proper handwashing.
- Remind students of the importance of proper observation and reporting.

PROCEDURE PRACTICE

- Demonstrate the steps for Procedure 19.18, Oral Hygiene—Ambulatory Patient, as many times as necessary, or ask students to demonstrate the steps. Have students practice and perform the procedure until they are competent.

Procedure 19.18 Oral Hygiene—Ambulatory Patient

BACKGROUND: A clean mouth and clean teeth help prevent oral problems, freshen the breath, and give an overall feeling of well-being.
ALERT: Follow Standard Precautions

Preprocedure

1. Wash hands.
2. Tell patient what you are going to do.

Procedure

3. Set up equipment at sink:
   a. Toothbrush
   b. Toothpaste
   c. Tablets or powder to soak dentures in, if necessary
   d. Towel
   e. Glass

Postprocedure

4. Rinse equipment and put away.
5. Wash hands.

Charting Example:

5/24/24 0745	
	Brushed teeth without assistance
	S. Gomez CNA

Procedure 19.19 Oral Hygiene—Denture Care

BACKGROUND: Food and bacteria collect under dentures causing discomfort due to tissue breakdown and mouth odor. Clean dentures protect against oral problems and refresh the mouth. Often patients are sensitive about removing their dentures. Provide privacy and encouragement for oral care. Learn the correct method of handling dentures so that you do not break them.
ALERT: Follow Standard Precautions

Preprocedure

1. Wash hands.
2. Assemble equipment:
   a. Tissues
   b. Paper towel or gauze squares
   c. Mouthwash
   d. Disposable denture cup
   e. Toothbrush or denture brush
   f. Denture paste or toothpowder
   g. Towel
   h. Disposable nonsterile gloves
   i. Emesis basin
3. Identify patient.
4. Explain what you are going to do.

Procedure

5. Pull privacy curtain.
6. Lower side rails.
7. Raise head of bed if allowed.
8. Place towel across patient's chest.
9. Prepare emesis basin by placing tissue, paper towel, or washcloth in bottom of basin.
10. Put on gloves.
11. Have patient remove his or her dentures.

(continued)

614 Chapter 19 | Measuring Vital Signs and Other Clinical Skills

Procedure Tip

19.19 Oral Hygiene—Denture Care

- Review the background information, emphasizing that dentures require special precautions.
- Emphasize the importance of following Standard Precautions.
- Review the preprocedure steps.
- Step 1: Emphasize the importance of proper handwashing.
- Steps 3 and 4: Emphasize the importance of effective communication techniques.
- Step 5: Emphasize the importance of privacy.
- Review the procedure steps.

Procedure 19.19 | **Oral Hygiene—Denture Care (continued)**

Procedure (cont)

12. Remove dentures if patient cannot.

Upper Denture

a. Explain what you are going to do.
b. Use a gauze square to grip upper denture.
c. Place your index finger between top ridge of denture and cheek.
d. Gently pull on denture to release suction.
e. Remove upper denture.

Lower Denture

a. Use a gauze square to grip lower denture.
b. Place your index finger between lower ridge and cheek.
c. Gently pull on denture to release suction.
d. Remove lower denture.

13. Place dentures in lined emesis basin and take to sink or utility room.
14. Remember to pull side rails up if you walk away from the bed.
15. Hold dentures firmly in palm of hand.
16. Put toothpowder or toothpaste on toothbrush.
17. Rinse dentures in cool water.
18. Hold dentures under cold running water and brush dentures on all surfaces until clean.
19. Rinse dentures under cold running water.
20. Remember to rinse denture cup with cold water before placing clean dentures in the cup.
21. Place in denture cup.
22. Place some mouthwash and cool water in cup.
23. Help patient rinse mouth with mouthwash; if food particles are between cheek and gumline, gently swab away with gauze. Clean gums with toothette.
24. Have patient replace dentures.
25. Place dentures in labeled denture cup next to bed, if dentures are to be left out.
26. Rinse equipment and put away.

Postprocedure

27. Remove gloves; dispose of in hazardous waste.
28. Wash hands.
29. Position patient.
30. Secure call bell within patient's reach.
31. Chart procedure and how it was tolerated.

NOTE: The patient may want to soak dentures overnight after PM care has been given. Place dentures in a solution in a denture cup and store in a safe place.

Charting Example:

7/07/24	*0725*
	Set out equipment for denture care
	Able to clean dentures
	Or: Removed dentures, cleaned,
	and freshened
	Provided oral hygiene
	No oral problems noted
	R. Johnson CNA

Measuring Vital Signs and Other Clinical Skills | Chapter 19 615

Procedure Tip

19.19 Oral Hygiene—Denture Care, continued

- Review the postprocedure steps.
- Step 28: Emphasize the importance of proper
- Step 31: Emphasize the importance of proper observation and reporting.

PROCEDURE PRACTICE

- Demonstrate the steps for Procedure 19.19, Oral Hygiene—Denture Care, as many times as necessary, or ask students to demonstrate the steps. Have students practice and perform the procedure until they are competent.

Procedure Tip

19.20 Oral Hygiene—For the Unconscious Patient

- Review the background information, emphasizing that this procedure is for the unconscious patient.
- Emphasize the importance of following Standard Precautions.
- Review the preprocedure steps.
- Step 1: Emphasize the importance of proper handwashing.
- Review the procedure steps.
- Review the postprocedure steps.
- Step 16: Emphasize the importance of proper handwashing.
- Step 17: Emphasize the importance of proper observation and reporting.

PROCEDURE PRACTICE

- Demonstrate the steps for Procedure 19.20, Oral Hygiene—For the Unconscious Patient, as many times as necessary, or ask students to demonstrate the steps. Have students practice and perform the procedure until they are competent.

Procedure 19.20 Oral Hygiene—For the Unconscious Patient

BACKGROUND: The unconscious patient often mouth breathes causing very dry lips and mucous membrane. Careful care and observation help prevent oral problems.
ALERT: Follow Standard Precautions

Preprocedure

1. Wash hands.
2. Tell patient what you are going to do. When patient is unconscious he or she may hear even if he or she cannot respond.
3. Provide privacy.
4. Assemble equipment:
   a. Emesis basin
   b. Towel
   c. Lemon glycerin swabs
   d. Tongue blades
   e. 4 × 4 gauze
   f. Lip moisturizer
   g. Disposable nonsterile gloves
5. Position bed at a comfortable working height.
6. Put on gloves.

Procedure

7. Position patient's head to side and place towel on bed under patient's cheek and chin.
8. Secure emesis basin under patient's chin.
9. Wrap a tongue blade with 4 × 4 gauze and slightly moisten. Swab mouth being certain to clean gums, teeth, tongue, and roof of mouth.
10. Apply lip moisturizer to lips and swab mouth with lemon and glycerin if available.
11. Remove towel and reposition patient.
12. Make sure side rails are up and bed is in low position.
13. Discard disposable equipment in hazardous waste.
14. Clean basin and put away.
15. Remove gloves and put in hazardous waste.

Postprocedure

16. Wash hands.
17. Report and document patient's tolerance of procedure.

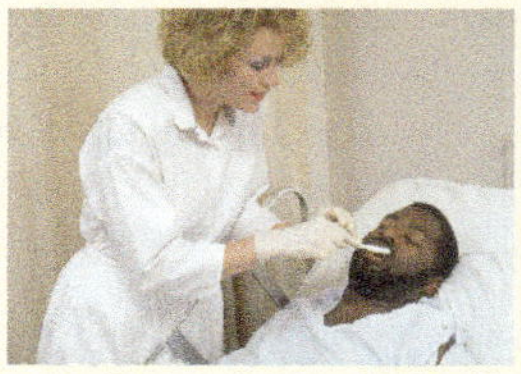

Charting Example:

6/16/24 1040
Cleaned teeth, moistened lips,
provided oral hygiene
Noted small canker sore on palate
Reported to team leader
S. Gomez CNA

616 Chapter 19 | Measuring Vital Signs and Other Clinical Skills

Offering the Urinal and/or Bedpan

Eliminating waste products from the body is necessary for good health. When patients are confined to bed, they must use a bedpan or urinal. Male patients use urinals to empty the bladder. Women use the bedpan for both urine and the elimination of solid waste (bowel movement). Men also use a bedpan for the elimination of solid waste. Solid waste is called *feces* or *stool.* When patients eliminate liquid waste, we call it *urinating* or *voiding.* Liquid bowel movements, such as diarrhea, may also be referred to as liquid waste.

If your patient does not eliminate liquid waste from the bladder, he or she may develop a urinary tract infection. This is very painful and serious. Small amounts of liquid elimination may indicate infection, dehydration, or fluid retention in the body.

If solid waste is not eliminated, large amounts of stool may cause an impaction. When a large amount of stool stays in the bowel it causes discomfort, and the patient experiences nausea and sometimes vomiting. This can be prevented by carefully recording bowel movements and letting the charge nurse know if a patient has not had a bowel movement. The charge nurse will give the patient a **laxative**, **suppository**, or enema, which is discussed later in this chapter.

laxative
(LAK suh tiv)
A medicine for relieving constipation.

suppository
(suh POZ i tawr ee)
A solid, conical mass of medicinal substance that melts upon insertion into the rectum.

Procedure 19.21 Elimination—Offering the Bedpan

BACKGROUND: Carefully placing the bedpan prevents discomfort. This procedure allows observations for skin breakdown and elimination.
ALERT: Follow Standard Precautions

Preprocedure

1. Wash hands.
2. Assemble equipment:
   a. Bedpan with cover
   b. Toilet tissue
   c. Soap and water
   d. Towel and washcloth
   e. Disposable nonsterile gloves (two pairs)
3. Ask visitors to wait outside room.
4. Provide privacy for patient with curtain, screen, or door.
5. Put on clean gloves before handling the bedpan.
6. Remove bedpan from storage space.
7. Warm metal bedpans by running warm water over them and drying.

Procedure

8. Lower head of bed if it is elevated.
9. Fold top covers back enough to see where to place the pan. Do not expose patient.
10. Ask patient to raise hips off bed. Help support patient by placing your hand at patient's midback:
    a. Roll the patient onto his or her side if the patient is unable to lift the hips.
    b. Place bedpan on buttocks. For a standard bedpan: Position bedpan so wider end of pan is aligned with patient's buttock; for a fracture pan: position bedpan with handle toward the foot of the bed.
    c. Hold in place with one hand and help patient roll back onto bedpan.
11. Slide bedpan into place.

(continued)

Measuring Vital Signs and Other Clinical Skills | Chapter 19 617

Teaching Tips

- Explain personal care equipment:
  - Urinals are available for men and women
  - Most often, men use a urinal for liquid waste and a bedpan for solid waste
  - Female urinals may be difficult to use
  - Women usually use a bedpan for both liquid and solid waste
- Explain how to determine when to offer a urinal or bedpan.
- Explain that an accurate record of bowel movements can help identify a number of problems:
  - Constipation
  - Impacted bowel
  - Cramping and gas
  - Nausea
  - Abdominal pain
  - Vomiting

TEAMWORK

In small groups, have students research the causes and symptoms of dehydration, and how dehydration might affect the body. Have them present their research to the class.

Procedure Tip

19.21 Elimination—Offering the Bedpan

- Review the background information.
- Emphasize the importance of following Standard Precautions.
- Review the preprocedure steps.
- Step 1: Emphasize the importance of proper handwashing.
- Steps 3 and 4: Emphasize the importance of privacy.
- Step 7: Emphasize the importance of comfort and consideration.
- Review the procedure steps.
- Step 9: Emphasize the importance of the patient's dignity.

Procedure Tip

19.21 Elimination—Offering the Bedpan, continued

- Step 13: Emphasize the importance of a comfortable position.
- Step 14: Emphasize the importance of comfort and dignity.
- Step 16: Emphasize the importance of proper handwashing.
- Step 17: Emphasize the importance of effective communication techniques.
- Step 18: Emphasize the importance of privacy.
- Review the postprocedure steps.
- Step 27: Emphasize the importance of proper handwashing.
- Step 36: Emphasize the importance of proper observation and reporting.

PROCEDURE PRACTICE

- Demonstrate the steps for Procedure 19.21, Elimination—Offering the Bedpan, as many times as necessary, or ask students to demonstrate the steps. Have students practice and perform the procedure until they are competent.

Procedure 19.21 | **Elimination—Offering the Bedpan (continued)**

Procedure (cont)

12. Cover patient again.
13. Raise head of bed for comfort.
14. Put toilet tissue within patient's reach.
15. Remove gloves.
16. Wash your hands.
17. Leave call light with patient and ask patient to signal when finished.
18. Leave room to provide privacy.
19. Watch for call light to signal patient's readiness to be removed from bedpan.
20. Put on gloves.
21. Assist patient as necessary to ensure cleanliness.
22. Lower head of bed before removing bedpan.
23. Remove bedpan and empty. Rinse bedpan and pour rinse into the toilet.
24. Use a paper towel to flush the toilet and wipe the faucet, with gloves still on.
25. Measure urine if on I & O.
26. Remove gloves and dispose of in biohazardous container.

Postprocedure

27. Wash hands.
28. Put on clean gloves.
29. Provide washcloth, water, and soap for patient to wash hands.
30. Dispose of soiled washcloth or wipes in proper container.
31. Provide comfort measures for patient.
32. Secure call light in patient's reach, make sure side rails are up and bed is in lowest position.
33. Remove and dispose of gloves in biohazardous container.
34. Wash hands.
35. Open privacy curtain.
36. Chart the following:
    a. Bowel movement amount, color, consistency
    b. Amount voided if on I & O

Charting Example:

4/10/24	0830
	Small, light brown, dry bowel
	Complained of discomfort when eliminating
	Noted small amount bright red blood
	Reported to team leader
	R. Johnson CNA

CUSTOMIZED INSTRUCTION

Less Advanced Students

Be sure to allow enough time for less advanced students to practice and become proficient at the procedures.

Procedure 19.22 **Elimination—Offering the Urinal**

BACKGROUND: Offering a urinal at the time of elimination allows the patient who is not able to go into the bathroom a way to stay in bed or in a chair and eliminate liquid waste. Remember to provide privacy to maintain the patient's dignity.

ALERT: Follow Standard Precautions

Preprocedure

1. Wash hands.
2. Assemble equipment:
   a. Urinal with cover
   b. Soap and water
   c. Towel and washcloth
   d. Disposable nonsterile gloves
3. Ask visitors to wait outside room.
4. Provide privacy for patient.

Procedure

5. Hand urinal to patient:
   a. Place call light at patient's side.
   b. Wash your hands.
   c. Leave room until patient signals with the call light.

   (If the patient is unable to place urinal, place penis in urinal. If necessary, stand and hold urinal until patient has finished voiding.) Wear gloves for this step.
6. Return to room when patient has finished voiding.
7. Put on gloves.
8. Offer washcloth for patient to wash their hands.
9. Place cover over urinal and carry it into bathroom.
10. Check to see if patient is on I & O or if a urine specimen is needed. (See I & O and specimen collection in this chapter.)
11. Observe urine color, consistency, and odor.
12. Empty into toilet.
13. Use a paper towel to turn on the faucet and flush the toilet, since still have gloves on. Rinse urinal with cold water.

Postprocedure

14. Cover and place in a convenient location for the patient.
15. Remove gloves and place in biohazard container.
16. Wash hands.
17. Secure call light in reach of patient.
18. Report and document unusual color, odor, or consistency of urine.
19. Record amount if on I & O.

Charting Example:

4/10/24 1030
Voided 250 cc.
Recorded on I & O sheet
——— R. Johnson CNA

Measuring Vital Signs and Other Clinical Skills | Chapter 19 619

Procedure Tip

19.22 Elimination—Offering the Urinal

- Review the background information, emphasizing that this procedure is used primarily for male patients.
- Emphasize the importance of following Standard Precautions.
- Review the preprocedure steps.
- Step 1: Emphasize the importance of proper handwashing.
- Steps 3 and 4: Emphasize the importance of privacy.
- Review the procedure steps.
- Step 5: Emphasize that this step is for patients who are able to care for themselves. Refer to parenthetical information for how to proceed if the patient is unable to care for himself.
- Review the postprocedure steps.
- Step 16: Emphasize the importance of proper handwashing.
- Steps 18 and 19: Emphasize the importance of proper observation and reporting.

PROCEDURE PRACTICE

- Demonstrate the steps for Procedure 19.22, Elimination—Offering the Urinal, as many times as necessary, or ask students to demonstrate the steps. Have students practice and perform the procedure until they are competent.

Procedure Tip

19.23 Elimination—Bedside Commode

- Review the background information, explaining that a commode is similar to a portable toilet, and that it is more comfortable than a bedpan.
- Emphasize the importance of following Standard Precautions.
- Review the preprocedure steps.
- Step 1: Emphasize the importance of proper handwashing.
- Steps 3 and 4: Emphasize the importance of effective communication techniques.
- Review the procedure steps.
- Step 5: If the commode has wheels, emphasize the importance of locking the wheels.
- Step 7: Emphasize the importance of privacy.
- Step 31: Emphasize the importance of proper handwashing.
- Step 33: Emphasize the importance of proper observation and reporting.

Procedure 19.23 Elimination—Bedside Commode

BACKGROUND: A bedside commode allows patients who cannot ambulate to the toilet to eliminate body waste by sitting on a chairlike device at the bedside. Patients generally have less difficulty eliminating waste when they use a commode instead of a bedpan.
ALERT: Follow Standard Precautions

Preprocedure

1. Wash hands.
2. Assemble equipment:
   a. Bedside commode
   b. Toilet tissue
   c. Washcloth
   d. Warm water
   e. Soap
   f. Towel
   g. Disposable nonsterile gloves
3. Identify patient.
4. Explain what you are going to do.

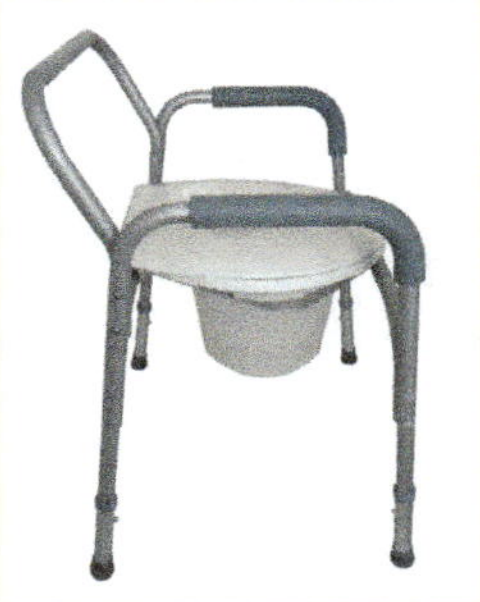

Procedure

5. Place commode chair next to bed facing head of bed.
6. Check to see if receptacle is in place under seat.
7. Provide privacy by pulling privacy curtains.
8. Lower bed to lowest position.
9. Lower side rail.
10. Help patient to sitting position.
11. Help patient swing legs over side of bed.
12. Put on patient's slippers and assist to stand.
13. Have patient place hands on your shoulders.
14. Support under patient's arms, pivot patient to right, and lower to commode. (See the procedure "Transferring—Pivot Transfer from Bed to Wheelchair.")
15. Place call bell within reach.
16. Place toilet tissue within reach.
17. Remain nearby if patient seems weak.
18. Return immediately when patient signals.
19. Put on gloves.
20. Assist patient to stand.
21. Clean anus or perineum if patient is unable to help self.
22. Remove gloves and put in hazardous waste.
23. Help patient wash hands. Remember to do this before you stand the patient up.
24. Assist back to bed and position comfortably.
25. Put up side rail if required.
26. Put on gloves.
27. Put down cover on commode chair and remove receptacle.
28. Empty contents, measuring if on I & O.
29. Empty and clean per hospital policy.
30. Remove gloves and put in hazardous waste.

(continued)

620 Chapter 19 | Measuring Vital Signs and Other Clinical Skills

Procedure 19.23 | **Elimination—Bedside Commode (continued)**

Postprocedure

31. Wash hands.
32. Replace equipment and tidy unit.
33. Record the following:
    a. Bowel movement
        (1) Amount
        (2) Consistency
        (3) Color
    b. Any unusual observations, such as
        (1) Weakness
        (2) Discomfort

Charting Example:

11/24/24	*1030*
	Eliminated moderate amount of brown,
	formed stool and 200 cc of urine. Returned
	to bed, positioned for comfort; Tolerated
	activity well
	________ S. Gomez CNA

Procedure 19.24 | **Assisting to Bathroom**

BACKGROUND: It is the nurse's responsibility to obtain an assessment of the patient's baseline functional status at the time that care for the patient is assumed. Understanding the baseline functional status of the patient enables the nurse to establish goals for activities of daily living. The goal must always be to maintain or improve the baseline function of the patient.

Institutionalization where staff may take over these activities promotes decreased self mobility and may contribute to the future dependency of the patient. Assisting the patient with toileting activities can maintain continence as well as provide opportunities for the patient to ambulate and build strength.

ALERT: Follow Standard Precautions

Preprocedure

1. Establish the baseline function of the patient. Determine the amount of assistance required (one nurse, two nurses).
2. Establish the need for devices such as cane, walker, or gait belt.
   NOTE: The use of a gait belt for any patient that is not fully independent is highly recommended. This a protective device for both the patient and the nurse.
3. Assure that the path to be used is clear of obstruction.
4. Explain to the patient what is to be done. Instruct the patient to alert the nurse of any lightheadedness or discomfort.

Procedure

5. Assist the patient to an erect position at the edge of the bed.
6. Pause at the edge of the bed (and again after the patient arises) to ensure that the patient feels steady. You should stand in front of and face the patient. Brace the patient's lower extremities. Place belt around the patient's waist.
7. Elevate the bed to a height that allows the patient's legs to rest firmly on the ground but not to have to lift his body from a low position as the patient rises.
8. With your hands under the gait belt, assist the patient to rise.

(continued)

PROCEDURE PRACTICE

- Demonstrate the steps for Procedure 19.23, Elimination—Bedside Commode, as many times as necessary, or ask students to demonstrate the steps. Have students practice and perform the procedure until they are competent.

Procedure Tip

19.24 Assisting to Bathroom

- Review the background information, emphasizing that this procedure is for a patient who is able to ambulate to the bathroom.
- Emphasize the importance of following Standard Precautions.
- Review the preprocedure steps.
- Step 4: Emphasize the importance of effective communication techniques.
- Review the procedure steps.
- Review the postprocedure steps.
- Step 15: Emphasize the importance of proper observation and reporting.

PROCEDURE PRACTICE

- Demonstrate the steps for Procedure 19.24, Assisting to Bathroom, as many times as necessary, or ask students to demonstrate the steps. Have students practice and perform the procedure until they are competent.

Teaching Tips

- Explain ambulation.
- Describe ways a nurse assistant may have to help a patient move:
  - Into a chair or wheelchair
  - Into bed from a chair or wheelchair
  - From bed to gurney
  - From gurney to bed
  - Transferring into a wheelchair
  - Transporting by gurney
  - Using a mechanical lift

Figure Focus

19.12 Mechanical lift. Under what circumstances would you use a mechanical lift for a patient?

Answer: Patients who are paralyzed can be easily transferred with a mechanical lift. Mechanical lifts allow patients who would otherwise be bedridden to be placed into a bathtub or chair.

Procedure 19.24 Assisting to Bathroom (continued)

Procedure (cont)

9. Patients who are fearful of walking may tend to bend forward and look at their feet. They will need to be reminded to stand erect and hold their head high.
10. Guide the patient to the bathroom with one hand under the gait belt at the patient's back and the other hand guiding the patient's free arm. Walk slightly behind and to one side of the patient for the full distance, while holding on to the belt. Assist with lowering the patient onto the toilet seat. For those patients who have functional disabilities it is advisable to obtain and use an elevated toilet seat. This will enable the patient to sit and rise with the least amount of energy use and the greatest degree of safety.
11. Instruct the patient on using the nurse call light to call for assistance after toileting is complete.
12. After toileting is complete assist the patient with completing personal hygiene as necessary.
13. Return the patient to the bedside and assist as necessary with positioning the patient back into bed.

Postprocedure

14. Assure that all needs are met and that the patient is comfortable prior to leaving the area.
15. Document in the medical record the patient's level of activity, any problems with independent function, and the level of assistance required.

Charting Example:

11/24/24 1030
Went to bathroom with assistance;
Tolerated activity well.
S. Gomez CNA

Movement and Ambulation of the Patient

You are responsible for moving , transferring, and lifting your patient in many different ways:

- Into a chair or wheelchair
- Into bed from a chair or wheelchair
- From bed to gurney
- From gurney to bed
- Transferring into a wheelchair
- Transporting by gurney
- Using a mechanical lift (Figure 19.12)
- Turning the patient for procedures or comfort
- Repositioning the patient for procedures, meals, and rest

Figure 19.12
Mechanical lift. Under what circumstances would you use a mechanical lift for a patient?

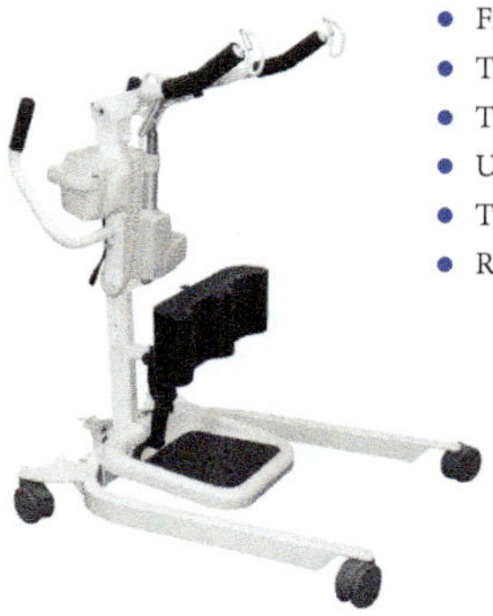

622 Chapter 19 | Measuring Vital Signs and Other Clinical Skills

TEAMWORK

Have an improvisation workshop. Divide the class into groups of four or five students, in which one student is the patient, one a family member, and two are health care workers. You provide a scenario in which the patient must either ambulate or be moved, giving details such as patient age, condition, size, and weight. The students must improvise a skit demonstrating how the health care workers would respond.

Procedure 19.25 Assist to Dangle, Stand, and Walk

BACKGROUND: Patients that have been immobile for a period of time may need assistance from the nurse to sit, stand, and walk. Determining what the patient's baseline activity level has been, any recent changes in mobility, and goals of care are the first steps to improving the patient's functional level.

The goal must always be to maintain or improve baseline function. A patient who has not been walking at all may have a goal of taking one independent step. One who has diminished tolerance of activity may have a goal of increasing the number of feet walked without an increase in fatigue. The goal should always be individualized to the particular patient.

ALERT: Follow Standard Precautions

Preprocedure

1. Assess the functional level of the patient. Include the patient when determining the plan of care and goals.
2. Explain the procedure to the patient.
3. Provide privacy for the patient.
4. Ensure a clear path for ambulation.
5. Place a chair midway of the distance to be traveled to facilitate a rest spot if necessary.

Procedure

6. Assist the patient to an erect position on the side of the bed. Pause to determine the patient's tolerance of the activity.
7. Place a gait belt around the patient's waist to ensure safety for the patient and the nurse.
8. Stand the patient at the bedside. Pause to determine the patient's tolerance of the activity.
9. With the nurses nearest hand placed under the gait belt at the patient's back and the other hand grasping the patient's nearest elbow: (a) Guide the patient forward; (b) Assess the patient's gait and tolerance of activity as the patient progresses forward.
10. If the patient should faint or begin to fall the nurse can use the gait belt to pull the patient towards the nurse and ease the patient to the ground.
11. Return the patient to the bedside and assist the patient into a chair or back into the bed. Assure that the patient is comfortable and has no further needs.
12. Reassure and encourage the patient to continue the mobility program for increasing functional status.

Postprocedure

13. Wash hands.
14. Document in observation note patient's gait, feet walked, and tolerance of activity.

NOTE: If the patient has numerous tethers and ambulation is problematic an alternative activity can be marching in place at the bedside.

Charting Example:

5/30/24	0945
	Assisted patient to standing position;
	patient was unsteady on his feet.
	R. Johnson CNA

Measuring Vital Signs and Other Clinical Skills | Chapter 19 623

Procedure Tip

19.25 Assist to Dangle, Stand, and Walk

- Review the background information, explaining baseline function.
- Emphasize the importance of following Standard Precautions.
- Review the preprocedure steps.
- Steps 1–3: Emphasize the importance of effective communication techniques.
- Review the procedure steps.
- Step 6: Explain that this is "dangle" as legs are dangling over the edge of the bed.
- Step 12: Emphasize the importance of encouragement and positive feedback.
- Review the postprocedure steps.
- Step 13: Emphasize the importance of proper handwashing.
- Step 14: Emphasize the importance of proper observation and reporting.
- Note: Explain that tethers include equipment such as monitors and IVs.

PROCEDURE PRACTICE

- Demonstrate the steps for Procedure 19.25, Assist to Dangle, Stand, and Walk, as many times as necessary, or ask students to demonstrate the steps. Have students practice and perform the procedure until they are competent.

Teaching Tips

- Discuss proper body mechanics.
- Explain that proper body mechanics insures the safety of the health care worker and the patient.
- Review body mechanics, covered in Section 18.4.
- Explain the importance of moving residents regularly:
  - Maintain stamina
  - Increase joint mobility
  - Improve muscle tone
  - Prevent lung congestion
  - Improve circulation
  - Help prevent blood clots
  - Maintain independence
  - Provide a sense of accomplishment
- Explain moving devices and techniques.
- Emphasize the importance of not disturbing tubes or catheters.

ACTIVITY

Have students create a chart or table comparing the different methods of moving a patient.

Be careful not to injure the patients or yourself when you move them. Always remember to evaluate whether you need help before you start to move the patient, and do not hesitate to ask someone to give you a hand.

When patients first try to get out of bed, they may feel dizzy. Help them sit on the side of the bed. Encourage the patient to swing his or her legs slightly back and forth until you determine that he or she is strong enough to stand and walk.

ambulation
(AM byoo lay shuhn)
Walking.

When your patients are able to walk, encourage them to do as much as they are capable of. They may seem slow, and it may take you a little extra time, but it is important for them. Walking (**ambulation**):

- Helps maintain stamina
- Increases joint mobility
- Improves muscle tone
- Helps prevent lung congestion
- Improves circulation
- Helps prevent blood clots
- Helps maintain independence
- Provides a sense of accomplishment

Your patients may need a device such as a cane, crutches, or walker. They may need a wheelchair much of the time but still be able to ambulate in a limited way.

Before patients are moved, check to see if there are tubes or catheters in place. You must be careful not to pull them out, crimp them, or put a strain on them. If patients have drainage equipment (e.g., Foley bag), do not raise the tubing above the level of insertion into the body. If they have an IV, do not allow the tubing to drop below the bed level.

Never let any tubing touch the floor. If you have any question about moving patients, ask the charge nurse before moving them.

Procedure 19.26 **Transferring—Pivot Transfer from Bed to Wheelchair**

BACKGROUND: Pivot transfer allows you to move the patient in one easy, safe motion into or out of a wheelchair. Use good body mechanics, explain each step, and reassure the patient of his/her safety.
ALERT: Follow Standard Precautions

Preprocedure

1. Wash hands.
2. Explain procedure to patient, speaking clearly, slowly and directly, maintaining face-to-face contact whenever possible.
3. Provide for patient's privacy during the procedure, using a curtain, screen, or door.
4. Make sure that wheels on bed are locked.
5. Lift foot rests or swing leg supports out of way.
6. Position wheelchair alongside bed. Lock wheels.

Procedure

7. Place bed at a safe and appropriate level for the patient. Support patient's back and hips and assist patient to sitting position with feet flat on the floor.
8. Move patient to edge of bed, with legs over side.
9. Before transferring patient, put non-skid footwear on patient and securely fasten.
10. Have patient dangle legs for a few minutes and take slow, deep breaths. Observe for dizziness.
11. Remember to use a gait belt. Stand in front of patient, positioning yourself to ensure your safety and that of your patient during transfer (e.g., knees bent, feet apart, back straight), place belt around patient's waist, and grasp belt.
12. Brace patient's lowest extremities to prevent slipping.
13. Count to three (or say other prearranged signal) to alert patient to begin transfer.
14. Support him or her at midriff and ask patient to stand, if patient is not dizzy.
15. Once standing, have patient pivot (turn) and hold onto armrest of wheelchair with both arms or one strong arm.
16. Gently ease patient into a sitting position.
17. Position yourself at back of wheelchair. Ask patient to push on the floor with feet as you lift gently under each arm to ease patient into a comfortable position against backrest. Make sure patient's hips are touching the back of the wheelchair and then remove the transfer belt, if used.
18. Return foot rests to normal position and place feet and legs in a comfortable position on rests. Make sure the signaling device is within the patient's reach.
19. Do not leave a patient who requires a postural support until it is in place.
20. Reverse above procedure to return patient to bed.

Postprocedure

21. Wash hands.

Charting Example:

5/30/24	0945
	Transferred from bed into wheelchair;
	Tolerated pivot transfer well.
	R. Johnson CNA

Measuring Vital Signs and Other Clinical Skills | Chapter 19 625

Procedure Tip

19.26 Transferring—Pivot Transfer from Bed to Wheelchair

- Review the background information, emphasizing the use of proper body mechanics.
- Emphasize the importance of following Standard Precautions.
- Review the preprocedure steps.
- Step 1: Emphasize the importance of proper handwashing.
- Step 2: Emphasize the importance of effective communication techniques.
- Step 3: Emphasize the importance of the patient's privacy.
- Steps 4 and 6: Emphasize the importance of locking the wheels.
- Review the procedure steps.
- Step 10: Emphasize importance of observation.
- Step 13: Emphasize importance of communication.
- Step 20: Review the procedure steps in reverse to explain how to return the patient to the bed.
- Review the postprocedure steps.
- Step 21: Emphasize the importance of proper handwashing.
- Remind students to document the procedure.

PROCEDURE PRACTICE

- Demonstrate the steps for Procedure 19.26, Transferring—Pivot Transfer from Bed to Wheelchair, as many times as necessary, or ask students to demonstrate the steps. Have students practice and perform the procedure until they are competent.

CUSTOMIZED INSTRUCTION

Special Needs Students

If you have disabled students with experience using a wheelchair, ask them to share personal stories about the difficulty of moving from one place to another, people's attitudes toward them when they are in a chair, and the importance of independence.

Procedure Tip

19.27 Transferring—Sliding from Bed to Wheelchair and Back

- Review the background information, emphasizing that this procedure is used to assist patients who are paralyzed from the waist down.
- Emphasize the use of proper body mechanics.
- Emphasize the importance of following Standard Precautions.
- Review the preprocedure steps.
- Step 1: Emphasize the importance of proper handwashing.
- Step 3: Emphasize the importance of effective communication techniques.
- Step 4: Emphasize the importance of the patient's privacy.
- Review the procedure steps.
- Step 5 and 7: Emphasize the importance of locking the wheels.
- Step 8: Emphasize the importance of proper positioning.
- Review the procedure steps in reverse for returning the patient from the wheelchair to the bed.
- Review the postprocedure steps.
- Step 13: Emphasize the importance of proper handwashing.
- Remind students to document the procedure.

PROCEDURE PRACTICE

- Demonstrate the steps for Procedure 19.27, Transferring—Sliding from Bed to Wheelchair and Back, as many times as necessary, or ask students to demonstrate the steps. Have students practice and perform the procedure until they are competent.

Procedure 19.27 Transferring—Sliding from Bed to Wheelchair and Back

BACKGROUND: Sliding transfer allows you to assist the patient who is paralyzed from the waist down to easily move in and out of a wheelchair. Use good body mechanics, explain each step, and reassure the patient of his or her safety.
ALERT: Follow Standard Precautions

Preprocedure

1. Wash hands.
2. Assemble equipment: wheelchair with removable arms.
3. Explain the procedure to the patient.
4. Provide privacy for the patient.

Procedure

5. Position wheelchair at bedside with back parallel to head of bed. Lock wheels. Move foot rests out of the way.
6. Remove wheelchair arm nearest to bedside.
7. Place bed level to chair seat height if possible. Lock bed wheels.
8. Raise head of bed so that patient is in sitting position.
9. Position yourself beside wheelchair and carefully assist patient to slide from bed to wheelchair.
10. Replace wheelchair arm and return foot rests to their normal position.
11. Position patient for comfort and apply postural supports.

Postprocedure

12. Make sure call bell is within reach.
13. Wash hands.

Charting Example:

5/30/24 0945
Transferred from bed into
wheelchair
Tolerated sliding transfer well
R. Johnson CNA

Procedure 19.28 Transferring—Two-Person Lift from Bed to Chair and Back

BACKGROUND: A person who is unable to bear his or her weight during a pivot transfer can be lifted by two people. Use good body mechanics, explain each step, and reassure the patient of his or her safety.
ALERT: Follow Standard Precautions

Preprocedure

1. Wash hands.
2. Assemble equipment: chair.
3. Ask one other person to help.
4. Tell patient what you are going to do.
5. Provide privacy for the patient.

Procedure

6. Position chair next to bed with back of chair parallel with head of bed. Lock wheels.
7. Position patient near edge of bed. Lock wheels of bed.
8. Position co-worker on side of bed near feet.
9. Position yourself behind chair at head of bed.
10. Place your arms under patient's axillae and clasp your hands together at patient's midchest.
11. Co-worker places hands under patient's upper legs.
12. Count to three. On the count of three, lift patient into chair.
13. Position for comfort and secure postural supports.

(continued)

626 Chapter 19 | Measuring Vital Signs and Other Clinical Skills

Procedure Tip

19.28 Transferring—Two-Person Lift from Bed to Chair and Back

- Review the background information, emphasizing that this procedure is used to assist patients who cannot bear their own weight.
- Emphasize the use of proper body mechanics.
- Emphasize the importance of following Standard Precautions.
- Review the preprocedure steps.
- Step 1: Emphasize the importance of proper handwashing.
- Steps 3 and 4: Emphasize the importance of effective communication techniques, including communication with the co-worker.
- Step 5: Emphasize the importance of the patient's privacy.
- Review the procedure steps.
- Steps 6 and 7: Emphasize the importance of locking the wheels.
- Steps 7–9: Emphasize the importance of proper positioning.

Procedure 19.28 **Transferring—Two-Person Lift from Bed to Chair and Back (continued)**

Postprocedure

14. Put call bell within reach of patient.
15. Wash hands.

Charting Example:

11/20/24 2100
Transferred per two-person lift from chair into bed, positioned for HS comfort
Tolerated transfer well
A. Chaplin, CNA

Procedure 19.29 **Transferring—Sliding from Bed to Gurney and Back**

BACKGROUND: A sliding transfer of a patient on and off a gurney is easily and safely accomplished with two people using a pull sheet. Use good body mechanics, explain each step, and reassure the patient of his or her safety.
ALERT: Follow Standard Precautions

Preprocedure

1. Wash hands.
2. Assemble equipment:
   a. Gurney
   b. Cover sheet
3. Ask a co-worker to help.
4. Explain what you are going to do and lock wheels on bed.
5. Provide privacy for the patient.

Procedure

6. Cover patient with sheet and remove bed covers.
7. Raise bed to gurney height: lower side rail and move patient to side of bed.
8. Loosen draw sheet on both sides so it can be used as a pull sheet.
9. Position gurney next to bed and lock wheels on gurney.
10. Position yourself on outside of gurney—one arm at the head, the other at the hips. Co-worker is on other side of bed.
11. Reach across gurney and securely hold edge of draw sheet. Pull patient onto gurney and cover. (If patient is large, a third person on the opposite side of bed may be necessary.)
12. Position patient for comfort.
13. Secure with safety straps or raise side rails.

Postprocedure

14. Wash hands.

Charting Example:

9/10/24 0900
Transferred to radiology via gurney following a sliding transfer from bed
Tolerated transfer well
A. Chaplin CNA

Measuring Vital Signs and Other Clinical Skills | Chapter 19 627

19.28 Transferring—Two-Person Lift from Bed to Chair and Back, continued

- Review the procedure steps in reverse for returning the patient from the wheelchair to the bed.
- Review the postprocedure steps.
- Step 15: Emphasize the importance of proper handwashing.
- Remind students to document the procedure.

PROCEDURE PRACTICE

- Demonstrate the steps for Procedure 19.28, Transferring—Two-Person Lift from Bed to Chair and Back, as many times as necessary, or ask students to demonstrate the steps. Have students practice and perform the procedure until they are competent.

Procedure Tip

19.29 Transferring—Sliding from Bed to Gurney and Back

- Review the background information, emphasizing that this procedure requires two people.
- Emphasize the use of proper body mechanics.
- Emphasize the importance of following Standard Precautions.
- Review the preprocedure steps.
- Step 1: Emphasize the importance of proper handwashing.
- Steps 3 and 4: Emphasize the importance of effective communication techniques, including communication with the co-worker.
- Step 5: Emphasize the importance of the patient's privacy.
- Review the procedure steps.
- Steps 6 and 8: Differentiate between the cover sheet and the draw sheet.
- Step 9: Emphasize the importance of locking the wheels.
- Steps 10–12: Emphasize the importance of proper positioning.
- Review the procedure steps in reverse for returning the patient from the gurney to the bed.
- Review the postprocedure steps.
- Step 14: Emphasize the importance of proper handwashing.
- Remind students to document the procedure.

PROCEDURE PRACTICE

- Demonstrate the steps for Procedure 19.29, Transferring—Sliding from Bed to Gurney and Back, as many times as necessary, or ask students to demonstrate the steps. Have students practice and perform the procedure until they are competent.

Procedure Tip

19.30 Transferring—Lifting with a Mechanical Lift

- Review the background information, emphasizing that this procedure is for patients who are paralyzed.
- Emphasize the use of proper body mechanics.
- Emphasize the importance of following Standard Precautions.
- Review the preprocedure steps.
- Step 1: Emphasize the importance of proper handwashing.
- Steps 4 and 6: Emphasize the importance of effective communication techniques, including communication with the co-worker.
- Step 6: Emphasize the importance of locking the wheels.
- Step 7: Emphasize the importance of the patient's privacy.
- Review the procedure steps.
- All procedure steps: Emphasize the importance of proper positioning.
- All procedure steps: Emphasize the proper use of the equipment.
- Step 14: Emphasize a positive, calming approach.

Procedure 19.30 Transferring—Lifting with a Mechanical Lift

BACKGROUND: Patients who are paralyzed can be easily transferred with a mechanical lift. Mechanical lifts allow patients who would otherwise be bedridden to be placed into a bathtub or chair.

Your ability to use the lift safely will provide important environmental and physical stimulation for the patient. Remember to ask a co-worker to double-check all connections and positions before moving the patient to ensure their safety.

ALERT: Follow Standard Precautions

Preprocedure

1. Wash hands.
2. Gather equipment:
   a. Mechanical lift
   b. Sheet or blanket for patient comfort
   c. Sling
3. Check all equipment to be sure it is in good working order and that the sling is not damaged or torn.
4. Ask one other person to help.
5. Prepare patient's destination:
   a. Chair
   b. Gurney
   c. Bathtub
   d. Shower
6. Lock wheels on bed and explain what you are going to do.
7. Provide privacy for the patient.

Procedure

8. Roll patient toward you.
9. Place sling on bed behind patient:
   a. Position top of sling at shoulders.
   b. Position bottom of sling under buttocks.
   c. Leave enough of sling to support body when the body is rolled back. Fan-fold remaining sling next to body. It will be pulled through when patient is rolled back.
10. Roll patient to other side of bed and pull fan-folded portion of sling flat. Remove all wrinkles and allow patient to lie flat on back.
11. Position lift over patient, being sure to broaden base of lift. This stabilizes the lift while raising patient.
12. Raise head of bed to a semi-Fowler's position.
13. Attach straps on lift to sling loops. Shorter straps must be attached to shoulder loops. Longer straps are attached to loops at hips. (Important: If you reverse the strap attachment, the patient's head will be lower than his or her hips.)
14. Reassure patient. Let patient know you will keep him or her from falling. Gently raise patient from bed with hand crank or pump handle.
15. Keep patient centered over base of lift as you move lift and patient to his or her destination. (It is helpful to have a helper stand by and steady patient while moving so that patient doesn't swing.)

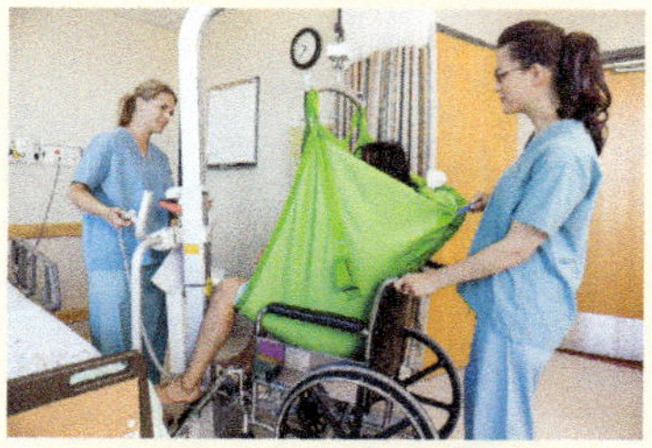

16. Position patient over chair, commode, bathtub, shower chair, etc. Ask a co-worker to steady chair.
17. Slowly lower patient into chair using foot-pedal positioning.
18. Unhook sling from lift straps and carefully move lift away from patient.
19. Provide all comfort measures for patient.
20. Secure postural supports, if necessary.
21. Return lift to storage area.

(continued)

628 Chapter 19 | Measuring Vital Signs and Other Clinical Skills

Procedure 19.30 Transferring—Lifting with a Mechanical Lift (continued)

Postprocedure

22. Wash hands.
23. Reverse procedure when returning patient to bed.

NOTE: The mechanical lift is an expensive item. Depending on the size of the facility you are in, there may be a limited number available. Always return the lift to its storage area so that it will be available for others to use.

Charting Example:

4/20/24 0830
Transferred via mechanical lift to bathtub
Tolerated bath well
Positioned in day chair and taken to patio
_______ *S. Gomez CNA*

Procedure 19.31 Transferring—Moving a Patient on a Gurney or Stretcher

BACKGROUND: Patients who are medicated or must stay in a reclined position can be moved throughout a facility on a gurney or stretcher. It is important to secure safety rails and wheel them in a safe manner.
ALERT: Follow Standard Precautions

Preprocedure

1. Wash hands.
2. Position bed to gurney height.
3. Lock all the brakes on gurney and bed.
4. Follow the procedure for transferring to and from a gurney.

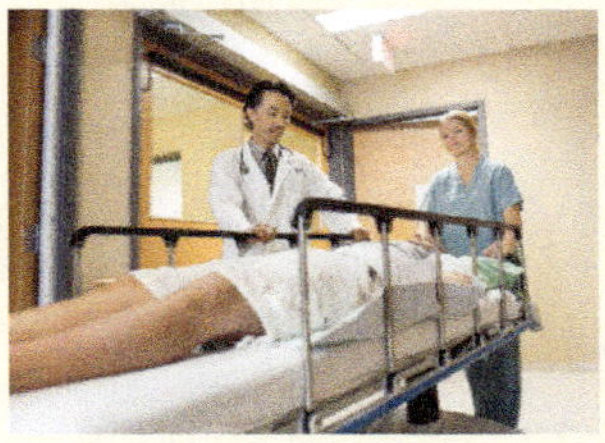

Procedure

5. Stand at the patient's head and push the gurney with patient's feet moving first down the hallway.
6. Slow down when turning a corner. Always check the intersection mirrors for traffic.
7. Enter an elevator by standing at patient's head and pulling gurney into elevator. The feet will be the last to enter elevator.
8. Leave elevator by carefully pushing the gurney out of elevator into corridor.
9. Position yourself at patient's feet, and back a patient on a gurney down a hill.
10. Never leave a patient unattended on a gurney.
11. Raise side rails and secure a safety strap.

Postprocedure

12. Wash hands.

Charting Example:

12/14/24 1320
Transferred via gurney to surgery
_______ *R. Johnson CNA*

PROCEDURE PRACTICE

- Demonstrate the steps for Procedure 19.30, Transferring—Lifting with a Mechanical Lift, as many times as necessary, or ask students to demonstrate the steps. Have students practice and perform the procedure until they are competent.

Procedure Tip

19.31 Transferring—Moving a Patient on a Gurney or Stretcher

- Review the background information, emphasizing that this procedure is for patients who must remain in a reclined position.
- Emphasize the importance of following Standard Precautions.
- Review the preprocedure steps.
- Step 1: Emphasize the importance of proper handwashing.
- Step 3: Emphasize the importance of locking the wheels.
- Review the procedure steps.
- Review the postprocedure steps.
- Step 13: Emphasize the importance of proper handwashing.
- Remind students to document the procedure.

PROCEDURE PRACTICE

- Demonstrate the steps for Procedure 19.31, Transferring—Moving a Patient on a Gurney or Stretcher, as many times as necessary, or ask students to demonstrate the steps. Have students practice and perform the procedure until they are competent.

Teaching Tips

- Discuss body alignment and positioning.
- Describe complications of poor body alignment:
  - Breathing problems
  - Added pressure to the bony areas, causing skin breakdown
  - Strain on the lumbar spine
  - Contractures
  - Decreased circulation
  - Discomfort and pain
  - Edema
  - Foot drop
- Describe actions to keep the patient's body in good alignment:
  - Pillow support at back for side lying
  - Pillow support from the knee to ankle to support upper leg
  - Trochanter support to prevent outward rotation
  - Footboard and padded splints to prevent foot drop

TEAMWORK

Working in pairs, have students practice positioning their partners using correct body alignment. Have them practice good alignment for lying down and sitting up.

Positioning and Body Alignment

alignment
(uh LINE muhnt)
Keeping a patient in proper position.

Always position your patients with the head in a straight line with the spine and the body in a comfortable, normal **alignment**. If a patient is bent in an unnatural position (slumped forward, rolled in a ball) the patient may experience:

- Breathing problems
- Added pressure to the bony areas, causing skin breakdown (decubiti)
- Strain on the lumbar spine
- Contractures, chronic loss of joint motion due to structural changes in non-bony tissue; these non-bony tissues include muscles, ligaments, and tendons
- Decreased circulation
- Discomfort and pain
- Edema
- Foot drop

Confining a patient to a bed should be avoided whenever possible. The hydraulic lift can be used to move the paralyzed patient out of the bed. This lift should only be used when there is no possibility of the patient ever becoming independently mobile. Otherwise, the patient should be encouraged to function at the highest possible level.

If a patient must be maintained on bed rest, all systems of the body will be affected. Respiratory, GI, Renal, skeletal-muscular function, and skin integrity will all be diminished by absolute bed rest. The patient will need the support of the caregiver for passive range of motion and positional changes. (Range of motion is covered in Procedure 21.4.) Specialty beds may be necessary.

The nurse must monitor the patient's functions frequently. These patients will be more prone to the development of pneumonia, urinary tract infections and diminished renal function, fecal impaction, decubiti, etc. The following nursing actions can promote optimal well being of the bedridden patient:

trochanter
(TROW kan ter)
One of the bony prominences toward the near end of the thigh bone (the femur).

- Pillow support at back for side lying
- Pillow support from the knee to ankle to support upper leg
- **Trochanter** support to prevent outward rotation
- Footboard and padded splints to prevent foot drop

Good body alignment is important at all times. This includes when the patient is lying in bed, sitting in a chair, and sitting in a wheelchair. When your patients are positioned in good body alignment, they look comfortable.

630 Chapter 19 | Measuring Vital Signs and Other Clinical Skills

Procedure 19.32 **Transferring—Moving a Patient in a Wheelchair**

BACKGROUND: Patients can easily be transferred from place to place in a wheelchair. It is important to move them safely and secure their transfer in and out of the wheelchair.
ALERT: Follow Standard Precautions

Preprocedure

1. Wash hands.
2. Position wheelchair.
3. Lock all brakes on wheelchair and bed.

Procedure

4. Follow procedure for transferring patient to and from a wheelchair.
5. Push wheelchair carefully into hallway, watching for others who may be near doorway.
6. Move cautiously down hallway, being especially careful at intersections.
7. Always back a patient in a wheelchair over bumps, doorways, and into or out of elevators.
8. Always back a patient in a wheelchair down a hill.
9. Check patient for comfort measures before leaving.
10. Always notify appropriate person that patient has arrived.

Postprocedure

11. Wash hands.

Charting Example:

10/10/24	1730	*Transferred via wheelchair to radiology*
		S. Gomez CNA

Procedure 19.33 **Moving—Helping the Helpless Patient to Move Up in Bed**

BACKGROUND: Keeping patients in good alignment helps prevent a decubitus, respiratory problems, and general discomfort. Following correct procedures when lifting and moving the patient prevents injury to the patient and the nurse assistant(s).
ALERT: Follow Standard Precautions

Preprocedure

1. Wash hands.
2. Ask a co-worker to help move patient. (Co-worker will work on opposite side of bed.)
3. Identify patient and explain what you are going to do. (Even if the patient seems unresponsive, he or she may be able to hear.) Provide privacy for the patient.

Procedure

4. Lock wheels of bed. Raise bed to comfortable working position, and lower side rails.
5. Remove pillow and place it at head of bed or on a chair.
6. Loosen both sides of draw sheet.
7. Roll edges toward side of patient's body.
8. Face head of bed and grasp rolled sheet edge with hand closest to patient.
9. Place your feet 12 inches apart with foot farthest from the edge of bed in a forward position.
10. Place your free hand and arm under patient's neck and shoulders, supporting head.

(continued)

Measuring Vital Signs and Other Clinical Skills | Chapter 19 631

Procedure Tip

19.32 Transferring—Moving a Patient in a Wheelchair

- Review the background information, emphasizing safety.
- Emphasize the use of proper body mechanics.
- Emphasize the importance of following Standard Precautions.
- Review the preprocedure steps.
- Step 1: Emphasize the importance of proper handwashing.
- Step 3: Emphasize the importance of locking the wheels.
- Review the procedure steps.
- Steps 7 and 8: Discuss situations when it is necessary to move pulling backwards.
- Step 10: Emphasize the importance of effective communication techniques, including communication with the co-worker.
- Review the postprocedure steps.
- Step 11: Emphasize the importance of proper handwashing.
- Remind students to document the procedure.

PROCEDURE PRACTICE

- Demonstrate the steps for Procedure 19.32, Transferring—Moving a Patient in a Wheelchair, as many times as necessary, or ask students to demonstrate the steps. Have students practice and perform the procedure until they are competent.

Procedure Tip

19.33 Moving—Helping the Helpless Patient to Move Up in Bed

- Review the background information, emphasizing problems that can arise when a patient is unable to move.
- Emphasize the use of proper body mechanics.
- Emphasize the importance of following Standard Precautions.
- Review the preprocedure steps.
- Step 1: Emphasize the importance of proper handwashing.
- Steps 2 and 3: Emphasize the importance of effective communication techniques, including communication with the co-worker.
- Step 3: Emphasize the importance of privacy, even for a non-responsive patient.
- Review the procedure steps.
- Step 4: Emphasize the importance of locking the wheels.

Procedure Tip

19.33 Moving—Helping the Helpless Patient to Move Up in Bed, continued

- Review the postprocedure steps.
- Step 16: Emphasize the importance of proper handwashing.
- Remind students to document the procedure.

PROCEDURE PRACTICE

- Demonstrate the steps for Procedure 19.33, Moving—Helping the Helpless Patient to Move Up in Bed, as many times as necessary, or ask students to demonstrate the steps. Have students practice and perform the procedure until they are competent.

Procedure Tip

19.34 Moving—Assisting Patient to Sit Up in Bed

- Review the background information, emphasizing patient comfort.
- Emphasize the use of proper body mechanics.
- Emphasize the importance of following Standard Precautions.
- Review the preprocedure steps.
- Step 1: Emphasize the importance of proper handwashing.
- Step 2: Emphasize the importance of effective communication techniques, including communication with the co-worker. Also emphasize the importance of privacy.
- Review the procedure steps.
- Step 3: Emphasize the importance of locking the bed.
- Review the postprocedure steps.
- Step 9: Emphasize the importance of proper handwashing.
- Remind students to document the procedure.

PROCEDURE PRACTICE

- Demonstrate the steps for Procedure 19.34, Moving—Assisting Patient to Sit Up in Bed, as many times as necessary, or ask students to demonstrate the steps. Have students practice and perform the procedure until they are competent.

Procedure 19.33 **Moving—Helping the Helpless Patient to Move Up in Bed (continued)**

11. Bend your hips slightly.
12. On the count of three, you and your co-worker will raise patient's hips and back with draw sheet, supporting head and shoulders, and move patient smoothly to head of bed.

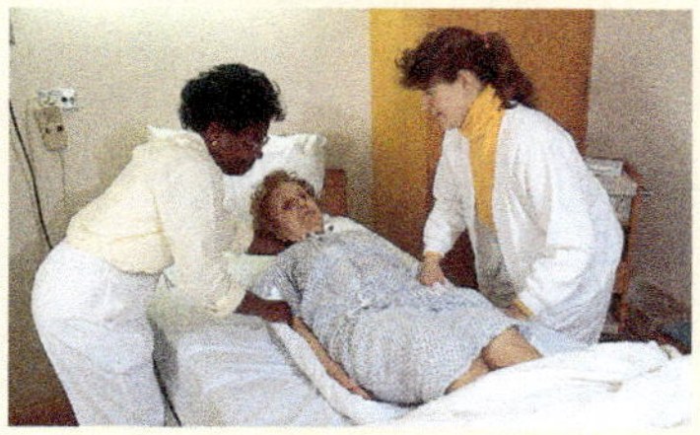

13. Replace pillow under patient's head and check for good body alignment.
14. Tighten and tuck in draw sheet and smooth bedding.
15. Raise side rails and lower bed.

Postprocedure

16. Wash hands.

Charting Example:

5/10/24	0850
	Helped to move patient up in bed
	No complaints of discomfort
	R. Johnson CNA

Procedure 19.34 **Moving—Assisting Patient to Sit Up in Bed**

BACKGROUND: Some patients are too weak to adjust themselves in bed. Sitting up comfortably helps prevent fatigue and poor body alignment. Using correct procedure prevents injury to the patient and the nurse assistant(s).
ALERT: Follow Standard Precautions

Preprocedure

1. Wash hands.
2. Identify patient and explain what you are going to do. Provide privacy for the patient.

Procedure

3. Lock bed and lower all the way down.
4. Face head of bed, keeping your outer leg forward.
5. Turn your head away from patient's face.
6. Lock your arm nearest patient with patient's arm. To lock arms, place your arm between patient's arm and body, and hold upper arm near shoulder. Have patient hold back of your upper arm.
7. Support patient's head and shoulder with your other arm.
8. Raise patient to sitting position. Adjust head of bed and pillows.

Postprocedure

9. Wash hands.

Charting Example:

5/10/24	0850
	Helped to sitting position
	No complaints of discomfort
	R. Johnson CNA

632 Chapter 19 | Measuring Vital Signs and Other Clinical Skills

Procedure 19.35 **Moving—Logrolling**

BACKGROUND: Maintaining alignment is essential to prevent injury. Logrolling helps prevent movement of the back following surgery.
ALERT: Follow Standard Precautions

Preprocedure

1. Wash hands.
2. Identify patient and explain what you are going to do.
3. Provide privacy by pulling privacy curtain.

Procedure

4. Lock wheels of bed. Raise bed to a comfortable working position.
5. Lower side rail on side you are working on.
6. Be certain that side rail on opposite side of bed is in up position.
7. Leave pillow under head.
8. Place a pillow lengthwise between patient's legs.
9. Fold patient's arms across chest.
10. Roll patient onto his or her side like a log, turning body as a whole unit, without bending joints.
11. Check for good body alignment.
12. Tighten and tuck in draw sheet and smooth bedding.
13. Tuck pillow behind back for support.
14. Raise side rails and lower bed.
15. Secure call light in patient's reach.

Postprocedure

16. Wash hands.
17. Chart position of patient and how procedure was tolerated.

Charting Example:

10/24/24	1145
	Logrolled to left side
	Moved every 2 hours
	Skin in good condition
	Complained of slight pain in left leg
	when moved
	Pillows placed behind back to maintain
	alignment
	Made comfortable with rails up
	A. Chaplin CNA

Measuring Vital Signs and Other Clinical Skills | Chapter 19 633

Procedure Tip

19.35 Moving—Logrolling

- Review the background information, explaining that logrolling helps keep the back still while the patient is being moved.
- Emphasize the use of proper body mechanics.
- Emphasize the importance of following Standard Precautions.
- Review the preprocedure steps.
- Step 1: Emphasize the importance of proper handwashing.
- Step 2: Emphasize the importance of effective communication techniques, including communication with the co-worker.
- Step 3: Emphasize the importance of privacy.
- Review the procedure steps.
- Step 4: Emphasize the importance of locking the bed.
- Review the postprocedure steps.
- Step 16: Emphasize the importance of proper handwashing.
- Step 17: Emphasize the importance of observation and documentation.

PROCEDURE PRACTICE

- Demonstrate the steps for Procedure 19.35, Moving—Logrolling, as many times as necessary, or ask students to demonstrate the steps. Have students practice and perform the procedure until they are competent.

Procedure Tip

19.36 Moving—Turning Patient Away from You

- Review the background information, discussing situations when this procedure is used.
- Emphasize the use of proper body mechanics.
- Emphasize the importance of following Standard Precautions.
- Review the preprocedure steps.
- Step 1: Emphasize the importance of proper handwashing.
- Step 2: Emphasize the importance of effective communication techniques, including communication with the co-worker; emphasize the importance of privacy.
- Review the procedure steps.
- Step 3: Emphasize the importance of locking the bed.
- Point out that the patient is moved to the center of the bed for safety prior to turning.
- Review the postprocedure steps.
- Step 17: Emphasize the importance of proper handwashing.
- Remind students to document the procedure.

PROCEDURE PRACTICE

- Demonstrate the steps for Procedure 19.36, Moving—Turning Patient Away from You, as many times as necessary, or ask students to demonstrate the steps. Have students practice and perform the procedure until they are competent.

Procedure 19.36 **Moving—Turning Patient Away from You**

BACKGROUND: Following correct procedure for turning patients away from you when bed changing, bathing, and positioning provides good alignment and prevents injury. As a safety measure, this procedure must be done before turning a patient onto his or her side. It ensures that the patient, when turned, is located in the center of the mattress.
ALERT: Follow Standard Precautions

Preprocedure

1. Wash hands.
2. Identify patient and explain what you are going to do. Provide privacy for the patient.

Procedure

3. Lock bed and elevate to a comfortable working height.
4. Lower side rail on side you are working from.
5. Place arm nearest head of bed under patient's shoulders and head. Place other hand and forearm under small of the patient's back. Bend your body at hips and knees, keeping your back straight. Pull patient toward you.
6. Place forearms under patient's hips and pull patient toward you.
7. Place one hand under ankles and one hand under knees and move ankles and knees toward you.
8. Bend the resident's farthest arm next to head and place the other arm across chest. Cross patient's leg closest to you over other leg at ankles.
9. Roll patient away from you by placing one hand under hips and one hand under shoulders.
10. Place one hand under patient's shoulders and one hand under patient's head. Draw patient back toward center of bed.
11. Place both hands under patient's hips and move hips toward center of bed.
12. Put a pillow behind patient's back to give support and keep patient from falling onto his or her back.
13. Be certain patient is in good alignment.
14. Place upper leg on a pillow for support.
15. Replace side rail on near side of bed and return bed to lowest height.
16. You may place a turning sheet under a helpless or heavy patient to help with turning. Use a folded large sheet or half sheet and place it so that it extends just above shoulders and below hips.

Postprocedure

17. Wash hands.

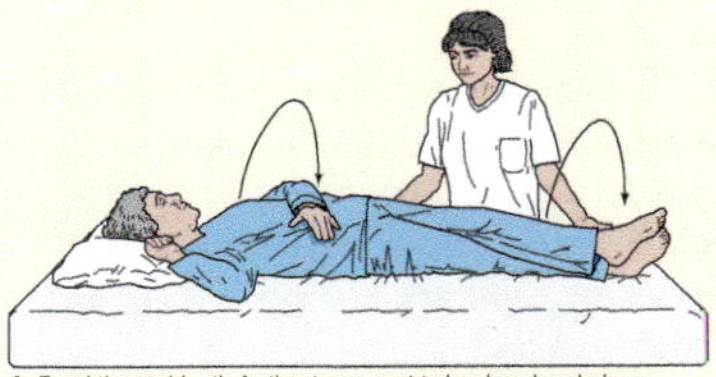

A Bend the resident's farthest arm next to her head and place the other arm across her chest. Cross her near leg over the other leg.

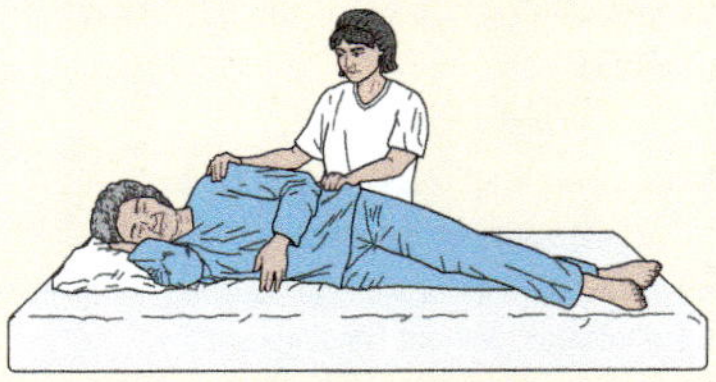

B Place one hand on the resident's shoulder and the other on her hip. Turn her away from you onto her side.

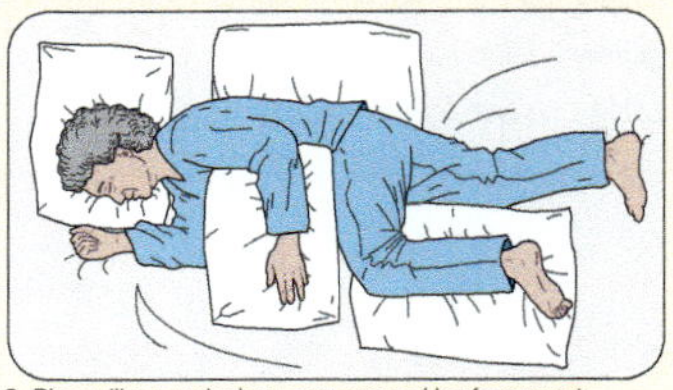

C Place pillows under her upper arm and leg for support.

Charting Example:

8/04/24 1145
Turned to left side
Pillows placed behind back to
maintain good body alignment
Resting comfortably
Side rails up
A. Chaplin CNA

634 Chapter 19 | Measuring Vital Signs and Other Clinical Skills

Procedure 19.37 Turning Patient on Side

BACKGROUND: The nurse's responsibility is to determine baseline function of the patient and to strive to maintain and/or improve function. Prolonged periods of bedrest are harmful to the overall status of the patient and must be avoided whenever possible. However, when a patient cannot turn in bed without assistance nurses need to use their knowledge of correct body mechanics and correct alignment to change the patient from one position to another.
ALERT: Follow Standard Precautions

Preprocedure

1. Wash hands.
2. Explain procedure to patient.
3. Provide privacy for the patient with curtain, screen, or door.

Procedure

4. Raise the bed to a height that allows the nurse to remain in an erect posture while moving patient. Adjust the bed to a flat position or as low as the patient can tolerate. Make sure side rails on side to which patient's body will be turned are raised. Lower the side rail nearest to nurse.
5. Use a pull sheet or pad for moving the patient in order to avoid the effects of friction on the patient's skin integrity.
6. Place the patient's arms across the chest and cross the patient's far leg over the near one. Grasping the pull sheet on the far side of the patient pull the patient towards the nurse.
7. Slowly roll patient onto side toward raised side rail while supporting patient's body.
8. Place a pillow under the head and the neck to prevent lateral flexion of the neck.
9. Place a pillow behind the patient's back to promote the side lying position. Ensure that the shoulders are aligned with the hips.
10. Place a pillow under the upper arm. The lower arm should be flexed and positioned comfortably. Make sure patient is not lying on their arm.
11. Use one or two pillows as needed to support the leg from the groin to the foot. Avoid having bony prominences resting against hard surfaces.
12. Assure that the two shoulders are aligned with the two hips.
13. For the completely immobile patient it is important that passive range-of-motion exercises by provided during the time used to reposition the patient. (See Procedure 21.4.)
14. Readjust the bed height and position and raise the side rail if appropriate. Put the bed in the lowest position.
15. Assure that the patient is comfortable and has no further needs before leaving the bedside.
16. Put the call signal within the patient's reach.

Postprocedure

17. Wash your hands.

Charting Example:

5/05/24	1000
	Repositioned on left side
	Skin care given
	Skin is clean and dry
	S. Gomez CNA

Measuring Vital Signs and Other Clinical Skills | Chapter 19 635

Procedure Tip

19.37 Turning Patient on Side

- Review the background information, discussing problems that might arise if patient is not able to move.
- Emphasize the use of proper body mechanics.
- Emphasize the importance of following Standard Precautions.
- Review the preprocedure steps.
- Step 1: Emphasize the importance of proper handwashing.
- Step 2: Emphasize the importance of effective communication techniques, including communication with the co-worker.
- Step 3: Emphasize the importance of privacy.
- Review the procedure steps.
- Step 13: Discuss importance of exercising the immobile patient.
- Review the postprocedure steps.
- Step 17: Emphasize the importance of proper handwashing.
- Remind students to document the procedure.

PROCEDURE PRACTICE

- Demonstrate the steps for Procedure 19.37, Turning Patient on Side, as many times as necessary, or ask students to demonstrate the steps. Have students practice and perform the procedure until they are competent.

Procedure Tip

19.38 Moving—Turning Patient Toward You

- Review the background information, discussing situations when the procedure might be used.
- Emphasize the use of proper body mechanics.
- Emphasize the importance of following Standard Precautions.
- Review the preprocedure steps.
- Step 1: Emphasize the importance of proper handwashing.
- Step 2: Emphasize the importance of effective communication techniques, including communication with the co-worker. Also emphasize the importance of privacy.
- Review the procedure steps.
- Step 12: Emphasize proper alignment.
- Step 14: Emphasize the importance of checking tubing.
- Review the postprocedure steps.
- Step 18: Emphasize the importance of proper handwashing.
- Remind students to document the procedure.

PROCEDURE PRACTICE

- Demonstrate the steps for Procedure 19.38, Moving—Turning Patient Toward You, as many times as necessary, or ask students to demonstrate the steps. Have students practice and perform the procedure until they are competent.

Procedure 19.38 Moving—Turning Patient Toward You

BACKGROUND: Following correct procedure for turning patients toward you when bed changing, bathing, and positioning provides good alignment and prevents injury.
ALERT: Follow Standard Precautions

Preprocedure

1. Wash hands.
2. Identify patient and explain what you are going to do. Provide privacy for the patient.

Procedure

3. Lock bed and elevate to a comfortable working height.
4. Lower side rail on side you are working from.
5. Cross patient's far leg over leg that is closest to you.
6. Place one hand on patient's far shoulder. Place your other hand on the hip.
7. Brace yourself against side of bed. Roll patient toward you in a slow, gentle, smooth movement.
8. Help patient bring upper leg toward you and bend comfortably (Sims position).
9. Put up side rail. Be certain it is secure.
10. Go to other side of bed and lower side rail.
11. Place hands under patient's shoulders and hips. Pull toward center of bed. This helps maintain side-lying position.
12. Be certain to align patient's body properly.
13. Use pillows to position and support legs if patient is unable to move self.
14. Check tubing to make certain that it is not caught between legs or pulling in any way if patient has an indwelling catheter.
15. Tuck a pillow behind patient's back. This forms a roll and prevents patient from rolling backward onto back.
16. Return bed to low position.
17. Secure call light in patient's reach.

Postprocedure

18. Wash hands.

Charting Example:

5/05/24	1000
	Repositioned on right side
	Skin care given
	Skin is clean and dry
	S. Gomez CNA

636 Chapter 19 | Measuring Vital Signs and Other Clinical Skills

Principles of Applying Restraints

The Omnibus Budget Reconciliation Act 1987 (OBRA) set forth regulations regarding the use of **restraints** in nursing homes. According to these guidelines, restraints cannot be used for convenience or discipline.

restraints
(ri STREYNT)
A piece of equipment or device that restricts a patient's ability to move.

Before restraints are used on a patient, the nurse must make an assessment and get a physician to agree that restraints are necessary and that all other alternatives have failed. The patient cannot be restrained until a health care professional explains to the patient, family member, or legal representative about the restraining device and that it will be used for a specified period of time. Every time a patient is restrained, they must be assessed and all methods must be documented.

Nurses must reassess a restrained person every 30 minutes and assess circulation to the hands, feet, and toes; skin for bruising; and activities for daily living such as eating, drinking, and toileting. All of this must be documented in the patient's chart.

Restraints can be beneficial to patients by preventing a patient from getting out of bed, moving arms or legs excessively, or preventing patient from hurting themselves or others. For example, restraints are often used to keep a patient from inflicting self-harm or injury (usually with suicidal patients); to prevent patients from removing medically necessary tubes, intravenous lines, and dressing; and to keep a child still during a surgical procedures, such as receiving stitches. In health care, the use of restraints should be a last resort.

The most commonly used physical restraints include:

- Soft wrist and ankle restraints
- Strap fastening vest (posey jacket)
- Seat belt with buckle (restraint belt)
- Mittens (restraint mitts)
- Leather wrist and ankle restraints

For a patient's safety, restraints should be tied/locked to the bed frame, not the bed rails. A quick-release knot should be used to allow for immediate release.

Restraints can cause complications to a patient, including injury to the restrained extremity (fracture, muscle strain, dislocation, or contusion) or numbness and tingling.

Postural Supports

Soft postural supports (soft cloth ties used on arms and legs, or vests) are used to protect elderly or disoriented patients from hurting themselves or someone else. It is much better if you do not have to use them. They can be used only if they are ordered by the doctor. Precautions must be taken when they are used as they may create the following conditions:

- Increased agitation
- Increased risk of pneumonia

Measuring Vital Signs and Other Clinical Skills | Chapter 19 637

Teaching Tips

- Review the Omnibus Budget Reconciliation Act 1987 (OBRA), which set forth regulations regarding the use of restraints in nursing homes.
- Explain that according to these guidelines, restraints cannot be used for convenience or discipline.
- Restraints may only be used if a physician agrees that restraints are necessary and that all other options have been tried and failed.
- Emphasize that a nurse must evaluate a restrained patient every 30 minutes.
- Emphasize the importance of documentation when observation and monitoring a restrained patient.
- Review reasons restraints may be used.
- Review problems that might occur due to the use of restraints.
- Describe the most common types of restraints:
  - Soft wrist and ankle restraints
  - Strap fastening vest (posey jacket)
  - Seat belt with buckle (restraint belt)
  - Mittens (restraint mitts)
  - Leather wrist and ankle restraints

Teaching Tips

- Emphasize that postural supports may only be used with a doctor's order.
- Identify postural supports:
  - Soft material with ties
  - Mittens
  - Vests
  - Limbs, waist
- Explain why they might be necessary:
  - Prevent patient from pulling out tubes and catheters
  - Prevent scratching or injuring self or others
  - Keep from falling out of bed or chair
- Explain problems that might arise from the use of supports:
  - Increased agitation
  - Immobilized patient
  - Increased risk of pneumonia
  - Skin breakdown
  - Decreased circulation
- Review steps that must be taken when supports are used.
- Describe postoperative care supportive devices and equipment:
  - Trochanter roll
  - Abduction splint
  - Abductor wedge
  - Footboard
  - Pillows

- Skin breakdown
- Decreased circulation

When postural supports are used, you must:

- Anticipate elimination needs
- Check for swelling above, below, and at the site of supports
- Release the supports periodically
- Provide for hydration by offering fluids
- Change position frequently

There are times when postural support must be used:

- To prevent patient from pulling out tubes and catheters
- To prevent patient from scratching or injuring self and others
- To keep patient from falling out of bed or chair

There must always be a valid reason for using the supports. Do not use them just because you are annoyed that the patient takes too much of your time.

Postoperative Care Supportive Devices and Equipment

Fractures and joint replacement are two major areas in sub-acute postoperative care. Keeping the patient in good *alignment* is very important. Poor alignment can cause a new hip joint to move out of the socket and cause improper healing of fractures. The following are some of the common supportive devices:

- **Trochanter roll.** A towel or small blanket is rolled and put next to the greater trochanter (femur). It keeps the hip from rotating outward and prevents permanent disability or difficulties with walking.
- **Abduction splint.** This is a device that keeps the thighs apart and keeps the hip joints in proper alignment.
- **Abductor wedge.** A wedge-shaped, spongy material is placed between the legs. The wedge is used to keep the hip that has been replaced or fractured away from the center of the body. This prevents excessive strain on the hip and prevents a dislocation of the repair.
- **Footboard.** A padded board is placed at the feet when the patient is in a prone or supine position. The feet naturally extend when lying in this position. If the feet are not aligned correctly, contractures occur and cause problems with walking.
- **Pillows.** Pillows of different sizes and shapes are placed to support joints and provide support for proper body alignment.

638 Chapter 19 | Measuring Vital Signs and Other Clinical Skills

ACTIVITY

Have students make a Dos and Don'ts list for using restraints and postural supports. This may done together as a class or individually.

TEAMWORK

In small groups, perform a skit demonstrating how a family member might react upon entering a room and seeing the patient in restraints or postural supports. Demonstrate how the health care worker should respond.

Procedure 19.39 Applying Restraints

BACKGROUND: Restraints should be used only as a last resort when alternative measures have failed, and the patient is at an increased risk for harming himself or others. Alternative measures might include: assuring that basic patient needs have been met; providing a sitter; providing distraction.

CAUTION: Physically restraining a patient can escalate the patient's confusion and their level of agitation.

ALERT: Follow Standard Precautions

Preprocedure

1. Determine the need for restraints and that alternative measures have been attempted.
2. Assess patient's physical condition, behavior, and mental status.
3. Determine the agency's policy for application of restraints. Secure a physician's order.
4. Explain the reason for use to patient and family. Clarify how the patient's needs will be met and that the use of restraints is only temporary.

Procedure

5. Wash your hands.
6. Apply restraints according to manufacturer's directions (each type of restraint may require a different type of application):
   a. Choose the least restrictive type of device that allows the greatest degree of mobility.
   b. Pad bony prominences. Ensure that two fingers can be inserted between the restraint and the patient's wrist or ankle.
   c. Maintain restrained extremity in normal anatomical position.
   d. Use a quick release tie for all restraints.
   e. Fasten restraint to bed not side rail.
   f. Remove restraint every two hours or according to agency policy and patient need.
   g. While removed, check for signs of decreased circulation, impaired function of limb, or impaired skin integrity.
   h. Perform range-of-motion exercises before reapplying.
   i. Reevaluate the need for use of physical restraints, alternative measures attempted before reapplying.
   j. Document procedure and rationale.
   k. Obtain a new physician's order for restraint every 24 hours if continued need.

Postprocedure

7. Assure that patient safety and comfort has been maintained throughout the period that restraints are in place.

Charting Example:

9/09/24	0930	
	Patient attempting to pull out tubes;	
	applied restraints.	
	________ *S. Gomez CNA*	

Measuring Vital Signs and Other Clinical Skills | Chapter 19 639

Procedure Tip

19.39 Applying Restraints

- Review the background information, emphasizing restraints should be a last resort. Discuss alternative measures.
- Emphasize the importance of following Standard Precautions.
- Review the preprocedure steps.
- Review the procedure steps.
- Step 3: Emphasize the need to follow facility's policies; emphasize the need for a physician's order.
- Step 4: Emphasize the need for effective communication.
- Step 5: Emphasize the importance of proper handwashing.
- Step 6f: Emphasize the importance of monitoring the patient regularly.
- Step 6j: Emphasize the importance of documentation.
- Step 6k: Emphasize the need to obtain a new physician's order.
- Review the postprocedure steps.
- Remind students to document the procedure.

PROCEDURE PRACTICE

- Using a mannequin, demonstrate the steps for Procedure 19.39, Applying Restraints, as many times as necessary, or ask students to demonstrate the steps. Have students practice and perform the procedure until they are competent.

Procedure Tip

19.40 How to Tie Postural Supports

- Review the background information, emphasizing that a quick-release knot is imperative in case of an emergency.
- Emphasize the importance of following Standard Precautions.
- Review the preprocedure steps.
- Step 1: Emphasize the importance of proper handwashing.
- Step 2: Review the types of postural supports.
- Review the procedure steps.
- Step 3: Explain that a double-knot, or any type of knot other than a quick-release knot, may not be used under any circumstances.
- Review the postprocedure steps.
- Step 5: Emphasize the importance of proper handwashing.
- Remind students to document the procedure.

PROCEDURE PRACTICE

- Demonstrate the steps for Procedure 19.40, How to Tie Postural Supports, as many times as necessary, or ask students to demonstrate the steps. Have students practice and perform the procedure until they are competent.

Procedure 19.40 How to Tie Postural Supports

BACKGROUND: Postural supports must be secured with a quick-release knot that allows the patient to be moved quickly in the event of an emergency.
ALERT: Follow Standard Precautions

Preprocedure

1. Wash hands.
2. Assemble equipment: a postural support that has been ordered.

Procedure

3. Tie a half-bow knot or quick-release knot. Tie the same way you tie a bow on a shoe. Once bow is in place, grasp one loop and pull end of tie through knot.
4. Knot can be easily released pulling end of loop.

NOTE: Half-bow knot/quick-release knot is always used when a restraint is attached to wheelchair or mattress support. This allows quick release if it is necessary to move patient in a hurry.

Postprocedure

5. Wash hands.

Charting Example:

9/09/24	*0930*
	Transferred to wheelchair
	Vest postural support applied and
	secured with a quick-release knot
	at back of chair
	S. Gomez CNA

640 Chapter 19 | Measuring Vital Signs and Other Clinical Skills

Procedure 19.41 **Postural Supports: Limb**

BACKGROUND: Postural supports for the limbs are necessary to prevent some patients from causing injury to themselves or others.
ALERT: Follow Standard Precautions

Preprocedure

1. Check for physician's order.
2. Wash hands.
3. Assemble equipment: a limb support.
4. Identify patient. Provide privacy for the patient by curtain, screen, or door.

Procedure

5. Explain what you are going to do, even if the patient is confused.
6. Place soft side of limb support against skin. Check to make sure the wrinkles are out.
7. Wrap around limb and put one tie through opening on other end of support.
8. Gently pull until it fits snugly around limb.
9. Buckle or tie in place so that support stays on limb.
10. Tie out of patient's reach (see Procedure 19.40, "How to Tie Postural Supports"):
    a. Tie to bed frame (not side rails).
    b. Tie to wheelchair (not to stationary chair).
11. Check for proper alignment and comfort of patient.
12. Check to be certain that knots or wrinkles are not causing pressure.
13. Check to be certain that support is snug but does not bind. (You should be able to put two fingers under edges.)
14. Place call light where it can be easily reached.

Postprocedure

15. Wash hands.
16. Circulation under restraint should be checked every 15–30 minutes and documented.
17. Check patient frequently and move at least every 2 hours. Restraints should be removed every 2 hours for at least 5–10 minutes.
18. Chart the following:
    a. Reason for use of support
    b. Type of support used
    c. When it was applied
    d. When it was released
    e. Times of repositioning
    f. How patient tolerated it
    g. Condition of skin

Charting Example:

10/14/24	0200
	Resident disoriented; swinging arms and
	legs against side rails
	Limb postural supports applied and
	secured with a quick-release knot
	to legs and arms, to prevent injury
	per physician's order
	R. Johnson CNA

Measuring Vital Signs and Other Clinical Skills | Chapter 19 641

Procedure Tip

19.41 Postural Supports: Limb

- Review the background information, emphasizing the reasons for using postural supports on limbs.
- Emphasize the importance of following Standard Precautions.
- Review the preprocedure steps.
- Step 1: Emphasize the importance of obtaining a physician's order.
- Step 2: Emphasize the importance of proper handwashing.
- Step 4: Emphasize the importance of patient privacy.
- Review the procedure steps.
- Step 5: Emphasize the importance of effective communication techniques.
- Step 10: Review locations of ties.
- Review the postprocedure steps.
- Step 15: Emphasize the importance of proper handwashing.
- Step 16: Emphasize the importance of monitoring patient every 15–30 minutes.
- Step 17: Emphasize importance of checking and moving patient and removing restraints at regular intervals.
- Step 18: Review the proper methods for documenting the use of restraints.

PROCEDURE PRACTICE

- Demonstrate the steps for Procedure 19.41, Postural Supports: Limb, as many times as necessary, or ask students to demonstrate the steps. Have students practice and perform the procedure until they are competent.

Procedure Tip

19.42 Postural Supports: Mitten

- Review the background information, emphasizing the reasons for using postural supports on hands.
- Emphasize the importance of following Standard Precautions.
- Review the preprocedure steps.
- Step 1: Emphasize the importance of obtaining a physician's order.
- Step 2: Emphasize the importance of proper handwashing.
- Steps 4 and 5: Emphasize the importance of effective communication techniques.
- Review the procedure steps.
- Step 9: Review the note, and discuss the difference between securing the support to the hand and securing the support to a bed or chair.
- Review the postprocedure steps.
- Step 14: Emphasize the importance of proper handwashing.
- Step 15: Emphasize the importance of monitoring patient every 15–30 minutes.
- Step 16: Emphasize importance of removing restraints at regular intervals.
- Step 17: Emphasize importance of checking and moving patient at regular intervals.
- Step 18: Review the proper methods for documenting the use of restraints.

Procedure 19.42 **Postural Supports: Mitten**

BACKGROUND: Mitten postural supports prevent the hands from grasping objects.
ALERT: Follow Standard Precautions

Preprocedure

1. Check for physician's order.
2. Wash hands.
3. Assemble equipment: a soft cloth mitten.
4. Identify patient.
5. Explain what you are going to do.

Procedure

6. Slip mitten on hand with padded side against palm and net on top of hand.
7. Lace mitten.
8. Gently pull until it fits snugly around wrist.
9. Tie with a double bow knot so that support stays on hand.

NOTE: Double bow knot helps secure the restraint to the patient. Use only a half-bow/quick-release knot to tie a postural support to a bed, wheelchair, or other furniture.

10. Check for proper alignment and comfort of patient.
11. Check to be certain knots or wrinkles are not causing pressure.
12. Check to be certain support is snug but does not bind. (You should be able to put two fingers under edges.)
13. Place call light where it can be easily reached.

Postprocedure

14. Wash hands.
15. Check circulation and document every 15–30 minutes.
16. Remove mitten restraint every 2 hours for at least 5–10 minutes.
17. Check patient frequently and move at least every 2 hours.
18. Chart the following:
    a. Reason for use of support
    b. Type of support used
    c. When it was applied
    d. When it was released
    e. Times of repositioning
    f. How patient tolerated it
    g. Condition of skin

Charting Example:

11/07/24	1400
	Bilateral mitten postural supports applied
	and secured with a quick-release knot to
	prevent the resident from removing
	abdominal dressing and IV per physician's
	order
	S. Gomez CNA

642 Chapter 19 | Measuring Vital Signs and Other Clinical Skills

PROCEDURE PRACTICE

- Demonstrate the steps for Procedure 19.42, Postural Supports: Mitten, as many times as necessary, or ask students to demonstrate the steps. Have students practice and perform the procedure until they are competent.

Procedure 19.43 | **Postural Supports: Vest or Jacket**

BACKGROUND: Vest postural support is necessary to prevent some patients from injuring themselves.
ALERT: Follow Standard Precautions

Preprocedure

1. Check for physician's order.
2. Wash hands.
3. Assemble equipment: a vest support.
4. Identify patient.
5. Explain what you are going to do.

Procedure

6. Put arms through armholes of vest with opening to back.
7. Cross back panels by bringing tie on left side over to right and right tie to left.
8. Carefully smooth material so that there are no wrinkles.
9. Tie where patient cannot reach (see the procedure "How to Tie Postural Supports"):
    a. Tie to bed frame (not side rails)
    b. Tie to wheelchair (not stationary chair)
10. Check for proper alignment and comfort of patient.
11. Check to be certain that knots or wrinkles are not causing pressure.
12. Check to be certain that support is snug but does not bind. (You should be able to put two fingers under edges.)
13. Place call light where it can be easily reached.

Postprocedure

14. Wash your hands.
15. Check skin condition and circulation every 15–30 minutes.
16. Remove restraint every 2 hours for 5–10 minutes.
17. Check patient frequently and move at least every 2 hours.
18. Chart the following:
    a. Reason for use of support
    b. Type of support used
    c. When it was applied
    d. When it was released
    e. Times of repositioning
    f. How patient tolerated it
    g. Condition of skin

Charting Example:

9/14/24 1700
Vest postural support applied to
protect resident from getting out of
bed and falling, per physician's order
A. Chaplin CNA

Measuring Vital Signs and Other Clinical Skills | Chapter 19 643

PROCEDURE PRACTICE

- Demonstrate the steps for Procedure 19.43, Postural Supports: Vest or Jacket, as many times as necessary, or ask students to demonstrate the steps. Have students practice and perform the procedure until they are competent.

Procedure Tip

19.43 Postural Supports: Vest or Jacket

- Review the background information, emphasizing the reasons for using vest postural support.
- Emphasize the importance of following Standard Precautions.
- Review the preprocedure steps.
- Step 1: Emphasize the importance of obtaining a physician's order.
- Step 2: Emphasize the importance of proper handwashing.
- Steps 4 and 5: Emphasize the importance of effective communication techniques.
- Review the procedure steps.
- Step 9: Review the locations of the ties.
- Review the postprocedure steps.
- Step 14: Emphasize the importance of proper handwashing.
- Step 15: Emphasize the importance of monitoring patient every 15–30 minutes.
- Step 16: Emphasize importance of removing restraints at regular intervals.
- Step 17: Emphasize importance of checking and moving patient at regular intervals.
- Step 18: Review the proper methods for documenting the use of restraints.

Teaching Tips

- Explain reasons for bathing the resident:
  - Removes perspiration and dirt
  - Removes odor
  - Increases circulation
  - Gives you an opportunity to observe the patient's skin
  - Provides relaxation
- Explain the four types of bathing:
  - Bed bath
  - Tub bath
  - Whirlpool bath
  - Shower
- Explain why a full bath may not be necessary every day.
- Explain the importance of cleaning the armpits and perineum every day.

ACTIVITY

Randomly distribute strips of paper with one of the four types of bathing written on them. Have students write down a description of the type of bathing on the slip he or she selected. Include reasons why this type might be used and the benefits it provides to the patient.

Bathing the Patient

Providing for your patients' cleanliness is an important responsibility. Bathing is important because it:

- Removes perspiration and dirt
- Removes odor
- Increases circulation
- Allows for some exercise
- Gives you an opportunity to observe the patients' skin
- Provides relaxation

You may be asked to give several different types of baths. This depends on the patient's condition. Always check the chart to see what type of bath is ordered. The following are types of baths:

- Bed bath
- Tub bath
- Whirlpool bath
- Shower

Patients may not have a complete bath every day. Sometimes they are bathed only twice a week. This is especially true of elderly patients, who have drier skin, less subcutaneous fat, and more fragile tissues.

Always wash the perineum (pericare) and the underarms every day. These areas tend to develop an odor because they have more bacteria and are not open to the air. Good pericare is especially important when there is a urinary catheter in place. Good pericare helps prevent infection. Back care should be provided as a part of the daily hygiene process. Even if the patient does not receive a complete bath, the provision of back care will promote the patient's comfort level.

644 Chapter 19 | Measuring Vital Signs and Other Clinical Skills

Procedure 19.44 **Giving a Bed Bath**

BACKGROUND: Providing a bed bath improves circulation, relaxes the patient, provides an opportunity to examine the skin, and enables you to interact with the patient.
ALERT: Follow Standard Precautions

Preprocedure

1. Wash hands.
2. Assemble equipment:
   a. Soap and soap dish
   b. Face towel
   c. Bath towel (at least 2)
   d. Washcloth (at least 2)
   e. Hospital gown or patient's sleepwear
   f. Lotion or powder
   g. Nailbrush and emery board
   h. Comb and brush
   i. Bedpan or urinal and cover
   j. Bed linen
   k. Bath blanket
   l. Bath basin, water at 105° F
   m. Disposable nonsterile gloves
3. Place linens on chair in order of use and place towels on overbed table.
4. Identify patient.
5. Explain what you are going to do.
6. Provide for privacy by pulling the privacy screen curtain, or door.

Procedure

7. Raise bed to a comfortable working height.
8. Offer bedpan or urinal. Empty and rinse before starting bath. Wash your hands. (Remember to wear gloves when handling urine.)
9. Lower headrest and knee gatch (raised knee area/bed) so that bed is flat.
10. Lower the side rail only on side where you are working.
11. Put on gloves.
12. Loosen top sheet, blanket, and bedspread. Remove and fold blanket and bedspread, and place over back of chair.
13. Cover patient with a bath blanket.
14. Ask patient to hold bath blanket in place. Remove top sheet by sliding it to foot of bed. Do not expose patient. (Place soiled linen in laundry container.)
15. Leave a pillow under patient's head for comfort.
16. Remove patient's gown and place in laundry container. If nightwear belongs to patient, follow hospital policy (i.e., send home with family or to hospital laundry).
17. To remove gown when the patient has an IV:

NOTE: Most facilities provide gowns with snaps for easy removal around existing intravenous tubing.
   a. Loosen gown from neck.
   b. Slip gown from free arm.
   c. Be certain that patient is covered with a bath blanket.
   d. Slip gown away from body toward arm with IV.
   e. Gather gown at arm and slip downward over arm and tubing. Be careful not to pull on tubing.
   f. Gather material of gown in one hand and slowly draw gown over tip of fingers.
   g. Lift IV free of stand with free hand and slip gown over bottle.
   h. Do not lower bottle. Raise gown.
18. Fill bath basin two-thirds full with warm water. Test water temperature and ensure it is safe and comfortable before bathing patients and adjust if necessary.
19. Help patient move to side of bed nearest you.
20. Fold face towel over upper edge of bath blanket. This will keep it dry.

(continued)

Procedure Tip

19.44 Giving a Bed Bath

- Review the background information, discussing the benefits of bathing the patient.
- Emphasize the importance of following Standard Precautions.
- Review the preprocedure steps.
- Step 1: Emphasize the importance of proper handwashing.
- Step 2: Review the list of necessary equipment.
- Steps 4 and 5: Emphasize the importance of effective communication techniques.
- Step 6: Emphasize the importance of patient privacy.
- Review the procedure steps.
- Step 8: Refer to Procedures 19.21 and 19.22.
- Step 11: Emphasize the importance of wearing gloves.
- Steps 13 and 14: Emphasize the importance of patient privacy.
- Step 17: Emphasize the importance of using care when handling tubes and catheters.

ACTIVITY

As a class, brainstorm problems that might arise while giving a patient a bed bath, and think of solutions you could use to solve or minimize the problems.

TEAMWORK

Most Americans bathe every day, but that is not true for people of all cultures. In small groups, use the Internet or reference books to find out the bathing habits or routines of three other cultural groups around the world. Make a chart or table comparing the three with Americans.

Procedure Tip

19.44 Giving a Bed Bath, continued

- Step 23: Review the importance of effective communication.
- Emphasize the importance of drying skin completely to avoid irritation.
- Step 31: Review reasons for changing water: dirt, temperature.
- Step 33e: Refer to Procedure 19.14.
- Step 34: Emphasize that the patient should wash their own genitals, if able.

ACTIVITY

As a class, discuss problems that might arise if the skin is not dried completely after a bath.

Procedure 19.44 Giving a Bed Bath (continued)

Procedure (cont)

21. Form a mitten by folding washcloth around your hand.

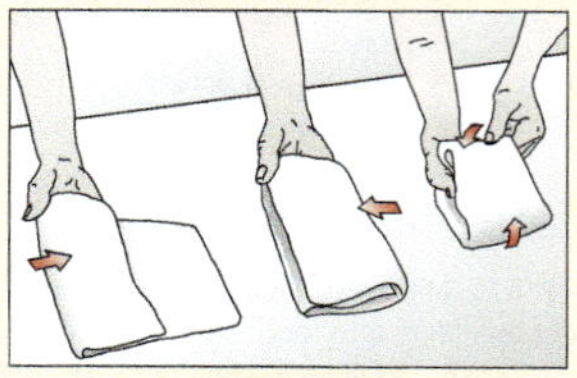

22. Wash patient's eyes from nose to outside of face. Use different corners of washcloth.
23. Ask patient if he or she wants soap used on the face. Gently wash and rinse face, ears, and neck. Be careful not to get soap in eyes. Dry face with towel, using a blotting motion.
24. To wash patient's arms, shoulders, axilla:
    a. Uncover patient's far arm (one farthest from you).
    b. Protect bed from becoming wet with a bath towel placed under arm. Wash with long, firm, circular strokes, rinse, and dry.
    c. Wash and dry armpits (axillae). Apply deodorant and powder.
25. To wash hand:
    a. Place basin of water on towel.
    b. Put patient's hand into basin.
    c. Wash, rinse, and dry and push back cuticle gently.
26. Repeat on other arm.
27. To wash chest:
    a. Place towel lengthwise across patient's chest.
    b. Fold bath blanket down to patient's abdomen.
    c. Wash chest. Be especially careful to dry skin under female breasts to prevent irritation. Dry area thoroughly.
28. To wash abdomen:
    a. Fold down bath blanket to pubic area.
    b. Wash, rinse, and dry abdomen.
    c. Pull up bath blanket to keep patient warm.
    d. Slide towel out from under bath blanket.
29. To wash thigh, leg, and foot:
    a. Ask patient to flex knee if possible.
    b. Fold bath blanket to uncover thigh, leg, and foot of leg farthest from you.
    c. Place bath towel under leg to keep bed from getting wet.
    d. Place basin on towel and put foot into basin.
    e. Wash and rinse thigh, leg, and foot.
    f. Dry well between toes. Be careful to support the leg when lifting it.
30. Follow same procedure for leg nearest you.
31. Change water. You may need to change water before this time if it is dirty or cold.
32. Raise side rail on opposite side if it is down.
33. To wash back and buttocks:
    a. Help patient turn on side away from you.
    b. Have patient move toward center of bed.
    c. Place a bath towel lengthwise on bed, under patient's back.
    d. Wash, rinse, and dry neck, back, and buttocks.
    e. Give patient a back rub. Help patient turn back on their back and make sure they are still covered with a bath blanket. Massage back for at least a minute and a half, giving special attention to shoulder blades, hip bones, and spine. Observe for reddened areas. (See the procedure "Skin Care—Giving a Back Rub.")
34. To wash genital area:
    a. Offer patient a clean, soapy washcloth to wash genital area.
    b. Give the person a clean, wet washcloth to rinse with and a dry towel to dry with.
35. Clean the genital area thoroughly if patient is unable to help. To clean the genital area:
    a. Put a towel or disposable pad under the patient's buttock.
    b. When washing a female patient always wipe from front to back.
    c. Separate the labia and use a clean area of the wash cloth for each side of the perineal area.

(continued)

Procedure 19.44 **Giving a Bed Bath (continued)**

Procedure (cont)

d. When washing a male patient, be sure to wash and dry penis, scrotum, and groin area carefully. Clean the tip of the penis using a circular motion and clean the shaft of the penis from top to bottom. Remember to pull back the foreskin if the patient is not circumcised.

e. Remove towel or disposable pad and discard appropriately.

f. Remove gloves and put in hazardous waste.

36. If range of motion is ordered, complete at this time.
37. Put a clean gown on patient.
38. If patient has an IV:
    a. Gather the sleeve on IV side in one hand.
    b. Lift bottle free of stand. Do not lower bottle.
    c. Slip bottle through sleeve from inside and rehang.
    d. Guide gown along the IV tubing to bed.
    e. Slip gown over the patient's hand. Be careful not to pull or crimp tubing.
    f. Put gown on arm with IV, then on opposite arm.
39. Comb or brush hair.
40. Follow hospital policy for towels and washcloths. Some have you hang them for later use; others have you place them in the laundry containers immediately.
41. Leave patient in a comfortable position and in good body alignment.
42. Place call bell within reach. Replace furniture and tidy unit.

Postprocedure

43. Wash hands.
44. Chart procedure and how patient tolerated it. Note any unusual skin changes or patient complaints.

Charting Example:

10/24/24	0945
	Completed bed bath
	Dime-sized red area on sacrum
	Reported to charge nurse
	No complaints of discomfort
	Resting quietly with rails up
	A. Chaplin CNA

Procedure Tip

19.44 Giving a Bed Bath, continued

- Step 40: Emphasize need to follow hospital policy for handling towels and washcloths.
- Review the postprocedure steps.
- Step 43: Emphasize the importance of proper handwashing.
- Step 44: Emphasize the importance of observation and documentation.

PROCEDURE PRACTICE

- Demonstrate the steps for Procedure 19.44, Giving a Bed Bath, as many times as necessary, or ask students to demonstrate the steps. Have students practice and perform the procedure until they are competent. If students will be using real water, remind them to bring bathing suits or quick-dry clothes to wear while practicing. Alternatively, use a mannequin.

Procedure Tip

19.45 Giving a Partial Bath (Face, Hands, Axillae, Buttocks, and Genitals)

- Review the background information, discussing the benefits of bathing the patient.
- Emphasize the importance of following Standard Precautions.
- Review the preprocedure steps.
- Step 1: Emphasize the importance of proper handwashing.
- Step 2: Review the list of necessary equipment.
- Steps 3 and 4: Emphasize the importance of effective communication techniques.
- Step 5: Emphasize the importance of patient privacy.
- Step 6: Refer to Procedures 19.21 and 19.22.
- Review the procedure steps.
- Steps 10 and 11: Emphasize the importance of patient privacy.
- Step 18: Emphasize the importance of patient independence.
- Step 21: Emphasize importance of wearing gloves.
- Emphasize the importance of drying skin completing to avoid irritation.
- Step 22: Review reasons for changing water: dirt, temperature.

Procedure 19.45 Giving a Partial Bath (Face, Hands, Axillae, Buttocks, and Genitals)

BACKGROUND: Providing a partial bath relaxes the patient and prevents odors. The interaction with the patient is important through communication and touch.
ALERT: Follow Standard Precautions

Preprocedure

1. Wash hands.
2. Assemble equipment:
   a. Soap and soap dish
   b. Face towel
   c. Bath towel
   d. Washcloth
   e. Hospital gown or patient's sleepwear
   f. Lotion or powder
   g. Nail brush and emery board
   h. Comb and brush
   i. Bedpan or urinal and cover
   j. Bath blanket
   k. Bath basin, water at 105°F
   l. Clean linen, as needed
   m. Disposable gloves
3. Identify patient.
4. Explain what you are going to do.
5. Provide privacy by pulling privacy screen, curtain, or door.
6. Offer bedpan or urinal. Empty and rinse before starting bath. (Wear gloves if handling body fluid.)
7. Raise headrest to a comfortable position, if permitted.
8. Lower side rails if permitted. If they are to remain up, lower only side rail on side where you are working.

Procedure

9. Loosen top sheet, blanket, and bedspread. Remove and fold blanket and bedspread and place over back of chair.
10. Cover patient with a bath blanket.
11. Ask patient to hold bath blanket in place. Remove top sheet by sliding it to the foot of bed. Do not expose patient. Place soiled linen in laundry container.
12. Leave a pillow under the patient's head for comfort.
13. Remove patient's gown and place in laundry container. If nightwear belongs to patient, follow hospital policy (i.e., send home with family or to hospital).
14. To remove gown when patient has an IV, see the procedure "Giving a Bed Bath."
15. Fill bath basin two-thirds full with warm water and place on overbed table. Test water temperature and ensure it is safe and comfortable before bathing patients; adjust if necessary.
16. Put overbed table where patient can reach it comfortably.
17. Place towel, washcloth, and soap on overbed table.
18. Ask patient to wash as much as he or she is able to and tell the person that you will return to complete bath.
19. Place call bell where patient can reach it easily. Ask patient to signal when ready.
20. Remove glove, wash your hands, and leave unit.
21. When patient signals, return to unit, wash your hands, and put on gloves.
22. Change water. Test water temperature and ensure it is safe and comfortable before bathing patients and adjust if necessary.
23. Complete bathing areas the patient was unable to reach. Make sure that face, hands, axillae, genitals, and buttocks are dry. To wash the genital area:
   a. Offer the patient a clean, soapy washcloth to wash genital area. Provide a clean, wet washcloth to rinse with and a dry towel to dry with. If patient is unable to help, you will need to clean the genital area thoroughly.
   b. When washing a female patient, always wipe from front to back.
   c. Separate the labia and use a clean area of the wash cloth for each side of the perineal area.

(continued)

648 Chapter 19 | Measuring Vital Signs and Other Clinical Skills

TEAMWORK

In small groups, prepare and perform a skit demonstrating how a health care worker should respond to a patient who does not want to be bathed.

Procedure 19.45 **Giving a Partial Bath (Face, Hands, Axillae, Buttocks, and Genitals) (continued)**

Procedure (cont)

d. When washing a male patient, be sure to wash and dry penis, scrotum, and groin area carefully. Clean the tip of the penis using a circular motion and clean the shaft of the penis from top to bottom. Remember to pull back the foreskin if the patient is not circumcised.

e. Remove gloves and put in hazardous waste. If range of motion is ordered, complete it at this time.

24. Give a back rub. (See the procedure "Skin Care—Giving a Back Rub.")
25. Put a clean gown on patient.
26. If patient has an IV, see the procedure "Giving a Bed Bath."
27. Assist patient in applying deodorant and putting on a clean gown.
28. Change bed according to hospital policy. Not all facilities change linen every day.
29. Put up side rails if required.
30. Leave patient in a comfortable position and in good body alignment.

Postprocedure

31. Remove and discard gloves.
32. Wash hands.
33. Place call bell within reach. Replace furniture and tidy unit.
34. Chart procedure and how it was tolerated.

Charting Example:

9/23/24	*0730*
	Partial bath
	No skin breakdown noted
	Complained of headache
	Reported to charge nurse
	S. Gomez CNA

Procedure 19.46 **Tub/Shower Bath**

BACKGROUND: Providing a relaxing tub/shower bath gives one-on-one time to the patient. It is an opportunity to check for skin and other problems. Careful observation is essential.
ALERT: Follow Standard Precautions

Preprocedure

1. Wash hands.
2. Assemble equipment on a chair near the tub:
   a. Bath towels
   b. Washcloths
   c. Soap
   d. Bath thermometer
   e. Wash basin
   f. Clean gown
   g. Bathmat
   h. Disinfectant solution
   i. Shower chair, if necessary
3. Identify patient and explain what you are going to do.
4. Provide privacy by pulling privacy curtain, screen, or door.

Procedure

5. Help patient out of bed.
6. Help with robe and slippers.

(continued)

Procedure Tip

19.45 Giving a Partial Bath (Face, Hands, Axillae, Buttocks, and Genitals), continued

- Step 24: Refer to procedure 19.14.
- Step 28: Emphasize need to follow hospital policy.
- Review the postprocedure steps.
- Step 32: Emphasize the importance of proper handwashing.
- Step 34: Emphasize the importance of observation and documentation.

PROCEDURE PRACTICE

- Demonstrate the steps for Procedure 19.45, Giving a Partial Bath (Face, Hands, Axillae, Buttocks, and Genitals), as many times as necessary, or ask students to demonstrate the steps. Have students practice and perform the procedure until they are competent. If students will be using real water, remind them to bring bathing suits or quick-dry clothes to wear while practicing. Alternatively, use a mannequin.

ACTIVITY

Bathing a patient is often the responsibility of a nurse assistant. However, responsibilities vary depending on the type of health care facility. Have students contact three different types of health care facilities in your area by phone, mail, or e-mail. Students should identify themself as a student studying health care occupations, and ask for information about the responsibilities of different health care workers in that facility. Discuss the responses as a class.

Procedure Tip

19.46 Tub/Shower Bath

- Review the background information, discussing the benefits of bathing the patient. Emphasize careful observation.
- Emphasize the importance of following Standard Precautions.
- Review the preprocedure steps.
- Step 1: Emphasize the importance of proper handwashing.
- Step 2: Review the list of necessary equipment.
- Step 3: Emphasize the importance of effective communication techniques.
- Step 4: Emphasize the importance of patient privacy.
- Review the procedure steps.

Procedure Tip

19.46 Tub/Shower Bath, continued

- Step 7: Emphasize the need to check with the head nurse.
- Step 11: Emphasize the importance of patient privacy.
- Note: Wear gloves.
- Step 14: Emphasize the importance of patient independence and privacy.
- Step 18: Emphasize importance of drying skin completing to avoid irritation.
- Step 21: Emphasize aseptic techniques.
- Review the postprocedure steps.
- Step 22: Emphasize the importance of proper handwashing.
- Step 23: Emphasize the importance of observation and documentation.

PROCEDURE PRACTICE

- Demonstrate the steps for Procedure 19.46, Tub/Shower Bath, as many times as necessary, or ask students to demonstrate the steps. Have students practice and perform the procedure until they are competent. If students will be using real water, remind them to bring bathing suits or quick-dry clothes to wear while practicing. Alternatively, use a mannequin.

Procedure 19.46 Tub/Shower Bath (continued)

Procedure (cont)

7. Check with head nurse to see if the patient can ambulate or if a wheelchair or shower chair is needed. If a shower chair is used, always do the following:
   a. Cover patient with a bath blanket or sheet so that patient is not exposed in any way.
   b. Provide adequate clothing for patient, such as a robe or extra cover.
8. Take patient to shower or tub room.
9. For tub bath, place a towel in bottom of tub to help prevent falling.
10. Fill tub with water or adjust shower flow (95–105°F).
11. Help patient undress. Give a male patient a towel to wrap around his midriff.
12. Assist patient into tub or shower. If shower, leave weak patient in shower chair.

NOTE: Remember to put on gloves.

13. Wash patient's back. Observe carefully for reddened areas or breaks in skin.
14. Patient may be left alone to complete genitalia area if feeling strong.

NOTE: If patient shows signs of weakness, remove plug from tub and drain water, or turn off shower. Allow patient to rest until feeling better.

15. Assist patient from tub or shower.
16. Wrap bath towel around patient to prevent chilling.
17. Remove gloves and put in biohazardous container.
18. Assist in drying and dressing.
19. Return to unit and make comfortable. Make sure call bell is within patient's reach.
20. Put away equipment.
21. Clean bathtub with disinfectant solution.

Postprocedure

22. Wash hands.
23. Chart procedure and how patient tolerated it.

NOTE: Use gloves if you are in contact with body fluids.

Charting Example:

7/07/24	0900	
	Assisted with shower	
	Taken to shower on shower chair	
	No skin problems noted	
	Tolerated well	
		A. Chaplin CNA

Procedure 19.47 Patient Gown Change

BACKGROUND: Changing a patient's gown makes the patient feel clean and refreshed. It also allows you to visually examine the skin.
ALERT: Follow Standard Precautions

Preprocedure

1. Wash hands.
2. Assemble equipment: clean patient gown.
3. Tell patient what you are going to do.
4. Provide privacy by pulling privacy curtain.
5. Put on gloves in case you come in contact with bodily fluids.

Procedure

6. Untie strings of gown at neck and midback. (It may be necessary to assist patient onto side.)
7. Pull soiled gown out from sides of patient.
8. Unfold clean gown and position over patient.
9. Remove soiled gown one sleeve at a time.
10. Leave soiled gown laying over patient's chest; insert one arm into sleeve of clean gown.
11. Fold soiled gown to one side as clean gown is placed over patient's chest.
12. Insert other arm in empty sleeve of gown.
13. Tie neck string on side of neck.
14. Tie midback tie if patient desires.
15. Remove soiled gown to linen hamper.
16. Slip gown under covers, being careful not to expose patient.
17. Position patient for comfort.
18. Raise side rails when necessary.
19. Place bedside stand and call light in patient's reach.

Postprocedure

20. Remove gloves and put in biohazardous container.
21. Wash hands.

Procedure 19.48 Perineal Care

BACKGROUND: Perineal care provides cleansing around areas where body waste is eliminated. The perineal area is dark, warm, and moist, providing an environment for bacterial growth. Keeping the perineum free of drainage and bacteria is an important preventive health measure and helps patients feel more comfortable.
ALERT: Follow Standard Precautions

Preprocedure

1. Wash hands.
2. Assemble equipment:
   a. Bath blanket
   b. Bedpan and cover
   c. Basin
   d. Solution, water, or other if ordered
   e. Cotton balls
   f. Waterproof protector for bed
   g. Disposable gloves
   h. Perineal pad and belt if needed
3. Identify patient.
4. Explain what you are going to do.
5. Provide privacy by pulling privacy curtain.

Procedure

6. Put warm water in basin.
7. Raise bed to a comfortable working height.
8. Lower side rail.
9. Put on disposable gloves.

(continued)

Measuring Vital Signs and Other Clinical Skills | Chapter 19 651

Procedure Tip

19.47 Patient Gown Change

- Review the background information, discussing the benefits of changing the patient's gown regularly.
- Emphasize the importance of following Standard Precautions.
- Review the preprocedure steps.
- Step 1: Emphasize the importance of proper handwashing.
- Step 3: Emphasize the importance of effective communication techniques.
- Step 4: Emphasize the importance of patient privacy.
- Step 5: Emphasize the importance of wearing gloves.
- Review the procedure steps.
- Steps 8–16: Emphasize the importance of patient privacy.
- Review the postprocedure steps.
- Step 21: Emphasize the importance of proper handwashing.
- Emphasize the importance of observation and documentation.

PROCEDURE PRACTICE

- Demonstrate the steps for Procedure 19.47, Patient Gown Change, as many times as necessary, or ask students to demonstrate the steps. Have students practice and perform the procedure until they are competent.

TEAMWORK

In small groups, research special bathing considerations for certain types of patients. For example, women who just gave birth and people who are recovering from invasive surgery might have different requirements. Report your findings to the class.

Procedure Tip

19.48 Perineal Care

- Review the background information, emphasizing the importance of cleaning the perineal every day.
- Emphasize the importance of following Standard Precautions.
- Review the preprocedure steps.
- Step 1: Emphasize the importance of proper handwashing.
- Step 2: Review the equipment list.
- Steps 3 and 4: Emphasize the importance of effective communication techniques.
- Step 5: Emphasize the importance of patient privacy.
- Review the procedure steps.

Procedure Tip

19.48 Perineal Care, continued

- Step 11: Emphasize the importance of patient privacy.
- Step 13: Emphasize importance of keeping bed dry.
- Review the postprocedure steps.
- Step 23: Emphasize the importance of proper handwashing.
- Emphasize the importance of observation and documentation.

PROCEDURE PRACTICE

- Using a mannequin, demonstrate the steps for Procedure 19.48, Perineal Care, as many times as necessary, or ask students to demonstrate the steps. Have students practice and perform the procedure using a mannequin until they are competent.

Teaching Tips

- Explain the importance of caring for a patient's hair and nails.
- Emphasize personal hygiene and comfort.
- Discuss methods of cleaning hair and scalp.
- Emphasize need for doctor's order to use chemical shampoos.
- Discuss the risks of long nails.
- Emphasize that patient's with diabetes must have their toenails cut by a podiatrist.
- Explain that diabetic patients tend to have poor circulation and do not heal well.
- This results in severe ulcerations if their skin is nicked or broken.
- Emphasize the importance of checking with the charge nurse prior to cutting a patient's nails.

Procedure 19.48 **Perineal Care (continued)**

Procedure (cont)

10. Remove spread and blanket.
11. Cover patient with bath blanket.
12. Have patient hold top of bath blanket, and fold top sheet to bottom of bed.
13. Place waterproof protector under patient's buttocks.
14. Pull up bath blanket to expose perineal area.
15. Provide male and female pericare:
    a. Circumcised male: Wipe away from urinary meatus as you wash with soap and water, rinse, and dry in a circular motion. Clean the shaft of the penis from top to bottom.
    b. Uncircumcised male: Gently move foreskin back away from tip of penis. Wash as directed in step a. After drying, gently move foreskin back over tip of penis.
    c. Female:
        (1) Instruct patient to bend knees with feet flat on bed.
        (2) Separate patient's knees.
        (3) Separate the labia and wipe from front to back away from the urethra as you wash with soap and water, rinse, and dry. Use a clean part of the washcloth for each stroke.
16. Remove waterproof protector from bed and dispose of gloves.
17. Cover patient with sheet and remove bath blanket.
18. Return top covers.
19. Return bed to lowest position and put up side rails if required.
20. Secure call bell within patient's reach.

Postprocedure

21. Clean equipment; dispose of disposable material according to hospital policy.
22. Discard gloves and put in biohazardous container.
23. Wash hands.

Charting Example:

4/14/24	1045
	Perineal care provided
	Observed a dime-sized reddened area
	on the interior left thigh approximately
	2 inches below the groin
	R. Johnson CNA

Care of Hair and Nails

Hair and nail care helps patients feel good about themselves. Good grooming adds to a feeling of well-being. Hair is always kept clean and neatly arranged. Style hair appropriately for the age of the patient. For example, ponytails are not a hairstyle that an elderly person would normally select. If patients can have a tub bath or shower, shampoo their hair at bath time.

It is important to keep your patients' hair clean even when they are on bed rest. Today there are chemical shampoos that remove oil and refresh the scalp. You will need a physician's order together with a facility policy that says you can use a chemical shampoo. To use a packaged chemical on the hair, always follow the directions on the package. To wash hair in bed with water and shampoo, carefully follow the steps below.

Keep nails trimmed and clean. Long nails may scratch the patient or someone else. They break more easily and are more difficult to clean when they are not kept short. Toenails may become very thick and hard. Often it is necessary to have a podiatrist (foot doctor) cut them.

652 Chapter 19 | Measuring Vital Signs and Other Clinical Skills

If the patient has diabetes, *do not cut the nails.* Diabetic patients tend to have poor circulation and do not heal well. This results in severe **ulcerations** if their skin is knicked or broken. Whenever you cut fingernails or toenails, check first with the charge nurse.

ulcerations (UHL suhr ay shuhns) Open areas, or sores.

Procedure 19.49 Shampooing the Hair in Bed

BACKGROUND: Clean hair makes a patient feel fresh and provides a sense of well-being. Your careful attention to the steps below will make this a pleasant experience for the patient and yourself.
ALERT: Follow Standard Precautions

Preprocedure

1. Wash hands.
2. Assemble equipment:
   a. Chair
   b. Basin of water (105°F)
   c. Pitcher of water (115°F)
   d. Paper or Styrofoam cup
   e. Large basin
   f. Shampoo tray or plastic sheet
   g. Waterproof bed protector
   h. Pillow with waterproof cover
   i. Bath towels
   j. Small towel
   k. Cotton balls
3. Identify patient.
4. Explain what you are going to do.
5. Provide privacy by pulling privacy curtain.

Procedure

6. Raise bed to a comfortable working position.
7. Place a chair at side of bed near patient's head.
8. Place small towel on chair.
9. Place large basin on chair to catch water.
10. Put cotton in patient's ears to keep water out of ears.
11. Have patient move to side of bed with head close to where you are standing.
12. Remove pillow from under head. Lower head of bed and remove pillows. Cover pillow with waterproof case.
13. Place pillow under patient's back so that when he or she lies down the head will be tilted back.
14. Place bath blanket on bed.
15. Have patient hold top of bath blanket, and pull top covers to foot.
16. Place waterproof protector under head.
17. Put shampoo tray under patient's head (i.e., plastic bag with both ends open).
18. Place end of plastic in large basin.
19. Have patient hold washcloth over eyes.
20. Put basin of water on bedside table with paper cup. Have pitcher of water for extra water. Test water temperature to ensure it is safe and comfortable before wetting patient's hair. Adjust if needed.
21. Brush patient's hair thoroughly.
22. Fill cup with water from basin.
23. Pour water over hair; repeat until completely wet.
24. Apply small amount of shampoo; use both hands to massage the patient's scalp with your fingertips. Be careful not to scratch the scalp with your fingernails.
25. Rinse soap off hair by pouring water from cup over hair. Have patient turn head from side to side. Repeat until completely rinsed.
26. Dry patient's forehead and ears.
27. Remove cotton from ears.
28. Lift patient's head gently and wrap with bath towel.
29. Remove equipment from bed.
30. Change patient's gown and be certain patient is dry.
31. Gently dry patient's hair with towel. (Use a hair dryer if allowed by your facility.)

(continued)

Measuring Vital Signs and Other Clinical Skills | Chapter 19 653

Procedure Tip

19.49 Shampooing the Hair in Bed

- Review the background information, explaining that clean hair can make a patient happier and more comfortable.
- Emphasize the importance of following Standard Precautions.
- Review the preprocedure steps.
- Step 1: Emphasize the importance of proper handwashing.
- Step 2: Review the equipment list.
- Steps 3 and 4: Emphasize the importance of effective communication techniques.
- Step 5: Emphasize the importance of patient privacy.
- Review the procedure steps.
- Step 13: Emphasize proper positioning.
- Step 16: Emphasize importance of keeping bed dry.
- Step 25: Emphasize importance of rinsing completely.
- Steps 30 and 31: Emphasize importance of drying completely.

PROCEDURE PRACTICE

- Demonstrate the steps for Procedure 19.49, Shampooing the Hair in Bed, as many times as necessary, or ask students to demonstrate the steps. Have students practice and perform the procedure until they are competent. If students will be using real water, remind them to bring bathing suits or quick-dry clothes to wear while practicing. Alternatively, use a mannequin.

Procedure Tip

19.50 Shampooing in Shower or Tub

- Review the background information, explaining that clean hair makes a patient happier and more comfortable.
- Emphasize the importance of following Standard Precautions.
- Review the preprocedure steps.
- Step 1: Emphasize the importance of proper handwashing.
- Step 2: Review the equipment list.
- Step 3: Emphasize the importance of patient privacy.
- Step 4: Emphasize the importance of effective communication techniques.
- Review the procedure steps.
- Step 5: Explain that patient is already in shower or tub.
- Step 9: Emphasize importance of rinsing completely.
- Steps 14 and 16: Emphasize importance of drying.

Procedure 19.49 Shampooing the Hair in Bed (continued)

Procedure (cont)

32. Comb or brush hair and arrange neatly.
33. Remove bath blanket and cover patient with top covers.
34. Make patient comfortable.
35. Lower bed to its lowest position.
36. Put up side rail if required.

Postprocedure

37. Return equipment.
38. Tidy unit.
39. Wash hands.
40. Record procedure.

Charting Example:

9/06/24	1130
	Hair washed while in bed
	There is a dime-sized red scaly area
	on scalp directly above left ear
	Resident denies pain or itching at site
	Notified charge nurse
	Hair dried with hair dryer and styled
	to suit resident
	R. Johnson CNA

Procedure 19.50 Shampooing in Shower or Tub

BACKGROUND: Clean hair makes a patient feel fresh and provides a sense of well-being. Your careful attention to the steps below will make this a pleasant experience for the patient and yourself.
ALERT: Follow Standard Precautions

Preprocedure

1. Wash hands.
2. Assemble equipment:
   a. Shampoo
   b. Washcloth
   c. Towel
   d. Cream rinse, if desired
3. Provide privacy by pulling curtain or door.
4. Explain what you are going to do.

Procedure

5. Instruct patient to tip head back.
6. Wet hair with water, being careful not to get eyes wet.
7. Give patient a washcloth to wipe his or her face as needed.
8. Apply a moderate amount of shampoo to hair. Massage head and hair until a lather develops. (Be careful not to use fingernails.)
9. Rinse hair with clean, clear water until shampoo has disappeared.
10. Repeat shampooing procedure a second time. When rinsing, be sure to remove all shampoo.
11. If a cream rinse is used, apply a small amount to hair, paying special attention to ends of hair.
12. Allow rinse to remain on hair for a few seconds before rinsing.
13. Rinse thoroughly with clean, clear water.
14. Towel dry.
15. Gently comb or brush hair to remove tangles.
16. Use a hair dryer to dry hair.
17. Arrange in an appropriate hairstyle for the patient's age and manner. (Remember that ponytails, pigtails, etc. are not appropriate for a 70-year-old patient.)

(continued)

654 Chapter 19 | Measuring Vital Signs and Other Clinical Skills

Procedure 19.50 Shampooing in Shower or Tub (continued)

Postprocedure

18. Return equipment.
19. Wash hands.
20. Record procedure.

Charting Example:

10/13/24 0830
Hair washed while in shower
Scalp is clean and there is no
evidence of sores or scratches present
Upon return to room, hair styled
according to resident's preference
A. Chaplin CNA

Procedure 19.51 Arranging the Hair

BACKGROUND: A patient's outward appearance plays a significant role in his or her self-image. Arranging the hair is a key part of the daily grooming routine for every patient. It is important to arrange your patient's hair according to their preferences.
ALERT: Follow Standard Precautions

Preprocedure

1. Wash hands.
2. Assemble equipment:
   a. Comb and/or brush
   b. Towel
3. Identify patient.
4. Explain what you are going to do.
5. Provide privacy by pulling privacy curtain.
6. Raise bed to a comfortable working height.

Procedure

7. Assist as needed.
8. If total assistance is needed:
   a. Section the hair, starting at one side, working around to other side.
   b. Comb or brush hair thoroughly, being careful not to pull it.
   c. Arrange hair neatly.
9. Lower bed to lowest position.
10. Put up side rail if required.
11. Secure call light in patient's reach.

Postprocedure

12. Clean and replace all equipment.
13. Wash hands.
14. Report procedure and observations (e.g., dry scalp, reddened areas).

Measuring Vital Signs and Other Clinical Skills | Chapter 19 655

Procedure Tip

19.50 Shampooing in Shower or Tub, continued

- Review the postprocedure steps.
- Step 19: Emphasize the importance of proper handwashing.
- Step 20: Emphasize the importance of observation and documentation.

PROCEDURE PRACTICE

- Demonstrate the steps for Procedure 19.50, Shampooing in Shower or Tub, as many times as necessary, or ask students to demonstrate the steps. Have students practice and perform the procedure until they are competent. If students will be using real water, remind them to bring bathing suits or quick-dry clothes to wear while practicing. Alternatively, use a mannequin.

Procedure Tip

19.51 Arranging the Hair

- Review the background information, explaining the benefits of a positive self-image.
- Emphasize the importance of following Standard Precautions.
- Review the preprocedure steps.
- Step 1: Emphasize the importance of proper handwashing.
- Steps 3 and 4: Emphasize the importance of effective communication techniques.
- Step 5: Emphasize the importance of privacy.
- Review the procedure steps.
- Step 7: Emphasize the importance of patient independence.
- Review the postprocedure steps.
- Step 13: Emphasize the importance of proper handwashing.
- Step 14: Emphasize the importance of observation and documentation.

PROCEDURE PRACTICE

- Demonstrate the steps for Procedure 19.51, Arranging the Hair, as many times as necessary, or ask students to demonstrate the steps. Have students practice and perform the procedure until they are competent.

Procedure Tip

19.52 Nail Care

- Review the background information, discussing the benefits of a daily grooming routine.
- Emphasize the importance of following Standard Precautions.
- Review the preprocedure steps.
- Step 1: Emphasize the importance of proper handwashing.
- Step 3: Emphasize the importance of effective communication techniques.
- Step 4: Emphasize the importance of patient privacy.
- Step 7: Emphasize the importance of wearing gloves.
- Review the procedure steps.
- Step 8: Emphasize the importance of drying hand completely.
- Step 9: Emphasize that nails should only be cut if approved by the charge nurse and facility policy.
- Review the postprocedure steps.
- Step 18: Emphasize the importance of proper handwashing.
- Step 19: Emphasize the importance of observation and documentation.

PROCEDURE PRACTICE

- Demonstrate the steps for Procedure 19.52, Nail Care, as many times as necessary, or ask students to demonstrate the steps. Have students practice and perform the procedure until they are competent.

Procedure 19.52 Nail Care

BACKGROUND: A patient's outward appearance plays a significant role in his or her self-image. Nail care is a key part of the daily grooming routine for every patient. Keeping nails clean and trimmed prevents sores from developing around the nail beds and eliminates unintentional scratches that could become infected.
ALERT: Follow Standard Precautions

Preprocedure

1. Wash hands.
2. Assemble equipment:
   a. Warm water
   b. Orange sticks
   c. Emery board
   d. Nail clippers

NOTE: Do not clip a diabetic patient's nails.

3. Identify the patient and explain the procedure.
4. Provide privacy for the patient by pulling a curtain or closing the door.
5. Test water temperature and ensure it is safe and comfortable before immersing patient's fingers in water; adjust if needed.
6. Place basin of water at a comfortable level for patients. Cleanse nails by soaking in water.
7. Put on gloves.

Procedure

8. Use slanted edge of orange stick to clean dirt out from under nails. Wipe orangewood stick on towel after each nail and dry patient's hand/fingers, including between fingers.
9. File nails with emery board to shorten. (Clip if permitted by your facility.)
10. Use smooth edge of emery board to smooth.
11. Apply lotion to help condition cuticle.
12. Massage hands and feet with lotion.
13. Make patient comfortable.
14. Raise side rail if required. Make sure call bell is within reach.

Postprocedure

15. Empty, rinse, and wipe basin.
16. Return equipment.
17. Remove and dispose of gloves in biohazardous container.
18. Wash hands.
19. Record procedure and any unusual conditions (e.g., hangnails, broken nails).

Charting Example:

12/10/24	0730
	Nails trimmed and filed.
	R. Johnson CNA

Procedure 19.53 **Foot Care**

BACKGROUND: Providing and assisting with foot care is an important part of total patient care. For elderly patients and the diabetic patient, improper foot care can lead to decreased mobility and even loss of mobility.

Both the elderly and the diabetic may experience decreased circulation and decreased sensation to the lower extremities. This makes it even more imperative that the condition of the feet are checked frequently for any change in status or acute problems.

ALERT: Follow Standard Precautions

Preprocedure

1. Wash hands.
2. Put on disposable gloves.
3. Explain procedure to patient and provide for patient privacy with curtain, screen, or door.

Procedure

4. Inspect the feet for any problems/change in skin integrity. Check for the presence of pulses and note their strengths. Assess for any patient complaints.
5. Test water temperature and ensure it is safe and comfortable before placing patient's foot in water and adjust if needed.
6. Place basin at a good position on protective barrier.
7. Completely submerge and soak foot in water
8. Bathe the feet thoroughly in tepid water with a mild soap. Be sure to clean the interdigital areas.
9. Dry the feet thoroughly, paying particular attention to the interdigital areas. Apply lotion to feet but avoid leaving lotion in the interdigital areas, as it could provide a moist environment for bacteria and fungal growth. Support foot and ankle throughout the procedure.
10. If nails are overgrown, use a file instead of scissors or clippers. If the patient is a diabetic and a file is not sufficient, refer the patient to a podiatrist for care.
11. Empty, rinse, and wipe bath basin and return to proper storage.
12. Dispose of soiled linens in proper container. Remove glove and place in biohazardous container.
13. Make sure the patient is comfortable and the call bell is within reach.
14. Discourage the patient from going barefoot. Decreased sensation may allow an injury to occur without the patient noting it.
15. Encourage the patient to use appropriate footwear. Ill-fitting shoes may contribute to skin breakdown. All new footwear should be broken in gradually over time. All shoes that are rough or worn or do not provide adequate foot support should be discarded.
16. Clean, dry socks that provide warmth, absorb perspiration, and protect the feet should be worn.

Postprocedure

17. Return equipment.
18. Remove and dispose of gloves in biohazardous container.
19. Wash hands.
20. Report any signs of foot problems to the physician. Early interventions will diminish the magnitude of any problems noted.

NOTE: It is always the caregiver's responsibility to provide education to the patient while providing care.

Charting Example:

12/10/24 0730
Toenails trimmed; patient complaining of callous on right heel.
R. Johnson CNA

Shaving the Patient

Men usually shave every day when they are able to care for themselves. Encourage them to shave themselves when possible. They will feel much better about themselves. If they are unable to shave themselves, take time to shave them.

Measuring Vital Signs and Other Clinical Skills | Chapter 19 657

PROCEDURE PRACTICE

- Demonstrate the steps for Procedure 19.53, Foot Care, as many times as necessary, or ask students to demonstrate the steps. Have students practice and perform the procedure until they are competent.

Procedure Tip

19.53 Foot Care

- Review the background information, emphasizing that foot care is more than just cosmetic, as foot problems can lead to decreased mobility and other serious issues.
- Emphasize the importance of following Standard Precautions.
- Review the preprocedure steps.
- Step 1: Emphasize the importance of proper handwashing.
- Step 2: Emphasize the importance of wearing gloves.
- Step 3: Emphasize the importance of effective communication techniques and patient privacy.
- Review the procedure steps.
- Step 4: Emphasize the importance of observation and documentation.
- Step 9: Emphasize the importance of washing and drying feet completely.
- Step 10: Emphasize that nails should not be cut.
- Steps 14 and 15: Discuss the importance of patient education.
- Review the postprocedure steps.
- Step 19: Emphasize the importance of proper handwashing.
- Step 20: Emphasize the importance of observation and documentation.

Procedure Tip

19.54 Shaving the Patient

- Review the background information, emphasizing the importance of a daily grooming routine.
- Emphasize the importance of following Standard Precautions.
- Review the preprocedure steps.
- Step 1: Emphasize the importance of proper handwashing.
- Step 2: Review the equipment list.
- Step 3: Emphasize the importance of effective communication techniques.
- Step 4: Emphasize the importance of patient privacy.
- Review the procedure steps.
- Step 8: Emphasize the importance of sufficient lighting.
- Step 9: Emphasize the importance of wearing gloves.
- Review the postprocedure steps.
- Step 12: Emphasize the importance of proper handwashing.
- Step 13: Emphasize the importance of observation and documentation.

PROCEDURE PRACTICE

- Demonstrate the steps for Procedure 19.54, Shaving the Patient, as many times as necessary, or ask students to demonstrate the steps. Have students practice and perform the procedure until they are competent.

Women tend to have facial hair when they age. This can be very distressing to the patient. Follow the procedures that your facility has to remove the facial hair. In some facilities it is plucked; in others it is shaved. Be certain to look in the procedure book.

Procedure 19.54 Shaving the Patient

BACKGROUND: A patient's outward appearance plays a significant role in his or her self-image. Shaving facial hair is a key part of the daily grooming routine for many patients. Carefully follow the steps below as you groom your patient each day.

ALERT: Follow Standard Precautions

Preprocedure

1. Wash hands.
2. Assemble equipment:
   a. Electric shaver or safety razor
   b. Shaving lather or an electric preshave lotion
   c. Basin of warm water
   d. Face towel
   e. Mirror
   f. Aftershave
   g. Disposable gloves
3. Identify patient and explain what you are going to do.
4. Provide privacy by pulling privacy curtains.

Procedure

5. Raise head of bed if permitted.
6. Place equipment on overbed table.
7. Place a towel over patient's chest.
8. Adjust light so that it shines on patient's face.
9. Shave patient.
   a. If you are using a safety razor:
      (1) Put on gloves.
      (2) Moisten face and apply lather.
      (3) Start in front of ear; hold skin taut and bring razor down over cheek toward chin. Use short firm strokes. Repeat until lather on cheek is removed and skin is smooth.
      (4) Repeat on other cheek.
      (5) Wash face and neck. Dry thoroughly.
      (6) Apply aftershave lotion or powder if desired.
      (7) Discard gloves according to facility policy.
   b. If you are using an electric shaver:
      (1) Put on gloves.
      (2) Apply preshave lotion.
      (3) Gently shave until beard is removed.
      (4) Wash face and neck. Dry thoroughly.
      (5) Apply aftershave lotion or powder if desired.
      (6) Remove gloves.
10. Lower bed if you raised it and make sure side rails are up.
11. Make sure patient is comfortable and call bell is within reach.

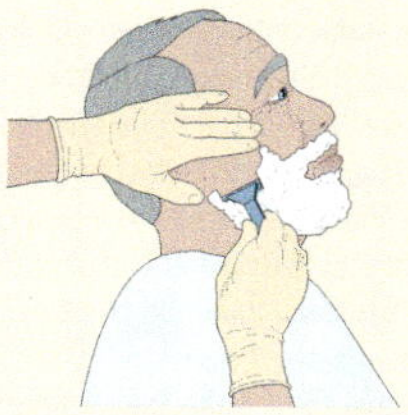

Postprocedure

12. Wash hands.
13. Chart procedure and how procedure was tolerated.

Charting Example:

12/10/24 0730
Face shaved with a safety razor
Skin is clear and free of irritation
R. Johnson CNA

658 Chapter 19 | Measuring Vital Signs and Other Clinical Skills

Dressing and Undressing the Patient

It is very important for the patient to be up and dressed. Patients must not remain in bed unless the doctor orders bedrest. Being up and dressed creates an attitude of wellness. Staying in bedclothes presents an attitude of "being sick." Be certain that patients are dressed nicely and that their clothes are in good repair. Match the clothing rather than just throwing on "anything that's handy."

For patients who have a handicap, take special care in how you put on their clothes. This is also true of patients who have an IV. The following are some rules to follow:

- Always dress the weak or most involved side first. A **limb** that does not function well slides into a sleeve or pant leg if you start on that side.
- Always undress the weak or most involved side last.
- If the patient has an IV, be very careful not to disturb or dislodge it.

Career Connect

Dealing with terminal care situations can be an extremely rewarding experience, but it is not for everyone. Volunteer at a hospice and shadow one of the health care professionals working there as they deal with terminal patients, the death of a patient, and the families left behind.

limb
(LIM)
Arm, leg.

Terminal and Postmortem Care

You might be called upon to provide care for someone who is dying. Always be gentle and respectful both before and after death. Before death occurs, gently wash away discharges that have accumulated. As death approaches, the muscles lose their tone and the body openings drain. Gently straighten the limbs and make the patient as comfortable as possible. After death occurs, you may be asked to prepare the body. Check the procedures of the facility you work in and follow the steps your facility provides.

The loss of a family member is a very significant time for loved ones. It is important that we provide as much time as necessary for the family to be with the patient preceding and immediately after death. Cleaning the deceased patient and placing the patient in a comfortable position for the family to view is an important part of a nurse's care.

Apply It

As a class, discuss how to appropriately interact with family members of a recently deceased patient. Once you are aware of the type of behavior you should exhibit and the kinds of things you should say, divide into groups and role play the scenario.

Procedure 19.55 Postmortem Care

BACKGROUND: Provides direction for the preparation of the body following death.
ALERT: Follow Standard Precautions

Preprocedure

1. Wash hands.
2. Assemble equipment:
   a. Wash basin with warm water
   b. Washcloth and towel
   c. Shroud/postmortem set:
      (1) Sheet or plastic container
      (2) Identification tags
      (3) Large container for personal belongings
      (4) Plastic pad

(continued)

Teaching Tips

- Explain proper dressing and undressing of the patient.
- Explain that dressing gets patient out of bed and ready for visitors.
- It also promotes well-being.
- Grooming should always be age appropriate.
- Resident should be allowed to select clothes.
- Review common rules:
  - Dress the weak or most involved side first
  - Undress the weak or most involved side last
  - Use extreme caution when dressing and undressing patients who have IVs
- Define and describe terminal and postmortem care.
- Explain that after death:
  - Muscles lose their tone
  - Body openings drain
- Discuss proper behavior:
  - Be gentle
  - Be respectful
  - Follow the facility's guidelines for postmortem care

Career Connect

- You may want to prepare a list of hospice facilities in the area.
- Only certain students will show an interest in this type of occupation; they should be encouraged.
- You may want to contact the hospice or other end-of-life specialist to set up visits or job shadows.
- Alternatively, prepare the student by practicing how he or she will contact the professional.
- If a job shadow or site visit is not possible, you might invite the professional to address the class.
- Alternatively, students may conduct telephone or e-mail interviews with the professional.

Apply It

- Guide students in a discussion that elicits appropriate comments and behavior to use with family members of deceased patients.
- Arrange for students to work in small groups for their role play.
- Allow time for students to complete their role play and discuss their responses to it.

Procedure Tip

19.55 Postmortem Care

- Review the background information, emphasizing the need for respect and consideration for the deceased and the family.
- Emphasize the importance of following Standard Precautions.
- Review the preprocedure steps.
- Step 1: Emphasize the importance of proper handwashing.
- Step 2: Review the equipment list.
- Step 3: Emphasize the importance for privacy as a sign of respect.
- Step 4: Emphasize the importance of wearing gloves.
- Review the procedure steps.
- Step 5: Emphasize proper positioning.
- Step 11: Emphasize the importance of cleaning the body.
- Step 13: Emphasize the importance of identification.
- Step 14: Follow facility's procedures.
- Step 16: Emphasize the importance of proper handwashing.
- Step 17: Emphasize the importance of caring for personal belongings
- Step 19: Emphasize importance of documenting personal belongings.
- Review the postprocedure steps.
- Step 21: Emphasize the importance of proper handwashing.
- Step 22: Emphasize the importance of observation and documentation.

Procedure 19.55 Postmortem Care (continued)

Preprocedure (cont)

   d. Gurney or morgue cart
   e. Nonsterile disposable gloves
3. Close privacy curtains.
4. Put on gloves.

Procedure

5. Position body in good alignment in supine position.
6. Keep one pillow under head.
7. Straighten arms and legs.
8. Gently close each eye. Do not apply pressure to eyelids.
9. Put dentures in mouth or in a denture cup. If placed in a denture cup, put cup inside shroud so that mortician can find.
10. Remove all soiled dressings or clothing.
11. Bathe body thoroughly.
12. Apply clean dressings where needed.
13. Attach identification tags to wrists and ankles. Tag is usually placed on the right great toe and also on the outside of the shroud. Fill in tags with:
    a. Name
    b. Sex
    c. Hospital ID number
    d. Age
14. Place body in a shroud, sheet, or other appropriate container. Do this in the following way:
    a. Ask for assistance from a co-worker.
    b. Logroll body to one side. Place shroud behind body leaving enough material to support body when rolled back. Fan-fold remaining shroud next to body.
    c. Place a plastic protection pad under buttocks.
    d. Roll body on its back and then to the other side.
    e. Pull fan-folded portion of shroud until flat.
    f. Roll body on its back.
    g. Cover entire body with shroud.
    h. Tuck in all loose edges of cover.
    i. Position a tie above elbows and below knees and secure around body.
    j. Attach ID tag to tie just above elbows.
15. Remove gloves and discard according to facility policy and procedure.
16. Wash hands.
17. Place all personal belongings in a large container. Label container with:
    a. Patient's name
    b. Age
    c. Room number
18. Place list of belongings in container and on patient's chart.
19. Follow your facility's procedure for transporting body and belongings through hallways.
20. Remove all linen and other supplies from room.

Postprocedure

21. Wash hands.
22. Report procedure completed to charge nurse.

Charting Example:

12/07/24	0430
	Postmortem care completed
	Belongings listed and placed in bag,
	given to family
	Charge nurse notified
	R. Johnson CNA

660 Chapter 19 | Measuring Vital Signs and Other Clinical Skills

ACTIVITY

Have students make sample "toe tag" postmortem identification tags.

Prosthetic Devices

A prosthesis or prosthetic device replaces or aids a body part that is injured, lost, or not working correctly. These include:

- Dentures
- Glasses/contact lenses
- Hearing aids
- Artificial limbs
- Artificial eyes
- Artificial breasts (after mastectomy)

These devices are very important to the well-being of the patient and are treated carefully. You need to learn the correct way to put them on. Your patient is an excellent source of information on how they fit. Always put them in the same place when the patient is not using them, so that they are not lost and the patient can find them.

Bedmaking

When bedding is wrinkled or wet, it causes irritation to the skin and is very uncomfortable. Keeping the bed smooth and dry prevents a decubitus, a severe breakdown of the skin (see the section "Skin Management" on page 608).

The number of times that you change the bed depends on whether or not the patient is continent. When the patient is in bed, check to be sure that the wrinkles are smoothed out and that the bed is dry.

The hospital bed has a small sheet, called a draw sheet that is placed in the midsection of the bed between the patient's knees and shoulders. This provides protection to the bottom sheet and can be changed easily without having to change the entire bottom sheet.

Often, a plastic cover is placed over the bottom sheet and under the draw sheet to prevent soiling. Be certain that the plastic sheet is always smooth.

There are several ways that hospital beds are made. If the patient is up and about, you make a closed bed. If the patient must remain in bed, you have to make an occupied bed. When the patient is in and out of bed during the day, you make an open bed.

Measuring Vital Signs and Other Clinical Skills | Chapter 19 661

Teaching Tips

- Define prosthetic device.
- Explain common and uncommon devices:
  - Dentures
  - Glasses/contact lenses
  - Hearing aids
  - Artificial limbs
  - Artificial eyes
  - Artificial breasts
  - Pacemakers
- Explain the importance of maintaining the devices and keeping them safe.
- Explain key principles of bedmaking:
  - Importance of keeping linen wrinkle-free and dry to prevent pressure sores
  - Draw sheet and how it is used
- Explain the types of beds:
  - Closed bed: Patient has been moved or discharged
  - Open bed: Patient is in and out of bed during the day
  - Occupied bed: Patient remains in bed

ACTIVITY

Make a table or chart comparing the three types of beds: closed, open, and occupied.

Procedure Tip

19.56 Making a Closed Bed

- Review the background information, emphasizing that a closed bed is when the patient has been moved or discharged.
- Emphasize the importance of following Standard Precautions.
- Review the preprocedure steps.
- Step 1: Emphasize the importance of proper handwashing.
- Step 2: Review the list of necessary equipment.
- Review the procedure steps.
- Have students refer to illustrations for proper procedure.
- Reinforce need to keep linens wrinkle-free.

ACTIVITY

Instruct students to write step-by-step procedures for how they make their beds at home.

Procedure 19.56 Making a Closed Bed

BACKGROUND: Clean linens help prevent the spread of bacteria in the health care environment. A closed bed is made ready for new admissions or when a patient is not expected to return to bed until evening. Neatly made beds create a sense of order.

ALERT: Follow Standard Precautions

Preprocedure

1. Wash hands.
2. Assemble equipment:
   a. Mattress pad, if used
   b. Fitted bottom sheet and one large sheet
   c. Draw sheet or large pad
   d Blankets as needed
   e. Spread
   f. Pillow
   g Pillowcase
3. Raise bed to a comfortable working height. Lock wheels on bed.

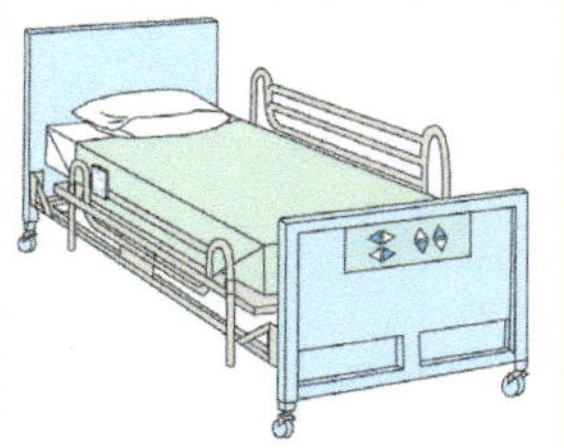

4. Place a chair at the side of bed.
5. Put linen on chair in the order in which you will use it. (First things you will use go on top.)

Procedure

6. Place the bottom sheet on top of the mattress pad. Unfold the sheet lengthwise. The center fold should be in the middle of the bed with the hem stitching facing the mattress pad (see Figure a). Pull the sheet up to align the bottom edge of the sheet with the bottom of the mattress. (If your facility uses a fitted bottom sheet, pull the corners of the sheet smoothly over the corners of the mattress.)
7. Smooth the sheet and tuck it tightly under the top of the mattress.
8. Make a mitered corner at the head of the bed by:
   a. Picking up the sheet hanging at the side of the bed, about 12 inches from the head of the bed, and forming a triangle (see Figure b).
   b. Placing the triangle (the folded corner) on top of the mattress (see Figure c).
   c. Tucking the hanging portion of the sheet well under the mattress (see Figure d).
   d. Bringing the triangle down over the side of the mattress while holding the fold at the edge of the mattress.
   e. Tucking the sheet under the mattress from head to foot (see Figure e).

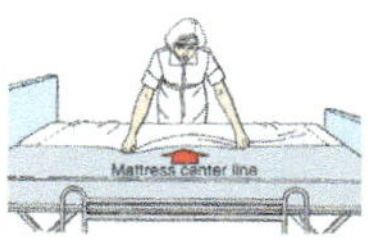

Figure a

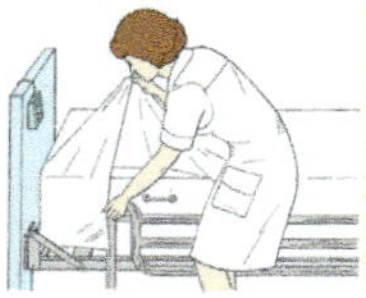

Figure b

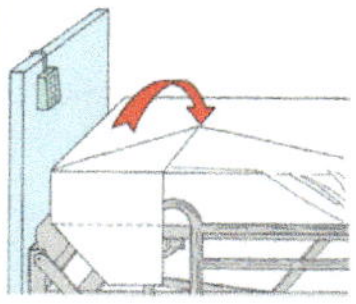

Figure c

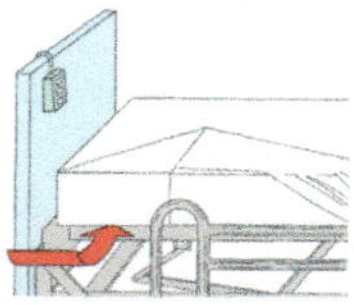

Figure d

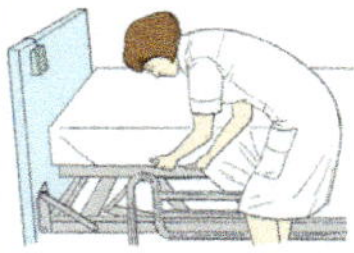

Figure e

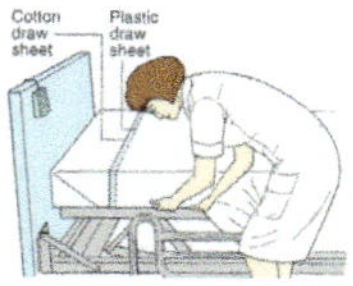

Figure f

(continued)

Procedure 19.56 **Making a Closed Bed (continued)**

Procedure (cont)

9. If used, place the plastic and cotton draw sheets with the upper edges about 14 inches from the head of the mattress and tuck them under one side. Be sure the cotton draw sheet completely covers the plastic one (see Figure f).
10. Apply the top sheet, wrong side up, with the hem even with the upper edge of the mattress.
11. Spread and center the blanket and bedspread over the top sheet and the foot of the mattress.
12. Tuck the top sheet, blanket, and bedspread under the mattress at the foot of the bed. Make a mitered corner at the foot of the bed. Do not tuck in the sides.
13. Go to the other side of the bed and fold the top linens to the center of the bed.
14. Tuck the bottom sheet under the head of the mattress and make a mitered corner.
15. Working from top to bottom, pull the sheet tight and tuck it under the mattress.
16. Pull the draw sheets tight and tuck them under the mattress separately.
17. Straighten the top sheet, blanket, and bedspread, and tuck them in at the foot of the bed. Make a mitered corner. (Note: Some beds are made with a toe pleat in the top covers [sheet, blanket, and bedspread]. This lessens the pressure of the covers on the feet. To create a toe pleat, make a 3- to 4-inch fold across the foot of the bed.)
18. Fold the top sheet back over the blanket at the top of the bed to make an 8-inch cuff (see Figure g).
19. Insert the pillow into the pillowcase by:
    a. Grasping the center of the outside of the pillowcase and seam and turning the case inside out over your hand.
    b. Grasping the pillow through the case and pulling the case down over the pillow (see Figure h). Tags or zippers should be on the inside of the pillowcase.
    c. Folding the extra material from the side seam of the pillowcase under the pillow.

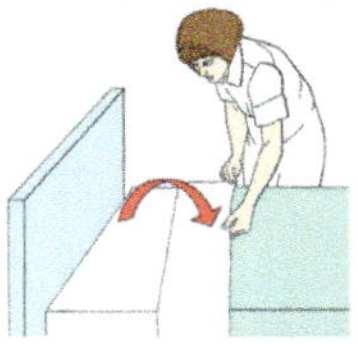

Figure g

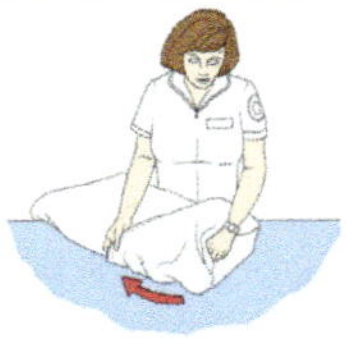

Figure h

20. Put bed in lowest position.

Postprocedure

21. Wash hands.

Charting Example:

11/16/24	1535
	Bed made/closed method
	_______ R. Johnson CNA

Procedure Tip

19.56 Making a Closed Bed, continued

- Step 19b: Refer to illustrations for proper technique for applying pillowcases.
- Step 20: Emphasize importance of leaving bed in lowest position.
- Review the postprocedure steps.
- Step 21: Emphasize the importance of proper handwashing.

PROCEDURE PRACTICE

- Demonstrate the steps for Procedure 19.56, Making a Closed Bed, as many times as necessary, or ask students to demonstrate the steps. Have students practice and perform the procedure until they are competent.

Procedure Tip

19.57 Making an Occupied Bed

- Review the background information, explaining that an occupied bed has a patient in it.
- Emphasize the importance of following Standard Precautions.
- Review the preprocedure steps.
- Step 1: Emphasize the importance of proper handwashing.
- Step 2: Review the equipment list.
- Step 3: Emphasize the importance of effective communication techniques.
- Step 4: Emphasize the importance of locking the wheels.
- Step 7: Emphasize the importance of patient privacy.
- Review the procedure steps.
- Step 9: Explain reasons for not shaking linens.
- Step 13: Emphasize the importance of patient privacy.

TEAMWORK

As a class, brainstorm problems that might arise while making an occupied bed that would not arise while making an open or closed bed. Brainstorm solutions to the problems, as well.

Procedure 19.57 Making an Occupied Bed

BACKGROUND: Clean linens help prevent the spread of bacteria in the health care environment. Making an occupied bed with fresh linen will provide cleanliness, comfort, and will help the patient maintain a healthy skin condition.
ALERT: Follow Standard Precautions

Preprocedure

1. Wash hands.
2. Assemble equipment:
   a. Draw sheet or large pad
   b. Two large sheets or fitted bottom sheet and one large sheet
   c. Two pillowcases
   d. Blankets as needed
   e. Bedspread (if clean one is needed)
   f. Pillow
   g. Disposable gloves if needed
3. Identify patient and explain what you are going to do.
4. Raise bed to comfortable working height. Lock wheels on bed.
5. Place chair at side of bed.
6. Put linen on chair in the order in which you will use it. (First things you will use go on top.)
7. Provide for privacy by pulling privacy curtain.

Procedure

8. Lower headrest and kneerest until bed is flat, if allowed.
9. Loosen linens on all sides by lifting edge of mattress with one hand and pulling out bedclothes with the other. Never shake linen: This spreads microorganisms.
10. Push mattress to top of bed. Ask for assistance if you need it.
11. Remove bedspread and blanket by folding them to the bottom, one at a time. Lift them from center and place over back of chair.
12. Place bath blanket or plain sheet over top sheet. Ask patient to hold top edge of clean cover if he or she is able to do so. If patient cannot hold the sheet, tuck it under patient's shoulders.
13. Slide soiled sheet from top to bottom and put in dirty linen container. Be careful not to expose patient.
14. Ask patient to turn toward the opposite side of bed. Have patient hold onto the side rail. Assist patient if he or she needs help. Patient should now be on far side of bed from you.

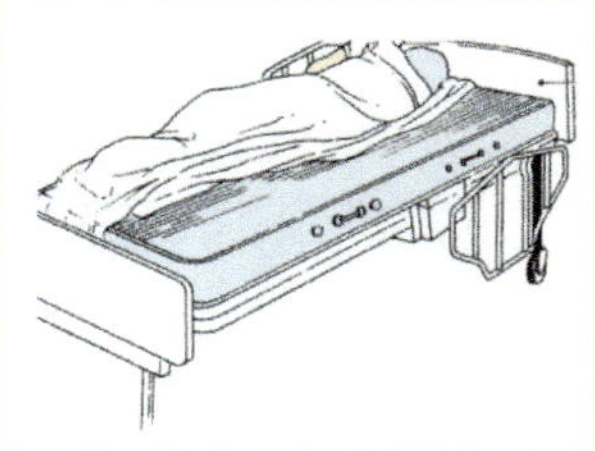

15. Adjust pillow for patient to make him or her comfortable.
16. Fan-fold soiled draw sheet and bottom sheet close to patient and tuck against patient's back. This leaves mattress stripped of linen.
17. Work on one side of bed until that side is completed. Then go to other side of bed. This saves you time and energy.
18. Take fitted bottom and fold it lengthwise. Be careful not to let it touch floor.
19. Place sheet on bed, still folded, with fold on middle of mattress.
20. Fold top half of sheet toward patient. Tuck folds against patient's back.
21. Miter corner at head of mattress. Tuck bottom sheet under mattress on your side from head to foot of mattress.

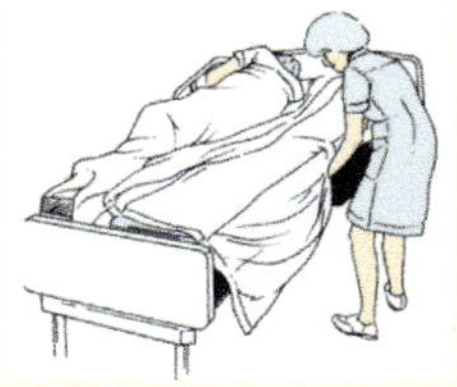

(continued)

664 Chapter 19 | Measuring Vital Signs and Other Clinical Skills

Procedure 19.57 | **Making an Occupied Bed (continued)**

Procedure (cont)

22. Place clean bottom draw sheet or large pad that has been folded in half with fold along middle of mattress. Fold top half of sheet toward patient. Tuck folds against patient's back.
23. Raise side rail and lock in place.
24. Lower side rail on opposite side.
25. Ask patient to roll away from you to other side of bed and onto clean linen. Tell patient that there will be a bump in the middle. (Be careful not to let patient become wrapped up in bath blanket.)
26. Remove old bottom sheet and draw sheet from bed and put into laundry container.
27. Pull fresh linen toward edge of mattress. Tuck it under mattress at head of bed.
28. Tuck bottom sheet under mattress from head to foot of mattress. Pull firmly to remove wrinkles.
29. Pull draw sheet very tight and tuck under mattress. If pad used, pull from patient and straighten.
30. Have patient roll on back, or turn patient yourself. Loosen bath blanket as patient turns.
31. Change pillowcase:
    a. Hold pillowcase at center of end seam.
    b. With your other hand turn pillowcase back over hand, holding end seam.
    c. Grasp pillow through case at center of end of pillow.
    d. Bring case down over pillow and fit pillow into corners of case.
    e. Fold extra material over open end of pillow and place pillow under patient's head.
32. Spread clean top sheet over bath blanket with wide hem at the top. Middle of sheet should run along middle of bed with wide hem even with top edge of mattress. Ask patient to hold hem of clean sheet. Remove bath blanket by moving it toward foot of bed. Be careful not to expose patient.
33. Tuck clean top sheet under mattress at foot of bed. Make toepleat in top sheet so that patient's feet can move freely. To make a toepleat, make 3-inch fold toward foot of bed in topsheet before tucking in sheet. Tuck in and miter corner.
34. Place blanket over patient, being sure that it covers the shoulders.
35. Place bedspread on bed in same way. Tuck blanket and bedspread under bottom of mattress and miter corners.
36. Make cuff:
    a. Fold top hem edge of spread over blanket.
    b. Fold top hem of top sheet back over edge of bedspread and blanket, being certain that rough hem is turned down.
37. Position patient and make comfortable.
38. Put bed in lowest position.
39. Open privacy curtains.
40. Raise side rails, if required.
41. Place call light where patient can reach it.

Postprocedure

42. Tidy unit.
43. Wash hands.
44. Chart linen change and how the patient tolerated procedure.

Procedure Tip

19.57 Making an Occupied Bed, continued

- Review the postprocedure steps.
- Step 43: Emphasize the importance of proper handwashing.
- Step 44: Emphasize the importance of observation and documentation.

PROCEDURE PRACTICE

- Demonstrate the steps for Procedure 19.57, Making an Occupied Bed, as many times as necessary, or ask students to demonstrate the steps. Have students practice and perform the procedure until they are competent.

Procedure Tip

19.58 Making an Open Bed

- Review the background information, explaining that an open bed is one that the patient has left temporarily.
- Emphasize the importance of following Standard Precautions.
- Review the preprocedure steps.
- Step 1: Emphasize the importance of proper handwashing.
- Review the procedure steps.
- Step 4: Emphasize the importance of keeping the linens wrinkle-free.
- Review the postprocedure steps.
- Step 5: Emphasize the importance of proper handwashing.

PROCEDURE PRACTICE

- Demonstrate the steps for Procedure: 19.58, Making an Open Bed, as many times as necessary, or ask students to demonstrate the steps. Have students practice and perform the procedure until they are competent.

Procedure 19.58 Making an Open Bed

BACKGROUND: Clean linens help prevent the spread of bacteria in the health care environment. An open bed provides easy access for patients returning to bed within a short period.
ALERT: Follow Standard Precautions

Preprocedure

1. Wash hands.

Procedure

2. Grasp cuff of bedding in both hands and pull to foot of bed.
3. Fold bedding back on itself toward head of bed. The edge of cuff must meet fold. (This is called fan-folding.)
4. Smooth the hanging sheets on each side into folds.

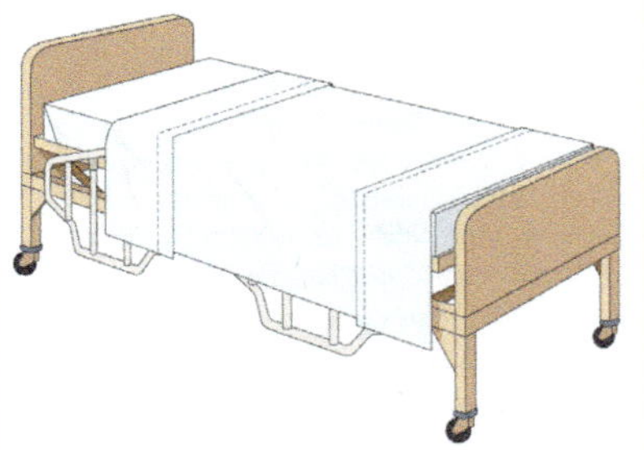

Postprocedure

5. Wash hands.

Procedure 19.59 Placing a Bed Cradle

BACKGROUND: There can be situations where having the top bed linens touching the patient's lower extremities could be harmful to the patient. In this case, an apparatus called a bed cradle can be used.

A cradle is usually a metal frame that supports the bed linens away from the patient while providing privacy and warmth. These cradles come in a variety of sizes and shapes. If used, the cradle should be fastened to the bed so that it does not slide or fall on the patient.

ALERT: Follow Standard Precautions

Preprocedure

1. Identify the patient requiring a bed cradle. Assess the extremity to be protected. Note any special requirements necessitated by the patient's condition.
2. Wash hands.
3. Explain the procedure to the patient.

Procedure

4. Address any needs for repositioning prior to placing the cradle.
5. Fold down the top covers off of the patient.
6. Place cradle over the patient's lower extremities.
7. Secure the cradle to the bed frame so that it will not collapse on to the patient.
8. Replace the top covers over the top of the cradle
9. Assure that no part of the cradle or the top covers are touching the patient's affected extremity.

Postprocedure

10. Assure that the patient is comfortable and has no further needs before leaving the area.
11. Wash hands.
12. Document the procedure noting any special findings or needs of the patient.
13. Check the patient frequently to assure the stability of the cradle and the comfort of the patient.

666 Chapter 19 | Measuring Vital Signs and Other Clinical Skills

Procedure Tip

19.59 Placing a Bed Cradle

- Review the background information, describing a bed cradle and explaining its use.
- Emphasize the importance of following Standard Precautions.
- Review the preprocedure steps.
- Step 1: Emphasize the importance of observation.
- Step 2: Emphasize the importance of proper handwashing.
- Step 3: Emphasize the importance of effective communication techniques.
- Review the procedure steps.
- Step 7: Emphasize the importance of securing the cradle.
- Review the postprocedure steps.
- Step 11: Emphasize the importance of proper handwashing.
- Step 12: Emphasize the importance of proper observation and documentation.

PROCEDURE PRACTICE

- Demonstrate the steps for Procedure 19.59, Placing a Bed Cradle, as many times as necessary, or ask students to demonstrate the steps. Have students practice and perform the procedure until they are competent.

Feeding the Patient

Mealtime can be a pleasant time for patients. It is often the most pleasurable event of the day. This should be an unhurried, enjoyable experience. Be certain that the patient is prepared for meals before the food arrives. The elderly patient may tolerate more small meals better than fewer large meals. Providing extra nourishments between meals may increase overall intake.

The preparation for the meal includes the following:

- Assisting patients or reminding them to wash their hands
- Removing any unpleasant items from the area, such as **emesis** basins and bedpans
- Offering the opportunity to use the bedpan or the bathroom
- Providing for the patient's comfort:
  - Raise the head of the bed
  - Position the patient in a chair
  - Transport the patient to the dining area
- Checking to be certain that you have the right tray for the patient and that it is the correct diet
- Always placing the food within reach
- Checking the tray to be certain that everything is there
- Preparing any item that the patient cannot manage
- Telling the patient where each item is according to the face of a clock if the patient is blind

emesis
(eh MUH suhs)
Vomit.

Teaching Tips

- Explain the importance of a pleasant mealtime.
- Discuss the importance of preparing a patient for the meal before the meal arrives.
- Explain the responsibilities of preparing the patient for a meal:
  - Assist patients to wash hands.
  - Offer the bedpan or the bathroom.
  - Remove unpleasant items from the area.
  - Position the patient for comfortable dining, or transport to the dining area.
  - Check that the tray is correct.
  - Place food within reach.
  - Prepare any item that the patient cannot manage.
  - Tell the patient where each item is according to the face of a clock if the patient is visually disabled.

Procedure Tip

19.60 Preparing the Patient to Eat

- Review the background information, emphasizing the need to make mealtimes pleasant.
- Emphasize the importance of following Standard Precautions.
- Review the preprocedure steps.
- Step 1: Emphasize the importance of proper handwashing.
- Step 4: Emphasize the importance of effective communication techniques.
- Review the procedure steps.
- Step 8: Emphasize the importance of providing the correct tray.
- Review the postprocedure steps.
- Step 13: Emphasize the importance of proper handwashing.
- Remind students of the importance of proper observation and documentation.

PROCEDURE PRACTICE

- Demonstrate the steps for Procedure 19.60, Preparing the Patient to Eat, as many times as necessary, or ask students to demonstrate the steps. Have students practice and perform the procedure until they are competent.

Procedure 19.60 Preparing the Patient to Eat

BACKGROUND: Preparing patients for a meal by providing clean, neat surroundings and encouraging toileting and washing hands before eating can help patients enjoy their meal and promote their appetites.
ALERT: Follow Standard Precautions

Preprocedure

1. Wash hands.
2. Assemble equipment:
   a. Bedpan or urinal, if necessary
   b. Toilet tissue, if necessary
   c. Washcloth
   d. Hand towel
3. Assist patient as needed to empty bladder, if necessary, and wash hands and face.
4. Explain that you are getting ready to give patient a meal.

Procedure

5. Clear bedside table.
6. Position patient for comfort and a convenient eating position.
7. Wash your hands.
8. Identify patient and check name on food tray to ensure that you are delivering the correct diet to patient.
9. Place tray in a convenient position in front of patient.

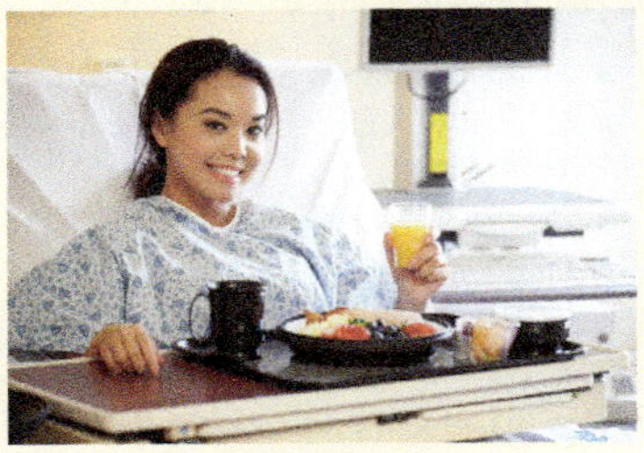

10. Open containers if patient cannot.
11. If patient is unable to prepare food, do it for patient:
    a. Butter the bread
    b. Cut meat
    c. Season food as necessary
12. Follow the procedure for feeding a patient if patient needs to be fed.

Postprocedure

13. Wash hands.

668 Chapter 19 | Measuring Vital Signs and Other Clinical Skills

Procedure 19.61 Preparing the Patient to Eat in the Dining Room

BACKGROUND: Eating in the dining room provides a more normal environment for patients, creating an opportunity to visit with others during the meal.
ALERT: Follow Standard Precautions

Preprocedure

1. Wash hands.
2. Help patient take care of toileting needs.
3. Assist with handwashing.
4. Take patient to dining room.

Procedure

5. Position patient in wheelchair at table that is proper height for wheelchair.
6. Be certain patient is sitting in a comfortable position.
7. Provide adaptive feeding equipment if needed.
8. Bring patient tray.
9. Identify patient.
10. Serve tray and remove plate covers.
11. Provide assistance as needed (e.g., cut meat, butter bread, open containers).
12. Remove tray when finished, noting what patient ate.
13. Assist with handwashing and take patient to area of choice.

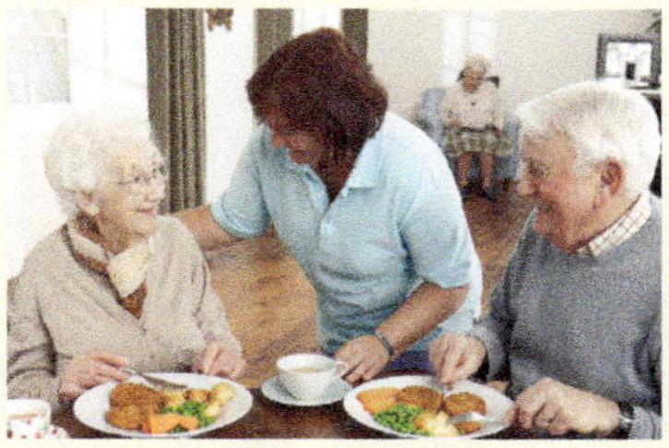

Postprocedure

14. Wash hands.
15. Record what patient ate.
16. Record I & O if necessary. (See the section "Measuring Intake and Output" on page 674.)

Charting Example:

8/10/24	0800
	Taken by wheelchair to dining room
	80% of breakfast eaten, and
	tolerated well
	S. Gomez CNA

Measuring Vital Signs and Other Clinical Skills | Chapter 19 669

Procedure Tip

19.61 Preparing the Patient to Eat in the Dining Room

- Review the background information, emphasizing the need to make mealtimes pleasant.
- Emphasize the importance of following Standard Precautions.
- Review the preprocedure steps.
- Step 1: Emphasize the importance of proper handwashing.
- Review the procedure steps.
- Step 6: Emphasize the importance of a comfortable position for eating.
- Steps 8 and 9: Emphasize the importance of providing the correct tray.
- Review the postprocedure steps.
- Step 14: Emphasize the importance of proper handwashing.
- Steps 15 and 16: Emphasize the importance of proper observation and documentation.

PROCEDURE PRACTICE

- Demonstrate the steps for Procedure 19.61, Preparing the Patient to Eat in the Dining Room, as many times as necessary, or ask students to demonstrate the steps. Have students practice and perform the procedure until they are competent.

Procedure Tip

19.62 Assisting the Patient with Meals

- Review the background information, emphasizing the need to encourage patients to eat.
- Emphasize the importance of following Standard Precautions.
- Review the preprocedure steps.
- Step 1: Emphasize the importance of proper handwashing.
- Step 2: Emphasize the importance of identifying the patient.
- Review the procedure steps.
- Steps 3 and 4: Emphasize the importance of effective communication techniques.
- Step 5: Emphasize the importance of a comfortable position for eating.
- Step 10: Emphasize the importance of encouraging patient independence.
- Step 12: Emphasize the importance of being sure food is chewed and swallowed.
- Step 15: Emphasize the social nature of eating.

Procedure 19.62 Assisting the Patient with Meals

BACKGROUND: Food is essential to maintain health. As a health care worker you are responsible to encourage patients to maintain their health by eating routine meals. Your attitude and willingness to assist patients who require your attention during meals can encourage their intake of a balanced diet.
ALERT: Follow Standard Precautions

Preprocedure

1. Wash hands.
2. Check patient's ID band with name on food tray to ensure that you will be feeding correct diet to patient.

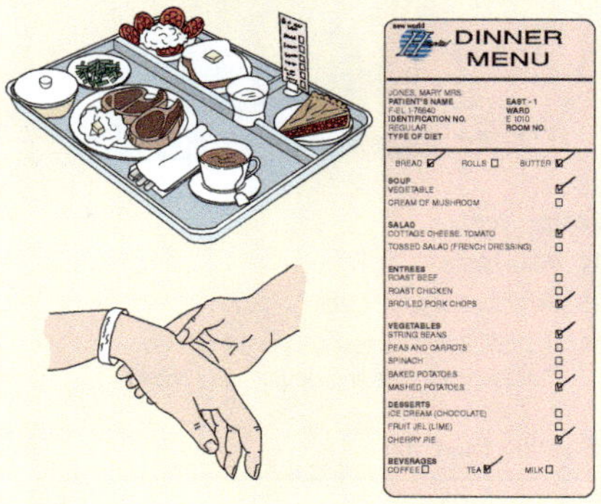

Procedure

3. Tell patient what food is being served.
4. Ask patient how he or she prefers food to be prepared (e.g., salt, pepper, cream or sugar in coffee).
5. Position patient in a sitting position, as allowed by physician. If ordered to lie flat, turn patient on side.
6. Position yourself in a comfortable manner, facing the patient, so that you won't be rushing patient because you are uncomfortable. (Do not sit on bed.)
7. Cut food into small bite-sized pieces.
8. Place a napkin or small hand towel under patient's chin.
9. Put a flex straw in cold drinks. Hot drinks tend to burn mouth if taken through a straw.
10. Use a spoon to feed patient small to average-sized bites of food. (Encourage patient to help self as much as possible.)

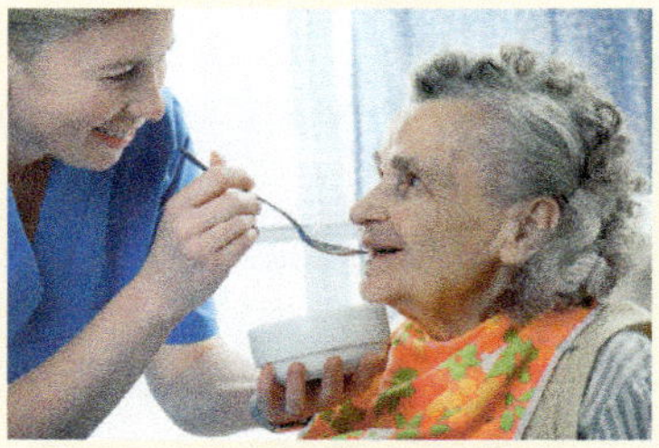

11. Always feed patient at a slow pace. It may take more time for him or her to chew and swallow than you think is necessary.
12. Always be sure that one bite has been swallowed before you give another spoonful to patient.
13. Tell patient what is being served and ask which item he or she prefers first, if patient cannot see food.
14. Offer beverages to patient throughout the meal.
15. Talk with patient during meal.
16. Encourage patient to finish eating, but do not force.
17. Assist patient in wiping face as necessary and when patient is finished eating.
18. Observe amount of food eaten.

(continued)

670 Chapter 19 | Measuring Vital Signs and Other Clinical Skills

Procedure 19.62 Assisting the Patient with Meals (continued)

Postprocedure

19. Remove tray from room.
20. Position patient for comfort and safety.
21. Place call light in a convenient place.
22. Wash hands.
23. Record amount of food eaten (half, three-fourths, one-fourth, etc.) on chart, and indicate if food was tolerated well or not.

Charting Example:

10/10/24 1800
50% of meal taken with assistance and tolerated well.
Resident stated that he doesn't like beef
Dietitian notified of resident's request for meat other than beef.
R. Johnson CNA

Procedure 19.63 Serving Food to the Patient in Bed (Self-Help)

BACKGROUND: As a health care worker you are required to identify the right diet for each patient and recognize what they need assistance with. Your opening packages and cartons or cutting food into bite-sized pieces may make the difference between a patient eating or refusing his or her food.

ALERT: Follow Standard Precautions

Preprocedure

1. Wash hands.
2. Assemble equipment:
   a. Food tray with diet card
   b. Flex straws
   c. Towel

Procedure

3. Assist patient with bedpan or urinal.
4. Place in a sitting position if possible.
5. Help patient wash hands and face.
6. Remove unsightly or odor-causing articles.
7. Clean overbed table.
8. Check tray with diet card for:
   a. Patient's name
   b. Type of diet
   c. Correct foods according to diet (e.g., diabetic, puréed, chopped, regular)
9. Set up tray and help with foods if needed (e.g., cut meat, butter bread, open containers). Do not add foods to the tray until you check on diet.
10. Encourage patient to eat all foods on tray.
11. Remove tray when finished and note what patient ate.
12. Help patient wash hands and face.
13. Position patient comfortably and make sure call bell is within reach.
14. Remove tray.
15. Be certain that water is within reach.

Postprocedure

16. Wash hands.
17. Record I & O if required.
18. Record amount eaten.

Charting Example:

11/03/24 1230
Lunch served with meat and vegetables cut into bite-sized pieces.
Mr. Axel struggled to butter the bread without assistance. He said, "I knew I could butter it without help." 90% of lunch eaten, tolerated well.
S. Gomez CNA

Measuring Vital Signs and Other Clinical Skills | Chapter 19 671

Procedure Tip

19.62 Assisting the Patient with Meals, continued

- Review the postprocedure steps.
- Step 22: Emphasize the importance of proper handwashing.
- Step 23: Emphasize the importance of proper observation and documentation.

PROCEDURE PRACTICE

- Demonstrate the steps for Procedure 19.62, Assisting the Patient with Meals, as many times as necessary, or ask students to demonstrate the steps. Have students practice and perform the procedure until they are competent.

Procedure Tip

19.63 Serving Food to the Patient in Bed (Self-Help)

- Review the background information, emphasizing that this procedure provides assistance to patients who need some assistance.
- Emphasize the importance of following Standard Precautions.
- Review the preprocedure steps.
- Step 1: Emphasize the importance of proper handwashing.
- Step 2: Review the equipment list.
- Review the procedure steps.
- Step 4: Emphasize the importance of a comfortable position for eating.
- Step 8: Emphasize the importance of identifying that the patient has received the correct meal.
- Review the postprocedure steps.
- Step 16: Emphasize the importance of proper handwashing.
- Steps 17 and 18: Emphasize the importance of proper observation and documentation.

PROCEDURE PRACTICE

- Demonstrate the steps for Procedure 19.63, Serving Food to the Patient in Bed, as many times as necessary, or ask students to demonstrate the steps. Have students practice and perform the procedure until they are competent.

Procedure Tip

19.64 Providing Fresh Drinking Water

- Review the background information, emphasizing the importance of fluid intake.
- Emphasize the importance of following Standard Precautions.
- Review the preprocedure steps.
- Step 1: Emphasize the importance of NOT providing fluids to a patient with restricted fluid intake.
- Step 2: Emphasize the importance of proper handwashing.
- Review the procedure steps.
- Review the postprocedure steps.
- Step 8: Emphasize the importance of proper handwashing.

PROCEDURE PRACTICE

- Demonstrate the steps for Procedure 19.64, Providing Fresh Drinking Water, as many times as necessary, or ask students to demonstrate the steps. Have students practice and perform the procedure until they are competent.

Procedure 19.64 Providing Fresh Drinking Water

BACKGROUND: Providing fluids for the patient is an integral part of the process of returning the patient to an optimal health status. The elderly patient may experience a diminished sense of thirst and may require additional encouragement and assistance to maintain adequate oral intake. Recording the volume of oral intake is the responsibility of the nurse assigned to the patient's care.
ALERT: Follow Standard Precautions

Preprocedure

1. Identify any patients whose fluids may be restricted as a medical necessity.
2. Wash hands.
3. Assemble equipment: the container to be used for patient's water supply.

Procedure

4. Collect and discard any of the containers previously used for the patient's water supply.
5. Establish the temperature of water preferred by the patient (i.e., iced, tepid, etc.).
6. Provide a clean container and fresh water for the patient.
7. Establish that the patient has no further needs before leaving the bedside.

Postprocedure

8. Wash hands.

Procedure 19.65 Feeding the Helpless Patient

BACKGROUND: Patients must routinely eat a balanced diet. You are required to feed patients who are not able to feed themselves. Your patience and willingness to feed them in a gentle, caring, compassionate manner could make the difference in their eating or not eating.
ALERT: Follow Standard Precautions

Preprocedure

1. Wash hands.
2. Bring patient's tray.
3. Check name on card with patient ID band.
4. Explain to patient what you are going to do.

Procedure

5. Sit comfortably, facing patient.
6. Tuck a napkin under patient's chin.
7. Season food the way patient likes it.
8. Use a spoon and fill only half full.
9. Give food from tip, not side of spoon.
10. Name each food as you offer it, if patient can't see it.
11. Describe position of food on plate (e.g., hot liquids in right corner, peas at the position of 3 o'clock on a clock) if patient cannot see but can feed self.
12. Tell patient if you are offering something that is hot or cold.
13. Use a straw for giving liquids.

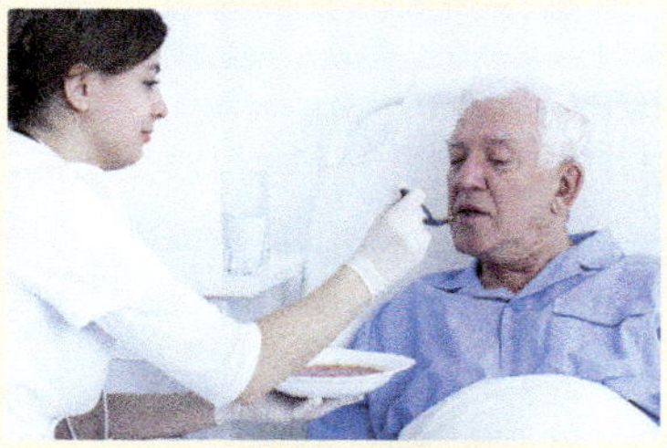

14. Feed patient slowly and allow time to chew and swallow. Offer beverages throughout the meal.

(continued)

672 Chapter 19 | Measuring Vital Signs and Other Clinical Skills

Procedure Tip

19.65 Feeding the Helpless Patient

- Review the background information, emphasizing that this procedure is for patients who are conscious, but unable to feed themselves.
- Emphasize the importance of following Standard Precautions.
- Review the preprocedure steps.
- Step 1: Emphasize the importance of proper handwashing.
- Steps 2 and 3: Emphasize the importance of identifying the patient and ensuring that the patient receives the correct tray.
- Step 4: Emphasize the importance of effective communication techniques.
- Review the procedure steps.
- Steps 10–12: Emphasize the importance of effective communication techniques.
- Step 13: Emphasize that hot liquids should not be given through a straw.

Procedure 19.65 Feeding the Helpless Patient (continued)

Procedure (cont)

15. Note amount eaten and remove tray when finished.
16. Help with washing hands and face.
17. Position patient comfortably and place call bell within reach.

Postprocedure

18. Wash hands.
19. Record amount eaten and I & O if required. See following pages for directions on recording I & O.

Charting Example:

12/12/24	*1830*
	Ate 60% of food and drank
	240cc of tea. Chokes easily when
	drinking liquids Reported choking
	incidents to team leader
	A. Chaplin CNA

INTAKE AND OUTPUT SHEET

Hospital #________ Patient Name ________

Date ________ Room #________

	INTAKE			OUTPUT			
				URINE		GASTRIC	
Time 7-3	BY MOUTH	TUBE	PARENTERAL	VOIDED	CATHETER	EMESIS	SUCTION
TOTAL							
Time 3-11							
TOTAL							
Time 11-7							
TOTAL							
24 HOUR TOTAL							
24 Hour Grand Total • Intake				24 Hour Grand Total • Output			

Additional Nourishments

Nourishments are usually served to patients who require additional nutrition. You are required to identify the right nourishment for patients and to recognize what they need assistance with. Telling the patient that the nourishment is served, making it ready to drink or eat, or feeding him or her if necessary makes it possible for the patient to receive the needed nourishment.

You may have a patient with a nasogastric (N/G) tube. The nasogastric tube is used when the patient has difficulty swallowing or has no swallow reflex. It is a soft, plastic tube that is inserted in the nostril and goes down the back of the throat through the esophagus to the stomach. The tube is taped to the patient's nose.

Fluids such as liquid food and medication are put into the tube. Another type of tube is the gastric tube. This tube enters the stomach through the abdominal wall. It is left in place and capped after each feeding. Be very careful not to pull out these tubes.

Measuring Vital Signs and Other Clinical Skills | Chapter 19 673

Procedure Tip

19.65 Feeding the Helpless Patient, continued

- Step 15: Emphasize importance of observation.
- Review the postprocedure steps.
- Step 18: Emphasize the importance of proper handwashing.
- Step 19: Emphasize the importance of proper observation and documentation.

PROCEDURE PRACTICE

- Demonstrate the steps for Procedure 19.65, Feeding the Helpless Patient, as many times as necessary, or ask students to demonstrate the steps. Have students practice and perform the procedure until they are competent.

Teaching Tips

- Explain the nourishment is provided for patients who require additional nutrition.
- Explain the use of a nasogastric tube.
- Explain the use of a gastric tube.

Procedure Tip

19.66 Serving Nourishments

- Review the background information, explaining that this procedure refers to snacks or nourishments between regular meals.
- Emphasize the importance of following Standard Precautions.
- Review the preprocedure steps.
- Step 1: Emphasize the importance of proper handwashing.
- Step 3: Emphasize the importance of identifying the patient and the correct nourishment.
- Review the procedure steps.
- Review the postprocedure steps.
- Step 9: Emphasize the importance of proper handwashing.
- Steps 8 and 10: Emphasize the importance of proper observation and documentation.

PROCEDURE PRACTICE

- Demonstrate the steps for Procedure 19.66, Serving Nourishments, as many times as necessary, or ask students to demonstrate the steps. Have students practice and perform the procedure until they are competent.

Procedure 19.66 Serving Nourishments

BACKGROUND: Between-meal nourishments are served to people who need additional nutrients to maintain or improve their health. People with diabetes need nourishments to maintain balanced glucose levels. Some may need protein to build and repair body tissue and others may need specific vitamins.
ALERT: Follow Standard Precautions

Preprocedure

1. Wash hands.
2. Assemble equipment:
   a. Nourishment
   b. Cup, dish, straw, spoon
   c. Napkin
3. Identify patient.

Procedure

4. Take nourishment to patient.
5. Help if needed.
6. After patient is finished, collect dirty utensils.

Postprocedure

7. Return utensils to dietary cart or kitchen.
8. Record intake on I & O sheet if required.
9. Wash hands.
10. Record nourishment taken.

Charting Example:

9/15/24	*1500*
	Took 50% of afternoon nourishment
	R. Johnson CNA

Measuring Intake and Output

One of your most important responsibilities is helping the patient with fluid balance. Normally, our bodies maintain this balance without our thinking about it. We take in fluids in our foods and liquids. About the same amount is eliminated by the kidneys (urine), respiration, and perspiration. However, in some patients, fluid balance becomes a very serious problem. Fluid imbalance occurs when fluid stays in the tissues, causing edema, or when there is excessive loss of fluid (dehydration).

dehydration
(dee HIE dray shuhn)
Severe loss of fluid from tissue and cells.

Dehydration is caused by:

- Diarrhea
- Vomiting
- Bleeding
- Poor fluid intake
- Excessive perspiration (diaphoresis)

If you notice any of the following symptoms of dehydration, report them immediately:

- Fever is present
- There is a decrease in urine
- Urine is concentrated
- Weight loss occurs
- Membranes are dry, and patient has difficulty swallowing
- Tongue is coated and thickened
- Skin becomes hard and cracks and is dry and warm

674 Chapter 19 | Measuring Vital Signs and Other Clinical Skills

Teaching Tips

- Introduce concepts of intake and output.
- Explain that monitoring intake and output helps maintain the patient's fluid balance.
- Define dehydration: an excessive loss of fluid.
- Explain causes of dehydration:
  - Diarrhea
  - Vomiting
  - Bleeding
  - Excessive perspiration (diaphoresis)
  - Poor fluid intake
- Explain symptoms of dehydration:
  - Fever
  - Decrease in urine
  - Urine is concentrated
  - Weight loss
  - Membranes are dry, and patient has difficulty swallowing
  - Tongue is coated and thickened
  - Skin becomes hard and cracks

Edema is serious; it is caused by:

- High salt intake
- Infections
- Injuries or burns
- Certain kidney diseases
- Certain heart diseases or heart inefficiencies
- Sitting too long in one position
- Infiltration of IV fluid

If you notice any of the symptoms of edema, report them immediately:

- Decrease in urine output
- Gain in weight
- Puffiness or swelling
- Sometimes shortness of breath

When any of these situations occur, the doctor writes an order to record intake and output (I & O). You record any fluid taken in and any fluid that is eliminated. To measure intake, record the amount of fluid consumed by mouth. Be sure to include the following:

- All liquid taken by mouth
- Any food item that turns to liquid at room temperature (e.g., gelatin, ice cream)
- All fluid taken by IV or tube feeding

Your facility will have a charting method for you to use. Record the amount of liquid taken at the time it is taken. This way, you do not forget this important task. You are probably most familiar with measuring liquid in ounces.

When you record liquid intake, you record it in cubic centimeters (cc's). This is a metric measure and is used in medical facilities. Most facilities have a chart that helps you determine how many cubic centimeters are in a serving. (**Table 19.7**) If you need to change ounces to cubic centimeters, use the formula below:

30 × (number of ounces) = number of cc

For example:

30 × 8 ounces = 240 cc

To measure patient output, measure all of the following:

- Urine
- Liquid stool
- Emesis (vomit)
- Suctioned secretio
- Drainage
- Excessive perspiration

Teaching Tips

- Define edema: fluid stays in the tissues.
- Explain causes of edema:
  - High salt intake
  - Infections
  - Injuries or burns
  - Certain kidney diseases
  - Certain heart diseases or heart inefficiencies
  - Sitting too long in one position
  - Infiltration of IV fluid
- Explain symptoms of edema:
  - Decrease in urine output
  - Gain in weight
  - Puffiness or swelling
  - Sometimes shortness of breath

Teaching Tips

- Review Table 19.7 together as a class.
- Remind students that cubic centimeters (cc) and milliliters (ml) are the same.
- Direct students to Sections 11.2 and 12.2 for information on the metric system and converting cubic centimeters to ounces.

Procedure Tip

19.67 Measuring Urinary Output

- Review the background information, emphasizing the importance of monitoring fluid balance.
- Emphasize the importance of following Standard Precautions.
- Review the preprocedure steps.
- Step 1: Emphasize the importance of proper handwashing.
- Step 2: Review the equipment list.
- Step 3: Emphasize the importance of wearing gloves.
- Review the procedure steps.
- Step 4: Display a graduate.
- Step 6: Emphasize importance of observation.

ACTIVITY

Ask students to bring pictures of food that make up a complete meal to class. Cut the pictures to create a partially eaten meal. Have students estimate how much was eaten. Have them document their observations.

Suctioned secretion and perspiration are estimated. It is a good idea to have an experienced person help you determine the amount. When you have measured input and output, record them on the chart provided. You may be asked to empty a urinary bag and measure the urine at the end of your shift. The totals are taken each 24 hours. If you notice any unusual recordings, be absolutely certain that you report it.

Table 19.7 Customary Liquid Measures and Their Equivalents*

Liquid Measurment	Equivalents
1 cc/1 mL	15 drops
1 cc/1 mL	1/4 teaspoon
5 cc/mL	1 teaspoon
15 cc/mL	1 tablespoon
30 cc/mL	1 oz
60 cc/mL	2 oz
120 cc/mL	4 oz
180 cc/mL	6 oz
240 cc/mL	8 oz (1 cup)
500 cc/mL	16 oz (1 pint)
1,000 cc/mL	32 oz (1 quart)
4,000 cc/mL	64 oz (1 gallon)

*cc, cubic centimeter; mL, milliliter; oz, ounce.

Procedure 19.67 Measuring Urinary Output

BACKGROUND: All body systems rely on fluid balance to maintain normal functioning. By measuring urinary output, you can determine the body's ability to maintain fluid balance and observe characteristics of urine that indicate normalcy or potential abnormalities.
ALERT: Follow Standard Precautions

Preprocedure

1. Wash hands.
2. Assemble equipment:
   a. Bedpan, urinal, or special container
   b. Graduate or measuring cup
   c. Disposable nonsterile gloves
3. Put on gloves.

Procedure

4. Pour urine into measuring graduate.
5. Place graduate on flat surface and read amount of urine.
6. Observe urine for:
   a. Unusual color
   b. Blood
   c. Dark color
   d. Large amounts of mucus
   e. Sediment

(continued)

676 Chapter 19 | Measuring Vital Signs and Other Clinical Skills

Procedure 19.67 **Measuring Urinary Output (continued)**

Procedure (cont)

7. Show the specimen and report to nurse immediately if you notice any unusual appearance.
8. Discard in toilet if urine is normal. Use a paper towel to flush toilet and turn on faucet.
9. Rinse graduate or pitcher and put away.

Postprocedure

10. Remove gloves and discard according to facility policy.
11. Wash hands.
12. Record amount of urine in cc's on I & O sheet.

Charting Examples:

11/23/24 1200
Voided 300 cc dark,
amber-colored urine
______ S. Gomez CNA

11/23/24 1600
Voided 100 cc pink-tinged urine
Complained of pain upon urination
Team leader notified
______ S. Gomez CNA

Special Procedures

Enemas

You may have the responsibility of giving the patient an enema. Fluid is run into the rectum to remove feces and gas from the bowel. The solution in the bowel causes the patient to feel uncomfortable and want to force the fluid out. Encourage him or her to retain the fluid as long as possible. This gives better results.

An enema is given only when there is a doctor's order. There are several different kinds of enemas. These include tap water, soap suds, saline, and prepackaged enemas. An oil retention enema is held in the bowel longer than the cleansing enema. Encourage the patient to retain the oil solution for 20 to 30 minutes.

Procedure Tip

19.67 Measuring Urinary Output, continued

- Review the postprocedure steps.
- Step 11: Emphasize the importance of proper handwashing.
- Step 12: Emphasize the importance of proper observation and documentation.

PROCEDURE PRACTICE

- Demonstrate the steps for Procedure 19.67, Measuring Urinary Output, as many times as necessary, or ask students to demonstrate the steps. Have students practice and perform the procedure until they are competent.

Teaching Tips

- Introduce the topic of special procedures.
- Discuss each type of enema, and simulate procedures:
  - Oil retention
  - Prepackaged
  - Tap water
  - Soap suds
  - Saline
- Emphasize that an enema requires a doctor's order.

Procedure Tip

19.68 Oil Retention Enema

- Review the background information, explaining the purpose of the enema.
- Emphasize the importance of following Standard Precautions.
- Review the preprocedure steps.
- Step 1: Emphasize the importance of proper handwashing.
- Step 2: Review the equipment list.
- Step 4: Emphasize the importance of patient privacy.
- Step 5: Emphasize the importance of effective communication techniques.
- Step 6: Emphasize the importance of wearing gloves.
- Review the procedure steps.
- Step 11: Explain the Sims position.
- Step 16: Reinforce the importance of effective communication.
- Step 22: Emphasize the importance of monitoring the patient.
- Step 28: Emphasize the importance of observation.

Procedure 19.68 Oil Retention Enema

BACKGROUND: Oil retention enema solutions stimulate the bowl and lubricate the colon and rectum, which facilitates the release of stool from the colon.
ALERT: Follow Standard Precautions

Preprocedure

1. Wash your hands.
2. Assemble equipment:
   a. Prepackaged oil retention enema
   b. Bedpan and cover
   c. Waterproof bed protector
   d. Toilet tissue
   e. Towel, basin of water, and soap
   f. Disposable gloves
3. Identify patient.
4. Ask visitors to leave the room. Provide privacy with curtain, screen, or door.
5. Explain what you are going to do.
6. Put on gloves.

Procedure

7. Cover patient with a bath blanket, and fan-fold linen to foot of bed.
8. Put bedpan on foot of bed.
9. Elevate the bed to a comfortable working height and lower the side rail on the side you are working on.
10. Place bed protector under buttocks.
11. Help patient into the Sims position.

NOTE: The Sims position is a position in which the patient lies on one side with the under arm behind the back and the upper thigh flexed.

12. Tell patient to retain enema as long as possible.
13. Open a prepackaged oil retention enema.
14. Fold the bath blanket back to expose the buttock.
15. Lift patient's upper buttock and expose anus.
16. Tell patient when you are going to insert prelubricated tip into anus. (Instruct patient to take deep breaths and try to relax.) Insert tip 2–4 inches into the rectum.
17. Squeeze container slowly and steady until all solution has entered rectum.
18. Remove container; place in original package to be disposed of in contaminated waste according to facility policy and procedure.
19. Instruct patient to remain on side and retain the solution for at least 30 minutes.
20. Lower the bed and pull the side rail up. Leave the call bell in place.
21. Remove gloves and discard according to facility policy.
22. Check patient every 5 minutes until fluid has been retained for at least 20 minutes. Usually it is at least 30 minutes.
23. Position patient on bedpan or assist to bathroom. Instruct patient not to flush toilet.
24. Raise head of bed, if permitted, if using a bedpan.
25. Place toilet tissue and call bell within easy reach.
26. Stay nearby if patient is in bathroom.
27. Put on gloves.
28. Remove bedpan or assist patient to return to bed. Observe contents of toilet or bedpan for:
    a. Color, consistency, unusual materials, odor
    b. Amount of return
29. Cover bedpan and dispose of contents. Use paper towel to flush toilet and turn on faucet.
30. Remove gloves and discard in biohazardous container.

(continued)

678 Chapter 19 | Measuring Vital Signs and Other Clinical Skills

ACTIVITY

Write the names of items that a nurse assistant might encounter during the course of his or her shift, such as linens, bedpans, charts, gurneys, etc. Have each student write down the item and the precautions he or she must use when handling it.

Procedure 19.68 Oil Retention Enema (continued)

Procedure (cont)

31. Replace top sheet and remove bath blanket and plastic bed protector.
32. Give patient soap, water, and towel for hands and face.

Postprocedure

33. Wash your hands.
34. Chart the following:
    a. Date and time
    b. Type of enema given
    c. Consistency and amount of bowel movement
    d. How the procedure was tolerated

Charting Example:

5/13/24	*1930*
	16 oz oil retention enema administered
	and retained 12 minutes. Passed large
	amount of dark brown formed stool
	________ R. Johnson CNA
6/07/24	*0800*
	Tolerated enema well
	Resting quietly
	________ S. Gomez CNA

Procedure 19.69 Prepackaged Enemas

BACKGROUND: Prepackaged enema solutions stimulate the bowel and facilitate the release of stool from the colon.
ALERT: Follow Standard Precautions

Preprocedure

1. Wash your hands.
2. Assemble equipment:
    a. Prepackaged enema
    b. Bedpan and cover
    c. Waterproof bed protector
    d. Toilet tissue
    e. Towel, basin of water, and soap
    f. Disposable gloves
3. Identify patient.
4. Ask visitors to leave room.
5. Explain what you are going to do and provide privacy with curtain, screen, or door.

Procedure

6. Cover patient with a bath blanket, and fan-fold linen to foot of bed.
7. Put on gloves.
8. Raise bed to comfortable working height and lower side rail.
9. Place bed protector under buttocks.
10. Put bedpan on foot of bed.
11. Help patient into the Sims position.

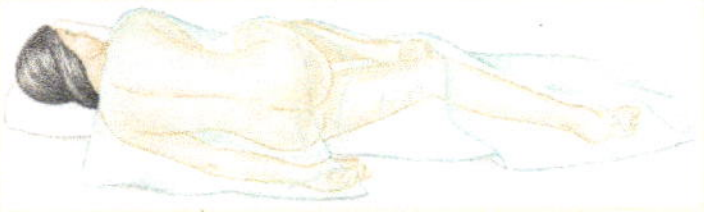

12. Fold back blanket and expose buttock.

(continued)

Measuring Vital Signs and Other Clinical Skills | Chapter 19 679

Procedure Tip

19.68 Oil Retention Enema, continued

- Review the postprocedure steps.
- Step 33: Emphasize the importance of proper handwashing.
- Step 34: Emphasize the importance of proper observation and documentation.

PROCEDURE PRACTICE

- Demonstrate the steps for Procedure 19.68, Oil Retention Enema, as many times as necessary, using a simulation or a mannequin, or ask students to demonstrate the steps. Have students practice and perform a simulated procedure until they are competent.

Procedure Tip

19.69 Prepackaged Enemas

- Review the background information, explaining the purpose of the enema.
- Emphasize the importance of following Standard Precautions.
- Review the preprocedure steps.
- Step 1: Emphasize the importance of proper handwashing.
- Step 2: Review the equipment list.
- Step 4: Emphasize the importance of patient privacy.
- Step 5: Emphasize the importance of effective communication techniques.
- Review the procedure steps.
- Step 7: Emphasize the importance of wearing gloves.
- Step 11: Explain the Sims position.

Procedure Tip

19.69 Prepackaged Enemas, continued

- Step 16: Reinforce the importance of effective communication.
- Step 27: Emphasize the importance of observation.
- Review the postprocedure steps.
- Step 32: Emphasize the importance of proper handwashing.
- Step 33: Emphasize the importance of proper observation and documentation.
- Demonstrate the steps as a simulated procedure.
- Have students practice and perform a simulated procedure.

PROCEDURE PRACTICE

- Demonstrate the steps for Procedure 19.69, Prepackaged Enemas, as many times as necessary, using a simulation or a mannequin, or ask students to demonstrate the steps. Have students practice and perform a simulated procedure until they are competent.

Procedure 19.69 Prepackaged Enemas (continued)

Procedure (cont)

13. Tell patient to retain enema as long as possible.
14. Open a prepackaged enema.
15. Lift patient's upper buttock and expose anus.
16. Tell patient when you are going to insert prelubricated tip into anus. (Have patient take deep breaths and try to relax.)
17. Squeeze container until all the solution has entered the rectum.
18. Remove container; place in original package to be disposed of according to facility policy.
19. Remove gloves and dispose of in biohazardous container.
20. Instruct patient to remain on side and to hold solution as long as possible. Have call bell in reach.
21. Put on gloves.
22. Position patient on bedpan or assist to bathroom. Instruct patient not to flush toilet.
23. Raise head of bed if permitted if patient is using a bedpan.
24. Place toilet tissue and call bell within easy reach.
25. Stay nearby if patient is in bathroom.
26. Remove bedpan or assist patient to return to bed.
27. Observe contents of toilet or bedpan for:
    a. Color, consistency, unusual materials, odor
    b. Amount of return
28. Cover bedpan and dispose of contents. Use paper towels to flush toilet and turn on facet.

Postprocedure

29. Remove gloves and dispose of according to facility policy.
30. Replace top sheet and remove bath blanket and plastic bed protector.
31. Give the patient soap, water, and towel for hands and face.
32. Wash hands.
33. Chart the following:
    a. Date and time
    b. Type of enema given
    c. Consistency and amount of bowel movement
    d. How the procedure was tolerated

Charting Example:

9/10/24	1430
	12 oz prepackaged enema
	administered and retained 5 minutes
	Complained of severe abdominal cramps.
	Passed 12 oz watery, tan-colored fluid.
	Reported to team leader
	________ A. Chaplin CNA
9/10/24	1515
	Restless
	Continues to complain about abdominal
	cramps
	Team leader notified
	________ A. Chaplin CNA

Procedure 19.70 **Tap Water, Soap Suds, Saline Enemas**

BACKGROUND: Tap water, soap suds, and saline solutions stimulate the bowel and facilitate the release of stool from the colon.
ALERT: Follow Standard Precautions

Preprocedure

1. Wash your hands.
2. Assemble equipment:
   a. Disposable gloves
   b. Disposable enema equipment:
      (1) Plastic container
      (2) Tubing
      (3) Clamp
      (4) Lubricant
   c. Enema solution as instructed by the head nurse, e.g.:
      (1) Tap water, 700–1,000 cc water (105°F)
      (2) Soap suds, 700–1,000 cc (105°F), one package enema soap
      (3) Saline, 700–1,000 cc water (105°F), 2 teaspoons salt
   d. Bedpan and cover
   e. Urinal, if necessary
   f. Toilet tissue
   g. Waterproof disposable bed protector
   h. Paper towel
   i. Bath blanket
3. Identify patient.

Procedure

4. Ask visitors to leave room
5. Tell patient what you are going to do.
6. Attach tubing to irrigation container. Adjust clamp to a position where you can easily open and close it. Close clamp.
7. Fill container with warm water (105° F):
   a. Add one package enema soap for soap suds enema.
   b. Add 2 teaspoons salt for saline enema.
   c. For tap water enema, do not add anything.
8. Provide privacy by pulling privacy curtain.
9. Raise bed to working level and put down side rail on the side you are working on.
10. Cover patient with a bath blanket. Remove upper sheet by fan-folding to foot of bed. Be careful not to expose patient.
11. Put on gloves.
12. Put waterproof protector under patient's buttocks.
13. Place bedpan on foot of bed.
14. Place patient in the Sims position.
15. Open clamp on enema tubing and let a small amount of solution run into bedpan. (This eliminates air in tubing and warms tube.) Close clamp.
16. Put a small amount of lubricating jelly on tissue. Lubricate enema tip. Check to be certain that the opening is not plugged.
17. Expose buttocks by folding back bath blanket.
18. Lift the upper buttock to expose anus.
19. Tell patient when you are going to insert lubricated tip into anus.
20. Hold rectal tube about 5 inches from tip and insert slowly into rectum.
21. Tell patient to breathe deeply through mouth and to try to relax.
22. Raise container 12 to 18 inches above patient's hip.

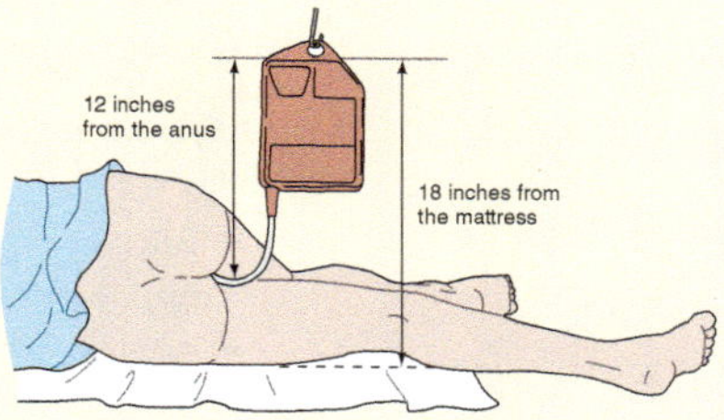

(continued)

Measuring Vital Signs and Other Clinical Skills | Chapter 19 681

Procedure Tip

19.70 Tap Water, Soap Suds, Saline Enemas

- Review the background information, explaining the purpose of the enemas.
- Emphasize the importance of following Standard Precautions.
- Review the preprocedure steps.
- Step 1: Emphasize the importance of proper handwashing.
- Step 2: Review the equipment list.
- Review the procedure steps.
- Step 4: Emphasize the importance of patient privacy.
- Step 5: Emphasize the importance of effective communication techniques.
- Steps 8 and 10: Reiterate the importance of patient privacy.
- Step 11: Emphasize the importance of wearing gloves.
- Step 12: Emphasize the importance of keeping the linens clean and dry.
- Step 14: Explain the Sims position.
- Step 19: reinforce the importance of effective communication.

ACTIVITY

Make a list of conditions that might require an enema as a treatment. Use the Internet or reference books to learn about the conditions.

Procedure Tip

19.70 Tap Water, Soap Suds, Saline Enemas, continued

- Step 28: Emphasize importance of monitoring the patient.
- Step 31: Emphasize the importance of observation.
- Review the postprocedure steps.
- Step 37: Emphasize the importance of proper handwashing.
- Step 38: Emphasize the importance of proper observation and documentation.

PROCEDURE PRACTICE

- Demonstrate the steps for Procedure 19.70, Tap Water, Soap Suds, Saline Enemas, as many times as necessary, using a simulation or a mannequin, or ask students to demonstrate the steps. Have students practice and perform a simulated procedure until they are competent.

Teaching Tips

- Define incontinence.
- Explain that it often makes a patient self-conscious and embarrassed.
- Explain some common causes of incontinence:
  - Infections
  - Surgical problems (e.g., prostate surgery)
  - Spinal cord injuries
  - Loss of sphincter control (muscle control)
  - Some diseases, such as multiple sclerosis and central nervous system damage
  - Disorientation

Procedure 19.70 **Tap Water, Soap Suds, Saline Enemas (continued)**

Procedure (cont)

23. Open clamp and let solution run in slowly. If patient complains of cramps, clamp tubing for a minute and lower bag slightly.
24. When most of solution has flowed into rectum, close clamp. Gently withdraw rectal tube. Wrap tubing with paper towel and place into enema can.
25. Ask patient to hold solution as long as possible.
26. Assist patient to bathroom and stay nearby if patient can go to bathroom. Ask patient not to flush toilet.
27. Help patient onto bedpan and raise head of bed if permitted.
28. Place call light within reach and check patient every few minutes.
29. Dispose of enema equipment while you are waiting for patient to expel enema. Follow hospital policy.
30. Remove bedpan or assist patient back to bed.
31. Observe contents for:
    a. Color, consistency, unusual materials
    b. Note amount (i.e., large or small)
32. Cover bedpan and remove bed protector.
33. Remove gloves and dispose of according to facility policy. Wash hands.
34. Replace top sheet and remove bath blanket.
35. Give patient soap, water, and a towel to wash hands.
36. Secure call light in patient's reach.

Postprocedure

37. Clean and replace all equipment used and wash your hands.
38. Chart the following:
    a. Date and time
    b. Type of enema given
    c. Results (amount, color, consistency) of bowel movement
    d. How the procedure was tolerated

Charting Example:

4/14/24	*1800*
	1,000 cc soap suds enema
	administered and retained 15 minutes
	Complained about severe abdominal
	cramps
	Passed large amount of brown, formed
	stool, brown-colored liquid, and loose
	brown stool particles
	______ S. Gomez CNA
4/14/24	*1845*
	Resting quietly in bed, no pain
	______ S. Gomez CNA

Incontinent Patient

When a patient is incontinent, he or she loses the ability to control the bowel or bladder or both. This is embarrassing to most patients. They are often irritable and depressed. You can help them by having a positive attitude and by being patient and kind. Some of the causes of incontinence are:

- Infections
- Surgical problems (e.g., prostate surgery)
- Spinal cord injuries
- Loss of sphincter control (muscle control)

- Some diseases, such as multiple sclerosis and central nervous system damage
- Disorientation

Bladder training is one method that is used to help relieve incontinence. This requires the cooperation of the health care workers and the patient. Your part in helping with the retraining of the bladder is to follow instructions carefully. They include the following:

- Keeping a careful intake and output record
- Giving fluids at specific times
- Taking the patient to void at specific intervals
- Watching for symptoms of bladder distension:
    - Restlessness
    - Dribbling
    - Distended lower abdomen
    - Sensation of pressure.
- **Residual** urine

residual
(REE sid yoo uhl)
Left over.

Staying on a schedule is the only way that bladder training can be successful. Everyone who cares for the patient must cooperate.

Indwelling foley catheters are a source of nosocomial infections and their use should be avoided whenever possible. If an indwelling catheter must be used it should be monitored and removed as soon as medically feasible.

When caring for the patient with an indwelling catheter, assess the urinary output in the collection bag. It should be:

- Clear, not cloudy
- Straw-colored, pale yellow (not deep in color)
- 1,200 to 1,500 cc per day; if less than 30 cc per hour, notify the charge nurse

If you notice anything unusual about the urine, report it immediately. This includes blood, mucus, or deep color.

NOTE: Never allow the urinary drainage bag to be higher than the hips of the patient. Keeping the bag lower provides drainage away from the urinary bladder. If the drainage bag were higher, urine could flow back into the bladder and cause an infection.

Figure 19.13
Urinary catheter. What symptoms might signal a potential problem?

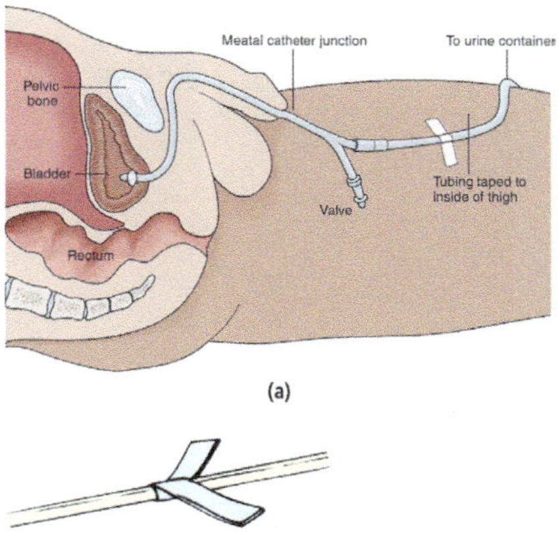

Measuring Vital Signs and Other Clinical Skills | Chapter 19 683

Teaching Tips

- Explain the reasons for bowel and bladder training:
    - Improve self-esteem
    - Reduce infection
    - Allow freer movements
- Describe procedures:
    - Keeping an intake and output record
    - Giving fluids at specific times
    - Taking the patient to void at specific intervals
    - Watching for symptoms of bladder distension
- Explain indwelling foley catheters.
- Describe what to look for in a urine collection bag:
    - Clear, not cloudy
    - Straw-colored, pale yellow (not deep in color)
    - 1,200 to 1,500 cc per day; if less than 30 cc per hour, notify the charge nurse
- Emphasize the importance of keeping the urinary drainage bag lower than the hips of the patient.
- Explain that keeping the bag lower provides drainage away from the urinary bladder. If the drainage bag were higher, urine could flow back into the bladder and cause an infection.

Figure Focus

19.13 Urinary catheter. What symptoms might signal a potential problem?

Answer: Symptoms that might signal a potential problem include cloudy urine that has a deep color. Also urine output that is less than 30 cc per hour.

ACTIVITY

Randomly assign each student a procedure covered in this chapter. Have the other students play twenty-questions to determine which procedure it is. Direct students to ask only yes/no questions, such as, "Does the procedure require contact with a patient?" or "Does the procedure use a thermometer?" Students get one point for each procedure they correctly identify within twenty questions.

Teaching Tips

- Explain that urine is often collected as a specimen for testing and to measure output.
- Describe the types of urine collection procedures: routine urine specimen, clean-catch urine specimen, fresh fractional urine, 24-hour urine specimen, and strained urine.
- Explain the importance of observing urine for color, clearness, and odor.

ACTIVITY

Read out loud symptoms or characteristics of a condition or illness. The first student who identifies the condition or illness correctly gets a point. Read out loud symptoms or characteristics of a condition or illness. The first student who identifies the condition or illness correctly gets a point.

Specimen Collection

Specimens that you collect from your patients are sent to the laboratory and tested. These tests give the physician information that helps him or her treat the patient. It is important that specimens be collected carefully and properly. They must also be labeled correctly.

Urine specimens are collected in different ways. The following are five common urine specimen collection procedures:

- Routine urine specimen
- Clean-catch urine specimen
- Fresh fractional urine
- 24-hour urine specimen
- Strained urine

When obtaining urine specimens, always observe and record:

- **Color**, which may range from light straw color to dark amber
- **Clearness**, **cloudiness**, or **particles**
- **Odor**, which may be normal, strong, or unusual

Use the urine specimen collection procedures to guide you in the correct way to collect useful specimens.

Other specimens commonly collected for testing include stool and sputum. The stool samples are examined for occult (hidden) blood and for microorganisms. Sputum samples help the physician determine what is causing an illness of the respiratory system.

When obtaining these specimens always observe and record:

- Color
- Consistency
- Odor

Use the correct specimen collection procedures to guide you when obtaining these specimens.

684 Chapter 19 | Measuring Vital Signs and Other Clinical Skills

Procedure 19.71 Disconnecting an Indwelling Catheter

BACKGROUND: Disconnecting an indwelling catheter from the drainage bag and plugging the catheter keeps urine from draining out of the body. This procedure is commonly followed when the physician wants to remove the catheter and bladder retraining is necessary; or to allow the patient to participate in activities without the urinary drainage bag.
ALERT: Follow Standard Precautions

Preprocedure

1. Wash hands.
2. Assemble equipment:
   a. Disinfectant (can use an alcohol or Betadine swab)
   b. Sterile gauze sponges
   c. Sterile cap or plug
   d. Disposable gloves
3. Identify patient and provide privacy with curtain, screen, or door.
4. Explain what you are going to do.
5. Put on gloves.

Procedure

6. Place a towel under the tubing where it connects to the catheter.
7. Disinfect connection between catheter and drainage tubing where it is to be disconnected by applying disinfectant with cotton or gauze.
8. Disconnect catheter and drainage tubing. Do not allow catheter ends to touch anything!
9. Insert a sterile plug in end of catheter. Place sterile cap over exposed end of drainage tube.
10. Carefully secure drainage tube to bed.

Postprocedure

11. Remove gloves and discard according to facility policy.
12. Wash hands.
13. Record procedure. Reverse procedure to reconnect.

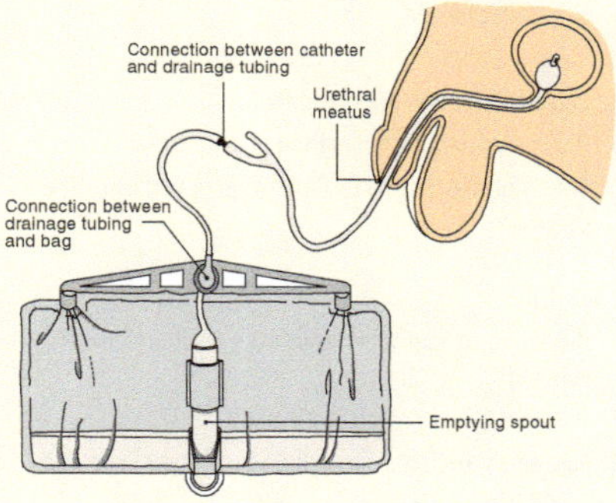

Charting Example:

5/11/24	1000
	Urinary catheter disconnected and
	plugged with a sterile plug
	S. Gomez CNA
5/11/24	1130
	Lower abdominal pain
	Catheter drained 400 cc of urine
	Plug reinserted
	S. Gomez CNA

Measuring Vital Signs and Other Clinical Skills | Chapter 19 685

Procedure Tip

19.71 Disconnecting an Indwelling Catheter

- Review the background information, explaining the situations when this procedure may be necessary.
- Emphasize the importance of following Standard Precautions.
- Review the preprocedure steps.
- Step 1: Emphasize the importance of proper handwashing.
- Step 2: Review the equipment list.
- Step 3: Emphasizing the importance of patient privacy.
- Step 4: Emphasize the importance of effective communication techniques.
- Step 5: Emphasize the importance of wearing gloves.
- Review the procedure steps.
- Steps 7 and 8: Emphasize the importance of aseptic techniques.
- Review the postprocedure steps.
- Step 12: Emphasize the importance of proper handwashing.
- Step 13: Emphasize the importance of proper observation and documentation.
- Review procedure steps in reverse for reconnecting.

PROCEDURE PRACTICE

- Demonstrate the steps for Procedure 19.71, Disconnecting an Indwelling Catheter, as many times as necessary, using a simulation or a mannequin, or ask students to demonstrate the steps. Have students practice and perform the procedure until they are competent.

Procedure Tip

19.72 Giving Indwelling Catheter Care

- Review the background information, explaining the importance of monitoring for infection.
- Emphasize the importance of following Standard Precautions.
- Review the preprocedure steps.
- Step 1: Emphasize the importance of proper handwashing.
- Step 2: Review the equipment list.
- Step 4: Emphasize the importance of effective communication techniques.
- Step 5: Emphasize patient privacy.
- Step 6: Emphasize the importance of wearing gloves.
- Review the procedure steps.
- Step 8: Emphasize the importance of keeping the bed clean and dry.
- Step 9: Review the importance of patient privacy.
- Step 10: Refer to Procedure 19.48.
- Step 15: Emphasize the importance of keeping the tube straight.
- Review the postprocedure steps.
- Step 22: Emphasize the importance of proper handwashing.
- Step 23: Emphasize the importance of proper observation and documentation.

Procedure 19.72 Giving Indwelling Catheter Care

BACKGROUND: Giving indwelling catheter care helps to prevent infection and provides an opportunity to observe the insertion site for irritation and to adjust catheter position to maximize efficient drainage.
ALERT: Follow Standard Precautions

Preprocedure

1. Wash hands.
2. Assemble equipment:
   a. Antiseptic solution or catheter care kits
   b. Waterproof bed protector
   c. Disposable nonsterile gloves
   d. Bath blanket
3. Identify patient.
4. Explain what you are going to do.
5. Provide privacy by pulling the privacy curtains.
6. Put on gloves. (Some facilities require you use sterile gloves.)

Procedure

7. Raise bed to comfortable working level and lower side rail.
8. Put waterproof protector on bed.
9. For female patients, have them bend their knee and drape them with the bath blanket, so that only the perineum is exposed. For males, pull covers back to knee and cover top half of body with bath blanket.
10. Carefully clean perineum.
11. Observe around catheter for sores, leakage, bleeding, or crusting. Report any unusual observation to nurse.
12. For females, separate labia with forefinger and thumb. Apply antiseptic solution around area where catheter enters the urethra. Wipe from front to back and place used applicator or gauze pad in biohazardous container. Use a clean applicator or gauze with antiseptic solution each time you wipe from back to front.
13. For males, pull back foreskin on uncircumcised patient and apply antiseptic to entire area. Wipe from the meatus down the shaft of the penis. Use a clean applicator or gauze with every stroke.
14. Apply antiseptic ointment (if allowed in your facility).
15. Position patient so catheter does not have kinks and is not pulling. Be sure the tubing is free of kinks and is draining.
16. Remove waterproof protector.
17. Cover patient.
18. Dispose of supplies according to facility policy.
19. Remove gloves and dispose of according to facility policy.
20. Position patient comfortably. Lower bed and raise side rail.
21. Secure call light within patient's reach.

Postprocedure

22. Wash hands.
23. Record procedure.

Charting Example:

11/02/24	0920
	Perineal care complete
	Catheter insertion site clean and free
	from irritation
	Catheter secured to left inner thigh to
	allow drainage
	________ R. Johnson CNA

686 Chapter 19 | Measuring Vital Signs and Other Clinical Skills

PROCEDURE PRACTICE

- Demonstrate the steps for Procedure 19.72, Giving Indwelling Catheter Care, as many times as necessary, using a simulation or a mannequin, or ask students to demonstrate the steps. Have students practice and perform the procedure until they are competent.

Procedure 19.73 External Urinary Catheter

BACKGROUND: An incontinent patient may use an external urinary catheter to control the flow of urine into a drainage bag in place of wearing a diaper. This is sometimes known as a condom catheter, because the device fits over the penis like a condom.
ALERT: Follow Standard Precautions

Preprocedure

1. Wash hands.
2. Assemble equipment:
   a. Basin warm water
   b. Washcloth
   c. Towel
   d. Waterproof bed protector
   e. Gloves
   f. Plastic bag
   g. Condom with drainage tip
   h. Paper towels
3. Identify patient.
4. Explain what you are going to do.

Procedure

5. Provide privacy by pulling privacy curtain.
6. Raise bed to comfortable working height.
7. Cover patient with bath blanket. Have patient hold top of blanket, and fold cover to bottom of bed.
8. Put on gloves.
9. Place waterproof protector under patient's buttocks.
10. Pull up bath blanket to expose genitals only.
11. Remove condom by rolling gently toward tip of penis.
12. Wash and dry penis.
13. Observe for irritation, open areas, bleeding.
14. Report any unusual observations.
15. Check condom for "ready stick" surface. If there is none, apply a thin spray of tincture of benzoin. Do not spray on head of penis.
16. Apply new condom and drainage tip to penis by rolling toward base of penis.
17. Reconnect drainage system.
18. Remove and dispose of gloves in biohazardous container.
19. Pull up top bedding and remove bath blanket.
20. Replace equipment.
21. Lower bed to lowest position.
22. Put up side rail if required.
23. Secure call light within patient's reach.

Postprocedure

24. Tidy unit.
25. Wash hands.
26. Record procedure.

Charting Example:

4/10/24	0730
	Shower taken and tolerated well
	Urinary condom drainage system
	applied and drains well
	A. Chaplin CNA

Measuring Vital Signs and Other Clinical Skills | Chapter 19 687

Procedure Tip

19.73 External Urinary Catheter

- Review the background information, explaining the device and how it is used.
- Emphasize the importance of following Standard Precautions.
- Review the preprocedure steps.
- Step 1: Emphasize the importance of proper handwashing.
- Step 2: Review the equipment list.
- Step 4: Emphasize the importance of effective communication techniques.
- Review the procedure steps.
- Step 5: Emphasize patient privacy.
- Step 8: Emphasize the importance of wearing gloves.
- Steps 13 and 14: Reinforce the importance of observation and reporting.
- Step 19: Emphasize the importance of keeping the bed clean and dry.
- Review the postprocedure steps.
- Step 25: Emphasize the importance of proper handwashing.
- Step 26: Emphasize the importance of proper observation and documentation.

PROCEDURE PRACTICE

- Demonstrate the steps for Procedure, 19.73, External Urinary Catheter, as many times as necessary, or ask students to demonstrate the steps using a simulation or mannequin. Have students practice and perform the procedure until they are competent.

Procedure Tip

19.74 Emptying the Urinary Drainage Bag

- Review the background information, emphasizing the opportunity to measure output.
- Emphasize the importance of following Standard Precautions.
- Review the preprocedure steps.
- Step 1: Emphasize the importance of proper handwashing.
- Step 2: Emphasize the importance of effective communication techniques.
- Step 3: Emphasize patient privacy.
- Step 4: Review the equipment list.
- Emphasize the importance of wearing gloves.
- Review the procedure steps.
- Step 7: Emphasize the use of aseptic techniques.
- Steps 9 and 10: Reinforce the importance of observation and reporting.
- Step 11: Remind students why graduate must be held at eye level.
- Review the postprocedure steps.
- Step 15: Emphasize the importance of proper handwashing.
- Step 16: Emphasize the importance of proper observation and documentation.

Procedure 19.74 Emptying the Urinary Drainage Bag

BACKGROUND: Emptying the urinary drainage bag provides an opportunity to:

1. Measure urinary output for a specific period of time
2. Observe characteristics of urine

ALERT: Follow Standard Precautions

Preprocedure

1. Wash hands.
2. Identify patient and explain procedure
3. Provide privacy with curtain, screen, or door.
4. Assemble equipment:
   a. Graduate or measuring cup
   b. Disposable gloves
   c. Paper towel
   d. An alcohol swab
5. Put on disposable gloves.

Procedure

6. Place towel on floor and set graduate cylinder on top of the towel.
7. Carefully open drain outlet on urinary bag. Do not allow container outlet to touch floor. This will introduce microorganisms into bag and can cause infection.
8. Drain bag into graduate and clean drain outlet with alcohol swab. Then reattach drainage outlet securely.
9. Observe urine for:
   a. Dark color
   b. Blood
   c. Unusual odor
   d. Large amount of mucus
   e. Sediment
10. Report any unusual observations to nurse immediately (do not discard urine).
11. Hold graduate at eye level and read amount of urine on measuring scale.
12. Discard urine if normal. Flush toilet and turn on faucet with paper towel.
13. Rinse graduate and put away.

Postprocedure

14. Remove gloves and discard in hazardous waste.
15. Wash hands.
16. Record amount of urine in cc's on the I & O record.

Charting Example:

10/10/24	0700
	15.00 Urinary drainage, 1,290 cc
	A. Chaplin CNA

688 Chapter 19 | Measuring Vital Signs and Other Clinical Skills

PROCEDURE PRACTICE

- Demonstrate the steps for Procedure 19.74, Emptying the Urinary Drainage Bag, as many times as necessary, or ask students to demonstrate the steps. Have students practice and perform the procedure until they are competent.

Procedure 19.75 Collect Specimen Under Transmission-Based Precautions

BACKGROUND: Concerns about the transmission of blood borne diseases, such as AIDS and the hepatitis B virus, and the increasing incidence of hospital acquired infections has caused a change in the focus of infection control programs. Since 1987 the CDC (Centers for Disease Control) has promoted the use of universal precautions.

It is recommended that health-care workers use gloves, gowns, masks, and protective eyewear when exposure to blood or body fluids is likely and that all patients be considered potentially infected. Universal precautions are used along with category-specific isolation systems when indicated.

Efforts have also been made to remove all sharps, such as needles, from the health-care system whenever possible, thus diminishing contamination from needle sticks. Collecting specimens requires some contact with body fluids so the prudent use of universal precautions becomes a critical part of the process.

ALERT: Follow Standard Precautions

Preprocedure

1. Collect the equipment necessary for obtaining the specimen (specimen cup, lab tubes, tourniquets, etc.).
2. Wash hands.
3. Put on disposable gloves, gowns, mask, and protective eyewear as may be required depending on the specimen to be collected.

Procedure

4. Provide an explanation to the patient regarding the specimen to be collected. Answer any questions the patient may have.
5. Collect the specimen using aseptic or sterile technique as required.
6. Label the specimen with the patient's name, date, and time of collection.
7. Place the specimen in a protective package as prescribed by the institution.
8. Assure that the patient has no further needs.
9. Dispose of any used supplies and any protective items used in the collection of the specimen in the appropriate manner, as determined by your institution.

Postprocedure

10. Wash hands.
11. Send the specimen to the laboratory.

Measuring Vital Signs and Other Clinical Skills | Chapter 19 689

PROCEDURE PRACTICE

- Demonstrate the steps for Procedure 19.75, Collect Specimen Under Transmission-Based Precautions, as many times as necessary, or ask students to demonstrate the steps. Have students practice and perform the procedure until they are competent.

Procedure Tip

19.75 Collect Specimen Under Transmission-Based Precautions

- Review the background information. Review Transmission-Based Precautions (Section 17.3) and Universal Precautions (Section 17.4).
- Emphasize the importance of following the indicated precautions.
- Review the preprocedure steps.
- Step 1: Discuss the equipment that might be required.
- Step 2: Emphasize the importance of proper handwashing.
- Review the procedure steps.
- Step 4: Emphasize the importance of effective communication techniques.
- Step 5: Review aseptic and sterile techniques (Section 17.1).
- Step 6: Emphasize the proper labeling procedures.
- Step 7: Emphasize the need to follow the facility's policies.
- Review the postprocedure steps.
- Step 10: Emphasize the importance of proper handwashing.
- Step 11: Emphasize the importance of knowing the procedure for sending the specimen to the lab.
- Review the importance of proper observation and documentation.

Procedure Tip

19.76 Routine Urine Specimen

- Review the background information, discussing situations when a urine specimen may be required.
- Emphasize the importance of following Standard Precautions.
- Review the preprocedure steps.
- Step 1: Emphasize the importance of proper handwashing.
- Step 2: Review the equipment list.
- Step 4: Emphasize the importance of effective communication techniques.
- Review the procedure steps.
- Step 5: Emphasize the proper labeling procedures.
- Step 6: Emphasize the importance of patient privacy.
- Step 7: Emphasize the importance of wearing gloves.
- Step 17: Emphasize the importance of washing the patient's hands.
- Review the postprocedure steps.
- Step 18: Emphasize the importance of proper handwashing.
- Step 19: Emphasize the importance of knowing the procedure for the lab.
- Step 20: Emphasize the importance of proper observation and documentation.

Procedure 19.76 Routine Urine Specimen

BACKGROUND: To evaluate the chemical structure of urine and determine the need for further testing.
ALERT: Follow Standard Precautions

Preprocedure

1. Wash hands.
2. Assemble equipment:
   a. Graduate (pitcher)
   b. Bedpan or urinal
   c. Urine specimen container
   d. Label
   e. Paper bag
   f. Disposable nonsterile gloves
3. Identify patient.
4. Explain what you are going to do.

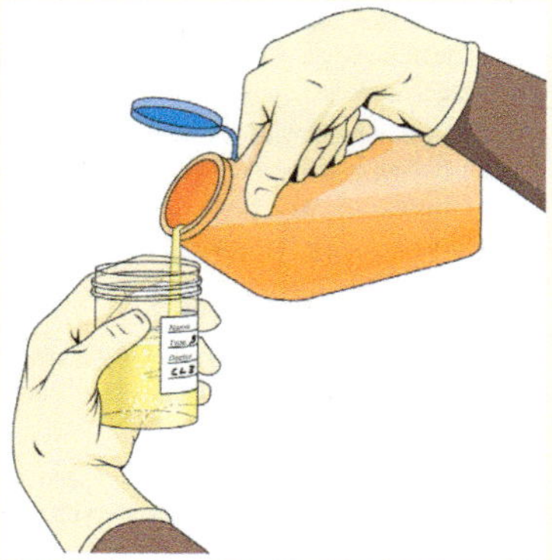

Procedure

5. Label specimen carefully:
   a. Patient's name
   b. Date
   c. Time
   d. Room number
6. Provide privacy by pulling privacy curtain.
7. Put on gloves.
8. Have patient void (urinate) into clean bedpan or urinal.
9. Ask patient to put toilet tissue into paper bag.
10. Pour specimen into graduate.
11. Pour from graduate into specimen container until about three-quarters full.
12. Place lid on container.
13. Discard leftover urine.
14. Clean and rinse graduate, bedpan, or urinal, and put away.
15. Remove gloves.
16. Position patient comfortably.
17. Assist patient to wash hands.

Postprocedure

18. Wash hands.
19. Store specimen according to direction for lab pickup.
20. Report and record procedure and observation of specimen.

690 Chapter 19 | Measuring Vital Signs and Other Clinical Skills

PROCEDURE PRACTICE

- Demonstrate the steps for Procedure 19.76, Routine Urine Specimen, as many times as necessary, or ask students to demonstrate the steps using a simulation or mannequin. Have students practice and perform the procedure until they are competent.

Procedure 19.77 Midstream Clean-Catch Urine, Female

BACKGROUND: A midstream clean-catch urine procedure provides a way to collect urine free of bacteria present at the urethral meatus at the beginning of urination, and in sediment in the urinary bladder, which drains at the end of urination.
ALERT: Follow Standard Precautions

Preprocedure

1. Wash hands.
2. Assemble equipment:
   a. Antiseptic solution or soap and water or towelettes
   b. Sterile specimen container
   c. Tissues
   d. Nonsterile gloves
3. Identify patient.
4. Explain what you are going to do.

Procedure

5. Label specimen:
   a. Patient's name
   b. Time obtained
   c. Date
6. If patient is on bedrest:
   a. Put on gloves.
   b. Lower side rail.
   c. Position bedpan under patient.
7. Have patient carefully clean perineal area if able; if not, you will be responsible for cleaning perineum:
   a. Wipe with towelette or gauze with antiseptic solution from front to back.
   b. Wipe one side and throw away wipe.
   c. Use a clean wipe for other side.
   d. Use another wipe down center.
   e. Then proceed with collecting midstream urine.
8. Explain procedure if patient can obtain own specimen:
   a. Have patient start to urinate into bedpan/toilet.
   b. Allow stream to begin.
   c. Stop stream and place specimen container to collect midstream.
   d. Remove container before bladder is empty.
9. Wipe perineum, if on bedpan.
10. Remove bedpan.
11. Rinse bedpan and put away.
12. Remove gloves and discard according to facility policy and procedure.
13. Raise side rail.
14. Secure call light in patient's reach.
15. Dispose of equipment. Never handle contaminated equipment without gloves.

Postprocedure

16. Wash hands.
17. Record specimen collection.
18. Report any unusual:
    a. Color
    b. Consistency
    c. Odor

Charting Example:

7/14/24	*1300*
	Clean-catch urine collected
	Urine was straw colored
	Labeled and sent to the laboratory
	R. Johnson CNA

Measuring Vital Signs and Other Clinical Skills | Chapter 19 691

Procedure Tip

19.77 Midstream Clean-Catch Urine, Female

- Review the background information, explaining the purpose of a clean-catch specimen.
- Emphasize the importance of following Standard Precautions.
- Review the preprocedure steps.
- Step 1: Emphasize the importance of proper handwashing.
- Step 2: Review the equipment list.
- Step 4: Emphasize the importance of effective communication techniques.
- Review the procedure steps.
- Step 5: Emphasize the proper labeling procedures.
- Review the postprocedure steps.
- Step 16: Emphasize the importance of proper handwashing.
- Steps 17 and 18: Emphasize the importance of proper observation and documentation.

PROCEDURE PRACTICE

- Demonstrate the steps for Procedure 19.77, Midstream Clean-Catch Urine, Female, as many times as necessary, or ask students to demonstrate the steps using a simulation or mannequin. Have students practice and perform the procedure until they are competent.

Procedure Tip

19.78 Midstream Clean-Catch Urine, Male

- Review the background information, explaining the purpose of a clean-catch specimen.
- Emphasize the importance of following Standard Precautions.
- Review the preprocedure steps.
- Step 1: Emphasize the importance of proper handwashing.
- Step 2: Review the equipment list.
- Review the procedure steps.
- Step 4: Emphasize the proper labeling procedures.
- Step 5: Emphasize the importance of effective communication techniques.
- Review the postprocedure steps.
- Step 9: Emphasize the importance of proper handwashing.
- Step 10: Emphasize the importance of proper observation and documentation.

PROCEDURE PRACTICE

- Demonstrate the steps for Procedure 19.78, Midstream Clean-Catch Urine, Male, as many times as necessary, or ask students to demonstrate the steps using a simulation or mannequin. Have students practice and perform the procedure until they are competent.

Procedure 19.78 Midstream Clean-Catch Urine, Male

BACKGROUND: A midstream clean-catch urine procedure provides a way to collect urine free of bacteria present at the urethral meatus at the beginning of urination, and in sediment in the urinary bladder, which drains at the end of urination.
ALERT: Follow Standard Precautions

Preprocedure

1. Wash hands.
2. Assemble equipment:
   a. Antiseptic solution or soap and water or towelettes
   b. Sterile specimen container

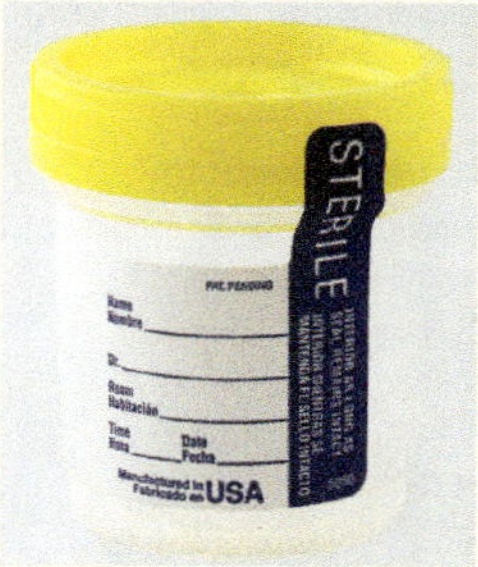

   c. Tissues
   d. Disposable gloves
3. Identify patient.

procedure

4. Label specimen:
   a. Patient's name
   b. Date
   c. Time obtained
5. Explain procedure (if possible allow patient to obtain his own specimen):
   a. Put on gloves.
   b. Cleanse head of penis in a circular motion with towelette or gauze and antiseptic. (If patient is uncircumcised, have him pull back foreskin before cleaning.)
   c. Have patient start to urinate into clean bedpan, urinal, or toilet. (If he is uncircumcised, have patient pull back foreskin before urinating.)
   d. Allow stream to begin.
   e. Stop stream and place specimen container to collect midstream.
   f. Remove container before bladder is empty.
6. Dispose of equipment according to facility policy.

Postprocedure

7. Remove and discard gloves according to facility policy and procedure.
8. Make patient comfortable and put call bell within reach.
9. Wash hands.
10. Record specimen collection.

Charting Example:

5/16/24 1300
Clean-catch urine collected
Urine was dark amber in color with
white sediment
Labeled and sent to the laboratory
A. Chaplin CNA

692 Chapter 19 | Measuring Vital Signs and Other Clinical Skills

Procedure 19.79 **HemaCombistix**

BACKGROUND: HemaCombistix detects the presence of blood in urine.
ALERT: Follow Standard Precautions

Preprocedure

1. Wash hands.
2. Assemble equipment:
   a. Bottle of HemaCombistix
   b. Nonsterile gloves
3. Identify patient.
4. Explain what you are going to do.
5. Put on gloves.

Procedure

6. Secure fresh urine sample from patient.
7. Take urine and reagent to bathroom.
8. Remove cap and place on flat surface. Be sure top side of cap is down.
9. Remove strip from bottle by shaking bottle gently. Do not touch areas of strip with fingers.
10. Dip reagent stick in urine. Remove immediately.
11. Tap edge of strip on container to remove excess urine.
12. Compare reagent side of test areas with color chart on bottle. Use time intervals that are given on bottle.

NOTE: Do not touch reagent strip to bottle.

13. Remove gloves and discard both strip and urine specimen according to facility policy and procedure. Need to discard specimen and then take off gloves.

Postprocedure

14. Replace equipment.
15. Wash hands.
16. Record results:
    a. Date and time
    b. Name of procedure used
    c. Results

Charting Example:

10/04/24	*1800*
	Urine specimen tested with a
	hemacombistix
	Results negative for blood
	R. Johnson CNA

Measuring Vital Signs and Other Clinical Skills | Chapter 19 693

Procedure Tip

19.79 HemaCombistix

- Review the background information, explaining the purpose of using HemaCombistix, and why blood in the urine might indicate a problem.
- Emphasize the importance of following Standard Precautions.
- Review the preprocedure steps.
- Step 1: Emphasize the importance of proper handwashing.
- Step 2: Review the equipment list.
- Step 4: Emphasize the importance of effective communication techniques.
- Step 5: Emphasize the importance of wearing gloves.
- Review the procedure steps.
- Step 6: Refer to Procedures 19.77 and 19.78.
- Step 9: Emphasize aseptic and/or sterile precautions.
- Review the postprocedure steps.
- Step 15: Emphasize the importance of proper handwashing.
- Step 16: Emphasize the importance of proper observation and documentation.

PROCEDURE PRACTICE

- Demonstrate the steps for Procedure 19.79, HemaCombistix, as many times as necessary, or ask students to demonstrate the steps. Have students practice and perform the procedure until they are competent.

Procedure Tip

19.80 Straining Urine

- Review the background information, defining kidney stones, and explaining why it might be necessary to collect them.
- Emphasize the importance of following Standard Precautions.
- Review the preprocedure steps.
- Step 1: Emphasize the importance of proper handwashing.
- Step 2: Review the equipment list.
- Review the procedure steps.
- Step 4: Emphasize the importance of effective communication techniques.
- Step 5: Emphasize the importance of wearing gloves.
- Step 12: Emphasize the importance of proper handwashing.
- Step 13: Emphasize the importance of proper labeling.
- Review the postprocedure steps.
- Step 17: Emphasize the importance of proper handwashing.
- Steps 18 and 19: Emphasize the importance of proper observation and documentation.

PROCEDURE PRACTICE

- Demonstrate the steps for Procedure 19.80, Straining Urine, as many times as necessary, or ask students to demonstrate the steps. Have students practice and perform the procedure until they are competent.

Procedure 19.80 Straining Urine

BACKGROUND: Pouring urine through a strainer allows calculi (kidney stones) to be collected.
ALERT: Follow Standard Precautions

Preprocedure

1. Wash hands.
2. Assemble equipment:
   a. Paper strainers or gauze
   b. Specimen container and label
   c. Bedpan or urinal and cover
   d. Laboratory request for analysis of specimen
   e. Sign for patient's room or bathroom explaining that all urine must be strained
   f. Nonsterile gloves
3. Identify patient.

Procedure

4. Tell the patient to urinate into a urinal or bedpan and that the nurse assistant must be called to filter each specimen. Tell patient not to put paper in specimen.
5. Put on gloves.
6. Pour voided specimen through a paper strainer or gauze into a measuring container.
7. Place paper or gauze strainer into a dry specimen container if stones or particles are present after pouring urine through.

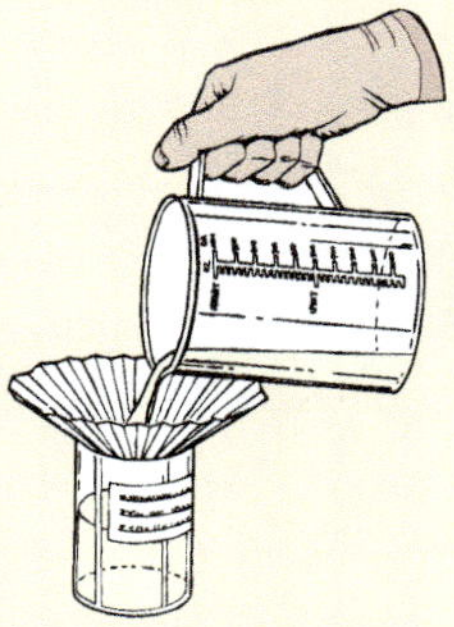

NOTE: Do not attempt to remove the particles from strainer.

8. Measure the amount voided and record on intake and output record.
9. Discard urine and container according to facility policy and procedure.
10. Clean urinal or bedpan and put away. Flush toilet and turn faucet on with a paper towel.
11. Remove gloves and discard according to facility policy and procedure.
12. Wash hands.
13. Label specimen:
    a. Patient's name
    b. Date
    c. Room number
    d. Time
14. Return patient to comfortable position.
15. Place call button within reach of patient.
16. Provide for patient safety by raising side rails when indicated or using postural supports as ordered.

Postprocedure

17. Wash hands.
18. Report collection of specimen to supervisor immediately.
19. Record specimen collection.

Charting Example:

6/20/24	*1400*
	300 cc strained
	Two small stones collected
	Given to team leader
	________ *S. Gomez CNA*

694 Chapter 19 | Measuring Vital Signs and Other Clinical Skills

Procedure 19.81 Stool Specimen Collection

BACKGROUND: Stool specimens are collected most frequently to determine if blood or parasites are present in the stool.

ALERT: Follow Standard Precautions

Preprocedure

1. Wash hands.
2. Assemble equipment:
   a. Stool specimen container with label
   b. Wooden tongue depressor
   c. Disposable gloves
   d. Bedpan and cover
3. Identify patient.
4. Explain what you are going to do.

Procedure

5. Be certain container is properly labeled with:
   a. Patient's name
   b. Time
   c. Date
   d. Room number
6. Provide privacy by pulling privacy curtains.
7. Put on gloves.
8. Take bedpan into bathroom after patient has had bowel movement.
9. Use tongue depressor to remove about 1 to 2 tablespoons of feces from bedpan.
10. Place specimen in specimen container.

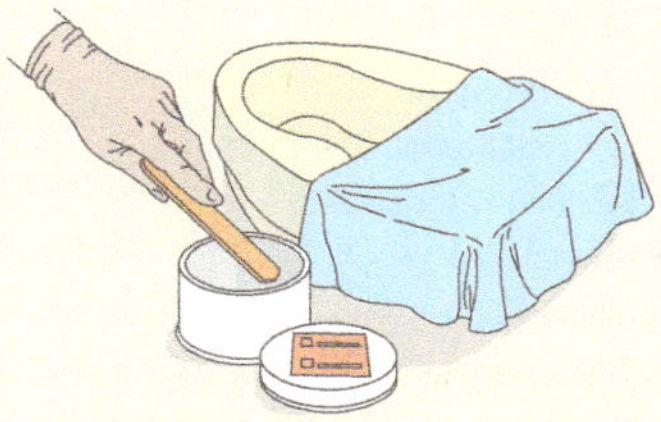

11. Cover container immediately.
12. Wrap tongue depressor in paper towel and discard as per facility rules.
13. Remove gloves and dispose of according to facility policy.

Postprocedure

14. Wash hands.
15. Follow instruction for storage of specimen for collection by lab.
16. Position patient comfortably with call bell in place.
17. Report and record procedure.

Charting Example:

12/14/24 1000
Soft, brown stool collected,
labeled, and sent to laboratory
R. Johnson CNA

Measuring Vital Signs and Other Clinical Skills | Chapter 19 695

Procedure Tip

19.81 Stool Specimen Collection

- Review the background information, discussing reasons why it might be necessary to collect a stool specimen.
- Emphasize the importance of following Standard Precautions.
- Review the preprocedure steps.
- Step 1: Emphasize the importance of proper handwashing.
- Step 2: Review the equipment list.
- Step 4: Emphasize the importance of effective communication techniques.
- Review the procedure steps.
- Step 5: Emphasize the importance of proper labeling.
- Step 6: Emphasize the importance of patient privacy.
- Step 7: Emphasize the importance of wearing gloves.
- Review the postprocedure steps.
- Step 14: Emphasize the importance of proper handwashing.
- Step 15: Emphasize the importance of properly preparing the specimen for the lab.
- Step 17: Emphasize the importance of proper observation and documentation.

PROCEDURE PRACTICE

- Demonstrate the steps for Procedure 19.81, Stool Specimen Collection, as many times as necessary, or ask students to demonstrate the steps. Have students practice and perform the procedure until they are competent.

Procedure Tip

19.82 Occult Blood Hematest

- Review the background information, explaining why blood in the stool might indicate a problem.
- Emphasize the importance of following Standard Precautions.
- Review the preprocedure steps.
- Step 1: Emphasize the importance of proper handwashing.
- Step 2: Review the equipment list.
- Step 4: Emphasize the importance of effective communication techniques.
- Step 5: Emphasize the importance of wearing gloves.
- Review the procedure steps.
- Step 6: Review Procedure 19.81.
- Review the postprocedure steps.
- Step 17: Emphasize the importance of proper handwashing.
- Step 18: Emphasize the importance of proper observation and documentation.

PROCEDURE PRACTICE

- Demonstrate the steps for Procedure 19.82, Occult Blood Hematest, as many times as necessary, or ask students to demonstrate the steps. Have students practice and perform the procedure until they are competent.

Language Arts Link—Portrayal of Health Care Workers on TV

- Discuss the current television shows that depict health care workers.

Procedure 19.82 Occult Blood Hematest

BACKGROUND: Occult blood Hematest reveals the presence of blood in a stool specimen.
ALERT: Follow Standard Precautions

Preprocedure

1. Wash hands.
2. Assemble equipment:
   a. Hematest Reagent filter paper
   b. Hematest Reagent tablet
   c. Distilled water
   d. Tongue blade
   e. Disposable gloves
3. Identify patient.
4. Explain what you are going to do.
5. Put on gloves.

Procedure

6. Secure stool specimen from patient.
7. Place filter paper on glass or porcelain plate.
8. Use tongue blade to smear a thin streak of fecal material on filter paper.
9. Place Hematest Reagent tablet on smear.
10. Place 1 drop distilled water on tablet.
11. Allow 5 to 10 seconds for water to penetrate tablet.
12. Add second drop, allowing water to run down side of tablet onto filter paper and specimen.
13. Gently tap side of plate to knock water droplets from top of tablet.
14. Observe filter paper for color change (2 minutes). Positive is indicated by blue halo on paper.
15. Dispose of specimen and equipment according to your facility's policy.
16. Remove gloves and dispose of according to your facility's policy.

Postprocedure

17. Wash hands.
18. Report and record results (e.g., date, time, procedure, and results).

Language Arts Link

Portrayal of Health Care Workers on TV

The number of TV shows about hospitals and health care professionals has increased significantly over the last several years. Many of the health care workers shown on TV appear as glamorous, caring, and dedicated professionals.

How do you feel the depiction of health care workers on TV effects what people expect when seeking health care services? Do the TV shows help or hurt the image of the health care professional?

Create a new document on the computer, or get a blank sheet of paper. In paragraph form, write how you feel about the portrayal of health care workers on TV. Include a title for your report and a thesis statement (a sentence stating your main ideas) in the opening paragraph. Develop your opinions fairly and thoroughly, with the most relevant information you have gathered, pointing out the strengths and weaknesses of the health care professional representations.

Check the spelling and grammar and correct any errors. Be sure to cite any sources that you use in the format required by your teacher. Exchange reports with a classmate. Provide feedback and corrections as necessary, and then exchange back. Read your classmate's comments and revise your report as necessary.

696 Chapter 19 | Measuring Vital Signs and Other Clinical Skills

- Remind students of the need to include a thesis statement, and to back it up with facts, or real-life examples.
- You might want to set a minimum and maximum number of words or pages.
- Encourage peer review by having students exchange reports to critique and edit.
- Evaluate the reports based on proper formatting, spelling, grammar, and content.

CUSTOMIZED INSTRUCTION

More Advanced Students

Assign more advanced students the opportunity to write a script for a TV show, movie, or play that centers around a health care situation. It might take place in a health care facility, have health care workers as the main characters, or depict a particular event that involves health care. Encourage them to be creative and original.

Procedure 19.83 **24-Hour Urine Test**

BACKGROUND: Routine urine tests were performed as early at 1821. Analysis of the patient's urine is useful for diagnosing renal disease or metabolic disease not related to the kidneys. For some laboratory studies, 24-hour urine specimens are required.
ALERT: Follow Standard Precautions

Preprocedure

1. Determine the laboratory test and any special requirements associated with the test. This could include altering the dietary intake, special collection containers, adding preservatives to the designated container, icing the container, etc.
2. The nurse should determine if any drugs affect the results of this test. Obtain a history of any drugs the patient is currently taking and advise the laboratory as necessary.
3. Obtain the appropriate container to be used for urine collection. Label the container with the patient's name, hospital number, date, and time of the urine collection.

Procedure

4. Explain the procedure to the patient. Provide a means for the patient to collect their urinary output, if the patient is able to participate in the procedure.
5. Post a sign that all urine is to be collected for a specified time. Assure that all staff providing care for this patient during this period of time are aware of the need to save all urine output.
6. When initiating the collection the patient will empty his or her bladder, and this specimen will be discarded. All urine produced after this time will be saved. At the end of the time period, the patient will again empty his or her bladder and this last specimen will be added to the specimen container.
7. If any urine is inadvertently discarded during the 24-hour collection, the test must be restarted.

Postprocedure

8. At the end of the test period, transport the labeled specimen to the laboratory.

Summary

It is important to a patient's well-being that he or she is clean and groomed. As a nursing assistant, you will need to know how to help patients undertake these activities. This may include assisting a patient with bathing, oral care needs, and hair and nail care. It is vital that the patient is as comfortable as possible. You may also be responsible for collecting patient specimens, so it's important that you learn these skills.

Community

At the completion of the chapter, assist at a health care clinic or assist the school nurse with taking and recording vital signs under direct supervision of a health care professional.

Section 19.3 Review Questions

1. Why is important to move patients every two hours?
2. List five ways to prevent pressure sores/decubiti.
3. Why is bathing a patient important?
4. Why is hair and nail care important?
5. List the five common urine specimen collection procedures.
6. What is the formula for converting ounces to cubic centimeters?
7. Under what conditions might you use restraints on a patient?

Measuring Vital Signs and Other Clinical Skills | Chapter 19 697

Procedure Tip

19.83 24-Hour Urine Test

- Review the background information, explaining that the procedure involves collecting urine for 24 hours.
- Emphasize the importance of following Standard Precautions.
- Review the preprocedure steps.
- Steps 1 and 2: Discuss the importance of proper preparation in order to assure the validity of the specimen.
- Step 3: Emphasize the importance of proper labeling.
- Review the procedure steps.
- Steps 4 and 5: Emphasize the importance of effective communication techniques.
- Step 7: Emphasize the importance of collecting all urine during the 24-hour period.
- Review the postprocedure steps.
- Step 8: Emphasize the importance of proper handling and preparation of the specimen for the lab.

PROCEDURE PRACTICE

- Demonstrate the steps for Procedure 19.83, 24-Hour Urine Test, as many times as necessary, or ask students to demonstrate the steps. Have students practice and perform the procedure until they are competent.

Teaching Tips

- Review the responsibilities of a nurse assistant.
- Review the objectives covered in Section 19.3.
- Ask students if there are any objectives they feel they need to spend more time on, and then do so.

Section 19.3 Review Questions

1. Answer: Patients should be moved every two hours to avoid pressure sores.
2. Answer: Change the patient's position at least every two hours. If patient is up in chair, ask the patient to shift their weight at least every two hours. Keep skin clean. Massage reddened areas over sharp, bony areas to increase circulation. Provide back rubs to increase circulation and relax the patient. Keep linen dry and free of wrinkles. Consider the use of specialized beds or gel-filled pads for the patient at high risk of a break in skin integrity.

Community

- You may want to contact health care facilities and/or the school nurse to identify locations that are receptive to allowing your students to assist.
- Remind them that they represent your school and to behave in a professional manner at all times.
- Allow class time to discuss the experience.

3. Answer: Removes perspiration and dirt; removes odor; increases circulation; gives you an opportunity to observe the patient's skin; and provides relaxation
4. Answer: Hair and nail care helps is important for patients because it makes them feel good.
5. Answer: Routine urine specimen; clean-catch urine specimen; fresh fractional urine; 24-hour urine specimen; and strained urine
6. Answer: 30 × (number of ounces) = number of cc
7. Answer: Restraints might be used on a patient to prevent a patient from inflicting self-harm or injury; prevent patients from removing medically necessary tubes, IV, and dressing; and to keep a small child still during a procedure.

CHAPTER 19 REVIEW

Chapter Review Questions

1. List three factors that may increase body temperature and three factors that may decrease body temperature. (19.1)
2. Where on the body is the most accurate temperature reading taken? Under what conditions is a patient's temperature taken at this site? (19.1)
3. At what site on the body is the apical pulse counted? What instrument is used to count an apical pulse? (19.1)
4. Name three factors that may cause a decreased pulse rate. (19.1)
5. What does a pulse oximeter measure? (19.1)
6. Vital signs are recorded in this order: TPR. Why is it important that you record vital signs in this order? (19.1)
7. What do vital signs tell us about homeostasis? (19.1)
8. Blood pressure depends on three factors. Name these three factors. (19.2)
9. Name five factors that can decrease blood pressure. (19.2)
10. What is a sphygmomanometer? (19.2)
11. What is hypotension? (19.2)
12. List ten responsibilities of a nurse or nurse assistant. (19.3)
13. Why is it important to encourage patients to walk? (19.3)
14. List three examples of when postural supports or restraints should be used. (19.3)
15. List the steps for preparing a patient for a meal. (19.3)
16. Compare the symptoms of dehydration and edema. (19.3)
17. List three causes of incontinence. (19.3)

Activities

1. Find your radial pulse on both arms. Record the number of beats per minute (bpm), using both paper and electronic formats. Then, do the same for two other sites, such as the carotid, brachial, or popliteal sites. Are the results the same in all locations?
2. Ask five people of various ages if you can practice counting their pulse and respiration. Prepare a chart similar to the one shown below. First write down the information and then create an electronic document to record the information. Fill in the information and submit the completed chart to your teacher.

Person	Age	Pulse	Pulse Characteristics	Respiratory Rate	Respiration Characteristics
1					
2					
3					
4					
5					

698 Chapter 19 | Measuring Vital Signs and Other Clinical Skills

CHAPTER 19 REVIEW

Chapter Review Questions

1. Answer: Factors that increase body temperature include: exercise, digestion of food, increased environmental temperature, illness, infection, excitement, and anxiety. Factors that decrease body temperature include: sleep, fasting, exposure to cold, certain illnesses, decreased muscle activity, mouth breathing, and depression.
2. Answer: Rectal temperature is the most accurate and can be taken if the patient is less than six years of age; has difficulty breathing; is extremely weak, confused, unconscious, or senile; is being given oxygen; is a mouth breather; or is experiencing partial paralysis of the face caused by a stroke or accident.
3. Answer: The apical pulse is taken at the pointed end of the heart, which is called the apex of the heart. A stethoscope is used to count an apical pulse.
4. Answer: A decreased pulse rate may be caused by high levels of aerobic activity, depression, medication, cardiac dysfunction, or sleep.
5. Answer: A pulse oximeter measures the oxygen (O_2) saturation of arterial blood.
6. Answer: It's important to record vital signs in TPR order because all health care professionals record vital signs in the same way.
7. Answer: Vital signs help provide a patient's health status, important for maintaining homeostasis (balance in the body).
8. Answer: Blood pressure depends on the volume of blood in the circulating system, the force of the heartbeat, and the condition of the arteries.
9. Answer: The following factors decrease blood pressure: hemorrhage, inactivity, fasting, suppressants, depression, and shock.
10. Answer: A device used to measure the pressure against the arteries of the body.

CHAPTER 19 REVIEW

3. Homeostasis, a constant balance within the body, is critical to good health and is affected in differing ways by each body system.
   a. Select two body systems and describe biological processes that maintain homeostasis and the interaction of the two systems selected to support the process.
   b. Select two body systems and describe chemical processes that maintain homeostasis and the interaction of the two systems to support the process.
4. Working with a partner, practice taking each other's vital signs. Then, pretend that your partner has a wound and demonstrate first aid techniques.

Case Studies

1. You are assigned a patient and you need to take vital signs. Mr. Marks is an elderly man and seems very agitated and upset. You know that his agitation affects his vital signs. What verbal and nonverbal communication skills can you use to reduce his anxiety? Write a brief description of how to help Mr. Marks relax so that you can take accurate vital signs.
2. Mr. Ames is on oxygen and cannot breathe comfortably when you remove his oxygen mask. It is time to take his vital signs. He has a severe infection, and an accurate temperature reading is extremely important. What is the correct location for taking his temperature? Explain why. What information is appropriate to give Mr. Ames before you take his temperature?

Thinking Critically

1. **Medical Terminology**—Define the following medical terms and explain why they are important when taking vital signs: arrhythmia, aural, axillary, Celsius, diastolic pressure, homeostasis, hypertension, pyrexia, systolic pressure, and thready.
2. **Safety Alert**—Never forget the safety aspects of procedures. For example, when using a glass thermometer, caution the patient not to bite down. Brainstorm with classmates on other specific industry standards related to safety. Create a poster that illustrates some of these safety alerts.
3. **Patient Education**—Write a short script for what you would say to a patient as you begin a blood pressure reading. Remember that many patients become frightened of the mounting pressure on their arm.

Measuring Vital Signs and Other Clinical Skills | Chapter 19 699

11. Answer: Hypotension is low blood pressure.
12. Answer: Responsibilities of a nurse or nurse assistant include:
    - Provide AM and PM care
    - Provide oral hygiene
    - Offer the bedpan and urinal
    - Monitor the patient's elimination functions
    - Assist with dressing and undressing
    - Bathe patients
    - Provide effective skin care
    - Follow the patient care plan
    - Perform range of motion
    - Provide body alignment and positioning
    - Care for hair and nails
    - Shave the patient
    - Apply hot and cold applications
    - Make the bed
    - Assist patients to move and ambulate
    - Apply prosthetic devices and supports
    - Assist with feeding the patient
    - Record intake and output
    - Care for the incontinent patient
    - Understand tubes and catheters
    - Collect specimens
    - Measure height and weight
    - Take seizure precautions
    - Give stoma care
    - Do postmortem care
13. Answer: Walking helps maintain stamina, increases joint mobility, improves muscle tone, helps prevent lung congestion, improves circulation, helps prevent blood clots, helps maintain independence, and provides a sense of accomplishment.
14. Answer: Restraints might be used on a patient to prevent a patient from inflicting self-harm; prevent patients from removing medically necessary tubes, IV, and dressing; and to keep a small child still during a procedure (e.g., receiving stitches).
15. Answer: The preparation for the meal includes the following:
    - Assisting patients or reminding them to wash their hands.
    - Removing any unpleasant items from the area, such as emesis basins and bedpans.
    - Offering the opportunity to use the bedpan or the bathroom.
    - Providing for the patient's comfort: Raise the head of the bed and position the patient in a chair.
    - Transport the patient to the dining area.
    - Checking to be certain that you have the right tray for the patient and that it is the correct diet.
    - Always placing the food within reach.
    - Checking the tray to be certain that everything is there.
    - Preparing any item that the patient cannot manage.
    - Telling the patient where each item is according to the face of a clock if the patient is blind.

16. Answer:
    - Symptoms of dehydration include: fever; decrease in urine; concentrated urine; weight loss; dry membranes; patient has difficulty swallowing; tongue is coated and thickened; skin becomes hard and cracks and is dry and warm.
    - Symptoms of edema include: decrease in urine output; weight gain; puffiness or swelling; and shortness of breath.
17. Answer:
    - Infections
    - Surgical problems (e.g., prostate surgery)
    - Spinal cord injuries
    - Loss of sphincter control (muscle control)
    - Some diseases, such as multiple sclerosis and central nervous system damage
    - Disorientation

Activities

1. Direct students to review Procedure 19.7 for counting a radial pulse. Direct students to record the measurements, and to write a report as if for a patient. You may want to allow students to work in pairs.
2. Direct students to set up the table on paper or using a computer program, first. Remind students to use "patients" of different ages.
3. a. Student answers will vary. Refer them to Chapter 13 to see how each body system's biological processes help maintain homeostasis.
   b. Student answers will vary. Refer them to Chapter 13 to see how each body system's chemical processes help maintain homeostasis.
4. Prior to these activities, have a discussion about body contact, appropriate vs. inappropriate touching, and consent. Have them practice asking for consent before touching another student.

CHAPTER 19 REVIEW

Portfolio Connection

As a health care worker, you are expected to observe patients for their state of health. You are obligated to report any unusual or abnormal signs or symptoms. Answer the following questions in report form. This report will demonstrate your evaluating, observing, and reporting skills.

Your patient has an elevated blood pressure of 210/140. Does this blood pressure cause concern? What is the medical term for this blood pressure? What are the possible causes of an elevated blood pressure? What can you observe about the patient that is important in your report to your supervisor? Should you report this blood pressure immediately or wait until you report at the end of your day? What are the key things that you must report? Follow your teacher's instructions on saving this report in your portfolio.

PORTFOLIO TIP

Taking a temperature is a vital procedure, but to many patients it seems a nuisance. Try to explain to the patient as you start the process what a change in temperature will tell the health care staff and how checking it will keep recovery on track.

Case Studies

1. Direct students to Section 19.2 for more information on how agitation affects vital signs. Remind students of the importance of effective and age-appropriate communication skills.
2. Direct students to Section 19.2 for information on recording temperature and other vital signs. Remind students of the importance of effective and age-appropriate communication skills. In addition to writing a specific and detailed plan, you may want to allow students to present skits demonstrating their response to this situation.

Thinking Critically

1. Direct students to Section 10.1 for information about word elements and medical terminology. Encourage students to create a dictionary using the specified words. Encourage them to include other terminology they think is appropriate.
2. You might have the students work in small groups for this activity. Encourage students to present their responses creatively. For example, they might create a safety brochure or poster.
3. Direct students to use effective communication techniques. They might want to write variations on the script for patients of different ages, conditions, or cultures. You might want to have the students act out their scripts.

Portfolio Connection

- Review proper observations and reporting procedures.
- Remind the students that this report will become part of their portfolio.
- Direct them to use proper spelling and grammar.
- Remind students to proofread and revise their work.
- Check to make sure that students have completed the assignment and added it to their portfolio.

CUSTOMIZED INSTRUCTION

English Language Learners

For the Thinking Critically 3 activity, have students read their script aloud to a partner.

ACTIVITY

Divide the class into teams of 8 to 12 students. Hold a "definition bee" in which you read a term introduced or used in this chapter, and ask one team to define it. If they succeed, they get a point; if not, the other team has a chance. The team with the most points at the end of the competition wins.

20 Medical Assisting and Laboratory Skills

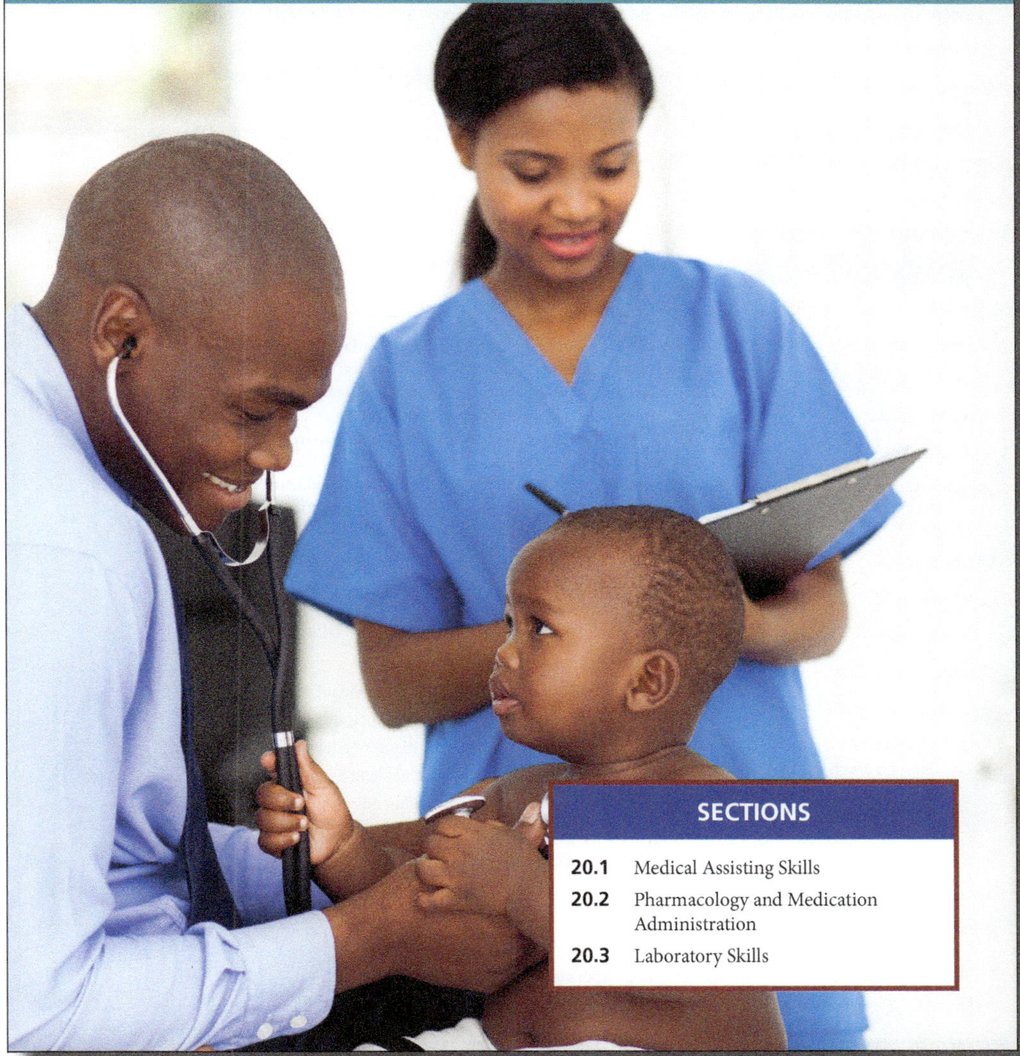

SECTIONS

CHAPTER 20 OVERVIEW

In Chapter 20, students learn common skills required for a medical assistant. They also learn about pharmacology, medication administration, and about specific laboratory skills.

Section 20.1: Section 20.1 explains the responsibilities of a medical assistant. It covers procedures such as admitting and discharging a patient, as well as measuring height and weight and assisting during an examination.

Section 20.2: Section 20.2 introduces students to pharmacology and medication administration. Students learn about prescriptions, drug dosage, safe handling and storing of medications, and how to administer medications.

Section 20.3: In Section 20.3, students learn about the responsibilities of a laboratory assistant. Skills such as how to use a microscope and how to test a urine specimen are covered. Students also learn about lab safety.

Advance Preparation	
Review	■ Chapter text for Sections 20.1, 20.2, and 20.3; and chapter procedures.
Contact	■ Medical, pharmacy, or laboratory assistants to address the class about the skills required for their position or demonstrate procedures. ■ Medical facilities or associations such as the American Society for Clinical Laboratory Science or the pharmacy association for your state to request brochures and other educational material about laboratory safety. ■ Medical laboratory, pharmacy, or physician's office to request tour or possibility of job shadows.
Prepare	■ Samples of admission checklists, registration and medical history forms, and different types of lab slips. ■ Materials for procedures including (but not limited to): urine cups and clinistix, graduates and other measuring devices, scales, measuring tape, pillows, and occult blood test kits. ■ A variety of drug reference books, including the *Physicians' Desk Reference* (PDR). ■ Pictures of medications; pictures of workers in a laboratory. ■ Magazine or newspaper articles about laboratory research.

FOCUS AND ENGAGE

Getting Started

- Explain "brown bagging."
- Direct students to make a table listing all medications, including the name, expiration date, and condition it treats.
- Direct students to bring the table to class. Emphasize that they should not bring the medications to class.
- Discuss the information as a class, including the risks of using expired medications, possible drug interactions, cost, generics, etc.

Introduce the Section

a. Review the content of the Background paragraph, reminding students of the role of a medical assistant.
b. Emphasize the importance of communicating with the patient to make the examination as pleasant an experience as possible.
c. Review section objectives.

Vocabulary Review

a. Direct students to the key terms.
b. Pronounce each word, and have the students repeat the pronunciation out loud.
c. Discuss each definition.

TEACH

Discuss

- Ask students to share stories of positive and negative experiences they have had visiting a physician.
- Discuss how a medical assistant can make a positive or negative first impression.

Reinforce and Review

- Review the descriptions and careers for a medical assistant in Chapter 3.

Getting Started

At home, "Brown Bag" all of the medications you can find in your home. You should include all over the counter medicines, herbal, and vitamin supplements. Inspect the medicines. Can you find any outdated medications? Any medications that are no longer prescribed? Any two medications that treat the same problem, but have a different name? If you are not sure what they are used for, look the medications up in the *Physicians' Desk Reference* (www.pdr.net/browse-by-drug-name).

Note: Everyone should inspect their medicine cabinets annually. Older patients should be encouraged to "brown bag" their medicines, including any over-the-counter medicines and bring them to their physician's office once a year to assure appropriateness and patient safety. Older patients are usually on more than five medications.

SECTION 20.1 Medical Assisting Skills

Background

Medical assistants are among the most dynamic and versatile members within the allied health care professions. As a profession, medical assisting careers originated in response to a severe shortage of nurses in private practice. As a medical assistant you will gain the knowledge and skills to perform both administrative and clinical procedures. Administrative duties include answering telephones, scheduling patient appointments, recording data in the patient's chart, as well as registering, admitting, and discharging patients from the doctors office, hospital, or other health facilities. Your clinical duties will range from monitoring vital signs, assisting with physical exams, injecting vaccinations, performing venipunctures, and preparing laboratory specimens.

Objectives

When you have completed this section, you will be able to do the following:

- Match key terms with their correct meanings.
- Explain the roles of patient registration and the medical history form.
- Describe the processes of patient admission, transfer, and discharge.
- Perform and record the weight and height for adults and children
- Perform and record infant weight, height, and head circumference.
- Identify the role of the basic examination positions
- Describe the physical examination techniques.
- Explain the Snellen Visual Acuity measurement

702 Chapter 20 | Medical Assisting and Laboratory Skills

CUSTOMIZED INSTRUCTION

Less Advanced Sudents

This is a lengthy chapter. Help less advanced students get a head start by providing vocabulary words and terminology in advance. They might benefit from a glossary, table, or flashcards to use as study aids.

CUSTOMIZED INSTRUCTION OVERVIEW	
Less Advanced Students	Page 702
More Advanced Students	Pages 746, 765
English Language Learners	Pages 704, 717
Special Needs Students	Pages 704, 752
At-Risk Students	Page 705

Registration

New patients must complete two basic forms when registering:

1. Patient information forms
2. Medical history forms

Patient Information Forms

The patient information form gives the following information:

- Patient's name, address, and phone number
- Birth date, sex, marital status, Social Security number
- Patient's employer name, address, and phone number
- Insurance company's name, address, and phone number
- Insured's employer name, address, and phone number
- If the patient is a minor, name of the responsible party

Medical History Forms

The medical history form, sometimes filled out by an RN or other licensed personnel, gives the provider the necessary information to evaluate the physical condition of the patient. The patient must give you the following information (Figure 20.1):

- Previous surgeries
- Allergies
- Chronic illness
- Medications taken
- General medical history
- Childhood diseases
- Persons to contact in case of medical emergency
- Nutritional status and any problems related to nutritional intake
- Activities of daily living and instrumental activities of daily living
- Family related medical history
- Any substance abuse history
- Mental health history
- Notation of any alterations in skin integrity (bruising, open areas, abnormal growths, etc.)

If a health care professional is taking or reviewing a patient's medical history, he/she might want to ask a series of questions about things that cannot be observed, such as:

- In general, how are you feeling?
- What is your biggest concern?
- Do you have any pains?

These types of questions should be asked in a non-leading way; for example: "How does your stomach feel?" rather than "Are you nauseous?" In addition to medications, health care professionals need to determine if the person is on any over the counter medications or supplements, such as herbs. Finally, they need to visually assess the overall physical and mental state of the patient—are they particularly stressed, nervous, out of breath, etc.

Medical Assisting and Laboratory Skills | Chapter 20 703

TEAMWORK

Divide the class into teams of five to seven students. Within a set time limit, such as two minutes, have each team write as many questions typically found on medical history forms that they can think of. When the time is up, see which team has the most correct behaviors. Award extra points for listing a question that other teams missed.

Teaching Tips

- Explain the forms usually used during the registration process.
- Review information required on a client/patient information form:
  - Name, address, phone number, birth date, sex, marital status, Social Security number
  - Employer name, address, phone
  - Insurance company's name, address, phone
  - Insured's employer name, address, phone
  - Name of person responsible for a minor
- Review information usually required on a medical history form:
  - Previous surgeries
  - Allergies
  - Chronic illness
  - Medications taken
  - General medical history including childhood diseases
  - Persons to contact in case of a medical emergency
  - Nutritional status
  - Activities of daily living and instrumental activities of daily living
  - Family-related medical history
  - Any substance abuse history
  - Mental health history
  - Notation of any alterations in skin integrity (bruising, open areas, abnormal growths)
- Review types of additional questions to ask:
  - How are you feeling?
  - Do you have concerns?
  - Are you in pain?

Teaching Tips

- Emphasize the importance of filling in all blanks on a medical history form.
- Explain the use of a notation such as "N/A" if the question is not applicable.

Figure Focus

20.1 Medical history form. Why are medical history forms important?

Answer: A medical history form gives the provider the necessary information to evaluate the physical condition of the patient/client. It is important because it provides information that the medical provider needs to accurately diagnose and treat the patient.

Figure 20.1
Medical history form. Why are medical history forms important?

GREEN VALLEY MEDICAL GROUP, INC.
MEDICAL HISTORY

NAME ______ DATE OF BIRTH ______
OCCUPATION ______ MARITAL STATUS: S M D W

ALLERGIES:
Are you allergic to:
Penicillin .... Yes ____ No ____
Sulfa .... Yes ____ No ____
Aspirin .... Yes ____ No ____
Codeine .... Yes ____ No ____
Tetanus Injections .... Yes ____ No ____
Iodine .... Yes ____ No ____
Foods .... Yes ____ No ____
Tape .... Yes ____ No ____
Other ______

MEDICATIONS:
List all medications, including over the counter, you are currently taking:
______

HABITS:
Do you:
Smoke? Yes ____ No ____ How Much ____
Drink Alcohol? Yes ____ No ____ How Much ____
Drink Beverages That Contain Caffeine?
Yes ____ No ____ How Much ____
Limit Cholesterol Yes ____ No ____
Use Other Substances Yes ____ No ____
What? ______

EXERCISE:
Do you on a regular basis:
Walk .... Yes ____ No ____
Run .... Yes ____ No ____
Bike .... Yes ____ No ____
Swim .... Yes ____ No ____
Aerobic Exercise .... Yes ____ No ____
Other .... Yes ____ No ____

MENSTRUAL HISTORY (FEMALES):
Date of last PAP & results ______
Date of last normal period ______
Date of last mammogram & results ______
Length of cycle (days) ______
Usual duration (days) ______
Number of pregnancies ______
Number of children ______

PRESENT COMPLAINTS:
Do you have:
Headaches .... Yes ____ No ____
Fever .... Yes ____ No ____
Cough .... Yes ____ No ____
Chest Pains .... Yes ____ No ____
Nausea .... Yes ____ No ____
Vomiting .... Yes ____ No ____
Diarrhea .... Yes ____ No ____
Constipation .... Yes ____ No ____
Black Stools .... Yes ____ No ____
Bloody Stools .... Yes ____ No ____
Painful Urination .... Yes ____ No ____
Recent Weight Gain or Loss ... Yes ____ No ____
Other Complaints ______

PAST ILLNESS:
Have you ever had:
High Blood Pressure .... Yes ____ No ____
Heart Trouble .... Yes ____ No ____
Pneumonia .... Yes ____ No ____
Hepatitis .... Yes ____ No ____
Cancer .... Yes ____ No ____
Diabetes .... Yes ____ No ____
Tuberculosis .... Yes ____ No ____
Asthma .... Yes ____ No ____
Ulcers .... Yes ____ No ____
Seizures .... Yes ____ No ____
Sexually Transmitted Disease .. Yes ____ No ____
Blood Disorder .... Yes ____ No ____
Other ______

OPERATIONS:
Have you had any surgery:
Appendix .... Yes ____ No ____
Tonsils .... Yes ____ No ____
Gallbladder .... Yes ____ No ____
Stomach .... Yes ____ No ____
Hemorrhoids .... Yes ____ No ____
Female Organs .... Yes ____ No ____
Thyroid .... Yes ____ No ____
Hernia .... Yes ____ No ____
Heart .... Yes ____ No ____
Other ______

704 Chapter 20 | Medical Assisting and Laboratory Skills

CUSTOMIZED INSTRUCTION

Special Needs Students

Spend time reviewing how to fill in a form completely so that special needs students understand the process. If possible, obtain or create forms with larger print and larger blank spaces to make it easier for special needs students to comply.

English Language Learners

With a partner, have students practice asking the questions on the medical history form shown in Figure 20.1. If desired, they may omit the Menstrual History section. Encourage them to practice clear annunciation.

Both the patient information form and the medical history form must be completed accurately and fully to serve the needs of both the patient and the provider. Do not leave any blanks on these forms. If it does not apply to the patient, you should write N/A or not applicable.

Admission

Since you are one of the first people to interact with the patient, it is very important to establish that the patient is not in any kind of acute distress. Inquire about their comfort level; quickly assess their general appearance for any kind of acute distress. If the patient appears to be in any kind of distress, quickly excuse yourself and notify the doctor or nurse on duty.

Be pleasant and try to put everyone at ease. (Figure 20.2) The facility where you work has a procedure for you to follow when you admit the patient. Do not rush the patient. Give the person time to adjust to the new environment. When a patient is admitted to the hospital, there are some basic procedures that are followed. (See Figure 20.3 for a sample of an admission checklist.) These include the following:

- Making a clothing list
- Making a list of personal items
- Requesting that the family take home valuables or see that they are put in a safe place
- Taking vital signs
- Weighing the patient
- Explaining the call light and routine
- Collecting urine specimens if required

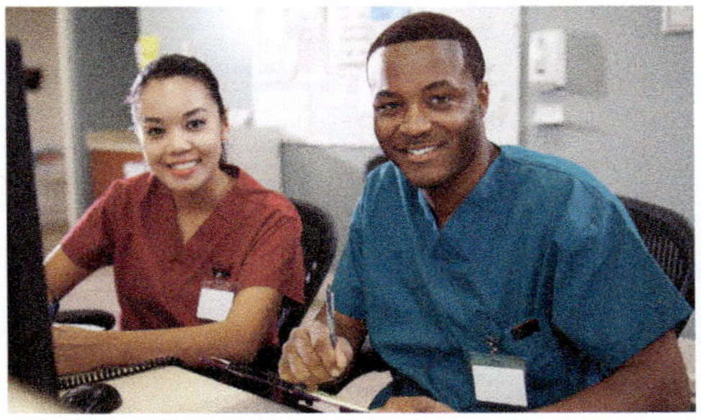

Figure 20.2
Why should you follow set procedures when admitting a patient?

NOTE: All medical records must be written in ink or electronically. Always remember to record date, time, personal care or treatment given, any complaints, problems reported to the team leader/head nurse, and any other required information. Complaints or patient statements should be put in quotes. Always sign with your name and certification.

Charting Flow Sheet

Many facilities provide a printed flow sheet for charting. The sheet includes activities of daily living (ADL), vital signs, diet, liquids, and type of care given. This checkoff list helps the charter provide all of the necessary information about patient care. (Figure 20.4) If your facility doesn't have a flow sheet, use the charting examples.

Medical Assisting and Laboratory Skills | Chapter 20 705

Teaching Tips

- Review the responsibilities of a medical assistant.
- Discuss areas where a medical assistant may be employed.
- Explain the difference between registration and admission.
- Explain the importance of making a patient feel at ease during admission.
- Discuss the importance of observation: to determine whether the patient requires urgent access to care.
- Explain that each facility has its own admission procedure.
- Review common admission procedures:
  - Clothing list
  - Personal items list
  - Securing valuables
  - Taking vital signs
  - Weighing the patient
  - Explaining the call light and routine
  - Collecting urine specimens if required
- Review the importance of documentation, and of using the proper procedure for documentation.

Figure Focus

20.2 Why should you follow set procedures when admitting a patient?

Answer: Following set procedures gives the patient a sense of well-being and security. It also protects the facility from errors in identification and loss of patients' belongings.

CUSTOMIZED INSTRUCTION

At-Risk Students

In small groups, have students discuss the importance of tone of voice, facial expressions, and body language when communicating with others. These factors greatly influence the message you send. As a group, students should prepare a list of factors that convey positive communication vs. those that are negative. Discuss the list with the class.

TEAMWORK

Divide the class into groups of four or five, with one student representing a patient, one representing the patient's family, and the others representing a health care team. You give the "patient" and the "family member" a slip of paper with an illness, an age, a culture, and an attitude written on it. The group should act out an admission procedure, with the "health care team" members responding to the actions of the "patient" and his or her family.

Teaching Tips

- Discuss how to use a checklist when admitting a patient.
- Review the types of questions that might be on an admission checklist, depending on the facility.
- Emphasize the importance of completing every question without skipping any.
- Explain that even if a question is not applicable, it is important to check it off using "N/A" or a similar notation.
- Explain the purpose of an Activities for Daily Living Checklist.

Figure Focus

20.3 Sample admission checklist. Why is it important to use an admission checklist when admitting a patient?

Answer: It is important to use a checklist because then you can be sure that you followed the correct procedure completely.

Figure Focus

20.4 Example of a flow chart. How and when should a flow chart be used?

Answer: A flow chart may be used to track patient care. All procedures, information, and observations should be recorded on the flow chart.

TEAMWORK

In groups of two or three, have students contact a local health care facility and request sample copies of registration, admission, and/or daily living checklist forms. Compare the forms and discuss the similarities and differences.

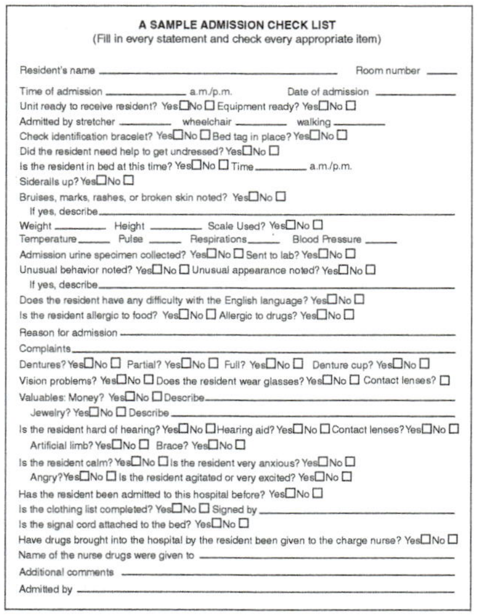

A SAMPLE ADMISSION CHECK LIST
(Fill in every statement and check every appropriate item)

Resident's name ______ Room number ______
Time of admission ______ a.m./p.m. Date of admission ______
Unit ready to receive resident? Yes☐No ☐ Equipment ready? Yes☐No ☐
Admitted by stretcher ______ wheelchair ______ walking ______
Check identification bracelet? Yes☐No ☐ Bed tag in place? Yes☐No ☐
Did the resident need help to get undressed? Yes☐No ☐
Is the resident in bed at this time? Yes☐No ☐ Time ______ a.m./p.m.
Siderails up? Yes☐No ☐
Bruises, marks, rashes, or broken skin noted? Yes☐No ☐
If yes, describe ______
Weight ______ Height ______ Scale Used? Yes☐No ☐
Temperature ______ Pulse ______ Respirations ______ Blood Pressure ______
Admission urine specimen collected? Yes☐No ☐ Sent to lab? Yes☐No ☐
Unusual behavior noted? Yes☐No ☐ Unusual appearance noted? Yes☐No ☐
If yes, describe ______
Does the resident have any difficulty with the English language? Yes☐No ☐
Is the resident allergic to food? Yes☐No ☐ Allergic to drugs? Yes☐No ☐
Reason for admission ______
Complaints ______
Dentures? Yes☐No ☐ Partial? Yes☐No ☐ Full? Yes☐No ☐ Denture cup? Yes☐No ☐
Vision problems? Yes☐No ☐ Does the resident wear glasses? Yes☐No ☐ Contact lenses? ☐
Valuables: Money? Yes☐No ☐ Describe ______
Jewelry? Yes☐No ☐ Describe ______
Is the resident hard of hearing? Yes☐No ☐ Hearing aid? Yes☐No ☐ Contact lenses? Yes☐No ☐
Artificial limb? Yes☐No ☐ Brace? Yes☐No ☐
Is the resident calm? Yes☐No ☐ Is the resident very anxious? Yes☐No ☐
Angry? Yes☐No ☐ Is the resident agitated or very excited? Yes☐No ☐
Has the resident been admitted to this hospital before? Yes☐No ☐
Is the clothing list completed? Yes☐No ☐ Signed by ______
Is the signal cord attached to the bed? Yes☐No ☐
Have drugs brought into the hospital by the resident been given to the charge nurse? Yes☐No ☐
Name of the nurse drugs were given to ______
Additional comments ______
Admitted by ______

Figure 20.3
Sample admission checklist. Why is it important to use an admission checklist when admitting a patient?

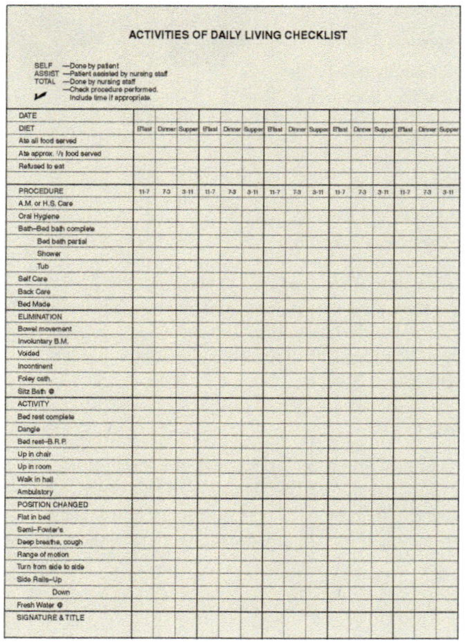

ACTIVITIES OF DAILY LIVING CHECKLIST

SELF —Done by patient
ASSIST —Patient assisted by nursing staff
TOTAL —Done by nursing staff
✔ —Check procedure performed. Include time if appropriate.

DATE															
DIET	B'fast	Dinner	Supper	B'fast	Dinner	Supper	B'fast	Dinner	Supper	B'fast	Dinner	Supper	B'fast	Dinner	Supper
Ate all food served															
Ate approx. 1/2 food served															
Refused to eat															
PROCEDURE	11-7	7-3	3-11	11-7	7-3	3-11	11-7	7-3	3-11	11-7	7-3	3-11	11-7	7-3	3-11
A.M. or H.S. Care															
Oral Hygiene															
Bath–Bed bath complete															
Bed bath partial															
Shower															
Tub															
Self Care															
Back Care															
Bed Made															
ELIMINATION															
Bowel movement															
Involuntary B.M.															
Voided															
Incontinent															
Foley cath.															
Sitz Bath @															
ACTIVITY															
Bed rest complete															
Dangle															
Bed rest–B.R.P.															
Up in chair															
Up in room															
Walk in hall															
Ambulatory															
POSITION CHANGED															
Flat in bed															
Semi-Fowler's															
Deep breathe, cough															
Range of motion															
Turn from side to side															
Side Rails–Up															
Down															
Fresh Water @															
SIGNATURE & TITLE															

Figure 20.4
Example of a flow chart. How and when should a flow chart be used?

706 Chapter 20 | Medical Assisting and Laboratory Skills

Procedure 20.1 **Admitting a Patient**

BACKGROUND: Carefully following the admitting procedure gives the patient a sense of well-being and security. It also protects the facility from errors in identification and loss of patients' belongings.
ALERT: Follow Standard Precautions

Preprocedure

1. Wash hands.
2. Assemble equipment:
   a. Admission checklist
   b. Admission pack (may be all disposable depending on facility):
      (1) Bedpan
      (2) Urinal
      (3) Emesis basin
      (4) Wash basin
      (5) Tissues
   c. Gown or pajamas
   d. Portable scale
   e. Thermometer
   f. Blood pressure cuff
   g. Stethoscope
   h. Clothing list
   i. Envelope for valuables

Procedure

3. Fan-fold bed covers to foot of bed. (See the procedure "Making an Open Bed.")
4. Put away patient's equipment.
5. Put gown or pajamas on foot of bed.
6. Greet patient and introduce yourself.
7. Identify patient by looking at arm band and asking name. Ask what they like to be called.
8. Introduce patient to roommates, if appropriate.
9. Explain:
   a. How call signal works
   b. How bed controls work
   c. Hospital regulations
   d. What you will be doing to admit him or her
   e. How telephone and television work
10. Provide privacy by pulling privacy curtains.
11. Ask patient to put on gown or pajamas.
12. Check weight and height. (You will find this skill later in this chapter.)
13. Help to bed if ordered. (Check with nurse.)
14. Put up side rails if required.
15. If patient has valuables:
    a. Make a list of jewelry, money, wallet, etc.
    b. Have patient sign list
    c. Have relative sign list
    d. Either have relative take home valuables or send to cashier's office in valuables envelope
16. Take and record the following:
    a. Temperature, pulse, respiration
    b. Blood pressure
    c. Urine specimen, if required

(continued)

Medical Assisting and Laboratory Skills | Chapter 20 707

Procedure Tip

20.1 Admitting a Patient

- Review the background information, emphasizing the importance of following the specific procedure for the facility where you work.
- Point out that Standard Precautions must be followed.
- Review the preprocedure steps.
- Step 1: Emphasize proper handwashing.
- Step 2: Review the list of equipment.
- Review the procedure steps.
- Steps 6–9: Emphasize effective communication techniques.
- Step 10: Emphasize the importance of patient privacy.
- Step 15: Discuss the importance of securing the patient's personal property.
- Step 16: Review proper recording procedures.

Procedure Tip

20.1 Admitting a Patient, continued

- Step 17: Review other procedures on the checklist.
- Steps 18 and 19: Reiterate the importance of communication.
- Review the postprocedure steps.
- Step 20: Emphasize importance of handwashing.
- Step 21: Emphasize importance of observation and reporting.

PROCEDURE PRACTICE

- Demonstrate the steps for Procedure 20.1, Admitting a Patient, as many times as necessary, or ask students to demonstrate the steps. Provide samples of an admission checklist. Have students practice and perform the procedure until they are competent.

Teaching Tips

- Discuss the importance of height and weight as a baseline.
- Discuss reasons height and weight are required:
  - Accurate dosing of medications
  - Nutritional status
  - Changes might indicate potential problems
- Review the different types of scales:
  - Standing scale
  - Bed scale
  - Infant scale
  - Scale with mechanical lift
  - Wheelchair scale
- Discuss digital scales, including their advantages and their use with patients and clients.

Procedure 20.1 | Admitting a Patient (continued)

Procedure (cont)

17. Complete admission checklist noting:
    a. Allergies
    b. Medications being taken
    c. Food preferences and dislikes
    d. Any prosthesis
    e. Skin condition
    f. Handicaps (e.g., deafness, sight, movement)

NOTE: This is usually done by a registered nurse.

18. Orient patient to meal times, visiting hours, and use of television and telephone.
19. Ask if patient has any questions regarding the information given.

Postprocedure

20. Wash hands.
21. Record information according to your facility's policy.

Charting Example:

10/04/24	*1500*
	VS 98–76–18 120/80
	Admitted and oriented to facility.
	Admission checklist completed.
	Sitting in chair.
	States "Wish I could stay at home."
	S. Gomez CNA

Height and Weight

Patients are weighed and measured for height when they are admitted. These measurements provide a baseline during the patient's stay. (Table 20.1) Measurements must be accurate, as they are important to the well-being of the patient. Accurate heights and weights are very important to the physician and the pharmacist for accurate dosing of any medications to be given. The patient's weight is important because it indicates:

- Nutritional status
- Any change (weight loss or gain) in condition, which *might* indicate potential physical or emotional problems, or other issues

There are several different types of scales and most are available digitally. Digital scales can measure with precision accuracy. Each type of scale is designed for ease in weighing patients with varying problems. Types of scales include:

- Standing scale
- Bed scale
- Infant scale
- Scale with mechanical lift
- Wheelchair scale

708 Chapter 20 | Medical Assisting and Laboratory Skills

- Review methods of measuring height:
  - If patient can stand, use measure on standing scale
  - If patient cannot stand, use measuring tape

ACTIVITY

Have students design and create their own admission checklist.

ACTIVITY

Have students make a table or chart comparing the different types of scales and explaining when a particular type of scale should be used.

Patients who are wheelchair-bound can be left in the wheelchair and weighed. Allowance is made for the weight of the wheelchair and platform by subtracting a certain amount from the weight or by having the scale adjusted to allow for the extra weight. You can also use a mechanical lift that has a scale. It is operated by using a hydraulic pump to raise and lower the patient.

Most facilities have in-bed scales available. The bed must be balanced prior to taking the patient's weight and the amount of bedding used should be consistent. This method makes weighing the patient much easier for both the patient and the nurse.

Height is used as an indicator of the ideal weight of the patient. You may have to measure the patient with a measuring tape if the person is unable to stand. If the patient can stand, use the measure on the standing scale.

Table 20.1 Height and Weight Table for Adults

Men					Women				
Height		Bone Structure (lbs)			Height		Bone Structure (lbs)		
ft. & in.	in. only	Small	Medium	Large	ft. & in.	in. only	Small	Medium	Large
5' 2"	62	128–134	131–141	138–150	4' 10"	58	102–111	109–121	118–131
5' 3"	63	130–136	133–143	140–153	4' 11"	59	103–113	111–123	120–134
5' 4"	64	132–138	135–145	142–156	5' 0"	60	104–115	113–126	122–137
5' 5"	65	134–140	137–148	144–160	5' 1"	61	106–118	115–129	125–140
5' 6"	66	136–142	139–151	146–164	5' 2"	62	108–121	118–132	128–143
5' 7"	67	138–146	142–154	149–168	5' 3"	63	111–124	121–135	131–147
5' 8"	68	140–148	145–157	152–172	5' 4"	64	114–127	124–138	134–151
5' 9"	69	142–151	148–160	155–176	5' 5"	65	117–130	127–141	137–155
5' 10"	70	144–154	151–163	158–180	5' 6"	66	120–133	130–144	140–159
5' 11"	71	146–157	154–166	161–184	5' 7"	67	123–136	133–147	143–163
6' 0"	72	149–160	157–170	164–188	5' 8"	68	126–139	136–150	146–167
6' 1"	73	152–164	160–174	168–192	5' 9"	69	129–142	139–153	149–170
6' 2"	74	155–168	164–178	172–197	5' 10"	70	132–146	142–156	152–173
6' 3"	75	158–172	167–182	176–202	5' 11"	71	135–148	145–159	155–176
6' 4"	76	162–176	171–187	181–207	6' 0"	72	138–151	148–162	158–179

Medical Assisting and Laboratory Skills | Chapter 20 709

Teaching Tips

- Discuss implications of body weight gain and loss:
  - Obesity
  - Edema
  - Glandular changes
  - Disease process in weight loss
- Review factors to consider when measuring weight:
  - Use same scale
  - Weigh at the same time of day
  - Note clothing weight for more closely monitored patient
- Review safety factors in weighing.
- Review Table 20.1 together as a class.
- Discuss the relationship between height and weight.
- Explain that height is used as an indicator of the ideal weight of the patient.
- Review the body mass index (Section 16.1).

ACTIVITY

Ask students to consider whether there is a difference between measuring height and weight (or body mass) for the purpose of a nutrition and wellness analysis, and measuring it for admission to a hospital. Have them write a one-page essay explaining their opinion. Remind them to include a thesis statement and supporting facts. Have them proofread and revise their work, or use peer review to improve it.

Procedure Tip

20.2 Measuring Weight on a Standing Balance or Digital Scale

- Review the background information, emphasizing that a baseline is for comparing future changes.
- Point out that Standard Precautions must be followed.
- Review the preprocedure steps.
- Step 1: Emphasize proper handwashing.
- Step 2: Review the equipment list.
- Step 4: Emphasize effective communication techniques.
- Step 5: Emphasize the importance of patient privacy.
- Review the procedure steps.
- Step 7: Explain that the paper towel is for the patient's protection.
- Step 9: Explain how to calibrate a balance scale and a digital scale.
- Step 13: Review how to read the scale.
- Step 14: Emphasize the importance of recording the weight immediately.
- Review the postprocedure steps.
- Step 17: Review powering off a digital scale.
- Step 18: Emphasize importance of handwashing.
- Step 19: Emphasize importance of observation and reporting.

Procedure 20.2 **Measuring Weight on a Standing Balance or Digital Scale**

BACKGROUND: Weighing the patient provides a weight baseline. This baseline is used to compare decreases or increases in the patient's weight. Changes in body weight may indicate a change in the patient's health.

ALERT: Follow Standard Precautions

Preprocedure

1. Wash hands.
2. Assemble equipment:
   a. Portable balance or digital scale
   b. Paper towel
   c. Paper and pencil/pen
3. Identify patient.
4. Explain what you are going to do and ask patient if they need to void before you weigh them.
5. Provide privacy with curtain, screen, or door.

Procedure

6. Take patient to scale or bring scale to patient's room.
7. Place paper towel on platform of scale (with standing scale).
8. Put both weights to the very left on zero. When using a digital scale, turn the scale on and wait for the display to show a reading; make sure the display reads "zero" before you begin weighing the patient.
9. Balance beam pointer must stay steady in middle of balance area. (If pointer does not center, turn balance screw until it remains centered.) The manufacturer's instructions for a digital scale will provide instructions on how to calibrate the scale, or bring the display to zero. There usually is a button to push for calibration.
10. Have patient remove shoes and assist to stand on scale.

NOTE: The balance bar raises to top of bar guide and pointer is not centered.

11. While keeping one hand near the patient's back, use other hand to move large weight to estimated weight of patient.
12. Move small weight to right until balance bar hangs free halfway between upper and lower bar guide.
13. The largest (lower) weight is marked in increments of 50 pounds; the smaller (upper weight) is marked in single pounds. The even-numbered pounds are marked with numbers (e.g., 2, 4, 6). The uneven pounds are unmarked long lines and the short line is one-fourth of a pound.
14. Write down weight on a notepad. Record weight displayed on a digital scale.
15. Help patient with shoes and make him or her comfortable.

Postprocedure

16. Discard towel.
17. Replace scale. With a digital scale, make sure the power is off.
18. Wash hands.
19. Chart weight. Report any unusual increases or decreases in weight.

Charting Example:

10/05/24	0900
	Standing scale weight 125; 10
	pounds less than last weight.
	No complaints of loss of appetite,
	pain, or other problems. Weight
	change reported to head nurse.
	S. Gomez CNA

710 Chapter 20 | Medical Assisting and Laboratory Skills

PROCEDURE PRACTICE

- Demonstrate the steps for Procedure 20.2, Measuring Weight on a Standing Balance or Digital Scale, as many times as necessary, or ask students to demonstrate the steps. Have students practice and perform the procedure until they are competent.

Procedure 20.3 | **Measuring Weight on a Chair Scale**

BACKGROUND: The chair scale provides a safe way to weigh a nonambulatory patient. Weighing the patient provides a weight baseline. This baseline is used to compare decreases or increases in the patient's weight. Changes in body weight may indicate a change in the patient's health.
ALERT: Follow Standard Precautions

Preprocedure

1. Wash hands.
2. Assemble equipment:
   a. Balance scale
   b. Paper towel
   c. Paper and pencil/pen
3. Identify patient.
4. Explain what you are going to do and ask patient if they need to void before you weigh them.
5. Provide privacy with curtain, screen, or door.

Procedure

6. Take patient to scale or bring scale to patient's room.
7. Put both weights to the very left on zero. If you are using a digital scale, make sure the display reads zero.
8. Balance beam pointer must stay steady in middle of balance area. (If pointer does not center, turn balance screw until it remains centered.) Calibrate a digital scale according to the manufacturer's instructions.
9. Have patient remove shoes and move patient to chair at the side of the scale.
10. Place wheelchair on scale and weigh it.
11. Assist patient back into wheelchair. Weigh wheelchair with patient in it.

NOTE: To determine weights, see previous procedure: "Measuring Weight on a Standing Balance or Digital Scale."

12. Determine patient weight by subtracting the weight in #10 above from the weight in #11.
13. Write down weight on a notepad. Record weight displayed on a digital scale.
14. Help patient with shoes and make him or her comfortable.

Postprocedure

15. Replace scale. With a digital scale, make sure the power is off before replacing it.
16. Wash hands.
17. Chart weight. Report any unusual increases or decreases in weight.

Charting Example:

05/03/24	0800
	Chair scale weight 125;
	no weight change.
	________ S. Gomez CNA

Medical Assisting and Laboratory Skills | Chapter 20 711

Procedure Tip

20.3 Measuring Weight on a Chair Scale

- Review the background information, emphasizing that a chair scale is used for a nonambulatory patient.
- Point out that Standard Precautions must be followed.
- Review the preprocedure steps.
- Point out that a chair scale may be digital; if so, follow steps for using a digital scale, as indicated in Procedure 20.2.
- Step 1: Emphasize proper handwashing.
- Step 2: Review the equipment list.
- Step 4: Emphasize effective communication techniques.
- Step 5: Emphasize the importance of patient privacy.
- Review the procedure steps.
- Steps 9 and 10: Explain that it is necessary to determine the weight of the chair without the patient in order to accurately determine the weight of the patient.
- Step 12: Explain that you determine the weight of the patient by subtracting the weight of the chair from the combined weight of the chair and patient.
- Step 13: Emphasize the importance of recording the weight immediately.
- Review the postprocedure steps.
- Step 16: Emphasize importance of handwashing.
- Step 17: Emphasize importance of observation and reporting.

PROCEDURE PRACTICE

- Demonstrate the steps for Procedure 20.3, Measuring Weight on a Chair Scale, as many times as necessary, or ask students to demonstrate the steps. Have students practice and perform the procedure until they are competent.

Procedure Tip

20.4 Measuring Weight on a Mechanical Lift

- Review the background information, emphasizing that a mechanical lift is used for weighing a bedridden patient.
- Point out that Standard Precautions must be followed.
- Review the preprocedure steps.
- Step 1: Emphasize proper handwashing.
- Step 2: Review the equipment list.
- Step 4: Emphasize effective communication techniques.
- Step 5: Emphasize the importance of patient privacy.
- Review the procedure steps.
- Step 7: Explain that the sling is part of the mechanical lift, and that the sheet is for comfort and cleanliness.
- Step 15: Explain that no part of the patient must be touching the bed in order for the patient to hang freely in the sling.
- Step 18: Explain that an electric scale automatically displays the weight digitally.
- Step 19: Review the steps in reverse for returning patient to bed.
- Review the postprocedure steps.
- Step 21: Emphasize importance of handwashing.
- Step 22: Emphasize importance of observation and reporting.

Procedure 20.4 Measuring Weight on a Mechanical Lift

BACKGROUND: The mechanical lift provides a safe method for weighing a bedridden patient. Weighing the patient provides a weight baseline. This baseline is used to compare decreases or increases in the patient's weight. Changes in body weight may indicate a change in the patient's health.
ALERT: Follow Standard Precautions

Preprocedure

1. Wash hands.
2. Assemble equipment:
   a. Mechanical lift
   b. Sling
   c. Clean sheet
3. Identify patient.
4. Explain what you are going to do.
5. Pull privacy curtain.

Procedure

6. Lower side rail on side you are working on.
7. Cover sling with clean sheet.
8. Help patient roll on side and place sling with top at shoulders and bottom at knees.
9. Fan-fold remaining sling.
10. Help patient roll to other side onto one half of sling and pull other half of sling through.
11. Broaden base of lift.
12. Wheel lift to side of bed with base beneath bed.
13. Position lift over patient.
14. Attach sling using chains and hooks provided. Keep open end of hook away from patient to avoid injury.
15. Use hand crank or pump handle to raise patient from bed. Make certain that buttocks are not touching bed.
16. Check to be certain that patient is in center of sling and is safely suspended.
17. To weigh patient:
    a. Swing feet and legs over edge of bed; move lift away from bed so that no body part contacts bed.
    b. If bed is low enough, raise patient above bed so that no body part contacts bed.
18. Adjust weights until the scale is balanced. (See the procedure "Measuring Weight on a Standing Balance Scale.") Remember that most mechanical lift scales these days are electric. Be sure the scale is on zero before measuring the patient's weight.
19. Return patient to bed by reversing steps.

Postprocedure

20. Replace mechanical lift.
21. Wash hands.
22. Note weight.

Charting Example:

02/26/24	1000
	Chair scale weight 250
	No changes since last weighing
	Tolerated well.
	Noted reddened area on left
	shoulder. Reported to head nurse
	S. Gomez CNA

712 Chapter 20 | Medical Assisting and Laboratory Skills

PROCEDURE PRACTICE

- Review the steps for Procedure 20.4, Measuring Weight on a Mechanical Lift, as many times as necessary, or ask students to demonstrate the steps. If possible, have students practice and perform the procedure until they are competent.

ACTIVITY

Ask students if they know how a veterinarian weighs animals. Have them create a chart or table listing different types of animals of all sizes, and then look up the types of scales used to weigh them.

Procedure 20.5 Measuring Height

BACKGROUND: Accurately measuring height provides a baseline to help determine the patient's ideal weight. A loss in height over a period of time may indicate osteoporosis.
ALERT: Follow Standard Precautions

Preprocedure

1. Wash hands.
2. Assemble equipment:
   a. Balance scale with height rod
   b. Paper towels
3. Identify patient and explain procedure.
4. Put paper towel on platform of scale.
5. Explain what you are going to do.
6. Have patient remove shoes.

Procedure

7. Raise measuring rod above head.
8. Assist patient onto the scale. Have patient stand with back against measuring rod.
9. Instruct patient to stand straight, with heels touching measuring rod.
10. Lower measuring rod to rest on patient's head.
11. Check number of inches indicated on rod. This number is found where the sliding rod enters the hollow post.
12. Assist patient off of the scale.
13. Record in meters, centimeters, or feet and inches according to hospital policy.

Postprocedure

14. Help patient with shoes.
15. Chart height.
16. Discard paper towel and wash hands.

Charting Example:

02/09/24 0700
Height 55 inches on admission.
S. Gomez CNA

Measuring Height, Weight, and Head Circumference: Infants and Toddlers (Under 3 Years of Age)

Infant and toddler growth is rapid and requires frequent monitoring. Infants are usually seen every 2 months to monitor growth and development patterns. Careful measuring and graphing of these patterns can help detect early changes that are important.

Measuring Head Circumference

Measuring head circumference screens infants and toddlers for abnormal head size. Watching head size can alert the provider if a problem such as **hydrocephaly** is present. Always place the measuring tape over the occipital bone on the back of the head and wrap forward just above the ears to center of forehead.

hydrocephaly
(hi DROW n sef awl ee)
Excessive accumulation of cerebrospinal fluid in the brain, often leading to increased brain size and other brain trauma.

Measuring Infant and Toddler Height

Infant and toddler heights indicate normal or abnormal growth patterns. Always use the same technique to measure their height and weight. Never estimate height. Use a tape measure or the ruler on the scale or tabletop.

Medical Assisting and Laboratory Skills | Chapter 20 713

Teaching Tips

- Reinforce the importance of carefully watching growth pattern of infants and toddlers.
- Explain head circumference: The length around the outside of the head.
- Explain that abnormal head circumference may indicate a problem, such as hydroencephaly.
- Explain proper placement of the measuring tape: Over the occipital bone on the back of the head and wrap forward just above the ears to center of forehead.

Procedure Tip

20.5 Measuring Height

- Review the background information, emphasizing that a baseline is for comparing future changes. Explain osteoporosis, if necessary.
- Point out that Standard Precautions must be followed.
- Review the preprocedure steps.
- Step 1: Emphasize proper handwashing.
- Step 2: Review the equipment list.
- Steps 3 and 5: Emphasize effective communication techniques.
- Step 4: Explain that the paper towel is for the patient's protection.
- Review the procedure steps.
- Step 11: Review how to read the measuring rod.
- Step 13: Explain that some facilities use standard measurements and some use metric.
- Review the postprocedure steps.
- Step 15: Emphasize importance of observation and reporting.
- Step 16: Emphasize importance of handwashing.

PROCEDURE PRACTICE

- Review the steps for Procedure 20.5, Measuring Height, as many times as necessary, or ask students to demonstrate the steps. Have students practice and perform the procedure until they are competent.

Procedure Tip

20.6 Measuring Height of Adult/Child (Over 3 Years of Age)

- Review the background information, emphasizing that accurate height measurement can help identify normal growth.
- Emphasize use of Standard Precautions.
- Review the preprocedure steps.
- Step 1: Emphasize proper handwashing.
- Step 3: Emphasize effective communication techniques and patient privacy.
- Review the procedure steps.
- Step 11: Review how to read the measuring rod.
- Review the postprocedure steps.
- Remind students of proper observation and reporting.

PROCEDURE PRACTICE

- Review the steps for Procedure 20.6, Measuring Height of Adult/Child (Over 3 Years of Age), as many times as necessary, or ask students to demonstrate the steps. Have students practice using a doll or mannequin, and perform the procedure until they are competent.

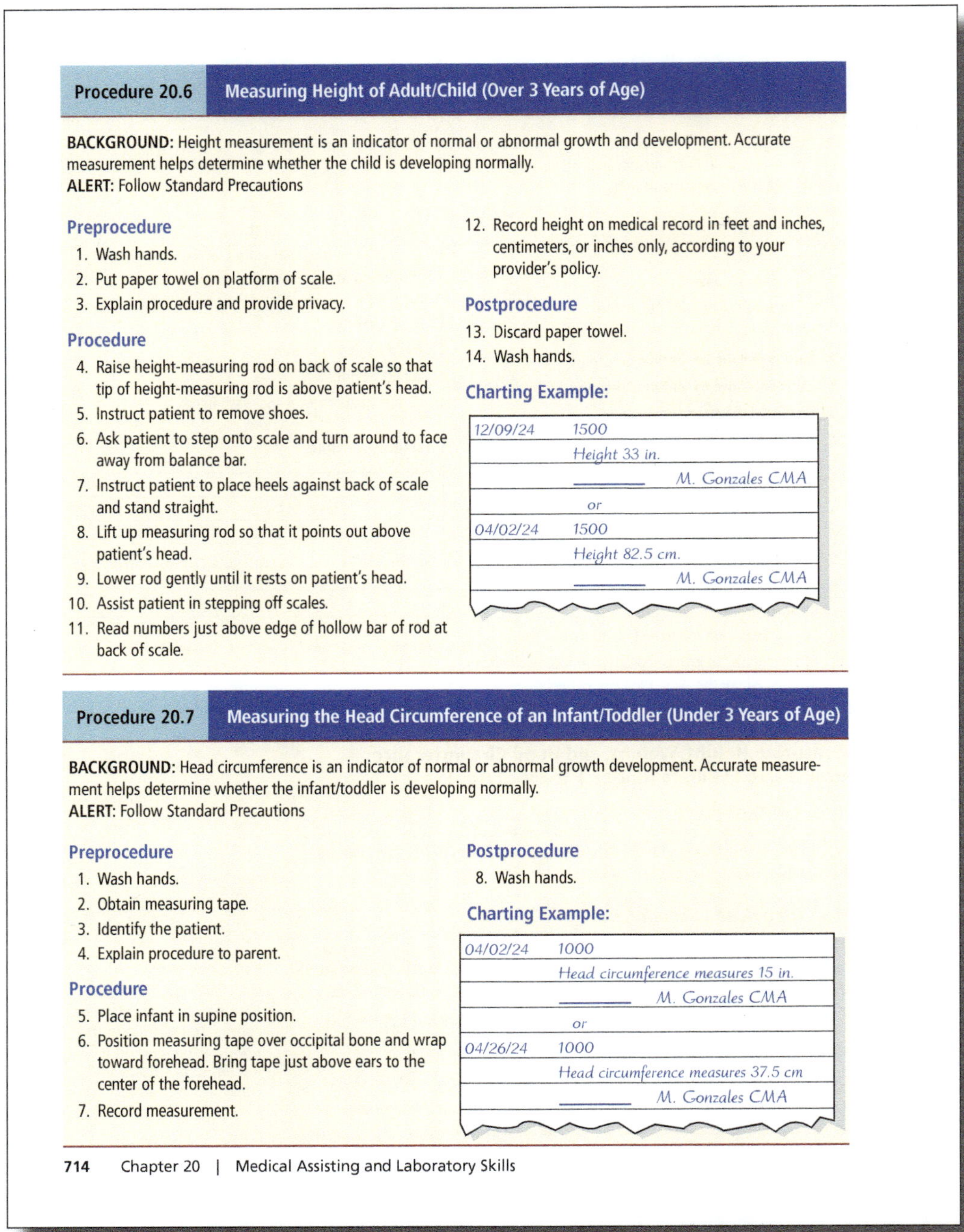

Procedure 20.6 Measuring Height of Adult/Child (Over 3 Years of Age)

BACKGROUND: Height measurement is an indicator of normal or abnormal growth and development. Accurate measurement helps determine whether the child is developing normally.
ALERT: Follow Standard Precautions

Preprocedure

1. Wash hands.
2. Put paper towel on platform of scale.
3. Explain procedure and provide privacy.

Procedure

4. Raise height-measuring rod on back of scale so that tip of height-measuring rod is above patient's head.
5. Instruct patient to remove shoes.
6. Ask patient to step onto scale and turn around to face away from balance bar.
7. Instruct patient to place heels against back of scale and stand straight.
8. Lift up measuring rod so that it points out above patient's head.
9. Lower rod gently until it rests on patient's head.
10. Assist patient in stepping off scales.
11. Read numbers just above edge of hollow bar of rod at back of scale.
12. Record height on medical record in feet and inches, centimeters, or inches only, according to your provider's policy.

Postprocedure

13. Discard paper towel.
14. Wash hands.

Charting Example:

12/09/24	1500	
	Height 33 in.	
	________	M. Gonzales CMA
	or	
04/02/24	1500	
	Height 82.5 cm.	
	________	M. Gonzales CMA

Procedure 20.7 Measuring the Head Circumference of an Infant/Toddler (Under 3 Years of Age)

BACKGROUND: Head circumference is an indicator of normal or abnormal growth development. Accurate measurement helps determine whether the infant/toddler is developing normally.
ALERT: Follow Standard Precautions

Preprocedure

1. Wash hands.
2. Obtain measuring tape.
3. Identify the patient.
4. Explain procedure to parent.

Procedure

5. Place infant in supine position.
6. Position measuring tape over occipital bone and wrap toward forehead. Bring tape just above ears to the center of the forehead.
7. Record measurement.

Postprocedure

8. Wash hands.

Charting Example:

04/02/24	1000	
	Head circumference measures 15 in.	
	________	M. Gonzales CMA
	or	
04/26/24	1000	
	Head circumference measures 37.5 cm	
	________	M. Gonzales CMA

714 Chapter 20 | Medical Assisting and Laboratory Skills

Procedure Tip

20.7 Measuring the Head Circumference of an Infant/Toddler (Under 3 Years of Age)

- Review the background information.
- Review the preprocedure steps.
- Step 1: Emphasize proper handwashing.
- Step 4: Emphasize effective communication techniques.
- Review the procedure steps.
- Step 5: Explain supine.
- Step 6: Review proper placement of measuring tape.
- Step 7: Emphasize proper observation and reporting.
- Review the postprocedure steps.
- Step 8: Emphasize proper handwashing.

PROCEDURE PRACTICE

- Review the steps for Procedures 20.7, Measuring the Head Circumference of an Infant/Toddler (Under 3 Years of Age), as many times as necessary, or ask students to demonstrate the steps. Have students practice using a doll or mannequin, and perform the procedure until they are competent.

Procedure 20.8 | **Measuring the Height of an Infant/Toddler**

BACKGROUND: Height is an indicator of normal or abnormal growth development. Accurate measurement helps determine whether the infant/toddler is developing normally.
ALERT: Follow Standard Precautions

Preprocedure

1. Wash hands.
2. Obtain tape measure or measuring bar.

Procedure

3. Place infant on flat surface.
4. Place zero mark of tape or measuring bar level with top of infant's head.
5. Ask parent or co-worker to hold top of head gently at zero mark.
6. Gently straighten legs.
7. Read measurement that is level with infant's heel.

NOTE: An alternative is to lay the infant on exam paper or sheet. Draw a line at the top of the infant's head. Have the parent hold on to the infant and stretch out the infant's leg. Draw another line at the infant's heel. Have parent pick up the infant, and then measure between the two lines.

Postprocedure

8. Wash hands.

Charting Example:

02/23/24	*1000*
	Height 21 in.
	_______ M. Gonzales CMA
	or
03/30/24	*1000*
	Height 52.5 cm
	_______ M. Gonzales CMA

Measuring Weight: Infant/Toddler

Infant and toddler weights are an important measure of growth patterns. Weight in an infant can change very quickly during an illness. Weight loss is an important indicator of dehydration. *Do not* change from weighing with clothes during one visit to weighing without clothes the next visit. Be consistent.

A large difference in the expected growth pattern may indicate a problem (for example, glandular imbalance or nutritional deficiency).

Medical Assisting and Laboratory Skills | Chapter 20 715

Procedure Tip

20.8 Measuring the Height of an Infant/Toddler

- Review the background information.
- Emphasize use of Standard Precautions.
- Review the preprocedure steps.
- Step 1: Emphasize proper handwashing.
- Review the procedure steps.
- Note that an alternative procedure is given.
- Review the postprocedure steps.
- Step 8: Emphasize proper handwashing.
- Remind students of the importance of proper observation and reporting.

PROCEDURE PRACTICE

- Review the steps for Procedure 20.8, Measuring the Height of an Infant/Toddler, as many times as necessary, or ask students to demonstrate the steps. Have students practice using a doll or mannequin, and perform the procedure until they are competent.

Teaching Tips

- Explain that because infants and toddlers are small, gaining or losing even a few ounces might be a significant proportion of body weight.
- Explain the importance of using consistent procedures during measurement.

Procedure Tip

20.9 Measuring the Weight of an Infant/Toddler

- Review the background information, emphasizing that accurate weight measurement can help identify normal growth.
- Emphasize use of Standard Precautions.
- Review the preprocedure steps.
- Step 1: Emphasize proper handwashing.
- Step 2 Review equipment list.
- Step 3: Emphasize effective communication techniques.
- Step 5: Emphasize the importance of balancing the scale with the towel in place so the weight of the towel is not included in the measurement.
- Review the procedure steps.
- Step 7: Emphasize the importance of not touching the patient.
- Review the postprocedure steps.
- Step 13: Emphasize proper handwashing.
- Step 14: Emphasize the importance of proper observation and reporting.

PROCEDURE PRACTICE

- Review the steps for Procedure 20.9, Measuring the Weight of an Infant/Toddler, as many times as necessary, or ask students to demonstrate the steps. Have students practice using a doll or mannequin, and perform the procedure until they are competent.

Procedure 20.9 Measuring the Weight of an Infant/Toddler

BACKGROUND: Infant weight is an indicator of normal or abnormal growth development. Accurate measurement helps determine whether the infant/toddler is developing normally.
ALERT: Follow Standard Precautions

Preprocedure

1. Wash hands.
2. Assemble equipment:
   a. Infant scale, either balance or digital
   b. Towel
   c. Growth chart
3. Ask parent to remove infant's clothing.
4. Place clean towel on scale cradle to decrease shock of cold metal against infant or to prevent friction on a plastic cradle.
5. Balance the scale at zero with towel in place. Calibrate a digital scale to zero with towel in place.

Procedure

6. Place infant face up on scale. Keep diaper or towel over infant's genital area in case of elimination.

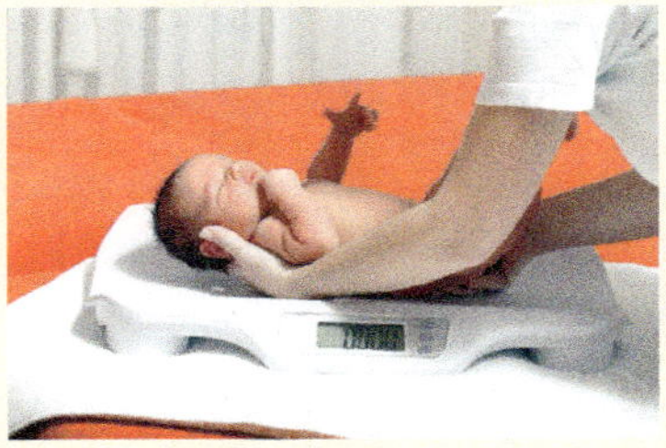

7. Place one hand over infant (almost touching) to give a sense of security.
8. Slide weight easily until scale balances or take measurement from digital reading.
9. Read scale in pounds and ounces or in kilograms.
10. Return infant to parent.

Postprocedure

11. Balance the scale at zero mark or power off a digital scale.
12. Discard towel.
13. Wash hands.
14. Record weight on growth chart and in patient's chart.

Charting Example:

04/29/24 0800
Measured on balance scale, wt. 25 lb.
M. Gonzales CMA
or
04/29/24 0800
Weighed mother and then mother and child to determine weight
Infant too distressed to weigh on infant balance scale
Wt. 25 lb.
M. Gonzales CMA

Language Arts Link

Working with Infants and Toddlers

Dealing with infants and toddlers can be very challenging. During the first two years of a child's life, when making an office visit, most parents feel anxious in determining if their toddler is unwell or simply fearful of the doctor's office. And, of course, the toddler typically cannot explain what is bothering them. When a toddler comes in for a routine checkup and starts to cry hysterically, you must still measure their height and weight and conduct normal procedures. As a health care professional, you will be expected to make both the parent and the child feel at ease.

Working with a partner, evaluate multiple sources of information, presented in diverse formats and media, to determine the education, certification, licensure or degree, along with the skills, needed to prepare for a pediatric career. If possible, include in your analysis an interview with a pediatric professional to identify how they became interested in this field, their current job responsibilities, and benefits of working in pediatrics. Ask about how they deal with uncooperative infants, toddlers, and distraught parents. What tips can they offer to someone considering that field?

After you've completed the research, create a checklist that can be used by a medical assistant, or other pediatric support staff, to calm a parent and deal with a crying infant or toddler.

Be sure to proofread your work to see if you can improve it by making it clearer, more concise, or more accurate. Check the spelling and grammar and correct any errors.

Transfer

When you assist in transferring the patient to another area, the patient may be unhappy about the move. Be calm and pleasant, and explain that you will make the move as easy as possible. Be certain that all of the patient's belongings are transferred to the new area and that the nurse assistant who is responsible for the patient knows that the patient has arrived. Follow the policies and procedures of your facility for transferring patients.

Discharge

A patient cannot be discharged without an order from his or her physician. If your patient plans to leave when it has not been ordered, report it to the head nurse immediately. Each facility has a policy and procedure for discharging the patient. Know what you are expected to do if you are asked to assist in discharging the patient. Be sure that the patient has all of his or her personal belongings. If the patient has valuables that were put away for safekeeping, remind the person to take them home. This is usually a happy time for the patient.

Medical Assisting and Laboratory Skills | Chapter 20 717

Language Arts Link—Working with Infants and Toddlers

- Discuss the issues involved in working with infants and toddlers.
- You might want to have a list of resources available, such as reference books, Web sites, and professionals willing to talk to the students.
- Direct students to use the admission checklist as a guide for creating their checklist.
- Encourage peer review by having students exchange reports to critique and edit.
- Evaluate the checklist based on proper formatting, spelling, grammar, and content.

Teaching Tips

- Discuss reasons for transferring a patient:
  - Change in condition
  - Room requirements
  - Cost
- Emphasize the need for effective communication and consideration of the patient during the move.
- Emphasize the need to keep track of patient's personal belongings.
- Explain discharge.
- Emphasize the need for a physician's order.
- Emphasize that each facility has its own discharge policies and procedures.

CUSTOMIZED INSTRUCTION

English Language Learners

For the Language Arts Link activity, have students read their checklist aloud to a partner and make changes as necessary.

TEAMWORK

In small groups, use a baby doll to practice safe handling of an infant. Lift, hold, and carry the doll. Pass the doll from one team member to another. Always use proper and safe techniques.

Procedure Tip

20.10 Moving Patient and Belongings to Another Room

- Review the background information, emphasizing that a transfer may be a time of stress, and that minimizing patient anxiety is important.
- Point out that Standard Precautions must be followed.
- Review the preprocedure steps.
- Step 1: Emphasize proper handwashing.
- Step 2: Review the list of equipment.
- Step 4: Emphasize effective communication techniques.
- Review the procedure steps.
- Step 5: Emphasize the importance of confirming the new room is ready before leaving the old room.
- Step 6: Explain the importance of verifying that all personal belongings are accounted for.
- Steps 9, 10, 13: Emphasize the importance of effective communication.
- Review the postprocedure steps.
- Step 14: Emphasize importance of handwashing.
- Steps 16 and 17: Emphasize importance of observation and reporting.

PROCEDURE PRACTICE

- Review the steps for Procedure 20.10, Moving Patient and Belongings to Another Room, as many times as necessary, or ask students to demonstrate the steps. Have students practice and perform the procedure until they are competent.

Procedure 20.10 Moving Patient and Belongings to Another Room

BACKGROUND: Following the transfer procedure provides a sense of security for the patient and ensures that personal belongings are not lost. Introduction to the new area, roommate, and caregiver reduces the stress and provides continuing care.
ALERT: Follow Standard Precautions

Preprocedure

1. Wash hands.
2. Assemble equipment:
   a. Patient's chart
   b. Nursing care plan
   c. Medications (Remember: Nursing assistants cannot transfer medications.)
   d. Paper bag
3. Identify patient.
4. Explain what you are going to do.

Procedure

5. Determine location to which patient is being transferred and see if new room is ready.
6. Gather patient belongings. (Check admission list.)
7. Determine how patient is to be transported:
   a. Wheelchair
   b. Stretcher
   c. Entire bed
   d. Ambulation
8. Transport patient to new unit.
9. Introduce to staff on new unit.
10. Introduce to new roommate.
11. Make patient comfortable.
12. Put away belongings.
13. Notify family members listed on patient's admission record of the move.

Postprocedure

14. Wash hands.
15. Give transferred medications, care plan, and chart to nurse.
16. Before leaving unit, record the following:
    a. Date and time of transfer
    b. How transported (e.g., wheelchair)
    c. How transfer was tolerated by patient
17. Return to original unit and report completion of transfer.

Charting Example:

07/14/24	1430
	Transferred in bed to room 20
	Introduced to roommate and
	caregiver. Resting quietly in bed.
	S. Gomez CNA

718 Chapter 20 | Medical Assisting and Laboratory Skills

Procedure 20.11	Discharging a Patient

BACKGROUND: Carefully following the discharge procedure ensures that the patient takes all medications and personal belongings and that final arrangements are completed.
ALERT: Follow Standard Precautions

Preprocedure

1. Check chart for discharge order.
2. Wash hands.
3. Identify patient.
4. Explain what you are going to do.
5. Provide privacy by pulling the privacy curtain.

Procedure

6. Check with the patient's nurse regarding discharge status prior to continuing process. The nurse will need to:
   a. Remove any tethers such as IV lines or indwelling catheters.
   b. Review the patient's medication list, especially new medications and their use.
   c. Notify the patient of any follow up appointments to be scheduled or already scheduled with the physician, or for follow up lab or diagnostics.
   d. Inform the patient of any restriction of activity or diet.
7. Help patient dress.
8. Collect patient's belongings. Check room carefully. Remember to check for hearing aids and dentures.
9. Check belongings against admission list.
10. Secure and return valuables:
    a. Verify with patient that all valuables are there.
    b. Have patient sign for them.
11. Check to see if patient has prescriptions and/or medications and discharge instructions to take home.
12. Check to see if any equipment is to be taken home.
13. Help patient into wheelchair.

NOTE: Patients may have to go by the financial office before leaving.

14. Help patient into car.

Postprocedure

15. Return to unit:
    a. Remove all items left in unit (e.g., basins, disposable items).
    b. Clean unit according to your facility's policy.
16. Wash hands.
17. Record discharge:
    a. Date and time
    b. Method of transport
    c. Whom patient left with

Charting Example:

08/31/24	*1100*
	Discharged by wheelchair with
	son, personal belongings,
	medications, and instructions
	________ S. Gomez CNA

Medical Assisting and Laboratory Skills | Chapter 20 719

Procedure Tip

20.11 Discharging a Patient

- Review the background information, emphasizing that it is important to keep track of personal belongings.
- Point out that Standard Precautions must be followed.
- Review the preprocedure steps.
- Step 1: Emphasize the importance of obtaining the discharge order.
- Step 2: Emphasize proper handwashing.
- Step 4: Emphasize effective communication techniques.
- Step 5: Emphasize the importance of patient privacy.
- Review the procedure steps.
- Step 6: Review nurse's responsibilities.
- Steps 8–10: Explain the importance of verifying that all personal belongings are accounted for.
- Steps 9, 10, 13: Emphasize the importance of effective communication.
- Review the postprocedure steps.
- Step 16: Emphasize importance of handwashing.
- Step 17: Emphasize importance of observation and reporting.

PROCEDURE PRACTICE

- Review the steps for Procedure 20.11, Discharging a Patient, as many times as necessary, or ask students to demonstrate the steps. Have students practice and perform the procedure until they are competent.

Teaching Tips

- Discuss the responsibilities of a medical assistant before and during an examination.
- Reinforce Standard Precautions with examinations.
- Emphasize that the assistant's assurance and communication skills help put the patient at ease.
- Review the basic setup for exams.
- Explain that the type of equipment required depends on the type of examination being performed.
- Review some of the common equipment items that might be required, and how they are used.

Figure Focus

20.5 Otoscope. Who would use an otoscope and why?

Answer: A health care provider might use an otoscope for a routine examination of the ear or if a patient/client has an ear injury.

Figure Focus

20.6 Percussion hammer. Why would a percussion hammer be used?

Answer: A health care provider might use a percussion hammer for examining a patient/client's body, especially the joints.

Assisting with Examinations

Patients need reassurance during a physical examination. The patient may not know what to expect and may feel anxious. To help put him or her at ease, be friendly and efficient.

Equipment

Set up equipment according to the provider's request and check all equipment to be sure it works properly. Equipment varies depending on the body areas to be examined. Learn to anticipate each provider's needs and have equipment and supplies ready before he or she asks for them. Basic equipment includes the following:

- Pen light
- Blood pressure cuff and sphygmomanometer
- Stethoscope
- Opthalmoscope
- Otoscope (**Figure 20.5**)
- Percussion hammer (**Figure 20.6**)
- Disposable gloves
- Basin/pan
- Tape measure (**Figure 20.7**)
- Tongue blade
- Speculums

You may need to set up additional equipment. The type of examination determines which equipment the provider will need.

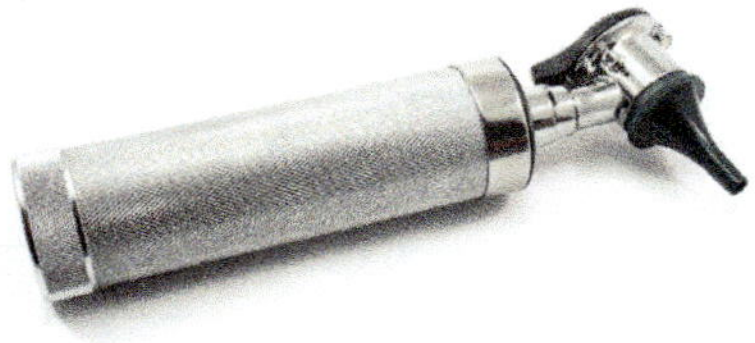

Figure 20.5
Otoscope. Who would use an otoscope and why?

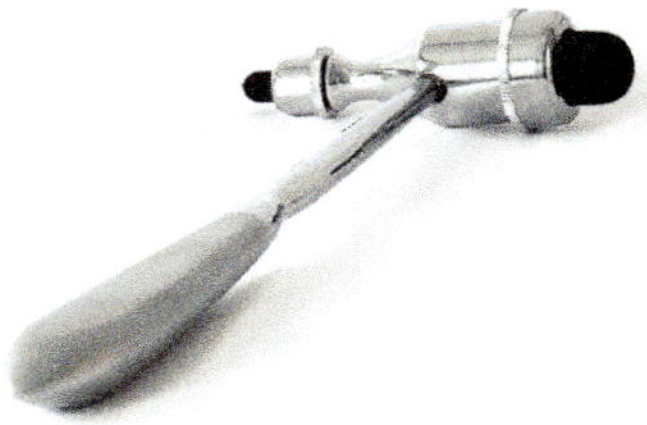

Figure 20.6
Percussion hammer. Why would a percussion hammer be used?

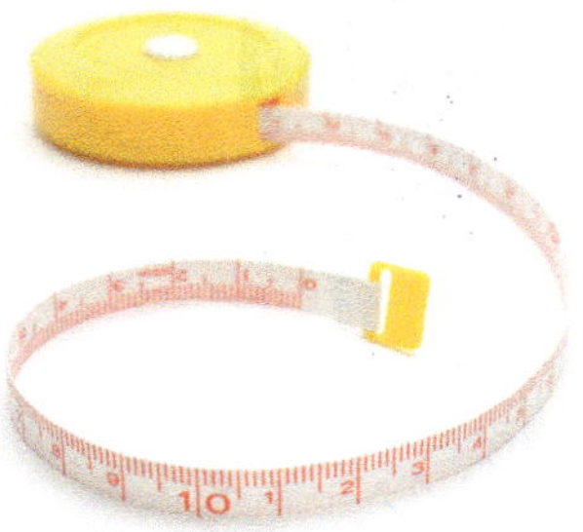

Figure 20.7
Tape measure. When would you use a tape measure with a patient?

Examination Positions

There are specific positions for each procedure. Putting the patient in the correct position makes the examination easier. Always protect the patient's privacy by positioning and draping according to the directions in each procedure.

- **Horizontal recumbent (supine) position.** Use this position for examination, treatment, and surgical procedures of the ventral (anterior) part of the body (for example, for abdominal pain, removal of stitches in chest).
- **Fowler's position.** This position relieves patients who are having trouble breathing (for example, asthma, chest pain). This position allows examination of the anterior and posterior chest (for example, listening to heart and lung sounds).
- **Trendelenburg position.** This position helps restore blood flow to the brain when the body experiences shock. This position also helps promote drainage of congested lungs.
- **Dorsal lithotomy position.** Use this position to examine or perform surgical procedures on the peritoneal and rectal areas (for example, vaginal exam, cystoscopy).
- **Prone position.** Use this position for examination, treatment, or surgical procedures of the dorsal (back) part of the body.
- **Left lateral position and left Sims position.** Use this position for minor rectal examinations, enemas, and treatments.
- **Knee-chest position.** Use this position for rectal examinations and surgical procedures. Some examination tables adjust to support the patient's abdomen and chest.
- **Jackknife.** Use this position for inserting a tube into the urethra.
- **Dorsal recumbent.** Use this position for the examination and treatment of the abdominal area and for vaginal or rectal exams.

Medical Assisting and Laboratory Skills | Chapter 20 721

Figure Focus

20.7 Tape measure. When would you use tape measure with a patient?

Answer: A tape measure might be used to measure the circumference of a baby's head or a baby's height.

Teaching Tips

- Review the examination positions and their usage:
  - Horizontal recumbent (supine) position
  - Fowler's position
  - Trendelenburg position
  - Dorsal lithotomy position
  - Prone position
  - Left lateral and left Sims position
  - Knee-chest position
  - Jackknife
  - Dorsal recumbent

TEAMWORK

Divide the class into teams of five or six students. For each team in turns, read symptoms of a condition, or name a type of procedure. The team must name the proper examination position to use. If they are correct, they get a point. If not, the question moves to the next team. At the end, the team with the most points wins.

Procedure Tip

20.12 Horizontal Recumbent (Supine) Position

- Review the background information, explaining that this position allows examination of the ventral part of the body.
- Point out that Standard Precautions must be followed.
- Review the preprocedure steps.
- Step 1: Emphasize proper handwashing.
- Step 2: Emphasize effective communication techniques.
- Review the procedure steps.
- Step 5: Explain that this is the examination position (refer to illustration).
- Step 6: Emphasize patient privacy.
- Review the postprocedure steps.
- Step 8: Emphasize importance of handwashing.

PROCEDURE PRACTICE

- Review the steps for Procedure 20.12, Horizontal Recumbent (Supine) Position, as many times as necessary, or ask students to demonstrate the steps. Have students practice and perform the procedure until they are competent.

Procedure 20.12 Horizontal Recumbent (Supine) Position

BACKGROUND: Placing the patient in the correct position for treatment, examinations, and for comfort measures is essential for safe and accurate care of the patient.
ALERT: Follow Standard Precautions

Preprocedure

1. Wash hands.
2. Explain to patient what you are going to do.

Procedure

3. Assist patient with gown.
4. Determine any problems associated with placing the patient in this position, such as increased respiratory distress, etc.
5. Assist patient to a position lying flat on his or her back with arms at side in good alignment, with a small pillow under the head.
6. Drape cover so that he or she is not exposed, leaving all edges of drape loose.

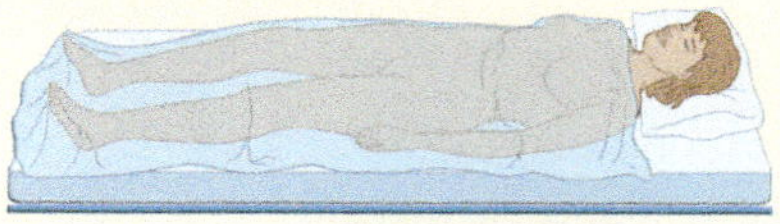

Postprocedure

7. After exam, assist patient off the table and with dressing if needed.
8. Wash hands.

Procedure 20.13 Fowler's Position

BACKGROUND: Placing the patient in the correct position for treatment, examinations, and for comfort measures is essential for safe and accurate care of the patient.
ALERT: Follow Standard Precautions

Preprocedure

1. Wash hands.
2. Explain to patient what you are going to do.
3. Assist patient with gown.

Procedure

4. Determine any problems associated with placing the patient in this position, such as increased back pain, etc.
5. Assist patient to a position lying flat on his or her back in good alignment with small pillow under their head.
6. Keep patient covered so that he or she is not exposed.
7. Flex knees slightly and support them with a pillow.
8. Adjust backrest to one of the following positions according to patient's or physician's needs: Low Fowlers 25°; Semi-Fowlers 45°; High Fowlers 90°. (See figure at top right.)
9. Drape cover so that patient is not exposed, leaving all edges of drape free.

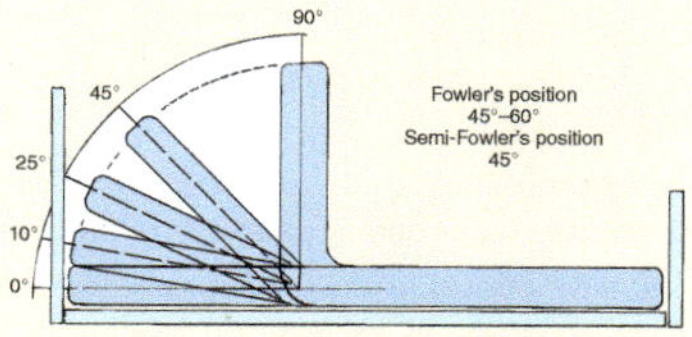

Postprocedure

10. After exam, assist patient off and table and with dressing, if needed.
11. Wash hands.

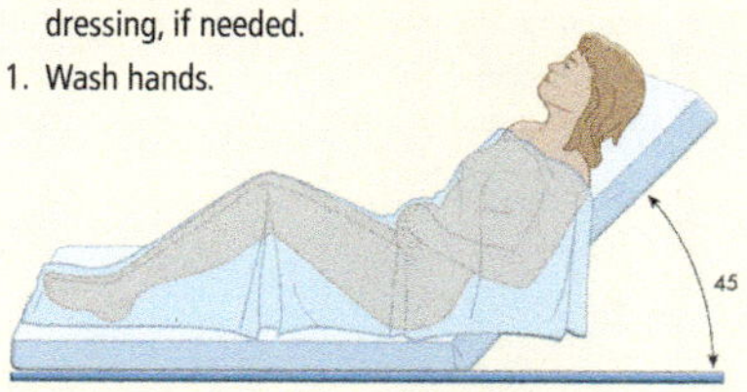

722 Chapter 20 | Medical Assisting and Laboratory Skills

Procedure Tip

20.13 Fowler's Position

- Review the background information, explaining that this position relieves patients who are having trouble breathing and allows examination of the anterior and posterior chest.
- Point out that Standard Precautions must be followed.
- Review the preprocedure steps.
- Step 1: Emphasize proper handwashing.
- Step 2: Emphasize effective communication techniques.
- Review the procedure steps.
- Steps 6 and 9: Emphasize patient privacy.
- Step 8: Review the difference between Low Fowler's, Semi-Fowler's, and High Fowler's.
- Review the postprocedure steps.
- Step 11: Emphasize importance of handwashing.

PROCEDURE PRACTICE

- Review the steps for Procedure 20.13, Fowler's Position, as many times as necessary, or ask students to demonstrate the steps. Have students practice and perform the procedure until they are competent.

Procedure 20.14 Trendelenburg Position

BACKGROUND: Placing the patient in the correct position for treatment, examinations, and for comfort measures is essential for safe and accurate care of the patient.
ALERT: Follow Standard Precautions

Preprocedure

1. Wash hands.
2. Explain to patient what you are going to do.
3. Assist patient with gown.
4. Determine any problems associated with placing patient in this position, such as increased respiratory distress, etc.
5. Assist patient to a position lying flat on his or her back in good alignment.

Procedure

6. Drape cover so that he or she is not exposed, leaving all edges of drape loose.
7. Lower the head of the table until the body is at a 45° angle. Legs may be bent or extended.

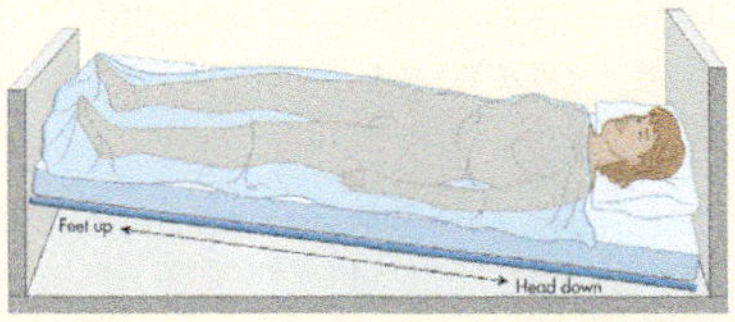

8. Reassure patient that he or she will not slide off table. Remain with patient at all times.

Postprocedure

9. After exam, assist patient off the table and with dressing, if needed.
10. Wash hands.

Procedure 20.15 Dorsal Lithotomy Position

BACKGROUND: Placing the patient in the correct position for treatment, examinations, and for comfort measures is essential for safe and accurate care of the patient.
ALERT: Follow Standard Precautions

Preprocedure

1. Wash hands.
2. Explain to patient what you are going to do
3. Assist patient with gown.

Procedure

4. Determine any problems associated with placing patient in this position, such as increased pain, etc.
5. Assist patient to a position lying flat on his or her back with arms at side.
6. Place pillow under head.
7. Cover patient so that he or she is not exposed.
8. Gently assist patient to bend knees.
9. Separate legs by placing each foot flat on bed about 2 feet apart or in stirrups attached to examination table.
10. Move patient's hips to edge of end of table when stirrups are available.
11. Drape with half-size sheet positioned with one corner toward head and opposite corners between legs. Secure side corner around legs.
12. Remain with the patient.

Postprocedure

13. After exam, assist patient off the table and with dressing, if needed.
14. Wash hands.

Medical Assisting and Laboratory Skills | Chapter 20 723

Procedure Tip

20.14 Trendelenburg Position

- Review the background information, explaining that this position helps restore blood flow to the brain if the patient is in shock, and also helps promote drainage of congested lungs.
- Point out that Standard Precautions must be followed.
- Review the preprocedure steps.
- Step 1: Emphasize proper handwashing.
- Step 2: Emphasize effective communication techniques.
- Step 5: Review good body alignment.
- Review the procedure steps.
- Step 6: Emphasize patient privacy.
- Step 7: Refer to the illustration.
- Step 8: Emphasize the importance of reassuring the patient.
- Review the postprocedure steps.
- Step 10: Emphasize importance of handwashing.

PROCEDURE PRACTICE

- Review the steps for Procedure 20.14, Trendelenberg Position, as many times as necessary, or ask students to demonstrate the steps. Have students practice and perform the procedure until they are competent.

Procedure Tip

20.15 Dorsal Lithotomy Position

- Review the background information, explaining that this position allows access to the peritoneal and rectal areas.
- Point out that Standard Precautions must be followed.
- Review the preprocedure steps.
- Step 1: Emphasize proper handwashing.
- Step 2: Emphasize effective communication techniques.
- Review the procedure steps.
- Step 7: Emphasize patient privacy.
- Review the postprocedure steps.
- Step 14: Emphasize importance of handwashing.

PROCEDURE PRACTICE

- Review the steps for Procedure 20.15, Dorsal Lithotomy Position, as many times as necessary, or ask students to demonstrate the steps. Have students practice and perform the procedure until they are competent.

Procedure Tip

20.16 Prone Position

- Review the background information, explaining that this position allows access to the dorsal (back) part of the body.
- Point out that Standard Precautions must be followed.
- Review the preprocedure steps.
- Step 1: Emphasize proper handwashing.
- Step 2: Emphasize effective communication techniques.
- Review the procedure steps.
- Steps 6 and 7: Refer to the illustration.
- Step 8: Emphasize patient privacy.
- Review the postprocedure steps.
- Step 10: Emphasize importance of handwashing.

PROCEDURE PRACTICE

- Review the steps for Procedure 20.16, Prone Position, as many times as necessary, or ask students to demonstrate the steps. Have students practice and perform the procedure until they are competent.

Procedure 20.16 Prone Position

BACKGROUND: Placing the patient in the correct position for treatment, examinations, and for comfort measures is essential for safe and accurate care of the patient.
ALERT: Follow Standard Precautions

Preprocedure

1. Wash hands.
2. Explain to patient what you are going to do.
3. Assist patient with gown.

Procedure

4. Determine any problems associated with placing patient in this position, such as increased pain or respiratory distress.
5. Turn patient toward self.
6. Position patient on the abdomen with arms flexed by head.
7. Position head to side on small pillow.
8. Cover patient so that he or she is not exposed and let drape hang loosely.

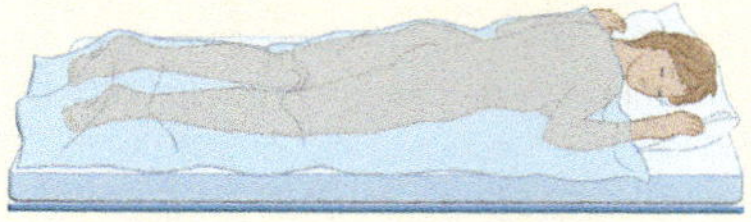

Postprocedure

9. After exam, assist patient off the table and with dressing, if needed.
10. Wash hands.

Procedure 20.17 Left Lateral Position and Left Sims Position

BACKGROUND: Placing the patient in the correct position for treatment, examinations, and for comfort measures is essential for safe and accurate care of the patient.
ALERT: Follow Standard Precautions

Preprocedure

1. Wash hands.
2. Explain to patient what you are going to do.
3. Assist patient with gown.

Procedure

4. Determine any problems associated with placing patient in this position, such as increased pain, respiratory distress, etc.
5. Assist patient to a position lying flat on his or her back.
6. Cover patient so that he or she is not exposed.
7. Assist patient to turn onto left side.
8. Position patient's left arm slightly behind him or her on bed and bend right arm in front of the body.
9. Turn head to side on small pillow.
10. Gently bend both knees.
11. Place right leg slightly forward of left leg for lateral position.
12. Bend right knee toward chest for Sims position.
13. Drape with one sheet; make sure drape is hung loosely.

Postprocedure

14. After exam, assist patient off table and with dressing, if needed.
15. Wash hands.

724 Chapter 20 | Medical Assisting and Laboratory Skills

Procedure Tip

20.17 Left Lateral Position and Left Sims Position

- Review the background information, explaining that this position is suitable for minor rectal examinations, enemas, and treatments.
- Point out that Standard Precautions must be followed.
- Review the preprocedure steps.
- Step 1: Emphasize proper handwashing.
- Step 2: Emphasize effective communication techniques.
- Review the procedure steps.
- Step 6: Emphasize patient privacy.
- Step 12: Explain the difference between the two positions.
- Review the postprocedure steps.
- Step 15: Emphasize importance of handwashing.

PROCEDURE PRACTICE

- Review the steps for Procedure 20.17, Left Lateral and Left Sims Position, as many times as necessary, or ask students to demonstrate the steps. Have students practice and perform the procedure until they are competent.

Procedure 20.18 Knee-Chest Position

BACKGROUND: Placing the patient in the correct position for treatment, examinations, and for comfort measures is essential for safe and accurate care of the patient.
ALERT: Follow Standard Precautions

Preprocedure

1. Wash hands.
2. Explain to patient what you are going to do.
3. Determine any problems associated with placing patient in this position such as increased pain, etc.
4. Assist patient to a position lying flat on his or her back.

Procedure

5. Cover patient so that he or she is not exposed.
6. Assist patient to turn onto his or her stomach, keeping patient covered.
7. Instruct patient to raise hips upward by kneeling on both knees.

NOTE: It is hard for the patient to stay in this position, so put them in it immediately prior to the procedure and stay with them.

8. Rest patient's head and shoulders on a pillow.
9. Flex arms slightly and have them at the side of their head.
10. Drape with a large sheet, allowing edges to hang free.

Postprocedure

11. After exam, assist patient off table and with dressing, if needed.
12. Wash hands.

Examination and Diagnostic Techniques

Examinations require four basic techniques:

1. **Observation/Inspection.** Here the provider looks at the patient for normal and abnormal appearance. Skin, eyes, hair, nails, movements, or actions that look unusual may be important in determining an illness. (**Figure 20.8**)

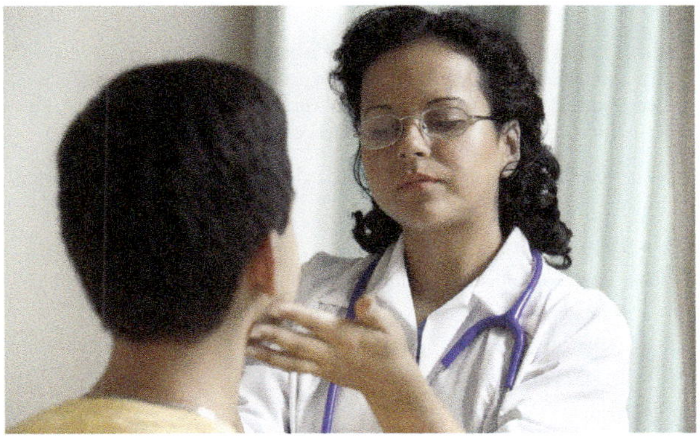

Figure 20.8
Why is it important to do a visual inspection of a patient?

Medical Assisting and Laboratory Skills | Chapter 20 725

Procedure Tip

20.18 Knee-Chest Position

- Review the background information, explaining that this position is suitable for rectal examinations and surgical procedures.
- Point out that Standard Precautions must be followed.
- Review the preprocedure steps.
- Step 1: Emphasize proper handwashing.
- Step 2: Emphasize effective communication techniques.
- Review the procedure steps.
- Step 5: Emphasize patient privacy.
- Review the note, and emphasize the need to respect the patient's comfort and dignity.
- Review the postprocedure steps.
- Step 12: Emphasize importance of handwashing.

PROCEDURE PRACTICE

- Review the steps for Procedure 20.18, Knee-Chest Position, as many times as necessary, or ask students to demonstrate the steps. Have students practice and perform the procedure until they are competent.

Figure Focus

20.8 Why is it important to do a visual inspection of a patient?

Answer: A visual inspection gives the provider clues about how the body is working and helps the provider determine the correct diagnosis.

Teaching Tips

- Review the four basic examination techniques:
  - Observation/inspection
  - Palpation
  - Percussion
  - Auscultation
- Discuss how the provider uses these techniques to reach a diagnosis.
- Discuss the clues that the provider assesses to help with a final diagnosis:
  - Patient/client history
  - Physical examination findings
  - Vital signs
  - Laboratory results
  - Diagnostic test results
  - Symptoms described by the patient
- Explain why a provider might need to rule out (R/O) some possible problems in order to reach a final diagnosis, and how this is accomplished.

Figure Focus

20.9 The stethoscope is one of the most widely recognized symbols of medicine. What do health care providers listen for through the stethoscope?

Answer: The stethoscope is a medical device used for listening to the internal sounds of an animal or human body. It is used to listen to lung sounds, heart sounds, intestines, and blood flow in arteries and veins.

2. **Palpation.** In this procedure, the provider feels parts of the body for unusual or abnormal conditions. Feeling and applying pressure also allow the provider to locate tender or painful areas.
3. **Percussion.** Providers use their fingers to tap over areas of the body. The sounds the provider hears during percussion indicate the fullness, emptiness, and size of internal organs.
4. **Auscultation.** The provider listens to body sounds through a stethoscope. Sounds of the heart and lungs, bowel sounds, and even the flow of blood through arteries can be heard. (Figure 20.9)

auscultation
(aw skuhl TEY shuh n)
The act of listening, either directly or through a stethoscope or other instrument, to sounds within the body as a method of diagnosis.

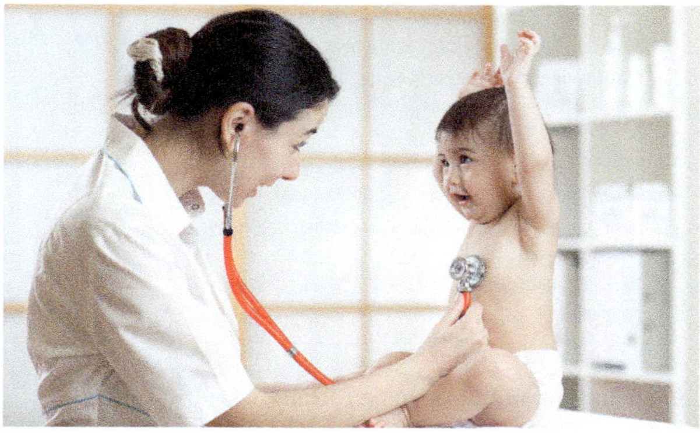

Figure 20.9
The stethoscope is one of the most widely recognized symbols of medicine. What do health care providers listen for through the stethoscope?

These four techniques give a provider clues about how the body is working. For example, if a patient complains of a chest cold, the provider listens to the chest with a stethoscope. Gurgling sounds or very little airflow in the lungs tell the provider that the lungs are congested with fluid. A chest x-ray confirms what auscultation indicated.

When a patient complains of pain or other problems, the provider uses the four basic examination techniques. Prepare each patient for observation, palpation, percussion, and auscultation. Tell patients what you want them to do. Remember that patients are often nervous. Show patience and understanding.

diagnosis
(dahy uh g NOH sis)
Identification of a disease or condition.

To determine a final **diagnosis** the physician looks for clues from the following sources:

- Patient history
- Physical examination findings
- Vital signs
- Laboratory results
- Diagnostic test results
- Symptoms described by the patient

726 Chapter 20 | Medical Assisting and Laboratory Skills

ACTIVITY

Make a poster showing the four basic methods of examination, providing an explanation of each method.

If there is more than one possible diagnosis, the provider needs to rule out each possible condition before determining a final diagnosis. For example, a patient complaining of abdominal pain may need additional tests to:

- Rule out (R/O) appendicitis
- Rule out (R/O) gastroenteritis
- Rule out (R/O) pelvic inflammatory disease (PID)

The provider makes a final diagnosis when tests rule out possible conditions and provide evidence of a specific disease.

Testing Visual Acuity

Vision acuity (clearness) testing helps the provider detect eye disease or injury. Vision acuity tests are usually part of a physical examination. A provider always does a vision acuity test when the patient complains of eye pain, itching, tenderness, or injury. The provider can identify changes and evaluate the treatment more effectively when there is a **baseline** acuity test.

baseline
(BEYS lahyn)
A number, graph, or indication to use as a guideline; A measurement taken at a later time may differ from the baseline, indicating a possible cause for concern.

Patients over age 65 should be encouraged to obtain annual eye exams for early diagnosis of disease and correction of common problems associated with the aging eye. Poor eyesight contributes to safety problems in the aged.

To read the result of the visual acuity test on a Snellen chart, find the fraction to the left of the line the patient is able to read. (**Figure 20.10**) For example, if the patient reads all the letters in the line marked 20/20 and is unable to read line 20/15, the patient's vision is 20/20. The top number means that the patient is 20 feet from the chart. The bottom number is the distance at which a patient with normal vision can read that row of letters. If line 20/50 is the last line read, the patient's vision is 20/50. This means that the patient is able to read at 20 feet what a person with normal vision sees at 50 feet.

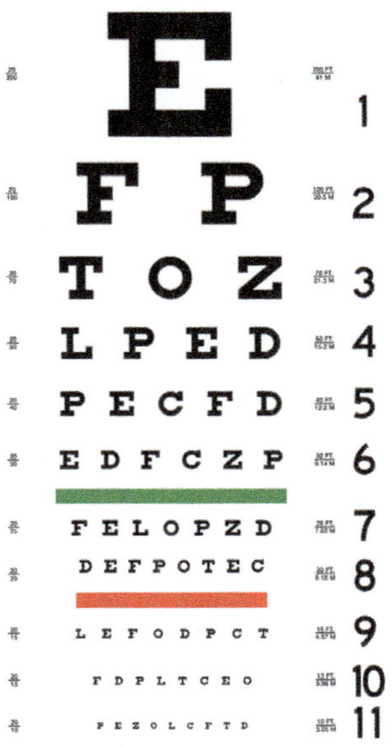

Figure 20.10
Snellen eye chart for English readers. If your instructor has a full-size copy of the eye chart, check to see what your vision is.

Teaching Tips

- Discuss visual acuity tests:
  - Used from early childhood
  - Provide a baseline for any indication of change over time
  - Taken whenever there are complaints related to the eye
  - Injury, illness, or medication might cause changes in acuity
- Explain that some patients receive annual eye exams from a specialist.
- Explain the use of a Snellen Chart.
- Discuss alternatives for patients who cannot read, such as non-English speakers or young children, such as using fingers to indicate direction of letter E.

Figure Focus

20.10 Snellen eye chart for English readers. If your instructor has a full-size copy of the eye chart, check to see what your vision is.

Allow class time for students to assess their own or each other's vision.

ACTIVITY

Create your own version of an eye chart that could be used by patients who cannot read English.

Procedure Tip

20.19 Testing Visual Acuity: Snellen Chart

- Review the background, explaining that this is a screening method. Problems would indicate further testing and an appointment with a specialist.
- Point out that Standard Precautions must be followed.
- Review the preprocedure steps.
- Step 1: Emphasize proper handwashing.
- Step 2: Emphasize the importance of proper positioning of the chart.
- Step 4: Emphasize the importance of effective communication techniques.
- Review the procedure steps.
- Step 5: Emphasize the importance of proper distance.
- Step 9: Emphasize the importance of proper recording.
- Review the postprocedure steps.
- Step 13: Emphasize importance of handwashing.

PROCEDURE PRACTICE

- Review the steps for Procedure 20.19, Testing Visual Acuity: Snellen Chart, as many times as necessary, or ask students to demonstrate the steps. Provide Snellen Charts, as necessary. Have students practice and perform the procedure until they are competent.

Procedure 20.19 **Testing Visual Acuity: Snellen Chart**

BACKGROUND: Vision affects all activities of daily living. Correct measurement of visual acuity is essential to determine whether patient has normal or abnormal eyesight.
ALERT: Follow Standard Precautions

Preprocedure

1. Wash hands.
2. Assure that the Snellen Chart is at patient's eye level and that the tape for them to stand on is 20 feet from the chart.
3. Identify patient.
4. Explain procedure to patient.

Procedure

5. Position patient 20 feet (6 meters) from Snellen chart. Have patient stand with heel on 20 foot mark.
6. Instruct patient to keep both eyes open during testing. Ask them to remove corrective lenses.
7. Ask patient to cover left eye with an occluder and read smallest line of letters that he or she can see.
8. Use a pointer and point to letters in the row in random order. Do not cover the letter or symbol with the pointer.
9. Record the distance patient is from the chart compared to the size of letters patient can see clearly (e.g., 20/20, 20/30, 20/40).
10. Repeat test with right eye covered.
11. Repeat test, allowing patient to use both eyes.
12. Repeat each test with patient wearing glasses (if he or she has prescription lenses).

Postprocedure

13. Wash hands.

Summary

The medical assisting skills of admitting, registering, transferring, and discharging a patient are important processes in a patient's health. You must interact with and make the patient feel at ease, as well as perform some basic tasks, such as measuring height and weight.

Section 20.1 Review Questions

1. When admitting a patient, what are the basic procedures?
2. What two forms must be completed by new patients when registering?
3. How would you measure an infant's head circumference?
4. List the five basic pieces of equipment used during examinations.
5. Why is it important to use a consistent method in weighing an infant?
6. Name and explain the purpose of three examination and diagnostic techniques.

728 Chapter 20 | Medical Assisting and Laboratory Skills

Section 20.1 Review Questions

1. Answer:
   - Make a clothing list.
   - Make a list of personal items.
   - Request that the family take home valuables or see that they are put in a safe place.
   - Take vital signs.
   - Weigh the patient.
   - Explain the call light and routine.
   - Collect urine specimens if required.
2. Answer: Patient information forms and medical history forms
3. Answer: Place the measuring tape over the occipital bone on the back of the head and wrap forward just above the ears to center of forehead.
4. Answer:
   - Pen light
   - Blood pressure cuff and sphygmomanometer
   - Stethoscope
   - Opthalmoscope
   - Otoscope
   - Percussion hammer
   - Disposable gloves
   - Basin/pan
   - Tape measure
   - Tongue blade
   - Speculums
5. Answer: You should be consistent when weighing an infant because a difference in expected growth pattern may indicate a medical problem.
6. Answer:
   - Observation/Inspection: Provider looks at the patient for normal and abnormal appearance. Skin, eyes, hair, nails, movements, or actions that look unusual may be important in determining an illness.

Pharmacology and Medication Administration

SECTION 20.2

Background

Medical assistants are responsible for understanding the guidelines for preparing and administering medications. There are a variety of resources commonly available to help answer their questions. In addition, medical assistants must be aware of the legal ramifications of controlling, using, and distributing various drugs.

Objectives

When you have completed this section, you will be able to do the following:

- Match key terms with their correct meanings.
- Match common prescription abbreviations with their meanings.
- Match controlled substances with their assigned schedule level.
- Name a few drug reference books.
- Describe methods to ensure safekeeping of medication.
- Write a formula for calculating medication dosage.
- Name the rights of medication administration.
- Recognize the guidelines for preparing and administering medications.
- Demonstrate all procedures in this chapter.

Responsibilities

Working with medication and administering medication are serious responsibilities. As a medical assistant you are responsible for the following:

- Administering medication
- Being aware of side effects
- Interpreting prescriptions
- Reinforcing the provider's instructions
- Recognizing adverse effects of medications
- Reporting accurate observations
- Using references to obtain directions

Common Prescription Abbreviations

Special abbreviations and symbols are used when working with medication. Abbreviations are commonly used when delivering medical care. Some of these are listed below. However, each facility may use a different set of accepted abbreviations. It is very important that you follow your facilities accepted list. Using abbreviations that are not considered acceptable in your facility can lead to errors in treatment that could be serious.

Medical Assisting and Laboratory Skills | Chapter 20 729

- Palpation: Provider feels parts of the body for unusual or abnormal conditions. Feeling and applying pressure also allows the provider to locate tender or painful areas.
- Percussion: Providers use their fingers to tap over areas of the body. The sounds the provider hears during percussion indicate the fullness, emptiness, and size of internal organs.
- Auscultation: The provider listens to body sounds through a stethoscope. Sounds of the heart and lungs, bowel sounds, and even the flow of blood through arteries can be heard.

FOCUS AND ENGAGE

Introduce the Section

a. Review the content of the Background paragraph, explaining that medication administration is often a responsibility of a medical assistant.
b. Emphasize the importance of safe and accurate medication administration for the health and well-being of the patient.
c. Review the objectives for the section.

Vocabulary Review

a. Direct students to the key terms.
b. Pronounce each word, and have the students repeat the pronunciation out loud.
c. Discuss the definition of each word.

TEACH

Discuss

- Ask students if they know the difference between prescription and over-the-counter (OTC) medications.
- Discuss the difference between legal and illegal substances.
- Point out that some OTC and prescription medications can be used for illegal purposes.
- Discuss the responsibilities of medical professionals in terms of monitoring the use of medications.

Reinforce and Review

- Review Sections 5.2 and 5.3 in Chapter 5, Understanding Your Legal Obligations.
- Review Section 12.2, Measurements, in Chapter 12, Measurement and the Scientific Process.
- Review Section 10.2, Abbreviations, in Chapter 10, Medical Terminology.

ACTIVITY

Have each student write the name of a medication on a slip of paper. Then, collect the slips, shuffle them, and redistribute them to the class. Go around the class and have each student read the medication and identify it as a prescription or over-the-counter drug.

Teaching Tips

- Review the responsibilities of a medical assistant when giving medication:
  - Administering medication
  - Being aware of side effects
  - Interpreting prescriptions
  - Reinforcing the provider's instructions
  - Recognizing adverse effects of medications
  - Reporting accurate observations
  - Using references to obtain directions
- Discuss risks of medication administration:
  - Wrong medication can cause death or injury
  - Wrong dosage can cause death or injury
- Emphasize that some facilities may use different abbreviations when prescribing medications.
- Explain that health care workers must familiarize themselves with the abbreviations used by the facility where they work.
- Review common prescription abbreviations.
- Emphasize that there are federal guidelines for regulating medication, monitored by the Drug Enforcement Agency (DEA) of the Department of Justice.
- Explain that there are also state regulations that are monitored and enforced by the local state government.

Abbreviation	Meaning	Abbreviation	Meaning
cap(s)	capsule(s)	Mcg	microgram
Dil	dilute	mEq	milliequivalent
Dr	dram	Mg	milligram
D/W	dextrose in water	Ml	milliliter
fl or fld	fluid	NS	normal saline
Gal	gallon	OD	right eye
gt or gtt	drop	Oint	ointment
IM	intramuscular	OS	left eye
IU	international units	OU	both eyes
IV	intravenous	Oz	ounce
Kg	kilogram	Pt	pint or patient
L	liter	Pulv	powder
Liq	liquid	SC, SQ, subc, or subq	subcutaneous
m or min	minim	tinc or tr or tinct	tincture

Legal Issues

There are federal guidelines and legislation regulating the manufacture, distribution, dispensing, and sale of medication. Federal regulations are monitored by the Drug Enforcement Agency (DEA) of the Department of Justice. State regulations are monitored by the State Department of Health and Human Services.

The medical assistant supports the provider by:

- Monitoring expiration dates of the physician's DEA registration
- Keeping records and inventory that are legally acceptable
- Controlling access to all drugs, controlled substances, and prescription pads
- Destroying medication when expired. Disposal of controlled substances must be witnessed

Drugs that can cause addiction and abuse are divided into five groups, called schedules. Each schedule names the drugs and explains their ability to become addicting and/or abused. (Table 20.2)

Prescriptions

Prescription drugs are medications that require monitoring by a licensed physician. The Federal Drug Administration determines which drugs must be prescribed by a physician. Prescriptions are instructions to a pharmacist to supply the patient with medication in a specified amount. The prescription also provides directions for taking medication. The prescription is a legal document. There are six parts to complete in a prescription:

730 Chapter 20 | Medical Assisting and Laboratory Skills

- Review the medical assistant's duties in controlling medication:
  - Monitor expiration dates of physician's DEA registration.
  - Keep legally acceptable records and inventory.
  - Control access to all drugs, controlled substances, and prescription pads.
  - Destroy expired medication. Disposal of controlled substances must be witnessed.
  - Explain prescription drug.

ACTIVITY

Have students make flashcards to use as a study aid in learning the medical abbreviations commonly used on medication prescriptions.

1. Patient information and superscription:
   - Date
   - Age, if child
   - Patient's name
   - Rx, meaning "recipe" or "take"
   - Patient's address
2. Inscription:
   - Name of medication
   - Amount of medication
3. Subscription:
   - Directions to pharmacist
4. Sig or signa:
   - Directions to patient
5. Physician's signature and address, registry number, and controlled substances approval number (BNDD).
6. Number of times, if any, the prescription can be refilled.

Table 20.2 Schedule of Controlled Substances

The drugs and drug products that come under the jurisdiction of the Controlled Substances Act are divided into five schedules. Some examples from each schedule are outlined below. For a complete listing of all of the controlled substances, contact any office of the Drug Enforcement Administration or log on to www.DEA.GOV and click on "Drug Scheduling."

Category	Description	Examples	
Schedule I	The substances in this schedule are those that have no accepted medical use in the United States and have a high abuse potential.	acetylmethadol dihydromorphine fenethylline heroin LSD marijuana* MDMA (Ecstasy)	mescaline methaqualone N-ethylamphetamine peyote psilocybin tilidine
Schedule II	The substances in this schedule have a high abuse potential with severe psychic or physical dependence liability. Schedule II controlled substances consist of certain narcotic, stimulant, and depressant drugs.	amobarbital amphetamine (Dexedrine) cocaine codeine dronabinol etorphine hydrochloride fentanyl (Sublimaze) hydromorphone (Dilaudid) meperidine (Demerol) methadone methamphetamine (Desoxyn) methylphenidate (Ritalin) morphine	nabilone opium oxycodone (Percodan) oxymorphone (Numorphan) pantopon pentobarbital phenmetrazine (Preludin) phenylacetone secobarbital sufentanil

* As of 2014 several states have authorized the legal use of marijuana for health purposes, and marijuana has been legalized in Colorado, Washington, Alaska, and Oregon.

(continued)

Medical Assisting and Laboratory Skills | Chapter 20 731

Teaching Tips

- Review and explain the six parts of a prescription:
  1. Patient information and superscription
  2. Inscription
  3. Subscription
  4. Sig or signa
  5. Physician's signature and address, registry number, and controlled substances
  6. Number of times the prescription can be refilled
- Explain that the Controlled Substances Act identifies drugs that are regulated because they can cause addiction and abuse.
- Emphasize that drugs that can cause addiction and abuse are divided by law into five groups, called "Schedules."
- Explain that each of the five schedules lists the drugs in that schedule, along with an explanation of how it can become addictive or abused.
- Review Table 20.2 together as a class.
- Point out that the Category column identifies the schedule, using roman numerals.
- Review roman numerals from 1 to 5 (I, II, III, IV, V), if necessary.
- Explain that Schedule I are the highest risk drugs, and that Schedule V are the lowest risk drugs.
- Ask a student to read the description of each schedule.

ACTIVITY

Write a piece of information that represents one part of a prescription on the board. Students must identify the correct prescription part.

Teaching Tips

- Review the examples of drugs in each schedule. Point out the brand names that are included in parentheses.
- Point out some of the more commonly known substances, such as marijuana in Schedule I, methylphenidate (Ritalin) in Schedule II, Tylenol with Codeine in Schedule III, and diazepam (Valium) in Schedule IV.
- If appropriate, discuss with students the use of medical marijuana.

TEAMWORK

In small groups, have students research the federal and state laws governing controlled substances. Have students learn what constitutes a felony, what constitutes a misdemeanor, and what the punishments are.

Table 20.2 Schedule of Controlled Substances (continued)

Category	Description	Examples	
Schedule III	The substances in this schedule have an abuse potential less than those in Schedules I and II, and include compounds containing limited quantities of certain narcotic drugs and non-narcotic drugs.	amobarbital compounds benphetamine chlorphentermine clortermine derivatives of barbituric acid nalorphine	paregoric pentobarbital compounds phendimetrazine secobarbital compounds Tylenol with Codeine
Schedule IV	The substances in this schedule have an abuse potential less than those listed in Schedule III.	alprazolam (Xanax) Barbital chloral hydrate chlordiazepoxide (Librium) clonazepam (Clonapin) clorazepate (Tranxene) detropropoxyphene (Darvon) diazepam (Valium) diethylpropion ethclorovynol (Placidyl) paraldehyde ethinamate (Valmid) fenfluramine flurazepam (Dalmane) halazepam (Paxipam) lorazepam (Ativan) mebutamate meprobamate (Equanil, Miltown) methohexital methylphenobarbital	midazolam (Versed) oxazepam (Serax) pentazocine (Talwin-NX) phenobarbital phentermine prazepam (Verstran) quazepam (Dormalin) temazepam (Restoril) triazolam (Halcion)
Schedule V	The substances in this schedule have an abuse potential less than those listed in Schedule IV and consist primarily of preparations containing limited quantities of certain narcotic and stimulant drugs generally for antitussive, antidiarrheal, and analgesic purposes.	buprenorphine propylhexedrine	

732 Chapter 20 | Medical Assisting and Laboratory Skills

Medication/drugs are described in three ways:

1. A brand name is assigned to a drug by the manufacturer. The brand name is commonly used in advertising a medication.
2. A generic name often describes the chemical makeup or classification of a drug. Generic names are adopted by the U.S. Adopted Name Council (USAN); Pharmacopia (USP), *a database catalog*; or the United States National Formulary (NF), *the dictionary of drug names.*
3. The chemical name reflects the chemicals in the drug and its structure.

The cost of generic medication is usually less than that of brand-name medication. Patients save money if the doctor prescribes the generic form or tells the patient that a generic medication is acceptable.

Drug Reference Books

There are so many medications available that it is difficult to remember all the important information. To determine the best medication for a patient, doctors often refer to reference books. Nurses must have knowledge of the use, common dosages, and side effects of every medication they administer.

Your facility will provide an up-to-date nurse reference book for use on the unit. No medication should be given until the nurse feels comfortable with her knowledge of the medication.

Whenever possible, the patient should be advised of the medication being delivered. If the patient questions the medication, the nurse should check the physician's order and the medication to assure that it is correct and then reassure the patient. Patients have the right to refuse medication as well as any other treatment being provided to them.

The following paragraphs briefly describe the most frequently used reference books.

The United States Pharmacopia (USP)–*National Formulary* (NF) is published every five years. The publication lists only official drugs, and it identifies drug standards. The NF chapter explains the ingredients of each drug. Drug information includes the following:

- Description of drug
- Standards for purity
- Strength and composition
- Storage
- Use
- Dosage

American Medical Association Drug Evaluations is a periodically revised book of officially established and recognized drug names and standards.

Medical Assisting and Laboratory Skills | Chapter 20 733

Teaching Tips

- Explain that medication is described in three ways:
  - A brand name is assigned to a drug by the manufacturer. The brand name is commonly used in advertising a medication.
  - A generic name often describes the chemical makeup or classification of a drug. Generic names are adopted by the U.S. Adopted Name Council (USAN); Pharmacopia (USP), a database catalog; or the United States National Formulary (NF), the dictionary of drug names.
  - The chemical name reflects the chemicals in the drug and its structure.
- Display several different drug reference books, including the PDR.
- Explain that different books provide different categories of information.
- Explain why the information in these books is essential to every medical assistant.
- Reinforce the importance of looking up a medication before giving it.
- Review the patient's right to refuse medication.

TEAMWORK

Divide the class into teams of four or five students. Hand out lists of brand name drugs. The team that identifies the generic and chemical names of each drug on their list first wins.

Teaching Tips

- Discuss the most frequently used drug reference books:
  - *United States Pharmacopia (USP)—National Formulary (NF):* Published every 5 years; lists official drugs; identifies drug standards; includes description of drug, standards for purity, strength and composition, storage, use, dosage
  - *American Medical Association Drug Evaluations:* Revised periodically; includes officially established and recognized drug names and standards
  - *American Hospital Formulary Services (AHFS):* Periodic supplements; unbiased information
  - *Physicians' Desk Reference (PDR):* Unofficial, but most commonly used; published annually; twice yearly supplements; includes comprehensive descriptions and classifications

American Hospital Formulary Services (AHFS) provides periodic supplements that maintain current information. This publication gives unbiased drug information. Drugs are listed by generic names according to their therapeutic or pharmacological class.

***Physicians' Desk Reference* (PDR)** A commonly used reference book that provides information about drugs, drug manufacturers, emergency phone numbers, and more.

***The Physicians' Desk Reference* (PDR)** is not an official drug reference book but it is the most commonly used. It is published annually; periodic (twice yearly) supplements provide information on newest medications. PDR information is also available at PDR.net. The PDR contains the following information:

- Manufacturers' Index (White Pages)
- Brand and Generic Name Index (Pink Pages)
- Generic Brand/Cross-Reference Table
- Product Category Index (Blue Pages)
- Key to Controlled Substances Schedule
- Key to FDA Use-in-Pregnancy Ratings
- U.S. Food and Drug Administration Telephone Directory
- Poison Antidotes
- Drugs Excreted in Breast Milk
- Product Identification Guide
- Healthcare Provider Resource Center
- Product Information
- Dietary Supplements
- Drugs That Should Not Be Used in Pregnancy
- Drugs That Should Not Be Crushed

It is important for MAs to understand how to use reference books. MAs are responsible for giving medication correctly. Drug reference books provide guidelines for responsible administration of prescribed medication. *The Physicians' Desk Reference* is the most available reference.

Using the Physicians' Desk Reference (PDR)

The PDR can be used in a variety of ways. To demonstrate this we will use the example of a patient who hands you an oval-shaped pill with "Wallace 200" stamped on it. You can take that pill to the PDR and compare it with the pictures. An exact comparison indicates that Wallace is the manufacturer and 200 is the dose. To become more familiar with the PDR, follow the steps in Procedure 20.20.

734 Chapter 20 | Medical Assisting and Laboratory Skills

TEAMWORK

Divide the class into teams of five or six students. Hand out descriptions or pictures of three or four specific medications to each team. See which team can identify all of the medications first. Specify the information they should obtain, such as manufacturer, strength, composition, dosage, etc.

Procedure 20.20 Using the *Physicians' Desk Reference* (PDR)

BACKGROUND: It is important for the health care worker to know details about medications. The PDR is an essential tool that provides information about medications the health care worker gives. Understanding how to use the PDR helps in finding information in a timely manner.

Procedure

1. Identify the name of the manufacturer; compare the tablet with pictures to identify the medication:
   a. Wallace is the manufacturer.
   b. Turn to the page where Wallace pills are displayed.
   c. Match the pill with pictures of pills displayed.
   d. A yellow oval pill marked "Wallace 200" matches "Soma Compound with Codeine 200 mg" in the display.
2. Turn to Section 2, the pink pages. Find "Soma Compound with Codeine 200 mg." Two page numbers are listed:
   a. The first page number refers to the picture of the medication.
   b. The second page number provides product information.
3. Turn to the page number indicated to find specific drug information:
   a. Description of drug
   b. Clinical pharmacology
   c. Indications and usage (describes the reasons for using the drug)
   d. Contraindications (reasons not to give this drug)
   e. Warnings
   f. Precautions
   g. Dosage and administration
   h. How supplied
   i. Storage recommendations
4. Go to Section 1 for more information about a drug. Find the manufacturer:
   a. Wallace Laboratories is listed with the W's in the alphabetical list.
   b. Write requests for information using the address supplied.
   c. Call for assistance using the professional services telephone number or night and weekend emergency number if available

Storage and Handling of Drugs

Medication requires special handling. To ensure the safekeeping of medications, always:

- Keep medications in a locked area away from other supplies.
- Keep medications in original containers.
- Refrigerate medications that require storage at lower than room temperatures.
- Rotate medications so that the oldest are used before expiration dates.
- Destroy expired medications. (Follow office policy when destroying medication.)
- Keep medications requiring darkness out of the light (in a dark cupboard or container).
- Be aware of medications that react with other materials (for example, some medications react with plastic so must be stored in glass).

Medical Assisting and Laboratory Skills | Chapter 20 735

Procedure Tip

20.20 Using the *Physicians' Desk Reference* (PDR)

- Review the background information, emphasizing the importance of knowing what a medication is before administering it.
- Use an actual PDR to demonstrate this procedure.
- Note that the steps refer to a tablet of Soma Compound with Codeine 200 mg.
- Step 2: Demonstrate how to use Section 2. Explain the page numbers.
- Step 3: Review the type of information that is available.
- Step 4: Demonstrate how to use Section 1 to learn more about the manufacturer, including how to contact the manufacturer for more information.

PROCEDURE PRACTICE

- Demonstrate the procedure steps to the class as many times as necessary, or ask students to demonstrate the steps. Provide descriptions or pictures of medications for them to look up. Have students practice and perform the procedure until they are competent.

Teaching Tips

- Explain federal law for storage and reporting of lost or stolen controlled substances.
- Explain the classification of medications for storage purposes.

Teaching Tips

- Review the precautions for safe storage and handling of drugs:
  - Keep medications in a locked area away from other supplies.
  - Keep medications in original containers.
  - Refrigerate medications that require storage at lower-than-room temperatures.
  - Rotate medications so that the oldest are used before expiration dates.
  - Destroy expired medications using office policy.
  - Keep medications requiring darkness out of the light.
  - Be aware of medications that react with other materials.
- Explain the importance of knowing how to calculate a dosage.

TEAMWORK

In small groups, create a public service poster, brochure, or presentation explaining the importance of safe handling and storage of all medications.

antibiotics
(anti bi ot ik)
Substances that slow growth of or destroy microorganisms.

contraceptives
(kon tre sept tivs)
Items that serve to prevent pregnancy.

diuretics
(die ret ik)
Drugs that increase urine output.

parenteral
(pa REN ter uhl)
Not in the digestive system (e.g., injections are parenterally administered).

topical
(TOP i kuhl)
Surface of the body.

formula
(FAWR myuh luh)
Accepted rule (e.g., a math formula and a baby formula are both guidelines or rules).

To organize the storage of drugs, use a simple, logical system. One example of a system is alphabetic arrangement by classification—for example, all **antibiotics** together, **contraceptives** together, **diuretics** together, etc. Within each classification, separate oral, **parenteral**, **topical**, and other medications. Federal law requires that you place all controlled substances (see **Table 20.2**) in a locked cabinet safely separated from other medications. Any controlled substances that are lost or stolen must be reported by the physician to the Drug Enforcement Agency.

Drug Dosage

Pharmacy calculations are an essential function of the Pharmacy Technician. In order to read, write, and fill out prescriptions, the health care professional must understand Roman Numerals. They are commonly used in pharmacology, especially in the directions (or Sig) on prescriptions. For instance, 3 tablets three times a day is often written as lll tabs t.i.d. It is expected that pharmacy technicians will understand the primary Roman Numerals and the rules for adding and subtracting them.

A basic list of the Roman Numerals is included below:

II or ii for 2	VIII or viii for 8
III or iii for 3	IX or ix for 9
IV or iv for 4	X for 10
V or v for 5	XI or xi for 11
VI or vi for 6	XXXII or xxxii for 32
VII or vii for 7	XLV or xlv for 45

Giving the right medication dosage is an important part of administering medication. Many medications are prepackaged and ready to give. Some medications require dosage calculation. A simple **formula** for calculating dosage is:

$$\text{dosage you want} = \frac{\text{dosage you give}}{\text{dosage you have}}$$

Example: The physician orders 200 mg (milligrams) of a medication. You have 100-mg tablets of the medication.

$$\frac{\text{dosage you want}}{\text{dosage you have}} = \frac{200 \text{ mg}}{100\text{-mg tablets}} = \text{dosage you give}$$

Divide 200 mg by 100 mg:

$$\begin{array}{r} 2 \\ 100\,\overline{)200} \\ 200 \end{array}$$

The patient needs to take two tablets to receive 200 mg of the ordered medicine.

736 Chapter 20 | Medical Assisting and Laboratory Skills

The medication that the doctor orders must be measured in the same terms as the medication you have on hand. For example, if the physician orders a medication in milligrams and you have doses measured in grams, you must convert milligrams to grams. To convert measures, see Table 20.3 or use the following easy steps:

- To convert grams to grains or grains to grams, you must learn that 1 g = 15 gr.
- To convert grams to grains, multiply the number of grams × 15. *Example:* 30 g × 15 = 450 gr
- To convert grains to grams, divide the number of grains by 15. *Example:* 450 gr ÷ 15 = 30 g
- To convert grams to milligrams, move the decimal three places to the right. *Example:* 1 g = 1,000 mg (1 g = 1,000 mg)
- To convert milligrams to grams, move the decimal three places to the left. *Example:* 1,000 mg = 1 g (1,000 mg = 1.000 g)

Table 20.3 Metric Dosage and Apothecary Equivalents

Liquid Measure		Weight	
Metric	**Approximate Apothecary Equivalents**	**Metric**	**Approximate Apothecary Equivalents**
1,000 mL	1 quart = 1 L	30 g	1 ounce
750 mL	1 1/2 pints	15 g	4 drams
500 mL	1 pint	10 g	2 1/2 drams
240 mL	8 fluidounces	7.5 g	2 drams
200 mL	7 fluidounces	6 g	90 grains
100 mL	3 1/2 fluidounces	5 g	75 grains
50 mL	1 3/4 fluidounces	3 g	45 grains
30 mL	1 fluidounce	2 g	30 grains (1/2 dram)
15 mL	4 fluidrams	1.5 g	22 grains
10 mL	2 1/2 fluidrams	1 g	15 grains
8 mL	2 fluidrams	0.75 g	12 grains
5 mL	1 1/4 fluidrams	0.6 g	10 grains
4 mL	1 fluidram	0.5 g	7 1/2 grains
3 mL	45 minims	0.4 g	6 grains
2 mL	30 minims	0.3 g	5 grains
1 mL	15 minims	0.25 g	4 grains
0.75 mL	12 minims	0.2 g	3 grains
0.6 mL	10 minims	0.15 g	2 1/2 grains
0.5 mL	8 minims	0.12 g	2 grains
0.3 mL	5 minims	0.1 g	1 1/2 grains
0.25 mL	4 minims	75 mg	1 1/4 grains
0.2 mL	3 minims	60 mg	1 grain
0.1 mL	1 1/2 minims	50 mg	3/4 grain

(continued)

Teaching Tips

- Review the primary roman numerals (I through X), and the rules for adding and subtracting them.
- Review the formula for calculating dosage.
- Review each step of the formula, reinforcing how to divide.
- Review Section 11.2, The Metric System, in Chapter 11, Medical Math, and Section 12.2, Measurements, in Chapter 12, Measurement and the Scientific Process, to help students remember how to calculate medical weights and measures.
- Explain the importance of metric and apothecary equivalents for accuracy and safety.
- Review the steps for converting milligrams, grams, and grains.
- Review Table 20.3 together as a class, spending enough time on it to be certain the students understand it.
- Explain the apothecary equivalents and how they are used.
- Explain that liquid measure and weight are the measurements usually used for calculating dosages.

Teaching Tips

- Point out the bottom of Table 20.3, which identifies measurement and equivalents for pouring medicines.
- Assign students to memorize the pouring equivalents.
- Explain why the equivalents are approximations.
- Review the following conversions:
  - Ounces (oz) to cubic centimeters (cc) or milliliters
  - Milliliters (mL) to ounces (oz)
  - Pounds (lb) to kilograms (kg)
  - Kilograms (kg) to pounds (lb)

Table 20.3 Metric Dosage and Apothecary Equivalents (continued)

Liquid Measure		Weight	
Metric	**Approximate Apothecary Equivalents**	**Metric**	**Approximate Apothecary Equivalents**
0.06 mL	1 minim	40 mg	2/3 grain
0.05 mL	3/4 minim	30 mg	1/2 grain
0.03 mL	1/2 minim	25 mg	3/8 grain
		20 mg	1/3 grain
		15 mg	1/4 grain
		12 mg	1/5 grain
		10 mg	1/6 grain
		8 mg	1/8 grain
		6 mg	1/10 grain
		5 mg	1/12 grain
		4 mg	1/15 grain
		3 mg	1/20 grain
		2 mg	1/30 grain
		1.5 mg	1/40 grain
		1.2 mg	1/50 grain
		1 mg	1/60 grain
		0.8 mg	1/80 grain
		0.6 mg	1/100 grain
		0.5 mg	1/120 grain
		0.4 mg	1/150 grain
		0.3 mg	1/200 grain
		0.25 mg	1/250 grain
		0.2 mg	1/300 grain
		0.15 mg	1/400 grain
		0.12 mg	1/500 grain
		0.1 mg	1/600 grain

Some measurements and equivalents* for pouring medicines (to be memorized):

04 mL (4–5 mL)	=	1 teaspoon	or	1 dram	or	60 drops (gtt)
01 mL	=	1/4 teaspoon	or	1/4 dram	or	15–16 drops (gtt)
02 mL	=	1/2 teaspoon	or	1/2 dram	or	30–32 drops (gtt)
15 mL	=	3 teaspoons	or	4 drams	or	1/2 ounce (oz)
30 mL	=	6 teaspoons	or	8 drams	or	1 ounce (oz)
1 tablespoon	=	3 teaspoons	or	15 mL	or	1/2 ounce (oz)
2 tablespoons	=	6 teaspoons	or	30 mL	or	1 ounce (oz)
6 fluidounces	=	1 teacupful	or	150–180 mL		
8 fluidounces	=	1 glassful	or	240–250 mL		
2 pints	=	1 quart	or	1,000 mL		
4 quarts	=	1 gallon	or	4,000 mL		

* These equivalents are approximate only. In practice, the cubic centimeter and the milliliter are equal. Actually, the cubic centimeter is less than the milliliter by 0.000028 cc.

738 Chapter 20 | Medical Assisting and Laboratory Skills

Review Chapter 11. This review will help you remember common medical weights and measures. Use the formulas in Chapter 11 to review and practice changing or converting the following:

- Ounces (oz) to cubic centimeters (cc) or milliliters
- Milliliters (mL) to ounces (oz)
- Pounds (lb) to kilograms (kg)
- Kilograms (kg) to pounds (lb)

Community

Volunteer to create a poster for a senior citizen's center that describes the parts of a prescription label. Part of the poster should be an enlargement of a standard prescription label from a local pharmacy, with each line identified and described.

Administering Medications

The safety and proper care of patients depends on your correct and careful handling of medications. To prevent mistakes and injury to the patient, always follow carefully the six "rights" of medication administration:

1. Right drug
2. Right dose
3. Right route of administration (**Figure 20.11**)
4. Right time
5. Right patient
6. Right documentation

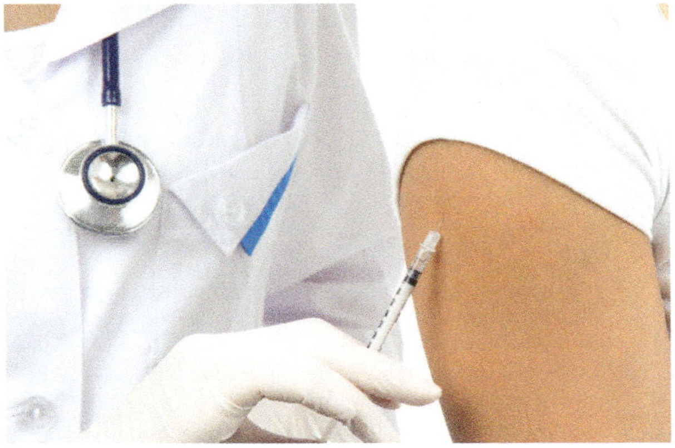

Figure 20.11
The safety and proper care of patients depends on your correct and careful handling of medications. Always confirm the six "rights" of medication administration.

Medical Assisting and Laboratory Skills | Chapter 20 739

Teaching Tips

- Review the six "rights" for administering medication:
  1. Right drug
  2. Right dose
  3. Right route of administration
  4. Right time
  5. Right patient
  6. Right documentation
- Reinforce the importance of following each step every time a medication is given, to prevent mistakes and injury to a patient.

Figure Focus

20.11 The safety and proper care of patients depends on your correct and careful handling of medications. Always confirm the six "rights" of medication administration.

Discuss with students why the six "rights" ensure that mistakes aren't made, such as giving the drug to the wrong patient, a wrong dose being used, or the drug being administered incorrectly.

ACTIVITY

Have students create a career ladder for job opportunities in a pharmacy. They should consult reference books, the Internet, or people who are currently employed in a pharmacy. Have students include job descriptions, educational requirements, and salary ranges.

Community

- You could divide the class into small groups for this activity, and have each group prepare a poster for a different senior center or care facility.
- Encourage students to use medications commonly taken by seniors as examples in the posters.
- Check the posters to be sure they include and identify the parts of the prescription accurately.
- Direct students to include additional information that the seniors might find helpful, such as the phone number of the closest pharmacy.
- Students might also want to include public service messages—such as messages that encourage seniors to ask questions about their medications or warn them to be aware of drug interactions—or list generic equivalents of brand name medications that might cost less.

Teaching Tips

- Review the guidelines for preparing and administering medications:
  1. Wash hands.
  2. Follow only written medication orders.
  3. Do not allow yourself to be distracted while preparing medication.
  4. Always read the medication label three times.
  5. Know the drug you are giving.
  6. Calculate the ordered dosage if necessary.
  7. Measure medications.
  8. Apply topical medications as directed.
  9. Never leave medication unattended.
  10. Never administer medication prepared by another person.
  11. Always verify the patient's name and the order on the chart.
  12. Check patient allergies before administering medication.
- Emphasize the need to read the label three times:
  - Taking from shelf
  - Measuring
  - Returning to shelf
- Emphasize that every guideline is important and must be followed.
- Emphasize the importance of using aseptic techniques and Standard Precautions as necessary.
- Discuss the importance of checking liquids before giving them.

Guidelines for Preparing and Administering Medications

1. Wash hands.
2. Follow only written medication orders.
3. Do not allow yourself to be distracted while preparing medication.
4. Always read the medication label three times:
   a. When taking it from the shelf (do not use medication that is not clearly labeled)
   b. Before measuring the ordered amount
   c. When returning the container to the shelf or discarding it
5. Know the drug you are giving. Look it up in one of the reference books to confirm the expected action, dosage, and route of administration. You need to know the side effects. For example, if the patient will have dry mouth, you might want to have hard candy available for them or make sure they had plenty of water to drink. Be sure to notify patients of any medications which may alter the color of their urine.
6. Calculate the ordered dosage if necessary. Verify calculations with a co-worker.
7. Measure medications.
   a. Measure solid medications such as pills, tablets, or capsules by dropping the medication from the package into a medicine cup.
   b. Observe liquid medications for:
      - Color change
      - Cloudiness
      - Sedimentation

      Note: If these conditions exist, discard the medication.
   c. Always have a second nurse verify order, dose, and measured medication in syringe when giving:
      - Insulin
      - Heparin
   d. Gently shake emulsions and suspensions to mix ingredients completely. Shaking distributes all of the ingredients equally. This allows you to give accurate amounts of all ingredients.
   e. When pouring liquids, place the label of the bottle in the palm of your hand to keep liquid from dripping on label.
   f. Pour the liquid into a medicine cup; hold at eye level to achieve an accurate measure.

740 Chapter 20 | Medical Assisting and Laboratory Skills

- Look for changes that might indicate a problem with the medication:
  - Color change
  - Cloudiness
  - Sedimentation
- Explain that there are different routes for administering medication.

ACTIVITY

Select 12 students. Have each write one of the twelve guidelines for preparing and administering medications on a large piece of paper, without including the number. Shuffle the papers and redistribute them to the same 12 students. Have them stand in front of the class displaying their papers. Have the other students arrange them into the correct order.

g. Clean the neck of the medication bottle before capping.
h. Never mix two or more medications unless ordered (check compatibility).

ALERT: Follow Standard Precautions.

8. Apply topical medications to the skin, mucous membrane (including vaginal creams and suppositories), or the cornea of the eye. Always follow the specific directions on the medication. Use aseptic technique to prevent contamination of medication.
9. Never leave medication unattended. Prepare medication and administer immediately. Watch the patient swallow oral medication.
10. Never administer medication prepared by another person.
11. Always verify the patient's name and the order on the chart to ensure that the right medication is given to the right patient.
12. Check patient allergies before administering medication. Look at allergies listed on patient's chart and ask patient if he or she is allergic to the medication.

Apply It

Form teams of two and play "Provide the Prescription." One person will suggest a prescription for a patient including the drug, dosage, and directions; the other will create the label for the prescription bottle. Then, change places and reverse the roles.

Table 20.4 Medication Administration Procedures

Administration Route	Type of Medication	Administration Procedure
Buccal	Tablets	Tablet placed between the gums and cheek of the mouth; absorbed as tablet dissolves
Inhalation	Medicated aerosols, mists, sprays, streams	Liquid medication inhaled through nebulizer, respirator, or inhalation device
Irrigation	Solutions	Solution washed through a body cavity or over a membrane
Installation	Solutions	Medication dropped into area requiring treatment, such as ear or eye
Injunction or topical	Liniments, lotions, ointments, powders, solutions, sprays, tinctures	Medication applied to skin (use gloves to apply)
Oral	Capsules, pills, solutions, spansules, tablets	Medication taken by mouth and swallowed
Parenteral	Sterile solutions	Medicated solution injected into body tissue and absorbed
Rectal	Suppositories, solutions	Medicated solution or suppository inserted into rectum
Sublingual	Tablets	Tablet placed under the tongue to dissolve
Vaginal	Creams, foams, liquids, ointments,	Medication applied, inserted, or irrigated (douche)

Teaching Tips

- Review Table 20.4 together as a class.
- Explain the table as follows:
  - The left column identifies the administration route, such as orally (taken by mouth) or parenteral (injection).
  - The middle column describes the form the medication is usually in when delivered via the specified route.
  - The right column describes the administration procedure.

Apply It

- Note that this activity is for pairs.
- Have the first student act as the physician, writing a prescription.
- Have the second student act as the pharmacist, creating the label for the prescription container.
- You might want to provide the illness or condition to be treated, and then verify that the prescription is correct.

ACTIVITY

Give students a list of different medications. Have them create a table or chart identifying the usual delivery route and administration procedure for each medication in the list.

Personal Wellness—Health Risks

- Review the information covered in Chapter 17, Controlling Infection, which describes the types of infections that might be transmitted in a health care facility.
- Review Standard Precautions, Transmission-Based Precautions, and Universal Precautions.
- Review aseptic techniques that help control the spread of infection.
- Point out that this feature is focusing on a health information technician's risk level.
- Discuss the types of health care workers who might be at greater or lesser risk of infection.
- Emphasize the most basic and effective method of preventing infection: proper handwashing techniques.

How does your health affect the health of patients? How can you protect them?

Answer: Whenever you are sick, you bring pathogens and the risk of infection to patients you come in contact with. You can protect patients by staying healthy yourself, by managing rather than ignoring signs of illness, and staying home if you have a contagious illness that can infect patients.

Personal Wellness

Health Risks

As a health information technician, your contact with patients will be casual. You will be talking to them, getting and giving information, but you will have little if any more physical contact. Nonetheless, anyone working in a health care environment is at some risk of infection. So how much at risk of infection are you and what can you do to reduce your risk?

Hepatitis B Virus (HBV) is one of the most serious infections. It is typically spread through sexual contact, by sharing needles among drug users, and by accidental needle sticks, which represent the greatest risk to health care workers. HBV cannot be contracted by casual contact with infected patients. Check with your supervisor. You may be entitled to an inoculation against HBV at no cost.

Human immunodeficiency virus (HIV) is primarily transmitted by sexual contact and intravenous drug use. It is not transmitted by casual contact, through contaminated food or water, or through the air.

Influenza is a common illness that often brings patients into the medical facility. To protect yourself from infection and to avoid spreading the flu to other patients, you should consider getting an annual flu vaccination. Check with your supervisor about the provider's policy.

The health information technician may be exposed to other microorganisms that can be spread through casual contact in the medical facility. The best precaution against infection is to regularly and frequently wash your hands. Keep your hands away from your mouth. If you develop any signs or symptoms of illness, report them immediately.

How does your health affect the health of patients? How can you protect them?

Summary

Medical assistants are responsible for working and administering medicines, so they must be knowledgeable about the legal issues associated with dispensing and administering medicines. In addition, medical assistants need to know how to handle and store prescriptions and convert dosages.

Section 20.2 Review Questions

1. Which agency monitors the federal guidelines for regulating the manufacturing, distribution, dispensing, and sales of medications?
2. What do the following prescription abbreviations mean: IV, dil, OU, OS, OD?
3. List two controlled substances in each of the five schedules (groups).
4. What types of information does the *Physician's Desk Reference* (PDR) contain?
5. List ways to ensure the safekeeping of medications.
6. Why are health care workers at risk for contracting the Hepatitis B Virus (HBV)?

742 Chapter 20 | Medical Assisting and Laboratory Skills

Teaching Tips

- Review the responsibilities of a medical assistant regarding the handling, storage, and administration of medications.
- Review the schedule levels used to monitor controlled substances.
- Review the most common drug reference books and how they are used.
- Review methods of storing and handling medications.
- Review the formula used for calculating medication dosage.
- Review the six rights of medication administration.
- Review the guidelines for preparing and administering medications.

Section 20.2 Review Questions

1. Answer: Drug Enforcement Agency (DEA) of the Department of Justice
2. Answer:
   - IV Intravenous
   - dil dilute
   - OU both eyes
   - OS left eye
   - OD right eye
3. Answers will vary. Refer to Table 20.2.
4. Answer:
   - Manufacturers' Index (White Pages)
   - Brand and Generic Name Index (Pink Pages)
   - Generic Brand/Cross-Reference Table
   - Product Category Index (Blue Pages)
   - Key to Controlled Substances Schedule
   - Key to FDA Use-in-Pregnancy Ratings
   - U.S. Food and Drug Administration Telephone Directory
   - Poison Antidotes
   - Drugs Excreted in Breast Milk

Laboratory Skills

SECTION 20.3

Background

Laboratory assistants are responsible for understanding laboratory guidelines and safety procedures. They also need to gather and test specimens, such as blood and urine, and ensure that appropriate quality controls are in place in the laboratory.

Objectives

When you have completed this section, you will be able to do the following:

- Match key terms with their correct meanings.
- Follow general laboratory guidelines.
- Practice laboratory safety.
- Demonstrate loading and operating an autoclave.
- List the types of specimen studies.
- Identify general rules for testing specimen.
- Discuss quality control in the laboratory.
- Label a diagram of a microscope.
- Identify steps to acquire a midstream clean-catch urine specimen for male and female.
- Identify items learned from a CBC.
- Explain why a hematocrit and hemoglobin test are important.
- Explain the importance of counting WBCs and RBCs.

Responsibilities of Laboratory Assistants/ Medical Assistants

Laboratory assistants/medical assistants run tests that assist in diagnosing an illness or disease. Some of the tests performed by laboratory assistants/medical assistants are highly technical. Their duties include the following:

- Cleaning laboratory equipment (**Figure 20.12**)
- Preparing cleaning solutions
- Drying glassware and instruments using a cloth, hot air dryer, or acetone bath
- Examining clean equipment for cracks or chips
- Operating an autoclave to sterilize equipment
- Preparing stains, solutions, and culture media
- Counting blood cells
- Separating plasma from whole blood using a centrifuge
- Incubating cultures
- Using computerized test equipment to test blood specimens

Medical Assisting and Laboratory Skills | Chapter 20 743

- Product Identification Guide
- Healthcare Provider Resource Center
- Product Information
- Dietary Supplements
- Drugs That Should Not Be Used in Pregnancy
- Drugs That Should Not Be Crushed

5. Answer:
   - Keep medications in a locked area away from other supplies.
   - Keep medications in original containers.
   - Refrigerate medications that require storage at lower than room temperatures.
   - Rotate medications so that the oldest are used before expiration dates.
   - Destroy expired medications.
   - Keep medications requiring darkness out of the light (in a dark cupboard or container).
   - Be aware of medications that react with other materials.
6. Answer: HBV can be spread by needles, so accidental needlesticks put health care workers at risk.

FOCUS AND ENGAGE

Introduce the Section

a. Review the content of the Background paragraph, explaining the responsibilities of a laboratory assistant.
b. Emphasize the importance of following laboratory guidelines and safety procedures.
c. Review the objectives for the section.

Vocabulary Review

a. Direct students to the key terms.
b. Pronounce each word, and have the students repeat the pronunciation out loud.
c. Discuss the definition of each word.

TEACH

Discuss

- Discuss the laboratory environment.
- If possible display pictures and/or articles depicting lab workers.
- Students may be able to relate to the environment, equipment, and materials used in science class labs.

Reinforce and Review

- Review specimen collection (Section 18.3).
- Reinforce the use of aseptic techniques (Section 17.1).

Teaching Tips

- Explain that laboratory assistants frequently run highly technical tests that help diagnose an illness or disease.

ACTIVITY

Make a list of different medical tests you have undergone during your lifetime. Include information about how the test was performed, and what the test was hoping to determine.

Figure Focus

Figure 20.12 Why is it important that all laboratory equipment is clean and sterile?

Answer: If the equipment isn't cleaned properly, the test results may not be accurate.

Teaching Tips

- Review the responsibilities of a laboratory assistant.
- Emphasize the importance of laboratory tests:
  - A valuable diagnostic tool
  - Monitoring blood level of medication
  - Measuring chemical balance
- Emphasize the importance of laboratory standards:
  - Uniformity
  - Accuracy
  - Improved outcomes
- Explain the Clinical Laboratory Improvement Amendment of 1988 (https://www.cms.gov/Regulations-and-Guidance/Legislation/CLIA/index.html): Sets standards and regulates laboratories, physicians' offices, and other labs that use human specimens.
- Explain that the CLIA monitors quality control by sending tests to labs for reading and then comparing the results against their own readings.
- Discuss the types of simple tests allowed in a small lab or medical office.

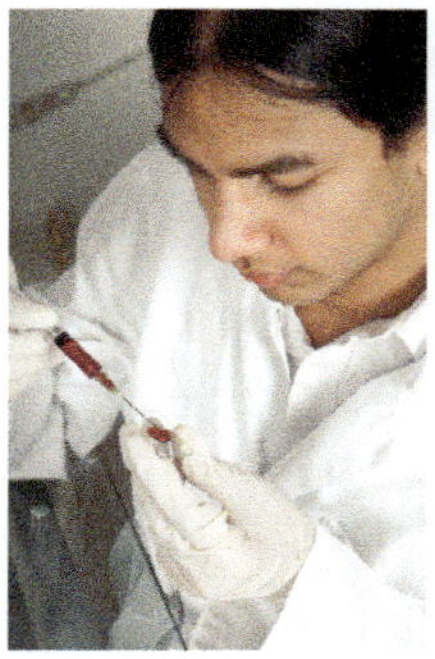

Figure 20.12
Why is it important that all laboratory equipment is clean and sterile?

- Performing venipuncture with a Vacutainer® and/or a needle and syringe
- Monitoring control tests
- Performing laboratory tests on stool, urine, blood, and sputum
- Preparing specimens for processing
- Giving patients instructions for specimen collection or self-testing

Importance of Laboratory Tests

Laboratory tests are important because they are:

- A valuable diagnostic tool
- Used to monitor the amount of medication a patient has in his or her system (therapeutic drug level)
- A measure of the body's chemical balance that compares blood and urine samples with normal test values
- A way to use blood and urine tests to diagnose a certain disease or condition

CLIA (see below) periodically sends tests to labs for reading. Tests are returned to CLIA to confirm the laboratory's readings. This is CLIA's quality control on laboratories.

Laboratory Standards

Medical laboratories and medical offices that perform lab tests on human specimens are regulated by a federal amendment called the Clinical Laboratory Improvement Amendment of 1988 (or CLIA). CLIA sets standards and regulates all laboratories, physicians' offices, and other labs that use human specimens to diagnose, prevent, or treat disease.

As a laboratory assistant/medical assistant you can perform simple tests allowed by CLIA. The lab or medical office must have a CLIA waiver certificate before you perform these tests. The tests include the following:

- Dipstick or tablet reagent urinalysis for bilirubin, glucose, hemoglobin, ketone, leukocytes, nitrite, pH, protein, urobilinogen, specific gravity.
- Ovulation tests: visual color test to tell if human luteinizing hormone is present.
- Urine pregnancy tests: visual color comparison test.
- Erythrocyte sedimentation rate (nonautomated).
- Hemoglobin copper sulfate (nonautomated).
- Fecal occult blood.
- Spun microhematocrit.
- Blood glucose by glucose monitoring devices cleared by the Food and Drug Administration for home use.

744 Chapter 20 | Medical Assisting and Laboratory Skills

- Emphasize that a student may not perform these steps unless the lab or medical office has a CLIA waiver certificate.
- Emphasize the importance of proper training before performing these tests.

ACTIVITY

Have students review and practice proper procedures of measuring using droppers, pipettes, flasks, and specimen cups. Have them record their observations and results.

Do not perform these tests unless you know that there is a waiver certificate and you have been trained properly.

Operating a laboratory with **uniformity** and maintaining standards of measure quality are important. People who work in the laboratory must follow the same guidelines that all laboratory workers follow. These guidelines are as follows:

uniformity
(yoo nuh FAWR mi tee)
A state of being all the same; does not vary.

- Clean and cover microscope daily according to manufacturer's guidelines.
- Maintain all infection control logs.
- Report all defective equipment immediately to your supervisor.
- Maintain and observe quality control logs.
- Follow all directions to ensure accurate results from each test:
  - Refrigerate promptly
  - Transport specimens in racks
  - Follow instructions when watching for serum separation
  - Instruct patients in proper collection of all specimens
  - Use appropriate technique with all specimen collections
- Check temperatures of appliances daily.
- Learn new techniques for testing new material or equipment changes.
- Check expiration dates of all reagents and testing kits weekly.
- Do quality control checks on all testing materials and equipment following manufacturer's directions and CLIA standards.
- Ask the supervisor for help when in doubt regarding any procedure or result.
- Recognize the importance of correct and accurate test results for doctors.
- Report all "stats" immediately.

The medical laboratory is an environment with hazards. The laboratory assistant/medical assistant or anyone working with laboratory tests must be aware of possible dangers. In the laboratory, you work with patient specimens that must be treated as **hazardous** materials. You also work with various chemicals that can react when mixed together. Some of these chemicals are harmful to the skin, eyes, and/or the respiratory system. To be safe in the laboratory:

hazardous
(HAZ er duhs)
Dangerous.

- Learn safety measures and follow them carefully.
- Always follow Standard Precautions.

General Safety Practice Guidelines: Personal Safety

The protective equipment you wear includes the following:

- A nonpermeable lab coat to protect your clothes
- Safety eye goggles/glasses to guard your eyes from splashes
- Gloves to keep you from being contaminated by infectious material
- A rubber apron to protect you from **acids** that can spill or splash
- Metal tongs when working with hot objects

acids
(as ids)
Substances that cause the urine to have an acid pH.

Medical Assisting and Laboratory Skills | Chapter 20 745

Teaching Tips

- Review guidelines for all laboratory workers:
  - Clean and cover microscope daily
  - Maintain infection control logs
  - Report defective equipment
  - Maintain and observe quality control logs
  - Follow directions
  - Check temperatures of appliances daily
  - Learn new techniques
  - Check expiration dates
  - Do quality control checks
  - Ask for help when in doubt
  - Recognize the importance of correct and accurate test results
  - Report all "stats" immediately
- Discuss safety hazards present in labs.
- Emphasize the use of Standard Precautions.
- Review protective equipment.
- Review additional safety considerations.

ACTIVITY

Make a poster about one safety hazard that might be encountered in a testing lab, including information about proper protective measures for that hazard.

Teaching Tips

- Emphasize the importance of fire prevention.
- Review fire prevention responsibilities:
  - Locate the fire extinguisher
  - Participate in fire drills
  - Report all potential electrical hazards to the supervisor immediately
  - Use grounded plugs for equipment
- Review additional safety practice guidelines.

Science Link—Acids and Bases

- Differentiate between acids and bases.
- Explain the pH scale, which is used to identify acids and bases:
  - Ranges from 0 to 14.0
  - A pH measurement between 0 and 7.0 indicates an acid
  - A pH measurement between 7.0 and 14.0 indicates a base
  - A pH measurement of 7.0 is a neutral solution.

How can you describe human blood plasma with a pH of 7.4 in terms of acids and bases?

Answer: Human blood with a pH measurement of 7.4 should be described as a weak base or slightly basic.

Other safety considerations are as follows:

- Never use your mouth to pipette.
- Do not eat, drink, or apply makeup in the laboratory area.
- Flush eyes first, then report eye contamination immediately to supervisor for eye treatment.
- Dispose of all broken glass, needles, or other sharp objects in a sharps container.
- Do not bend, break, or recap needles.
- Follow Standard Precautions and consider all specimens as highly infectious.
- Disinfect counters, surfaces, and equipment daily.

Fire Prevention

- Locate the fire extinguisher.
- Participate in fire drills.
- Report all potential electrical hazards to the supervisor immediately.
- Use grounded plugs for equipment.

Additional Safety Practice Guidelines

reagents
(re a jents)
Chemical substances that react to the presence of other substances in the blood and urine.

- Clearly label and date all **reagents**.
- Label all waste containers with a biohazard symbol.
- Complete incident reports. These are used to report any unusual or dangerous occurrences—for example, an accident, an injury, a hazardous spill or fire—to supervising personnel.

Science Link

Acids and Bases

Some substances break up into parts called ions when added to water. An ion is an atom that has lost or gained negatively charged electrons. If the ions produced by a compound in solution are hydrogen ions (H+), the compound is an acid. If the ions are hydroxide ions (OH-), the compound is a base.

The pH scale is used to measure the concentration of H+ ions in solution. The pH scale spans from 0 to 14. If there is a high concentration of H+ ions, the solution is very acidic and the pH value is low. Solutions with pH values lower than 7.0 are acids.

If there is a high concentration of OH- ions, the concentration of H+ ions must be low and the pH value is high. Solutions with pH values higher than 7.0 are bases. A solution with a pH value of 7.0 is neither an acid nor a base: It is a neutral solution.

How can you describe human blood plasma with a pH of 7.4 in terms of acids and bases?

If the body were at pH neutrality (equilibrium) how would it affect your sense of wellbeing?

What might be the results of a pH value of 6.8 or 8.0?

746 Chapter 20 | Medical Assisting and Laboratory Skills

CUSTOMIZED INSTRUCTION

More Advanced Students

Provide pH testing kits to more advanced students and ask them to test various substances. They should create a table or chart depicting the results and present their findings to the class.

- Keep trash from building up in any area.
- Keep all posters and decorations away from lights and vents.
- Inspect areas where heating elements are used for possible fire hazards.
- Keep spills wiped up and use a disinfectant when necessary.
- Discard any rag with a flammable substance on it in a metal container with a self-closing lid.

Sterilization

You must sterilize all items in the laboratory that have contact with body tissue or fluids. The most effective way to sterilize equipment is in an autoclave. (Figure 20.13) The autoclave produces steam under pressure. The high heat of the steam kills organisms that cause disease. Keep items that you are sterilizing in the autoclave for the specified length of time to ensure that all microorganisms are killed.

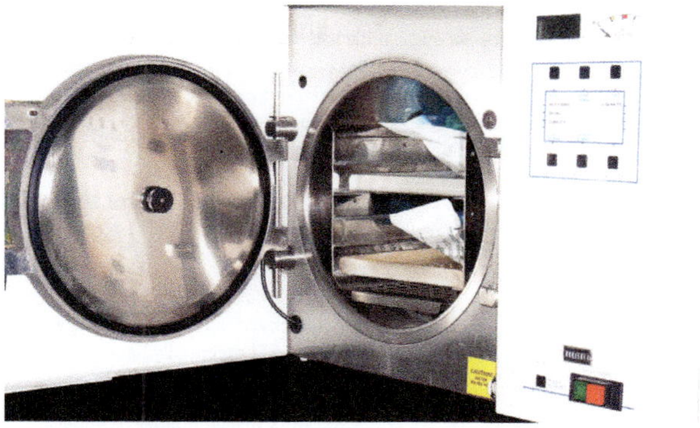

Figure 20.13
Autoclave. Why is an autoclave used in a laboratory?

CAUTION: The autoclave is a heavy piece of equipment with a chamber that withstands high degrees of temperature and a great deal of pressure. Steam under pressure can burn skin, hair, and eyes. Always follow these basic rules when operating an autoclave:

1. Read the directions for the autoclave you are using.
2. Use protective gloves when placing articles in an autoclave or taking them out.
3. In order to maintain sterility of surgical instruments, use sterilization wraps. Current popular wrapping products use a layered design consisting of three thermally bonded layers, which provide strength and a barrier to microbial contaminations. To further minimize contamination, many hospitals double wrap instruments.

Teaching Tips

- Emphasize the importance of sterilization of equipment.
- Review the Standard Precautions.
- Review aseptic techniques.
- Review the methods of sterilization:
  - Steam
  - Gas
  - Chemical
  - Safety precautions to prevent burns
- Review the basic rules for operating an autoclave.
- Emphasize the types of items that should never be placed in an autoclave: Any item that you cannot reuse.
- Emphasize the importance of disposing of hazardous waste properly:
  - Body tissue
  - Body fluid
  - Any item that has been in contact with body tissue or body fluid

Figure Focus

20.13 Autoclave. Why is an autoclave used in a laboratory?

Answer: An autoclave is used to sterilize any items that have come in contact with body tissues or fluids.

Teaching Tips

- Explain the purpose of the OSHA safety guidelines.
- Explain the use of material safety data sheets (MSDS).
- Describe contaminated/hazardous waste: Articles that have contacted blood, body fluids, or body tissue.
- Emphasize the importance of Standard Precautions.
- Review the importance of disposing of contaminated/hazardous waste in specially designated containers—not in the regular trash.
- Describe biohazardous waste containers.
- Review proper handling of biohazardous waste.
- Review the most common types of specimens used in testing:
  - Urine
  - Blood
  - Sputum
  - Stool
- Review the importance of lab tests:
  - Diagnose illness
  - Determine cause of illness
  - Confirm diagnosis
  - Evaluate progress
  - Regulate treatment
  - Establish a baseline for future tests

Figure Focus

20.14 Handle all contaminated/hazardous materials according to OSHA guidelines. Why are these guidelines so important?

Discuss with students reasons why these guidelines are so important.

4. Protect yourself if the autoclave is hot from recent use.
5. Do not overload. If you pack material into the autoclave too tightly, the steam cannot circulate and the items will not be sterilized.
6. Allow the temperature and pressure to return to normal before opening the autoclave when sterilization is complete.
7. Clean the autoclave according to the manufacturer's directions.

Items that you cannot reuse are not sterilized. Never put body tissue, body fluid, or any article that has been in contact with blood, body fluids, or tissues in the regular trash. Dispose of them in a biohazard container following your facility's policies. All health care workers have the responsibility to protect themselves and others.

The increased concerns over hazardous and/or toxic materials in all areas of work create the need for strict guidelines to protect people. The federal Occupational Safety and Health Administration (OSHA) provides guidelines to help ensure safety. Your laboratory supervisor will have these guidelines in a notebook with material safety data sheets. The MSDS forms follow OSHA guidelines by explaining how to dispose of and handle hazardous materials safely. The sheets also describe possible physical symptoms of overexposure and proper first-aid treatment if exposed. Ingredients of the hazardous product are also identified on MSDS forms. It is important to follow the general guidelines above and check the MSDS for specific information on each substance.

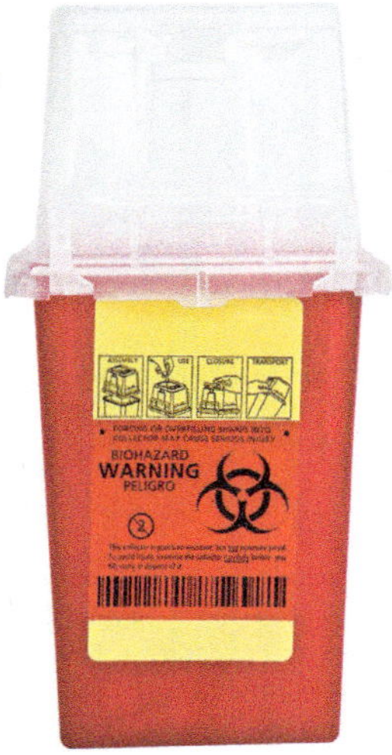

Figure 20.14
Handle all contaminated/hazardous materials according to OSHA guidelines. Why are these guidelines so important?

Contaminated/Hazardous Material

Specimens being analyzed in the laboratory come from patients. The physician often does not know what is causing a patient's illness, so you must treat every specimen as though it is contaminated and potentially hazardous. *Always follow Standard Precautions.*

When you work in a laboratory or medical office, you must practice good aseptic technique at all times. The most important steps include washing your hands before and after each procedure. Always wear gloves when working with specimens.

Biohazardous Waste Containers

In the medical setting, you must dispose of all contaminated biohazardous materials in biohazardous waste containers. The laboratory containers are lined with red plastic. (Figure 20.14) Put all discarded contaminated/biohazardous materials in the red-lined containers marked "Biohazard."

748 Chapter 20 | Medical Assisting and Laboratory Skills

TEAMWORK

Divide the class into groups of three students. Have one student write down the name of a lab test that requires preparation. The second student then instructs the third student in the correct test preparation.

Empty all containers at the end of each shift or when full. Carefully tie the bag and be certain that it will stay closed. Mark the tied bag "Biohazardous." Reline the container with a new red bag. Place the marked bag in a red sealed container for pickup. Handle all contaminated/hazardous materials according to OSHA guidelines. Never mix them with ordinary trash.

Laboratory Tests

Laboratory workers are responsible for testing specimens. The most common specimens include urine, blood, sputum, and stool. The results of these tests provide information about the patient's health. This information helps:

- Diagnose the illness
- Determine the cause of the illness
- Confirm a diagnosis
- Evaluate progress
- Regulate treatment
- Establish a baseline for future tests

Guidelines for Laboratory Tests

When you receive a laboratory request, check it for all information. This information includes:

- Patient's name and address
- Patient's age and sex
- Name of test requested
- Time and date of collection
- Physician's name and address
- Method of collection
- Possible diagnosis
- Type and source of specimen
- Medications the patient is taking
- Stat or routine tests

Preparation of Patients

There are many different kinds of laboratory tests. Some of the tests require very specific preparation. The results of some tests are affected by medication, food, time of day, and type of activity. Know the advance preparation for each test. If you are not certain about preparation, look it up in the procedures manual. Instruct the patient to follow the preparation orders exactly. Advance preparation may include:

- **Fasting.** Eating before some tests changes the results of the test (e.g., fasting blood sugar [FBS], glucose tolerance test [GTT], SMA-12 profile). During fasting, patients must not eat or drink fluid (except water). They usually fast for 12 to 14 hours before the test.

Medical Assisting and Laboratory Skills | Chapter 20 749

Teaching Tips

- Explain the use of lab slips.
- Point out that there are different types of lab slips, but that they all must include the same information:
  - Patient's name and address
  - Patient's age and sex
  - Name of test requested
  - Time and date of collection
  - Physician's name and address
  - Method of collection
  - Possible diagnosis
  - Type and source of specimen
  - Medications the patient is taking
  - Stat or routine tests
- Discuss the importance of proper client preparation for completing the test and obtaining accurate results.
- Explain that incorrect preparation may result in the need to repeat a test.
- Review types of client preparation:
  - Fasting
  - Medication restriction
- Explain the different types of specimens and discuss each test.

TEAMWORK

Divide the class into groups of four or five students. Provide examples of lab slips to each group. Assign each group a specific test, or series of tests, and have them make up lab slips with all of the correct information. Exchange the slips with other groups for evaluation.

Teaching Tips

- Review the general rules to follow when testing a specimen.
- Emphasize accuracy in conducting each step in testing and in recording all information.
- Explain that most facilities have their own standard procedures that must be followed.
- Discuss the three methods for testing specimens:
  - Manual
  - Automatic equipment
  - Semi-automatic equipment
- Discuss quality control.
- Explain why quality control is important:
  - Uniformity
  - Accuracy
- Review common quality control methods:
  - Discarding outdated reagents
  - Following the procedure for exact testing
  - Routinely verifying that laboratory equipment is reading specimens accurately
  - Maintaining equipment by having it serviced routinely
  - Maintaining accurate logs

TEAMWORK

In small groups, have students plan and present skits that demonstrate problems that might arise from a lack of quality control in a testing laboratory.

- **Medication restriction.** Many medications can change the chemical and physical qualities of the specimen. The patient needs special instruction if taking medications that can change test results. Medication affects urine specimens more than it affects blood. If the patient can be off the medication without causing injury, the medication is stopped 48 to 72 hours before the tests. The physician makes this decision.

Analyzing Specimens

There are many different studies that help identify and diagnose physical problems:

- **Urinalysis.** Examines urine chemically, physically, and microscopically.
- **Hematology.** Examines blood for disease conditions.
- **Microbiology.** Identifies pathogens in the body.
- **Histology.** Studies body tissues microscopically to detect diseased tissues.
- **Cytology.** Examines cells microscopically to discover abnormal cells.
- **Clinical chemistry.** Examines substances in body fluids, feces, tissues.
- **Serology and blood banking.** Studies antigen-antibody reactions to discover presence of foreign substance or disease.
- **Parasitology.** Determines parasite that is causing illness.

General Rules for Testing the Specimen

There are basic steps to follow for testing all specimens:

1. Measure the amount of specimen required for the test carefully. This is very specific.
2. Combine the correct chemical reagent for the test with the specimen.
3. Process the specimen correctly (e.g., centrifuge, heat in a water bath, incubate, heat fix, etc.).
4. Assess the sample by manual or automatic method.
5. Calculate results by hand or machine.
6. Record all the information on the lab report sheet, including:
   a. Patient's name
   b. Age and sex
   c. Time and date
   d. Source of specimen
   e. Name of test completed
   f. Results of test

Always follow the approved procedure in your facility.

Methods of Testing Specimens

The *manual method* requires carefully following a series of steps. Some small labs and physicians' offices use manual methods for simple tests (e.g., urinalysis).

750 Chapter 20 | Medical Assisting and Laboratory Skills

Semiautomated analysis is a combination of manual and automated testing (e.g., glucose monitor). To perform a glucose test, you stick the finger to get blood. The glucose monitor measures the glucose in the blood.

Automatic analyzers can do more than one specimen at a time. These analyzers measure the specimen, add reagent, process the specimen, and give the results.

Quality Control for Specimen Testing

There must be a method for quality control when performing laboratory tests. Performing these test controls tells you that the test is accurate. Quality control helps ensure that the test result is a true picture of the patient's condition. Some tests have the control built in. When the information is reliable, the physician can make a diagnosis. Quality control methods include:

- Discarding outdated reagents
- Following the procedure for exact testing
- Routinely verifying that lab equipment is reading specimens accurately
- Maintaining equipment by having it serviced routinely

Quality control includes keeping accurate logs. The log includes important information about the test (e.g., expiration date, lot number, date tested, and pass/fail of control). You must initial each test in the log.

Figure 20.15
Microscope. What is the purpose of using a microscope in the laboratory?

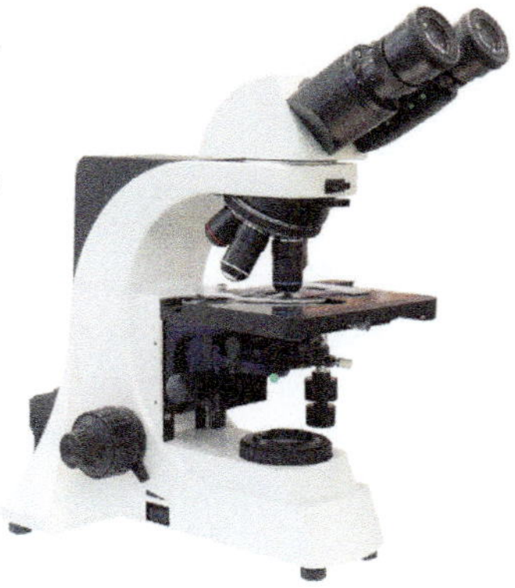

Laboratory Equipment

There are many kinds of laboratory equipment. The simple microscope and centrifuge are found in all laboratories. Some equipment is more complicated than others; for example, some labs use very advanced computers and analyzers.

Microscope

The microscope is an important tool that magnifies and enlarges objects. (**Figure 20.15**) You use it to see microorganisms and other components that are too small to see without magnification. The ability to see these components helps find the cause of illnesses. Learning to use the microscope is necessary for laboratory workers.

How to Use a Microscope

There are different types of microscopes. Some microscopes have one eyepiece. These are **monocular** microscopes. Microscopes with two eyepieces are **biocular.**

monocular
(muh NOK yuh ler)
Having one eyepiece.

binocular
(buh NOK yuh ler)
Having two eyepieces.

Basic Parts of the Microscope

- **Base.** Supports the microscope; it keeps the microscope from falling over.
- **Arm.** Supports the eyepiece and is used to carry the microscope.
- **Stage.** Holds slides that are put on the stage after you prepare them.

Medical Assisting and Laboratory Skills | Chapter 20 **751**

Teaching Tips

- Discuss some of the equipment commonly found in a laboratory.
- Explain that every lab worker must be able to use a microscope.
- Explain magnification, and how it is multiplied by increasing power.
- Differentiate between monocular and binocular microscopes.
- Review the basic parts of a microscope:
  - Base
  - Arm
  - Stage
  - Slide clips
  - Iris diaphragm
  - Mirror or illumination light
  - Eyepiece
  - Objectives
  - Body tube
  - Revolving nosepiece

Figure Focus

20.15 Microscope. What is the purpose of using a microscope in the laboratory?

Answer: A microscope is used to magnify or enlarge small objects. A microscope might be used to study the microorganisms or pathogens responsible for a disease or illness.

ACTIVITY

Have students make a poster or diagram of a microscope, labeling each part correctly.

Teaching Tips

- Explain the formula for determining how many times the specimen is magnified: Power of eyepiece multiplied by the power of the objective equals the total magnification.
- Explain the difference between coarse adjustment and fine adjustment:
  - Coarse adjustment: Upper knob on the arm, which moves the objectives up and down. This helps you put the specimen in rough focus.
  - Fine adjustment: Lower, smaller knob, which moves the objective more slowly. This helps you have a clear image of the specimen.
- Emphasize the importance of proper labeling and documentation of the test.
- Review the steps for taking care of the microscope:
  - Use special lens paper to clean the eyepiece.
  - Watch the objectives when you move them up and down.
  - Cover the microscope when you are not using it.
  - Keep the microscope in a safe place where it cannot be knocked to the floor.

- **Slide clips.** Hold the prepared slide in place.
- **Iris diaphragm.** Adjusts the amount of light that enters the microscope through the opening in the stage.
- **Mirror or illumination light.** Provides light so that you can see the object on the slide. You control the amount of light with the iris diaphragm. When you use a mirror, you turn the mirror to pick up a light source and *reflect* it into the microscope.
- **Eyepiece.** Lets you see the object on the slide. Some microscopes have eyepieces that magnify to 10 times (10×), others to 20 times (20×).
- **Objectives.** Magnify what you have on the slide. Most microscopes have three objectives. The most common objectives are:
  - High-power objectives that magnify the objects 40 times (40×).
  - Medium-power objectives that magnify the object 10 times (10×).
  - Low-power objectives that magnify 4 times (4×).
  - Oil immersion objective magnifies 95× to 100×. You put a drop of oil on a specimen that is dark and hard to see. The oil concentrates the light and makes the specimen easier to see.
- **Body tube.** Connects the eyepiece to the objectives, which are on the revolving nosepiece.
- **Revolving nosepiece.** The objectives are attached to the revolving nosepiece. You turn it to place the objective over the specimen.

How to Determine Total Magnification of the Specimen

Specimens are very small samples. It is important to know how many times the specimen is magnified. To determine how many times the specimen is magnified, multiply the power of the eyepiece by the power of the objective. For example:

Power of eyepiece 10×

Power of objective 4×

$10 \times 4 = 40$

This means that the specimen is enlarged 40 times its actual size.

NOTE: Always remember to record patient's name, account number, date, time, physician's name, type of test, and results of test. Always sign with your name and certification.

There are both a coarse adjustment and a fine adjustment on the microscope:

- **Coarse adjustment.** Upper knob on the arm, which moves the objectives up and down. This helps you put the specimen in rough focus.
- **Fine adjustment.** Lower, smaller knob, which moves the objective more slowly. This helps you have a clear image of the specimen.

CAUTION: Turning the adjustments too quickly can cause the glass slide to break. Turn each knob slowly. Begin with the coarse adjustment and then focus the image with the fine adjustment.

752 Chapter 20 | Medical Assisting and Laboratory Skills

CUSTOMIZED INSTRUCTION

Special Needs Students

You may be able to obtain equipment such as microscopes that are customized for use by special needs students.

Procedure 20.21	Using a Microscope

BACKGROUND: Proper care and use of the microscope prevents errors.
ALERT: Follow Standard Precautions

Preprocedure

1. Assemble equipment:
   a. Microscope
   b. Lens paper
   c. Slides and slide cover
   d. Specimen
   e. Oil if using oil immersion
   f. Gloves if specimens have been contaminated by blood or body fluids
2. Wash hands.
3. Place specimen (e.g., hair, scraping from under nails, scraping from tooth) on clean slide (one drop only if liquid specimen).
4. Add required solution.
5. Drop clean slide cover over specimen. Hold cover at an angle and let it drop. Make sure there are no air bubbles between the slide and cover slip. If there are bubbles, must do again.
6. Clean eyepiece with lens paper.
7. Clean objectives with lens paper.
8. Turn on illuminating light.
9. Open iris diaphragm.
10. Turn revolving nosepiece to low-power objective.

Procedure

11. Place slide on stage under slide clips. Avoid getting finger prints on the slide.
12. Turn coarse adjustment knob to move objective close to slide. Do not look into eyepieces while doing this, as you could crack the slide.
13. Look into eyepiece and slowly turn coarse adjustment to move tube upward until you focus specimen.
14. Turn fine-adjustment knob until specimen is clear and focused.
15. Continue steps 12 through 14 using the fine adjustment until you have best possible focus for specimen.
16. Observe specimen. If setup is for technician or physician, tell that person that slide is ready.

Postprocedure

17. Remove slide after it is read.
18. Discard slide according to procedure in your facility.
19. Clean lens and objective with lens paper.
20. Turn off illuminating light.
21. Put cover back on microsope
22. Wash hands
23. Fill out lab slips according to your facility's policies.

Medical Assisting and Laboratory Skills | Chapter 20 753

PROCEDURE PRACTICE

- Demonstrate the steps for Procedure 20.21, Using a Microscope, as many times as necessary, or ask students to demonstrate the steps. Provide samples of prepared slides for students to look at, such as hair, fingernail scrapings, water, etc. Have students practice and perform the procedure until they are competent.

Procedure Tip

20.21 Using a Microscope

- Review the background information, emphasizing the importance of preventing errors in order to achieve accurate test results.
- Emphasize the importance of following Standard Precautions.
- Review the preprocedure steps.
- Step 1: Review the equipment list.
- Step 2: Emphasize the importance of proper handwashing.
- Steps 3 and 5: Review proper slide preparation.
- Step 4: Discuss the solutions which might be used.
- Steps 6 and 7: Emphasize the importance of using lens paper.
- Review the procedure steps.
- Step 11: Explain the use of proper handling of slide to avoid fingerprints.
- Step 12: Emphasize the importance of moving the objective closer to slide while not looking through microscope, to avoid cracking the slide.
- Step 16: Emphasize the use of proper communication techniques.
- Review the postprocedure steps.
- Step 22: Emphasize importance of handwashing.
- Step 23: Review responsibilities for observation and reporting.

Teaching Tips

- Explain the purpose of routine urinalysis.
- Discuss guidelines for urine collection:
  - Clean, dry container
  - Collect on-site for immediate testing
  - Refrigerate specimen if necessary to hold for two hours or more
- Describe reagent strips.
- Review the guidelines for using reagent strips:
  - Check for expiration date.
  - Keep bottle in a cool, dry area with the top tightly closed. (Do not refrigerate.)
  - Do not use strips if they have changed color.
  - Use a clean-catch specimen for determining leukocytes.
  - Use a first urine in the morning specimen for determining nitrates.
  - Match colors on strips to the color chart on the label. Follow the times on the label carefully.
  - Write the type of strips used when recording the type of test.
- Explain importance of urinary sediment:
  - Epithelial cells
  - Casts
  - Miscellaneous structures

The microscope must be taken care of. Remember to:

- Use special lens paper to clean the eyepiece, or you will scratch the lens.
- Watch the objectives when you move them up and down. This prevents damaging the objectives or breaking the slide.
- Cover the microscope when you are not using it. This keeps out dust.
- Keep the microscope in a safe place where it cannot be knocked to the floor.

Urinalysis

A routine urinalysis provides information about the patient. The urinalysis gives the physician information about the physical, chemical, and microscopic characteristics of the urine. This information tells many different things about the patient's health: Is a woman pregnant? Is a urinary tract infection present? Does the urine show high levels of protein, which could be an indicator of kidney disease?

Urine Collection

Proper urine collection is important. The way you collect the urine affects the test. The following are some general guidelines for urine collection:

- Use a clean, dry container.
- A specimen over 32 hours old may give inaccurate test results.
- Refrigerate the specimen and write the collection time on the label if it is necessary to keep a specimen over two hours.
- If possible, collect on-site for immediate testing.

Reagent Strips

Your facility may use reagent strips and/or other individual tests. Always follow the procedures of your facility.

Reagent strips have small pads that react to a specific substance. When you dip the strip in a fresh urine sample, there is a chemical reaction. Carefully match the reagent strip with the color chart on the container label. The procedure for using all reagent strips is similar.

Guidelines for Using Reagent Strips

- Check the bottle for an expiration date.
- Keep the bottle in a cool, dry area with the top tightly closed. (Do not refrigerate.)
- Check the strips for a change in color. A tan-to-brown color change indicates deterioration. Do not use the strips.
- Keep the specimen container clean.
- Use freshly voided urine. Urine over 2 hours old gives poor results. Refrigerate if it stands more than 2 hours.

754 Chapter 20 | Medical Assisting and Laboratory Skills

TEAMWORK

Divide the class into groups of four or five students. Hand out jars of reagent strips. Have each team examine the jar and write down important information, such as the type of strip, the expiration date, and whether the strips appear to be in good condition. Have them note the times that should be used with the strips, and what the colors indicate.

- A clean-catch urine is best for determining leukocytes.
- First urine in the morning is best for determining nitrates.
- Match colors on strips to the color chart on the label. Follow the times on the label carefully.
- Write the type of strips used when recording the type of test.

Microscopic Examination of the Urine

Urinary sediment contains the solid materials in the urine. There are many components in the sediment that help the **provider** confirm or determine a diagnosis. The sediment may contain renal or kidney cells, casts, crystals, bacteria, parasites, mucus, or other substances. The sediment settles to the bottom of a centrifuged urine specimen. A small sample of the sediment is placed on a slide for the provider to look at. The provider looks for a cause of illness (e.g., bacteria causing a bladder infection, renal cells indicating renal damage, or red blood cells from irritation). Spinning urine (centrifuging) may be one of your duties.

provider
(pruh VAHY der)
Physician, physician assistant, nurse practitioner.

Procedure 20.22 Using Reagent Strips to Test Urine

BACKGROUND: Careful testing with reagent strips and accurate reporting of information are essential to reach a correct diagnosis. Always use the proper techniques to prevent contamination of the specimen.
ALERT: Follow Standard Precautions

Preprocedure

1. Wash hands.
2. Assemble equipment:
   a. Reagent strips and bottle
   b. Laboratory report slip
   c. Watch
   d. Urine specimen
   e. Disposable nonsterile gloves
3. Complete laboratory slip:
   a. Name
   b. Sex
   c. Age
   d. Physician
   e. Date
   f. Type of test
4. Put on gloves.

Procedure

5. Hold specimen to light and observe:
   a. Color (colorless, yellow, light yellow, brown, orange, etc.)
   b. Clarity (clear, hazy, cloudy)
6. Write color and clarity on lab slip.
7. Open reagent jar and remove one strip:
   a. Note expiration date. *Do not use if expired.*
   b. Replace jar cover immediately.
8. Hold strip by clear end and immerse in urine.
9. Remove strip immediately by pulling gently over lip of tube to remove excess urine.
10. Hold strip in horizontal position to prevent mixing of chemicals.
11. Hold strip close to color blocks on bottle label and match carefully. Note time.

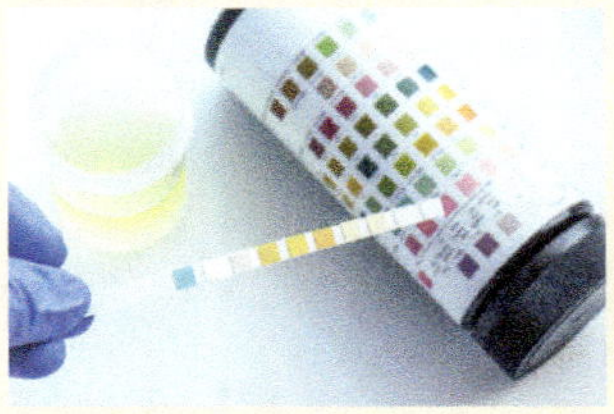

12. Read strip at time indicated and record results.
13. Discard reagent strip in biohazard waste.

(continued)

Medical Assisting and Laboratory Skills | Chapter 20 755

Procedure Tip

20.22 Using Reagent Strips to Test Urine

- Review the background information, emphasizing the importance of preventing contamination.
- Emphasize the importance of following Standard Precautions.
- Review the preprocedure steps.
- Step 1: Emphasize the importance of proper handwashing.
- Step 2: Review the equipment list.
- Step 3: Review the information that must be included on the lab slip.
- Step 4: Emphasize the importance of wearing gloves.
- Review the procedure steps.
- Step 5: Review the importance of observing the specimen.
- Step 6: Review the procedure for recording observations.
- Step 8: Review methods of identifying top and bottom of strip.
- Step 10: Emphasize importance of holding strip in proper position.
- Step 11: Review methods of matching color.
- Step 12: Review the procedure for recording the results.
- Step 13: Emphasize importance of disposing strip in biohazardous waste container.

Procedure Tip

20.22 Using Reagent Strips to Test Urine, continued

- Review the postprocedure steps.
- Step 14: Emphasize importance of properly cleaning equipment.
- Step 16: Emphasize importance of handwashing.
- Steps 17 and 18: Review responsibilities for observation and reporting.

PROCEDURE PRACTICE

- Demonstrate the steps for Procedure 20.22, Using Reagent Strips to Test Urine, as many times as necessary, or ask students to demonstrate the steps. Provide reagent strips so students can test samples of their own urine. Have students practice and perform the procedure until they are competent.

Teaching Tips

- Describe specific gravity: Identifies the dilution of urine.
- Review the methods of measuring specific gravity.
- Explain the normal range of specific gravity of urine: 1.010 to 1.025
- Review abnormal readings:
    - High specific gravity: Above 1.025; may be caused by dehydration, diabetes mellitus, kidney disease.
    - Low specific gravity: Below 1.010; may be caused by diabetes insipidus, diuretic medications, kidney disease.
- Explain how a urine test for a pregnancy test works.
- Review guidelines for performing an accurate pregnancy test.

Procedure 20.22 Using Reagent Strips to Test Urine (continued)

Postprocedure

14. Clean and replace equipment.
15. Remove gloves.
16. Wash hands.
17. Record required information.
18. Report any abnormal results to supervisor immediately.

Charting Example:

1/03/24	*0700*
	Reagent strip test, pH 7,
	Protein: Pos., Glucose: 1%, Ketones: Tr.,
	Blood: Neg. Positive protein and
	trace blood reported to health care
	provider
	G. Jones Lab Asst.

Special Urine Tests

Measuring Specific Gravity

You can measure specific gravity on a reagent stick. The urinometer is another simple way to check specific gravity. Specific gravity gives the dilution of urine. The normal range for specific gravity of urine is 1.010 to 1.025. An abnormal reading that is not within the range indicates possible problems. High specific gravity is above 1.025. Concentrated (heavy) urine may be caused by dehydration, sugar in the urine from diabetes mellitus, and too many substances in the urine due to kidney disease. Low specific gravity is below 1.010. Diluted urine may be caused by diabetes insipidus, diuretic medications, and kidney disease when unable to concentrate the urine. Specific gravity can also be measured with a refractometer.

Pregnancy Tests

A common test for determining pregnancy is a simple urine test. The test is performed on a concentrated urine specimen. The urine is tested for a hormone called human chorionic gonadotropin (HCG). This hormone is produced by the developing fertilized egg. Some of the hormone is secreted into the urine and blood. It is very important to read the manufacturer's instructions carefully before completing a pregnancy test.

To perform an accurate pregnancy test, follow these guidelines:

- Use clean urine containers to collect urine.
- Use the first voided morning specimen for the highest accumulation of HCG.
- Check the specific gravity. If it is less than 1.010, the urine is too diluted.

756 Chapter 20 | Medical Assisting and Laboratory Skills

ACTIVITY

Provide the results of five different specific gravity tests. Have students identify the results as high, low, or normal, and explain the implications of the results.

- Have the urine specimen at room temperature.
- Follow the manufacturer's instructions for storing the reagents.
- Do not use reagents after the expiration date.
- Do not contaminate the specimen.

Procedure 20.23 Measuring Specific Gravity with Urinometer

BACKGROUND: Careful testing of specific gravity and accurate reporting of information are essential to reach a correct diagnosis. Always use proper techniques to prevent contamination of the specimen.
ALERT: Follow Standard Precautions

Preprocedure

1. Wash hands.
2. Assemble equipment:
   a. Disposable gloves
   b. Glass cylinder (5 inches high)
   c. Urinometer (this is a float with a stem that is calibrated in thousands: 1.000, 1.001, 1.002, etc.)
   d. Fresh urine specimen; do not refrigerate
3. Put on gloves.

Procedure

4. Pour urine into cylinder to about one inch from the top.
5. Place urinometer in urine.
6. Spin urinometer gently. You must not touch side or bottom.
7. Place cylinder with lower line of meniscus at eye level.

NOTE: In glass containers, which curve at the edges, the curvature is called the meniscus. You measure the level at the horizontal center or inside part of the meniscus.

With water in glass, the meniscus will curve up at the edges and down in the center so we say you read the bottom of the meniscus.

8. Read specific gravity:
   a. Look at point where lowest part of meniscus crosses urinometer scale.
   b. Read gauge on nearest line.
9. Record reading to enter in computer or on lab slip.
10. Discard urine according to facility's contaminated waste policy.
11. Rinse urinometer with water and dry.
12. Rinse cylinder with water and dry.
13. Remove gloves and discard in contaminated waste.

Postprocedure

14. Wash hands.
15. Record specific gravity in computer or on lab list.
16. Document according to facility procedure.

Charting Example:

1/01/24 0800
Sp Gr 1.011
S. Jones MA

Procedure Tip

20.23 Measuring Specific Gravity with Urinometer

- Review the background information, describing a urinometer.
- Emphasize the importance of following Standard Precautions.
- Review the preprocedure steps.
- Step 1: Emphasize the importance of proper handwashing.
- Step 2: Review the equipment list.
- Step 3: Emphasize the importance of wearing gloves.
- Review the procedure steps.
- Step 6: Review method of spinning urinometer correctly.
- Step 7: Review the importance of viewing at eye level.
- Step 8: Review method of reading gauge correctly.
- Step 9: Review the procedure for recording the results.
- Steps 10 and 13: Emphasize importance of using biohazardous waste container.
- Review the postprocedure steps.
- Step 14: Emphasize importance of handwashing.
- Steps 15 and 16: Review responsibilities for observation and reporting.

PROCEDURE PRACTICE

- Demonstrate the steps for Procedure 20.23, Measuring Specific Gravity with Urinometer, as many times as necessary, or ask students to demonstrate the steps. If possible, have students test samples of their own urine. Have students practice and perform the procedure until they are competent.

Procedure Tip

20.24 Measuring Specific Gravity with Refractometer

- Review the background information.
- Emphasize the importance of following Standard Precautions.
- Review the preprocedure steps.
- Step 1: Emphasize the importance of proper handwashing.
- Step 2: Review the equipment list.
- Step 3: Emphasize the importance of wearing gloves.
- Review the procedure steps.
- Steps 4–6: Explain method of calibrating refractometer.
- Step 9: Review method of reading measurement correctly.
- Step 10: Review the procedure for recording the results.
- Step 11: Emphasize importance of using biohazardous waste containers.
- Review the postprocedure steps.
- Step 12: Reinforce importance of cleaning equipment properly.
- Step 14: Emphasize importance of handwashing.
- Step 15: Review responsibilities for observation and reporting.

PROCEDURE PRACTICE

- Demonstrate the steps for Procedure 20.24, Measuring Specific Gravity with Refractometer, as many times as necessary, or ask students to demonstrate the steps. If possible, have students test samples of their own urine. Have students practice and perform the procedure until they are competent.

Procedure 20.24 Measuring Specific Gravity with Refractometer

BACKGROUND: Careful testing of specific gravity and accurate reporting of information are essential to reach a correct diagnosis. Always use proper techniques to prevent contamination of the specimen.
ALERT: Follow Standard Precautions

Preprocedure

1. Wash hands.
2. Assemble equipment:
   a. Disposable gloves
   b. Refractometer
   c. Distilled water
   d. Fresh urine sample; do not refrigerate
   e. Will need eye dropper or pipette to get drop of water and/or urine
3. Put on gloves.

Procedure

4. Place one drop of distilled water on the glass plate.
5. Close lid.
6. Look through eyepiece to read specific gravity.

Note: Make sure it reads 1.000. If reading is not 1.000, follow manufacturer's directions to recalibrate refractometer.

7. Transfer one drop of well-mixed urine onto glass plate of refractometer.
8. Close lid.
9. Look through eyepiece to read specific gravity.
10. Record reading to enter in computer or on lab slip.
11. Discard urine according to facility's contaminated waste policy.

Postprocedure

12. Clean refractometer according to manufacturer's directions.
13. Remove gloves and discard in contaminated waste.
14. Wash hands.
15. Record specific gravity in computer or on lab list.

Charting Example:

10/10/24	0800
	Sp. gravity 1.040, reported to lab tech
	S. Jones Lab Asst.

Career Connect

Complete a job shadow experience at a local pharmacy. Determine the different career opportunities available, the services each provides, and the preparation and licensure required for each.

Testing Urine for Drugs

The collection of urine to determine drug use is becoming more and more common. Some reasons for drug testing:

- Employer requests a preemployment test
- Department of Transportation requires testing of pilots, truck drivers, and others
- Employer requests test for employee suspected of using drugs

There are many strict rules that you *must* adhere to when you collect urine for drug testing. Follow the instructions and proceed step by step. *Be very exact.*

758 Chapter 20 | Medical Assisting and Laboratory Skills

Career Connect

- If you are unable to arrange a pharmacy job shadow, students may be able to interview a pharmacy worker on the phone or by e-mail.
- Allow class time to discuss the experience.

Teaching Tips

- Explain that drug testing has many monitored steps to ensure proper handling.
- Review reasons for drug testing.

Clean-Catch Collection

Clean-catch midstream urine collection has a specific procedure. The physician may order a clean-catch urine when he or she suspects that a urinary infection is present or for any urine test. The clean-catch method reduces possible contamination of the specimen. Clean the area around the meatus carefully to remove microorganisms.

Collect the urine in a sterile cup using medical aseptic techniques. Pour off part of the specimen for the dipstick test and for spinning down when you collect a clean-catch urine. This leaves the urine in the specimen container uncontaminated. If necessary, you can use it for culture and sensitivity testing.

There are other urine specimen tests that may be ordered. Your facility will have a procedure manual with instructions for each test that your lab performs. Follow the instructions for collection carefully.

Procedure 20.25 Centrifuging a Urine Specimen

BACKGROUND: Careful centrifuging ensures that urine is properly concentrated for testing. Specimens must be properly prepared in order to achieve accurate results.
ALERT: Follow Standard Precautions

Preprocedure

1. Wash hands.
2. Assemble equipment:
   a. Centrifuge
   b. Two centrifuge tubes
   c. Microscope slide (number slide)
   d. Coverslip
   e. Pipette
   f. Disposable nonsterile gloves
   g. Urine specimen; it's best to use the first voiding in AM, as it is more concentrated
3. Fill in lab slip:
   a. Name
   b. Date
   c. Time
4. Put on gloves.

Procedure

5. Mix urine to suspend sediment by rolling specimen container gently between your hands.
6. Pour 10 mL of urine into centrifuge tube.
7. Put tube with urine into centrifuge.

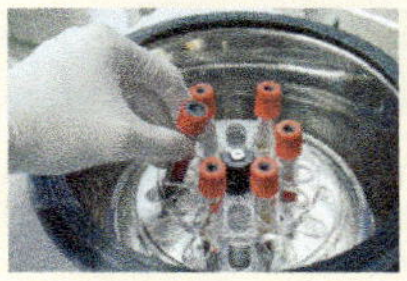

8. Pour 10 mL of water into second centrifuge tube.
9. Place in centrifuge opposite the tube with urine. This is very important for balance.
10. Secure centrifuge lid.
11. Set centrifuge timer for 4 to 5 minutes. (Allow it to stop on its own.)
12. Remove tube with urine.
13. Carefully invert urine centrifuge tube quickly over sink to pour 9 mL of urine into sink.
14. Turn tube right side up immediately. (About 1.0 cc will remain in tube.)
15. Mix sediment by snapping end of centrifuge tube with finger or gently shaking.

(continued)

Teaching Tips

- Explain clean-catch urine collection: Reduces possibility of contamination by bacteria.
- Emphasize reasons for ordering a clean-catch specimen:
  - Possibility of urinary tract infection
  - Maintain integrity of specimen for testing
- Review methods of ensuring clean-catch specimen.

Procedure Tip

20.25 Centrifuging a Urine Specimen

- Review the background information, explaining the purpose of centrifuging.
- Emphasize the importance of following Standard Precautions.
- Review the preprocedure steps.
- Step 1: Emphasize the importance of proper handwashing.
- Step 2: Review the equipment list.
- Step 3: Review the proper procedure for filling out lab slip.
- Step 4: Emphasize the importance of wearing gloves.
- Review the procedure steps.
- Steps 6 and 8: Emphasize importance of measuring accurately.
- Step 9: Emphasize importance of proper positioning of tubes to balance centrifuge.

Procedure Tip

20.25 Centrifuging a Urine Specimen, continued

- Step 16: Review procedure for using pipette.
- Step 17: Remind students of importance of properly preparing slide.
- Step 19: Review method of focusing microscope.
- Step 21: Review method of reading slide correctly.
- Review the postprocedure steps.
- Step 27: Reinforce importance of cleaning equipment properly.
- Step 28: Emphasize importance of handwashing.
- Steps 29 and 30: Review responsibilities for observation and reporting.

PROCEDURE PRACTICE

- Demonstrate the steps for Procedure 20.25, Centrifuging a Urine Specimen, as many times as necessary, or ask students to demonstrate the steps. If possible, have students test samples of their own urine. (This requires a centrifuge and a microscope.) Have students practice and perform the procedure until they are competent.

Procedure 20.25 Centrifuging a Urine Specimen (continued)

Procedure (cont)

16. Pipette 1 drop of urine on numbered slide. A pipette works by creating a vacuum above the liquid-holding chamber and then selectively releasing this vacuum to draw up and dispense liquid.
17. Put on coverslip. (Redo if air bubbles appear under coverslip.)
18. Put slide on microscope stage.
19. Use 10× objective with coarse adjustment to focus on slide. Watch while moving course adjustment, so that slide does not break.
20. Adjust light source.
21. Follow your facility's policy for reading slide. (If setup is for technician, tell him or her that slide is ready.)
22. Remove slide after it is read.
23. Discard slide according to facility procedure.
24. Clean lens and objective with lens paper.
25. Cover microscope.

Postprocedure

26. Clean equipment and replace equipment.
27. Remove gloves, and dispose of according to facility policy.
28. Wash hands.
29. Record results if you read the specimen.
30. Document according to facility procedure.

Charting Example:

1/20/24	*0745*	
	Microscopic Exam: epithelial:	
	few/1pf. WBCs: 2-3, /hpf.	
	RBCs: few/hpf. casts: neg.,	
	crystals: few/hpf	
		B Smith MA

Procedure 20.26 Midstream Clean-Catch Urine, Female

BACKGROUND: Careful instruction of the patient helps prevent contaminating the specimen. A clean-catch specimen is essential to accurately diagnose and treat the patient.
ALERT: Follow Standard Precautions

Preprocedure

1. Wash hands.
2. Assemble equipment:
   a. Sterile urine container for clean catch
   b. Label
   c. Disposable antiseptic towelettes
   d. Disposable nonsterile gloves; wear if you handle cup with specimen

Procedure

3. Label container.
4. Instruct patient to:
   a. Wash hands.
   b. Remove container lid and place on counter with inside of lid facing up.
   c. Separate labia to expose meatus.
   d. Take towelette and wipe on side of urinary meatus from front to back.
   e. Dispose of towelette.
   f. Repeat with new towelette on other side.
   g. Wipe directly over meatus with new towelette.
   h. Continue to hold labia open.
   i. Urinate small amount into toilet.
   j. Stop stream.
   k. Place sterile container under meatus and void into container (60 cc).

(continued)

760 Chapter 20 | Medical Assisting and Laboratory Skills

Procedure Tip

20.26 Midstream Clean-Catch Urine, Female

- Review the background information, explaining the purpose of a clean-catch specimen.
- Emphasize the importance of following Standard Precautions.
- Review the preprocedure steps.
- Step 1: Emphasize the importance of proper handwashing.
- Step 2: Review the equipment list.
- Review the procedure steps.
- Step 3: Emphasize the proper labeling procedures.
- Step 4: Emphasize the importance of effective communication techniques. Provide students with the following additional steps or refer them to Procedure 19.77:
  - j. Stop stream.
  - k. Place sterile container under meatus and void into container (60 cc).
  - l. Stop stream.
  - m. Remove container carefully.
  - n. Empty bladder.
  - o. Carefully replace lid.
  - p. Wipe outside of container with paper towel.
  - q. Transport the specimen to the laboratory within 30 minutes of collection or else refrigerate.
- Step 5: Emphasize the importance of wearing gloves.

Procedure 20.26	Midstream Clean-Catch Urine, Female (continued)

l. Stop stream.
m. Remove container carefully.
n. Empty bladder.
o. Carefully replace lid.
p. Wipe outside of container with paper towel.
q. Transport the specimen to the laboratory within 30 minutes of collection or else refrigerate.

5. Put on gloves.
6. Finish testing as ordered (e.g., dipstick, set up microscopic exam, drug test).

Postprocedure

7. Document procedure according to facility procedure.
8. Wash hands.

Charting Example:

03/26/24 0800
Instructed in correct procedure
for collecting clean catch
S. Jones CNA

Procedure 20.27	Midstream Clean-Catch Urine, Male

BACKGROUND: Careful instruction of the patient helps prevent contaminating the specimen. A clean-catch specimen is essential to accurately diagnose and treat the patient.
ALERT: Follow Standard Precautions

Preprocedure

1. Wash hands.
2. Assemble equipment:
   a. Sterile container for clean catch
   b. Label
   c. Disposable antiseptic towelettes
   d. Disposable nonsterile gloves; wear if handling container with specimen.

Procedure

3. Label container.
4. Instruct patient to:
   a. Wash hands.
   b. Remove container lid and place on counter with inside of lid facing up.
   c. Cleanse head of penis in a circular motion with towelette. (If uncircumcised, pull back foreskin before cleaning.)
   d. Urinate into toilet. (If uncircumcised, pull back foreskin while urinating.)
   e. Allow stream to begin.
   f. Stop stream and place specimen container to collect midstream. (Fill about half way full or 60 mL.)
   g. Remove container before bladder is empty.
   h. Empty bladder into toilet.
   i. Carefully replace lid.
   j. Wipe outside of container with paper towel.
   k. Transport the specimen to the laboratory within 30 minutes of collection or else refrigerate.
5. Put on gloves.
6. Finish testing as ordered (e.g., dip stick, set up microscopic exam, drug test).

(continued)

Medical Assisting and Laboratory Skills | Chapter 20 761

Procedure Tip

20.26 Midstream Clean-Catch Urine, Female, continued

- Review the postprocedure steps.
- Step 7: Emphasize the importance of proper observation and documentation.
- Step 8: Emphasize the importance of proper handwashing.

PROCEDURE PRACTICE

- Review the steps for Procedure 20.26, Midstream Clean-Catch Urine, Female, as many times as necessary, or ask students to demonstrate the steps. If possible, have students practice by instructing a partner and then collecting their own samples. Have students practice and perform the procedure until they are competent.

Procedure Tip

20.27 Midstream Clean-Catch Urine, Male

- Review the background information, explaining the purpose of a clean-catch specimen.
- Emphasize the importance of following Standard Precautions.
- Review the preprocedure steps.
- Step 1: Emphasize the importance of proper handwashing.
- Step 2: Review the equipment list.
- Review the procedure steps.
- Step 3: Emphasize the proper labeling procedures.
- Step 4: Emphasize the importance of effective communication techniques.
- Step 5: Emphasize the importance of wearing gloves.
- Review the postprocedure steps.
- Step 7: Emphasize the importance of proper observation and documentation.
- Step 8: Emphasize the importance of proper handwashing.

PROCEDURE PRACTICE

- Review the steps for Procedure 20.27, Midstream Clean-Catch Urine, Male, as many times as necessary, or ask students to demonstrate the steps. If possible, have students practice by instructing a partner and then collecting their own samples. Have students practice and perform the procedure until they are competent.

Procedure Tip

20.28 Collecting Urine from an Infant

- Review the background information, explaining the importance of preventing contamination.
- Emphasize the importance of following Standard Precautions.
- Review the preprocedure steps.
- Step 1: Emphasize the importance of proper handwashing.
- Step 2: Review the equipment list.
- Steps 3–5: Emphasize the importance of effective communication techniques.
- Review the procedure steps.
- Step 6: Emphasize the importance of wearing gloves.
- Step 9: Review the bag and proper positioning.
- Step 12: Emphasize the importance of monitoring the infant regularly.
- Review the postprocedure steps.
- Step 17: Emphasize the proper labeling procedures.
- Step 18: Emphasize the importance of proper observation and documentation.
- Step 19: Emphasize the importance of proper handwashing.

PROCEDURE PRACTICE

- Review the steps for Procedure 20.28, Collecting Urine from an Infant, as many times as necessary, or ask students to demonstrate the steps. Have students practice the procedure using a doll, if possible. Have students practice the procedure until they are competent.

Procedure 20.27 Midstream Clean-Catch Urine, Male (continued)

Postprocedure

7. Document procedure according to facility procedure.
8. Wash hands.

Charting Example:

06/17/24 0800
Instructed in correct procedure
for collecting clean catch
S. Jones CNA

Procedure 20.28 Collecting Urine from an Infant

BACKGROUND: Using the proper technique prevents leakage around the bag and thus prevents contamination of the specimen.
ALERT: Follow Standard Precautions

Preprocedure

1. Wash hands.
2. Assemble equipment:
   a. Specimen container
   b. Disposable urine collector (small plastic bag with opening and sticky area)
   c. Disposable nonsterile gloves
3. Identify patient.
4. Explain to parents what you are going to do.
5. Tell child what you are going to do even if you think that he or she is too young to understand. Children often understand.

Procedure

6. Put on gloves.
7. Remove diaper.
8. Make certain that skin is clean and dry in genital area.
9. Remove outside cover that is around opening of bag. This has a sticky area that is applied to vulva or around penis. Place over vulva or penis.
10. Replace diaper.
11. Remove gloves and dispose of according to facility procedure.
12. Check every half hour to see if bag has urine in it.
13. Remove bag when specimen is collected.
14. Rinse, clean, and dry genital area.
15. Replace diaper.
16. Put specimen in specimen container for lab.

Postprocedure

17. Label with:
    a. Patient's name
    b. Time of collection
    c. Date
    d. Room number
18. Record collection of specimen.
19. Wash hands.

Charting Example:

10/25/24 1030
Urine bag applied
Specimen successfully collected
for testing
Sent to lab
H. Martinez CNA

762 Chapter 20 | Medical Assisting and Laboratory Skills

Laboratory Cultures

Physicians need a culture of the microorganism that is causing an illness. Knowing what organism is causing the problem helps with the diagnosis and the treatment. Microorganisms that cause strep throat, staph infections, and other illnesses can be treated when they are identified. You need to know how to:

- Obtain a specimen
- Place the specimen on the medium, where it can grow and reproduce
- Stain a sample of the culture

Take a specimen for the culture from the affected body sites. These sites include any skin lesion, such as an open, draining sore. Cultures are also taken from any body opening, such as eyes, ears, nose, throat, and vagina. You must be careful when you take a specimen for culturing. Poor technique may cause a false test result. You must use a sterile swab to secure the specimen and be careful not to contaminate the sample.

A specimen may be placed on a slide immediately. This is a direct smear. When the technician or doctor reads the smear, he or she can identify the organism. Prepare a direct smear slide following the procedure for using a microscope.

The physician may also request that the microorganism be grown on an *agar plate*. (**Figure 20.16**) The agar in the plate provides food and moisture. The organisms grow and multiply when you place the agar plate in a warm incubator, at 36° to 37° Celsius (97° to 99° Fahrenheit) for 24 to 36 hours.

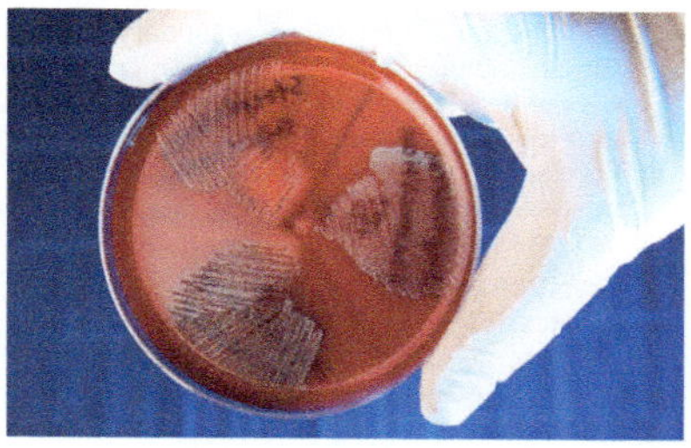

Figure 20.16
Why are bacteria grown on agar plates?

A common test is called a culture and sensitivity test. This test identifies the antibiotic that kills the organism. It also identifies the antibiotics to which the organisms are **resistant**. This information helps the physician decide which medication to prescribe. To do a culture and sensitivity test, place paper disks coated with antibiotic on an agar plate streaked with a specimen. If the organism is resistant to the antibiotic, it continues to grow around the disk. If the specimen is sensitive to the antibiotic, the colony around the disk dies. The physician then knows which antibiotic to prescribe for the patient.

resistant
(ri ZIS tuh nt)
Able to protect itself.

Gram Stain

Gram staining is a process that dyes and fixes microorganisms. The stain helps make the organism more visible in the microscope. It helps to identify the organism, thus allowing the doctors to chose the correct treatment. The slide can be kept and reviewed if necessary. To prepare a slide from colonies grown in an agar plate for staining, a small colony of organisms is taken from the agar plate. These organisms are placed on a slide and stained.

ACTIVITY

Have students make a table or chart comparing a direct smear with an agar plate culture.

Teaching Tips

- Explain the purpose of a laboratory culture.
- Discuss the common sites for laboratory cultures:
  - Blood
  - Body fluids
  - Ears
  - Eyes
  - Cerebrospinal fluid
  - Nasal passage
  - Sputum
  - Stool
  - Throat
  - Urine
  - Vagina or cervix
  - Wounds
- Display types of culture kits.
- Explain the importance of correctly collecting a culture in order to obtain accurate test results.
- Explain a direct smear: Specimen is collected using a sterile swab and placed on a microscope slide immediately.
- Explain the use of an agar plate:
  - Specimen is collected using a sterile swab and placed on an agar plate.
  - Plate is placed in a warm incubator so organism can grow and multiple.
- Explain a culture and sensitivity test.
- Explain a gram stain.

Figure Focus

20.16 Why are bacteria grown on agar plates?

Answer: The agar in the plate provides food and moisture.

What's New?—Rapid Medical Tests

- Discuss why it might be important to obtain results quickly:
  - Start treatment
  - Prevent the spread of illness
  - Limit secondary infections
  - Identify when an antibiotic is not warranted
- Review the rapid strep test procedure.
- Explain that a negative test does not guarantee that strep is not present.
- Discuss other types of rapid medical tests.
- Point out that many are available over-the-counter, and can be used at home without a physician's order.

What is one advantage and one disadvantage of a rapid strep test over a throat culture?

Answer: One advantage is that the rapid strep test is fast, which enables patients who test positive to start a course of antibiotics quickly. This prevents complications and further spread of the infection. One disadvantage is that the test is not as reliable as the throat culture and may produce false negative results. That is why if the test is negative, a throat culture should be obtained to verify that strep is not present.

Teaching Tips

- Introduce blood and blood testing.
- Reinforce guidelines:
  - When to use Standard Precautions
  - When to use Transmission-Based Precautions
  - When to use Universal Precautions

What's New?

Rapid Medical Tests

Years ago, it took days or even longer to obtain the results from common medical tests. Now, results are often produced within minutes. One of the most commonly used tests is the rapid strep test. This test is used to determine whether a patient has pharyngitis that is due to a group A *streptococcal* infection. A *streptococci* cause pharyngitis in 5–15 percent of adults and 15–30 percent of children.

It is important that strep infections be identified as quickly as possible and treated with antibiotics. Strep throat is contagious and can spread to close contacts, especially among children. In addition, if the infection is not treated, secondary complications including rheumatic fever (which can damage the heart) and glomerulonephritis (which affects the kidneys) can develop. At the same time, it is essential that patients are not prescribed antibiotics to treat the common viruses that can also cause sore throats.

A rapid strep test produces results in just 5–10 minutes. If the results are positive, further testing is not needed. The person carries the infection and a health care provider will most likely prescribe antibiotic therapy. However, if the rapid strep test is negative, a culture to grow the bacteria should be done to confirm the results. Up to one-third of negative rapid strep test results are false. This means that in up to one-third of the cases in which a rapid strep test produces negative results, the person actually has a strep throat infection. A throat culture is more accurate than the rapid strep test, but takes several days to produce results.

Because sensitivity reports can take several days to provide results, the patient will probably be on a broad-based antibiotic already. If the patient is receiving an antibiotic and the sensitivity report indicates that the identified bacteria is not sensitive to this particular antibiotic, the physician must be notified. The physician will want to prescribe an antibiotic to which the bacteria is sensitive.

Other rapid tests are becoming equally as common, and many of them are being sold for use in the home. These include pregnancy tests, ovulation kits, drug tests, as well as tests to identify certain medical conditions such as tuberculosis. As with the rapid strep tests, results are not always 100 percent reliable and should not only be repeated, but also interpreted by a qualified health care provider.

What is one advantage and one disadvantage of a rapid strep test over a throat culture?

Blood, Blood Composition, and Blood Testing

Components of Blood

Whole blood has many formed elements that are suspended in a clear yellow liquid called *plasma*. Plasma makes up 55 percent of the whole blood. The other 45 percent has the formed elements. These elements are:

- **Erythrocytes.** A cell that contains hemoglobin and can carry oxygen to the body. Also called a red blood cell (RBC).
- **Leukocytes.** White Blood Cells that help the body fight infections and other diseases.
- **Thrombocytes.** Platelets, which are crucial to normal blood clotting.

The average adult has six to eight quarts of blood.

764 Chapter 20 | Medical Assisting and Laboratory Skills

- Review the composition of blood and how each component affects the body:
  - Erythrocytes: Red blood cells carry oxygen to cells and carbon dioxide away from cells.
  - Leukocytes: White blood cells protect against infection and disease.
  - Thrombocytes: Platelets start the clotting process.

TEAMWORK

In groups of two or three, have students visit a retail store that sells do-it-yourself medical testing kits. Students should make a list of the types of kits that are available without a provider's prescription.

Personal Wellness

Triglycerides

It is important to understand the chemistry of blood. One important commonly measured quantity is the level of triglycerides, which are the chemical form of animal and vegetable fats. In the human body, these are carried through the blood plasma, and unused molecules are stored in the body as fat. Triglycerides are later released from fat tissue to meet the body's needs for energy between meals.

An excess of triglycerides in plasma is called hypertriglyceridemia. This condition is directly linked to coronary artery disease in some people. Like cholesterol, increases in triglyceride levels can be detected by plasma measurements. These measurements should be made after an overnight food and alcohol fast.

What can you do if you have high triglycerides? Changes in lifestyle habits may be the answer. You should consider the following:

- Cut down on calories to reach your ideal body weight.
- Reduce your dietary intake of saturated fat, trans fat, and cholesterol.
- Consume more fruits and vegetables.
- Reduce your intake of alcohol.
- Stop smoking if you do so.
- Get at least 30 minutes of physical activity each day.
- Substitute fish high in omega-3 fatty acids for high-fat meats.

Keep in mind that triglycerides do not only result from the consumption of fats, but also from the consumption of carbohydrates. Most carbohydrates are naturally turned into triglycerides by the body. Therefore, even if you follow a diet that is low in fat, but high in carbohydrates, you may still be increasing your triglyceride level.

In some cases, drugs may be required in addition to dietary management and exercise. People with high triglycerides should follow the specific plans prescribed by their health care providers.

Why shouldn't foods that result in the production of triglycerides be completely eliminated from the diet?

Blood Tests

Physicians order blood tests for routine checkups and to help diagnose an illness. There are many blood tests available. This chapter covers the blood tests that the physician orders frequently. (See **Table 20.5**, which gives you the important reasons for the tests you are doing.)

The laboratory most often uses capillary/peripheral blood and venous blood. You usually obtain capillary blood from the finger and sometimes from the earlobe. You use a heel stick for infants. The amount of blood is limited to a few drops. This is enough blood to do the following:

- Complete blood count (CBC)
- Hematocrit/microhematocrit
- Some bleeding and coagulation times
- Some chemical and **agglutination** tests

agglutination
(uh gloot n EY shuhn)
Clumping together (e.g., red blood cells clump together).

When you need a larger amount of blood, you draw venous blood from the veins with a Vacutainer or syringe and needle. Some states and schools do not allow students to perform blood tests. Your teacher will tell you what you can do. *Never* practice these tests without training.

Medical Assisting and Laboratory Skills | Chapter 20 765

CUSTOMIZED INSTRUCTION

More Advanced Students

Assign more advanced students the opportunity to learn more about triglycerides. Have them prepare a presentation, poster, or brochure to education others about the risks of high triglyceride levels and steps for keeping the levels low.

Personal Wellness—Triglycerides

- Explain triglycerides: The chemical form of animal and vegetable fats.
- Explain hypertriglyceridemia.
- Review methods of lowering triglyceride levels.

Why shouldn't foods that result in the production of triglycerides be completely eliminated from the diet?

Answer: The body needs triglycerides as a source of energy to conduction normal activities. A person would suffer from malnutrition if triglycerides were eliminated. Problems arise when there is an excess of triglycerides.

Teaching Tips

- Explain when physician's order blood tests, and why.
- Review the difference between peripheral or capillary blood and arterial blood:
  - Peripheral/capillary blood obtained from finger, earlobe, or heel. Only a few drops are necessary.
  - Arterial blood is drawn from a vein, usually in the inner arm, when a larger amount is required.
- Explain that a few drops of blood are enough for many tests, including:
  - Complete blood count
  - Hematocrit or microhematocrit
  - Some bleeding or coagulation tests
  - Some chemical and agglutination tests

Teaching Tips

- Emphasize that training is necessary before performing any blood tests.
- Discuss your school and state rules for students performing blood tests.
- Explain the components of a complete blood count:
  - RBC (red blood cell) count
  - WBC (white blood cell) count
  - Hemoglobin determination
  - Hematocrit determination
  - Differential white blood cell count
  - Estimate of the number of platelets
  - RBC morphology (size and shape)
- Explain a hematocrit/ microhematocrit test: Measures the volume of packed red blood cells in the blood.
- Explain a hemoglobin test: Measure the oxygen-carrying capacity of the blood.
- Review Table 20.5 together as a class.
- Explain the common blood tests.
- Review the abbreviations. Explain why the abbreviations are important (might be on the test order).
- Review the implications of high or low readings for each test.

Complete Blood Count

The laboratory worker performs many different types of blood tests. (**Table 20.5**) The most frequently ordered test is a complete blood count. The complete blood count (CBC) gives a lot of information about the patient's condition. It includes the following:

- RBC (red blood cell) count
- WBC (white blood cell) count
- Hemoglobin determination
- Hematocrit determination
- Differential white blood cell count
- Estimate of the number of platelets
- RBC morphology (size and shape)

Hematocrit/Microhematocrit

heparinized (HEP uh rin eyesd) Containing heparin, an anticoagulant.

polycythemia (pol e si theme a) Condition of having too much blood.

A hematocrit measures the volume of packed red blood cells in the blood. When you do this test you separate cell elements from the plasma. You perform this test with a few drops of capillary blood. Collect the blood in a **heparinized** capillary tube from a finger or earlobe stick for adults. In infants collect the blood from a heel stick. Centrifuge the blood to pack the cells. Low hematocrit readings tell the physician that there is a problem (e.g., anemia). High hematocrit readings provide important information (e.g., **polycythemia**).

Table 20.5 Common Blood Tests

			Examples of Possible Diagnosis	
Test	**Abbreviation**	**Normal Range**	**Increase**	**Decrease**
White blood cell count	WBC	5000–10,000 mm^3	Acute infection, leukemia, mononucleosis	Viral infections, bone marrow depression
Red blood cell count	RBC	Female: 4–5 million/mm^3 Male: 5–6 million/mm^3	Polycythemia, poisoning, pulmonary fibrosis	Anemia, multiple myeloma, lupus erythemia
Differential white blood cell count	Diff	Neutrophils 50–70%	*Neutrophilia:* acute bacterial infections, parasitic infections, liver disease	*Neutropenia:* acute viral infections, blood diseases, hormone diseases
		Eosinophils 1–4%	*Eosinophilia:* allergic conditions, parasitic infections, lung and bone cancer	*Eosinopenia:* infectious mononucleosis, congestive heart failure, aplastic, and pernicious anemia
		Basophils 0–1%	*Basophilia:* leukemia, hemolytic anemia, Hodgkin's disease	*Basopenia:* acute allergic reactions, hyperthyroidism, steroid therapy
		Lymphocytes 20–35%	*Lymphocytosis:* acute and chronic infections, carcinoma, hyperthyroidism	*Lymphopenia:* cardiac failure, Cushing's disease, Hodgkin's disease
		Monocytes 3–8%	*Monocytosis:* viral infections, bacterial and parasitic nfections, collagen diseases, cirrhosis	*Monocytopenia:* prednisolone treatment, hairy cell leukemia

(continued)

766 Chapter 20 | Medical Assisting and Laboratory Skills

ACTIVITY

Have students make a table or chart explaining what type of tests are included in a complete blood count. They should include information about why a complete blood count might be ordered, and what a provider might learn from it.

TEAMWORK

Divide the class into groups of three. Have one student act as the patient, describing symptoms of an illness or condition. Have the second student act as the provider, ordering tests necessary for diagnosis. Have the third student act as the laboratory assistant, preparing the test. As a group, have them write or present what they did and why.

Table 20.5 Common Blood Tests (continued)

			Examples of Possible Diagnosis	
Test	**Abbreviation**	**Normal Range**	**Increase**	**Decrease**
Hemoglobin	Hgb	Female: 12–16 g/100 mL Male: 14–18 g/100 mL	Congestive heart failure (CHF), chronic obstructive pulmonary disease(COPD), severe burn	Hodgkin's disease, hyperthyroidism, cirrhosis
Hematocrit/ microhematocrit	Hct, HCT	Female: 40–54% Male: 37–47%	Shock, dehydration, burns	Anemia, leukemia, acute blood loss
Prothrombin time	PT	11–16 sec	Anticoagulant therapy, liver disease, biliary obstruction	Diuretics, pulmonary embolism, multiple myeloma
Erythrocyte sedimentation rate	ESR	(According to method used)	Collagen disease, inflammatory disease, rheumatoid arthritis	Sickle cell anemia, CHF, polycythemia
Platelet count		200,000–400,000/mm^3	Cancer, leukemia, splenectomy	Bone-marrow-depressant drug, pneumonia infection

Hemoglobin

Hemoglobin (Hgb) tests measure the oxygen-carrying capacity of the blood. Hemoglobin has the *heme*, which carries iron, and *globin*, which is the protein in the red blood cell. Hemoglobin picks up oxygen in the lungs and transports it to the cells. It also helps carry waste product, CO_2, from the body cells back to the lungs. One way to measure hemoglobin is with a hemoglobinometer.

Summary

Laboratory assistants are responsible for understanding what laboratory tests are important and why, following laboratory guidelines, knowing how to test specimens, knowing how to use a microscope, and understanding blood and blood tests.

Section 20.3 Review Questions

1. What are the responsibilities of a laboratory assistant?
2. As a lab assistant, what kinds of protective equipment would you wear in a laboratory?
3. Why are laboratory tests important?
4. What are the four methods of quality control when testing specimens?
5. Describe the basic parts of the microscope?
6. What types of information does a complete blood count (CBC) provide?

Medical Assisting and Laboratory Skills | Chapter 20 767

Teaching Tips

- Review the responsibilities of a laboratory assistant.
- Review the general laboratory guidelines.
- Review laboratory safety rules and guidelines.
- Review the importance of using an autoclave to sterilize reusable equipment.
- Review the importance of properly disposing of biohazardous waste material.
- Review common types of specimen studies.
- Review the general rules for testing specimens.
- Review the importance of quality control in a laboratory, and ways in which quality control can be implemented.
- Review the parts of a microscope.
- Review the procedure for clean-catch urine specimen collection for both males and females.
- Review the types of common blood tests, and what information can be learned from each.
- Ask students if there are any objectives they feel they need to spend more time on, and then do so.

Section 20.3 Review Questions

1. Answer:
   - Cleaning laboratory equipment
   - Preparing cleaning solutions
   - Drying glassware and instruments using a cloth, hot air dryer, or acetone bath
   - Examining clean equipment for cracks or chips
   - Operating an autoclave to sterilize equipment
   - Preparing stains, solutions, and culture media
   - Counting blood cells
   - Separating plasma from whole blood using a centrifuge
   - Incubating cultures
   - Using computerized test equipment to test blood specimens
   - Performing venipuncture with a Vacutainer and/or a needle and syringe
   - Monitoring control tests
   - Performing laboratory tests on stool, urine, blood, and sputum
   - Preparing specimens for processing
   - Giving patients instructions for specimen collection or self-testing

ACTIVITY

Have students create a table comparing the skills and requirements of a medical assistant, a pharmacy technician, and a laboratory assistant.

CHAPTER 20 REVIEW

Chapter Review Questions

1. List four basic diagnostic techniques and their purpose. (20.1)
2. What type of information is gathered when completing a patient's medical history form? (20.1)
3. List the factors that determine which Standard Precautions employees should take to avoid infection? (20.1)
4. Describe the different examination positions. (20.1)
5. As a medical assistant, what would your responsibilities be in working with and administering medications? (20.2)
6. Explain each of the five schedules of controlled substances. (20.2)
7. What is the formula for dosage calculation? (20.2)
8. What are the six "rights" of medication administration? (20.2)
9. Which tests require a laboratory or medical office to have a CLIA waiver certificate before a lab assistant can perform the test? (20.3)
10. Why is it important to follow the rules when operating an autoclave? (20.3)
11. List the six general rules for testing specimens. (20.3)
12. How much blood does the average adult have in their body? (20.3)

Activities

1. Imagine that you are writing questions for a quiz show. Write ten questions that relate to Standard Precautions. After writing your questions, exchange them with your classmates to see how well you do.
2. Use the Internet or visit a local Biotechnology Lab and prepare a presentation or poster citing the steps in preparing a new drug for marketing, including the number and types of trials.
3. Create a checklist of hospital procedures for admission, transfer, and discharge. With a group of classmates, role play the health care staff as you move through these stages with a student pretending to be a patient.
4. Your friend is considering a career as a medical assistant, and she wants your advice. Write a letter to her identifying the basic skills required to be successful in this career.

Case Studies

1. Mr. Grey needs to be admitted to a hospital for a routine procedure and is a little nervous. He asks you to explain exactly what will occur when he is admitted, discharged, and transferred. What do you tell him?
2. A new coworker is a little unsure about collecting blood and urine specimens. What general safety practice guidelines can you tell her to follow?

768 Chapter 20 | Medical Assisting and Laboratory Skills

2. Answer:
   - A nonpermeable lab coat to protect your clothes
   - Safety eye goggles/glasses to guard your eyes from splashes
   - Gloves to keep you from being contaminated by infectious material
   - A rubber apron to protect you from acids that can spill or splash
   - Metal tongs when working with hot objects
3. Answer:
   - Diagnose the illness
   - Determine the cause of the illness
   - Confirm a diagnosis
   - Evaluate progress
   - Regulate treatment
   - Establish a baseline for future tests
4. Answer:
   - Discarding outdated reagents
   - Following the procedure for exact testing
   - Routinely verifying that laboratory equipment is reading specimens accurately
   - Maintaining equipment by having it serviced routinely
5. Answer:
   - Base: Supports the microscope; it keeps the microscope from falling over.
   - Arm: Supports the eyepiece and is used to carry the microscope.
   - Stage: Holds slides that are put on the stage after you prepare them.
   - Slide clips: Holds the prepared slide in place.
   - Iris diaphragm: Adjusts the amount of light that enters the microscope through the opening in the stage.
   - Mirror or illumination light: Provides light so that you can see the object on the slide. You control the amount of light with the iris diaphragm; when you use a mirror, you turn the mirror to pick up a light source and reflect it into the microscope.
   - Eyepiece: Lets you see the object on the slide. Some microscopes have eyepieces that magnify to 10 times (10×); others to 20 times (20×).
   - Objectives: Magnify what you have on the slide. Most microscopes have three objectives.
   - Body tube: Connects the eyepiece to the objectives, which are on the revolving nosepiece.
   - Revolving nosepiece: The objectives are attached to the revolving nosepiece. You turn it to place the objective over the specimen.
6. Answer:
   - RBC (red blood cell) count
   - WBC (white blood cell) count
   - Hemoglobin determination
   - Hematocrit determination
   - Differential white blood cell count
   - Estimate of the number of platelets
   - RBC morphology (size and shape)

CHAPTER 20 REVIEW

Thinking Critically

1. **Communication**—Create a poster explaining the "Safety First" procedures that health care professionals need to follow in the laboratory setting; for example, why you must wash your hands and use gloves.
2. **Patient Education**—A patient is complaining of a variety of flu-like symptoms. She is unhappy that the doctor isn't prescribing a series of medications to address each of the symptoms. Describe how you would explain to her about drug interactions.
3. **Computers**—Advances in medicine are continually changing the way health care workers protect themselves and treat infections. Explain how computers help keep the medical community informed about the latest medical progress. Describe ways you can access this information if you do not own a computer.

Portfolio Connection

Special abbreviations and symbols are used when working with medication. It's very important for health care workers to be able to easily identify these so as to eliminate any possibility of misinterpretation or errors in treatment.

Using the Internet, library, and other resources, create a comprehensive list of abbreviations and symbols used in pharmacology and medication administration. Use the list on p. 730 of some of the more common abbreviations as a guide. Place the list in the "Personal Tips and Reminders" section of your portfolio.

PORTFOLIO TIP

Create your list in a table in either your word processing or spreadsheet program. The table should have two columns: one for the abbreviation or symbol and the other for its meaning. Insert any symbols electronically or leave space for them and hand-draw them on a hard-copy printout of your list. Format the table so it is attractive and easy to read.

CHAPTER 20 REVIEW

Chapter Review Questions

1. Answer:
   - Observation/Inspection
   - Palpation
   - Percussion
   - Auscultation
2. Answer:
   - Patient's name, address, and phone number
   - Birth date, sex, marital status, Social Security number
   - Patient's employer name, address, and phone number
   - Insurance company's name, address, and phone number
   - Insured's employer name, address, and phone number
   - If the patient is a minor, name of the responsible party
3. Answer:
   - Is an infectious agent present?
   - Is there a susceptible host with a source of entry receptive to the agent?
   - Is there a mode of transmission for the agent?
   - Remember that all blood, bodily fluids, excretions (except sweat), secretions, and nonintact skin and mucous membranes may contain infectious agents. NOTE: Standard Precautions are referenced in this chapter. Students should recall this information from Chapter 17.
4. Answer:
   - Horizontal recumbent (supine) position: Use this position for examination, treatment, and surgical procedures of the ventral (anterior) part of the body (for example, for abdominal pain, removal of stitches in chest).
   - Fowler's position: This position relieves patients who are having trouble breathing (for example, asthma, chest pain). This position allows examination of the anterior and posterior chest (for example, listening to heart and lung sounds).

4. *(continued)*
   - Trendelenburg position: This position helps restore blood flow to the brain when the body experiences shock. This position also helps promote drainage of congested lungs.
   - Dorsal lithotomy position: Use this position to examine or perform surgical procedures on the peritoneal and rectal areas (for example, vaginal exam, cystoscopy).
   - Prone position: Use this position for examination, treatment, or surgical procedures of the dorsal (back) part of the body.
   - Left lateral position and left Sims position: Use this position for minor rectal examinations, enemas, and treatments.
   - Knee-chest position: Use this position for rectal examinations and surgical procedures. Some examination tables adjust to support the patient's abdomen and chest.
   - Jackknife: Use this position for inserting a tube into the urethra.
   - Dorsal recumbent: Use this position for the examination and treatment of the abdominal area and for vaginal or rectal exams.
5. Answer:
   - Administering medications
   - Being aware of side effects
   - Interpreting prescriptions
   - Reinforcing the provider's instructions
   - Recognizing adverse effects of medications
   - Reporting accurate observations
   - Using references to obtain directions

6. Answer:
   - Schedule I: These substances have no accepted medical use (except for the legal use of medical marijuana in some states) in the United States and have a high abuse level.
   - Schedule II: High abuse level with severe psychic or physical dependence liability.
   - Schedule III: Abuse potential is less than Schedule I or II and includes certain compounds containing limited quantities of certain narcotic drugs and non-narcotic drugs.
   - Schedule IV: Abuse potential less than in Schedule III.
   - Schedule V: Abuse potential less than IV; consists primarily of preparations containing limited quantities of certain narcotic and stimulant drugs generally for antitussive, antidiarrheal, and analgesic purposes.
7. Answer: $\frac{\text{dosage you want}}{\text{dosage you have}} = \text{dosage you give}$
8. Answer:
   - Right drug
   - Right dose
   - Right route of administration
   - Right time
   - Right patient
   - Right documentation
9. Answer:
   - Dipstick or tablet reagent urinalysis for bilirubin, glucose, hemoglobin, ketone, leukocytes, nitrite, pH, protein, urobilinogen, specific gravity
   - Ovulation tests: visual color test to tell if human luteinizing hormone is present
   - Urine pregnancy tests: visual color comparison test
   - Erythrocyte sedimentation rate (nonautomated)
   - Hemoglobin copper sulfate (nonautomated)
   - Fecal occult blood
   - Spun microhematocrit
   - Blood glucose by glucose monitoring devices cleared by the Food and Drug Administration for home use
10. Answer: The steam from the autoclave can burn skin, hair, and eyes.
11. Answer:
    - Measure the amount of specimen required for the test carefully. This is very specific.
    - Combine the correct chemical reagent for the test with the specimen.
    - Process the specimen correctly (e.g., centrifuge, heat in a water bath, incubate, heat fix, etc.).
    - Assess the sample by manual or automatic method.
    - Calculate results by hand or machine.
    - Record all the information on the lab report sheet, including:
      - Patient's name
      - Age and sex
      - Time and date
      - Source of specimen
      - Name of test completed
      - Results of test
12. Answer: Six to eight quarts

Activities

1. Direct students to review Section 17.2 for information about Standard Precautions. You might want to allow class time to play a quiz-show game using the students' questions.
2. Direct students to select a specific drug, and then research the number and types of trials it had to go through in order to reach market. Alternatively, students may report on one phase of testing. Encourage students to prepare a presentation or poster to display their research.
3. Have the students think about the importance of each step. You can even "erase" a step in the process and have the students evaluate the effects.
4. You can also have the students do a self-assessment of their strengths and weaknesses with respect to these skills.

Case Studies

1. Direct students to Section 20.1 for more information on admission and registration procedures. Remind students of the importance of effective and age-appropriate communication skills.
2. Direct students to Section 20.3 for information on collecting blood and urine specimens and on safety guidelines. Remind students of the importance of effective and age-appropriate communication skills.

Thinking Critically

1. Direct students to Section 20.3 for information about laboratory safety. Prepare a display of all the posters in the classroom, a science lab, or in a public area of the school.
2. Direct students to Section 20.2 for information about medications. You might consider allowing students to perform skits to demonstrate their responses to this situation.
3. Encourage students to write a complete essay, including a thesis statement supported by facts and real-life examples.

Portfolio Connection

- Encourage students to be as comprehensive as possible in creating the list of abbreviations and symbols.
- Encourage students to use peer review to see if there are any abbreviations and symbols missing from the lists.
- Check to make sure that students have completed the assignment and added it to their portfolio.

TEAMWORK

Divide the class into teams of 8 to 12 students. Hold a "definition bee" in which you read a term introduced or used in this chapter, and ask one team to define it. If they succeed, they get a point; if not, the other team has a chance. The team with the most points at the end of the competition wins.

21 Therapeutic Techniques and Sports Medicine

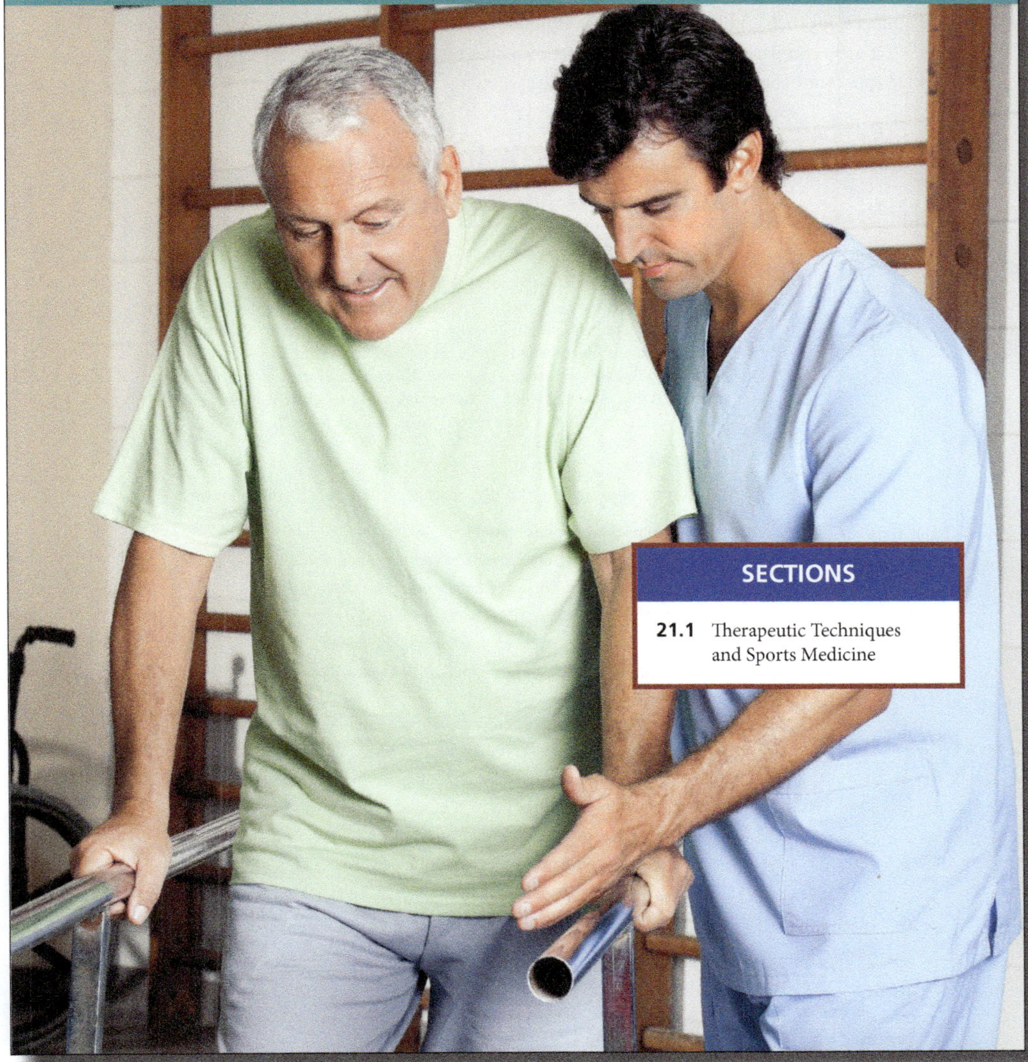

SECTIONS

CHAPTER 21 OVERVIEW

Chapter 21 provides information about the fields of physical therapy and sports medicine.

Section 21.1: Section 21.1 introduces students to therapeutic techniques and the responsibilities of a physical therapy aide. It covers common treatments and procedures, including preparing soaks and compresses, range-of-motion exercises, guarding techniques, and how to use ambulation devices.

Advance Preparation	
Review	■ Chapter text for Section 21.1, and chapter procedures.
Contact	■ A physical therapist or sports medicine specialist to address the class. ■ A physical therapy department or clinic to request a tour. ■ A physical therapy department or clinic to request brochures and other educational material.
Prepare	■ Magazine and newspaper articles about sports medicine. ■ Equipment needed for procedures, such as hot and cold compresses and ambulation devices. ■ A list of Web sites that provide information about physical therapy and sports medicine—such as sportsmed.org and apta.org.

FOCUS AND ENGAGE

Getting Started

- Divide the class into small groups of four or five students to complete this activity.
- Assign each group three different sports to research, so the class can compare the results when the work is complete.
- Direct the students to contact sports associations to request the statistics or to use an Internet search engine to search for statistics about injuring in their assigned sport.

Introduce the Section

a. Review the content of the Background paragraph, explaining that physical therapy is often used as an alternative to surgery, or in combination with surgery.

b. Emphasize that the goal of physical therapy is to restore function so the patient can be as independent as possible.

c. Review the objectives for the section.

Vocabulary Review

a. Direct students to the key terms.

b. Pronounce each word, and have the students repeat the pronunciation out loud.

c. Discuss the definition of each word.

TEACH

Discuss

- Ask students to share personal stories of sports-related injuries that may have required physical therapy.
- Discuss the types of physical therapy occupations.

Getting Started

Many injuries occur due to improper preparation for participating in athletic events. Back injury is often the result of improper lifting, bending, and turning. There are other injuries that occur as well. Participate as a member of a team to complete the following exercise:

- Select three different individual or team sports and determine the most common injuries for each and the percentage of athletes that sustain each injury.
- Prepare a comparison chart or graph that displays your findings.
- Display your completed chart/graph in the classroom.

SECTION 21.1 Therapeutic Techniques and Sports Medicine

Background

Physical therapy, sometimes known as physiotherapy, is a medical treatment of injuries or disorders using methods such as exercise, massage, or the application of water, light, or heat. Physical therapy helps condition muscles. It also restores strength and movement when people are injured, recovering from surgery, or have a physical disability such as cerebral palsy. That way, they can learn or relearn to do normal things such as walk, get out of bed, or throw a ball. A physical therapist also can prescribe splints, canes, special shoes, and other assistive devices.

Objectives

When you have completed this section, you will be able to do the following:

- Describe the responsibilities of a physical therapy aide.
- Describe the responsibilities of a sports medicine aide.
- Define *ultraviolet light* and name conditions treated with it.
- Describe conditions treated with diathermy.
- List conditions commonly treated by ultrasound.
- Document the most important question to ask a patient when preparing for an ultrasound treatment.
- Identify kinds of thermotherapy and the conditions they treat.
- Identify ways to give cryotherapy and conditions they treat.
- Define *hydrotherapy* and list reasons hydrotherapy is used.
- Explain the purpose of range of motion.
- Define *guarding technique* and *guarding belt*.
- List some commonly used ambulation devices.
- List some transporting devices commonly used.
- Demonstrate range of motion.
- Demonstrate each procedure in this chapter.

772 Chapter 21 | Therapeutic Techniques and Sports Medicine

ACTIVITY

Locate an article in a magazine, newspaper, or Web site that discusses an injury suffered by a professional athlete. Identify the type of injury, how it occurred, and the treatment required. Bring in the article and discuss it with the class.

CUSTOMIZED INSTRUCTION OVERVIEW

Less Advanced Students	Pages 776, 795
More Advanced Students	Pages 777, 779
English Language Learners	Page 773
Special Needs Students	Page 773
At-Risk Students	Pages 775, 802

The Physical Therapy Department

The physical therapy department is made up of a number of trained people who work as a team to assist and direct patients in the rehabilitation process. Their main goal is to reduce pain, prevent deformity, and promote healing. They also attempt to restore function or assist patients by teaching them new ways to adjust to their disabilities.

The entry-level job title for this department is "physical therapy aide." Physical therapy aides may be employed in the following facilities and agencies:

- Acute care facilities
- Long-term care facilities
- Rehabilitation centers
- Schools that educate disabled persons
- Public health agencies
- Home health-care agencies
- Sports medicine centers
- Professional or school sports teams

Responsibilities of a Physical Therapy Aide

As a physical therapy aide, you may be required to do the following tasks:

- Prepare equipment (e.g., **hydrotherapy** pools)
- Assist patients:
  - With walking and gait training
  - To dress and undress
  - To position themselves
  - To remove and replace braces, splints, and slings
- Change linens on beds and tables
- Fold linens
- Clean equipment and work area
- May inventory materials and supplies

hydrotherapy
(hahy druh THER uh pee)
The use of water (hot, cold, steam, or ice) to relieve discomfort and promote physical well-being.

Sports Medicine Aide/Athletic Trainer

One subspecialty of working as a physical therapy aide is working as a sports medicine aide. Sports medicine is one of the fastest growing fields in medicine. It includes working with professional sports teams, high school and college athletes, and individuals with sports-related injuries. Sports medicine aides perform the duties of physical therapy aides but deal with the practical aspects of sports injury prevention, recognition, and treatment of sports-related injuries.

Therapeutic Techniques and Sports Medicine | Chapter 21 773

Teaching Tips

- Discuss the personnel who work in a physical therapy department.
- Point out that it is part of the therapeutic services sector.
- Discuss the types of facilities that have physical therapy departments.
- Emphasize that the goal is to assist and direct patients in the rehabilitation process.
- Review the responsibilities of a physical therapy aide:
  - Prepare equipment
  - Assist patients as necessary
  - Change linens on beds and tables
  - Fold linens
  - Clean equipment and work area
  - Inventory materials and supplies
- Emphasize that different facilities have different policies regarding what aides are allowed to do.

CUSTOMIZED INSTRUCTION

Special Needs Students

Some special needs students may have experience with physical therapy. Ask them to share their personal stories with the class.

English Language Learners

Have students write each key term and its pronunciation on one side of an index card and its definition on the other side. Have them read each term and definition aloud to a partner.

Teaching Tips

- Differentiate between a sports therapy aide and a physical therapy aide: A sports therapy aide is a physical therapy aide who specializes in treating patients with sports-related injuries.
- Review the responsibilities of a sports therapy aide:
  - Perform all the duties of a physical therapy aide
  - Prepare equipment
  - Assist in injury treatments, evaluations, and rehabilitation of athletes
  - Assist or perform taping, wrapping, protective bracing, and equipment fitting
  - Help out in pre-practice preparations and post-practice follow-up
  - Be on hand to assist during event coverage
- Discuss the use of massage therapy in sports medicine.
- Explain that massage is the practice of manipulating the soft tissues of the human body in order to prevent injury, or aid in the recovery from injury.
- Emphasize that most states regulate massage certification.
- Refer to information on Alternative Health Care in Section 7.1.

Apply It

- Divide the class into teams of soccer players and health care advisors.
- The soccer players should each have a complaint or injury to report.
- The health care advisors should respond to each player in turn.
- Encourage students to put the diagnosis and treatment plan in writing.

Responsibilities of a Sports Medicine Aide/Athletic Trainer

As a sports medicine aide, you may be required to do the following tasks:

- Perform all the duties of a physical therapy aide
- Prepare equipment (e.g., massage tables)
- Assist in injury treatments, evaluations, and rehabilitation of athletes
- Assist or perform taping, wrapping, protective bracing, and equipment fitting
- Help out in pre-practice preparations and post-practice follow-up
- Be on hand to assist in event coverage

Apply It

Set up a "team" of health care advisors to work with a "mock" soccer team. As each soccer player complains of a specific problem, develop a potential diagnosis and treatment plan.

Massage Therapy Techniques in Sports Medicine

Massage therapy plays an important role in sports medicine. Massage is the practice of manipulating the soft tissues of the human body in order to prevent injury, or aid in the recovery from injury. There are more than two hundred varieties of massage.

Some practitioners use several different techniques such as stroking, kneading, tapping, compression, friction, and pressure. (**Figure 21.1**) Oils, lotions, and powders may also be included to reduce friction on the skin. In professional settings, the patient is treated while lying on a massage table, lying on a pad on the floor, or sitting upright in a massage chair.

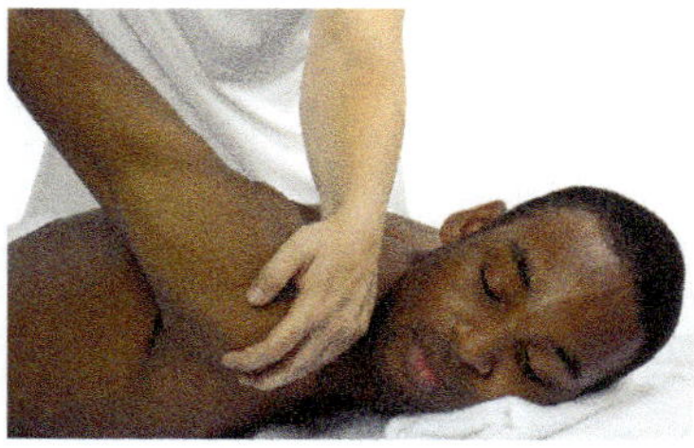

Figure 21.1
What skills and interests do you think might be necessary to become a massage therapist?

The benefits of massage are an accepted part of many physical rehabilitation programs, especially in sports medicine. Massage therapy is helpful for several chronic conditions including lower back pain, arthritis, bursitis, and fatigue. In sports medicine, massage helps prevent injury and restores mobility to injured muscle tissue.

Massage therapists can only massage. They are not allowed to diagnose, prescribe, manipulate, or adjust the human skeletal structure. You need a specific state license in order to practice branches of medicine such as orthopedics, physical therapy, podiatry, chiropractic, osteopathy, psychotherapy, or acupuncture.

Figure Focus

21.1 What skills and interests do you think might be necessary to become a massage therapist?

Student responses will vary.

ACTIVITY

Make a chart or table comparing a sports therapy aide to a physical therapy aide. Include specifics such as responsibilities, career ladder, salary range, typical patients, and facilities where they might be employed.

Personal Wellness

Overuse Injuries

One of the leading problems requiring physical therapy is overuse injuries, also known as cumulative trauma disorders. These are particularly common among participants in sports. Certain ailments are simply known as "tennis elbow," "golfer's elbow," and "runner's knee." However, overuse injuries are common in many fields; musicians get tendonitis, dancers sustain stress fractures, and people who work with computers develop carpal tunnel syndrome.

The term "overuse injury" refers to many different diagnoses, and there is no clear medical definition. Nonetheless, a sports medicine aide certainly will see numerous examples of the disorder.

An overuse injury occurs when any biological tissue, such as muscle, bone, ligament, or tendon, is stressed beyond its physical limit. Tissues are able to adapt to the stresses placed on them over time.

However, overuse injuries develop when repeated physical challenges are followed by insufficient recovery time. As the tissues attempt to adapt to the demands placed on them, they can become injured unless they have enough time to heal. These injuries are usually microscopic tears that lead to small amounts of bleeding and swelling in the injured area.

Overuse injuries can occur suddenly from one hard training session or become progressively worse over a long period. It is impossible to estimate the precise number of overuse injuries in the United States. However, one study showed that about two-thirds of runners develop injuries every year.

Athletes with repetitive stress injuries do not always seek medical attention because they are afraid the doctor will advise them to give up their sport temporarily or permanently. Instead, they try to avoid pain in training by changing their body mechanics. This usually does even more damage. Eventually, the injury gets so bad that the pain is unavoidable. By the time the athlete does seek help, there are usually multiple problems that need rehabilitation.

The simplest way to avoid an overuse injury is to allow for sufficient recovery time between workouts or stress. This is not always easy. Data entry clerks cannot simply decide to skip work. Psychological factors might keep athletes from scheduling rest days in their workout schedule. However, it is important to remind patients of something that they have probably already learned—overuse injuries are much easier to prevent than to cure.

Preparing Patients for Therapy

As an aide in the physical therapy department, you assist the therapist and prepare:

- The patient
- Supplies
- Equipment

There are various types of therapy, and each requires a slightly different preparation.

Ultraviolet-light therapy is used to treat various diseases, especially those of the skin. It is used to treat the following:

- Acne
- Pressure sores

ultraviolet light
(uhl truh VAHY uh lit lahyt)
An invisible band of radiation at the upper end of the visible light spectrum.

Therapeutic Techniques and Sports Medicine | Chapter 21 775

Personal Wellness—Overuse Injuries

- Explain that overuse injuries are common among athletes and casual sports participants.
- Review common overuse injuries:
  - Tennis elbow
  - Golfer's elbow
  - Runner's knee
- Emphasize that overuse injuries are also common among anyone who repeats the same motion frequently, including keyboarders, musicians, and those working on an assembly line.
- Review the cause of overuse injury.
- Review the problems that might arise from ignoring an overuse injury.
- Review methods of treating an overuse injury.

Athletes with repetitive strain injuries may be reluctant to seek medical attention. What could you tell an athlete that might encourage him or her to obtain the proper treatment?

Answer: Explain that even though he or she might be worried that a doctor will say to give up the sport temporarily or permanently, it is riskier over the long term to avoid treatment. He or she might end up doing more serious damage. Finally, overuse injuries are much easier to prevent than to cure.

CUSTOMIZED INSTRUCTION

At-Risk Students

Ask students to think of an injury they have sustained. This can be a recent injury or one from months or years ago, and it can be any type, ranging from a minor cut to a broken bone. Have them share with the class how they sustained the injury, and what, if anything, they could have done to prevent it.

ACTIVITY

Create a public service poster about an overuse injury that is common among student athletes. Display the poster in an appropriate place, such as the gym, the trainer's office, or the nurse's office.

Teaching Tips

- Review common types of treatments that aids might participate in.
- Explain that ultraviolet light uses rays like the sun.
- Emphasize that the light can burn the skin.
- Explain that ultraviolet light is used to treat skin conditions:
  - Psoriasis
  - Pressure sores
  - Wound infections
  - Acne
- Reinforce ultraviolet light safety measures.
- Discuss conditions treated with diathermy:
  - Arthritis
  - Bursitis
  - Tendonitis
  - Muscle problems
- Reinforce safety measures for diathermy:
  - Patient must remove all metal objects
  - Aide must report if patient has metal implanted in body
- Discuss conditions treated with ultrasound:
  - Pain
  - Muscle spasms
  - Circulation problems
- Emphasize that aides must ask patient if he or she has any metal implants, and report the answer to the therapist immediately.

- Psoriasis
- Wound infections

This treatment can cause severe burning. For this reason, the patient cannot be left unobserved in the room during a treatment.

CAUTION: Do not turn on the light before the therapist is ready to start the treatment.

diathermy
(DAHY uh thur mee)
The use of electric currents to produce heat in body tissues, usually as an aid to healing.

Diathermy is a heat-inducing treatment that increases the circulation in the treated area. It is often used to treat the following:

- Muscle problems
- Arthritis
- Bursitis
- Tendonitis

Metal attracts heat during this procedure, so it is your responsibility to do the following:

- Have the patient remove all metal jewelry, belts, hairpins, and so on.
- Ask the patient if they have any metal implants in joints or in other parts of the body. If they do, report it to the therapist right away.

ultrasound
(UHL truh sound)
Medical therapy that uses sound frequencies (above 20 kHz) beyond the limits of human hearing to treat hard-to-reach body areas.

Ultrasound uses high-frequency sound waves to penetrate deep tissues. It is most commonly used to treat:

- Pain
- Muscle spasms
- Problems in circulation

Ultrasound is also used to diagnose specific conditions. However, physical therapy uses ultrasounds only in a therapeutic mode. Because ultrasound vibrates tissues, caution has to be taken with patients with joint implants. Always ask patients during the preparation if they have any joint implants. If so, report it to the therapist.

thermotherapy
(thur moh THER uh pee)
Medical therapy involving the application of heat.

Thermotherapy refers to heat treatments. Heat is used to speed up the healing process. Heat causes the blood vessels to expand (dilate). This allows more blood to circulate to the area and helps the healing process. The blood brings oxygen and food needed for healing. If the area is swollen and/or inflamed, the blood helps absorb and carry away the extra fluid. This type of treatment is used to do the following:

- Relieve pain
- Promote muscle relaxation
- Reduce muscle spasms
- Reduce inflammation
- Treat skin ulcers

776 Chapter 21 | Therapeutic Techniques and Sports Medicine

CUSTOMIZED INSTRUCTION

Less Advanced Students

Provide additional tools for less advanced students to learn the vocabulary in this chapter. They might benefit from making flashcards or a glossary.

- Treat perineal lacerations
- Reduce swelling
- Promote drainage

There are two kinds of thermotherapy. One type is *moist heat*. The other type is *dry heat*. Moist heat is applied with the following:

- Hot soaks
- Hot compresses
- Hot packs

Dry heat is applied with:

- Heat lamps
- Infrared lights
- Standard electric bulbs
- Heating pads

Science Link

Ultraviolet Light

Ultraviolet (UV) light is an invisible band of radiation at the upper end of the visible light spectrum. The name means "beyond violet" (from the Latin word *ultra* meaning "beyond") because violet has the shortest wavelengths of visible light. UV rays were first identified in1801 by Johann Wilhelm Ritter, a German physicist. UV rays have wavelengths from 10 to 400 nm. In the light spectrum, they begin at the end of visible light and end at the beginning of x-rays.

The main source of ultraviolet light is the sun. Sunlight contains two main types of ultraviolet light: UVA and UVB. UVA rays have longer wavelengths that penetrate deep into the skin. Limited exposure to UVA rays causes the skin to tan. The wavelengths of UVB rays are much shorter and affect the outermost layers of skin. UVB rays cause sunburn and are sometimes known as the "burning rays."

Ultraviolet light has been used as a medical treatment since the early 1900s. A so-called "sunlamp" can produce UV rays artificially. The rays can be used to help people generate vitamin D in their bodies. Vitamin D helps prevent rickets and various bone disorder conditions.

Ultraviolet light is also useful as a disinfectant. UV rays can kill bacteria and so they are sometimes used to sterilize the air in operating rooms. They can also be used to treat skin disease, such as psoriasis, and seasonal affective disorder (SAD).

CAUTION: Prolonged exposure to UV radiation can result in acute and chronic health effects on the eyes, skin, and immune system.

Project 1

What is a suntan? What does sunscreen do? What is an SPF number? Use the Internet or other resources to locate information, and write a brief report on the nature of tanning and skin protection. Make sure you discuss ultraviolet rays in your report.

Project 2

Use the Internet to examine the use of ultraviolet light in tanning beds and sun lamps. List two arguments supporting and two arguments disputing the safety of artificial tanning. Cite your sources so the reader can judge if they are reliable.

Explain the difference between UVA and UVB. Which do you think is more dangerous?

Evaluate and report on the validity and reliability of claims in published materials of the effects of electromagnetic radiation on living tissue.

Therapeutic Techniques and Sports Medicine | Chapter 21 777

CUSTOMIZED INSTRUCTION

More Advanced Students

Assign more advanced students one or both of the example research problems included in the Science Link feature.

Teaching Tips

- Emphasize that thermotherapy uses heat to speed up healing by increasing blood flow and circulation.
- Explain that thermotherapy:
  - Relieves pain
  - Promotes muscle relaxation
  - Reduces muscle spasms
  - Reduces inflammation
  - Treats skin ulcers
  - Treats perineal lacerations
  - Reduces swelling
  - Promotes drainage
- Explain that moist heat is applied using:
  - Hot soaks
  - Hot compresses
  - Hot packs
- Explain that dry heat is applied using:
  - Heat lamp
  - Infrared lights
  - Standard electric bulbs
  - Heating pads
- Discuss safety issues and signs of problems.

Science Link—Ultraviolet Light

- Review the types of ultraviolet light.

Explain the difference between UVA and UVB. Which do you think is more dangerous?

Answer: UVA rays have longer wavelengths that penetrate deep into the skin. Limited exposure to UVA rays causes the skin to tan but can also cause irreparable damage that leads to skin cancer. The wavelengths of UVB rays are much shorter and affect the outermost layers of skin. UVB rays are the cause of sunburn.

Procedure Tip

21.1 Preparing Moist Hot Soaks

- Review the background information, emphasizing the need to use the proper temperature.
- Emphasize the importance of following Standard Precautions.
- Review the preprocedure steps.
- Step 1: Emphasize the importance of carefully reading the physician's order.
- Step 2: Emphasize the importance of proper handwashing.
- Step 3: Review the equipment list.
- Step 5: Emphasize the importance of effective communication techniques.
- Step 6: Emphasize the importance of patient privacy.
- Review the procedure steps.
- Step 10: Emphasize that the pad should never be applied directly to exposed skin.
- Step 12: Emphasize the importance of proper handwashing.
- Step 13: Emphasize the importance of monitoring and observing the patient.
- Review the postprocedure steps.
- Step 16: Emphasize the importance of proper handwashing.
- Step 17: Review proper observation and reporting procedures.

Procedure 21.1 Preparing Moist Hot Soaks

BACKGROUND: You can prevent injury by using the correct temperature for the hot moist pads. Make sure you carefully observe the treated area to watch for irritation or excessive redness.

ALERT: Follow Standard Precautions

Preprocedure

1. Check physician's orders.
2. Wash hands.
3. Assemble equipment:
   a. **Hydroculator pad**
   b. Towel
4. Identify patient.
5. Explain what you will be doing and reassure patient that procedure is painless.
6. Provide privacy.
7. Cover warm hydroculator pad with towel.
8. Expose site to be treated.
9. Position patient for comfort.

Procedure

10. Apply covered warm hydroculator pad to appropriate site. (Never put warm hydroculator pad directly on the skin, unless it is covered.)
11. Make sure call bell is in reach.
12. Wash hands.
13. Recheck patient frequently—every 5 minutes when heating device is on skin. Look for:
    a. Severely reddened areas
    b. Irritated areas
    c. Painful areas
14. Remove soaks as ordered.

Postprocedure

15. Position patient for comfort and make sure call bell is in reach.
16. Wash hands.
17. Report and record patient's tolerance of treatment and any changes in condition you observed.

Charting Example:

11/20/24	1100
	Hot, moist pads applied for 15 minutes
	Rechecked skin at site
	No reddened or irritated areas
	Patient states: Pain is better after
	treatment but returns in about an hour
	______ A. Cantina CNA

hydroculator pad (HI droc u la tor pad) A moist heat pack treatment.

You need to prepare hot packs so that they are ready when needed. Always check the skin for signs of extreme redness or burning. If a patient complains of discomfort, remove the packs immediately.

Cryotherapy means cold therapy. Cold therapy causes the blood vessels to get smaller (contract). This slows the flow of blood to the area. This reduces the amount of fluid and helps reduce pain. Cold application is used to:

- Relieve pain
- Reduce body temperature
- Control bleeding
- Reduce inflammation
- Prevent edema

778 Chapter 21 | Therapeutic Techniques and Sports Medicine

PROCEDURE PRACTICE

- Demonstrate the steps for Procedure 21.1, Preparing Moist Hot Soaks, as many times as necessary, or ask students to demonstrate the steps. Have students practice and perform the procedure until they are competent.

ACTIVITY

Describe a patient's response to a moist hot soak. Have students report the response as they would if they were caring for the patient in a physical therapy department of a hospital.

Cryotherapy can be given in two ways: dry cold and moist cold. *Dry cold* includes the use of:

- Ice bags
- Ice collars

Moist cold includes the use of:

- Cold compresses
- Cold packs
- Ice massage

Prepare cold packs for cryotherapy (cold, moist, or dry treatments) so that they are ready when needed. Always check the skin for signs of whiteness (blanching) or bluishness. If these occur, stop the treatment immediately.

What's New?

Acupuncture

Acupuncture certainly is not new. The practice of inserting needles in the human body to ease pain and aid recovery is at least 2,500 years old. What is new is acupuncture's increasing acceptance in mainstream medicine.

Not so long ago, Americans viewed acupuncture as a strange therapy, not unlike voodoo. Now, it is increasingly recognized as an effective treatment for some disorders and a common accompaniment to physical therapy, a massage, or a trip to the orthopedist.

The World Health Organization (WHO) recommends acupuncture as an effective treatment for more than 40 medical problems. In the United States, more than 2 million people use acupuncture each year, and an estimated 8.2 million adults have used it as a therapy.

Acupuncture involves the insertion and manipulation of sharp, thin needles in the body at very specific points. This process is believed to adjust and alter the body's energy flow (which the Chinese call "chi") into healthier patterns. Scientists are still studying how effective acupuncture is and why it works.

However, the U.S. National Institutes of Health now states that, "promising results have emerged, showing efficacy of acupuncture, for example, in adult postoperative and chemotherapy nausea and vomiting . . . . There are other situations—such as . . . stroke rehabilitation . . . tennis elbow . . . osteoarthritis, low-back pain, carpal tunnel syndrome, and asthma—in which acupuncture may be useful as an adjunct treatment or an acceptable alternative . . . . "

For example, knee osteoarthritis is a common condition seen by physical therapists in which changes in the knee joints lead to pain. Treatments include physical therapy, exercise, and drugs to decrease pain and inflammation. Recently, a study showed that acupuncture provided pain relief for people with knee osteoarthritis and would serve as an effective complement to standard care.

As a physical therapy aide, you might find yourself making sure acupuncture needles are sterile and setting up disinfectants for acupuncture treatments.

Why do you think the U.S. medical establishment was reluctant to recognize acupuncture as a possible medical treatment therapy?

Therapeutic Techniques and Sports Medicine | Chapter 21 779

Teaching Tips

- Emphasize that cryotherapy uses cold to constrict blood flow.
- Explain that cryotherapy:
  - Relieves pain
  - Reduces body temperature
  - Controls bleeding
  - Reduces inflammation
  - Prevents edema
- Explain that moist cold is applied using:
  - Cold compresses
  - Cold packs
  - Ice massage
- Explain that dry cold is applied using:
  - Ice bags
  - Ice collars
- Discuss safety issues and signs of problems.

What's New?—Acupuncture

- Explain acupuncture.
- Emphasize that it may be used in combination with physical therapy to treat certain conditions.
- Refer to Section 7.1, Holistic Health, for more information.

Why do you think the U.S. medical establishment was reluctant to recognize acupuncture as a possible medical treatment therapy?

Answer: The U.S. medical establishment might have been reluctant to recognize acupuncture as a possible medical treatment therapy because they cannot document how it works.

ACTIVITY

Use the Internet to look up some of the medical problems for which the World Health Organization recommends using acupuncture as a treatment. List the problems along with the traditional medical treatment.

Procedure Tip

21.2 Moist Cryotherapy (Cold) Compresses

- Review the background information, emphasizing the need to use the proper temperature.
- Emphasize the importance of following Standard Precautions.
- Review the preprocedure steps.
- Step 1: Emphasize the importance of carefully reading the physician's order.
- Step 2: Emphasize the importance of proper handwashing.
- Step 3: Review the equipment list.
- Review the procedure steps.
- Step 4: Emphasize the importance of effective communication techniques.
- Step 8: Emphasize the importance of proper handwashing.
- Step 9: Emphasize the importance of monitoring and observing the patient.
- Review the postprocedure steps.
- Step 11: Emphasize the importance of drying the skin thoroughly.
- Step 13: Emphasize the importance of proper handwashing.
- Step 14: Review proper observation and reporting procedures.

Procedure 21.2 **Moist Cryotherapy (Cold) Compresses**

BACKGROUND: You can prevent injury by using the correct temperature for moist cryotherapy. Make sure you carefully observe the treated area to watch for any pain or irregularities. Using correct temperature for moist cryotherapy and careful observation of the treated area prevents injury.

ALERT: Follow Standard Precautions

Preprocedure

1. Check doctor's orders.
2. Wash hands.
3. Assemble equipment:
   a. Cool, wet cloth
   b. Plastic cover
   c. Dry towel

Procedure

4. Explain procedure to client/patient.
5. Apply cool, wet cloth to patient as ordered.*

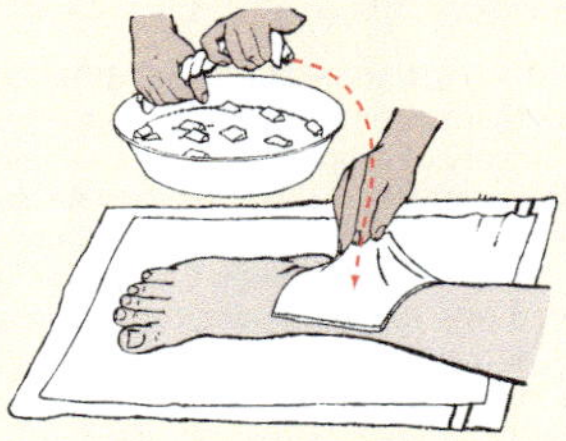

6. Cover wet area with plastic cover.
7. Cover plastic with dry towel.
8. Wash hands.
9. Recheck frequently for:
   a. Coolness of cloth
   b. Position
   c. Patient's comfort needs (reapply PRN)
10. Remove as ordered.

Postprocedure

11. Dry skin.
12. Dispose of supplies and clean area.
13. Wash hands.
14. Report and document effects of treatment.

Charting Example:

11/20/24	1100
	Moist, cold towels applied for 15
	minutes
	Rechecked skin at site
	No reddened or irritated areas
	Patient states: Pain is better
	after treatment but returns in
	about an hour
	A. Cantina CNA

* Wear gloves if there are broken areas on the skin.

780 Chapter 21 | Therapeutic Techniques and Sports Medicine

PROCEDURE PRACTICE

- Demonstrate the steps for Procedure 21.2, Moist Cryotherapy (Cold) Compress, as many times as necessary, or ask students to demonstrate the steps. Have students practice and perform the procedure until they are competent.

ACTIVITY

Compare the procedures for moist cryotherapy and dry cryotherapy. Document the differences and similarities. Include information about the conditions they treat.

Procedure 21.3 Dry Cryotherapy: Ice Bags/Ice Collars

BACKGROUND: Using the correct temperature for dry cryotherapy and careful observation of the treated area prevents injury.

ALERT: Follow Standard Precautions

Preprocedure

1. Check physician's orders.
2. Wash hands.
3. Assemble equipment:
   a. Ice bag or commercial cold compress
   b. Ice
   c. Cover for ice bag
4. Fill bag with ice. (Run water over cubes to soften sharp edges.)
5. Remove air from bag by pressing sides together.
6. Close end and check for leaks.
7. Cover bag with cloth or towel. (Never apply bag directly to skin; it may stick, burn, and tear skin when removed.)
8. Identify patient by checking order and name with patient's armband or patient chart.

Procedure

9. Explain procedure to patient.
10. Gently position ice bag as ordered. (The metal cap cannot touch the skin.)*
11. Secure bag so that it does not move away from affected area.
12. Provide needed comfort measures for patient. Make sure call bell is in reach.
13. Wash hands.
14. Return frequently to check for:
    a. Coolness of ice bag
    b. Position of ice bag
    c. Color of skin (remove ice if skin is white or bluish in color or if patient reports numbness and report)
15. Remove ice bag at ordered time.
16. Make sure patient is comfortable and call bell is in reach.

Postprocedure

17. Wash hands.
18. Recheck skin, and report and document effects of treatment.
19. Wash hands.
20. Empty bag, dry, and return to appropriate area for cleaning.

Charting Example:

11/20/24 1100
Dry, cold compress applied for15 minutes
Recheck skin at site
No reddened or irritated areas
Patient states: Pain is better after
treatment but returns in about an hour
A. Cantina CNA

* Wear gloves if there are broken areas on the skin.

Therapeutic Techniques and Sports Medicine | Chapter 21 781

Procedure Tip

21.3 Dry Cryotherapy: Ice Bags/Ice Collars

- Review the background information, emphasizing the need to use the proper temperature.
- Emphasize the importance of following Standard Precautions.
- Review the preprocedure steps.
- Step 1: Emphasize the importance of carefully reading the physician's order.
- Step 2: Emphasize the importance of proper handwashing.
- Step 3: Review the equipment list.
- Step 6: Emphasize the importance of checking for leaks.
- Step 7: Emphasize the importance of not applying the bag to exposed skin.
- Review the procedure steps.
- Step 9: Emphasize the importance of effective communication techniques.
- Step 13: Emphasize the importance of proper handwashing.
- Step 14: Emphasize the importance of monitoring and observing the patient.
- Review the postprocedure steps.
- Step 18: Review proper observation and reporting procedures.
- Step 19: Emphasize the importance of proper handwashing.

ACTIVITY

Draw a flowchart illustrating how cryotherapy affects the treated area.

PROCEDURE PRACTICE

- Demonstrate the steps for Procedure 21.3, Dry Cryotherapy: Ice Bags/Ice Collars, as many times as necessary, or ask students to demonstrate the steps. Have students practice and perform the procedure until they are competent.

Teaching Tips

- Explain that hydrotherapy—or water therapy—is used to:
  - Apply soothing medication
  - Promote relaxation
  - Improve circulation and mobility of an injured limb
  - Loosen and remove dead skin
- Discuss environments for hydrotherapy:
  - Tubs ranging from small basins to swimming pools
  - Usually in a whirlpool
- Review safety concerns, including the importance of aseptic techniques to clean equipment.
- Explain that range-of-motion exercises are used to:
  - Stimulate circulation
  - Encourage flexibility and mobility of the joints
  - Prevent contractures
  - Prevent mineral loss
  - Prevent other problems caused by lack of movement
- Differentiate between active ROM (patients move themselves), and passive ROM (therapist or aide moves patient).
- Explain the use of antiembolism hose.

TEAMWORK

In small groups, prepare a skit demonstrating problems that might occur in a patient who has not moved his or her muscles in a long time.

Hydrotherapy is water therapy. Hydrotherapy is usually given in a whirlpool. The whole body may be treated or just a limb. This treatment is used to:

- Apply soothing medication
- Promote relaxation
- Improve circulation and mobility of an injured limb
- Loosen and remove dead skin

This treatment is accomplished in various-sized tubs ranging from small basins to a swimming pool. Your responsibility is to:

- Assist the patient in disrobing or exposing the area to be treated.
- Ensure that the water temperature is correct (95° F to 105° F).
- Secure the patient to ensure there is no danger of injury.
- Disinfect and clean the equipment.
- Assist the patient when large areas of the body are to be submerged.
- Clean the tub after each treatment.

Range of Motion

range-of-motion (ROM)
(reynj uhv MOH shuhn)
Measurement of the achievable distance between the flexed position and the extended position of a particular joint or muscle group.

flexibility
(FLEK suh buhl itee)
The ability to easily bend.

contraction
(kuh n TRAK shuhn)
One that occurs when a muscle fiber lengthens or shortens.

Range-of-motion (ROM) exercises are very important for the resident who has limited movement. ROM exercises are given to:

- Stimulate circulation to decrease chance of blood clots or decubitus ulcers
- Encourage **flexibility** and mobility of the joints
- Prevent contractures (permanent **contraction** of the muscle)
- Prevent mineral loss
- Prevent other problems such as poor appetite, constipation, urinary infections, respiratory problems, and hypostatic pneumonia

Residents are encouraged to move each joint to the best of their ability. This is active ROM. When you do passive ROM for your residents, you move the joints for them.

Antiembolism Hose

Antiembolism hose are used to prevent blood from pooling in the legs. This reduces the possibility of developing phlebitis and blood clots. Elasticized hose are called TEDS or antiembolism hose. Sometimes elastic bandages are used. These extend from the ankle or foot to calf or midthigh. They are applied after surgery and when there is danger of a clot forming and causing thrombophlebitis. They must be applied so that they are smooth and even and do not cut off the circulation. Be certain to remove them and reapply them at least once every 8 hours.

782 Chapter 21 | Therapeutic Techniques and Sports Medicine

Procedure 21.4 Range of Motion

BACKGROUND: Correct ROM provides exercise to the joints and muscles, preventing contractures and immobility.

Note: The use of passive and active range of motion (ROM) is related to resident's ability level.

- **Active ROM**—Resident is able to perform all movements without assistance.
- **Passive ROM**—Health care worker moves body parts for resident.

ALERT: Follow Standard Precautions

Preprocedure

1. Wash hands.
2. Assemble equipment:
   a. Sheet or bath blanket
   b. Treatment table or bed
   c. Good lighting
3. Identify resident.
4. Explain what you are going to do.
5. Ask visitors to wait outside, and provide privacy.

Procedure

6. Place resident in a comfortable position. (For all but the head motions, the resident should be in a supine position on bed or treatment table.) Only expose affected area. Instruct resident to do the following movements at least five times each or to tolerance.

Head Flexion and Extension

7. Bend head until chin touches chest (flexion), then gently bend backward (extension).

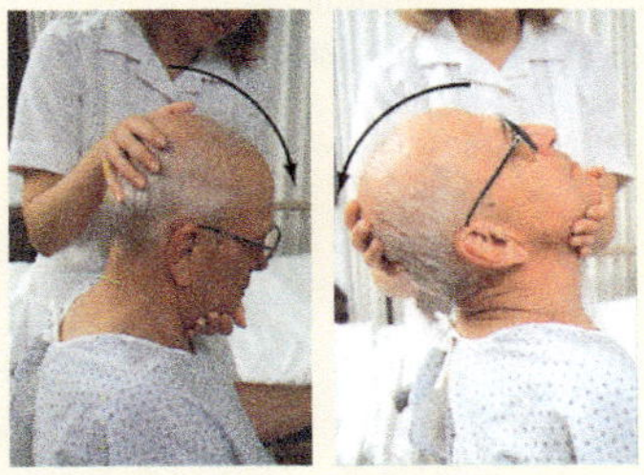

Right/Left Rotation

8. Turn head to right (right rotation), then turn head to left (left rotation).

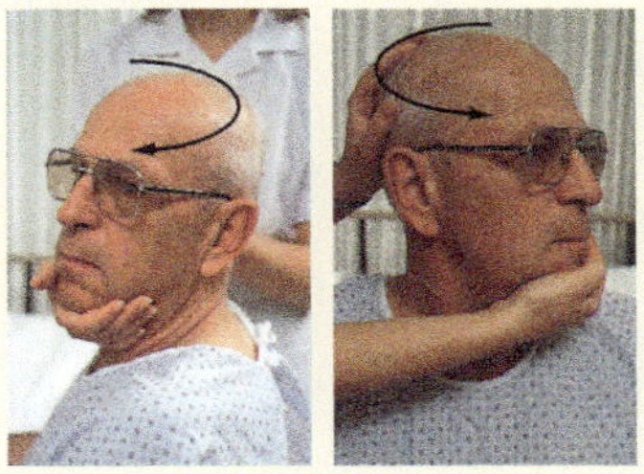

Right/Left Lateral Flexion

9. Move head so that right ear moves toward right shoulder (right lateral flexion), then move head to central position and continue moving head so that left ear moves toward left shoulder (left lateral flexion).

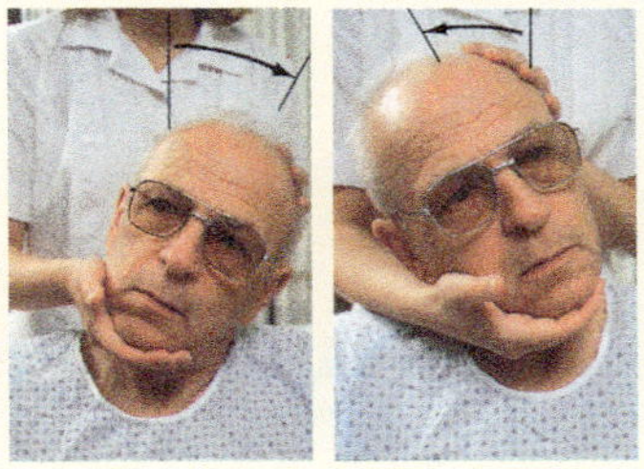

(continued)

Therapeutic Techniques and Sports Medicine | Chapter 21 783

Procedure Tip

21.4 Range of Motion

- Review the background information, emphasizing the purpose of range-of-motion exercises.
- Review the difference between active ROM and passive ROM.
- Emphasize the importance of following Standard Precautions.
- Step 1: Emphasize the importance of proper handwashing.
- Step 2: Discuss the equipment that may be required.
- Step 4: Emphasize the importance of effective communication techniques.
- Step 5: Emphasize the importance of patient privacy.
- Step 6: Discuss what is meant by tolerance.
- Review the procedures for moving the head:
  - Head flexion and extension
  - Right/left rotation
  - Right/left flexion
  - Hyperextension and extension (p. 784)

ACTIVITY

Practice the head movements yourself, as if you were engaged in active ROM.

Procedure Tip

21.4 Range of Motion, continued

- Review the procedures for moving the shoulders:
  - Shoulder flexion and extension
  - Shoulder abduction and adduction
  - Internal and external rotation of the shoulder
- Review the procedures for moving the elbows:
  - Elbow flexion and extension
  - Forearm pronation and supination
- Review the procedures for moving the wrist:
  - Wrist flexion and extension
  - Ulnar and radial deviation (p. 785)

ACTIVITY

Make a glossary of terms used to describe range of motion procedures. Break the terms into their word elements and include definitions. Terms that should be in the glossary include flexion, extension, pronation, supination, abduction, adduction, internal rotation, and external rotation. Include other terms as well.

Procedure 21.4 Range of Motion (continued)

Procedure (cont)

Hyperextension and Extension

10. Place the pillow under the shoulders and gently support the head in a backward tilt and return to straight position. Readjust pillow under head when finished.

Shoulder Flexion and Extension

11. Raise one arm overhead keeping elbow straight. Return to side position. Repeat with other arm.

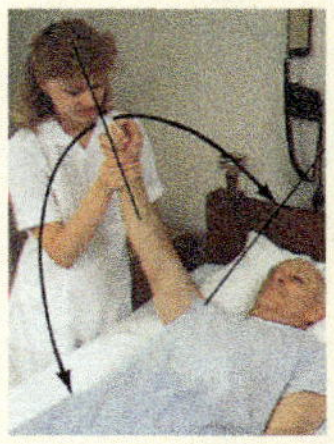

12. With the shoulder in abduction, flex the elbow and raise the entire arm over the head.

Shoulder Abduction and Adduction

13. Raise arm overhead, then lower, keep arm out to side. Repeat with other arm.

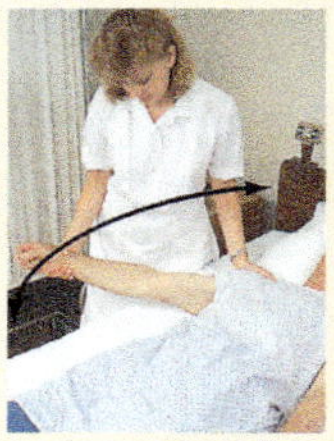

14. With the shoulder in abduction, flex the elbow and raise the arm over the head.

Internal and External Rotation of Shoulder

15. Roll entire arm toward body and away.

Elbow Flexion and Extension

16. Bend one hand and forearm toward shoulder (flexion) and straighten (extension). Repeat with other arm.

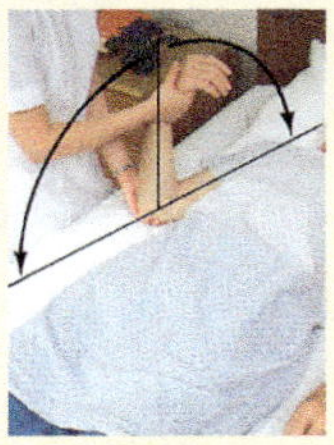

Forearm Pronation and Supination

17. Bend arm at elbow and rotate hand toward body (pronation), then rotate away from body (supination). Repeat with other arm.

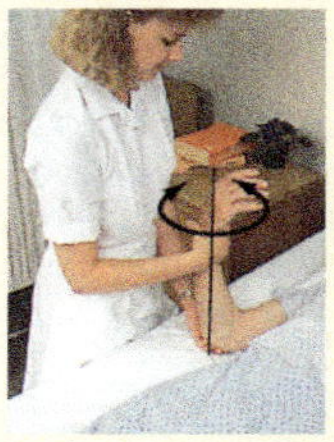

Wrist Flexion and Extension

18. Bend hand at wrist toward shoulder (flex), then gently force backward past a level position with arm (extension) to below arm level (hyperextension). Repeat with other hand.

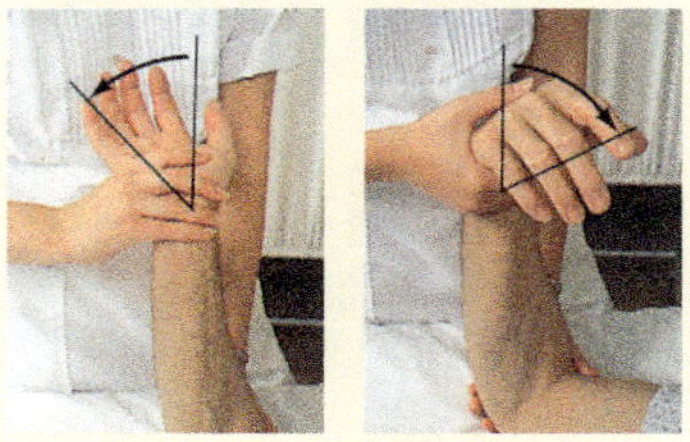

(continued)

Procedure 21.4 **Range of Motion (continued)**

Procedure (cont)

Ulnar and Radial Deviation

19. Holding hand straight, move toward thumb (radial deviation), then move hand toward little finger (ulnar deviation). Repeat with other hand.

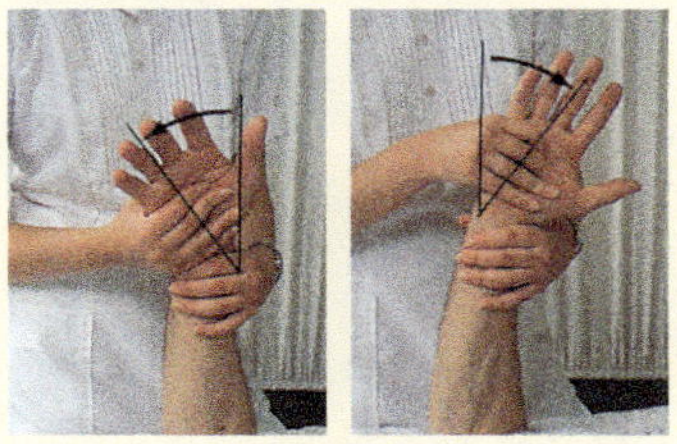

Finger Flexion and Extension

20. Bend thumb and fingers into hand making a fist (flexion), then open hand by straightening fingers and thumb (extension). Repeat with other hand.

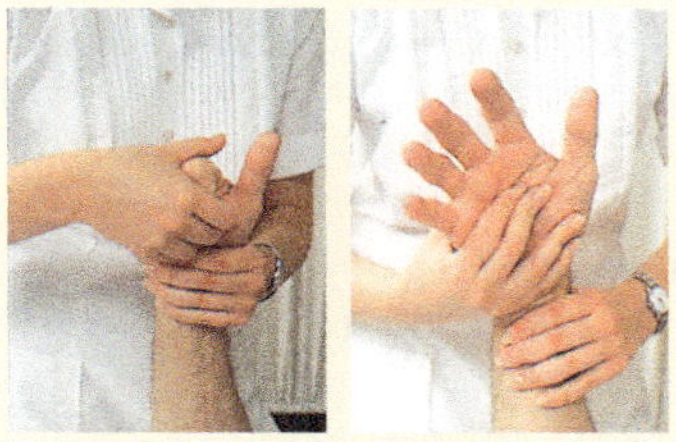

21. Move thumb away from hand (abduct), then toward hand (adduct). Repeat with other hand.

Finger/Thumb Opposition

22. Move thumb toward little finger, touch tips. Touch tip of thumb to each finger. Open hand each time. Repeat with other hand.

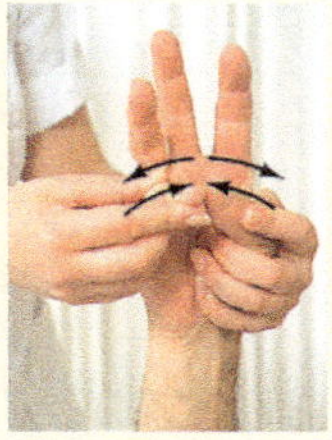

Finger Adduction and Abduction

23. Keeping fingers straight, separate them (abduction), then bring them together (adduction). Repeat with other hand.

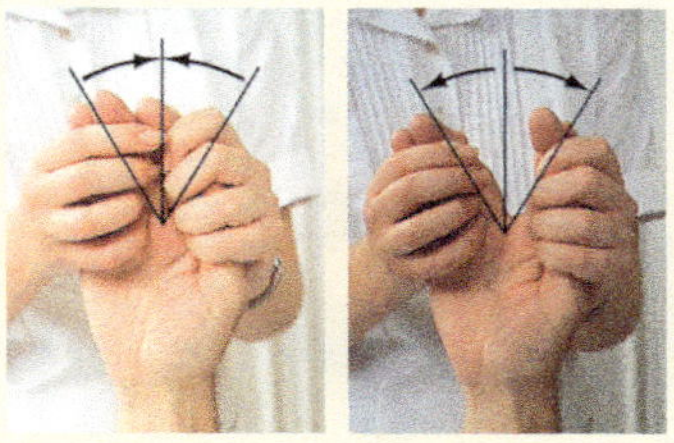

Hip/Knee Flexion and Extension

24. Raise leg, bend knee, then return to bed straightening knee. Repeat with other leg.

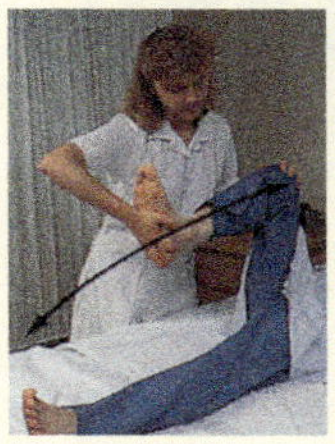

Straight Leg Raising

25. Keep knee straight. Slowly raise and lower leg. Repeat with other leg.

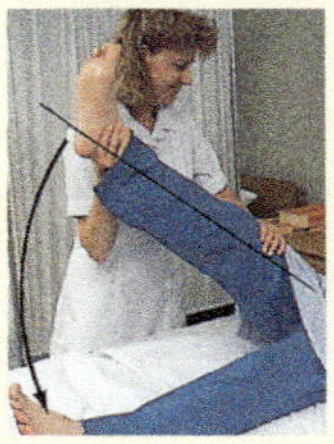

(continued)

Procedure Tip

21.4 Range of Motion, continued

- Review the procedures for moving the fingers:
  - Finger flexion and extension
  - Finger/thumb opposition
  - Finger adduction and abduction
- Review the procedures for moving hips and knees:
  - Hip/knee flexion and extension
  - Straight leg raising
  - Hip abduction and adduction (p. 786)
  - Lateral and medial hip rotation (p. 786)

Procedure Tip

21.4 Range of Motion, continued

- Review the procedures for moving the ankles, feet, and toes:
  - Ankle dorsiflexion and plantar flexion
  - Toe flexion and extension
- Step 36: Emphasize the importance of proper handwashing.
- Step 37: Emphasize the importance of monitoring and observing the patient.

PROCEDURE PRACTICE

- Demonstrate the steps for Procedure 21.4, Range of Motion, as many times as necessary, or ask students to demonstrate the steps. Have students practice and perform the procedure until they are competent.

ACTIVITY

Make a chart or table listing the different range-of-motion activities and a condition for which each one might be used.

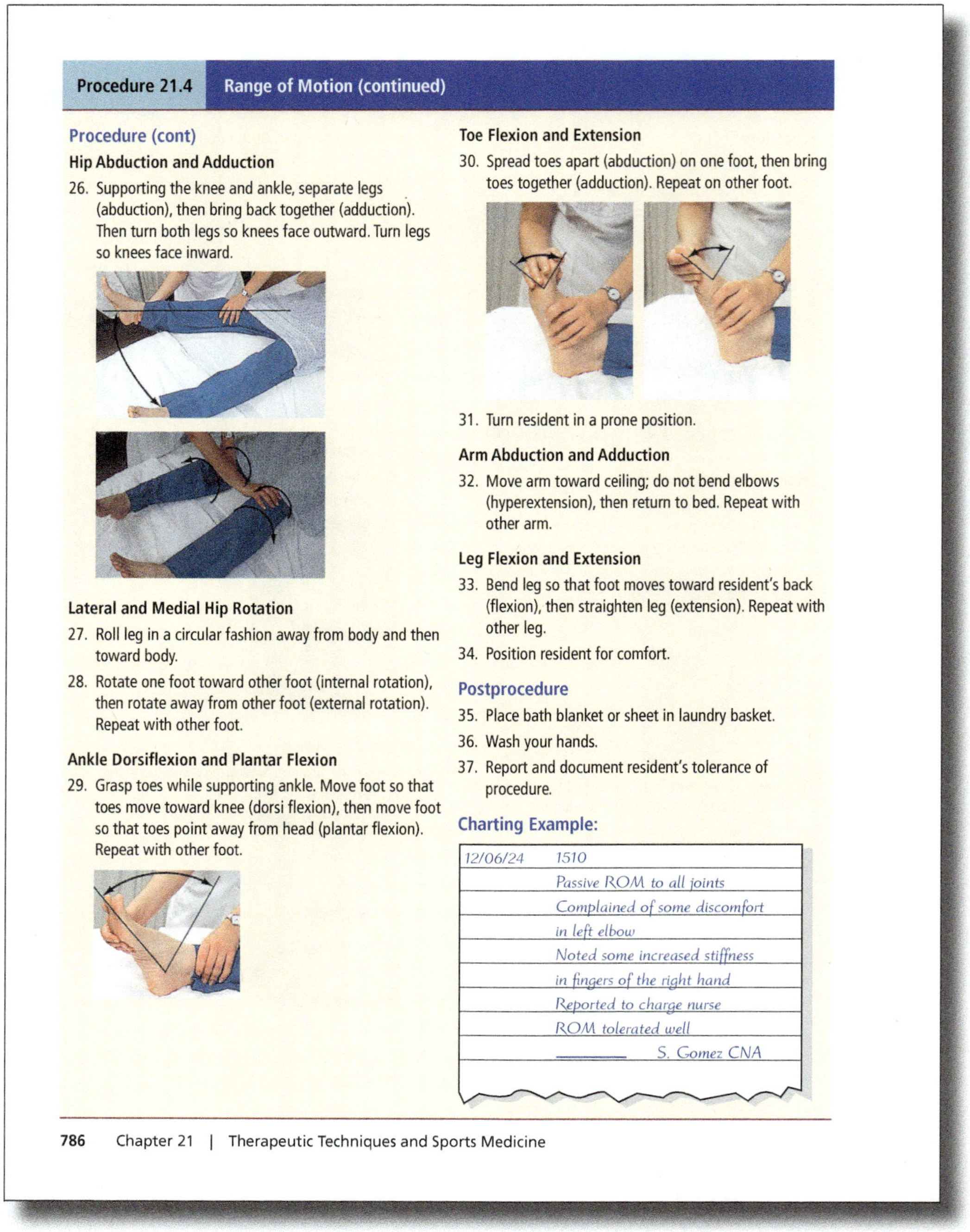

Procedure 21.4 Range of Motion (continued)

Procedure (cont)

Hip Abduction and Adduction

26. Supporting the knee and ankle, separate legs (abduction), then bring back together (adduction). Then turn both legs so knees face outward. Turn legs so knees face inward.

Lateral and Medial Hip Rotation

27. Roll leg in a circular fashion away from body and then toward body.
28. Rotate one foot toward other foot (internal rotation), then rotate away from other foot (external rotation). Repeat with other foot.

Ankle Dorsiflexion and Plantar Flexion

29. Grasp toes while supporting ankle. Move foot so that toes move toward knee (dorsi flexion), then move foot so that toes point away from head (plantar flexion). Repeat with other foot.

Toe Flexion and Extension

30. Spread toes apart (abduction) on one foot, then bring toes together (adduction). Repeat on other foot.
31. Turn resident in a prone position.

Arm Abduction and Adduction

32. Move arm toward ceiling; do not bend elbows (hyperextension), then return to bed. Repeat with other arm.

Leg Flexion and Extension

33. Bend leg so that foot moves toward resident's back (flexion), then straighten leg (extension). Repeat with other leg.
34. Position resident for comfort.

Postprocedure

35. Place bath blanket or sheet in laundry basket.
36. Wash your hands.
37. Report and document resident's tolerance of procedure.

Charting Example:

12/06/24	1510
	Passive ROM to all joints
	Complained of some discomfort
	in left elbow
	Noted some increased stiffness
	in fingers of the right hand
	Reported to charge nurse
	ROM tolerated well
	S. Gomez CNA

786 Chapter 21 | Therapeutic Techniques and Sports Medicine

Procedure 21.5 Wrapping/Taping an Ankle

BACKGROUND: Tape and elastic bandages are used to provide support and strength for a joint such as the ankle, elbow, wrist, or shoulder. Tape may be used for support in an athletic setting but caution must be used to avoid constriction of the circulatory system or worsening of any swelling that might be present in an injured joint.

The bandage is a continuous strip of elasticized material that is wound on itself to form a cylinder or roll. The common name used for these bandages is **Ace**. These bandages vary in width from 1 to 6 inches.

ALERT: Follow Standard Precautions

Preprocedure

1. Identify the patient and joint which requires the use of a supportive bandage. Check the physician's order for any special instructions. Gather the appropriate bandage.
2. Wash hands. Put on gloves.
3. Explain the procedure to the patient. Assist the patient to a comfortable position that provides easy access to the affected joint.

Procedure

4. Remove any old bandage and discard. If the bandage is to be reused, it may be unwound by keeping the loose end together and passing it as a ball from one hand to the other while unwinding it. Assess the joint for mobility and pain.
5. Clean the area before reapplying bandage. Make sure skin is dry before re-wrapping.
6. To begin, the free end of the bandage roll is held in place with one hand while the other hand passes the roll around the top middle of the ankle and then around the back of the Achilles tendon. After the bandage is anchored, the roll is passed or tolled around the ankle.
7. After the bandage is anchored, the roll is passed or rolled under the foot and back up the outside of the ankle, taking care to exert equal tension in all turns. There should be even overlapping of one-half to two-thirds the width of each bandage, except for the circular turn.
8. The figure-of-eight turn is most effective for use around joints such as the ankle. The figure-of-eight turns consists of making oblique overlapping turns that ascend and descend alternatively.

Postprocedure

9. Assure that the patient is comfortable and has no other needs before leaving the area.
10. Wash hands.
11. Document the appearance of the joint, any discomfort present and the application of the new bandage.

Charting Example:

12/06/24	1300
	Reapplied bandage to left ankle
	Joint appears swollen
	Slight discomfort was reported
	during the process
	Reported to charge nurse
	S. Gomez CNA

Therapeutic Techniques and Sports Medicine | Chapter 21 787

Procedure Tip

21.5 Wrapping/Taping an Ankle

- Review the background information, explaining that wrapping an ankle provides support for the injured joint.
- Emphasize the importance of not wrapping too tightly.
- Emphasize the importance of following Standard Precautions.
- Review the preprocedure steps.
- Step 1: Emphasize the importance of carefully reading the physician's order.
- Step 2: Emphasize the importance of proper handwashing and wearing gloves.
- Step 3: Emphasize the importance of effective communication techniques.
- Review the procedure steps.
- Step 4: Explain what is meant by "assess the joint."
- Step 5: Emphasize the importance of wrapping dry skin.
- Review the postprocedure steps.
- Step 10: Emphasize the importance of proper handwashing.
- Step 11: Review proper observation and reporting procedures.

ACTIVITY

Teach a friend or family member how to correctly wrap an ankle.

PROCEDURE PRACTICE

- Demonstrate the steps for Procedure 21.5, Wrapping/Taping an Ankle, as many times as necessary, or ask students to demonstrate the steps. Have students practice and perform the procedure until they are competent.

Procedure Tip

21.6 Elastic Hose (Antiembolism Hose)

- Review the background information, explaining the importance of keeping blood from pooling in the legs.
- Emphasize the importance of following Standard Precautions.
- Review the preprocedure steps.
- Step 1: Emphasize the importance of proper handwashing.
- Step 2: Discuss the importance of using the correct size hose.
- Step 3: Emphasize the importance of effective communication techniques.
- Step 4: Emphasize the importance of patient privacy.
- Review the procedure steps.
- Step 9: Emphasize the importance of there being no wrinkles.
- Review the postprocedure steps.
- Step 12: Emphasize the importance of proper handwashing.
- Step 13: Review proper observation and reporting procedures.
- Step 14: Emphasize the importance of removing and reapplying the hose periodically.

PROCEDURE PRACTICE

- Demonstrate the steps for Procedure 21.6, Elastic Hose (Antiembolism Hose), as many times as necessary, or ask students to demonstrate the steps. Have students practice and perform the procedure until they are competent.

Procedure 21.6 Elastic Hose (Antiembolism Hose)

BACKGROUND: Elastic hose help prevent blood from pooling in the legs, thus reducing the possibility of developing phlebitis.

ALERT: Follow Standard Precautions

Preprocedure

1. Wash hands.
2. Select elastic hose. Check to be sure that they are the correct size and length.
3. Identify resident and explain procedure to patient.
4. Provide for patient 's privacy.
5. Have resident lie down; expose one leg at a time.

Procedure

6. Hold the hose with both hands at top and roll toward toe end. Turn stockings inside-out, at least to heel area.
7. Place hose over toes, positioning opening at base of toes unless toes are to be covered. The raised seams should be on outside.
8. Pull top of stocking over foot, heel, and leg. Move patient's foot and leg gently and naturally. Avoid forcing and overextending limbs and joints.
9. Check to be sure that the stocking is applied evenly and smoothly. There must be no wrinkles.

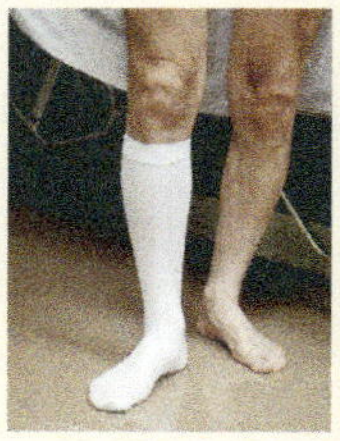

10. Repeat on opposite leg.

Postprocedure

11. Make patient comfortable, lower bed and raise side rails. Make sure call bell is within reach of patient.
12. Wash hands.
13. Record the following in the medical record:
    a. Date and time applied
    b. Any skin changes, temperature change, or swelling
14. Remove and reapply at least once every 8 hours, or more often if necessary.

Charting Example:

12/06/24	*1300*
	Elastic hose applied to right leg
	No skin changes
	S. Gomez CNA

788 Chapter 21 | Therapeutic Techniques and Sports Medicine

ACTIVITY

Use the Internet or a reference book to identify two or three conditions that might require the patient to wear an antiembolism hose. Explain the condition, and how the hose might help in treatment.

Guarding Techniques

Use **guarding techniques** when moving patients from place to place. These techniques protect the patient while transferring a patient from the bed to a **gurney** or chair, chair to a chair, chair to a toilet, or commode and back again. You use a variety of techniques to transfer the patient:

- **Pivot technique.** (Figure 21.2) You generally use this technique when moving a patient who can bear weight on at least one foot. It works best when moving from a bed or chair to a chair, toilet, or commode and back again. Normally this technique involves one person, using a transfer belt to help the patient.

guarding techniques
(GARD ing TEK neek)
Ways to protect a patient when he or she is being moved.

gurney
(ger NEE)
A metal stretcher with wheeled legs, often used in hospitals to transport patients.

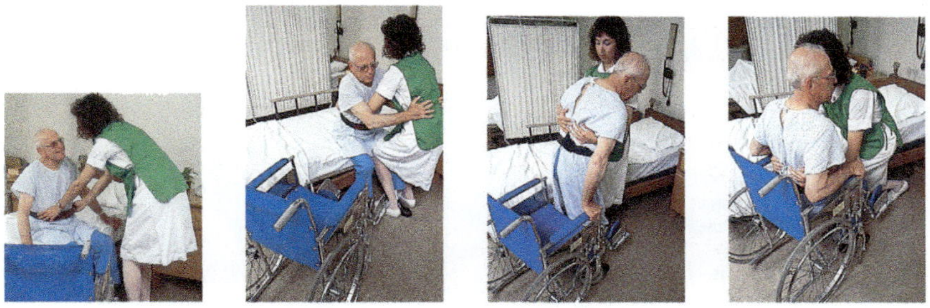

Figure 21.2
Transferring a patient from a bed to a wheelchair using the pivot technique. Why would you use the pivot technique?

- **Sliding technique.** You use sliding when a patient needs to be moved and cannot get up or bear weight on either foot. It works best when moving from bed to gurney, chair, commode, or toilet and back again. Paraplegic and quadriplegic patients may use a flat boardlike device to slide on. This provides security and decreases the chance of separation between chairs and bed and so on.

  Slide boards/transfer boards should be used when transferring between equal height surfaces. Slide boards should also be used to facilitate transfer to a wheelchair and for a patient with excessive weakness in their lower limbs.
- **Lifting technique.** Use this technique when there is ample help and strength to support the patient fully while moving him or her from one support to another. Make sure you keep your back straight, avoid twisting, stay close to the patient and keep a smooth flow of action (no jerking motions).

You also use guarding techniques when the patient is ambulating. All patients who can support themselves are encouraged to walk alone or with the assistance of another person. Patients who are uncomfortable usually resist having to move. Your encouragement is needed to keep their body functions as normal as possible. There are a variety of techniques you may use:

Teaching Tips

- Explain that guarding techniques are used when moving a patient from place to place, such as:
  - Bed to gurney or chair
  - Chair to bed
  - Gurney to bed
  - Chair to chair
  - Chair to a toilet
  - Back to a chair
- Explain that guarding techniques protect both the client and the health care worker.
- Discuss the main types of guarding techniques:
  - Pivot: Patient can bear weight on at least one foot
  - Sliding: Patient cannot get up or bear weight on either foot
  - Lifting: Patient cannot get up or bear weight, and there is enough help and strength to safely support patient fully

Figure Focus

21.2 Transferring a patient from a bed to a wheelchair using the pivot technique. Why would you use the pivot technique?

Answer: You would use the pivot technique to move a patient if the patient is able to bear weight on at least one foot. You would use a guarding technique to protect the patient and the health care worker.

ACTIVITY

Use the Internet or a reference book to identify two or three problems that might affect the health care worker if he or she does not use proper guarding techniques when moving a patient.

Teaching Tips

- Explain the guarding techniques used during ambulation:
  - A guarding belt (walking or gait belt)
  - Some patients may need to hold on to you
  - Some patients may require two people to assist them
  - Patients may benefit from walking next to a rail
- Emphasize safety and the importance of injury prevention.
- Have a discussion with students on the necessary precautions.

Figure Focus

21.3 Some patients may need to hold on to you. Just your hand may be enough to steady them in those first few steps after a lengthy stay in bed. What precautions should you take when walking with a patient?

Answer: You should walk slowly, and continually observe and monitor how the patient is doing.

- A guarding belt (walking or gait belt) supports and helps the patient feel secure. You may support the patient by placing one hand on the side of the gait belt and the other hand behind the patient holding onto the belt.
- Some patients may require two people to assist them. One person on each side of the patient should hold each arm and hold the person securely around the waist.
- Walking next to a rail is helpful. Patients often feel insecure when they are dependent on another person for support. A solid railing provides the extra security they need.

Safety is very important at all times. (**Figure 21.3**) The patient may lose his or her balance, feel faint, or the legs can collapse. If the patient falls, prevent injury by helping the resident to the floor. Protect yourself from injury by using good body mechanics. Stay with the patient and call for help. A licensed nurse should evaluate the patient before moving him or her. Ask for help when lifting a patient from the floor.

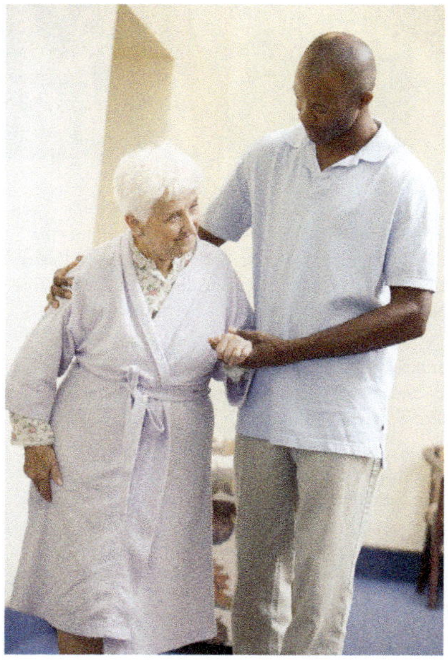

Figure 21.3
Some patients may need to hold on to you. Just your hand may be enough to steady them in those first few steps after a lengthy stay in bed. What precautions should you take when walking with a patient?

790 Chapter 21 | Therapeutic Techniques and Sports Medicine

Procedure 21.7 **Ambulating with a Gait Belt**

BACKGROUND: Using a **gait belt** protects the patient from falling when ambulating. It ensures the safety and security of the patient. Gait belts also decrease caregiver injuries and enable the caregiver to assist heavy patients they would not be able to assist otherwise.

Note: Caregivers are sometimes seen assisting a patient by holding them at the axillary area and without a gait belt. This type of assistance could result in the subluxation (partial dislocation) of the shoulder joint. If a patient cannot ambulate independently, a gait belt should always be used.

ALERT: Follow Standard Precautions

Preprocedure

1. Wash hands.
2. Assemble equipment:
   a. Gait belt/walking belt (correct size)
   b. Patient's robe
   c. Patient's footwear
3. Identify patient.
4. Explain what you are going to do.
5. Provide for privacy and lower side rail.
6. Assist patient to sitting position on side of bed.
7. Encourage patient to take a few deep breaths and ask if he or she feels dizzy. (If dizziness is present, let the patient sit a while before walking.)
8. Assist patient with robe and slippers.
9. Secure gait belt around patient's waist over clothing.
10. Tighten belt and buckle securely. Position buckle/clasp slightly off center. Check to see if patient can breathe easily and that breasts are above the belt. (Belt is too tight if you cannot put two fingers under it.)

Procedure

11. Stand in front of patient with broad base of support.
12. Instruct patient to put hands on your shoulder. Position yourself to ensure the safety of both yourself and the patient during transfer (e.g., knees bent, feet apart, back straight). Place hands under side of belt. Give signal for patient to stand.
13. Ease patient to a standing position and hold handgrip securely at back of belt.
14. Keep your back straight /straighten knees as patient stands. Move to position behind patient. Keep one hand on side of belt and other hand should grasp the back of the belt.

    TIP: If patient is confused, grip the gait belt from underneath in the back, holding the patient's arm nearest the caregiver, and pointing the patient's arm in the direction you want to move. This helps the patient move with you instead of against you.
15. Ambulate patient as ordered.
16. Observe patient for weakness or discomfort.
17. Return patient to room and make comfortable.
18. Remove belt, help take off robe and slippers, position patient in bed, raise siderails, and make sure call bell is in place.

Postprocedure

19. Document and report patient's tolerance of procedure.
20. Return gait belt to storage area so that it will be available for the next procedure.
21. Wash hands.

gait belt
(geyt belt)
A safety device used to move a patient from one place to another; also used to help hold up a weak person while they walk.

Therapeutic Techniques and Sports Medicine | Chapter 21 791

ACTIVITY

Create a poster showing the proper way to use a gait belt with an ambulatory patient.

PROCEDURE PRACTICE

- Demonstrate the steps for Procedure 21.7, Ambulating with a Gait Belt, as many times as necessary, or ask students to demonstrate the steps. Have students practice and perform the procedure until they are competent.

Procedure Tip

21.7 Ambulating with a Gait Belt

- Review the background information, explaining the importance of using a gait belt when assisting a patient to ambulate.
- Emphasize the importance of following Standard Precautions.
- Review the preprocedure steps.
- Step 1: Emphasize the importance of proper handwashing.
- Step 2: Review the equipment list.
- Step 4: Emphasize the importance of effective communication techniques.
- Step 5: Emphasize the importance of patient privacy.
- Steps 9 and 10: Emphasize the importance of fitting and securing the gait belt correctly.
- Review the procedure steps.
- Step 11: Explain and demonstrate "broad base of support."
- Step 16: Emphasize the importance of observation and monitoring of the patient during ambulation.
- Review the postprocedure steps.
- Step 19: Review proper observation and reporting procedures.
- Step 21: Emphasize the importance of proper handwashing.

Teaching Tips

- Discuss the types of commonly used rehabilitation equipment:
  - Ambulation devices assistant patients to walk
  - Transporting devices assist in moving patients from one place to another
  - Adaptive-assistive devices assist patients in performing everyday tasks
- Discuss commonly used ambulation devices:
  - Canes
  - Crutches
  - Walkers
  - Braces
  - Prosthetics

Figure Focus

21.4 Ambulation devices. What is one advantage and one disadvantage to having a walker with wheels?

Answer: A wheeled walker is much easier to use because a person with limited arm strength does not have to continually pick up the walker to move forward. However, it is possible for a wheeled walker to "run away" from the patient, which might cause the patient to fall.

Rehabilitation Equipment

Ambulation Devices

ambulation
(AM byuh lay shun)
The ability to walk and move around freely.

Ambulation devices assist patients to walk. (**Figure 21.4**) Some of the most common devices include canes, crutches, walkers, braces, and prosthetic devices.

Canes provide a third base of support for patients who are slightly unstable on their feet. Use a cane when patients are:

- Slightly weaker on one side
- Easily thrown off balance
- Insecure walking alone

Special considerations to keep in mind when preparing a cane for use include the following:

- The patient's height
- Use of a single-foot cane or multifoot cane
- Condition of rubber tips
- Weight and appearance of the cane

crutch
(kruhch)
A support used by physically disabled people as an aid in walking. It usually fits under the armpit and is often used in pairs.

Crutches provide support and stability by promoting use of the hands and arms more than the legs. Use them when patients are able to bear weight:

- On one foot or leg
- Only partially on one leg or on both feet and legs

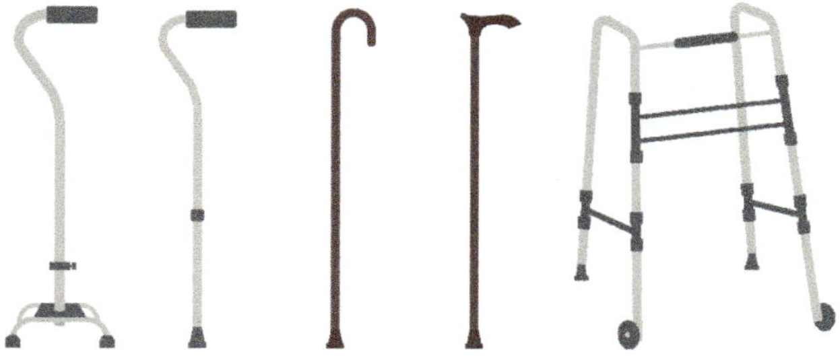

Figure 21.4
Ambulation devices. What is one advantage and one disadvantage to having a walker with wheels?

TEAMWORK

Divide the class into teams of five to seven students. Have each team create signs showing the name of the three types of commonly used rehabilitation equipment (ambulatory devices, transporting devices, adaptive-assistance devices). You read a device name out loud, and each team has 10 seconds to hold up the sign indicating the type of device it is. Award a point to each team that holds up the correct sign.

Procedure 21.8 Walking with a Cane

BACKGROUND: Safe canes, if correctly sized, and careful safety instruction protect the patient from falls or injuries.
ALERT: Follow Standard Precautions

Preprocedure

1. Wash hands.
2. Assemble equipment:
   a. Cane in good repair and with rubber tip
   b. Patient's/client's footwear
   c. Patient's/client's robe
3. Identify patient.
4. Assist patient with shoes and robe.
5. Explain what you are going to do.
6. Provide privacy as appropriate.
7. Assist to sitting position, feet resting on floor. Secure gait belt snug enough to provide support and loose enough to provide comfort. Place cane in reach.
8. Position patient in a standing position (have a co-worker help you if necessary).
9. Check height of cane. Top of cane should be at the patient's hip joint.

Procedure

10. Check arm position at side of body and hold top of cane. Arm should be bent at a 25 to 30° angle.
11. Have patient hold cane in hand on strongest side of body (unaffected side). Walk mostly beside, but slightly to the rear of the patient, while grasping gait belt to provide support. Observe for discomfort or weakness.
12. Assist patient as needed while ambulating. Most physicians order a standard gait procedure:
    a. With cane in hand on strongest side, move cane and weakest foot forward.
    b. Place body weight forward on cane and move strongest foot forward. (Patient will have cane's maximum support when this procedure is used when walking on flat surface, hill, or stairs. Remember: Weak leg and cane move together.)
13. When you have completed ordered ambulation, return patient to the starting place.

Postprocedure

14. Provide for patient's comfort.
15. Place cane in proper location. If patient is capable and physician permits ambulation without assistance, leave cane in a convenient place for patient.
16. Wash hands.
17. Report/document patient's tolerance of procedure.
    a. Date
    b. Time
    c. Ambulated with cane (e.g., 15 minutes in hall)
    d. How tolerated
    e. Signature and classification

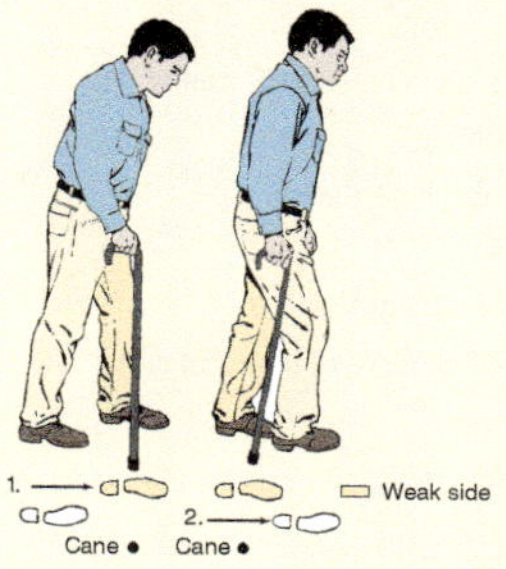

Charting Example:

11/03/24	2100
	Height of cane correct
	Checked for safety
	Instructions given with emphasis
	on using the cane on the
	affected side
	Ambulated without difficulty 15
	minutes in hall
	Tolerated well
	J. Munoz student

Therapeutic Techniques and Sports Medicine | Chapter 21 793

Procedure Tip

21.8 Walking with a Cane

- Review the background information, emphasizing the importance of safety consideration.
- Emphasize the importance of following Standard Precautions.
- Review the preprocedure steps.
- Step 1: Emphasize the importance of proper handwashing.
- Step 2: Review the equipment list.
- Step 5: Emphasize the importance of effective communication techniques.
- Step 6: Emphasize the importance of patient privacy.
- Step 7: Point out the use of a gait belt.
- Step 9: Emphasize the importance of fitting the cane to the patient.
- Review the procedure steps.
- Step 10: Emphasize the importance of proper positioning.
- Step 11: Emphasize the importance of observation and monitoring of the patient during ambulation.
- Review the postprocedure steps.
- Step 16: Emphasize the importance of proper handwashing.
- Step 17: Review proper observation and reporting procedures.

ACTIVITY

Imagine that you notice an elderly friend or relative having trouble with balance. Write a letter to this person, explaining why you think he or she should consider using a cane. Remember to use proper letter formatting, as well as effective communication techniques.

PROCEDURE PRACTICE

- Demonstrate the steps for Procedure 21.8, Walking with a Cane, as many times as necessary, or ask students to demonstrate the steps. Have students practice and perform the procedure until they are competent.

Procedure Tip

21.9 Walking with Crutches

- Review the background information, emphasizing the importance of safety.
- Emphasize the importance of following Standard Precautions.
- Review the preprocedure steps.
- Step 1: Emphasize the importance of proper handwashing.
- Step 2: Review the equipment list.
- Step 4: Emphasize the importance of effective communication techniques.
- Step 5: Emphasize the importance of patient privacy.
- Review the procedure steps.
- Step 6: Emphasize the importance of fitting the crutches to the patient.
- Step 7: Emphasize the importance of educating the patient on proper usage.

Special considerations when preparing crutches for use include the following:

- Adjusting their height for the patient. Keep in mind:
  - Axillary pressure—too much pressure causes injury
  - Hand level—position the handgrips to allow a slight bend of the elbows, like they are when you walk normally
- The patient's footwear (slippery soles, open toes, etc.)
- Condition of rubber tips, hand pads, and axillary pads
- Securing all joints on the crutches

Procedure 21.9 Walking with Crutches

BACKGROUND: Measuring crutches to fit properly and careful instruction in how to use crutches safely prevents injury.

ALERT: Follow Standard Precautions

Preprocedure

1. Wash hands.
2. Assemble equipment:
   a. Crutches in good repair with rubber tips
   b. Patient's footwear
   c. Patient's robe, if necessary
3. Identify patient.
4. Explain what you are going to do.
5. Help patient with shoes and robe. Provide privacy if needed.

Procedure

6. Check fit of crutches to patient:
   a. Have patient stand with crutches in place. (Ask a co-worker to assist if necessary.)
   b. Position foot of crutches about 4 inches to side of patient's foot and slightly forward of foot.
   c. Check distance between underarm and crutch underarm rest. It should be about 2 inches.
   d. Check angle of patient's arm. When hand is on hand rest bar and crutches are in walking position, arms should be at a 30° angle.
7. Remind patient that the hands support most of the body weight, not the underarms (axilla).
8. Assist patient to ambulate following gait method ordered. There are a variety of crutch walking gaits. The following will provide guidelines to the most commonly used:
   a. Three-point gait (beginners):
      (1) One leg is weight-bearing.
      (2) Place both crutches forward along with non-weight-bearing foot. Weight will be supported primarily by weight-bearing foot.
      (3) Shift weight to hands on crutches and move weight-bearing foot forward.

(continued)

794 Chapter 21 | Therapeutic Techniques and Sports Medicine

TEAMWORK

Bring in—or have students bring in—multiple pairs of crutches of different sizes. Practice fitting them to the students in the class.

Procedure 21.9 | **Walking with Crutches (continued)**

Procedure (cont)

b. Four-point gait (beginners) (see following figure):
   (1) Both legs are weight-bearing.
   (2) Place one crutch forward.
   (3) Move foot on opposite side of body forward, parallel with forward crutch.
   (4) Place other crutch forward and parallel with first crutch.
   (5) Move other foot forward so that it rests next to first foot.

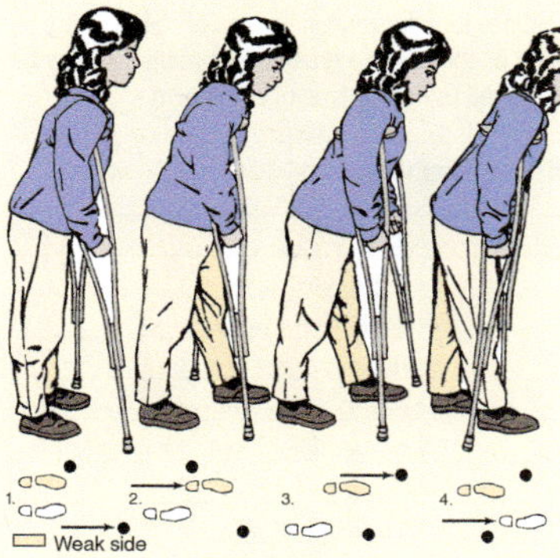

Four-point crutch gait

c. Two-point gait (advanced) (see following figure):
   (1) Both legs are weight-bearing.
   (2) Place one crutch forward and move opposite foot forward with it.
   (3) Place other crutch forward and parallel with first crutch. Then move opposite foot forward so that it is even with other foot.

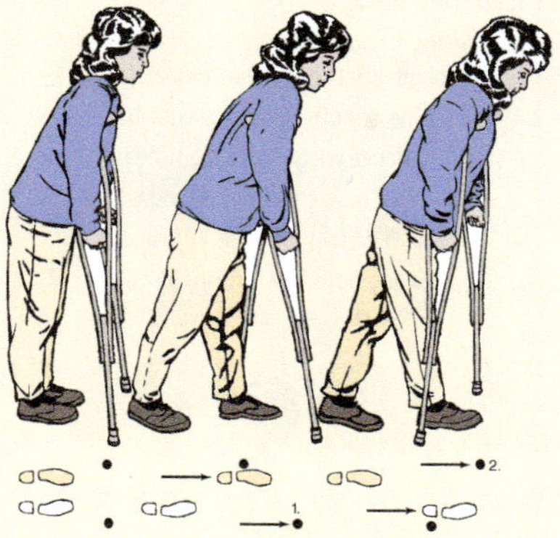

Two-point crutch gait

d. Swing-to gait (arm and shoulder strength are needed) (see following figure):
   (1) One or both legs are weight-bearing.
   (2) Balance weight on weight-bearing limb.
   (3) Place both crutches forward.
   (4) Shift weight to hands on crutches.
   (5) Swing both feet forward until parallel with crutches.

CAUTION: Placing crutches too far forward can result in a fall!

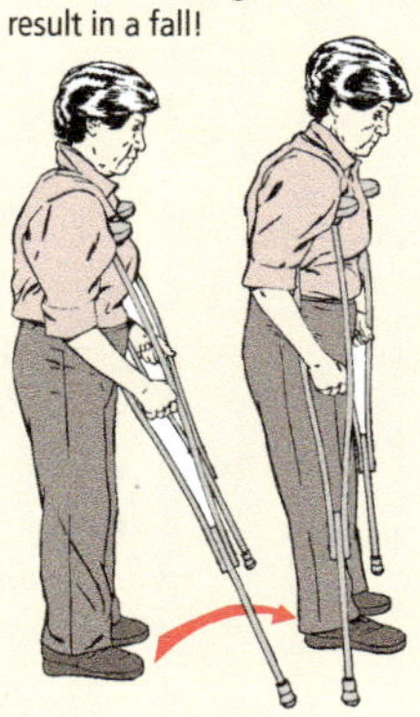
Swing-to gait

(continued)

Therapeutic Techniques and Sports Medicine | Chapter 21 795

Procedure Tip

21.9 Walking with Crutches, continued

- Step 8: Review the different crutch walking gaits:
  - Three-point gait (beginners)
  - Four-point gait (beginners)
  - Two-point gait (advanced)
  - Swing-to gait (must have shoulder and arm strength)
  - Swing-through gait (advanced; must have shoulder and arm strength)

CUSTOMIZED INSTRUCTION

Less Advanced Students

Be sure to allow adequate time for less advanced students to practice and demonstrate the correct procedures.

Procedure Tip

21.9 Walking with Crutches, continued

- Review the postprocedure steps.
- Step 11: Emphasize the importance of proper handwashing.
- Step 12: Review proper observation and reporting procedures.

PROCEDURE PRACTICE

- Demonstrate the steps for Procedure 21.9, Walking with Crutches, as many times as necessary, or ask students to demonstrate the steps. Have students practice and perform the procedure until they are competent.

Procedure 21.9 **Walking with Crutches (continued)**

Procedure (cont)

e. Swing-through gait (advanced: arm and shoulder strength are needed) (see following figure):
   (1) One or both legs are weight-bearing.
   (2) Balance weight on weight-bearing limb(s).
   (3) Place both crutches forward.
   (4) Shift weight to hands on crutches.
   (5) Swing both feet forward just ahead of crutches.

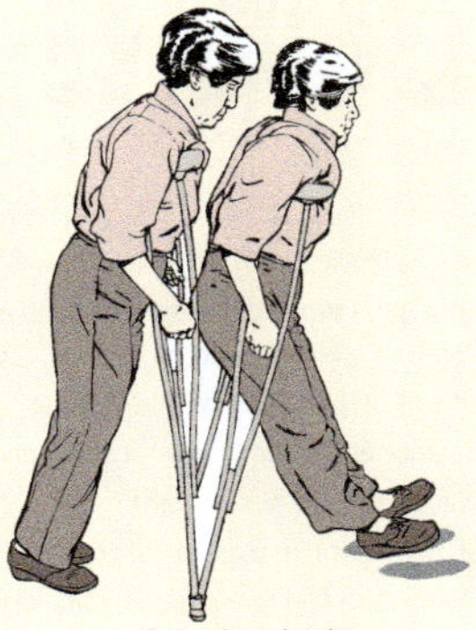

Swing-through gait

9. Return to room.

Postprocedure

10. Ensure that patient is comfortable.
11. Wash hands.
12. Record the following:
    a. Date
    b. Time
    c. Distance ambulated
    d. How tolerated
    e. Signature and classification

NOTE: Patients with memory loss (dementia) are not good candidates for education in the use of canes, crutches, or walkers as they cannot retain information and may be endangered using this type of equipment.

Charting Example:

12/10/24 2000
Measured crutches for
correct size and safety
Instructed patient in safe
use to prevent additional injury
Ambulated for 15 minutes in hallway
Tolerated well
J. Munoz CNA

walker
(WAH ker)
A waist-high four-legged framework of lightweight metal, for use by a weak or disabled person as a support while walking.

Walkers provide support and stability. Use them when patients are:

- Relearning to walk
- On limited weight-bearing
- Unstable on their feet

Special considerations to keep in mind when preparing walkers for patient use include the following:

- Adjusting the walker to the patient's height
- Assuring that the patient wears supportive shoes
- Securing all joints on walker
- Condition of rubber tips

To use a walker, the patient must be able to use their hands and arms to adapt properly to these devices. However, if the patient has paralysis of one side of their body (hemi paralysis) there are hemiwalkers made specifically for their use.

796 Chapter 21 | Therapeutic Techniques and Sports Medicine

ACTIVITY

Make a chart or table comparing ambulation devices. Include information about the type of patient each device would be suitable for, safety precautions, and considerations for fitting the devices properly.

Procedure 21.10 Walking with a Walker

BACKGROUND: It is important to measure a walker to fit properly and give the patient careful safety instruction in order to prevent injury.

ALERT: Follow Standard Precautions

Preprocedure

1. Wash hands.
2. Assemble equipment:
   a. Walker in good condition
   b. Patient's footwear
   c. Patient's robe if necessary
3. Identify patient.
4. Tell patient what you are going to do.
5. Check walker for safety.
6. Help put on proper and safe footwear and robe if necessary.
7. Assist to sitting position with feet resting on the floor.
8. Secure gait belt snug enough to provide support and loose enough to provide comfort. Place walker within reach.

Procedure

9. Stand patient up with walker. (Ask a co-worker to help if necessary.) Remind patient to stand as straight as possible.
10. Check to see if walker fits patient properly:
    a. Walker's handgrips should be at top of patient's leg or bend of leg at hip joint.
    b. Arm should be at a 25 to 30° angle.
11. Gripping gait belt from behind, assist patient to ambulate as ordered. Basic guidelines for walking with a walker are as follows:
    a. Patient begins by standing inside walker frame.
    b. Patient lifts walker (never slides) and places back legs of walker parallel with toes (never ahead of toes).
    c. Patient shifts weight onto hands and walker (for balance and support).
    d. Patient then walks into walker.
    e. Place yourself just to the side and slightly behind patient. This position will allow you to observe and be close enough to assist if necessary.
    f. Ambulate as ordered, observing for correct use of walker.
12. When you have completed the ordered ambulation, return patient to his or her starting place.

Postprocedure

13. Provide for patient's comfort with call signal in reach.
14. Place walker in proper location. If patient is capable and physician permits ambulation without assistance, leave walker in a convenient place for patient.
15. Wash hands.
16. Report/document patient's tolerance of procedure.
17. Record the following:
    a. Date
    b. Time
    c. Distance and amount of time ambulated
    d. How tolerated
    e. Signature and classification

Charting Example:

12/04/24 0800
Checked walker for safety measures
Instructed patient in correct use
of walker
Ambulated in hallway for 10 minutes
Patient complained of dizziness
initially
Dangled from bed until dizziness subsided
Tolerated with some difficulty with fatigue
Patient stated "I feel really tired
after using the walker."
J. Munoz P.T. Aide

Therapeutic Techniques and Sports Medicine | Chapter 21 797

Procedure Tip

21.10 Walking with a Walker

- Review the background information, emphasizing the importance of proper fit for safety.
- Emphasize the importance of following Standard Precautions.
- Review the preprocedure steps.
- Step 1: Emphasize the importance of proper handwashing.
- Step 2: Review the equipment list.
- Step 4: Emphasize the importance of effective communication techniques.
- Step 5: Review safety considerations.
- Step 8: Point out the use of a gait belt.
- Review the procedure steps.
- Step 10: Emphasize the importance of proper fit and positioning.
- Review the postprocedure steps.
- Step 15: Emphasize the importance of proper handwashing.
- Steps 16 and 17: Review proper observation and reporting procedures.

PROCEDURE PRACTICE

- Demonstrate the steps for Procedure 21.10, Walking with a Walker, as many times as necessary, or ask students to demonstrate the steps. Have students practice and perform the procedure until they are competent.

TEAMWORK

Divide the class into two teams and have a debate about whether patients should use walkers with wheels or walkers without wheels. Remind students of the purpose and format of a debate. You be the judge, or invite another class in to judge the debate. If possible, allow class time for teams to research and prepare their arguments.

Teaching Tips

- Review reasons a limb brace might be required:
  - Weakened joints or muscles
  - Injuries that need to be stabilized
- Review precautions for putting on a brace:
  - Braces are not meant to be shared
  - Braces may require padding
  - There is only one way to apply a brace
- Discuss types of prostheses:
  - Artificial limbs
  - Dentures
  - Glasses
  - Hearing aids
- Discuss precautions for putting on a prosthesis:
  - Have the right device
  - Rest the padded end against the patient
  - Check condition: clean, undamaged
  - Report irritations

Language Arts Link—Sports Medicine Careers

- You may want to provide a list of resources such as Web sites or local facilities that students can use to research this project.
- Remind students about your school's Internet policy, how to recognize a reputable online source, and to keep a list of sources for a bibliography.
- For evaluation, you should verify that the information is correct, and you should mark spelling and grammatical errors.

Some additional devices that aid in ambulation include the following:

Braces provide specific support for weakened muscle joints or immobilize an injured joint. Patients use them when they have:

- Weakened joints or muscles
- Injuries that need to be stabilized

Special considerations to keep in mind when preparing braces for a patient include the following:

- They are custom-made for each patient; they are not meant to be shared.
- They may require padding to protect the skin.
- There is only one way to apply a brace; be sure you know the correct way.

prosthesis
(pros thee sis)
An artificial body part such as a limb, tooth, or eye, used to replace a natural body part and minimize a disability.

A **prosthesis** is an artificial body part or an aid to a part of the body that minimizes a disability. When a body part is missing, the prosthesis gives a natural appearance and provides maximum usability for the person. The prosthesis most commonly dealt with in physical therapy is the artificial arm or leg. Special considerations to keep in mind when preparing a prosthesis for a patient include the following:

- You must have the right device.
- The end resting against the patient is padded.
- All straps must be in good condition.
- It is clean and the overall appearance is natural.
- Report tender areas at attachment site.

Language Arts Link

Sports Medicine Careers

Sports medicine is the specialty that deals with the diagnosis and treatment of injuries caused by exercise or sports. The injuries are often to the joints and muscles. A whole team of specialists deal with these types of injuries. They include athletic trainers, exercise physiologists, orthopedic surgeons, physical therapists, strength and conditioning specialists, and even dietitians.

Working with a partner, research the education, certification, licensure or degree, continuing education requirements, and salary potential for a sports medicine career. If possible, include in your analysis an interview with a sports medicine professional to identify how they became interested in this field, their current job responsibilities, and benefits of working in a sports medicine career.

After you've completed your research, create a document with several paragraphs on each career that you learned about. Be sure to proofread your work to see if you can improve it by making it clearer, more concise, or more effective. Check the spelling and grammar and correct any errors.

798 Chapter 21 | Therapeutic Techniques and Sports Medicine

Personal Wellness

Back Injuries

As a medical assistant, you will be called upon to support and to lift patients. It is essential that you always protect your back in the process.

You can often assist patients by yourself. Many times standby assistance for safety is all that is required. If you are unsure of patient status it is always best to ask another assistant to stand by to help if necessary when moving the patient.

Always use a gait belt if there are any doubts as to the patient's ability to ambulate independently. Explain to the patient that you are protecting the patient and yourself through this action. Be aware, that occasionally patients may unexpectedly fall or collapse, requiring you to support their entire weight. If a gait belt is in place you can gently lower the patient to the floor using good body mechanics:

- Take a wide stance to give yourself as much stability as possible. Use your legs, not your back, when lifting. Bend your knees and let your knees do the lifting.
- Try to avoid bending, leaning, stooping, and reaching. These positions make you vulnerable to injury.
- Keep your back straight. Don't twist it. If you need to turn the patient, swivel your hips or, better still, turn your feet.
- If you are lifting someone to or from a bed or wheelchair, make sure the wheels are locked before attempting the lift.

When you must lift a patient to assist the person in moving or in an emergency when the patient falls, think safety first. If something happens and you drop a patient, the person can be badly injured. If you attempt a lift and the weight is too much for you, you can seriously injure yourself.

What should you do if you know a patient is weak and unsteady and is too heavy for you to safely lift by yourself?

Transporting Devices

Transport devices include equipment to move patients from one place to another. The most common transporting devices are wheelchairs and gurneys. Gurneys and wheelchairs make it easy to move patients who are unable to walk.

Adaptive-Assistive Devices

Adaptive-assistive devices include equipment that helps a person perform daily activities. These devices range from special holders for silverware to devices that help people put on socks or button clothing.

Community

With a team of three others, visit an elementary or middle school class and show the students how to properly lift, bend, and turn to help reduce back injuries. Create a poster showing some of these techniques.

Oxygen Therapy

Some residents require oxygen to help them breathe. Concentrated oxygen helps these residents breathe more easily. The following are common ways to give oxygen therapy:

- **Nasal cannula.** A two-pronged tube that fits into the nostrils and is secured with an elastic strap that stretches around the back of the head.
- **Mask.** A plastic see-through mask that fits over the nose and mouth and is secured with an elastic strap that stretches around the back of the head.

Therapeutic Techniques and Sports Medicine | Chapter 21 799

CUSTOMIZED INSTRUCTION

More Advanced Students

Assign more advanced students to research developments in artificial limbs. Topics should include materials, computer chips, and movement. They should present their findings to the class.

Personal Wellness—Back Injuries

- Discuss importance of checking physician's orders before beginning any activity with a patient.
- Review the meaning of baseline function and current functional status.
- Review safety considerations, and emphasize that they protect the health care worker as well as the patient.
- Refer to Section 18.4 for more information on body mechanics.

What should you do if you know a patient is weak and unsteady and is too heavy for you to safely lift by yourself?

Answer: Ask another assistant to help when moving the patient. Use a gait belt during ambulation, and ask the other assistant to stand by to help in case you must lift the patient off the floor.

Teaching Tips

- Review the common ways of delivering oxygen therapy:
  - Nasal cannula
  - Mask

Community

- Encourage students to practice their presentation before visiting the other class.
- Remind students to prepare a presentation that is appropriate for the age of the students who will be in the audience.

Procedure Tip

21.11 Respiratory Therapy

- Review the background information, emphasizing that respiratory therapy should always be implemented by a trained respiratory therapist.
- Review the requirements and responsibilities of a respiratory therapist.
- Emphasize the importance of following Standard Precautions.
- Review the preprocedure steps.
- Step 1: Emphasize the importance of determining the respiratory baseline function.
- Step 2: Emphasize the importance of reviewing the physician's order.
- Step 3: Emphasize the importance of determining the health care worker's responsibilities.
- Review the procedure steps.
- Step 8: Emphasize the importance of patient education.
- Step 9: Emphasize the importance of monitoring the patient.
- Review the postprocedure steps.
- Steps 10 and 11: Review proper observation and reporting procedures.

PROCEDURE PRACTICE

- Demonstrate the steps for Procedure 21.11, Respiratory Therapy, as many times as necessary, or ask students to demonstrate the steps. Have students practice and perform the procedure until they are competent.

Procedure 21.11 Respiratory Therapy

BACKGROUND: Respiratory therapy is the provision of care dedicated to improving the pulmonary function of the patient. The provision of respiratory therapy has developed into a stand-alone discipline because of the specialized learning required to provide this care.

A respiratory therapist is trained in techniques that improve pulmonary function and oxygenation. Respiratory therapists may also be responsible for administering a variety of tests that measure lung function and for educating the patient about the use of various devices and machines prescribed by the physician.

The health care professional must have knowledge of respiratory physiology, the variables, and diseases that affect respiratory function. In some cases, the health care professional will be responsible for using specific equipment and protocols necessary to diagnose and treat respiratory problems.

ALERT: Follow Standard Precautions

Preprocedure

1. Determine the baseline function of the patient's respiratory system.
2. Consult the physician's orders to determine any specific respiratory treatment prescribed for the patient.
3. Determine the health care professional's responsibility for administering/supporting the treatment.

Procedure

4. Assess the patient's current respiratory status.
5. Review available documentation to determine when specific respiratory treatments were last delivered, and when they will be due again.
6. Determine what the health care professional's role is to be in assisting/promoting respiratory therapy.
7. Consult with the respiratory therapist for any necessary instructions on the use of equipment or procedures.
8. Encourage the patient to use good pulmonary techniques such as deep breathing, coughing, and incentive spirometry.

   NOTE: Incentive spirometry works to mimic natural sighing or yawning by encouraging the patient to take long, slow, deep breaths.
9. Provide continuous monitoring of the patient's respiratory status so that any decline in function can be addressed early and successfully.

Postprocedure

10. Collaborate with the physician and the respiratory therapist if there is a decline in the patient's respiratory status.
11. Document the respiratory assessment and any ongoing problems and their resolution in the medical chart.

800 Chapter 21 | Therapeutic Techniques and Sports Medicine

ACTIVITY

Research the career ladder of a respiratory therapist in your state. Look up the local educational requirements and certification policies. Using the information, write a want ad for a respiratory aide or respiratory therapist, including a starting salary.

You have specific responsibilities when you care for a resident on oxygen therapy, including the following:

- Ensuring that all oxygen safety rules are followed
- Checking the face and behind the ears to see if the strap is chafing and is a firm fit
- Cleaning the cannula, catheter, or mask and checking the skin for irritation
- Providing oral hygiene by moistening the lips and mouth frequently. Encourage fluid intake if allowed
- Keeping tubing free of kinks or blockage
- Checking flow rate and oxygen humidifier frequently
- Immediately reporting to supervisor any changes or problems, e.g., cyanosis (condition of having blue skin due to a lack of oxygen) or dyspnea (shortness of breath)

Career Connect

If possible, interview either a physical therapist, rehabilitation therapist, or a sports medicine physician. Prepare a list of questions you would like to ask regarding preparation and licensure for the career and processes and procedures they perform.

Summary

Physical therapy is a health-care profession that deals with prevention and management of movement disorders arising from conditions and diseases occurring throughout the lifespan. Physical therapists provide services that restore function, improve mobility, relieve pain, and prevent or limit permanent physical disabilities. They restore, maintain, and promote overall fitness and health.

Section 21.1 Review Questions

1. What tasks are required of physical therapy aides?
2. Compare moist heat and dry heat.
3. What is the purpose of range-of-motion (ROM) exercises?
4. When would antiembolism hose be used on a patient?
5. Explain the pivot, sliding, and lifting techniques.
6. When preparing a prosthesis for a patient, what considerations should you keep in mind?

Section 21.1 Review Questions

1. Answer: Prepare equipment (e.g., hydrotherapy pools); assist patients with walking and gait training, to dress and undress, to position themselves, and to remove and replace braces, splints, and slings; change linens on beds and tables; fold linens; clean equipment and work area; and may inventory materials and supplies.
2. Answer: Moist heat is applied with hot soaks, hot compresses, and hot packs. Dry heat is applied with heated lamps, infrared lights, standard electric bulbs, and heating pads.
3. Answer: Range-of-motion exercises stimulate circulation to decrease the chance of blood clots or decubitus ulcers, encourage flexibility and mobility of the joints, prevent contractures, prevent mineral loss, and prevent other problems such as poor appetite, constipation, urinary infections, respiratory problems, and hypostatic pneumonia.
4. Answer: Antiembolism hose are used on patients to prevent blood from pooling in the legs.
5. Answer: The pivot technique is used when moving a patient who can bear weight on at least one foot, possibly moving from a bed or chair to a chair, toilet, or commode and back again. The sliding technique is used when a patient needs to be moved and cannot get up or bear weight on either foot. The lifting technique is used when there is ample help and strength to support the patient fully while moving him or her from one support to another.
6. Answer: When preparing a prosthesis for a patient, keep in mind that you must have the right device, that the end resting against the patient is padded, that all straps must be in good condition, that it is clean and the overall appearance is natural, and that the patient can report tender areas at attachment site.

Teaching Tips

- Review the responsibilities of an aide caring for a patient on oxygen therapy:
  - Ensuring that all oxygen safety rules are followed
  - Checking the face and behind the ears to see if the strap is chafing and is a firm fit
  - Cleaning the cannula, catheter, or mask and checking the skin for irritation
  - Providing oral hygiene by moistening the lips and mouth frequently
  - Encouraging fluid intake if allowed
  - Keeping tubing free of kinks or blockage
  - Checking flow rate and oxygen humidifier frequently
  - Immediately reporting to supervisor any changes or problems (e.g., cyanosis, dyspnea, shortness of breath)

Career Connect

- Direct students to Chapter 3 for information on careers in physical therapy, rehabilitation therapy, and sports medicine.
- If students cannot arrange a class visit, students may be able to visit a facility to observe the professionals.
- Alternatively, they may be able to conduct a telephone or e-mail interview with a professional.
- Allow class time to prepare and approve questions.

CHAPTER 21 REVIEW

Chapter Review Questions

1. Answer: Ultraviolet light, diathermy, ultrasound, thermotherapy
2. Answer: UV therapy can cause severe burning.
3. Answer: Adjusting their height for the patient. Keep in mind: Axillary pressure—too much pressure causes injury; Hand level—position the handgrips to allow a slight bend of the elbows, like they are when you walk normally; the patient's footwear (slippery soles, open toes, etc.); condition of rubber tips, hand pads, and axillary pads; securing all joints on the crutches
4. Answer: Thermotherapy is heat treatments, used to speed up the healing process. It's primarily used to reduce pain, promote muscle relaxation, reduce muscle spasms, reduce inflammation, treat skin ulcers, treat perineal lacerations, reduce swelling, and promote drainage.
5. Answer: Overuse injuries are difficult to prevent because patients often do not allow enough recovery time between workouts or are subject to continual stress. They may have a job that makes recovery time difficult or psychological factors might keep athletes from scheduling rest days.
6. Answer: 95° F to 105° F
7. Answer: Acupuncture adjusts and alters the body's energy flow.
8. Answer: Sliding technique
9. Answer: You may support the patient by placing one hand on the side of the gait belt and the other hand behind the patient holding onto the belt.

CHAPTER 21 REVIEW

Chapter Review Questions

1. List four types of therapy you might encounter as a physical therapy aide? (21.1)
2. What is one of the problems associated with UV therapy? (21.1)
3. What are the steps to fit crutches for a patient? (21.1)
4. What is thermotherapy and for what is it primarily used? (21.1)
5. Why are overuse injuries difficult to prevent? (21.1)
6. What is the standard temperature for water in hydrotherapy treatment? (21.1)
7. According to its supporters, what is the main principle behind acupuncture? (21.1)
8. Which guarding technique is best for paraplegics? (21.1)
9. What is the standard gait procedure for walking with a cane? (21.1)
10. What is a prosthesis? (21.1)

Activities

1. Review and expand your personal plans for exercise and good body mechanics. You cannot help patients if you are not in fit condition yourself. What do you need to change? What interim steps will you take?
2. Use the Internet to make a list of three common running injuries. Then, suggest one or two possible physical therapy options that might prove useful to alleviate pain and restore mobility.
3. With a group of classmates, role play the health care staff as you demonstrate skills related to assisting patients with activities of daily living, such as dressing, undressing, grooming, bathing, and feeding. If available, practice using gait belts, wheelchairs, crutches, or walkers with your "patient." How would you determine the type of ambulatory device your "patient" would need?

Case Studies

1. Mr. Watkins has an exercise program designed by his physical therapist to restore full ROM after his complex leg fracture. The exercises cause some discomfort and he wants to stop exercising, insisting that a limited, shuffling gait is good enough. How would you explain to him the importance of his ROM exercises and the restoration of normal functioning? Find a partner and role-play how you would overcome his objections.
2. Ms. Starr has very bad arthritis that keeps her from doing some of the things she loves such as gardening and playing bridge. The physical therapist has decided to try diathermy to see if it can alleviate her pain. Before the treatment, you notice Ms. Starr has a wedding ring on. When you ask her to remove it, she refuses, telling you that "she never takes the ring off because it reminds her of her dear departed husband." What would you do?

802 Chapter 21 | Therapeutic Techniques and Sports Medicine

10. Answer: A prosthesis is an artificial body part such as a limb, tooth, or eye, used to replace a natural body part and minimize a disability.

Activities

1. Direct students to Section 7.1 for information about physical fitness. Direct students to write a diagnoses and treatment plan for themselves regarding their current state of physical fitness and the steps they should take to improve it.

CUSTOMIZED INSTRUCTION

At-Risk Students

For Activity 1, it may be helpful to prepare a list of fitness and healthy lifestyle resources at your school or within the community that at-risk students can consult with at no charge.

CHAPTER 21 REVIEW

Thinking Critically

1. **Communication**—Describe what you would say to a patient who was going to have his first hydrotherapy treatment. What special precautions would you take? What would you tell the patient about the possible outcome of his treatment?
2. **Legal**—Explain what it means to "know your limitations" as a physical therapy aide working in the physical therapy department.
3. **Ethical**—Use the Internet to look up the "Guide for Conduct of the Physical Therapist Assistant" issued by the American Physical Therapy Association (APTA). Take any standard or sub-standard in the guide and invent a hypothetical ethical dilemma that pertains to that standard. Make sure you give your solution to the problem quoting from the guide.

Portfolio Connection

A physical therapist's main goal is to reduce patient pain and increase mobility. Therapists are often an important part of rehabilitation and treatment of patients with chronic conditions or injuries.

Write a paper describing some of the challenges that a physical therapist might encounter on the job, and ways that the therapist can deal with these challenges. For example, interacting with patients who are experiencing pain is never an easy job. Are there any techniques the therapist can use to make this aspect of the job easier? Using your word processing program, write a brief report discussing some of the challenges a physical therapist may encounter and techniques that they can use to cope with these challenges. Include this document in your portfolio.

PORTFOLIO TIP

Before you file your portfolio sample, check that you have addressed all of the main challenges that you have outlined. It will make your report clear and logical. Be sure to keep your files neat and organized so you can easily locate a document or information.

Therapeutic Techniques and Sports Medicine | Chapter 21 803

2. Remind students of your school's Internet policy. Direct students to use reputable Web sites and to keep a list of sources.
3. Remind the students about consent and appropriate touching. You can also have the students think about how they would modify their strategies for patients with different mental or mobility impairments.

Case Studies

1. Remind students to use effective, age-appropriate communication techniques. In addition to role-playing their responses, direct them to write a specific and detailed explanation.
2. Remind students to use effective, age-appropriate communication techniques. In addition to writing a specific and detailed plan, you may want to allow students to present skits demonstrating their responses to this situation.

Thinking Critically

1. Direct students to p. 782 for information about hydrotherapy. Encourage students to describe the specific patient they are addressing, including age, culture, etc. Remind students of the importance of using appropriate communication techniques.
2. Direct students to review Chapter 5, Understanding Your Legal Obligations.
3. Direct students to review Chapter 6, Medical Ethics.

TEAMWORK

Divide the class into teams of five to seven students. You name the age, gender, and physical problem of a patient. Each team confers and writes down the type of physical therapy treatment that they think would be most effective. Allow teams to defend their response by presenting reasons they believe the treatment would be successful. Award a point to each team that answers correctly.

Portfolio Connection

- Remind students to proofread and revise their work.
- Encourage students to use peer review to find ways to improve the documents.
- Check to make sure that students have completed the assignments and added them to their portfolio.

22 Responsibilities of a Dental Assistant

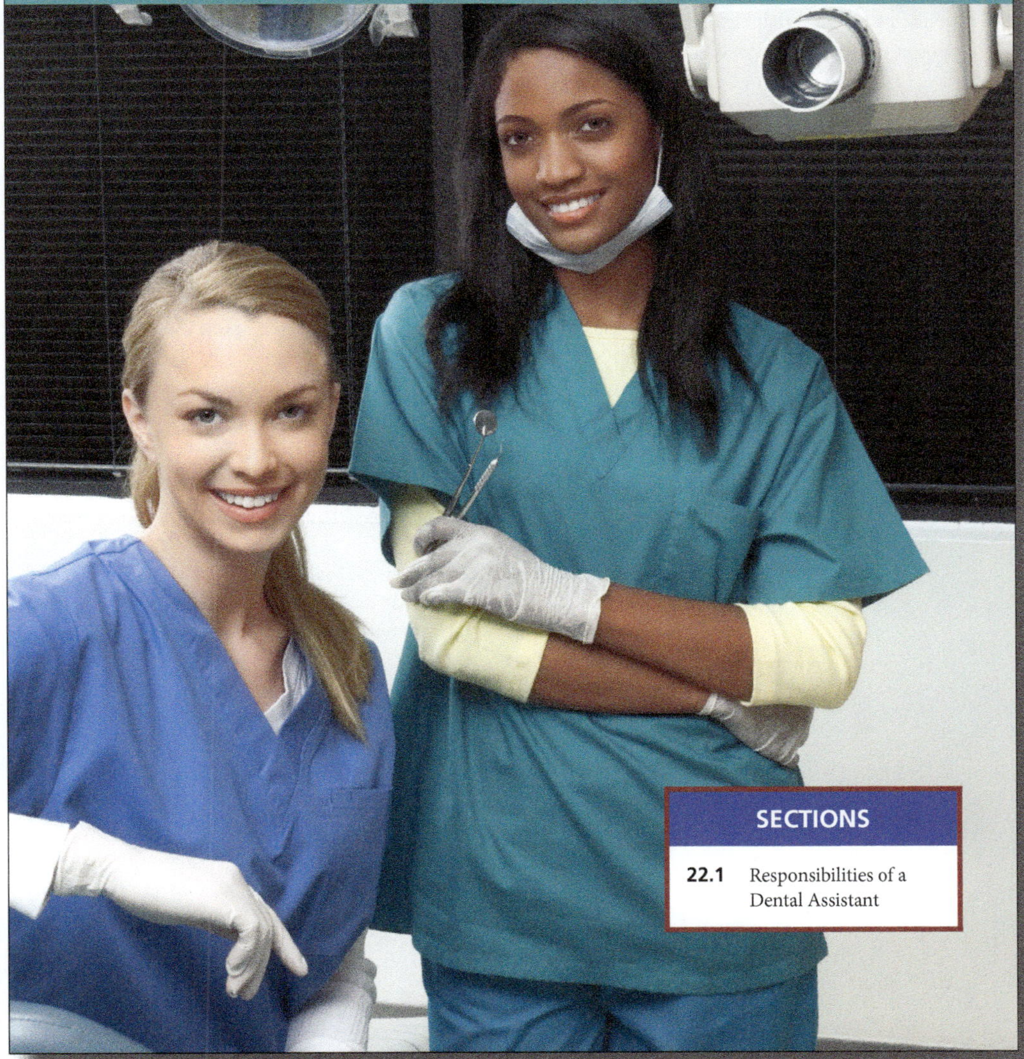

SECTIONS

CHAPTER 22 OVERVIEW

Chapter 22 reviews skills and practices of a dental assistant.

Section 22.1: This section discusses responsibilities of a dental assistant as well as information about the function, placement, and identification of teeth.

Advance Preparation	
Review	■ Chapter text for Section 22.1, and chapter procedures.
Contact	■ Local dental offices and elementary schools to arrange visits. ■ Dental assistants to act as guest speakers.
Prepare	■ Magazine and newspaper articles about dental health and treatments. ■ A list of Web sites that provide information about the dental profession—such as ada.org (American Dental Association) and adha.org (American Dental Hygienists' Association).

FOCUS AND ENGAGE

Getting Started

- This activity is designed to teach students the importance of correct brushing and flossing techniques.

Introduce the Section

a. Review the content of the Background paragraph, making sure to differentiate between a dental assistant and a dental hygienist.

b. Discuss the objectives for the section.

c. Have students look ahead into the section to find necessary key terms.

Vocabulary Review

a. Direct students to the key terms.

b. Pronounce each word, and have the students repeat the pronunciation out loud.

c. Discuss the definition of each word.

TEACH

Discuss

- Ask students what they know about the role of a dental assistant. As a class, discuss the responsibilities of a dental assistant.

ACTIVITY

Invite a dental assistant to speak to the class about the role of a dental assistant. Ask the speaker to talk about the best and worst days on the job, and the difference between working in a clinic and a single-dentist office.

Getting Started

You probably already know that poor oral hygiene can lead to cavities and bad breath, but did you know it can lead to much more serious problems, such as cardiovascular disease, dementia, respiratory infections, and diabetic complications? Under the guidance of a health care professional, practice correct brushing and flossing to promote good oral health. Test your process with a disclosing tablet that highlights any area that retains bacteria or any other substance. Create a poster demonstrating good oral hygiene techniques.

SECTION 22.1 Responsibilities of a Dental Assistant

Background

Dental assistants work closely and under the direction of a dentist. Dental assistants provide different types of patient care, office duties, and laboratory duties. They do not perform the same duties as a dental hygienist, but they need to be skilled in patient care, preparing and cleaning dental rooms, and setting up and sterilizing equipment and instruments. They need to be knowledgeable about the tooth: function, placement, identification, and anatomy.

Objectives

When you have completed this section, you will be able to do the following:

- Match key terms with their correct meanings.
- Describe the responsibilities of dental assistants.
- Differentiate between posterior and anterior teeth and their functions.
- Identify the following:
  - Deciduous and permanent teeth by name on a diagram.
  - Surfaces of a tooth.
  - Dental office equipment and instruments by name.
- Label the following:
  - Parts of the oral cavity on a diagram.
  - Teeth on a diagram using the universal method.
  - Anatomical structure of a tooth on a diagram.
- Teach the following:
  - How to use disclosing tablets/solutions.
  - The Bass toothbrushing technique.
  - Dental flossing techniques.

806 Chapter 22 | Responsibilities of a Dental Assistant

CUSTOMIZED INSTRUCTION

Less Advanced Students

Provide additional time for less advanced students to learn the vocabulary.

CUSTOMIZED INSTRUCTION OVERVIEW

Less Advanced Students	Pages 806, 809
More Advanced Students	Pages 812, 813, 818, 821, 824
English Language Learners	Page 807
Special Needs Students	Pages 810, 815
At-Risk Students	Pages 810, 820

Duties of a Dental Assistant

Dental assistants are valued members of the dental health care team. Their primary duty is chairside assisting during oral care procedures. Their basic duty is to maintain **visibility** in the mouth. They also provide instruments and materials as the dentist needs them to complete the dental treatment. Constant observance and consideration of the patient's/client's comfort level and health status are important in the role of a dental assistant. The responsibilities of a dental assistant include the following:

visibility
(vis uh BIL it tee)
Ability to see.

- Working directly with the dentist in the treatment room
- Preparing and cleaning dental treatment rooms following infection control guidelines
- Preparing necessary equipment and instrumentation for dental procedures
- Processing and mounting dental x-rays
- Caring for and maintaining dental equipment
- Teaching patients oral hygiene methods
- Taking and pouring study models (may be an expanded role in your state)
- Possibly performing some front office duties
- Exposing x-rays (radiographs) (requires completion of a state-approved radiology course or examination)

What's New?

Teeth Whitening

In recent years, teeth whitening has become a popular practice. Consumers can now buy toothpaste that whitens teeth as well as at-home bleaching kits. Dental offices also provide patients with the opportunity to whiten their teeth. Dental assistants may likely assist with such procedures.

Teeth whitening that is done in a dentist's office may require more than one office visit. Each visit may take 30 minutes to one hour. First, a dentist applies either a gel to the gums or a rubber shield to protect the oral soft tissues. Then a bleaching agent—hydrogen peroxide in concentrations ranging from 25 percent to 40 percent—is applied to the teeth. A special light or laser may be used to enhance the action of the agent.

Dentists may also provide patients with a teeth-whitening agent to take home. These whiteners contain peroxide and often come in a gel. The patient places the gel in a mouth guard that the dentist custom fits to the patient's teeth. Some products are used twice a day for two weeks, and others are used overnight for one to two weeks. Dentist-dispensed and over-the-counter tooth whitening bleaches are eligible for the ADA Seal of Acceptance.

How might a dental assistant assist a dentist with the teeth-whitening procedure?

What's New?—Teeth Whitening

- Have students find out about teeth whitening procedures offered at their dental offices. Ask students to consider such questions as:
    - How is the procedure done?
    - How long or how many visits does it require?
    - What is the cost?
    - Is it covered by dental insurance?
    - Is the whitening permanent?
- Discuss the role of the dental assistant in teeth whitening.

How might a dental assistant assist a dentist with the teeth-whitening procedure?

Answer: The dental assistant might prepare the patient for treatment, sterilize instruments, pass instruments to the dentist during the procedure, and hold suction devices.

TEAMWORK

Have students find out about training for dental assistants at local schools. Ask students to gather printed material or download information from those school Web sites. Allow students to share what they have found.

CUSTOMIZED INSTRUCTION

English Language Learners

Have students write each key term and its pronunciation on one side of an index card and its definition on the other side. Have them read each term and definition aloud to a partner.

Teaching Tips

- Describe the role of teeth.
- Explain how dentists examine patients.
- Explain how an examination of the oral cavity can show signs of diseases elsewhere in the body.
- Explain how a dental assistant will help the dentist during restorative care.
- Introduce students to the maxillary and mandibular arches.

accessory
(ak SES uh ree)
Helping.

masticate
(MAS ti keyt)
Chew.

primary
(PRAHY mere e)
First.

deciduous
(di SIJ oo uhs)
Falling out (e.g., primary teeth fall out to make room for permanent teeth).

erupt
(I RUHPT)
Push through.

dentition
(den TISH uhn)
Natural teeth in the dental arch.

Odontology

Odontology is the study of teeth. Teeth are **accessory** organs that help **masticate** food. There are two sets of teeth. They are the **primary** or **deciduous** (baby) teeth and the permanent teeth. When a baby is born it has 44 tooth buds. The tooth buds begin to **erupt** when the baby is about 6 months old. Deciduous teeth are the 20 baby teeth (primary teeth). Each tooth has a specific function in processing food and acting as a guide for a permanent tooth.

When the child is between 5 and 12 years old, the deciduous teeth begin to fall out and the permanent teeth erupt through the gingiva/gums. Permanent teeth are the 32 adult teeth. The child who has some deciduous teeth and some permanent teeth has mixed **dentition**.

Introduction to the Teeth and Oral Cavity

Teeth are identified by name, number, and the function they perform in the digestion of food. The following information teaches you how to identify teeth, where the teeth are located, and the anatomy of a tooth.

Face and Oral Cavity

When dentists examine patients they look at the face first. Dentists ask themselves:

- Is the bone structure normal and balanced?
- Do the skin and lips (labia) look healthy?

Next, the dentist does an oral examination. (Figure 22.1) This examination tells the dentist things about the patient's health and habits (for example, whether he or she practices good oral care). Often, a nondental disease shows up in the oral cavity first and is identified during the examination. For example, signs of periodontal disease or bacteria may indicate a previously undiagnosed heart condition or diabetes. A routine oral health exam also can uncover signs and symptoms of osteoporosis and low bone mass; eating disorders, such as anorexia nervosa and bulimia, which can be detected by thin tooth enamel and a red mouth; and HIV, which often shows signs in the mouth first.

restorative
(ri STAWY uh tiv)
To return to as close to normal conditions as possible.

The complete oral examination is one of the most important procedures that a dentist performs. As a dental assistant, you help the dentist during this examination and during **restorative** care. To assist the dentist, you need to know the following:

- Simple anatomy of the face and oral cavity
- Tooth numbers, parts, surfaces, and structures

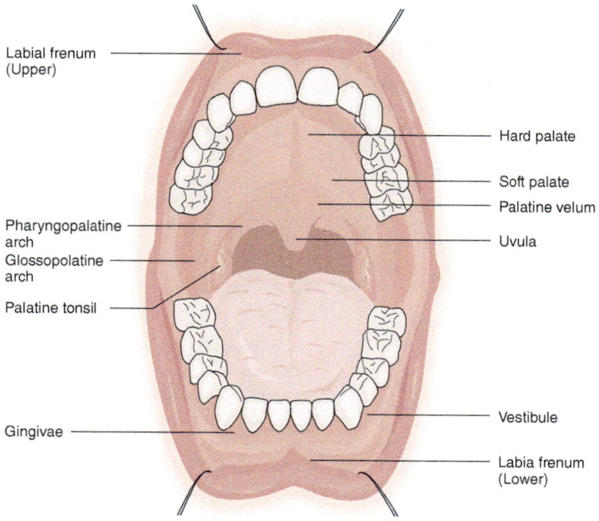

Figure 22.1
Mouth and oral cavity. Why is it important for a dental assistant to know the parts of the mouth and oral cavity?

Maxillary and Mandibular Arches

Refer to **Figure 22.2**, an illustration of the skull:

- **Maxilla**. The arched bone in the face where the roots of the upper teeth fit into the sockets (alveolus).
- **Mandible**. The arched lower bone (jawbone), where the roots of the lower teeth fit into the alveolus.
- **Median line** or **midline**. Divides the teeth into left and right sides.

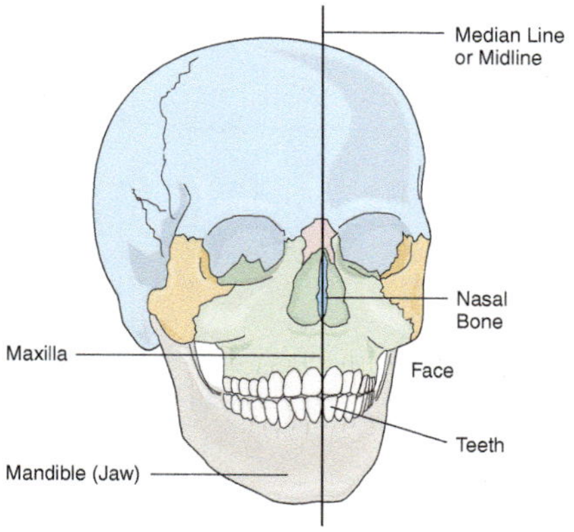

Figure 22.2
Skull. What does the median line or midline do?

Responsibilities of a Dental Assistant | Chapter 22 809

Figure Focus

22.1 Mouth and oral cavity. Why is it important for a dental assistant to know the parts of the mouth and oral cavity?

Answer: A dental assistant needs to be able to help a dentist perform an examination and therefore needs to know the parts of the mouth and oral cavity.

Figure Focus

22.2 Skull. What does the median line or midline do?

Answer: It divides the teeth into left and right sides.

Teaching Tips

- Review the parts of the skull in the diagram.

CUSTOMIZED INSTRUCTION

Less Advanced Students

Have students create a labeled diagram of the mouth and oral cavity. Ask students to present the diagrams to the class, briefly describing the function of each part.

Figure Focus

22.3 Location of posterior and anterior teeth. What are the two types of anterior teeth?

Answer: Incisors and cuspids/canines are anterior teeth.

Figure Focus

22.4 Universal method of identifying permanent teeth. How many permanent teeth are in the dentition?

Answer: There are 32 permanent teeth.

Teaching Tips

- Point to each tooth in the figures and identify it by name.
- Review the Maxillary and Mandibular Arches.
- Explain the difference between anterior and posterior teeth.
- Differentiate among incisors, cuspids/canines, premolars, and molars.

ACTIVITY

Write the terms maxilla, mandible, and midline on separate sheets of paper multiple times. Have students draw pieces of paper at random. As a student selects a paper, ask the student to describe the term and identify it on a skull.

Placement and Function of Teeth

The following are the anterior teeth (Figure 22.3):

- **Incisors.** Located in the very front of the mouth. Their thin cutting edge cuts food by biting pieces. They include the central and lateral incisors.
- **Cuspids/canines.** Located next to the lateral incisors. Their sharp points/cusps tear food that is too tough for the incisors to cut. Cuspids have the longest roots of all teeth.

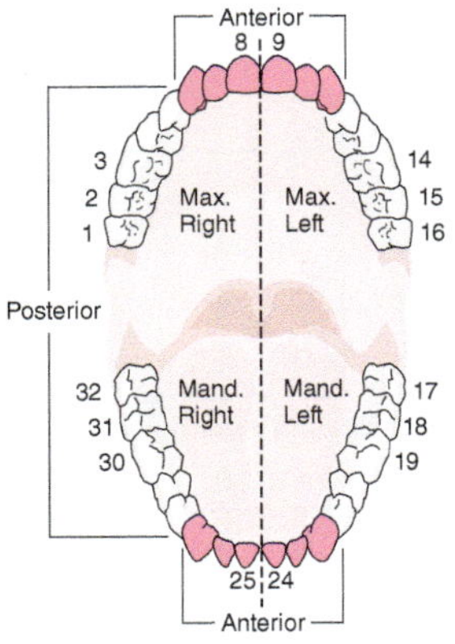

Figure 22.3
Location of posterior and anterior teeth. What are the two types of anterior teeth?

cusps
(kusps)
Pointed or rounded raised areas on the surface of the tooth.

The following are the posterior teeth (Figure 22.3):

- **Premolars.** Located next to the cuspids/canines. They are also called *bicuspids* because they have two **cusps** for tearing and grinding.
- **Molars.** Located next to the bicuspids. These are the largest teeth in the mouth. They have broad grinding surfaces that grind down large chunks of food.

Identification of Teeth by Name and Location

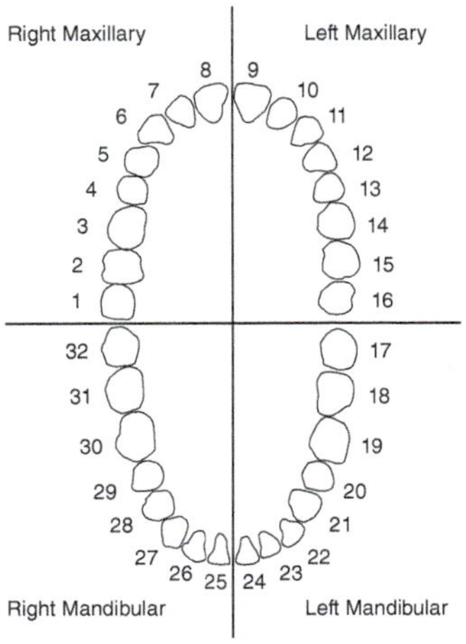

Figure 22.4
Universal method of identifying permanent teeth. How many permanent teeth are in the dentition?

ala
(ey luh)
Outer side of the nostril.

There are 32 permanent teeth (also known as secondary teeth) in the dentition. (Figure 22.4) The following are the maxillary teeth:

- 2 central incisors in the center next to the midline (8, 9)
- 2 lateral incisors next to the central incisors (7, 10)
- 2 cuspids under the **ala** next to the lateral incisors (6, 11)
- 2 first premolar/bicuspids next to the cuspids (5, 12)
- 2 second premolar/bicuspids next to the first bicuspids (4, 13)
- 2 first molars next to the second bicuspid (3, 14)

810 Chapter 22 | Responsibilities of a Dental Assistant

CUSTOMIZED INSTRUCTION

Special Needs Students

Some students may benefit from handling a physical model of the mouth. Allow students to handle a model and relate it to the diagram in the text.

At-Risk Students

Divide students into two teams. One team will be the "Right" team and the other will be the "Left." On a poster board or large sheet of plain white paper, have the "Right" team draw a picture of the right maxillary and right mandibular teeth, numbering and labeling each. Have the "Left" team do the same with the left maxillary and left mandibular teeth. Make sure both teams use the same size poster board or paper. When they are finished, assemble the drawings side-by-side and hang in the classroom.

- 2 second molars next to the first molar (2, 15)
- 2 third molars or "wisdom teeth" in the back of the mouth. Not everyone has these molars. Some remain under the gingiva/gums line or in the alveolar bone and are often removed if the mouth does not have room for them. (1, 16)

The mandibular teeth:

- 2 central incisors in the center next to the midline (24, 25)
- 2 lateral incisors next to the central incisors (23, 26)
- 2 cuspids under the corner of the nose next to the lateral incisors (22, 27)
- 2 first premolar/bicuspids next to the cuspids (21, 28)
- 2 second premolar/bicuspids next to the first bicuspids (20, 29)
- 2 first molars next to the second bicuspid (19, 30)
- 2 second molars next to the first molar (18, 31)
- 2 third molars or "wisdom teeth" in the back of the mouth. Not everyone has these molars. Some molars remain under the gingiva/gums line and are often removed if the mouth does not have room for them. (17, 32)

Apply It

With your classmates, play a game of "tooth fairy." Using a tooth chart, identify the 32 permanent teeth. Define the name, number, and the function they perform in the digestion of food.

There are 20 deciduous teeth in the dentition (**Figure 22.5**):

- 2 central incisors in the center next to midline (E, F)
- 2 lateral incisors next to the central incisors (D, G)
- 2 cuspids just under the ala wing of the nose (C, H)
- 0 There are no bicuspids in the deciduous dentition
- 2 primary first molars (L, S)
- 2 primary second molars (K, T)

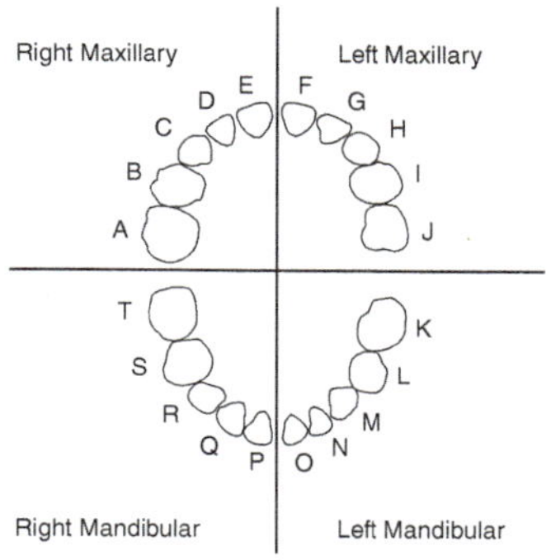

Figure 22.5
Universal method of identifying deciduous teeth. How does the method of identifying deciduous teeth differ from the method of identifying permanent teeth?

The mandibular arch:

- 2 central incisors in the center next to midline (O, P)
- 2 lateral incisors next to the central incisors (N, G)
- 2 cuspids just under the ala wing of the nose (M, R)
- 0 There are no bicuspids in the deciduous dentition
- 2 primary first molars (L, S)
- 2 primary second molars (K, T)

Teaching Tips

- Differentiate between deciduous and permanent teeth.
- Explain that deciduous means "to fall or drop."
- Deciduous teeth are also known as "baby teeth."
- Explain the universal system of naming teeth.
- Point to each tooth in the figures and identify it by name.

Figure Focus

22.5 Universal method of identifying deciduous teeth. How does the method of identifying deciduous teeth differ from the method of identifying permanent teeth?

Answer: Deciduous teeth are identified by letter and permanent teeth are identified by number.

Apply It

- Have a tooth chart of the permanent teeth ready.
- You may want to place numbers in a bag and have students draw them to select teeth.
- Conversely, you can use a blank chart and assign specific teeth to students.

Teaching Tips

- Describe the anatomical structures of a tooth: crown, cervix, and root.
- Review the parts and functions of each tooth.

Figure Focus

22.6 Sections of a tooth. Which part of the tooth can people see in their mouths?

Answer: Refer to the diagram to make sure students know that people see the crown.

ACTIVITY

Ask a local dentist or oral surgeon for a tooth or teeth to show in class. Or have students bring in teeth of their own that they may have saved. Point out the parts of the teeth and let students examine them. Make sure that anyone who handles the teeth wears gloves and washes their hands immediately afterward.

Identification of Teeth by Letter and Number

One method of identifying teeth is the *universal method.* In this method, deciduous/primary teeth are identified by letter, and permanent teeth are identified by number.

When identifying deciduous teeth, begin lettering with the right second molar in the maxillary arch. (Figure 22.5) It is labeled A. Continue lettering from upper right to upper left, then lower left to lower right. The last molar on the right mandibular arch is labeled T.

When identifying permanent teeth, begin numbering with the right third molar in the maxillary arch. (Figure 22.4) It is numbered 1. Continue numbering from upper right to upper left, then lower left to lower right. The last third molar on the mandibular arch is numbered 32. A tooth that has not erupted or is missing is still counted.

Anatomy of the Tooth

The dental assistant works directly with the dentist. It is important to communicate with the dentist during **intraoral** procedures. You must know the anatomy of the tooth to communicate effectively with the dentist.

intraoral
(in tra or el)
Within the oral cavity.

Sections of the Tooth

A tooth is divided into three main sections (Figure 22.6):

- **Crown.** Covered with enamel. The enamel is the white part of the tooth that we can see in our mouth.
- **Cervix.** Neck of the tooth. It begins where the enamel stops and the **cementum** begins. Dentists call this the CEJ (cemento-enamel junction).
- **Root.** Covered with cementum, lies below the gingiva/gums. It holds the tooth in the bony sockets of the jaw. A tooth may have more than one root, depending on where it is in the mouth:
  - Mandibular molars have two roots.
  - Maxillary molars have three roots.

cementum
(si MEN tuh m)
Hard, thin covering or shell covering root of tooth.

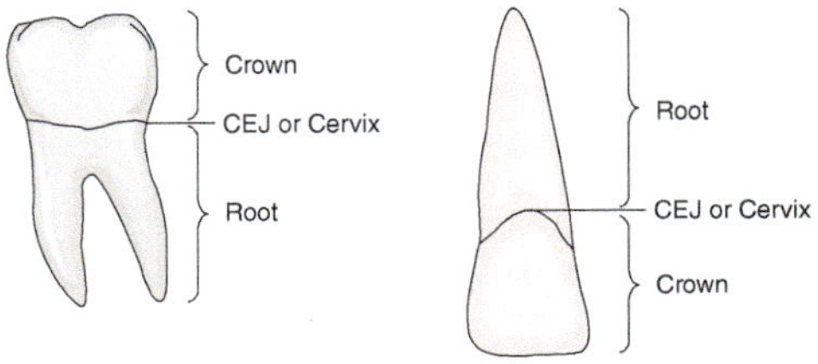

Figure 22.6
Sections of a tooth. Which part of the tooth can people see in their mouths?

812 Chapter 22 | Responsibilities of a Dental Assistant

CUSTOMIZED INSTRUCTION

More Advanced Students

Fillings are often visible in a person's mouth. Ask students to research or interview a dentist to find out about the composition of fillings and how they have changed over time.

Parts of the Tooth

Each tooth has several parts (Figure 22.7):

- **Enamel.** The hardest tissue in the body. It covers the crown section of the tooth. Enamel is a protective sheet made of calcium and phosphorus that protects the dentin of the tooth.
- **Dentin.** Harder than bone but softer than enamel. Dentin makes up the bulk of a tooth. It does not have nerves but it senses pain caused by **decay**, temperature, and chemical changes. Dentin may grow a second layer or wall of defense to try to keep decay from entering the pulp or nerve of the tooth.
- **Cementum.** The hard, thin covering or shell that covers the root.
- **Periodontal ligaments/periodontal membranes.** Small fibers that are anchored in the cementum and attached to the bone socket. They act as a shock absorber for the tooth and help the tooth withstand **functional stress**.
- **Pulp.** The soft tissue inside the hard wall of enamel and dentin. It has veins, arteries, and nerve tissue that nourish the tooth and sense pain.
- **Apex.** The very tip of each root. The blood vessels and nerves of the tooth enter through the **apical foramen** in the apex of the tooth.

decay
(di KEY)
Breaking down; rot.

functional stress
(FUHNGK shuh nl stress)
Stress to tooth caused by its normal function (e.g., force of pressure when biting something hard).

apical foramen
(EY pi kuhl fuh REY muhn)
Opening in the apex.

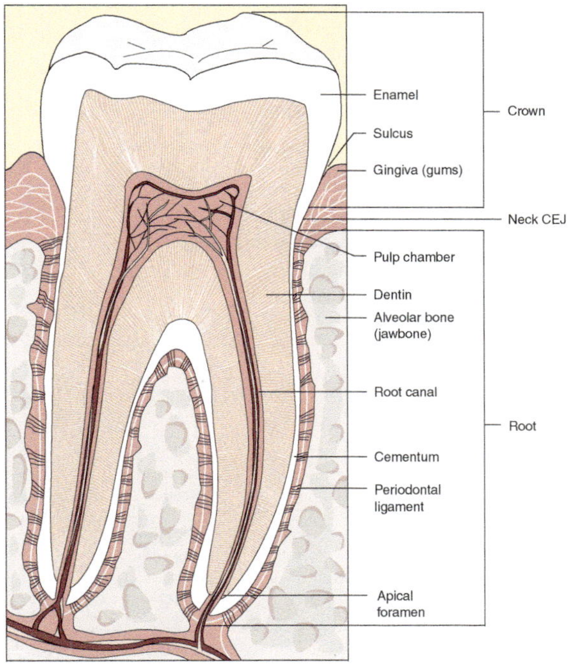

Figure 22.7
Parts of the tooth. Which part makes up the bulk of the tooth?

Responsibilities of a Dental Assistant | Chapter 22 813

Teaching Tips

- Discuss the tissues surrounding the teeth.
- Describe tooth surfaces.

Figure Focus

22.7 Parts of the tooth. Which part makes up the bulk of the tooth?

Answer: Direct students to the diagram of the tooth so they can see that the bulk of the tooth consists of the root(s).

Teaching Tips

- Discuss some of the facts of gum disease with students:
  1. Eighty percent of U.S. adults have some form of gum disease.
  2. These diseases range from simple inflammation (gingivitis) to serious disease that damages the bone (periodontitis).
  3. Smokers are much more likely than nonsmokers to have deeper pockets between the teeth and gums and lose more of the bone and tissue that support the teeth.
  4. Bleeding gums are one of the signs of gum disease.
  5. Good oral hygiene, proper diet, and not smoking are the best ways to prevent gum disease.

CUSTOMIZED INSTRUCTION

More Advanced Students

Have students review the definition of tissue. Ask students to relate tissue to organs and identify types of tissue in the body.

Figure Focus

22.8 Surfaces of the anterior and posterior teeth. Which surfaces are found on both anterior and posterior teeth?

Answer: Both anterior and posterior teeth have lingual, distal, and mesial surfaces.

Teaching Tips

- Find ways to help the students identify what can happen to their teeth.
- Tooth decay is second only to the common cold in terms of health disorders:
  - Bacteria are normally present in the mouth.
  - The bacteria convert all foods—especially sugar and starch—into acids.
  - Bacteria, acid, leftover food particles, and saliva combine in the mouth to form plaque (which "sticks" to the teeth).
  - Plaque begins to accumulate on teeth within 20 minutes after eating.
  - If this plaque is not removed, tooth decay will begin.
  - The acids in plaque dissolve the enamel surface of the tooth and create holes in the tooth (cavities).
  - Cavities are usually painless until they grow very large inside the tooth and destroy the nerve and blood vessels in the tooth.

Tissues Around the Teeth

The structures that surround the teeth are also important. They are as follows:

- **Alveolar processes (bone).** Form the sockets that hold and support teeth in their position.
- **Gingiva/gums.** Cover the alveolar bone, protecting the tooth and deeper tissues from injury or infection.
- **Gingival sulcus.** The open space between gingiva/gums and a tooth. This is the area where dental floss is applied to remove bacteria and food particles.

sulcus
(SUHL kuhs)
Depression, groove, area where gingival tip meets tooth enamel.

Surfaces of the Teeth

Dentists use terms that specify surfaces (sides of the tooth) to record information about the condition of each tooth. To chart conditions of the teeth, the dental assistant must know the crown surfaces. Each tooth has a crown and root. Each tooth also has four sides and a biting or chewing surface (**Figure 22.8**):

- **Anterior teeth.** Central and lateral incisors and the cuspids
- **Posterior teeth.** Bicuspids and molars

The surfaces of the anterior teeth are called:

- **Labial.** Surface that touches the lips
- **Lingual.** Surface facing toward the tongue
- **Incisal.** Edge of the tooth that we bite with
- **Distal.** Surface away from midline, toward the back
- **Mesial.** Surface toward the midline

The surfaces of the posterior teeth are called:

- **Buccal.** Surface that touches the cheeks
- **Lingual.** Surface facing toward the tongue
- **Occlusal.** Large chewing surface where food is ground
- **Distal.** Surface away from midline
- **Mesial.** Surface toward the midline

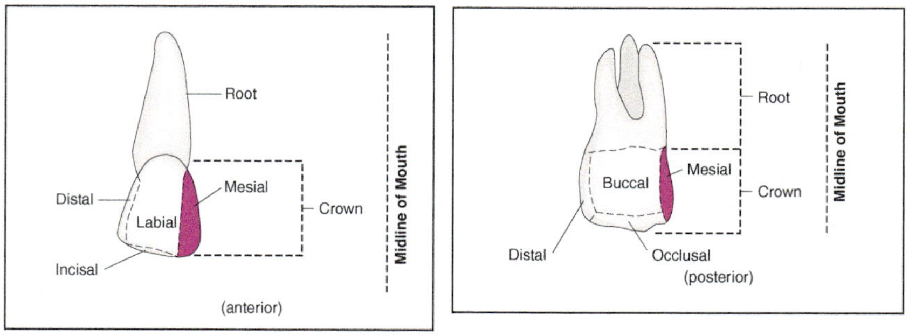

Figure 22.8
Surfaces of the anterior and posterior teeth. Which surfaces are found on both anterior and posterior teeth?

814 Chapter 22 | Responsibilities of a Dental Assistant

Language Arts Link

Dental Health Care Team

The dental team is comprised of highly trained health care professionals who specialize in treating conditions that affect structures in the mouth. There are many specialized careers within the team including general dentists, orthodontists, oral surgeons, dental hygienists, dental assistants, and dental laboratory technicians.

Working with a partner, research the education, certification, licensure or degree, continuing education requirements, and salary potential for a career in dental health. If possible, include in your analysis an interview with a dental health professional to identify how they became interested in this field, their current job responsibilities, and the benefits of working in a dental health career.

After you've completed the research, create several paragraphs that describe your findings. Use precise language and dental health career-specific vocabulary for each career investigated. Be sure to proofread your work for spelling, grammar, clarity, conciseness, and effectiveness.

All teeth have mesial and distal sides that touch each other. The mesial side of one tooth touches the distal side of the tooth next to it. These sides are **proximal** to each other and are called proximal surfaces.

proximal (PROK suh muhl) Nearest or next to.

Dental Equipment

A dental treatment (operatory) room is designed and organized to ensure that the dentist and assistant perform procedures in a safe and time-efficient manner. Treatment room equipment includes the following:

- Dental chair
- Dental unit
- Operational light
- Mobile carts or cabinets
- Operatory stools
- X-ray machine and view box

The type of equipment varies depending on the office. As a dental assistant, you are responsible for learning how to use the various types of equipment. Dental equipment is costly and requires special care. It is important that you follow the manufacturers' cleaning and operating instructions.

Dental Chair

Parts of a dental chair are as follows. (**Figure 22.9**) The body of the chair includes the backrest, seat, and leg support:

- The armrest is usually movable.
- The headrest supports the patient's head and is movable.

Responsibilities of a Dental Assistant | Chapter 22 **815**

Language Arts Link—Dental Health Care Team

- You may want to have students draft an outline, story web, or list questions they need to answer to organize their ideas.
- Remind students about your school's Internet policy before having them go online to find information. Emphasize that they should use reputable Web resources, such as sites sponsored by the government or educational institutions.
- Remind them to keep a list of sources to use for a bibliography.
- If students do not have access to the Internet, be sure to direct them to other resources, such as books, periodicals, or videos.
- For evaluation, verify that the information is correct and in the correct order, and you should mark spelling and grammatical errors.

Teaching Tips

- Show basic dental office equipment, explaining each item's function and how to operate it.
- Describe the dental chair and its function.

CUSTOMIZED INSTRUCTION

Special Needs Students

If possible, arrange for students to manipulate a dental chair. Help students relate the controls and functions of the chair to the needs of the dentist.

Figure Focus

22.9 What are the basic parts of a dental chair?

Answer: Armrest, headrest, control panel, and swivel lever

ACTIVITY

Arrange a tour of a local dental office. Ask the dental assistant at the office to point out the equipment. If students cannot go as a class, have the students go individually to their own dental offices.

- The control panel is on the side or back of the chair. Foot pedals are attached to base of chair or rest on the floor. These are used to move the chair into either a sitting or reclining (supine) position.
- The swivel lever is at the base of the chair, which allows the chair to rotate.

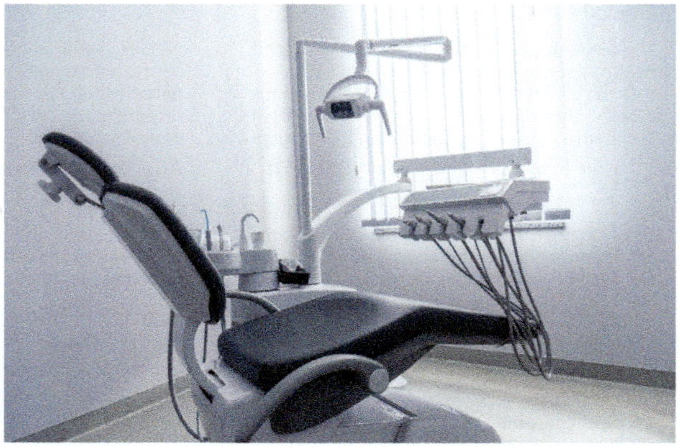

Figure 22.9
What are the basic parts of a dental chair?

Dental Unit

A dental unit is attached to the dental chair or to a separate movable cart. The basic parts of a dental unit are as follows:

- Master switch/control for:
  - Water and air
  - Handpiece
- Dental handpiece with burs or drills:
  - High speed
  - Slow speed
- Foot control (**rheostat**), which provides power to the handpiece.
- Air/water syringe to rinse and dry teeth.
- Oral **evacuation** system to **aspirate** saliva and drainage from the mouth. This system has two hoses attached to:
  - A suction tip
  - A small saliva ejector
- Cuspidor, the bowl that patients spit into (modern offices use suction in place of a cuspidor).

rheostat
(REE uh stat)
Control for flow of electric current.

evacuation
(i vak yoo EY shuhn)
Removal.

aspirate
(AS puh reyt)
Remove substances.

Dental Tools

Some common tools used by dental assistants include the following:

- **Mouth mirror**. To reflect light to see the surfaces of the teeth to inspect teeth, tongue, gingival, and oral cavity.
- **Explorer**. To feel teeth for decay or other problems. Explorers are sharp, pointed metallic instruments.
- **Non-locking cotton pliers**. To pick up gauze/cotton to dry areas of mouth/teeth. Cotton pliers are tong-like and metallic.
- **Scalers**. Locate and remove plaque especially between the teeth. When a scaler is used, a patient may experience pain.
- **Excavators**. Remove small amounts of decay close to the nerve. There are two types: spoons and hoes.
- **Carvers**. Used to carve amalgam filling to the shape of the tooth. A cleoid carver is a claw-shaped dental instrument used to remove carious material from a cavity. A discoid carver does the same but is flat and circular.
- **Root elevator**. A screwdriver-shaped instrument with a grooved and beveled blade, used to break the periodontal membrane and elevate and remove the root.
- **Surgical forceps**. A two-bladed instrument with a handle for compressing or grasping tissues in surgical operations, and for handling sterile dressings, etc.

Operational Light

The operational light is attached to the chair or the ceiling. It has handles to move the light. The light must focus on the site where the dentist is working.

Personal Protective Equipment

Standard precautions should be followed for work in a dental office. Dental workers should use appropriate personal protective equipment including gloves, gowns, masks, and eye protection.

Dental Mobile Carts or Cabinets

The dental cart/cabinet provides storage for a small number of sterile instruments, treatment trays, dental materials, and supplies. Large amounts of supplies are stored in areas away from the patient treatment room.

Operatory Stools

Operatory stools vary in design. There may be a footrest ring near the base on some stools, but all include the following:

- Padded seat
- Five casters at the base to prevent tipping

Responsibilities of a Dental Assistant | Chapter 22 817

Teaching Tips

- Display common instruments with their name label.
- Explain what each of the dental tools are used for.
- Explain how these tools are cleaned in between patients.
- Comment on any recent changes in these instruments; for example, have any of the students had their teeth cleaned using laser dentistry?

Teaching Tips

- Discuss with students the ALARA ("as low as [is] reasonably achievable") principles. Why are these important?

ACTIVITY

Have students report on the various dental specialties, such as endodontist, oral surgeon, orthodontist, or periodontist.

- Height-adjustment lever to position:
  - Dental assistant four to six inches above the dentist
  - Dentist stabilized below the assistant, with thighs parallel to floor when feet are flat on the floor
- Adjustable back support

Dental Radiology Equipment

The field of dentistry relies on the use of x-ray images, which involve radiation exposure for the patients and health care workers alike. Therefore, as a member of the dental team, you must be familiar with the different types of imaging equipment, understand the composition and function of x-ray radiation, and be knowledgeable and compliant with federal, state, and local safety guidelines and standards. You must also be trained to perform the manufacturer's recommendations for equipment operation, maintenance, and storage.

Patient Safety is guided by the ALARA ("as low as [is] reasonably achievable") principles, which means that all radiation exposure to humans should be limited to the lowest levels necessary to achieve the clinical goals (i.e., produce high quality x-ray images for the doctors to use in diagnosing and treating patients). Safety guidelines require that you:

- Follow the principles of ALARA.
- Use lead shields (i.e., protect gonads/reproductive organs).
- Reduce repeat radiation exposure by double checking the requisition, patient name, part to be x-rayed, the correct position, and x-ray settings.
- Ensure proper use of collimation (use the smallest radiation field that will cover the area of clinical interest—the radiation field must never be larger than the size of the film).
- Pregnant patients must consult with their physicians to weigh the risks and benefits of x-rays.
- Utilize personnel dosimeters to monitor radiation exposure levels.
- Remain within the Total Effective Dose Equivalent limits (TEDE), which determines the upper limits of radiation exposure that workers can be exposed to. The goal of TEDE is to ensure that the safety of radiation workers is the same as workers in other fields.
- Pregnant radiation workers must notify their employer of their pregnancy because radiation exposure can cause miscarriages, birth defects, and cancers in childhood. The pregnant woman's employer must make sure she stays below the TEDE limit.

overexposure
(OH ver ik SPOH zher)
Too much contact with radiation.

periodic
(peer ee OD ik)
Occurring at regular intervals.

State regulations tell how to prevent **overexposure** to radiation and provide safety guidelines for machine operations for conventional x-rays and imaging systems. These regulations require the following:

- Registration of each radiology machine
- **Periodic** inspection of equipment to ensure safe operation
- A licensed person to operate a radiology machine

818 Chapter 22 | Responsibilities of a Dental Assistant

CUSTOMIZED INSTRUCTION

More Advanced Students

Have advanced students research the regulations in your state.

Imaging Systems include:

- **Computed Tomography scanning (CT scanning).** Utilized for implant surgeries and to locate lesions within the oral cavity.
- **Magnetic Resonance Imaging (MRI).** Allows dentists to view soft tissues.
- **Digital imaging.** Is expected to replace traditional radiography methods. It is a computerized system that allows the dentist to take and review radiographs on the computer screen using pixels instead of analog images like those used in conventional radiographs.

Oral Hygiene

Human teeth are meant to last a lifetime. Remember that enamel is the hardest tissue in the body. Why, then, do we lose teeth? The bacteria that live in everyone's mouth cause disease. There are two main reasons why we lose teeth:

- Disease of the gingiva/gums, periodontal tissues, and/or the alveolar process (bony socket)
- Holes in the enamel and/or dentin (cavities)

Proper toothbrushing and flossing plus good nutrition can help prevent disease and destruction.

Dental assistants explain and demonstrate proper toothbrushing and flossing techniques to their patients. The instruction must be clear and meet each patient's needs (for example, working around a bridge). Correct flossing and brushing helps:

- Remove **plaque**
- Prevent bad breath (halitosis)
- Prevent periodontal infection
- Prevent bleeding gingiva/gums

plaque
(plak)
Soft deposit of bacteria and bacterial products on teeth.

Teaching Oral Hygiene

Your dentist may ask you to use disclosing tablets or solution to show the patient that there is plaque in the mouth. The disclosing tablets are usually red and stain the plaque to help the patient see the areas where plaque has formed. Patients can see that even when they think plaque is removed, it may not be. This is a very good way to help patients understand that correct brushing and flossing are important.

There are several types of brushing techniques. Use the technique your dentist prefers. The Bass technique is a common one.

Teaching Tips

- Describe oral hygiene.
- Review methods for teaching oral hygiene.

ACTIVITY

Have students create a checklist explaining the importance of correct toothbrushing and flossing. Ask them to specify how these activities prevent plaque, infections, and bad breath.

Personal Wellness—Oral Hygiene and Your Overall Health

- Have students visit the Web site of the American Dental Association at ada.org for recommendations on oral hygiene.
- Ask students to select a topic related to oral hygiene, such as how procedures change with age or how much toothpaste is appropriate. Have students present a brief oral presentation on their topic.
- Discuss actions students can take to improve their health and prevent disease by practicing good oral hygiene.

Common abbreviations for charting patient education:

- **OHI**. Oral hygiene instruction, complete cleansing of oral cavity
- **TBI**. Toothbrushing instruction
- **DFI**. Dental floss instruction

interproximal surfaces (in ter prok semal SUR fis) Sides between teeth.

Flossing removes the plaque from the **interproximal surfaces** (between teeth). It removes plaque and food. Flossing cleans areas where brushing cannot reach. Correct flossing is very important because tooth decay often begins on the interproximal surfaces.

Personal Wellness

Oral Hygiene and Your Overall Health

Your mouth can be a clue about your body's overall health. Ingesting, chewing, and swallowing food is the first step in the process of digestion and nutrition. Poor dentition puts the patient at risk for malnutrition because the patient will select soft foods often high in sugars and carbohydrates and low in nutrients.

Also, patients with loss of dentition or ill-fitting dentures will suffer diminished caloric intake due to the effort necessary to properly chew food. They frequently tire before adequate calorie intake is achieved.

The first sign of a disease may shows up in your mouth. In addition, infections in your mouth such as gum disease can cause problems in other areas of your body.

Many times, symptoms of a disease will first appear in your mouth. A person with diabetes has an increased risk of gum disease, cavities, tooth loss, or dry mouth. Also, people with AIDS may experience severe gum infections or unusual white spots or lesions on their tongues. While taking routine dental x-rays, a dentist may first notice osteoporosis. Certain cancers, eating disorders, syphilis, gonorrhea, and substance abuse can also show early symptoms in the mouth.

Not only can diseases first show themselves in your mouth, but diseases in your mouth can cause problems in other parts of your body. Your mouth is full of bacteria. However, good oral hygiene helps to control the bacteria. Your saliva also has enzymes that play an important role against bacteria and viruses. Sometimes harmful bacteria grow out of control and lead to serious gum infections. This gum disease provides bacteria a place to enter your bloodstream.

Some researchers believe that these bacteria in your bloodstream can lead to cardiovascular disease, premature birth, or difficulty with controlling diabetes. Bacteria from gum disease enter your bloodstream and travel to the arteries in your heart. This can affect the overall health of the cardiovascular system. In addition, research shows that these bacteria can end up in the placenta or amniotic fluid, possibly causing premature birth. These infections cause your blood sugar to rise, requiring diabetic patients to use more insulin to keep their levels under control.

What can you do daily to improve your health and prevent disease?

820 Chapter 22 | Responsibilities of a Dental Assistant

CUSTOMIZED INSTRUCTION

At-Risk Students

If your school provides free dental screenings, make sure to share information about the program with students.

Procedure 22.1 | **Bass Toothbrushing Technique**

BACKGROUND: Correct brushing is essential for healthy teeth and gums. Explain the importance of correct brushing and show a patient how good technique helps protect against dental problems.
ALERT: Follow Standard Precautions

Preprocedure

1. Wash hands.
2. Assemble equipment:
   a. Tooth model (if using a model for teaching)
   b. Protective wear (if brushing patient's teeth or if there is contact with saliva), including gloves, mask, and goggles
   c. Toothbrush

Procedure

3. Explain importance of toothbrushing.
4. Demonstrate correct brushing using model or on patient:
   NOTE: Put on gloves if demonstrating on patient.
   a. Place soft brush on upper right molars (maxillary).
   b. Position brush at 45° angle to teeth.
   c. Gently move bristles into gingival sulcus.
   d. Move brush in short strokes at least 10 to 20 times, keeping brush in place (wiggle-jiggle motion).
   e. Move brush to next two or three teeth and repeat until all buccal/labial surfaces are brushed.
   NOTE: Place brush in vertical or horizontal position for anterior teeth.
   f. Repeat technique beginning at upper right molars until all maxillary teeth are brushed.
   g. Use short, vibrating motion to scrub occlusal surfaces.
   h. Repeat this procedure for lower teeth (mandibular).
5. Ask client if he or she has any questions.

Postprocedure

6. Remove and clean equipment.
7. Remove protective wear.
8. Wash hands.
9. Chart TBI (toothbrushing instruction).

Responsibilities of a Dental Assistant | Chapter 22 821

Teaching Tips

- Assign Procedure 22.1.

Procedure Tip

22.1 Bass Toothbrushing Technique

- Review the background information, discussing the importance of correct brushing.
- Explain the preprocedure steps.
- Explain the procedure steps.
- Explain the postprocedure steps.

PROCEDURE PRACTICE

- Demonstrate the steps for Procedure 22.1, Bass Toothbrushing Technique, as many times as necessary, or ask students to demonstrate the steps. Have students practice and perform the procedure until they are competent.

CUSTOMIZED INSTRUCTION

More Advanced Students

Ask students to investigate different types of toothbrushes. Have them conduct their own research, and interview dentists and/or dental hygienists to get their opinions. Students should present their findings to the class along with a few examples, if possible.

Teaching Tips

- Assign Procedure 22.2.

Procedure Tip

22.2 Dental Flossing

- Review the background information, discussing the importance correct flossing to prevent decay and gum disease.
- Explain the preprocedure steps.
- Explain the procedure steps.
- Explain the postprocedure steps.

PROCEDURE PRACTICE

- Demonstrate the steps for Procedure 22.2, Dental Flossing, as many times as necessary, or ask students to demonstrate the steps. Have students practice and perform the procedure until they are competent.

Procedure 22.2 **Dental Flossing**

BACKGROUND: Correct dental flossing is essential for healthy teeth and gums. Explaining the importance of correct flossing and showing a patient good technique help protect against dental problems.
ALERT: Follow Standard Precautions

Preprocedure

1. Wash hands.
2. Assemble equipment:
   a. Tooth model (if using a model for teaching)
   b. Gloves, mask, and goggles (if flossing patient's teeth or if there is contact with saliva)
   c. Dental floss (waxed or unwaxed according to policy)

Procedure

3. Explain importance of flossing.
4. Demonstrate correct flossing technique using model or patient:
   NOTE: Put on protective wear if demonstrating on patient.
   a. Cut floss 18 inches (measure from finger to elbow).
   b. Wrap floss around middle or index finger of both hands, leaving 1 to 2 inches between fingers.
   c. Stretch floss between fingers and gently guide floss in between teeth. Do not snap floss; it can damage gingiva/gums.
   d. Pass floss through contacts (where teeth touch) and wrap it around tooth in a C shape.
   e. Move floss up and down several times on sides of each tooth.
   NOTE: Make sure that floss goes beneath gingiva/gums into the sulcus.

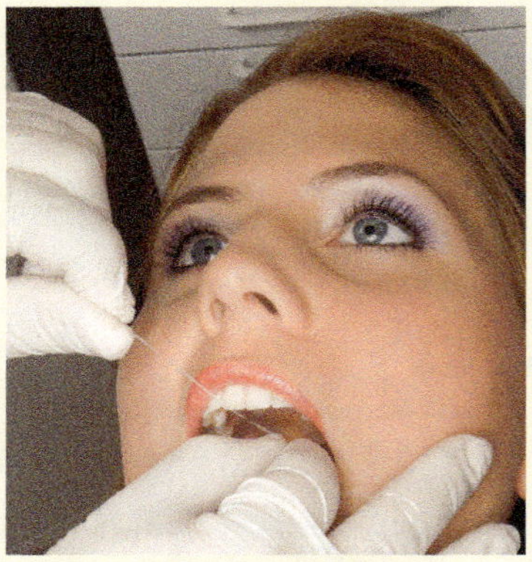

   f. Unroll new floss from one hand and wrap used floss around middle finger of other hand.
   g. Repeat for each tooth until all teeth in maxilla and mandible are completed.
5. Explain that there may be some bleeding of the gingiva/gums the first few times the patient does this procedure.
6. Ask patient if he or she has any questions.

Postprocedure

7. Remove protective wear.
8. Remove and clean equipment.
9. Wash hands.
10. Chart DFI (dental flossing instruction).

822 Chapter 22 | Responsibilities of a Dental Assistant

Dental Radiographs

Dental assistants must have special training before they can take radiographs of the mouth. (Check with your state dental board or association for information.) As an entry-level dental assistant, you may mount dental radiographs after they are developed. To mount radiographs correctly, you need some basic information.

Dental radiographs are photographs of the teeth. The radiographs allow the dentist to see between the teeth, the pulp of each tooth, and the bone (for example, caries, metallic restorations, poorly fitted crowns, root end infection, **resorption** of alveolar bone). Radiographs allow the dentist to identify problems and make repairs before the problems cause further damage.

resorption
(ri SAWP shuhn)
Loss of substance or bone.

Radiography Terminology

- *Radiopaque* structures do not allow radiation to pass through. Enamel, metallic restorations, and dentin are radiopaque. They are very white on the film.
- *Radiolucent* structures allow rays to penetrate through them. Pulp and caries are radiolucent. They are dark areas on the film.
- *Periapical* films (PA) show two or three teeth and their surrounding bone structure.
- *Bite wings* (BWX) show the crowns of the maxillary and mandibular teeth. These are often called the cavity detector films.
- *Occlusal* (OCC) is a large film that shows the whole arch from the occlusal view.
- *Panographic* (PANX) is a long film taken from outside the mouth (extra oral) by a special machine. It shows all structures and teeth. (Figure 22.10)

Career Connect

Spend a day job shadowing a dental professional. Consider specialty offices such as orthodontics, pedodontics, oral surgery, prosthodontics, and endodontics as well as general dental practice. Explore the various careers represented by those performing the services including preparation and licensure requirements.

The radiographs serve as a guide that helps determine the treatment plan. After the radiograph is taken, it must be developed and mounted. Mounting film may be one of your duties.

Some dentist offices have started to replace traditional x-rays with digital radiography. The dentist or dental assistant inserts a sensor into the patient's mouth to capture images of the teeth. The digital sensor is electronic and connected to a computer. Once the X-ray is taken, the image is projected on a computer screen for the dentist to view.

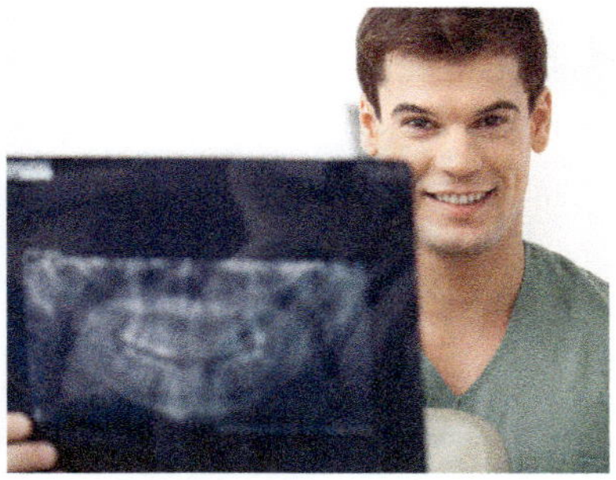

Figure 22.10
Panoramic survey. In what situation would a dentist want a panoramic survey?

Teaching Tips

- Explain what a radiograph is.
- Review radiography terminology.

Figure Focus

22.10 Panoramic survey. In what situation would a dentist want a panoramic survey?

Answer: The long film taken from outside the mouth covers a wider area than a conventional x-ray. It provides more information about the nasal area, maxillary sinuses, tooth positioning, and gum and bone irregularities.

Career Connect

- Discuss with students specialties in which they might be interested.
- Work with students to arrange shadowing days in appropriate offices.
- Have students present an oral report on what they did and learned.
- Make sure students follow up with a letter of thanks.

ACTIVITY

Obtain, or have students obtain, x-rays from a dental office. Review the x-rays and what they show as a class.

Teaching Tips

- Discuss types of mounts.
- Explain how to mount full-mouth and bite-wing x-rays.
- Assign Procedure 22.3.

Procedure Tip

22.3 Mounting Dental Films

- Review the background information, discussing how films help the dentist assist the patient's needs and treatment.
- Explain the preprocedure steps.
- Explain the procedure steps.
- Explain the postprocedure steps.

PROCEDURE PRACTICE

- Demonstrate the steps for Procedure 22.3, Mounting Dental Films, as many times as necessary, or ask students to demonstrate the steps. Have students practice and perform the procedure until they are competent.

Community

- Have students practice their instruction on you before working with young students.
- Arrange a visit with an elementary school.
- Make sure students have the proper supplies prepared in advance.

Procedure 22.3 Mounting Dental Films

BACKGROUND: Correct mounting of dental films helps the dentist assess whether the patient needs treatment.
ALERT: Follow Standard Precautions

Preprocedure

1. Wash hands.
2. Assemble equipment:
   a. Developed x-rays
   b. X-ray mounts
   c. View box

Procedure

3. Turn on view box.
4. Lay out x-rays. (Make certain that raised dot is facing upward.)
5. Arrange film on view box before placing into mount.
6. Mount the two or four bite-wing films.

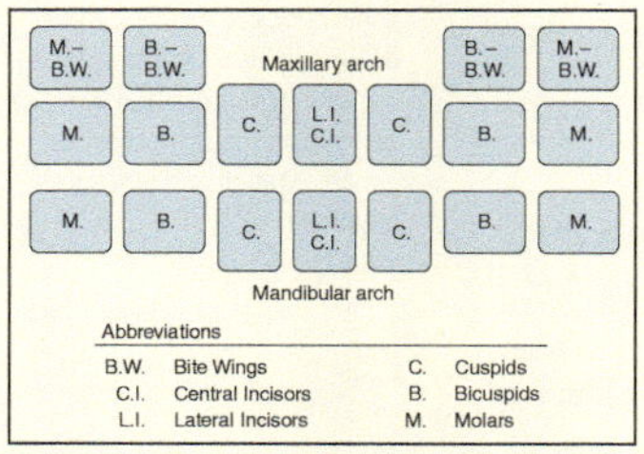

NOTE: Bicuspid views are closest to the center of the mount.

7. Mount two central (CI) and lateral (LI) incisor films. Place mandibular films with roots downward and maxillary films with roots upward.
8. Mount the four cuspid (C) films. The two longest cuspids are maxillary teeth.
9. Mount the four bicuspid (BC) films.
10. Mount the four molars (M) films. The molars with three roots are the maxillary molars.
11. Review the anatomical charts to check mount for accuracy.
12. Turn off view box.

Postprocedure

13. Clean and replace equipment.
14. Wash hands.
15. Record the following on patient chart and dental x-ray mount:
    a. Patient's name
    b. Date x-rays were taken
    c. Name of person who took x-rays
    d. Dentist's name and address

Community

As a member of a team, help teach elementary students how to brush and floss to promote good oral health.

Types of Mounts

Mounts come in different sizes. They may have 1, 2, 4, 7, 14, 16, 18, 20, and 28 windows. Bite-wing mounts have 2 or 4 windows. Common periapical mounts have 16 or 18 windows. When mounting films, you must remember the following:

- Periapical films show the crown and roots.
- Maxillary molars have three roots.
- Maxillary cuspids are the longest teeth in the mouth.
- Maxillary lateral incisors are larger than mandibular lateral incisors.
- Maxillary central incisors are larger than mandibular central incisors.
- Mandibular molars have two roots.
- Mandibular lateral incisors are wider than mandibular central incisors.

824 Chapter 22 | Responsibilities of a Dental Assistant

CUSTOMIZED INSTRUCTION

More Advanced Students

Have students contact a dental office or insurance company to find out about payment for dental x-rays. Some types of x-rays are covered by insurance policies on a schedule, such as every six months. Others are covered in specific situations. Ask students to report on what they find out.

- The center of the mount is the median line.
- If the distal portion is on the right margin, it is the left-hand side of the dental arch.
- If the distal portion is on the left margin, it is the right-hand side of the dental arch.
- Dental film has a raised dot on a corner of the film.
- Place all films with the dot facing upward, which is a convex view.
- **Convex** is a facial surface view.
- Concave is a lingual surface view.
- A full-mouth series usually includes 14 periapical films plus two or four bite wings.

convex
(kon VEKS)
Raised.

Summary

Dental assistants help dentists provide efficient dental care. Dental assistants have a responsibility to be considerate of the patent and make the patient feel comfortable. It is important for dental assistants to be familiar with standard concepts, practices, and procedures related to the field of the dentistry.

Section 22.1 Review Questions

1. What are the responsibilities of a dental assistant?
2. How many permanent teeth do adults have?
3. Explain the Bass technique of toothbrushing.
4. What is the difference between primary and secondary teeth?
5. What are the two main reasons we lose teeth?
6. What is the oral evacuation system?

Responsibilities of a Dental Assistant | Chapter 22 825

Teaching Tips

- Review the aspects of various types of teeth that would require different types of mounts.
- Review the main responsibilities of a dental assistant.

Section 22.1 Review Questions

1. Answer:
   - Working directly with the dentist in the treatment room
   - Preparing and cleaning dental treatment rooms following infection control guidelines
   - Preparing necessary equipment and instrumentation for dental procedures
   - Processing and mounting dental x-rays
   - Caring for and maintaining dental equipment
   - Teaching patients oral hygiene methods
   - Taking and pouring study models (may be an expanded role in your state)
   - Possibly performing some front office duties
   - Exposing x-rays (radiographs) (requires completion of a state-approved radiology course or examination)
2. Answer: Adults have 32 permanent teeth.
3. Answer:
   - Place soft brush on upper right molars (maxillary).
   - Position brush at 45° angle to teeth.
   - Gently move bristles into gingival sulcus.
   - Move brush in short strokes at least 10 to 20 times, keeping brush in place (wiggle-jiggle motion).

3. *(continued)*
   - Move brush to next two or three teeth and repeat until all buccal/labial surfaces are brushed. Place brush in vertical or horizontal position for anterior teeth.
   - Repeat technique beginning at upper right molars until all maxillary teeth are brushed.
   - Use short, vibrating motion to scrub occlusal surfaces.
   - Repeat this procedure for lower teeth (mandibular).
4. Answer: Primary teeth (baby teeth) are the 20 baby teeth. Secondary teeth are the 32 permanent teeth.
5. Answer: Disease of the gingiva/gums, periodontal tissues, and/or the alveolar process (bony socket); Holes in the enamel and/or dentin (cavities)
6. Answer: The oral evacuation system removes saliva and drainage from the mouth.

CHAPTER 22 REVIEW

Chapter Review Questions

1. Answer:
   - Anterior—incisors cut food for chewing; cuspids/canines tear food that is too tough to chew
   - Posterior—premolars tear and grind; molars grind down large chunks of food
2. Answer: In the universal method, deciduous/primary teeth are identified by letter, and permanent teeth are identified by number.
3. Answer: Crown, cervix, and root
4. Answer: Enamel, dentin, cementum, periodontal ligaments/membranes, pulp, apex
5. Answer:
   - Anterior teeth:

     Central and lateral incisors and the cuspids

     Labial: Surface that touches the lips

     Lingual: Surface facing toward the tongue

     Incisal: Edge of the tooth that we bite with

     Distal: Surface away from midline, toward the back

     Mesial: Surface toward the midline
   - Posterior teeth:

     Bicuspids and molars

     Buccal: Surface that touches the cheeks

     Lingual: Surface facing toward the tongue

     Occlusal: Large chewing surface where food is ground

     Distal: Surface away from midline

     Mesial: Surface toward the midline

CHAPTER 22 REVIEW

Chapter Review Questions

1. List the anterior and posterior teeth and their functions. (22.1)
2. Explain the universal method for identifying teeth. (22.1)
3. What are the three sections of a tooth? (22.1)
4. Describe the six parts of a tooth. (22.1)
5. Identify the surfaces of anterior and posterior teeth. (22.1)
6. What equipment would you find in a dental treatment room? (22.1)
7. What does the abbreviation "ALARA" stand for and what is its goal regarding radiation safety? (22.1)
8. Which imaging system is expected to replace conventional radiography and allows images to be viewed on computer screens? (22.1)
9. Describe the following dental instruments: mouth mirror, scalers, spoon excavator, and cleoid and discoid carvers. (22.1)
10. Explain the dental flossing technique. (22.1)

Activities

1. Imagine that you are writing questions for a quiz show. Write ten questions that relate to the basic skills required of a dental assistant. After writing your questions, exchange them with your classmates to see how well you do.
2. Use the Internet or visit a local dental group and prepare a display on oral hygiene that can be used in elementary schools.

Case Studies

1. You are preparing the room for a patient who is coming in for a routine cleaning. As a dental assistant, what are your responsibilities before, during, and after the procedure?
2. A patient needs dental x-rays. He wants to understand why they are necessary, what you look for, and who does what during the process. How do you answer his questions?

826 Chapter 22 | Responsibilities of a Dental Assistant

6. Answer: Dental chair; dental unit; operational light; mobile carts or cabinets; operatory stools; and x-ray machine and view box
7. Answer: ALARA stands for "as low as [is] reasonably achievable." These principles are designed to protect workers from radiation exposure.
8. Answer: Digital imaging
9. Answer:
   - Mouth mirror: To reflect light to see the surfaces of the teeth to inspect teeth, tongue, gingival, and oral cavity; and for retraction (hold the cheek back)
   - Scalers: Locate and remove plaque especially between the teeth; when a scaler is used, a patent may experience pain
   - Excavators: Remove small amounts of decay close to the nerve; there are two types: spoons and hoes

CHAPTER 22 REVIEW

Thinking Critically

1. **Communication**—The dental assistant may work directly with the dentist during routine procedures. Mrs. Smith, a new client, is upset by the precautions taken in the dental office—masks, gloves, etc. How do you explain to her why this is necessary?
2. **Medical Terminology**—An 8-year-old boy fell off of his bike and knocked his top two front teeth out. Using appropriate terminology and identifiers, write a description for a dental record of the dentition on this boy.
3. **Patient Education**—Describe what you would tell a patient about the need for and benefits of brushing and flossing. How would you show a patient where plaque is building up?
4. **Computers**—Describe ways computers are used in dental care.

Portfolio Connection

The dental assistant plays an important role on the dental team. He or she helps the dentist deliver quality oral health care. A good dental assistant needs to be patient, attentive, and good working with his or her hands.

Research dental assistant education, certification, and training requirements. Write a brief paper on your findings and include it in your portfolio.

PORTFOLIO TIP

If you are interested in a career as a dental assistant, set up a database or spreadsheet that lists dental programs in your area. Include information on costs, pre-requisites, and admission polices.

Responsibilities of a Dental Assistant | Chapter 22 827

- Carvers: Used to carve amalgam filling to the shape of the tooth; a cleoid carver is a claw-shaped dental instrument used to remove carious material from a cavity; a discoid carver does the same but is flat and circular

10. Answer:
    - Cut floss 18 inches (measure from finger to elbow).
    - Wrap floss around middle or index finger of both hands, leaving 1 to 2 inches between fingers.
    - Stretch floss between fingers and gently guide floss in between teeth.
    - Do not snap floss; it can damage gingiva/gums.
    - Pass floss through contacts (where teeth touch) and wrap it around tooth in a C shape.
    - Move floss up and down several times on sides of each tooth.
    - Make sure that floss goes beneath gingiva/gums into the sulcus.
    - Unroll new floss from one hand and wrap used floss around middle finger of other hand.
    - Repeat for each tooth until all teeth in maxilla and mandible are completed.

Activities

1. You may wish to discuss the formats of some popular quiz shows in advance. Have students decide on a format to use. Encourage students to be creative when writing their questions. If time allows, have the class play the game as a quiz show.
2. Tell students to use the information they have learned in the text along with any additional information they can gather. Remind students that their displays should be attractive so as to catch students' attention, but also be accurate. If possible, have students ask a dentist to review their displays.

Case Studies

1. Students should clearly outline their responsibilities. Students may separate their role during all three parts of the visit.
2. Students should provide clear, well thought out responses. The responses should be accurate and presented in a way that someone unfamiliar with the dental profession can easily understand.

Thinking Critically

1. Students should clearly describe the need for cleanliness in a way that is reassuring rather than threatening.
2. Students should use correct medical terminology in describing the patient's condition.
3. Students should use correct terminology to strongly urge the patient to brush and floss correctly. Answers should indicate the consequences of ignoring the advice.
4. Students should describe several uses of computers in dental care. Examples include anything from tracking patients' charts to recording and examining radiographs.

Portfolio Connection

- Check to make sure that students have completed the written assignments and added them to their portfolio.
- Encourage students to use computer programs to organize and update data.

Appendix A CDC Recommendations for Standard Precautions

In 2007, the Centers for Disease Control updated and expanded the 1996 Guidelines for Isolation Precautions in Hospitals. This Appendix provides a summary of the New Elements in the 2007 CDC Standard Precautions.

Go to *www.cdc.gov/hicpac/2007IP/2007isolation Precautions.html* for the complete text of the 2007 CDC Standard Precautions and any updates to the guidelines.

III.A.1. New Elements of Standard Precautions
Infection control problems that are identified in the course of outbreak investigations often indicate the need for new recommendations or reinforcement of existing infection control recommendations to protect patients. Because such recommendations are considered a standard of care and may not be included in other guidelines, they are added here to Standard Precautions.

Three such areas of practice that have been added are: Respiratory hygiene/Cough Etiquette, safe injection practices, and use of masks for insertion of catheters or injection of material into spinal or epidural spaces via lumbar puncture procedures (e.g., myelogram, spinal or epidural anesthesia). While most elements of Standard Precautions evolved from Universal Precautions that were developed for protection of health care personnel, these new elements of Standard Precautions focus on protection of patients.

III.A.1.a. Respiratory Hygiene/Cough Etiquette
The transmission of SARSCoV in emergency departments by patients and their family members during the widespread SARS outbreaks in 2003 highlighted the need for vigilance and prompt implementation of infection control measures at the first point of encounter within a health care setting (e.g., reception and triage areas in emergency departments, outpatient clinics, and physician offices). The strategy proposed has been termed Respiratory Hygiene/Cough Etiquette and is intended to be incorporated into infection control practices as a new component of Standard Precautions.

The strategy is targeted at patients and accompanying family members and friends with undiagnosed transmissible respiratory infections, and applies to any person with signs of illness including cough, congestion, rhinorrhea, or increased production of respiratory secretions when entering a health care facility. The term cough etiquette is derived from recommended source control measures for M. tuberculosis. The elements of Respiratory Hygiene/Cough Etiquette include:

1) education of health care facility staff, patients, and visitors;
2) posted signs, in language(s) appropriate to the population served, with instructions to patients and accompanying family members or friends;
3) source control measures (e.g., covering the mouth/nose with a tissue when coughing and prompt disposal of used tissues, using surgical masks on the coughing person when tolerated and appropriate);
4) hand hygiene after contact with respiratory secretions; and
5) spatial separation, ideally >3 feet, of persons with respiratory infections in common waiting areas when possible.

Covering sneezes and coughs and placing masks on coughing patients are proven means of source containment that prevent infected persons from dispersing respiratory secretions into the air. Masking may be difficult in some settings (e.g., pediatrics), in which case, the emphasis by necessity may be on cough etiquette.

Physical proximity of <3 feet has been associated with an increased risk for transmission of infections via the droplet route (e.g., N. meningitidis and group A streptococcus) and therefore supports the practice of distancing infected persons from others who are not infected. The effectiveness of good hygiene practices, especially hand hygiene, in preventing transmission of viruses and reducing the incidence of respiratory infections both within and outside health care settings is summarized in several reviews.

These measures should be effective in decreasing the risk of transmission of pathogens contained in large respiratory droplets (e.g., influenza virus, adenovirus, B. pertussis and Mycoplasma pneumoniae). Although fever will be present in many respiratory infections, patients with pertussis and mild upper respiratory tract infections are often afebrile. Therefore, the absence of fever does not always exclude a respiratory infection.

Patients who have asthma, allergic rhinitis, or chronic obstructive lung disease also may be coughing and sneezing. While these patients often are not infectious, cough etiquette measures are prudent. Health care personnel are advised to observe Droplet Precautions (i.e., wear a mask) and hand hygiene when examining and caring for patients with signs and symptoms of a respiratory infection. Health care personnel who have a respiratory infection are advised to avoid direct patient contact, especially with high-risk patients. If not possible, a mask should be worn while providing care.

III.A.1.b. Safe Injection Practices The investigation of four large outbreaks of HBV and HCV among patients in ambulatory care facilities in the United States identified a need to define and reinforce safe injection practices. The four outbreaks occurred in a private medical practice, a pain clinic, an endoscopy clinic, and a hematology/oncology clinic. The primary breaches in infection control practice that contributed to these outbreaks were 1) reinsertion of used needles into a multiple-dose vial or solution container (e.g., saline bag) and 2) use of a single needle/syringe to administer intravenous medication to multiple patients. In one of these outbreaks, preparation of medications in the same workspace where used needle/syringes were dismantled also may have been a contributing factor.

These and other outbreaks of viral hepatitis could have been prevented by adherence to basic principles of aseptic technique for the preparation and administration of parenteral medications. These include the use of a sterile, single-use, disposable needle and syringe for each injection given and prevention of contamination of injection equipment and medication.

Whenever possible, use of single-dose vials is preferred over multiple-dose vials, especially when medications will be administered to multiple patients. Outbreaks related to unsafe injection practices indicate that some health care personnel are unaware of, do not understand, or do not adhere to basic principles of infection control and aseptic technique. A survey of U.S. health care workers who provide medication through injection found that 1% to 3% reused the same needle and/or syringe on multiple patients.

Among the deficiencies identified in recent outbreaks were a lack of oversight of personnel and failure to follow-up on reported breaches in infection control practices in ambulatory settings. Therefore, to ensure that all health care workers understand and adhere to recommended practices, principles of infection control and aseptic technique need to be reinforced in training programs and incorporated into institutional polices that are monitored for adherence.

III.A.1.c. Infection Control Practices for Special Lumbar Puncture Procedues In 2004, CDC investigated eight cases of post-myelography meningitis that either were reported to CDC or identified through a survey of the Emerging Infections Network of the Infectious Disease Society of America. Blood and/or cerebrospinal fluid of all eight cases yielded streptococcal species consistent with oropharyngeal flora and there were changes in the CSF indices and clinical status indicative of bacterial meningitis.

Equipment and products used during these procedures (e.g., contrast media) were excluded as probable sources of contamination. Procedural details available for seven cases determined that antiseptic skin preparations and sterile gloves had been used. However, none of the clinicians wore a face mask, giving rise to the speculation that droplet transmission of oralpharyngeal flora was the most likely explanation for these infections.

Bacterial meningitis following myelogram and other spinal procedures (e.g., lumbar puncture, spinal and epidural anesthesia, intrathecal chemotherapy) has been reported previously. As a result, the question of whether face masks should be worn to prevent droplet spread of oral flora during spinal procedures (e.g., myelogram, lumbar puncture, spinal anesthesia) has been debated. Face masks are effective in limiting the dispersal of oropharyngeal droplets and are recommended for the placement of central venous catheters.

In October 2005, the Health Care Infection Control Practices Advisory Committee (HICPAC) reviewed the evidence and concluded that there is sufficient experience to warrant the additional protection of a face mask for the individual placing a catheter or injecting material into the spinal or epidural space.

Source: Centers for Disease Control.

Appendix

B Clinical Internship

Whether you are participating in a clinical rotation, internship, or mentorship, your attitude and performance will determine whether it is a positive experience for you.

It is your responsibility to ensure that learning takes place. You must communicate to the health care staff what knowledge and skills you bring to the clinical opportunity. Ask questions of health care staff and seek out learning opportunities. When you show initiative, your clinical rotation will be more meaningful to you.

Getting Ready for the Clinical Experience

1. Research the facility and/or particular unit where you will be working during the rotation.
2. Investigate what type of uniform or professional clothing is required and purchase them, if necessary. Remember to include footwear.
3. Obtain a name tag. (Many health care facilities require a picture ID.)
4. Read and complete any orientation materials the facility requires.
5. Gather immunization records and have a Tuberculosis Test. (Some facilities also require a physical within the past year.)
6. Arrange transportation to the facility.

Dress Code for the Clinical Experience

1. Uniform or professional clothing should be neat, clean, and pressed.
2. Shoes should be clean, comfortable leather shoes with socks or stockings.
3. Hair should be clean and cut in a conservative style. If long, it should be pulled away from the face.
4. Jewelry should be limited to a watch with a second hand, one small pair of stud earrings (for women), and no more than one ring.
5. Fingernails should be trimmed with no artificial nails and clear nail polish only.
6. Cosmetics should be minimal and used to enhance appearance. Avoid wearing perfumes, colognes, or aftershaves.
7. While in your clinical uniform, you should avoid chewing gum and being around cigarette smoke.

Having a Positive Clinical Experience

1. Be on time each day. (Getting there 10 minutes early is even more impressive.) If you will not be able to attend that day or you are running late, notify the clinical site AND your instructor.
2. Bring a black pen and small notepad to make notes about your experiences.
3. Turn cell phones off and do not make personal phone calls or send text messages during your clinical experience.
4. Never leave your assigned area without notifying the health professional you are working with.
5. Perform only the skills you have learned to perform in your classroom.
6. Show initiative and seek out learning opportunities. Be self directed and ask questions.
7. Use critical thinking skills and practice infection control and standard precaution concepts appropriately.
8. Respect the property of others and care for the equipment and supplies in the health care facility.
9. Obey all safety rules of the facility.
10. Report ANY accidents or incidents that occur in the clinical area to your mentor and instructor. Complete appropriate reports if needed.
11. Behave professionally toward employees, patients, and fellow students. Discuss problems in an appropriate manner.
12. Avoid discussing your personal life in the clinical area.
13. Respect the Patient's Bill of Rights and patient confidentiality.
14. Be flexible and positive. Things are always changing in the health care environment. Embrace the unexpected as a learning opportunity.

The Post-Clinical Experience

1. Complete assignments and/or journal as assigned by your instructor. Continue to respect patient confidentiality when writing about your experiences.
2. Send a thank you note to your mentor or the clinical facility.
3. Reflect on the clinical experience.
   - What did you learn?
   - What did you do well?
   - What could you improve?
   - What do you want to learn more about?

Completing a Clinical Journal

Print out and complete the following Journal worksheet while you are working as a clinical intern.

Name: ______________________________ Date: ______________________

Clinical Site: ___________________________ Area: ______________________

Summary of clinical experience:

____

____

____

____

Describe two things you learned today and explain how you will be able to use them in the future.

1. ____

____

2. ____

____

Describe one procedure or treatment you saw today and the patient's response:

____

____

____

____

List one new medical term you learned today and explain what it means:

____

____

I performed these hands-on-skills today:

____

____

____

____

Name one positive and one negative experience you had in your clinical rotation today:

____

____

____

____

Feelings, Smells, Sounds:

I felt ____

I smelled ____

I heard ____

Glossary

Numbers/Symbols

24-hour time/military time (MIL i ter ee TIEM) Method of telling time by counting each hour consecutively for 24 hours (i.e, 11, 12, 13.).

A

abbreviations (uh bree vee AY shun) Words that have been shortened.

abdominal thrust or Heimlich maneuver (HYM lik muh noo ver) Forceful thrust on the abdomen, between the sternum and the navel, in an upward motion toward the head.

ability (uh BIL i tee) Something a person does well.

absorption (ab SAWRP shuhn) Passage of a substance through a body surface into body fluids and tissues (e.g., nutrients from digested food pass through the wall of the small intestine into the blood); To take up liquid or other matter.

academic plan (ak uh DEM ik plan) A document that you use to set goals for the things you want to accomplish while you are in school.

accessible (ak SES uh buhl) Available to obtain.

accessory (ak SES uh ree) Helping.

accredited (a KRED dit ted) Attested and approved as meeting prescribed standards.

accuracy (AK yuhr uh see) How close a measurement is to the actual value.

accurate (AK yer it) Exact, correct, or precise.

acids (as ids) Substances that cause the urine to have an acid pH.

acquired immunodeficiency syndrome (AIDS) (uh KWAHY uhrd i myoo noh dih FIHSH uhn see SIHN droem) Late stages of HIV infection; characterized by secondary infections.

actin (AK tin) A protein present in all cells and in muscle tissue; plays a role in contraction.

active immunity (AK tiv im YOO ni tee) Protection that occurs when a body produces its own antibodies.

adapt (uh dapt) To change, to become suitable, to adjust.

adaptation (ad uhp TEY shuhn) Changing to work better.

adequate (AD uh kwit) Enough, sufficient.

adolescent (ad l ES uhnt) The period of life between childhood and maturity.

aerobic (ai ROH bik) Requiring oxygen.

afebrile (ey FEE bruhl) Referring to temperature within a normal range.

agency (EY juhn see) An organization that helps people in a particular way.

agent (EY juh nt) A person or business authorized to act on another's behalf.

agglutination (uh gloot n EY shuhn) Clumping together (e.g., red blood cells clump together).

airborne (EHR born) Articles that float in the air.

ala (ey luh) Outer side of the nostril.

alignment (uh LAHYN ment) Keeping the body in proper position—in a straight line without twisting.

alimentary canal (al uh MEN tuh-ree kuh NAL) Long muscular tube beginning at the mouth and ending at the anus.

alleles (uh LEEL) Forms of a gene that influence a trait or set of traits.

alveolar-capillary (al VEE uh ler KAP uh ler ee) Pertaining to air sacs in the lungs.

Alzheimer's disease (AWL sie muhrs DUH seez) Type of dementia that causes the death of brain cells and subsequent impairment of thinking and memory.

ambulation (AM byuh lay shun) The ability to walk and move around freely.

ambulation devices (am byoo LAY shun duh VYS iz) Canes, crutches, walkers, or other equipment that help a patient to walk.

ambulatory (AM buhlu tor ee) Serving patients who are able to walk.

amino acids (ah MEE no a sid) Any of a large number of compounds found in living cells that contain carbon, oxygen, hydrogen, and nitrogen, and join together to form proteins.

amniotic fluid (am nee AH tihk FLOO ihd) Liquid that surrounds the fetus during pregnancy.

amplify (AM pluh feye) To increase or elevate a sound (e.g., the ossicles of the ear amplify sound waves).

amylase (AM me layz) An enzyme in saliva and pancreatic juice that breaks down starch into simple sugars.

anaerobic (an uh ROH bik) Able to grow and function without oxygen.

anatomical position (ann e TOM ik el pozi shun) The position with the body erect with the arms at the sides and the palms forward.

anatomy (uh NAT uh mee) The science dealing with the structure of humans, animals, and other living organisms.

anesthesia (an uhs THEE zhuh) Loss of feeling or sensation.

annoyance (uh NOI uhns) Irritation (e.g., to feel irritated with a co-worker or patient).

anorexia nervosa (an uh REK see uh nur VOH suh) Loss of appetite with serious weight loss. It is considered a mental disorder.

antagonist (an TAG uh nist) Something that works against.

anterior (ann TEER ee uhr) Located in the front; opposite of posterior (e.g., the abdominal wall is anterior to the back).

antibiotics (anti bi ot ik) Substances that slow growth of or destroy microorganisms.

antibodies (ANN tuh bah dees) Substances made by the body to produce immunity to an antigen.

antigen (ANN tuh jin) Foreign matter that causes the body to produce antibodies.

antiseptic (an tuh SEP tik) Substance that slows or stops the growth of microorganisms.

anus (EY nuhs) Outlet from which the body expels solid waste.

anxiety (ang ZIE i tee) A feeling of worry and fear that causes physical symptoms, such as sweating, and stress.

anxiety disorder (ang ZIE i tee DIS ohr duhr) A mental illness in which a person feels too much anxiety, often in response to everyday situations.

apex (AY peks) Pointed end of something (for example, the pointed end of the heart is called the apex of the heart).

apical foramen (EY pi kuhl fuh REY muhn) Opening in the apex.

apparatus (ap uh RAT uhs) Equipment needed to perform a task. For example, blood pressure apparatus includes a blood pressure cuff and a stethoscope.

appearance (uh PEER ents) The way someone or something looks.

appendicular (ap pen DIK you ler) Pertaining to any body part added to the axis (e.g., arms and legs are attached to the axis of the body).

applicant (AP lih kent) A person applying for a job.

appropriate (uh PROH pree it) Suitable, correct.

arrhythmia (uh RITH mee uh) An irregular pulse rate.

arteriosclerosis (ahr teer ee oh skluh ROH sis) Condition of hardening of the arteries.

asepsis (uh SEP sis) Sterile condition, free from all germs.

aseptic technique (ay SEP tihk tek NEEK) Method used to make the environment, the worker, and the patient as germ-free as possible.

aspirate (AS puh reyt) Remove substances.

asymptomatic (ey simp tuh MAT ik) Without visible symptoms.

atherosclerosis (ath uh roh skluh ROH sis) Condition of hardening of the arteries due to fat deposits that narrow the space blood flows through.

attachment (uh TACH muhnt) A file linked to an e-mail message.

attention deficit hyperactivity disorder (AH ten shuhn DEF uh sit HIE puhr ak tiv uh tee DIS ohr duhr) A mental illness characterized by inattention, hyperactivity, and impulsiveness; diagnosed most often in children.

audiology (o dee A luh gee) The study of hearing disorders.

auscultation (aw skuhl TEY shuh n) The act of listening, either directly or through a stethoscope or other instrument, to sounds within the body as a method of diagnosis.

autoclaves (AH toh klayvz) Sterilizers that use steam under pressure to kill all forms of bacteria on fomites (objects that pathogens live on and can transfer infection).

axes (AKS ees) Reference lines that mark the borders of a graph; graphs may have two or more axes (singular, axis).

axial (AX ee uhl) Pertaining to the central structures of the body (e.g., vertebrae, skull, ribs, and sternum).

B

baseline (BEYS lahyn) A number, graph, or indication to use as a guideline; A measurement taken at a later time may differ from the baseline, indicating a possible cause for concern.

benefits (BEN a fi ts) Payment and assistance based on an agreement.

biases (BAHY uhs ez) Tendencies; prejudices.

binocular (buh NOK yuh ler) Having two eyepieces.

biohazard (BAYH o haz uhrd) Biological materials or infectious agents that may cause harm to human, animal, or environmental health.

bioscience (BI o si ence) Any science that deals with the biological aspects of living organisms.

bipolar disorder (BIE puhl uhr DIS ohr duhr) A mental illness that causes unusual shifts in a person's mood, energy, and ability to function; also known as manic-depressive disorder.

blind carbon copy (blahynd KAHR buhn KOP ee) An e-mail feature that allows a person to send an e-mail to multiple people without them seeing the other receivers' e-mail addresses.

blood pressure (BP) (bluhd PRESH er) Highest and lowest pressure of the blood pushing against the walls of the arteries.

bloodborne (BLUHD born) Carried in the blood.

bolus (BOW less) A soft rounded ball, especially of chewed food.

bounding (BAUND ing) Leaping, strong, or forceful pulse.

bradycardia (brad i KAHR dee uH) Pulse rate below 60 beats per minute.

brittle (BRIT uhl) Fragile, easy to break.

budget (BUH jet) An amount of money allocated for a particular purpose.

bulk (bulk) A greater amount.

C

calcify (CAL si fy) To harden by forming calcium deposits.

calibration (KAL i bray-shun) Standard measure (e.g., each line on a thermometer or a ruler is a calibration).

calorie (KAL uh ree) Unit of measurement of the fuel value of food.

carbon copy (KAHR buhn KOP ee) An e-mail feature that allows a person to send a copy of an e-mail to another person.

carbon dioxide (car buhn die OX eyed) A gas, heavier than air; a waste product from the body.

cardiac (KAR dee ack) Relating to the heart.

cardiopulmonary (kahr dee oh PUHL muh ner ee) Having to do with the heart and lungs.

career (kuh REER) A profession; a person's life work.

career plan (kuh REER plan) A tool that shows you how to achieve your career goals.

cartilage (CAR tuh lij) Tough connective tissue; forms pads at end of bones, is found in the nasal septum and external ear, and forms the major portion of the embryonic skeleton.

catheters (KAHTH uh tuhrs) Tubes inserted into body opening or cavity.

cell (SELL) Smallest structural unit of the body that is capable of independent functioning.

cellulose (SEL yo loz) The primary component of plant cell walls, which provides the fiber and bulk necessary for optimal functioning of the digestive tract.

Celsius (SEHL see uhs) Measure of heat; in medicine a Celsius thermometer is sometimes used to measure body heat. Also called centigrade.

cementum (si MEN tuh m) Hard, thin covering or shell covering root of tooth.

central processing unit (SEN truhl pros es ing yoo nit) The part of a computer that interprets and carries out instructions.

cerebrospinal fluid (suh ree broh SPAHYN uhl FLOO ihd) Liquid that flows through and around brain tissue.

certification (ser tuh fi KAY shun) A process by which an individual is evaluated and recognized as meeting certain predetermined criteria and standards.

certified (SER ti fide) A person who has received a certificate that shows he or she demonstrates understanding.

chain of infection (CHAY in ove in FEC shun) A chain of events all interconnected is required for an infection to spread.

chart (CHART) To write observations or records of patient care.

chiropractic (KI ruh prak tik) The method of adjusting the segments of the spinal column.

cholesterol (kuh LES tuh rawl) A type of lipid, or fat, found in the body; produced by the liver or eaten in food.

chromosomes (KROM uh some) Structures that contain coiled and condensed portions of the cell's DNA.

chronic (KRA nik) Continuing over many years and for a long time (e.g., chronic illness).

chyme (KIME) Creamy semifluid mixture of food and digestive juices.

cilia (SYL ee ah) Hairlike projections that move rhythmically.

circulation (sur kyuh LEY shuhn) Continuous one-way movement of blood through the heart and blood vessels to all parts of the body.

civil law (SI vel loh) The body of law governing certain relationships between people, such as marriage, contracts, and torts (injuries).

coding (KOH ding) Identifying items to be filed according to particular categories, such as surgical or laboratory.

cohesiveness (koh HEE siv niss) State of being well-integrated or unified.

co-insurance (koh in SHOOR uhns) A percentage the subscriber is required to pay of every medical bill.

colitis (kuh lahy tis) Inflammation of the colon.

collaborate (kuh LAB uh reyt) To work together.

commitment (kuh MIT ment) A pledge or promise.

communicable (kuh MYOO ni kuh buhl) Capable of passing directly or indirectly from one person or thing to another.

communication (kuh myoo ni KAY shuhn) Act of exchanging information.

compensation (kom puhn SEY shuhn) Payment.

comply (kum PLAHY) To follow directions, do what you are asked to do.

components (kom PO nent s) Parts or elements of a whole; an ingredient.

composed (kuhm POHZD) Formed by putting many parts together.

compressions (kuhm PRESH uhns) The act of pressing on the chest to pump blood through the body of a cardiac arrest.

compromise (KOM pruh mahyz) A settlement of differences between parties by each party agreeing to give up something that it wants.

compromising (KOM pruh mahyz) Giving up something important.

compulsions (cuhm PUHL shuhns) In obsessive-compulsive disorder, behaviors or rituals that develop in response to the anxiety caused by obsessive thoughts.

conception (kuhn SEP shuhn) Occurs when the male sperm fertilizes the female ovum and a new organism begins to develop.

concisely (kuhn SICE lee) In a brief manner; to express in a few words.

confidential (kon fi DEN shuhl) Limited to persons authorized to use information or documents.

confidentiality (kon fuh den chee AL uh tee) A promise to keep certain information secret.

conflict (KON flikt) A contradiction, fight, or disagreement.

congenital conditions (kon JEN i tull kon DI shuns) Existing at or before birth usually through heredity, as a disorder.

connective tissue (cuh NEK tiv TISH yew) Tissue specialized to bind together and support other tissues.

constipation (kon stuh PEY shuhn) Infrequent or difficult emptying of the bowel.

consultant (kuhn SUHL tnt) A person who gives professional or expert advice.

contaminated (kuhn TAM uh nayt uhd) Soiled, unclean, not suitable for use.

contingency (kuhn TIN juhn see) Event that may occur but is not intended or likely to happen.

continuity of care (KON te noo it tee of kaar) Process by which the patient and the physician are cooperatively involved in ongoing health care management.

continuum (kuhn TIN yoo uhm) Progression from start (birth) to finish (death).

contraceptives (kon tre sept tivs) Items that serve to prevent pregnancy.

contract (con TRAKT) To shorten, to draw together; muscles shorten when you flex a body part.

contraction (ken TRAK shun) A tightening or narrowing of a muscle, organ, or other body part.

contracts (KON trackt s) A legally binding exchange of promises or an agreement between parties that the law will enforce.

controlled experiments (kuhn TRULD eks PEER uh muhnts) Experiments in which only one factor, or variable, is changed.

contusion (cuhn TOO shuhn) Condition in which the skin is bruised, swollen, and painful, but is not broken.

convalescence (kon vu LES nts) The gradual recovery of health and strength after illness.

convents (KON vents) Establishments of nuns.

converse (KUHn vurs) Talk, have a conversation.

convex (kon VEKS) Raised.

coordination (koh awr dn EY shuhn) State of harmonized action, such as eye and hand coordination.

co-payment (koh PEY muhnt) A set amount the subscriber pays for each medical service.

courteous (KUR tee uhs) Polite; considerate toward others.

cover letter (KUH ver LEH tuhr) A letter that introduces you to a potential employer.

cover page (KUHV er peyj) The first page of a fax.

credible (KRED uh buhl) Worthy of belief or confidence; trustworthy.

criminal law (KRI me nell loh) Body of law that defines criminal offenses; deals with the apprehension, charging, and trial of suspected persons; and sets penalties applicable to convicted offenders.

crouch (KROWCH) To stoop, using the large muscles of the legs to help maintain balance.

crutch (kruhch) A support used by physically disabled people as an aid in walking. It usually fits under the armpit and is often used in pairs.

cultural competence (kulch-ral kam-pe-tens) Ability to interact effectively with people of different cultures and socioeconomic backgrounds.

cusps (kusps) Pointed or rounded raised areas on the surface of the tooth.

custodial (kuh STOH dee uhl) Marked by watching and protecting rather than seeking to cure.

cystitis (sis TAHY tihs) Inflammation of the urinary bladder.

cytoplasm (SIGH toe plaz um) The liquid within the cell that surrounds the nucleus and other parts of the cell.

D

data (DA tuh) Information.

debilitating (di BIL I teyt ing) Causing weakness or impairment.

decade (DEK eyd) Period of 10 years.

decay (di KEY) Breaking down; rot.

deciduous (di SIJ oo uhs) Falling out (e.g., primary teeth fall out to make room for permanent teeth).

decimal (DEH sim uhl) A number containing a decimal point.

decompose (dee kuhm POES) To decay, to break down.

deductible (di DUHK tuh buhl) An amount the subscriber must pay before the insurance begins to pay.

defamatory (dee FAM uh tor ee) Statement that causes injury to another's reputation.

defecation (deaf uh KAY shun) The pushing of solid material from the bowel.

defibrillator (dee FIB ruh lay ter) A device that administers an electric shock to restore normal heartbeat.

deficiency (di FISH uhn see) Shortage.

deficient (di FISH uhnt) Lacking something (e.g., a deficient diet causes the body to function poorly because it is missing an important element).

definitive (di FIN i tiv) Clear, without question, exacting (e.g., when giving emergency care, each treatment should be done in a definitive manner).

dehydration (dee HIE dray shuhn) Severe loss of fluid from tissue and cells.

delegation (del i gat shun) To give another person responsibility for doing a specific task.

denominators (di NOM uh ney ters) The bottom numbers of fractions.

dentition (den TISH uhn) Natural teeth in the dental arch.

deoxyribonucleic acid (dee AHKS ee rye bow new KLAY ik ASS id) A molecule found in all living cells that contains information for building proteins and influencing traits.

designated (DEZ ig nay ted) Chosen for a specific purpose.

deteriorate (dee TEER ee or ate) Break down.

diabetes mellitus (dahy uh BEE teez mel uh thus) Condition that develops when the body cannot change sugar into energy; there is an insufficient amount of insulin, leading to an increased amount of sugar in the blood.

diagnosis (die ug NO sis) The identification of a medical condition.

diagnostic (dahy uhg NOS tik) Pertaining to the determination of the nature of a disease or injury by examining (e.g., using x-ray and laboratory tests).

dialect (di e lekt) Language peculiar to a specific region or social group.

dialysis (die AL iss sus) Process of removing waste from body fluids.

diarrhea (dahy uh REE uh) Passage of watery stool at frequent intervals.

diastolic pressure (DIE es tahl ic) Lowest pressure against the blood vessels of the body. It is measured between contractions.

diathermy (DAHY uh thur mee) The use of electric currents to produce heat in body tissues, usually as an aid to healing.

digestion (di JES chuh n) The process of making food absorbable by dissolving it and breaking it down into simpler chemical compounds that occur in the living body chiefly through the action of enzymes secreted into the alimentary canal.

digestion (dye JES chun) Process of breaking down food mechanically and chemically.

dignity (DIG nih tee) The quality of value and worth.

directive (de REK tiv) Something that serves to guide or impel towards an action or goal.

discharging (dis CHAHRJ ing) The act of releasing or allowing to leave.

discipline (DIS uh plin) A branch of instruction or learning, such as cardiology.

disinfection (dis ihn FEHKT shuhn) Process of freeing from microorganisms by physical or chemical means.

disorientation (dis AWR ee uhn tey shuh n) State of being confused about time, place, and identity of persons and objects.

dispense (di SPENS) To distribute or pass out.

dissection (di SEK shuhn) Act or process of dividing, taking apart.

distal (DISS tuhl) Farthest from the point of attachment.

distress (di STRES) Great pain or suffering.

diuretics (die ret ik) Drugs that increase urine output.

division (di VIZH uhn) The process of separating into parts; the operation opposite of multiplication.

documentation (dok yuh men TEY shuhn) A record of something, such as a patient's progress.

dominant (DOM uh nuhnt) Shows influence or control.

dressings (DRES ing) Gauze pads that are used to cover a wound.

droplet (DRAWP leht) A small drop of fluid.

drug (DRUHG) Any chemical substance that changes a person's physical or psychological state.

drug addiction (DRUHG AH dikt shuhn) The uncontrolled use of a drug.

duct (DUHKT) Narrow, round tube that carries secretions from a gland.

durable power of attorney (DYUR e bul pou r of e tur nee) A type of advance medical directive in which legal documents provide the power of attorney (the authorization to act on someone else's behalf in a legal or business matter) to another person in the case of an incapacitating medical condition.

dynamics (di NAM ic s) Motivating or driving forces.

dysfunction (dis FUHNGK shuhn) Impaired or abnormal functioning.

E

edema (eh DEE muh) Swelling; abnormal or excessive collection of fluid in the tissues. Usually, the swelling is in the hands, ankles, legs, or abdomen.

efficiency (ee FISH uhn see) Ability to accomplish a job with the least possible difficulty.

elastic (ee LAS tik) Easily stretched.

elements (EL e ment s) Regulate the activity of the heart, nerves, and muscles. Build and renew teeth, bones, and other tissues.

eligibility (e li ja BI la tee) The quality or state of being qualified.

elimination (i lim uh NEY shuhn) Process of expelling or removing, especially of waste products from the body.

embryo (EM bree oh) Living human being during the first eight weeks of development in the uterus.

embryonic (em bree ON ik) Pertaining to the embryo.

emesis (eh MUH suhs) Vomit.

endometrium (en doh MEE tree um) Interlining of the uterus.

endowments (in DAU munts) Gifts of property or money given to a group or organization.

enterotoxin (ehn tuhr oh TAHKS uhn) Poisonous substance that is produced in, or originates in, the contents of the intestine.

entrepreneur (ahn truh pruh NUR) A person who organizes and manages a business.

environment (en VAHY ruhn muhnt) Surroundings we live in. Environmental disease can occur in any area around us (e.g., hospital, restaurants, public places, home, school).

environmental sanitation (in VI run men tel sa ne TA shun) Methods used to keep the environment clean and to promote health.

enzyme (EN zahym) Substance that causes a change to occur in other substances.

epidemics (ep i DEM iks) Diseases affecting many people at the same time.

epidermis (ep ih DER mus) Outer layer of skin.

epigastric (ep uh GAS trik) Pertaining to the area over the pit of the stomach.

episodes (EP i sod s) Events in a series.

epithelial (e pi THEE lee uhl) Pertaining to tissue that covers the internal and external organs of the body.

equilibrium (ee kwah LIB ree um) State of balance.

ergonomic (erg uh NOM ik) An object or practice designed to reduce injury.

erupt (I RUHPT) Push through.

essential (uh SEN shuhl) Necessary (e.g., certain food elements are necessary for the body's functions).

estimate (EH stuh muhnt) Determine approximate value of a number.

estrogen (ESS tro jen) Female hormone.

ethics (ETH iks) Social values; conduct; description of what is right and wrong.

etiquette (ek-i-kit) Rules of acceptable social behaviors.

evacuated (i VAK yoo yet) Emptied out.

evacuation (i vak yoo EY shuhn) Removal.

excellence (EK sell ence) The quality of having outstanding qualities.

excreted (ik SKREE ted) When waste matter is discharged from the blood, tissues, or organs.

excretion (ex SKREE-shun) The process of eliminating waste material.

exempt (egg ZEM p t) To be free or released from some liability or requirement to which others are subject.

exorcise (EK sawr sahyz) To force out evil spirits.

expiration/exhalation (ex pur AY shun/ex hull AY shun) Process of forcing air out of the body during respiration.

exposed (eks POEZD) Left unprotected.

expressed contracts (IK spres d KON trackts) Contracts in which terms are written out in the document.

extract (EK strakt) Identify and take out or emphasize.

extremities (ex TREM uh tees) Arms, legs, hands, and feet.

F

facilitator (fuh SIL i tey ter) A person responsible for leading or coordinating a group.

facilities (fuh SIL i teez) Places designed or built to serve a special function (e.g., hospital, clinic, doctor's office).

facsimile/fax machine (faks muh SHEEN) A device that sends and receives printed pages or images as electronic signals over telephone lines.

Fahrenheit (FEHR uhn hite) Measure of heat; in medicine a Fahrenheit thermometer is often used to measure body heat.

fairness (FAYR nes) Applying good rules equally to all people.

febrile (FEE bruhl) Referring to elevated temperature.

feces (FEE sees) Solid waste that is evacuated from the body through the anus.

feedback (FEED bak) Information received as a result of something done or said.

fetus (FEE tus) Infant developing in the uterus after the first three months until birth.

fixation (fik SEY shuhn) Repair or fix.

flammable (FLAM uh buhl) Catches fire easily or burns quickly.

flatulence (FLA chu lens) Excessive gas in the stomach and intestines that causes discomfort.

flexibility (FLEK suh buhl itee) The ability to easily bend.

flexible (FLEK suh buhl) Able to bend easily.

flushed (flush d) Showing reddening of the skin.

formula (FAWR myuh luh) Accepted rule (e.g., a math formula and a baby formula are both guidelines or rules).

fracture (FRAK cher) Broken bone.

frayed (frayd) Worn or tattered (e.g., electrical cords may be worn, causing wires to be exposed).

full time (FUHL time) Describes a job requiring between 32 and 40 hours per week.

function (FUHNGK shuhn) Action or work of tissues, organs, or body parts (e.g., the heart's function is to pump blood).

functional stress (FUHNGK shuh nl stress) Stress to tooth caused by its normal function (e.g., force of pressure when biting something hard).

G

gait belt (geyt belt) A safety device used to move a patient from one place to another; also used to help hold up a weak person while they walk.

ganglia (GANG glee ah) Mass of nerve tissue composed of nerve cell bodies. Ganglia lie outside the brain and spinal cord.

gastrointestinal (gas troh in TES tuh nuhl) Pertaining to the stomach and intestine.

gauge (GAYJ) Standard scale for measurement.

generalized (JEN uhr uhl ahyzd) Affecting all of the body.

genes (JEENZ) A portion of DNA that contains instructions for a trait.

genome (JEE nohm) The complete copy of the body's DNA.

geriatric (jer ee A trik) A branch of medicine that deals with the problems and diseases of old age and aging people.

gestures (JES cherz) Motions of a part of the body to express feelings or emotions (e.g., nodding yes or no).

graphic chart (GRAF ik charct) A visual record of data in graphic or tabular form.

gravity (GRAV i tee) Natural force or pull toward the earth. In the body, the center of gravity is usually the center of the body.

Greenwich time (GREN ich TIEM) Standard time, a 12-hour clock.

guarding techniques (GARD ing TEK neek) Ways to protect a patient when he or she is being moved.

gurney (ger NEE) A metal stretcher with wheeled legs, often used in hospitals to transport patients.

H

harass (huh RASS) To behave in an offensively annoying or manipulative way.

hazardous (HAZ er duhs) Dangerous.

Health Insurance Portability and Accountability Act (HIPAA) A law that includes regulations ensuring the privacy of patient information.

HEDIS Healthcare Effectiveness Data and Information Set; an organization that provides quality care guidelines.

heel (HEEL) Part of the hand between the palm and the wrist.

hemoglobin (HEE muh gloh bin) An iron-containing protein in red blood cells that combines reversibly with oxygen and transports it from the lungs to body tissues.

hemorrhage (HEM er rij or HEM-rij) Large amount of bleeding.

heparinized (HEP uh rin eyesd) Containing heparin, an anticoagulant.

hepatitis B (HBV) (hep uh TAHY tuhs BEE) Bloodborne viral disease that affects the liver; transmitted by blood exposure, sexual contact, sharing needles, or from infected mother to infant.

hepatitis C (HVC) (hep uh TAHY tuhs SEE) Bloodborne viral disease that affects the liver; transmitted by blood exposure, sharing needles, or from infected mother to infant; rarely transmitted by sexual contact.

hereditary (huh RED i ter ee) Passed from parent to child.

hernial (HUR nee uh) Pertaining to projection through an abnormal opening in the wall of a body cavity.

heterogeneous (ahet er uh JEE nee uhs) Different in kind; unlike.

holistic (hoh LIST tik) Pertaining to the whole; considering all factors.

homeostasis (hoh mee uh STEY sis) Constant balance within the body. This balance is maintained by the heartbeat, blood-making mechanisms, electrolytes, and hormone secretions.

hormones (HOR moans) Protein substances secreted by an endocrine gland directly into the blood.

horseplay (HAWS play) Rowdy behavior; acting inappropriately in a work environment.

HOSA-Future Health Professionals The student organization for health occupation students at the secondary, postsecondary, adult, and college level.

host (ho st) The organism from which a microorganism takes nourishment. The microorganism gives nothing in return and causes disease or illness.

human immunodeficiency virus (HIV) (HYOO man i MYOO noe dih FIHSH uhn see VAHY ruhs) Virus that infects cells of the immune system, reducing the immune system's ability to fight disease; transmitted by blood exposure, sexual contact, sharing needles, or from infected mother to infant.

hydroculator pad (HI droc u la tor pad) A moist heat pack treatment.

hydroencephaly (hi DROW n sef awl ee) Excessive accumulation of cerebrospinal fluid in the brain, often leading to increased brain size and other brain trauma.

hydrotherapy (hahy druh THER uh pee) The use of water (hot, cold, steam, or ice) to relieve discomfort and promote physical well-being.

hygiene (HI jean) The practice of keeping clean.

hypertension (hi per TEN shun) Elevation of the blood pressure.

hypotension (hahy puh TEN shuhn) Low blood pressure.

hypothermia (hahy puh THUR mee uh) Below-normal temperature.

hypothesis (HIE poth uh sis) An explanation for an observation that is based on scientific research and that can be tested.

I

ileitis (il ee AHY tis) Inflammation of the ileum (the lower three-fifths of the small intestine).

immunizations (im yuh nuh ZEY shuhns) Substances given to make disease organisms harmless to the patient; may be given orally or by injection (e.g., tetanus, polio).

impatience (im PEY shuh ns) Intolerance, edginess.

impending (im PEN ding) About to happen.

implement (IM pluh ment) To carry out a rule or procedure.

implied contracts (im PLY d KON trackts) Contracts in which some terms are not specifically stated, but are understood by the parties based on the nature of the transaction.

incontinent (in KAHNT uh nuhnt) Unable to control the bowel or bladder.

indexing (in desk sing) Organizing items in the order they are to be filed.

inferior (in FEER ee er) Lower, second-rate, substandard (e.g., one product is inferior in quality to another product).

infirmity (in FIR mi tee) Unsound or unhealthy state of being.

inflated (in FLEY tid) To swell or fill up with air.

informed consent (in FORMD kun SENT) The legal condition in which a person agrees to terms, after he or she understands all the facts and implications of an action or event.

infuses (in FYOO z) Flows into the body by gravity (e.g., IV drips through a tube into the body).

ingestion (in JES chuhn) Take in by mouth.

input (IN poot) To enter data into a computer for processing.

inspiration/inhalation (in spur AY shun/in hull AY shun) Process of breathing in air during respiration.

insulin (IN sel in) Hormone secreted by the pancreas; essential for maintaining the correct blood sugar level.

insulin shock (IN suh lin shok) Condition caused by too much insulin.

interdependent (in ter di PEN duh nt) Depending on each other.

interdisciplinary (in ter DIS uh pluh ner ee) Involving two or more disciplines.

interests (IN ter ists) Something that concerns, draws the attention of, or arouses the curiosity of a person.

Internet (IN ter net) A worldwide computer network with information on many subjects.

interproximal surfaces (in ter prok semal SUR fis) Sides between teeth.

interstitial (in tur STISH uhl) Space between tissues.

interstitial fluid (ihnt uhr STIHSH uhl FLOO ihd) Liquid that fills the space between most of the cells of the body.

intervention (in tur VEN shun) The act of interfering to modify an outcome.

intoxication (in tok si KEY shuhn) State of poisoning or becoming poisoned.

intraoral (in tra or el) Within the oral cavity.

intravenously (in truh VEE nuhs lee) Directly into a vein.

invasive (in VEY siv) Entering the body.

involuntary (IN vol en tar ee) Not under control (e.g., muscle twitching).

isolated (AHY suh leyt ed) Limited in contact with others.

J

jaundice (JAWN dis) Yellowing of the whites of the eyes, skin, and mucous membranes.

job outlook (job OUT look) The expectation or prospect of a particular job in the future.

K

keywords (KEE WUHRDZ) Significant or descriptive words.

L

labeling (LEY buhl ing) Describing a person with a word that limits them (e.g., lazy, stupid).

laceration (las uh RAY shuhn) Wound or tear of the skin.

lacrimal (LAK rim uhl) Pertaining to tears.

lactation (lak TEY shuhn) Body's process of producing milk to feed newborns.

lateral (LAT ur uhl) Relating to the sides or side of.

lawsuits (LA soots) A legal action started by one person against another based on a complaint that the person failed to perform a legal duty.

laxative (LAK suh tiv) A medicine for relieving constipation.

leadership (LEED uhr ship) Ability to influence or lead.

legal disability (LEE gull diss e BILL e tee) A person has a disability for legal purposes if he or she has a physical or mental impairment which has a substantial and long-term adverse effect on his or her ability to carry out normal day-to-day activities.

legible (LEJ uh buhl) Capable of being read easily.

legislation (le jus LA shun) A law or body of laws.

leisure (LEE zher) Time free from the demands of work.

length (LENGTH) The measure of something from end to end.

liable (LAHY uh bul) Legally responsible.

licensing (LAHY suhn sing) Giving an agency or person permission to carry on certain activities and defining the activities they are authorized to do.

licensure (LIE sen sher) A process by which a governmental agency or other authority gives permission to a person or health care organization to operate or to work in a profession.

limb (LIM) Arm, leg.

lipid (LIP id) Fat.

lipids (LIP id z) Any of a group of organic compounds, including the fats, oils, triglycerides, etc. that—together with carbohydrates and proteins—constitute the principal structural material of living cells.

living will (LIV ing will) A will in which the signer requests not to be kept alive by medical life-support systems in the event of a terminal illness.

load (LOHD) Weight of an object or person that is to be moved.

localized (LOH kuhl ahyzd) Affecting one area of the body.

lymphocyte (LIM fo sites) Type of white blood cell.

M

maintain (meyn teyn) Keep up.

major depressive disorder (MAY juhr DEE pres iv DIS ohr duhr) Mental illness characterized by a combination of symptoms that include prolonged sadness and that interfere with a person's ability to undertake everyday activities.

malfunctioning (mal fungk shen ing) Not working as it is supposed to.

malignant (mah LIG nent) Cancerous.

malnutrition (mal noo TRISH un) Poor nutrition caused by an insufficient or poorly balanced diet or by a medical condition.

malpractice (mal PRAK tis) Failure of a professional person, such as a physician, to render proper services through ignorance or negligence or through criminal intent, especially when injury or loss follows.

managed care (MAN ijd kair) A health care plan or system that seeks to control medical costs by contracting with a network of providers and by requiring preauthorization for visits to specialists.

mandates (MAN dayts) Orders or commands.

mass (MAS) The amount of matter in an object.

masticate (MAS ti keyt) Chew.

maternal (MA ter nel) Relating to the mother or from the mother.

matures (me TCHOOR) Becomes fully developed.

mechanism (MEK uh niz uhm) Process or a series of steps that achieve a result.

memorandum (mem e RAN dum) A short note written to help a person remember something or to remind a person to do something.

meninges (mi NIN jeez) Lining of the brain.

menstruation (men stroo AY shun) Cyclic deterioration of the endometrium.

mental illness (MEN tuhl IL nuhs) Health condition that changes a person's thoughts, emotions, and behavior and that affects the person's ability to undertake daily functions.

mentor (MEN tore) An experienced person who can offer advice and guidance.

metabolic (met uh BOL ik) Pertaining to the total of all the physical and chemical changes that take place in living organisms and cells.

metabolism (mi TAH buh lih zum) Collection of chemical reactions that takes place in the body's cells to convert the fuel in the food we eat into the energy needed to power everything we do.

metabolize (mi TAB e liz) To break down substances in cells to obtain energy.

meterstick (MEE ter STIK) A measuring stick one meter long that is marked off in centimeters and usually millimeters.

microbiology (mahy kroh bahy OL uh jee) The branch of biology dealing with the structure, function, uses, and modes of existence of microscopic organisms.

microns (MAHY krohns) Units equaling one millionth of a meter.

microorganisms (mie kroh ORG uhn izms) Tiny organism, such as a fungi, protists, or bacteria, that can only be seen under a microscope.

microscopic (mahy kruh SKOP ik) Too small to be seen by the eye but large enough to be seen through a microscope.

millimeters (MILL ih mee tehr) Measure of length.

minor (MAHY ner) Under the legal age of full responsibility.

minute (my NEWT) Exceptionally small.

misrepresentations (mis rep ri zen TAY shuns) Untruths; lies.

mission statement (MISH uhn STEYT muhnt) A summary describing the aims, values, and overall plan of an organization or individual.

mixed numbers (mikst NUHM bers) Numbers with whole numbers and a fraction (e.g., 6¼, 7½).

monasteries (MON uh ster ees) Homes for men following religious standards.

monocular (muh NOK yuh ler) Having one eyepiece.

monocytes (MAWN o sites) Large single-nucleus white blood cells.

multiplication (muhl tuh pli KEY shuhn) Finding the product of two numbers.

myosin (MI essin) A protein in muscles that helps them contract.

N

narrative (NAR uh tiv) A story or account of events.

nephron (NEF rawn) Functional part of the kidney that filters liquid waste.

networking (NET wur king) Sharing information about yourself and your career goals with personal contacts.

neurological (noor uh LOG I kuhl) Pertaining to the nervous system.

neuron (NUR awn) Nerve; includes the cell and the long fiber coming from the cell.

noninvasive (non in VEY siv) Not involving penetration of the skin.

nonpathogenic (nahn path oh JEN ik) Not disease causing.

nonwhole numbers (non HOHL NUHM bers) Numbers with decimals (e.g., 6.25, 9.85).

nosocomial infection (nohs uh KOH mee uhl ihn FEHKT shuhn) An infection acquired while in a health care setting, such as a hospital.

notation (noh TEY shuhn) The act of noting, marking, or setting down in writing.

nucleotides (NEW klee oh tyde) Subunits of DNA that each contain a phosphate, sugar, and base.

nucleus (NEW klee iss) The part of a cell that is vital for its growth, metabolism, reproduction, and transmitted characteristics.

numerators (NOO muh rey ters) The top numbers of fractions.

nutrients (NOO tree ent) Substances that the cell needs in order to function.

O

obesity (oh BEE sih tee) Extreme fatness; abnormal amount of fat on the body.

objective (ahb JEK tiv) Relating to a symptom or condition perceived by someone other than the person affected.

obligation (ob li GEY shuhn) Moral responsibility.

observant (ob ZUR vent) Quick to see and understand.

observation (ob zur VEY shuhns) Something that is noted or recorded.

observations (AHBS uhr vay shuhns) Using the senses and other means to get information about surroundings.

obsessions (ahb SESH uhns) In obsessive-compulsive disorder, undesirable thoughts that occur constantly, causing anxiety.

obstetrics (ub STE triks) The branch of medical science concerned with childbirth.

obstruction (ub STRUK shun) Blockage or clogging.

occupation (ok yuh PEY shuhn) A person's job to earn a living.

occupational therapy (ock you PAY shun l) Helps to give people skills for the job of living satisfying lives, such as dealing with job-related injuries.

ombudsman (OM budz muhn) A social worker, nurse, or trained volunteer who ensures that patients are properly cared for and respected.

opportunistic infections (op er too NIS tik in FEK shen) Infections that occur when the immune system is weakened. Common organisms that the body normally resists cause infection.

oral (AWR uhl) Referring to the mouth.

orthopedics (or tho PE diks) The medical specialty concerned with correcting problems with the skeletal system.

ossicles (OSS ik uhls) Three small bones in the middle ear: incus, stapes, and malleus.

outpatients (aout PAY shunts) Patients/clients who do not require hospitalization but are under a physician's care.

output (OUT poot) To produce information; turn out.

overexposure (OH ver ik SPOH zher) Too much contact with radiation.

ovum (OH vum) Female reproductive cell that when fertilized by the male develops into a new organism.

oxidation (ok si DAY-shun) The mixing of oxygen and another element.

oxygen (OX uh jin) Element in the atmosphere that is essential for maintaining life in most organisms.

oxygenated (OX uh jin ate ed) Containing oxygen.

P

paranoia (PAIR ah noy uh) Unfounded or irrational distrust of other people.

parasites (PARE uh sahyts) Organisms obtaining nourishment from other organisms they are living in or on.

parasitic (pare uh SIT ik) Pertaining to an organism that lives in or on another organism, taking nourishment from it.

parenteral (pa REN ter uhl) Not in the digestive system (e.g., injections are parenterally administered).

part time (PAHRT time) Describes a job requiring fewer than 32 hours per week.

passive immunity (PASS iv im YOO ni tee) Protection that occurs when a body receives antibodies from another source.

pasteurization (PAS chuh rahyz ay shuhn) To heat food for a period of time to destroy certain microorganisms.

pathogenic (path oh JEN ik) Disease causing.

pathway (PATH wa) Related job, industry, and occupation types within a career cluster.

penetrates (PEN i trayts) Enters or passes through (e.g., a fractured bone passes through the skin).

percentages (per SEN tij es) Portions in relation to a whole (e.g., 65%, 22%).

periodic (peer ee OD ik) Occurring at regular intervals.

peripheral (per IF er uhl) Situated away from a central structure.

peristalsis (pear is STALL sus) Progressive, wavelike motion that occurs involuntarily in hollow tubes of the body.

peritoneal cavity (pear it tun EEL kav it ee) Area of the body containing the liver, stomach, intestines, kidneys, urinary bladder, and reproductive organs.

peritoneal fluid (per ih toh NEE uhl FLOO ihd) Liquid in the peritoneal cavity.

pertinent (PUR tn uh nt) Relating directly to the matter at hand; relevant.

phagocytes (FAY go sites) Cells that surround, ingest, and digest microorganisms and cellular waste.

philosophy (fi LOS uh fee) Theory; a general principle used for a specific purpose.

phobia (FOH bee uh) An irrational fear of an object or event that poses little or no actual risk.

Physicians' Desk Reference (PDR) A commonly used reference book that provides information about drugs, drug manufacturers, emergency phone numbers, and more.

physiological (fiz ee uh LOJ I kuhl) Pertaining to normal body functions.

physiology (fiz ee OL uh jee) The branch of biology dealing with the functions and activities of living organisms and their parts.

pigmentation (pig men TAY shun) Natural color of the skin.

pigmented (PIG men ted) Colored; relating to various parts of the body (e.g., iris of the eye, lips, moles, freckles).

plane (PLAYN) A flat surface determined by the position of three points in space.

plaque (plak) Soft deposit of bacteria and bacterial products on teeth.

plasma (PLAZ muh) Watery, colorless fluid containing leukocytes, erythrocytes, and platelets.

pleural fluid (PLOOR uhl FLOO ihd) Liquid that surrounds the lungs.

podiatry (po DI u tree) The diagnosis and treatment of foot disorders.

pollutants (puh LEW tents) Things that contaminate (e.g., smoke, smog).

polycythemia (pol e si theme a) Condition of having too much blood.

porous (POUR iss) Filled with tiny holes.

posterior (poss TEER ee uhr) Behind, to the rear, toward the back (e.g., the heel is posterior to the toes).

postmortem (POHST mor tuhm) After death.

post-traumatic stress disorder (PTSD) (POHST TRAW mat ik STRES DIS ohr duhr) A mental illness that develops after a terrifying incident that involved physical harm or the threat of harm.

postural supports (POS chuh ruhl suh PORTS) Soft restraints used to protect residents.

potential (puh TEN chul) Possible.

pouch (POWCH) Small bag or sac.

precision (PREE si shuhn) For multiple measurements of the same thing, how close the values of the measurements are to each other.

predators (PRED uh ters) Organisms or beings that destroy.

prejudge (pree JUHJ) To decide or make a decision before having the facts.

prejudices (PREJ uh dis ez) Judgments or opinions formed before the facts are known.

premium (PREE mee uhm) The periodic payment to Medicare, an insurance company, or a health care plan for health care or prescription drug coverage.

preventive (pri VEN tiv) Intended to keep from happening.

primarily (pry MARE uh lee) For the most part; chiefly.

primitive (PRIM i tiv) Ancient or prehistoric.

principal (prins si PULL) First or among the first in importance or rank.

principles (PRIN suh puhl) Codes of behavior.

priorities (prah AWR i tee) Those things that are most important.

prioritize (prahy AWR i tahyz) To put in order of importance.

prioritizing (prahy AWR itahyz) Arranging or dealing with in the order of importance.

priority (pry OR it ee) A quality of importance; tasks of high priority are more urgent than items of low priority.

productivity (proh duhk TIV i tee) The power to reach goals and get results.

professional (pro FESH uh nuhl) One who is paid for their work.

professional development (pro FESS shun ul dee VEL up ment) Education for people who have already begun their careers to help them continue to grow.

progressive (pruh GRES iv) Moving forward, following steps toward an end product.

project (pruh JEKT) To show or reflect.

prone (PROHN) Lying on the stomach.

propensity (pro PEN sit tee) A natural inclination or tendency.

proportions (pruh POR shuhns) Parts of a whole.

prosthesis (pros thee sis) An artificial body part such as a limb, tooth, or eye, used to replace a natural body part and minimize a disability.

prosthetics (pros THE tiks) Artificial parts made for the body (e.g., teeth, feet, legs, arms, hands, eyes, breasts).

protein (PROH teen) Complex compound found in plant and animal tissues, essential for heat, energy, and growth.

protist (PRO tis t) An organism belonging to the kingdom that includes protozoans, bacteria, and single-celled algae and fungi.

protrusion (proh TROO shuhn) Pushing through.

provider (pruh VAHY der) Physician, physician assistant, nurse practitioner.

proximal (PROK suh muhl) Nearest or next to.

prudent (PRU dent) Careful or cautious.

psychiatric (sahy kee A trik) Pertaining to the mind.

psychiatrist (SIE kie uh trist) A medical professional who specializes in the prevention, diagnosis, and treatment of mental illness; has a medical degree (M.D.) and can prescribe medication as part of treatment.

psychiatry (si KAHY ut tree) The practice or science of diagnosing and treating mental disorders.

psychological (sahy kuh LOJ I kuhl) Pertaining to the mind.

psychologist (SIE kahl uh jist) A medical professional who specializes in the prevention, diagnosis, and treatment of mental illness; can only use talk therapy for treatment.

psychology (sahy KOL uh jee) The science of the mind or of mental states and processes.

psychotherapy (SIE koh ther uh pee) Treatment method in which a mental health professional and a patient discuss problems and feelings related to a mental illness.

pulse oximetry (puhls ok SIM I tree) Procedure used to determine the oxygen concentration in the hemoglobin of the arterial blood.

pyrexia (pahy REK see uh) Above-normal temperature.

pyrogenic (pahy ruh JEN ik) Producing fever.

Q

quackery (kwak uh ree) Practice of pretending to cure diseases.

quality of respirations (KWOL i tee ofres puh REY shuhn) The amount of air taken into the body and expelled from the body and the effort it takes to do this.

R

range-of-motion (ROM) (reynj uhv MOH shuhn) Measurement of the achievable distance between the flexed position and the extended position of a particular joint or muscle group.

rate of respirations (reyt of resp puh REY shuhn) The number of respirations per minute.

reagents (re a jents) Chemical substances that react to the presence of other substances in the blood and urine.

receptors (ree SEP torz) Nerves that respond to stimuli.

recessive (ri SES iv) Passive or hidden.

recipient (ri SIP ee uhnt) A person or thing that receives.

recommendations (rek uh men DAY shuns) Suggestions.

recreational therapy (rek ree A shun l) Uses play, recreation, and leisure activities to improve physical, cognitive, social, and emotional functioning; the primary goal is to develop lifetime leisure skills.

rectal (REK tl) Referring to the far end of the large intestine just above the anus.

refer (ri FER) To send to.

registration (rej uh STRAY shun) A list of individuals on an official record who meet the qualifications for an occupation.

regulate (REG yuh leyt) To control or adjust.

rehabilitation (ree huh BIL i tey shuhn) Process that helps people who have been disabled by sickness or injury to recover as many of their original abilities for activities of daily living as possible.

relevant (REL uh vuhnt) Pertaining to, or having to do with, the patient/client.

reliable (ri LAHY uh buhl) Dependable, accurate, honest.

remainder (ri MEYN der) The amount left over after division that is less than a whole number.

replicate (REP li kate) To reproduce or make an exact copy.

reprimanded (REP ree man did) Punished.

residual (REE sid yoo uhl) Left over.

resistance (ri ZIS tuhns) The ability of the body to protect itself from disease.

resistant (ri ZIS tuh nt) Able to protect itself.

resorption (ri SAWP shuhn) Loss of substance or bone.

respiration (res puh REY shuhn) Taking oxygen into the body and expelling carbon dioxide from the body.

respiratory (RES per uh tawr ee) Pertaining to or serving for breathing.

restorative (ri STAWY uh tiv) To return to as close to normal conditions as possible.

restraints (ri STREYNT) A piece of equipment or device that restricts a patient's ability to move.

restrict (ree STRIKT) To keep within limits; to confine.

resultant (ri ZUHL tunt) Resulting from an action.

resume (REZ oo mey) A document that provides details about your work history and accomplishments.

resuscitation (ri suhs i TAY shuhn) Bringing back to life, reviving.

retention (ri TEN shuhn) Keeping elements within the body that are normally eliminated (e.g., waste products such as urine and feces).

rheostat (REE uh stat) Control for flow of electric current.

rhythm of respirations (RITH uh m of res puh REY shuhn) The regularity, or irregularity, of breathing.

rickettsiae (rih KET see ee) Parasitic microorganisms that live on another living organism and cause disease.

roles (rol s) A position, responsibility, or duty.

S

sacral region (SAY chruhl ree jun) The area where the sacrum is located; forms the tail end of the spinal column.

salmonella (sal muh NEL uh) A rod-shaped bacterium found in the intestine that can cause food poisoning, gastroenteritis, and typhoid fever.

saprophytes (SAP ruh fahyts) Organisms that live on dead organic matter.

saturated (SACH uh reyt id) Soaked; filled to capacity.

scales (SKEYLZ) Instruments with marks that help to determine weight or mass.

scattering (SKAT e ring) Spreading in many directions, dispersing.

schizophrenia (SKIT soh fren ee uh) Mental illness in which a person loses touch with reality; often characterized by hallucinations, such as voices that other people cannot hear, and delusions.

scientific methods (SIE uhn tif ik METH uhds) Processes scientists use to answer questions.

scope of practice (SKOHP uv PRAK tis) A legal set of directives developed by a state board that governs practice for a health care professional.

sebaceous (seh BAY shus) Pertaining to fatty secretions.

secretion (si KREE shuhn) Producing and expelling a special substance (e.g., sebaceous glands secrete oil; salivary glands secrete saliva).

sedentary (SED n ter ee) Immobilized; does not move around very much.

self-esteem (SELF i STEEM) Belief in oneself.

semen (SEE mun) Fluid from the testes, seminal vesicles, prostate gland, and bulbourethral glands. Contains water, mucin, proteins, salts, and sperm.

service (SUHR viss) Caring for others.

sex cells (SEX sel) Cells that allow reproduction to occur.

shock (SHAHK) Convulsion of muscles and extreme stimulation of nerves when an electric current passes through the body.

slang (slanNG) Language of informal words and phrases; typically restricted to a particular context or group of people.

sloughed (SLUFFED) Discarded; separated from (e.g., to shed dead cells, as from the outer skin).

soft skills (soft skilz) Cluster of personality traits—communication, language, personal habits, friendliness, and optimism— that characterize relationships with other people.

soluble (SOL yuh buhl) Able to break down or dissolve in liquid.

sorting (SAWR ting) Separating items to be filed according to the filing system being used, such as alphabetical, numerical, color, chronological, and geographical.

specialties (SPESH uhl teez) Fields of study or professional work (e.g., pediatrics, orthopedics, obstetrics).

spermatozoa (spur mat uh ZOH uh) Male sex cells.

sphincter (SVING ter) Circular muscle that allows the opening and closing of a body part (e.g., anus, pylorus).

Sphygmomanometer (sfig moh muh NOM i ter) A device used to measure the pressure against the arteries of the body.

spirochetes (SPAHY ruh keets) Slender, coil-shaped organisms.

spontaneous (spon TEY nee uhs) Occurring naturally without apparent cause.

spurts (SPURTZ) Forces out in a burst; squirts.

stamina (STAM uh nuh) Body's strength or energy.

stance (stans) The way you stand.

Standard Precautions (STAN derd prih KAW shuhn) Guidelines designed to reduce the risk of transmission of microorganisms from recognized and unrecognized sources of infection in the hospital.

sterilized (STEHR uhl ahyzd) Made free from all living microorganisms.

stethoscope (STETH uh skohp) Instrument used to hear sound in the body (e.g., heartbeat, lung sounds, bowel sounds).

stimuli (STIM you lie) Elements in the external or internal environment that are strong enough to set up a nervous impulse.

stoma (STOH muh) Opening, e.g., opening in abdomen in an ostomy.

structure (STRUHK cher) The way that parts of the body are put together.

subcutaneous (sub kyu TAIN ee us) Beneath the skin.

subjective (suhb JEK tiv) Relating to a symptom or condition perceived by the patient and not by the examiner.

subsidized (SUB se dizd) Having partial financial support from public funds.

subtraction (suhb TRAK shuhn) Taking a number away from another number; the operation opposite of addition.

sufficient (suh FISH suhnt) Enough.

sulcus (SUHL kuhs) Depression, groove, area where gingival tip meets tooth enamel.

superstitious (soo per STISH uhs) Trusting in magic or chance.

supine (soo PAHYN) Lying on the back.

suppository (suh POZ i tawr ee) A solid, conical mass of medicinal substance that melts upon insertion into the rectum.

surgical (SUR ji kuhl) Repairing or removing a body part by cutting.

susceptible (suh SEHP tuh buhl) Capable of being affected or infected (e.g., body can be attacked by microorganisms and become ill).

swathe (SWOTH) Bandage.

symptom (SIMP tuhm) A sign or indication of something.

syndrome (SIN drohm) A number of symptoms occurring together.

systems (SIS tems) Coordinated bodies of methods or plans of procedure.

systolic pressure (sis TAHL ic) Highest pressure against blood vessels. It is represented by first heart sound or beat heard when taking a blood pressure.

T

tachycardia (tak i KAHR dee uh) Pulse rate over 100 beats per minute (for adults).

tasks (task) A function to be performed; job.

teamwork (TEEM work) Cooperative effort from a group of people working together for a common purpose.

telemedicine (TEL uh med uh sin) Using electronic communications to exchange medical information from one site to another for the health and education of the patient or health care provider.

terminal (TUR muh nl) Last or ending.

terminology (ter muh NOL uh jee) Specialized terms used in any occupation.

testosterone (tess TOSS ter own) Male hormone.

therapeutic (ther uh PYOO tik) Pertaining to the treatment of disease or injury (e.g., physical therapy, radiology, diet, nursing).

thermotherapy (thur moh THER uh pee) Medical therapy involving the application of heat.

thready (THRED ee) Weak, barely felt pulse; thin, like a thread.

tickler file (TIK ler fayhl) Special file kept to remind you of tasks that need to be done at a certain time.

tissues (TISH yews) Groups of cells of the same type that act together to perform a specific function.

tomography (tuh MOG ruh fee) X-ray technique that produces film of detailed cross sections of tissue.

tone (TOHN) Firmness or tightness.

topical (TOP i kuhl) Surface of the body.

tort (TORT) Under civil law, a wrong committed by one person against another.

toxins (TAHKS ihns) Poisonous substances.

TPR (TEE PEE R) An abbreviation that stands for "temperature, pulse, respiration."

traditional (truh DISH uh nl) Customary beliefs passed from generation to generation.

traits (TRAYTS) Genetically determined characteristics or conditions.

transcription (tran SKYRAHYB) A written copy.

translate (trans LEYT) To make understandable.

transmitting (trahnz MIHT ihng) Causing to go from one person to another person.

transversely (trans VURS lee) In a cross direction.

trephining (TRAY fin ing) Surgically removing circular sections (of bone, for example).

Trochanter (TROW kan ter) One of the bony prominences toward the near end of the thigh bone (the femur).

U

ulcerations (UHL suhr ay shuhns) Open areas, or sores.

ultrasound (UHL truh sound) Medical therapy that uses sound frequencies (above 20 kHz) beyond the limits of human hearing to treat hard-to-reach body areas.

ultraviolet light (uhl truh VAHY uh lit lahyt) An invisible band of radiation at the upper end of the visible light spectrum.

uniformity (yoo nuh FAWR mi tee) A state of being all the same; does not vary.

Universal Precautions (yoo nuh VER suhl pree KAHW shuhns) A set of precautions that prevents the transmission of HIV, HBV, HCV, and other bloodborne pathogens when providing health care.

unoxygenated (UN ox uh jin ate ed) Lacking oxygen.

urethritis (yoor uh THRAHY tihs) Inflammation of the urethra.

urology (yew RO le gee) The study of the urine and urinary organs in health and disease.

username (YOO zer naym) A unique identifier composed of alphanumeric characters, used as a means of initial identification to gain access to a computer system or Internet Service Provider.

vaccines (VAK seenz) A weakened bacteria or virus given to a person to build immunity against a disease.

V

value (VAL yoo) The importance that you place on various elements in your life.

variables (VAR ee uh buhls) Any factor that can change or be present in varying amounts.

vessels (VES el) Tubes that carry blood in the body.

villi (VIL eye) Tiny projections.

viruses (VAHY ruhs es) Genetic material that is surrounded by a protective coat and that can only reproduce inside a host cell; can only be seen under a microscope.

visibility (vis uh BIL it tee) Ability to see.

vitality (vahy TAL i tee) The ability of an organism to go on living.

vitamins (VAHY tuh min s) Group of substances necessary for normal functioning and maintenance of health.

Vocational portfolio (voh KA shuh nl pawrt FOH lee oh) A collection of materials that shows your knowledge, abilities, skills, and insights as they pertain to a particular occupation, business, or profession.

volume (VAHWL yoom) The amount of space that an object or liquid takes up.

voluntary (VOL en tar ee) Under the control of the person (e.g., you voluntarily raise your arm; it does not rise automatically).

W

wages (WEYJ s) Money that is paid or received for work or services.

walker (WAH ker) A waist-high four-legged framework of lightweight metal, for use by a weak or disabled person as a support while walking.

waste products (WAYST praw dukts) Elements that are unfit for the body's use and are eliminated from the body.

Web site (WEB sahyt) A group of pages on the Internet developed by a person or organization about a topic.

weight (WAIT) Measures the force of gravity on an object; varies due to distance between objects and mass.

whole numbers (HOHL NUHM bers) Numbers that do not contain decimals or fractions (e.g., 1, 2, 3).

withdrawal (with DRAW uhl) Uncomfortable physical and psychological symptoms that arise when a drug addict stops using a drug.

work ethic (werk e-thik) Values based on hard work and diligence.

written consent (RIT en kon scent) A person knowingly, without duress or coercion, clearly and explicitly consents to the proposed therapy in writing.

Z

zygote (ZAHY goht) Any cell formed by the coming together of two reproductive (sex) cells.

Index

A

B

C

D

E

F

G

H

I

J

K

L

N

O

P

V

W

X

Y

Z

Photo Credits

Part 1 Opener: p 1 wavebreakmedia/Shutterstock

Chapter 1: p 3 Maridav/Fotolia; p 6 Pakhay Oleksandr/Fotolia; p 8 Reeed/Shutterstock; p 13 PinkSony/Fotolia; p 14 John Kropewnicki/Fotolia; p 19 apops/Fotolia

Chapter 2: p 27 Monkey Business Images/Shutterstock; p 29 George Wada/Fotolia; p 41 Monkey Business/Fotolia

Chapter 3: p 45 duckman76/Fotolia; p 48 Monkey Business Images/Shutterstock; p 51 dotshock/Shutterstock; p 55 sudok1/Fotolia; p 56 Kadmy/Fotolia; p 57 Goodluz/Shutterstock; p 57 iceteastock/Fotolia; p 59 laviejasirena/Fotolia; p 59 Michael Heron/Pearson Education/PH College; p 60 StockLite/Shutterstock; p 62 Tyler Olson/Shutterstock; p 62 Monkey Business/Fotolia; p 63 Carolina K. Smith MD/Shutterstock; p 64 Dmitry Kalinovsky/Shutterstock; p 64 Spencer Grant/PhotoEdit Inc.

Chapter 4: p 71 Maridav/Shutterstock; p 73 Monkey Business Images/Shutterstock; p 84 michaeljung/Shutterstock; p 87 HOSA-Future Health Professionals; p 94 Monkey Business Images/Shutterstock; p 95 StockLite/Shutterstock

Chapter 5: p 99 Andresr/Shutterstock; p 105 Tyler Olson/Shutterstock; p 107 Diego Cervo/Shutterstock; p 115 Alexander Raths/Shutterstock

Chapter 6: p 119 Brian A Jackson/Shutterstock; p 121 Lighthunter/Shutterstock; p 122 Minerva Studio/Shutterstock

Chapter 7: p 133 stefanolunardi/Shutterstock; p 136 USDA; p 141 Monkey Business Images/Shutterstock; p 142 wavebreakmedia/Shutterstock; p 143 Robert Kneschke/Shutterstock; p 149 Monkey Business Images/Shutterstock; p 159 Helder Almeida/Shutterstock

Chapter 8: p 171 Andresr/Shutterstock; p 175 Rido/Shutterstock; p 178 Monkey Business Images/Shutterstock

Chapter 9: p 183 Dragon Images/Shutterstock; p 185 michaeljung/Shutterstock; p 189 V.C.L./ Getty Images, Inc.; p 195 Monkey Business Images/Shutterstock; p 198 forestpath/Shutterstock; p 199 Milkovasa/Shutterstock; p 203 K. Miri Photography/Shutterstock; p 205 beerkoff/Shutterstock; p 207 James Steidl/Shutterstock; p 217 Monkey Business Images/Shutterstock; p 220 racorn/Shutterstock; p 221 JohnKwan/Shutterstock; p 224 val lawless/Shutterstock

Part 2 Opener: p 233 Monkey Business Images/Shutterstock

Chapter 10: p 235 apops/Fotolia; p 245 Cheryl Casey/Shutterstock; p 251 pabijan/Fotolia

Chapter 11: p 255 Stauke/Fotolia

Chapter 12: p 279 dotshock/Shutterstock; p 281 Monkey Business/Fotolia; p 286 Zhil-anna/Fotolia; p 286 VIPDesign/Fotolia; p 286 Blueringmedia, Fotolia

Chapter 13: p 295 (c) Dorling Kindersley; p 297 Designua/Shutterstock; p 298 Network Graphics/Pearson Education/PH College; p 306 gwimages/Fotolia; p 316 Alila Medical Media/Shutterstock; p 317 Peter Atkins/Fotolia; p 325 wellphoto/Fotolia; p 332 Kadmy/Fotolia; 344 sudok1/Fotolia; p 352 nicoletaionescu/Fotolai; p 358 Tyler Olson/Fotolia; p 362 sneksy13/Fotolia; p 370 Trish23/Fotolia; p 379 Monkey Business/Fotolia; p 384 WavebreakmediaMicro/Fotolia; p 385 nobeastsofierce/Shutterstock; p 386 Mateusz Kopyt/Shutterstock; p 388 Monkey Business/Fotolia

Chapter 14: p 393 Lisa F. Young/Fotolia; p 415 yeyen/Fotolia; 418 Ocskay Bence/Fotolia

Chapter 15: p 425 Rawpixel/Fotolia; p 428 Monkey Business/Fotolia; p 428 hxdbzxy/Shutterstock; p 430 lefata/Fotolia; p 431 Tyler Olson/Fotolia; p 438 wavebreakmedia/Shutterstock

Chapter 16: p 445 Maridav/Fotolia; p 449 Paulista/Fotolia, p 450 yvdavid/Fotolia; p 450 kichigin19/Fotolia; p 450 danielskyphoto/Fotolia; p 450 hsagencia/Fotolia; p 450 larcobasso/Fotolia; p 450 amphaiwan/Fotolia; p 450 Mara Zemgaliete/Fotolia; p 451 USDA; p 461 sergo1972/Shutterstock

Chapter 17: p 467 Tyler Olson/Shutterstock; p 469 Pablo Calvog/Shutterstock; p 473 Centers for Disease Control and Prevention; p 482 Piotr Marcinski/Shutterstock; p 482 Tyler Olson/Shutterstock; p 484 JPC-PROD/Fotolia; p 486 Tyler Olson/Fotolia; p 495 Vladimir Melnik/Shutterstock; p 499 Michael G Smith/Shutterstock

Chapter 18: p 505 Jules Selmes/Pearson Education Ltd; p 513 spotmatikphoto/Fotolia; p 522 Barnaby Chambers/Shutterstock; p 525 aceshot1/Shutterstock; p 527 bst2012/Fotolia; p 534 aceshot1/Shutterstock; p 535 Ruth Jenkinson (c) Dorling Kindersley; P 536 Photographee.eu/Fotolia; p 539 Vvoe/Fotolia; p 539 F.C.G./Fotolia; p 542 Ruth Jenkinson (c) Dorling Kindersley; p 546 Alila Medical Media/Shutterstock; p 549 Michal Heron; p 564 wellphoto/Fotolia; p 569 Baloncici/Shutterstock

Chapter 19: p 573 iofoto/Shutterstock; p 578 Suppakij1017/Shutterstock; p 579 JPC-PROD/Shutterstock; p 580 Michal Heron; p 581 Patrick Watson; p 587 michaeljung/Shutterstock; p 589 LeventeGyori/Shutterstock; p 591 toysf400/Shutterstock; p 598 hxdbzxy/Shutterstock; p 620 romarti/Fotolia; p 622 daseaford/Shutterstock; p 628 Tyler Olson/Fotolia; p 629 Tyler Olson/Fotolia; p 668 Monkey Business/Fotolia; p 669 Monkey Business Images/Shutterstock; p 670 Alexander Raths/Shutterstock; p 672 Lisa F. Young/Fotolia; p 692 Charles Cloutier/Shutterstock

Chapter 20: p 701 Antonio Gravante/Fotolia; p 705 Monkey Business/Fotolia; p 716 Beneda Miroslav/Shutterstock; p 720 Keith Bell/Shutterstock; p 720 VIPDesign/Fotolia; p 721 Hayati Kayhan/Fotolia; p 725 JPC-PROD/Fotolia; p 726 Photographee.eu/Fotolia; p 727 Germán Ariel Berra/Fotolia; p 739 Dmitry Lobanov/Shutterstock; p 744 Anneka/Shutterstock; p 747 Chris Pole/ Shutterstock; p 748 Stephanie Frey/Shutterstock; p 751 Vereshchagin Dmitry/Shutterstock; p 755 Sébastien Eich/Fotolia; p 759 Suthep/Shutterstock; p 763 Monika WisniewskaShutterstock

Chapter 21: p 771 Eric Simard/Fotolia; p 774 Gianfranco Bella/Fotolia; p 790 Monkey Business/Fotolia; p 792 Vector pro/Shutterstock

Chapter 22: p 805 Michał Nowosielski/Fotolia; p 816 Howard Shooter (c) Dorling Kindersley; p 822 hightowernrw/Shutterstock; p 823 apops/Fotolia